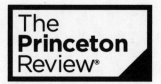

The Princeton Review

DAT® PREP

3rd Edition

The Staff of The Princeton Review

Penguin
Random
House

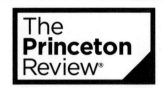

The Princeton Review
110 East 42nd Street, 7th floor
New York, NY 10017

Published in the United States by Penguin Random House LLC, New York.

ISBN: 978-0-593-51741-3
ISSN: 2163-601X

DAT is a registered trademark of the American Dental Association, which is not affiliated with The Princeton Review.

The Princeton Review is not affiliated with Princeton University.

The material in this book is up-to-date at the time of publication. However, changes may have been instituted by the testing body in the test after this book was published.

If there are any important late-breaking developments, changes, or corrections to the materials in this book, we will post that information online in the Student Tools. Register your book and check your Student Tools to see if there are any updates posted there.

Editor: Orion McBean
Production Artist: Jason Ullmeyer
Production Editors: Emma Parker and Nina Mozes

Printed in the United States of America.

10 9 8 7 6 5 4 3 2 1

3rd Edition

The Princeton Review Publishing Team

Rob Franek, Editor-in-Chief
David Soto, Senior Director, Data Operations
Stephen Koch, Senior Manager, Data Operations
Deborah Weber, Director of Production
Jason Ullmeyer, Production Design Manager
Jennifer Chapman, Senior Production Artist
Selena Coppock, Director of Editorial
Orion McBean, Senior Editor
Aaron Riccio, Senior Editor
Meave Shelton, Senior Editor
Chris Chimera, Editor
Patricia Murphy, Editor
Laura Rose, Editor

Penguin Random House Publishing Team

Tom Russell, VP, Publisher
Alison Stoltzfus, Senior Director, Publishing
Brett Wright, Senior Editor
Emily Hoffman, Assistant Managing Editor
Ellen Reed, Production Manager
Suzanne Lee, Designer
Eugenia Lo, Publishing Assistant

For customer service, please contact **editorialsupport@review.com**, and be sure to include:

- full title of the book
- ISBN
- page number

CONTRIBUTORS

The Princeton Review would like to thank the following for their contributions to this edition: Jessica Adams, Rachel Abramczuk, Neil Adams, Heidi Borenstein, Melissa Chan, Jane Feng, Jennifer Gorman, Erin Grennell, Jenny Jun, Michelle Kuah, Michelle Lim, Dave MacKenzie, Alexandra Malinowski, Augusto Matarazzo, Matthew Smithdeal, Dorothy Vandermolen, and Ryman Yeung.

The Princeton Review would also like to thank the following for their contributions to previous editions: Jessica Adams, Neil Adams, Jeremy Belch, Heidi Borenstein, Natalie Gelman, Dave MacKenzie, Augusto Matarazzo, Archana Murali, Nandini Raghuram, Graham Skelhorne-Gross, Christoper Stobart, David Stradley, Stephanie Tantum, Allison Uniacke, Dorothy Vandermolen, Tom Watts, Judene Wright, and Katherine Wright.

CONTENTS

DAT TEAR-OUT REVIEW GUIDE

Get More
(Free) Content
at **PrincetonReview.com/prep**

As easy as 1·2·3

1 Go to PrincetonReview.com/prep or scan the **QR code** and enter the following ISBN for your book: **9780593517413**

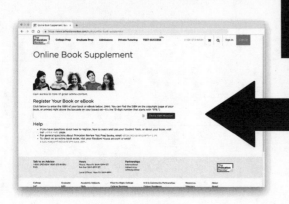

2 Answer a few simple questions to set up an exclusive Princeton Review account. *(If you already have one, you can just log in.)*

3 Enjoy access to your **FREE** content!

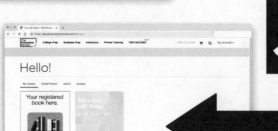

Once you've registered, you can...

- Access two full-length, scorable, online American DATs

- Access the Canadian versions of the same tests as downloadable PDFs

- Practice and prepare with an assortment of drill questions for all DAT sections

- Read helpful articles about dental school, dental careers and curriculum and lists of dentistry schools by program

- Check for any test updates released by the ADA and/or book corrections for this edition

Need to report a potential **content** issue?

Contact **EditorialSupport@review.com** and include:

- full title of the book
- ISBN
- page number

Need to report a **technical** issue?

Contact **TPRStudentTech@review.com** and provide:

- your full name
- email address used to register the book
- full book title and ISBN
- Operating system (Mac/PC) and browser (Chrome, Firefox, Safari, etc.)

Look For These Icons Throughout The Book

 ONLINE ARTICLES

 ONLINE PRACTICE TESTS

 PROVEN TECHNIQUES

 APPLIED STRATEGIES

 OTHER REFERENCES

Chapter 1
Introduction

1.1   SO YOU WANT TO BE A DENTIST

If you're reading this book, there's a pretty strong chance that you are giving serious thought to becoming a dentist. Maybe your parents are dentists and you always knew that you would grow up to be a dentist. Maybe you were pre-health in college and flirted with the idea of becoming a doctor or a nurse before you decided that becoming a dentist would suit you better. However you've come to this point, you've taken the required pre-dentistry classes, and now all that remains before you can apply is to take the Dental Admission Test (DAT).

Just the DAT

The DAT is a long, complex, detailed exam of much of the basic biology and chemistry that you learned in your pre-dental courses, together with math that you may not have seen since high school, reading comprehension that only vaguely resembles any kind of reading that you've done before, and perceptual ability that may not at all resemble anything that you've ever done before. And it's this monstrosity that is standing between you and dental school.

Understandably, you may feel somewhat daunted. The path to a good DAT score is not necessarily as straightforward as the path to a good GPA or to a good letter of recommendation. While much of the DAT is about recalling facts that you learned at some point in school, much of it is not, and the test is as much about how you apply what you know as it is about what you know.

However, we would like to help. This book is the complete package: we describe the test in detail, eliminating the mystery about what is tested and how it appears, and then we describe in detail the content and strategies that you should know to do well on this test. This means that we will review all the biology, general and organic chemistry, and math that you are expected to know for the test, but we won't just stop there. We will also discuss test-taking techniques for all of the subjects, including reading comprehension and perceptual ability. In short, everything that you should know for the DAT is in this book, no more and no less.

It's all here, because you want to be a dentist. And we want to help.

What is the DAT...Really?

Many students approach studying for the DAT like studying for a final exam in college. This can mean cramming lots and lots of science and math facts into your head in the few days leading up to the exam and hoping just to regurgitate what you've memorized on test day. This might have worked in college (although even then it probably wasn't the best way to go about taking a test), but it generally leads to disappointing results on the DAT.

The DAT is not a purely content-based, fact-recall test. If dental school admission committees wanted that, they could just look at your transcript. What they want to see is both how much you know and how well you think under the intense pressure of a timed admission exam. The combination of the two is what they will try to determine from your DAT score.

The nature of the test impacts how you must study for it. Making lots of flashcards to memorize Ochem reactions (or whatever) will help you prepare for this exam, but it will only get you part of the way. After all, there are no facts to memorize for reading comprehension or perceptual ability, and even on the sciences and math, you must be able to apply your knowledge to (potentially) new situations. So what else do you have to do to study for this exam, other than memorize lots of facts?

You must also practice applying the knowledge that you have to DAT-style questions. Taking the DAT is a skill in itself, and this skill, like any other, requires practice. This is much like learning to play a musical instrument or speak a foreign language; you learn to play the piano by practicing for an hour or two every day, not by reading about playing the piano all day before a big recital. This book contains a great many practice questions inside, and many more are available online. Other questions are available from the makers of the test, the American Dental Association (ADA), directly. Practice as much as you can, because it is through practice that you will get better and your score will improve. A good general rule is to spend no more than half your study time on reviewing and learning content, then the rest on practice problems and practice tests.

1.2 HOW TO USE THIS BOOK

Hopefully, you've picked this book up at the beginning of your DAT preparation, and you have at least two or three months to study before you take the test. If you're planning to take the test in a very short time, such as a week from now, it is unlikely that you will be able to read the whole text and do all of the practice that comes with it. Thus, how you use this book will depend on where you are in relation to your test date.

Long-Term Prep

If the test is still at least a month from now, try to read this book cover to cover. Begin with the introduction, and progress through the sections on the different subjects in a staggered fashion (that is, read a little bit of Biology, then a bit of Gchem, then a bit of Ochem, and so on, until you come back to Bio). Work the chapter-end practice questions as you go, since these are important to solidify the information that you're reviewing, and read the solutions both for questions you get right and questions you get wrong, so that you can make sure you understand the proper reasoning for the questions. Don't forget to use the online questions you have access to!

Access the online practice material as soon as you can, because the most important thing you can do is take the tests that come with this book and determine your strengths and weaknesses. If you're scoring a 25 in a subject, you probably don't need to practice it much (if at all), but if you're scoring a 15, it needs some serious shoring up before you take the test, and you don't know which subjects are which until you take a practice test. Thus, you should not leave both tests until the end of your practice. Take one in the middle to gauge your status, and one near the end for another assessment.

Shortly before the test you should read the introduction again, because you'll want to remind yourself of test-day procedures, and frankly, you should read the dental admissions information because you want to get excited for the test! You will do better if you think of this as your first step on the road to a great career in the field of dentistry than if you think of this as a horrible, time-consuming, draining, boring, standardized test (which it probably is, but it's better not to think of it that way!).

1.3

Short-Term Prep

If the test is very soon (e.g., a week from now), then read the introduction (you could skip the dental admissions information if you want, although, as noted above, it might be best not to), and take one of the online practice tests. Use this to identify your areas of weakness, which could be as general as "I'm not good enough at OChem" or as specific as "I forget how to use sine and cosine in math," and read up on those areas. Make sure that you work some of the practice questions in those subjects.

If you don't feel comfortable with these topics even after some practice, you might consider postponing your test date to give yourself a little more time to do more detailed review and additional practice. However, don't postpone indefinitely, because then you'll never be able to go to dental school. Choose a specific test date to move to, and prepare for that date. If you learn everything that is in this book and study the practice questions carefully, you will not be surprised by anything on the test, and you should be able to do your best. Good luck!

1.3 DAT NUTS AND BOLTS

Sections (Sub-Tests)

There are four timed groups of questions on the DAT. These groups of questions are called "tests" by ADA, but we will usually call them "sections." Before these sections is a tutorial, in the middle is a break, and after is a survey, so the overall structure of the test is as follows. The tutorial, the break, and the survey are all optional, but we highly recommend you take the break! More on this shortly.

Section	Number of Questions	Time
Tutorial		15 minutes

Survey of Natural Sciences (SNS)
  Biology
  General Chemistry
  Organic Chemistry
	100 total
	40
	30
	30
		90 minutes total

Perceptual Ability Test (PAT)	90	60 minutes
Break		30 minutes
Reading Comprehension Test (RCT)	50	60 minutes
Quantitative Reasoning Test (QRT)	40	45 minutes
Survey		15 minutes

Head to PrincetonReview.com to read helpful articles and check out information about the DAT.

The sections are always in this order. The test is a computer-based test (CBT), though it is fixed-form (not adaptive). You can move around within a section at your discretion, and the questions in any given test form are set before the test begins, just as on a pencil-and-paper exam. In total, the DAT is five hours and 15 minutes long, including the optional sections.

Every question on the DAT will be multiple choice. Most questions in SNS, RCT, and QRT will have five answer choices for you to pick from, but every once in a while, these sections have a three- or four-option question. Questions in the PAT will have either four or five options, depending on the type of question. This will be discussed more in the PAT chapters of this book.

Scoring

Every correct answer on the DAT is weighted the same, which means each question is scored as correct or incorrect. There is only one correct answer for each question; you cannot select more than one answer to a question. You receive eight scores after taking the DAT, six for different subjects and two multi-subject scores. Each score ranges from 1 to 30. Individual scores are reported for Biology, General Chemistry, Organic Chemistry, Perceptual Ability Test, Reading Comprehension Test, and Quantitative Reasoning Test. Next, you receive a separate overall score for the Survey of Natural Sciences. Finally, the scores for Biology, General Chemistry, Organic Chemistry, RCT, and QRT are combined into another score called the Academic Average (AA).

Typically, dental schools care most about the Academic Average and your PAT score, which is not part of your Academic Average. Some also look at your Biology score. They will also look for any outlier scores within the Academic Average. For example, you could have an AA of 20 with good science scores, an excellent RCT score and only a 10 in QRT; this low QRT score could draw negative attention.

However, if the difference is minor, schools will generally overlook it. For example, if your Academic Average is 21 and your QRT score is 19, it is unlikely that any school will give that small difference a second thought.

Thus, the ideal set of DAT scores fits the following criteria:

- A high Academic Average
- A high PAT score
- A high Biology score
- No individual scores significantly below the Academic Average (though small deviations are fine)

You might ask, "What's a 'high' Academic Average? What about a PAT score?" These questions are not as easy to answer as you might imagine. They do vary somewhat from school to school. However, a score between 20 and 22 is competitive for most schools, and for any more detail, you should consult the specific schools to which you would like to apply. You may also consult the following percentile chart to determine how a score compares to the scores other test-takers receive.

1.3

Score[1]	Biology	General Chemistry	Organic Chemistry	SNS	PAT	RCT	QRT	AA
1	0.0%	0.0%	0.1%	0.0%	0.0%	0.0%	0.0%	0.0%
2	0.0%	0.0%	0.1%	0.0%	0.0%	0.0%	0.0%	0.0%
3	0.0%	0.0%	0.1%	0.0%	0.0%	0.0%	0.0%	0.0%
4	0.0%	0.0%	0.1%	0.0%	0.0%	0.0%	0.0%	0.0%
5	0.0%	0.0%	0.1%	0.0%	0.0%	0.0%	0.0%	0.0%
6	0.0%	0.0%	0.1%	0.0%	0.0%	0.0%	0.0%	0.0%
7	0.0%	0.1%	0.1%	0.0%	0.0%	0.0%	0.1%	0.0%
8	0.1%	0.1%	0.1%	0.0%	0.0%	0.1%	0.1%	0.0%
9	0.1%	0.2%	0.3%	0.0%	0.0%	0.1%	0.3 %	0.0%
10	0.2%	0.5%	0.6%	0.1%	0.1%	0.1%	0.5%	0.1%
11	0.6%	1.4%	1.8%	0.3%	0.3%	0.2%	1.5%	0.2%
12	1.9%	2.7%	3.5%	1.4%	1.1%	0.6%	3.7%	0.6%
13	4.2%	5.6%	7.1%	3.7%	2.6%	1.4%	7.7%	2.0%
14	8.1%	10.3%	12.3%	8.2%	5.7%	2.7%	14.9%	5.0%
15	16.9%	17.0%	19.1%	15.0%	11.1%	5.5%	24.1%	10.2%
16	27.1%	24.8%	26.6%	25.1%	18.9%	9.7%	35.0%	18.6%
17	40.2%	36.1%	34.9%	36.5%	29.2%	16.2%	50.4%	30.3%
18	53.6%	48.0%	45.5%	50.2%	43.4%	24.6%	62.2%	44.3%
19	67.4%	58.6%	56.2%	64.1%	57.6%	35.9%	72.5%	59.4%
20	79.4%	71.3%	66.8%	75.4%	69.1%	49.5%	78.3%	71.7%
21	86.8%	78.4%	75.2%	84.7%	78.8%	62.3%	84.9%	81.5%
22	92.5%	86.4%	83.3%	91.1%	87.1%	71.5%	90.0%	88.5%
23	95.8%	87.5%	89.5%	94.8%	92.7%	80.0%	93.6%	93.7%
24	97.8%	92.6%	91.5%	97.6%	94.8%	85.6%	95.3%	96.8%
25	98.7%	94.4%	92.6%	98.6%	97.4%	91.0%	96.9%	98.5%
26	99.1%	96.4%	96.9%	99.2%	98.2%	94.1%	97.8%	99.5%
27	99.3%	97.0%	97.8%	99.6%	99.1%	96.3%	98.8%	99.9%
28	99.7%	99.0%	97.8%	99.8%	99.4%	97.2%	99.0%	100.0%
29	99.7%	99.0%	98.1%	99.9%	99.5%	98.2%	99.0%	100.0%
30	100.0%	100.0%	100.0%	100%	100.0%	100.0%	100.0%	100.0%

---

[1] n = 12,501; data from Dental Admission Test (DAT) User's Manual 2019 Data, © 2021 by American Dental Association.

You might notice that the overwhelming majority of students fall in a fairly narrow range between 1 and 30. For example, on the Academic Average only 5% of test-takers score below a 15, but 59.4% of students score below a 20. This means that a little more than 50% of test-takers score in the range 15–19.

Why does this matter to you? Well, it means that moving your Academic Average even one or two points can change how you look to admission committees. They get an astonishing number of applicants with an 18, but fewer with a 19, and even fewer with a 20. Those two points can put you ahead of nearly a quarter of test-takers, and that much more likely to get in.

There is an enormous premium, therefore, on eking out every last point that you can, and we will discuss how to do this.

Non-Scored Questions

The ADA says[2]: "Some questions on the test are experimental and are not scored. Data collected on unscored questions are used to determine whether those questions pass psychometric standards and would be appropriate for use in future test administrations. Unscored questions look the same to candidates as scored questions."

What does this mean for you? Well, certain questions will not count toward your score. There is no way to know how many or which ones. However, it does mean that you should not spend too much time on any one question, because it may not even count. As a rule of thumb, you should never spend more than three times as long on any one question as you average on the other questions. For example, if you average about 1 minute per QRT question, you should never spend more than 3 minutes on any one QRT question, unless you've already finished every other question in the section.

Registration and The Test Experience

The DAT is created by the American Dental Association, or ADA, and you can register at the ADA DAT website. It is offered by appointment at Prometric computer testing centers, which also offer many other tests; fact, other test-takers in the room with you will be taking other tests, unrelated to the one you are taking. Appointments are available for a variety of different dates and times, usually including mornings, afternoons, and evenings. Some weekend dates may be available. Convenient locations and dates often fill up well in advance, so you should sign up early (ideally at least a month or two before you are planning to take the test, just in case). The DAT is available year-round.

The testing center contains two parts, a waiting room and a secured computer area. In the waiting room, you are greeted by an administrator who checks your identification and signs you in. You must have two forms of identification. Your primary ID must be government issued with a signature and photograph (such as a driver's license or passport); your secondary ID can be anything with a signature (such as a credit card). Expired identification cannot be used. Test-takers are checked in as they arrive, so you may have to wait a short time before being checked in.

---

[2] Data from Dental Admission Test (DAT) 2022 Candidate Guide, © 2022 by American Dental Association.

You will be given a small locker in which to store whatever items you brought with you (such as a small snack). Literally everything that you brought with you, other than your clothing and your IDs, must go into your locker, including books, dental instruments, calculators, cell phones, bags of any kind, writing implements, or food. (The ADA specifically notes that, among other things, "good luck charms, statues, religious or superstitious talismans" cannot be brought into the computer room.) The ADA is very explicit about the items that can and can't be brought and when they can be accessed, so make sure to read their guidelines before you go.

The security verifications during check-in can be somewhat involved and intimidating, but they are nothing to worry about. Prometric testing centers are equipped with video and audio recording devices that can see and hear every part of the center, and you will be asked to sign in and out every time you enter and exit the computer room. You may also be asked to turn out your pockets, and other basic security procedures may be followed. Don't worry; they're standard.

During check-in, you will likely be provided with noteboards and two dry-erase markers. You may or may not be given an eraser. These noteboards are typically two sheets of laminated, letter-sized graph paper. The two dry-erase markers are fine-tipped, usually pencil-sized but sometimes larger. The eraser works, but the noteboards often don't erase very cleanly on the first swipe without pressing fairly hard, so don't plan to erase a great deal during the middle of a section. You can, however, get a fresh set of noteboards during the break in the middle of the test, so feel free to fill up the sheets during the SNS and PAT. Most students aim to use one noteboard (front and back) for each section of the DAT. Over the last few years, some test centers have switched to using scratch paper booklets (usually 4–6 pieces of paper) and pencils. Either way, you will have something to write on during the test. If you're worried about this, visit or call your test center ahead of time and ask what you will be given.

Once you are checked in, you will be allowed to enter the computer room. You will be taken to a seat and asked to verify that your name is on the computer screen. At the computer will be a screen, a keyboard, a mouse, and noise-canceling headphones (which are bulky but very effective). Most test centers also offer disposable, foam earplugs, available by request. The mouse will have two buttons. Once you sit down and click forward, the tutorial will begin.

During the test, other test-takers will be checking in and taking breaks sporadically. Test-takers are checked in one-by-one, so even if someone else has exactly the same appointment time as you, they will start the test before or after you, and most other test-takers do not have the same appointment time (and are not even taking the same test). Thus, don't worry about anyone else at the center. They are completely irrelevant to your test.

Each question of the DAT will be on a separate screen. To navigate between questions, you will use "Previous" and "Next" buttons. Before test day, you should work through the free DAT tutorial, available on the Prometric website. This is a good way to preview what the computer-based test interface will look like.

After the test, your scores pop up on the screen instantly, so steel yourself mentally when you finish the QRT. You are also given a printout of your scores. These printouts are technically unofficial, since the ADA must review them before they become official, though this step is usually just a formality.

1.4 TEST STRATEGIES

Strategy will be discussed at length in each the following chapters devoted to each subject, but there are a few overall test strategies that you should be familiar with at the outset.

CBT Tools

You will have several resources at your disposal on test day, in addition to the noteboards mentioned above. It is important to make good use of these resources. Here are some suggestions.

Keep your **noteboards** neat and organized. Here are some additional suggestions on how and when to use your noteboards:

- Summarize a question stem or take key notes, if you need help understanding what a question is asking
- Write down equation manipulations or calculations in Gchem or QRT
- Write down molecules, reactions and/or mechanisms in Ochem
- Use 4×4 grids on the graph paper for Hole Punching in PAT
- Map out cube stacks in Cube Counting of PAT
- Generate your passage maps in RCT

A **Mark** button is available for each question and allows you to flag a question as one you would like to review later, if time permits. When clicked, the "Mark" button turns red and says "Marked."

A **Review** button is found near the bottom of the screen, and when clicked, brings up a new screen showing all questions in the current section and their status (either "answered" or "unanswered," and "marked" or not). You can then choose one of three options: "review all," "review unanswered," or "review marked." You can only review questions in the section of the DAT you are currently taking. If you click a question on the Review screen, you will be taken directly to that question. Because of this, the Review screen is a good way to quickly navigate through a section.

For the most part, you will use the Mark and Review buttons for the "Two-Pass Technique" described below. No matter what, as time runs short in a section, use the Review button to make sure that you have selected an answer for every question before time runs out. You should never, ever, ever leave a question blank on the DAT, as the "Guessing" discussion below will explain.

Clicking the **Exhibit** button on the SNS will open a periodic table. The periodic table is large and covers most of the screen. However, this window can be resized so you can see the questions and a portion of the periodic table at the same time. The table text will not decrease, but scroll bars will appear on the window so you can center the section of the table of interest in the window. On the QRT, this button says **"Calculator"** instead, and it pops up the on-screen calculator. This calculator will be discussed in detail later, when we discuss the QRT. Note that a calculator is only available for the QRT; you will not have access to a calculator for the SNS.

You can **highlight** words in question stems and can also highlight RCT passages. To do this, click and drag over text, or double click to select a single word. Once you have some text selected, an icon shows up below the text and after clicking the icon, the word(s) you have selected are highlighted yellow. These markings will be retained for the entire section, even if you navigate around. You can remove highlighting by clicking it again. If you are struggling to understand what a question is asking, you should highlight some key words in the question stem. Many students answer questions more accurately if they highlight words in the question stem such as *least, most, not, except, true,* or *false.* Highlighting RCT passages will be discussed in Chapter 37.

You can also electronically **strikeout** answer options when you are doing process of elimination (POE), discussed below. To do this, right click on a word in an answer option, and that answer option will change to having a line through it, like this:

A. ~~An example of striking out~~

If you right click the answer option again, the strikeout will be removed, and if you left click, the strikeout will be removed and the option will be selected as the correct answer. Finally, strikeouts are retained as you navigate around a section of the DAT.

Process of Elimination

Since the DAT is a multiple-choice test, knowing that one answer is right is helpful, but knowing that all of the other answers are wrong is equally helpful. You might not be sure what the primary purpose of the first paragraph of a reading passage is, but you might be able to tell what it's not, and whatever is left over after you eliminate what it cannot possibly be must be the right answer. The same is true throughout the SNS, PAT, RCT, and QRT.

As you are doing **Process of Elimination (POE)**, strike out answers you are sure are definitely wrong. Leave answers that you are not sure about or that you don't understand. Hopefully, on your first pass through the answers, you will eliminate between 2 and 4 options. If you only have one answer left, read it quickly to make sure it makes sense; then select it and move on. Beware that you will see questions on test day where you are sure four answers are wrong but you're not sure why the option that is left is correct. If the other answers are definitely wrong, the last answer must be right, so don't waste time worrying about it and move on.

If you have more than one answer left, slow down a little and focus. Try to find something that is true and answers the question. If you're working on the RCT, the correct answer should also be supported by the passage. You can also compare the remaining answer choices to each other, to help you spot differences between them. Once you've decided on the best answer, select it and move on.

Over the last few years, the DAT has started to include content that is outside the scope of the test in question stems and answer choices. For example, you could see a biology question stem on astrocytes or an answer choice talking about Oomycota. Both of these are beyond the scope of the DAT and as a consequence, are not covered in this book. However, you are still expected to be able to answer questions like this by analyzing the other information you have and relying on content that is within the scope of the DAT (i.e., content reviewed in this book). Overall, you will see weird and unexpected stuff on test day, but focusing on what you know and relying on POE are your best strategies for succeeding on even these advanced and stressful questions.

Guessing

There are no penalties for wrong answers, so you should never leave blanks; a blank question is treated the same as a wrong answer, but a question with a guessed answer could be right. On some questions, you can eliminate answers and guess among the remaining choices. For the rest, choose your favorite guessing letter. We call this the **Letter of the Day.** Select your Letter of the Day for any question you can't or don't have time to answer. No letter is more often right than any other letter, but there is a statistical advantage to guessing consistently. Thus, if your Letter of the Day is A, guess A for every question you skip or can't answer in every section of the test. Finally, keep in mind that most questions on the SNS, RCT, and QRT will have five options (A through E), but some may have only three or four. Some sections of the PAT have four option questions and others have five options (which will be discussed more in Chapter 30). If E is your Letter of the Day, you may have to choose option D or even C on some questions.

Scoring and Pacing

Many students approach the DAT the way that they would approach tests in school: they attempt to answer every question to the best of their abilities, which in the DAT usually amounts to rushing at top speed through most sections. They expect that they will get almost all of the questions right, and that this is what they need to do to get a good score. Then they are shocked by what their actual score is.

The reason for this is that the DAT is not scored like tests in school. If you are accustomed to getting at least an A– (or possibly a B+) in most classes, and if you normally needed about 90% right on tests to achieve this score, prepare for a shock. A score between 20 and 22 is competitive for most dental schools, and you typically need between 75% and 85% correct to get a 20, and between 85% and 90% correct to get a 22. Combine this with the fact that there are likely to be some questions that, no matter how much time you spend on them, you just don't know how to answer them, and you come to the realization that you have to approach this test differently than other tests you've taken in your life.

Consider the following scoring grid, which converts numbers of questions answered correctly into scaled, standard scores. (This grid changes slightly from test to test, by the way, but it is often much like this one.)

1.4

STD Score	Raw Score (i.e., how many questions you answered correctly)							
	Biology [/40]	General Chem [/30]	Organic Chem [/30]	SNS [/100]	PAT [/90]	RCT [/50]	QRT [/40]	AA [/190]
30	40	30	30	100	90	50	40	190
29	–	–	–	99	89	49	–	189
28	39	–	–	98	88	–	39	188
27	–	29	29	97	–	48	–	186–187
26	38	–	–	96	87	–	38	184–185
25	–	–	–	95	86	47	–	181–183
24	37	28	28	94	84–85	46	37	178–180
23	–	–	–	92–93	82–83	45	–	174–177
22	36	27	27	90–91	79–81	44	–	169–173
21	35	26	26	87–89	75–78	42–43	36	163–168
20	34	25	25	83–86	70–74	40–41	34–35	155–162
19	32–33	24	24	78–82	65–69	37–39	32–33	146–154
18	30–31	23	22–23	71–77	59–64	33–36	30–31	136–145
17	28–29	21–22	20–21	64–70	53–58	29–32	28–29	124–135
16	25–27	19–20	18–19	57–63	46–52	27–28	25–27	114–123
15	22–24	15–18	15–17	50–56	40–45	25–26	22–24	99–113
14	19–21	12–14	12–14	42–49	34–39	22–24	19–21	85–98
13	14–18	9–11	9–11	34–41	28–33	18–21	16–18	72–84
12	10–13	7–8	7–8	27–33	23–27	15–17	13–15	59–71
11	7–9	6	6	22–26	18–22	13–14	11–12	47–58
10	5–6	5	5	18–21	15–17	11–12	8–10	38–46
9	4	4	4	14–17	11–14	9–10	6–7	31–37
8	3	3	3	10–13	8–10	7–8	5	24–30
7	–	2	2	7–9	7	5–6	4	18–23
6	2	–	–	5–6	5–6	–	3	13–17
5	–	1	1	4	4	4	–	9–12
4	–	–	–	3	3	3	2	6–8
3	1	–	–	2	2	2	–	3–5
2	–	–	–	1	1	1	1	1–2
1	0	0	0	0	0	0	0	0

Skip-Some Strategy

Now, let's do some calculations with the above numbers, specifically with the PAT for the sake of discussion. To get a competitive score around a 20 on the PAT you need about 70 questions correct. You could answer all 90 questions in the time allotted, at an average speed of 40 seconds per question, and hope to get 78% (70 questions) correct. This is certainly a possibility, and it is what many test-takers try to do.

However, it is not the only way to get this score. Consider slowing down and skipping some questions instead. If you completed only 70 of the 90 questions, you would have more time per question (an extra 10–12 seconds on average). You can get a few of the 70 wrong because if you guess on the 20 hardest questions, you would probably get about 3 or 4 of those questions right. Remember, if you guess consistently, you have a 1 in 4, or 1 in 5 chance of getting the question correct, depending on how many answer choices there are.

Now, a difference of 10–12 seconds per question may not sound like very much. However, bear in mind that if you guess on 20 questions, you get to skip questions that you don't know how to do. You could skip the entire Orthographic Projections section! Or the hardest 3 questions in every section of the PAT! You will have more time to answer the questions you do know how to do, instead of rushing through everything. If you're answering fewer questions, your accuracy rate has to increase, but this is likely going to happen anyhow if you're skipping the hardest questions and focusing on your strengths.

Overall then, pacing yourself to finish all the questions in every section may not be the best strategy for you. Instead, make pacing goals for each DAT section of each practice test (or section) you complete. A pacing goal is a total number of questions to attempt in a given section, perhaps combined with goals for times at which to finish each group of questions (e.g., finish the first 15 questions in 8 minutes, then the next 15 in 10 minutes, and so on). For example, if you just scored a 14 on the PAT (meaning you got 34 to 39 questions right out of 90), it's fairly unlikely that you will immediately jump to getting all 90 questions right. On your next practice test, you should try to gain a few scaled points, perhaps 2, which means that your total pacing goal should be to answer about 50 questions and guess on the rest. This is an achievable goal, and it will improve your score. Once you score a 16, you can pace yourself to answer more questions, and more, and more, until you get to your desired final score.

Similar advice applies to each of the other sections as well. On the RCT, answering all the questions on two passages completely and finishing about half of a third passage with a similar accuracy will result in 40 questions correct and a score of 20. To get a 20 on the SNS sections, you can miss about 6 biology questions and 5 questions from each chemistry section. Instead of rushing through everything, mark questions that you can't answer or questions that will take a long time to answer. If you have time for these at the end of the section, great. If not, answer them using your Letter of the Day. Keep in mind that Biology, General Chemistry, and Organic Chemistry are scored individually as well as together, and that you must complete all three in 90 minutes total. Many students find the chemistry questions more difficult than the biology questions, so you will probably need more time per question for the 60 chemistry questions than the 40 biology questions.

Two-Pass Technique

In the SNS, QRT, and PAT, you should move through the section in two passes. On the first pass, categorize questions as Now, Later, or Never. Now questions are those that you know how to answer quickly and accurately. Later questions are those that you can probably figure out how to answer, but they will take more time. Never questions are those that you probably don't know how to answer at all, at least not within a few minutes (and you should not spend more than a few minutes on any one question on the test).

While you are categorizing questions on the first pass, complete the Now questions as soon as you see them, and mark the Later questions in some way (either on your noteboard or with the Mark button) so that you can come back to them. Select your Letter of the Day for the Never questions, because you don't want to spend any more time thinking about them. On your practice exams, make some indication on your simulated noteboard that you guessed on a question, so that you will know on review why you chose your answer, although this is not necessary on the real DAT.

Then, on the second pass, come back for the Later questions. At this point, you can have a good idea how much time you have left for each remaining question. For example, if you categorize 25 QRT questions as Now and 10 as Later (with 5 Never questions), and if you finish the Now questions in 25 minutes (which is fast), then you know that you have 20 minutes left for the remaining 10 Later questions and should spend about 2 minutes on each question. On the other hand, if you just tried to complete the Later questions as you came to them, you would not know whether 2 minutes was too long to spend on a single question.

Strategy Summary

In essence, much of this advice boils down to four simple words: accuracy first, speed second. Getting questions wrong quickly is not much better than getting questions wrong slowly; first, get them right, and then you can worry about getting them right quickly. Students who rush through easier questions, to questions that are hard (or impossible) for them, often make preventable mistakes on the easy questions. First you must focus on answering the questions that you know how to answer, and then you can work on answering the rest of the questions.

More Great Books

Are you seeking anatomy or biology review content that's a bit different than your average textbook? Check out *Anatomy Coloring Workbook, 4th Edition* and *Biology Coloring Workbook, 2nd Edition,* our beautiful coloring books that help you review while you color.

Of course, if you do get to the point where you are consistently scoring a 20 or higher on a section and are shooting for an extremely high score, you need to answer all of the questions and get pretty much all of them right. (To give some frame of reference, on many sections you need about 95% correct on all the questions in order to score a 25 or above.) In that case, you don't need to worry about guessing letters, but you will still probably want to take the section in two passes and follow much of the rest of the advice above. Even if you answer all of the questions, there is an advantage to having the last few questions you work be the hardest questions, so that you know exactly how much time you can allot to working them. This might, in extreme cases, mean that your first pass consists of about 35 questions, and the second pass consists of about 5 questions; just make sure that your question sequence makes sense.

Thinking of Taking the Canadian DAT?

The Canadian DAT is very similar to the American DAT, but there are some important differences. For information on this test and the manual dexterity soap-carving section, check out the Canadian DAT supplement available online, when you register this book.

1.5 DENTAL OVERVIEW

Pre-Dental Curriculum

Before you take the DAT, you have to take certain classes in college. These are the pre-dental prerequisites. These may vary somewhat from school to school, but in general, you are required to take at least a year of English, general chemistry, organic chemistry, physics, and biology. Schools may also require classes in calculus, biochemistry, or other fields, such as psychology or statistics.

Most schools require you to have completed a bachelor's degree in some subject from an accredited college or university, though most do not recommend any particular major over any other, as long as you complete your prerequisite coursework. You will also find it useful in the long term to take classes that develop your interpersonal communication, business, and intensive science knowledge. Thus, in addition to advanced courses in biology, chemistry, and physics, you may find it useful to take courses that require extensive reading, writing, and analytical thinking, as well as courses in statistics, anatomy, physiology, accounting, and economics. Such courses are not required for admission to dental school, but they are useful to dental students as well as dentists beyond the world of education. In addition, picking up a hobby that develops manual dexterity could also be of benefit in preparation for the years ahead of developing hand skills. Hobbies such as woodworking, carving, drawing, and knitting may help develop your hand–eye coordination. These hobbies are also topics that can be brought up during a dental school interview.

As you are choosing your undergraduate courses, bear in mind that rigorous courses are viewed very positively in admissions. While GPA is important, schools also consider the context in which you earned your GPA. The strength of your overall course history is a very significant factor, perhaps as significant as your personal statement or recommendations. If you took GPA-boosting easy classes, while another student took challenging and rigorous classes, then the other student may get the benefit of the doubt even on a slightly lower GPA.

Also, sometimes students pursue graduate degrees before applying to dental school. Such degrees are helpful, even though your undergraduate GPA will be the primary GPA considered, not your graduate GPA. Having a Masters or PhD is definitely a modest advantage in admissions, in part because it shows additional academic ability.

Dental Admissions Information

Applications for dental school are usually processed through the American Association of Dental Schools Application Service (AADSAS), which is sort of like a common portal for dental schools. All components of a primary application go through this service. This application usually becomes available in June each year, and you must fill it out in the year before you intend to matriculate. Admissions is rolling at most dental schools, so applying in the summer, especially early in the summer, is advantageous.

The components of a dental school application include several numbers (termed "hard factors") and a variety of information ("soft factors" or "softs"). The main hard factors are your undergraduate GPA, potentially with emphasis on your science or major GPA, and your DAT scores, potentially with emphasis on your Academic Average and PAT scores. The soft factors include a personal statement, letters of recommendation (often three), and a resume.

Dental admission is typically holistic, meaning that no single factor is conclusive either way. For example, even if you have a great GPA, if your DAT is low and your personal statement is written poorly, you will likely be denied admission at most schools. Likewise, if you have an excellent overall application but one portion is a little worse than the others, that weak aspect may not hold you back. However, some dental schools do have minimum numbers for GPA or DAT scores, so be sure to check the specific schools' admission standards to make sure that you are eligible for admission.

Despite holistic admissions, the hard factors are usually the first consideration in evaluating an applicant. If your GPA and DAT scores are above average for what the school usually accepts, you have a very good chance, but if they are both below average for the school, your chances are low. Once admission committees have examined your numbers, they will also scrutinize the rest of your application. Many also request more information through a secondary application.

If you are in serious consideration after many applications are sifted and many candidates are eliminated, you will likely be asked to interview at the school. The interview usually involves going to the school, meeting with current students and faculty, and being asked extensive personal questions about your career goals and many other topics, sometimes including specific aspects of your application. (If there are any specific weaknesses or if there is anything unusual in your application, be prepared to address it.) Being granted an interview at all is a very good sign, though it does not guarantee admission.

The interview season lasts through late fall and winter after you have submitted your application. Regular decisions (acceptance, rejection, or waitlist) are usually completed by March or April of the year in which you intend to matriculate, although some may not be given until later.

Overview of Dental School

There are more than 60 different dental schools in the United States at some level of accreditation, and their educational methods are diverse, but some generalizations can be made. Dental school programs are typically four years long, like medical school programs. Like medical schools, dental schools grant two different degrees, but unlike the two medical school degrees (the M.D. and the D.O.), the two dental degrees are identical, with no difference in emphasis. Schools that grant degrees with names in English grant Doctor of Dental Surgery (D.D.S.) degrees, while schools that prefer Latin degree names grant degrees called Dentariae Medicinae Doctor (D.M.D., which in English is Doctor of Dental Medicine).

The first two years of the program are usually more focused on classroom instruction in core science and dental concepts, along with hands-on instruction in a "simulation learning–type" lab environment for various dental subjects. The third and fourth years typically introduce dental students to the clinic, beginning their experience in treating actual patients. Some dental schools share resources with medical schools, which are often located on the same campus, so some classes or activities may include both dental and medical students, especially in the first two years.

The DAT is not the last major standardized test that you must take if you want to become a dentist. You also get to look forward to taking the national boards during your third year of dental school, as well as regional boards and possibly other tests, too, should you decide to further your education in a dental specialty.

After graduating from general dental school, some students decide to pursue specialties. The ADA recognizes nine specialties, namely Dental Public Health, Endodontics, Oral and Maxillofacial Pathology, Oral and Maxillofacial Radiology, Oral and Maxillofacial Surgery, Orthodontics and Dentofacial Orthopedics, Pediatric Dentistry, Periodontics, and Prosthodontics. These specialties typically require several years of additional school.

Another option that students may pursue is a dual degree. Many dental schools are within or near universities that also offer other graduate degrees (such as a PhD, an MBA, or an MPH) and students may pursue both a dental degree and one of these other degrees simultaneously. A joint degree in dentistry and business or dentistry and public health is usually completed in four or five years (that is, not much longer than a dental degree by itself), while a joint dental degree and PhD may take as many as eight years or more (much longer than a dental degree by itself). Other joint degrees may be available, and a complex variety of interdisciplinary options may be available in a dental degree itself, so you should consult specific schools of interest if you want to learn more.

After Graduation

Dentists practice in a wide variety of contexts and locations. There are dentists in urban, suburban, and rural areas. Many dentists work in private practice, either in a smaller and usually self-owned practice or as part of a larger group. Some teach and do research at universities. Some work in hospitals alongside doctors and other specialists. Some work in public health, which can be anything from advocating for dental health policy in a political context to providing dental care in a Coast Guard base under the auspices of the U.S. Public Health Service. Thus, "being a dentist" can mean a lot of different things, depending on your interests.

In general, dentists are extremely well compensated. The American Dental Education Association (ADEA) says, "[I]n 2018, the average net income for an independent private general practitioner who owned all or part of their practice was $190,440. For dental specialists, it was $330,180."[3] This is tempered somewhat by the fact that dental school graduates often have substantial student debt. The ADEA estimates the average debt per dental school graduate in 2020 was $304,824.[4] Limited financial aid may be available, but due to the high expected salaries upon graduation, most dental schools expect students to borrow substantially to finance their education, and most dental students do not have difficulty paying back these loans with the income from their practices.

---

[3] www.adea.org, Aug 2022.

[4] www.ada.org and www.adea.org, Aug 2022.

Biology

Chapter 2
Biological
Macromolecules

2.1 INTRODUCTION TO THE SNS

What is the SNS?

SNS is the first section of the DAT and includes 40 Biology questions, 30 General Chemistry (Gchem) questions, and 30 Organic Chemistry (Ochem) questions. The questions will always show up in that order (Biology questions first, Ochem questions last). There are 100 questions in total and this section is 90 minutes long. Every question in the SNS will be a stand-alone multiple-choice question. Most will have five answer choices (A to E), but you may see a four-option question (A to D) or even a three-option questions (A to C).

SNS Content Breakdown

Generally speaking, the content you must know for the SNS is very broad, but not very deep. This means you literally have to know a little bit of everything, across a wide collection of content areas. The biology you should be familiar with spans most typical first- and second-year undergraduate courses. DAT Gchem covers most of first-year chemistry (a full-year course, or two semesters), while Ochem tests most of second-year Ochem (again, a full year course, or two semesters). While that may sound intimidating, the good news is we've collected the content you need to know for the DAT in this book. If you read it here, you should be familiar with it for the DAT. If something is not in this book, the probability of you needing background information on that topic is low.

That said, you will absolutely see new and unexpected content on test day. Over the last few years, the ADA has started including some pretty intimidating questions in the SNS section, especially biology. You may see content you've never heard of before in either a question stem or an answer choice. Don't panic! Between relying on the content in this book, using POE, and applying information they give you in the question stem, you'll be able to narrow down your options and likely make a solid guess at the best answer. Some of these intimidating questions will count toward your score, but a few are likely experimental questions that won't. As we saw in Chapter 1, every version of the DAT contains experimental questions that won't affect your score. No matter what, don't spend too long on any one question. If all else fails, guess using your Letter of the Day and move on.

Pace, Two-Pass Technique, and the Letter of the Day

Speaking of pace, many students aim to answer the 40 Biology questions in about 20 to 25 minutes, saving time for the chemistry questions. This is because you'll have to do equation work and calculations in Gchem (which take time) and work mechanisms and synthesis questions in Ochem (which also take time). Because Bio, Gchem, and Ochem are all part of the same section, you can spend time wherever you want, and you can answer the questions in whatever order you choose. Most test takers work through the SNS in order (Bio then Gchem then Ochem), and we suggest you do this in two passes.

On your first pass, work efficiently but don't rush. Answer the most doable questions, mark trickier questions so you can come back to them and select your Letter of the Day for the more challenging questions that are a big waste of time. Then take inventory of your section and your time. Go back through the section again on your second pass. This time, slow down, read carefully, and work on the more challenging questions. Don't spend more than 1–2 minutes on any one question; it is not worth it. You must know when to move on to avoid wasting time on one challenging question. Remember, every question is worth 0 or 1 point, no matter how long you spend on it.

Like all the other sections of the DAT, very few people spend time on every question. Accuracy is more important than speed! You can get a very respectable DAT score by skipping questions. For example, if you have high accuracy on the questions you're answering, you can get a score of 19–20 by skipping up to 5–6 questions! For this to work, make sure you're skipping the hardest questions and still answering them using your Letter of the Day. There are no penalties for wrong answers and a big advantage to guessing consistently.

Path to Score Improvement

There are six major steps you should take to see maximum score improvement on the SNS:

1. Get familiar with the SNS section: first, you need to know what you're preparing for. You have access to two online computer-based DAT practice tests by purchasing this book. They're waiting for you in your online tools. We suggest you take one of these tests soon, and the other 1–2 weeks before your DAT.
2. Go through the content in this book, reacquainting yourself with content and maybe even learning a few new things.
3. Once you've been through the content, go through it again in more detail, focusing on understanding. Make and review study notes. Draw out summary diagrams. Make a small number of flashcards to help you memorize some key pieces of information you often forget. Find a study partner and explain some concepts to them out loud. Go back and review content you've forgotten or don't quite understand yet.
4. Do *lots* of practice problems. You should spend more than half your study time doing practice questions. If you're working in a book, answer questions on a separate piece of paper so you can go back and redo questions you struggled with. Use the strategies in this book on every question. Finally, pay attention to which questions are easy for you and which are hard.
5. Review your work! It is not enough to do practice questions; you must spend time going through the solution for every question and learning from your mistakes. More specifically, if you spend 1 hour working on questions, you should spend 1 hour reviewing your work. Ask yourself questions like:
   - Did I answer the question the best way possible?
   - Did I eliminate the wrong answers for the right reasons?
   - Did I select the right answer for the right reason?
   - Could I have saved time on this question?
   - What could I have done differently?
   - Did I miss anything?
6. Finally, redo questions you got wrong, didn't understand, found tricky, or struggled with. Flag these questions and do them again a few days later. Then return to them again in a week, and maybe again a week after that. You understand a question well enough once you can explain it to a study friend (or your parent, or your pet, or your partner, or your neighbor… you get the idea).

Introduction to Biology

The SNS has a predictable content breakdown. In Biology, about a third of the questions will test cell and molecular biology. About a quarter of the questions will test structure and function of systems, which is a fancy way of saying vertebrate anatomy and physiology. Next, you will see about 5–6 questions on genetics. The rest of the section will test diversity of life, evolution, and ecology.

In 2022, the ADA added some new biology content to the DAT, which is included in this book. The new content includes viruses, Archaebacteria, genomics, gene expression, and epigenetics. They also formally added questions they're calling "integrated relationships," which are questions that test multiple content areas in one question.

Your success in the Biology section will affect your Biology, SNS, and AA scores. In addition, many dental schools consider your Biology score important when they're making admissions decisions. Knowing this, let's jump into biology content.

2.2 AMINO ACIDS

Proteins are biological macromolecules that act as enzymes, hormones, receptors, antibodies, and support structures inside and outside cells. Proteins are composed of twenty different **amino acids** linked together in polymers. The composition and sequence of amino acids in the **polypeptide** chain is what makes each protein unique and enables it to fulfill its special role in the cell. In this section, we will start with amino acids, the building blocks of proteins, and work our way up to three-dimensional protein structure and function.

Amino Acid Structure and Nomenclature

Understanding the structure of amino acids is key to understanding both their chemistry and the chemistry of proteins. The generic formula for all 20 amino acids is shown below.

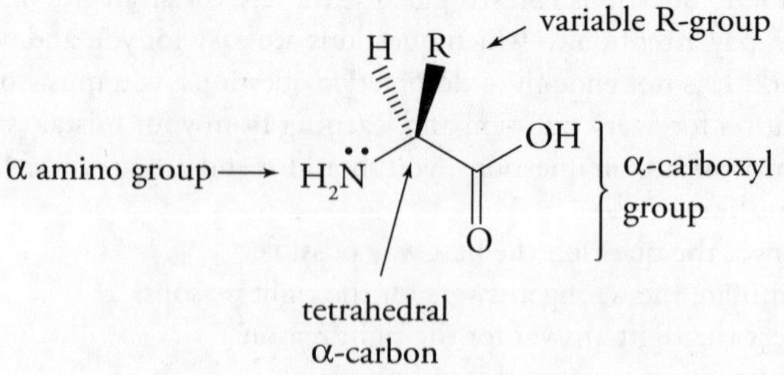

Figure 1   Generic Amino Acid Structure

All 20 amino acids share the same nitrogen-carbon-carbon (or N–C–C) backbone. The unique feature of each amino acid is its **side chain** (variable R-group), which gives it the physical and chemical properties that distinguish it from the other 19 amino acids.

Classification of Amino Acids

Each of the 20 amino acids is unique because of its side chain. Each amino acid has a three-letter abbreviation and a one-letter abbreviation, which you do NOT need to memorize. Though they are all unique, many amino acids have similar chemical properties. It is also NOT necessary to memorize all 20 side chains, but you should know the general structure of an amino acid (as above) and should recognize the four structures below. In addition, it is important to understand the chemical properties that characterize the 20 amino acids; the important properties of side chains include their varying polarity, size, shape, charge, ability to **hydrogen bond**, and ability to act as acids or bases. These R-group properties are important in the structure of proteins.

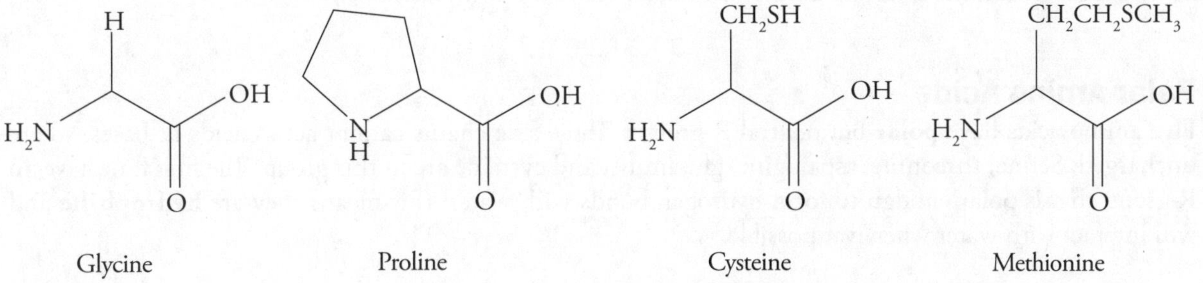

Glycine   Proline   Cysteine   Methionine

Figure 2   Important Amino Acids for the DAT

Hydrophobic Amino Acids

Amino acids are often classified based on their polarity. Hydrophobic amino acids have either aliphatic (alkyl) or aromatic side chains. Amino acids with aliphatic side chains include glycine, alanine, valine, leucine, isoleucine, proline, and methionine. Amino acids with aromatic side chains include phenylalanine, tyrosine, and tryptophan. **Hydrophobic** residues tend to associate with each other rather than with water, and therefore are found on the interior of folded globular proteins, away from water. The larger the hydrophobic group, the greater the hydrophobic force repelling it from water. Glycine is the smallest amino acid, as it has only a hydrogen atom for its R-group. As a consequence, glycine is a really flexible amino acid and can fit into all sorts of small spaces in proteins. The side chain of **proline** forms a secondary amino group, since the R-group loops around and covalently bonds to the nitrogen atom of the amino end. This creates a distinctive ring structure. As a consequence, proline is a very rigid amino acid, and it cannot be found in some protein regions/shapes (more on this shortly).

Hydrophilic Amino Acids

The hydrophilic, or water-loving, side chains are categorized into three distinct categories: acidic, basic, and neutral polar residues.

Acidic Amino Acids

Glutamic acid and aspartic acid are the only amino acids with carboxylic acid functional groups ($pK_a \approx 4$) in their side chains, thereby making the side chains acidic. Thus, there are three functional groups in these amino acids that may act as acids or bases—the two backbone groups and the R-group. You may hear the terms glutam*ate* and aspart*ate*—these refer to the anionic (unprotonated) form of the molecule.

Basic Amino Acids

Lysine, arginine, and histidine have basic R-group side chains. The pK_as for the side chains in these amino acids are 10 for Lys, 12 for Arg, and 6.5 for His. Histidine is unique in having a side chain with a pK_a so close to physiological pH. At pH 7.4 histidine may be either protonated or deprotonated—we put it in the basic category, but it often acts as an acid, too. This makes it a readily available proton acceptor *or* donor, explaining its prevalence at protein active sites (discussed below). A mnemonic is "His goes both ways." This contrasts with amino acids containing –COOH or –NH_2 side chains, which are *always* anionic (RCOO⁻) or cationic (RNH$_3^+$) at physiological pH. (By the way, *histamine* is a small molecule that has to do with allergic responses, itching, inflammation, and other processes. You've likely heard of antihistamine drugs. Histamine is not an amino acid; don't confuse it with *histidine*.)

Polar Amino Acids

Five amino acids have **polar** but neutral R-groups. These side chains cannot act as acids or bases, so are uncharged. Serine, threonine, asparagine, glutamine, and cysteine are in this group. The first four have an R-group that is polar enough to form hydrogen bonds with water; this means they are **hydrophilic** and will interact with water whenever possible.

Additional Classifications

In addition to being classified as nonpolar and polar, R-groups can be assigned additional groupings based on the atoms they contain.

Sulfur-Containing Amino Acids

Amino acids with sulfur-containing side chains include cysteine and methionine. Cysteine, which contains a thiol group (also called a sulfhydryl—like an alcohol that has an S atom instead of an O atom), is actually fairly polar, and methionine, which contains a thioether (like an ether that has an S atom instead of an O atom), is fairly nonpolar. Cysteine is the only amino acid able to participate in disulfide bonds, and methionine is coded by the AUG start codon. You'll learn more about these amino acids in the next few sections and chapters.

Hydroxyl-Containing Amino Acids

Serine, threonine, and tyrosine have terminal hydroxyl groups. These are often modified by regulatory enzymes, which can attach a phosphate group (a process called **phosphorylation**). The result is a change in structure due to addition of a hydrophilic phosphate group. This modification is an important means of regulating protein activity. In some cases, histidine can also be covalently modified by phosphorylation, even though it doesn't contain an OH-group.

Tyrosine is a bit of a tricky amino acid. It has a nonpolar aromatic ring, but a polar hydroxyl group. Note that we've drawn it here for you, but you don't need to memorize this structure. Tyrosine is usually classified as polar, but in some instances, can interact with more hydrophilic environments.

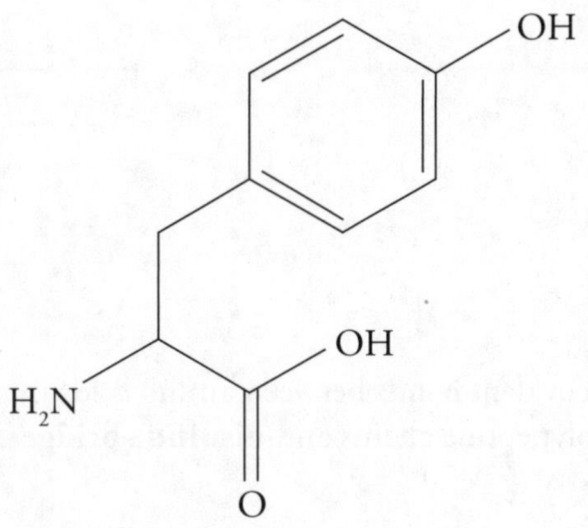

Figure 3   Tyrosine

Hydrophobic	Hydrophilic		
Nonpolar	Polar	Acidic	Basic
Glycine	Serine	Aspartic acid	Lysine*
Alanine	Threonine*	Glutamic acid	Arginine
Valine*	Asparagine		Histidine
Leucine*	Glutamine		
Isoleucine*	Cysteine		
Proline			
Methionine*			
Phenylalanine*			
Tyrosine			
Tryptophan*			
*Denotes one of the eight **essential amino acids**, those that cannot be synthesized by adult humans and must be obtained from the diet.			

Table 1   Summary Table of Amino Acids

- Which of these amino acids is most likely to be found on the interior of a protein at pH 7.0?[1]
  - A. Alanine
  - B. Glutamic acid
  - C. Phenylalanine
  - D. Glycine
  - E. Valine

---

[1]   Glutamic acid is incorrect, since this amino acid is charged at a pH of 7. Of the four remaining, phenylalanine has the largest hydrophobic group, and is therefore the most likely to be found on the interior of a protein. The answer is **C**.

- Which of the following amino acids is most likely to be found on the exterior of a protein at pH 7.0?[2]
  A. Leucine
  B. Alanine
  C. Serine
  D. Isoleucine
  E. Tyrosine

2.3 PROTEINS

There are two common types of covalent bonds between amino acids in proteins: the **peptide bonds** that link amino acids together into polypeptide chains and **disulfide bridges** between cysteine R-groups.

Peptide Bond

Polypeptides are formed by linking amino acids together in peptide bonds. A peptide bond is formed between the carboxyl group of one amino acid and the α-**amino group** of another amino acid with the loss of water. The figure below shows the formation of a dipeptide from the amino acids glycine and alanine.

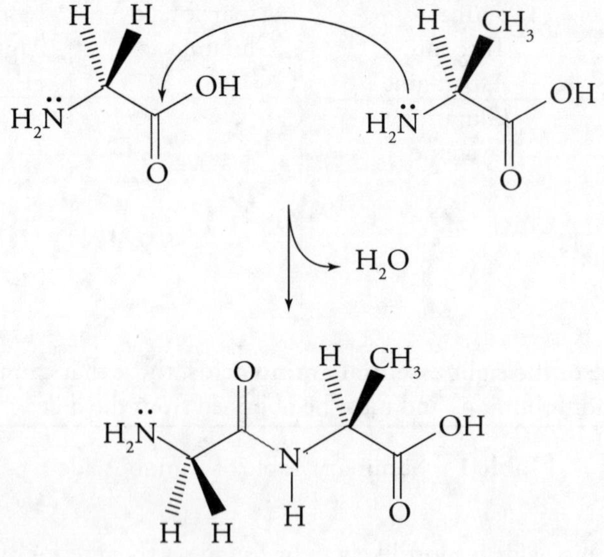

Figure 4 Peptide Bond (Amide Bond) Formation

---

[2] Leucine, alanine, and isoleucine are all hydrophobic residues more likely to be found on the interior than the exterior of proteins. Serine (**C**), which has a hydroxyl group that can hydrogen bond with water, is the correct answer. While Tyrosine has a polar OH group, it also has a hydrophobic aromatic ring, making serine a better answer.

Disulfide Bond

Cysteine is an amino acid with a reactive thiol (sulfhydryl, SH) in its side chain. The thiol of one cysteine can react with the thiol of another cysteine to produce a covalent sulfur-sulfur bond known as a **disulfide bond**, as illustrated. The cysteines forming a disulfide bond may be located in the same or different polypeptide chain(s). The disulfide bridge plays an important role in stabilizing tertiary protein structure; this will be discussed below. Once a cysteine residue becomes disulfide-bonded to another cysteine residue, it is called *cystine* instead of cysteine.

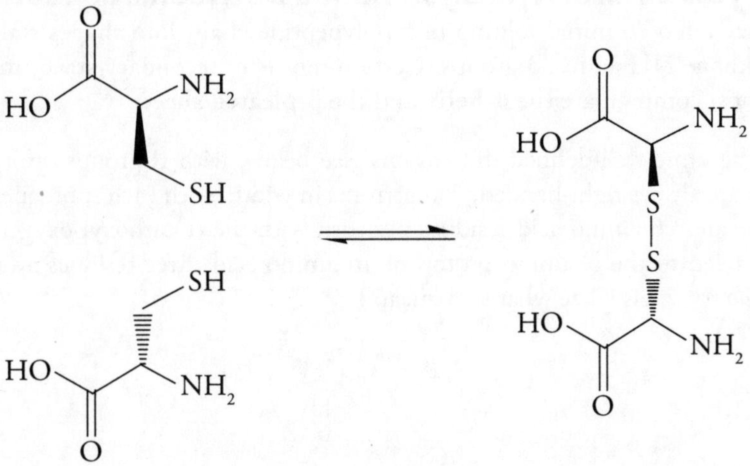

Figure 5   Formation of the Disulfide Bond

- Is disulfide bond formation an example of reduction or oxidation?[3]

Protein Structure in Three Dimensions

Each protein folds into a unique three-dimensional structure that is required for the protein to function properly. There are up to four levels of protein folding that contribute to the final three-dimensional structure. Each level of structure is dependent upon a particular type of bond, as discussed in the following sections.

Protein folding is tightly regulated and controlled by a family of proteins called **chaperones**. Improperly folded proteins are typically non-functional, as are denatured proteins. **Denaturation** is an important concept; it refers to disruption of a protein's shape without breaking peptide bonds. Proteins can be denatured by urea (which disrupts hydrogen bonds), extreme pH, extreme temperatures, or changes in salt concentration (or tonicity).

---

[3]   Disulfide bond formation is associated with a loss of hydrogen atoms; it is therefore an oxidation reaction. Breaking a disulfide bond is a reduction reaction. More on this shortly!

Primary [1°] Structure: The Amino Acid Sequence

The simplest level of protein structure is the order of amino acids bonded to each other in the polypeptide chain. This linear ordering of amino acid residues is known as **primary structure**. Primary structure is the same as **sequence**. The bond which determines 1° structure is the peptide bond, because this is the bond that links one amino acid to the next in a polypeptide.

Secondary [2°] Structure: Hydrogen Bonds Between Backbone Groups

Secondary structure refers to initial folding of a polypeptide chain into shapes stabilized by hydrogen bonds between backbone NH and CO groups. Certain motifs of secondary structure are found in most proteins. The two most common are the **α-helix** and the **β-pleated sheet**.

All α-helices have the same well-defined dimensions (see below, with R-groups omitted for clarity). The α-helices of proteins are always right-handed, 5 angstroms in width, with each subsequent amino acid rising 1.5 angstroms. There are 3.6 amino acid residues per turn with the α-carboxyl oxygen of one amino acid residue hydrogen-bonded to the α-amino proton of an amino acid three residues away. (*Don't* memorize these numbers, but *do* try to visualize what they mean.)

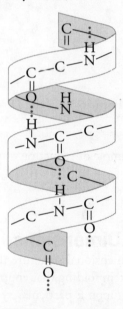

Figure 6   α-Helix

The unique structure of **proline** forces it to kink the polypeptide chain; hence proline residues never appear within an α-helix.

Proteins such as hormone receptors and ion channels are often found with α-helical transmembrane regions integrated into the hydrophobic membranes of cells. The α-helix is a favorable structure for a hydrophobic transmembrane region because all polar NH and CO groups in the backbone are hydrogen bonded to each other on the inside of the helix, and thus don't interact with the hydrophobic membrane interior. α-Helical regions that span membranes also have hydrophobic R-groups, which radiate out from the helix, interacting with the hydrophobic interior of the membrane.

β-Pleated sheets are also stabilized by hydrogen bonding between NH and CO groups in the polypeptide backbone. In β-sheets, however, hydrogen bonding occurs between residues distant from each other in the chain or even on separate polypeptide chains. Also, the backbone of a β-sheet is extended, rather than coiled, with side groups directed above and below the plane of the β-sheet. There are two types of β-sheets, one with adjacent polypeptide strands running in the *same* direction (**parallel** β-pleated sheet) and another in which the polypeptide strands run in *opposite* directions (**antiparallel** β-pleated sheet).

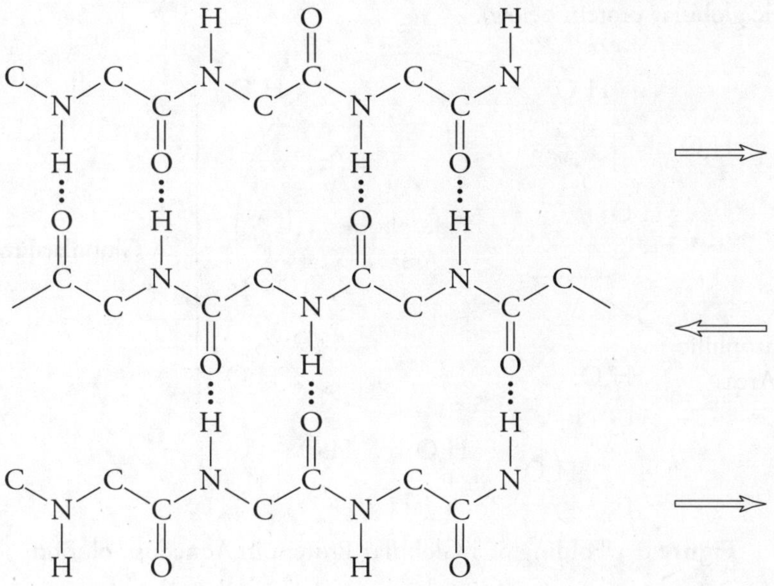

Figure 7 β-Pleated Sheet

- If a single polypeptide folds once and forms a β-pleated sheet with itself, would this be a parallel or antiparallel β-pleated sheet?[4]
- What effect would a molecule that disrupts hydrogen bonding, e.g., urea, have on protein structure?[5]

---

[4] It would be antiparallel because one participant in the β-pleated sheet would have a C to N direction, while the other would be running N to C.

[5] Putting a protein in a urea solution will disrupt H-bonding, thus disrupting secondary structure by unfolding α-helices and β-sheets. It would not affect primary structure, which depends on the much more stable peptide bond. Remember, disruption of 2°, 3°, or 4° structure without breaking peptide bonds is *denaturation*.

2.3

Tertiary (3°) Structure: Hydrophobic/Hydrophilic Interactions

The next level of protein folding, **tertiary structure**, concerns interactions between amino acid residues located more distantly from each other in the polypeptide chain. Folding of secondary structures, such as α-helices, into higher order tertiary structures is driven by interactions of R-groups with each other and with the solvent (almost always water). Hydrophobic R-groups tend to fold into the interior of the protein, away from the solvent, and hydrophilic R-groups tend to be exposed to water on the surface of the protein (shown for a generic globular protein below).

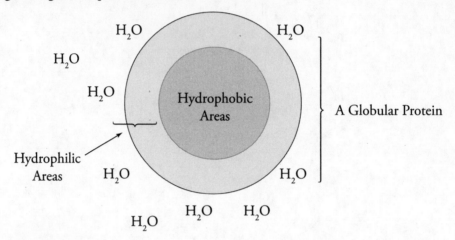

Figure 8   Folding of a Globular Protein in Aqueous Solution

Under the right conditions, the forces driving hydrophobic avoidance of water and hydrogen bonding will fold a polypeptide spontaneously into the correct conformation, the lowest energy conformation.

The disulfide bridge is a unique part of 3° structure because it is a covalent bond, not a hydrophobic interaction. However, because the disulfide is formed after 2° structure and before 4° structure, it is usually considered part of 3° folding.

- Which of the following may be considered an example of tertiary protein structure?[6]
  A.   van der Waals interactions between two phenylalanine R-groups located far apart on a polypeptide
  B.   Hydrogen bonds between backbone amino and carboxyl groups
  C.   Covalent disulfide bonds between cysteine residues located far apart on a polypeptide
  D.   More than one of the above
  E.   None of the above

- What effect would dissolving a globular protein in a hydrophobic organic solvent such as hexane have on tertiary protein structure?[7]

---

[6]   Choice A is a good example of 3° structure. Choice B describes 2°, not 3°, structure. Choice C describes the disulfide bond, which is part of tertiary folding because of when it is formed, despite the fact that it is a covalent bond. Overall, choice **D** is correct.

[7]   The protein would be turned inside out.

Quaternary (4°) Structure: Various Bonds Between Separate Chains

The highest level of protein structure, **quaternary structure**, describes interactions between polypeptide subunits. A **subunit** is a single polypeptide chain that is part of a large complex containing many subunits (a **multisubunit complex**). The arrangement of subunits in a multisubunit complex is what we mean by quaternary structure. For example, mammalian RNA polymerase II contains 12 different subunits. Both hemoglobin (or Hb, the protein that carries oxygen around in your blood) and immunoglobulins (also called antibodies, proteins crucial to your immune response) contain four peptide chains per protein. Interactions between subunits are instrumental in protein function, as in the cooperative binding of oxygen by each of the four subunits of hemoglobin.

The forces stabilizing quaternary structure are generally the same as those involved in secondary and tertiary structure—non-covalent interactions (hydrogen bonds, hydrophobic interactions, and van der Waals interactions). However, covalent bonds may also be involved in quaternary structure. For example, antibodies are large protein complexes with disulfide bonds holding the subunits together. It is key to understand, however, that there is one covalent bond that may not be involved in quaternary structure—the peptide bond—because this bond defines sequence (1° structure).

- What is the difference between a disulfide bridge involved in quaternary structure and one involved in tertiary structure?[8]

Here is a summary of protein structure:

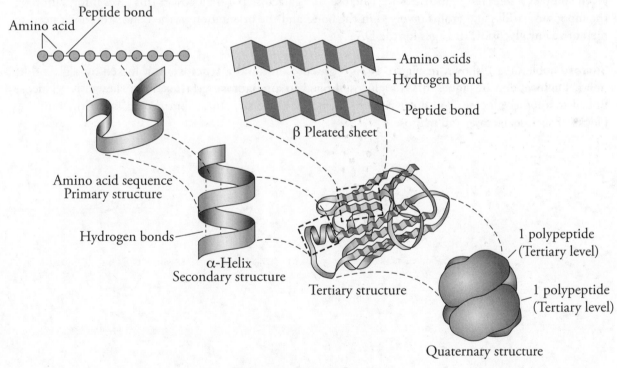

Figure 9 Protein Structure

---

[8] Quaternary disulfides are bonds that form between chains that aren't linked by peptide bonds. Tertiary disulfides are bonds that form between residues in the same polypeptide.

2.4 CARBOHYDRATES

Carbohydrates are chains of hydrated carbon atoms with the molecular formula $C_nH_{2n}O_n$. The chain usually begins with an aldehyde or ketone and continues as a polyalcohol in which each carbon has a hydroxyl substituent. Carbohydrates are produced by photosynthesis in plants and by biochemical synthesis in animals. Carbohydrates can be broken down to CO_2 in a process called **oxidation**, which is also known as burning or combustion. Because this process releases large amounts of energy, carbohydrates serve as the principle energy source for cellular metabolism. Glucose in the form of the polymer cellulose is also the building block of wood and cotton. Understanding the nomenclature, structure, and chemistry of carbohydrates is essential to understanding cellular metabolism. This chapter will also help you understand key facts such as why we can eat potatoes and cotton candy but not wood and cotton T-shirts, and why milk makes some adults flatulent.

Structure and Nomenclature

A single carbohydrate molecule is a **monosaccharide** (meaning "single sweet unit"), also known as a simple sugar. A pair bonded together form a **disaccharide**, a few form an **oligosaccharide**, and many form a **polysaccharide**. The bond between two sugar molecules is called a **glycosidic linkage**. This is a covalent bond, formed in a dehydration reaction that requires enzymatic catalysis. Glycosidic linkages are given complex names like "glucose α-1,2 fructose" or "galactose β-1,4 glucose". This gives information on the monosaccharides and atoms involved in the bond and the orientation of the bond. You don't need to memorize any glycosidic linkages for the DAT.

Sucrose (table sugar), shown in Figure 10, is a **glucose** unit and a **fructose** unit linked by a glycosidic bond. **Lactose**, also in Figure 10, is a glucose linked to a **galactose**. **Maltose**, not shown, is a glucose linked to another glucose. You don't need to memorize these structures, but should know the building blocks of sucrose, lactose, and maltose.

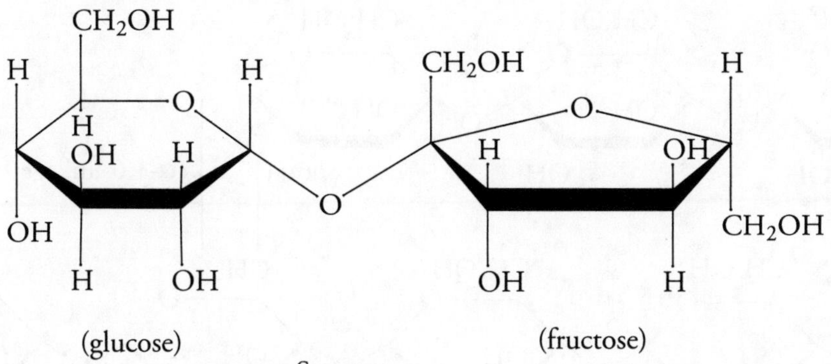

Sucrose

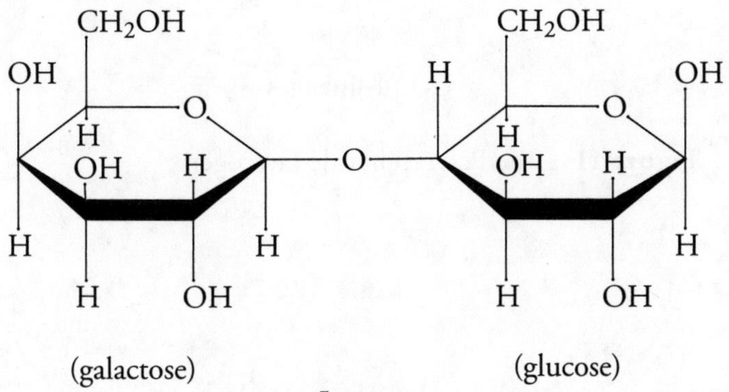

Lactose

Figure 10 Disaccharides

Polymers made from these disaccharides form important biological macromolecules. **Glycogen** (on the following page) serves as an energy storage carbohydrate in animals and is composed of thousands of glucose units joined together. **Starch** is the same as glycogen (except that the branches are a little different), and serves the same purpose in plants. **Cellulose** is a polymer of glucose, however the glycosidic bonds are slightly different and allow the polymer to assume a long, straight, fibrous shape. Wood and cotton are made of cellulose. Cellulose is also the main component of the plant cell wall.

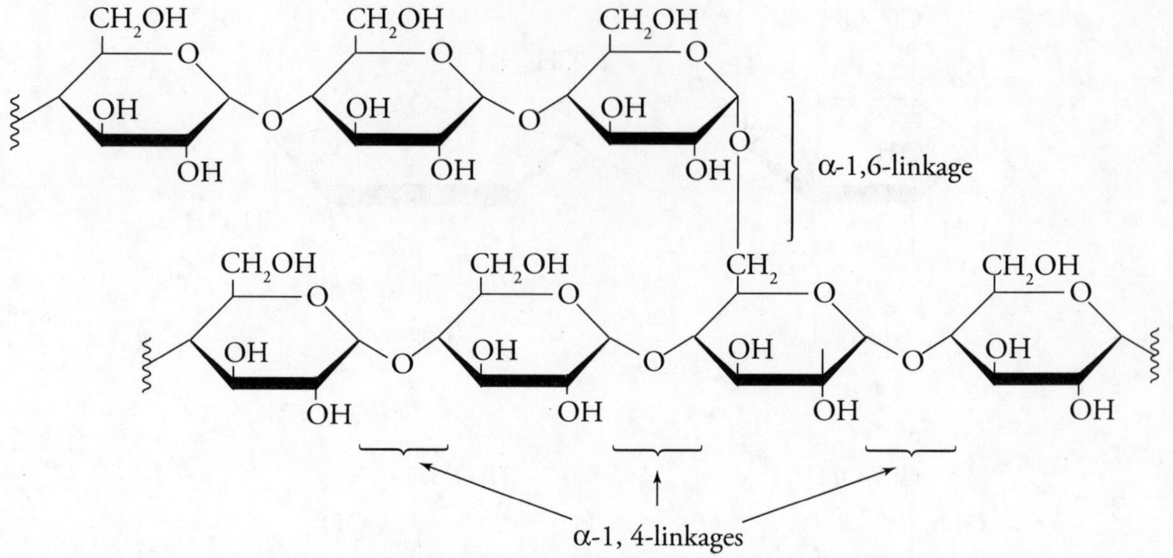

α-1,6-linkage

α-1, 4-linkages

Figure 11 The Polysaccharide Glycogen

2.5 LIPIDS

Lipids are oily or fatty substances that play three physiological roles, summarized here and discussed below.

- In cellular membranes, **phospholipids** constitute a barrier between intracellular and extracellular environments.
- In adipose cells, triglycerides (fats) store energy.
- Finally, cholesterol is a special lipid that serves as the building block for the hydrophobic steroid hormones.

The cardinal characteristic of a lipid is its **hydrophobicity**. Hydrophobic means *water-fearing*. It is important to understand the significance of this. Since water is very polar, polar substances dissolve well in water; these are known as *water-loving*, or **hydrophilic** substances. Carbon-carbon bonds and carbon-hydrogen bonds are nonpolar. Hence, substances that contain only carbon and hydrogen will not dissolve well in water. Some examples: table sugar dissolves well in water, but cooking oil floats in a layer above water or forms many tiny oil droplets when mixed with water. Cotton T-shirts become wet when exposed to water because they are made of glucose polymerized into cellulose, but a nylon jacket does not become wet because it is composed of atoms covalently bound together in a nonpolar fashion. A synonym for hydrophobic is **lipophilic** (which means lipid-loving); a synonym for hydrophilic is **lipophobic**. We'll return to these concepts below.

Fatty Acid Structure

Fatty acids are composed of long unsubstituted alkanes that end in a carboxylic acid. The chain is typically 14 to 18 carbons long, and because they are synthesized two carbons at a time from acetate, only *even-numbered* fatty acids are made in human cells. A fatty acid with no carbon-carbon double bonds is said to be **saturated** with hydrogen because every carbon atom in the chain is covalently bound to the maximum number of hydrogens. **Unsaturated** fatty acids have one or more double bonds in the tail, and thus do not bind to the maximum number of hydrogens.

Saturated fatty acid

Unsaturated fatty acid

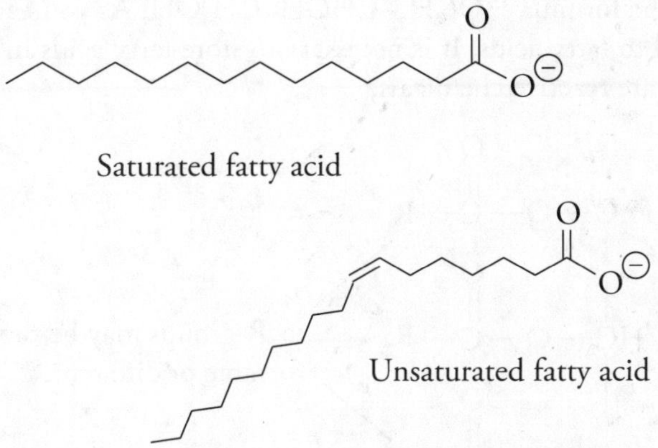

Figure 12   Fatty Acids

- How does the shape of an unsaturated fatty acid differ from that of a saturated fatty acid?[9]
- If fatty acids are mixed into water, how are they likely to associate with each other?[10]

The drawing below illustrates how free fatty acids interact in an aqueous solution; they form a structure called a **micelle**. **Soaps** are the sodium salts of fatty acids ($RCOO^-Na^+$). They are **amphipathic**, which means both hydrophilic and hydrophobic.

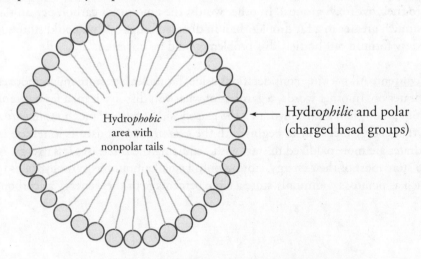

Hydro*phobic* area with nonpolar tails

Hydro*philic* and polar (charged head groups)

Figure 13   A Fatty Acid Micelle

- How does soap help to remove grease from your hands?[11]

---

[9] An unsaturated fatty acid is bent, or "kinked," at the *cis* double bond.

[10] The long hydrophobic chains will interact with each other to minimize contact with water, exposing the charged carboxyl group to the aqueous environment.

[11] Grease is hydrophobic. It does not wash off easily in water because it is not soluble in water. Scrubbing your hands with soap causes micelles to form around the grease particles. This allows the grease to dissociate from your hands and be swept away with water.

Triacylglycerols (TG)

The storage form of the fatty acid is fat. The technical name for fat is **triacylglycerol** or **triglyceride** (shown below). A triglyceride is composed of three fatty acids bonded to a glycerol molecule. Glycerol is a three-carbon triol with the formula $HOCH_2–CHOH–CH_2OH$. As you can see, it has three hydroxyl groups that can be bonded to fatty acids. It is necessary to store fatty acids in the relatively inert form of fat because free fatty acids are reactive chemicals.

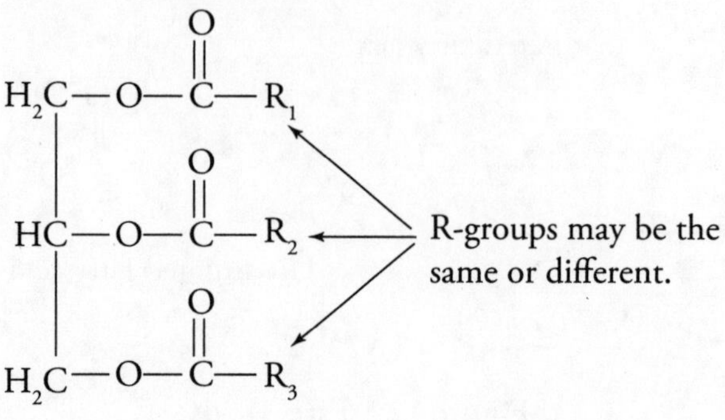

Figure 14   Triglyceride (Fat)

Triacylglycerols are stored in fat cells as an energy source. Fats are more efficient energy storage molecules than carbohydrates for two reasons: packing and energy content.

> **Packing:** Their hydrophobicity allows fats to pack together much more closely than carbohydrates. Carbohydrates carry a great amount of water-of-solvation (water molecules hydrogen bonded to their hydroxyl groups). In other words, the amount of carbon per unit area or unit weight is much greater in a fat droplet than in dissolved sugar. If we could store sugars in a dry powdery form in our bodies, this problem would be obviated.

> **Energy content:** All packing considerations aside, fat molecules store much more energy than carbohydrates do. In other words, regardless of what you dissolve it in, a fat has more energy carbon-for-carbon than a carbohydrate. The reason is that fats are much more *reduced*. Remember that energy metabolism begins with the *oxidation* of foodstuffs to release energy. Since carbohydrates are more oxidized to start with, oxidizing them releases less energy. Animals use fat to store most of their energy, storing only a small amount as carbohydrates (glycogen). Plants such as potatoes commonly store a large percentage of their energy as carbohydrates (starch).

Lipid Bilayer Membranes

Membrane lipids are **phospholipids** derived from diacylglycerol phosphate or DG-P (see Figure 15). For example, phosphatidyl choline is a phospholipid formed by the esterification of a choline molecule to the phosphate group of DG-P. Phospholipids are **detergents**, substances that efficiently solubilize oils while remaining highly water-soluble. Detergents are like soaps, but stronger.

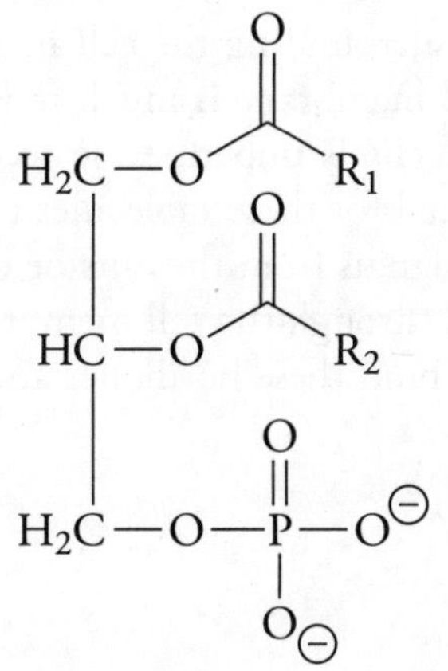

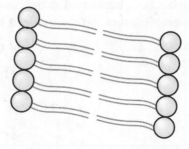

Figure 15   A Phosphoglyceride (Diacylglycerol Phosphate, or DGP)

We saw above how fatty acids spontaneously form micelles. Phospholipids also minimize their interactions with water by forming an orderly structure—in this case, it is a **lipid bilayer** (below). Hydrophobic interactions drive the formation of the bilayer, and once formed, it is stabilized by van der Waals forces between the long tails.

Figure 16   A Small Section of a Lipid Bilayer Membrane

- Would a saturated or an unsaturated fatty acid residue have more van der Waals interactions with neighboring alkyl chains in a bilayer membrane?[12]

A more precise way to give the answer to the question above is to say that double bonds (unsaturation) in phospholipid fatty acids *tend to increase membrane fluidity*. Unsaturation prevents the membrane from solidifying by disrupting the orderly packing of the hydrophobic lipid tails. This decreases the melting point. The right amount of fluidity is essential for function. Decreasing the *length* of fatty acid tails also increases fluidity. The steroid **cholesterol** (discussed in the next section) is a third important modulator of membrane fluidity. At low temperatures, it increases fluidity in the same way as kinks in fatty acid tails; hence, it is known as membrane antifreeze. At high temperatures, however, cholesterol attenuates (reduces) membrane fluidity. Don't ponder this paradox too long; just remember that cholesterol keeps fluidity at an *optimum level*. Remember, the structural determinants of membrane fluidity are degree of saturation, tail length, and amount of cholesterol.

---

[12] The bent shape of the unsaturated fatty acid means that it doesn't fit in as well and has less contact with neighboring groups to form van der Waals interactions. Unsaturation makes the membrane less stable, less solid.

The lipid bilayer acts like a plastic bag surrounding the cell in the sense that it seals the interior of the cell from the exterior. However, the cell membrane is much more complex than a plastic bag. Since the plasma bilayer membrane surrounding cells is impermeable to charged molecules such as Na⁺, protein gateways such as ion channels are required for these molecules to enter or exit cells. Proteins that are integrated into membranes also transmit signals from the outside of the cell into the interior. For example, certain hormones (peptides) cannot pass through the cell membrane due to their charged nature; instead, protein **receptors** in the cell membrane bind these hormones and transmit a signal into the cell in a **second messenger cascade**.

Steroids

Steroids are included here because of their hydrophobicity, and, hence, similarity to fats. Their structure is otherwise unique. All steroids have the basic tetracyclic ring system (see below), based on the structure of **cholesterol**. You should recognize this general tetracyclic ring structure on test day, but don't worry about memorizing the other structures we've shown below.

As discussed above, the steroid cholesterol is an important component of the lipid bilayer. It is obtained from the diet and synthesized in the liver. It is carried in the blood packaged with fats and proteins into **lipoproteins**. One type of lipoprotein has been implicated as the cause of atherosclerotic vascular disease, which refers to the build-up of cholesterol "plaques" on the inside of blood vessels.

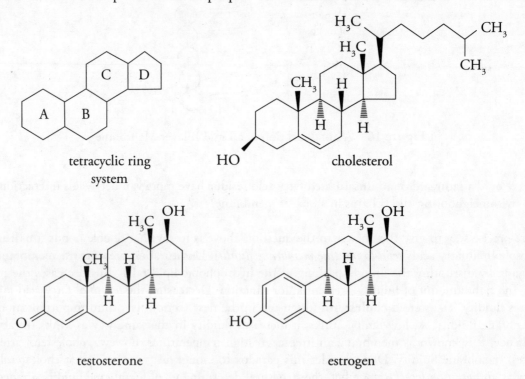

Figure 17 Cholesterol-Derived Hormones

Steroid hormones are made from cholesterol. Two examples are **testosterone** (an androgen or male sex hormone) and **estradiol** (an estrogen or female sex hormone). There are no receptors for steroid hormones on the surface of cells. Because steroids are highly hydrophobic, they can diffuse right through the lipid bilayer membrane into the cytoplasm. The receptors for steroid hormones are located within cells rather than on the cell surface. This is an important point! You must be aware of the contrast between *peptide* hormones, such as insulin, which exert their effects by binding to receptors at the cell-surface, and *steroid* hormones, such as estrogen, which diffuse into cells to find their receptors. We'll talk about this more when we review the endocrine system.

2.6   NUCLEIC ACIDS

We will introduce nucleic acids here and return to them in Chapter 4. Before we can talk about nucleic acids, we must first briefly review some background.

Phosphorus-Containing Compounds

Phosphate is also known as **orthophosphate**. Two orthophosphates bound together via an **anhydride linkage** form **pyrophosphate**. The P–O–P bond in pyrophosphate is an example of a **high-energy phosphate bond**. This name is derived from the fact that the hydrolysis of pyrophosphate is thermodynamically extremely favorable (shown below). In the cell, $\Delta G°$ for the hydrolysis of pyrophosphate is about –12 kcal/mol or –50 kJ/mol. This means it is a very favorable reaction.

There are three reasons phosphate anhydride bonds store so much energy:

1. When phosphates are linked together, their negative charges repel each other strongly.
2. Orthophosphate has more resonance forms and thus a lower free energy than linked phosphates.
3. Orthophosphate has a more favorable interaction with the biological solvent (water) than linked phosphates.

The details are not crucial. What is essential is that you fix the image in your mind of linked phosphates acting like compressed springs, just waiting to fly open and provide energy for an enzyme to catalyze a reaction.

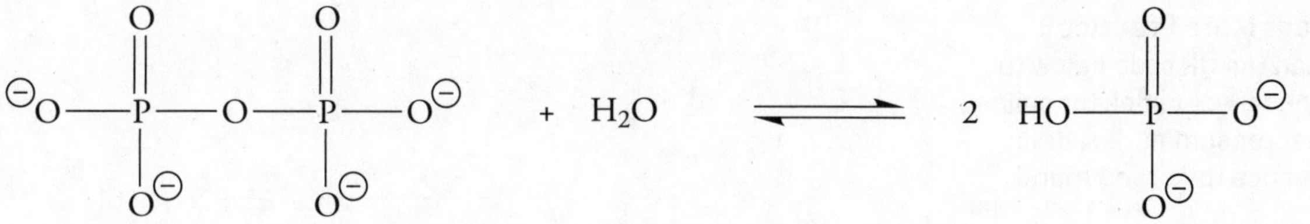

Figure 18   Hydrolysis of Pyrophosphate

Nucleotides

Nucleotides are the building blocks of nucleic acids (RNA and DNA). Each nucleotide contains a **ribose** (or **deoxyribose**) **sugar** group; a **purine** or **pyrimidine base** joined to carbon number one of the ribose ring; and one, two, or three **phosphate units** joined to carbon five of the ribose ring. The nucleotide **ad**enosine **tri**phosphate (ATP) plays a central role in cellular metabolism in addition to being an RNA precursor. **DNA** is a double-stranded molecule that forms a helix; **RNA** is a single-stranded molecule. There are three main types of RNA; mRNA, tRNA, and rRNA. (DNA and RNA structure and function will be discussed in more depth later.)

ATP is the universal short-term energy storage molecule. Energy extracted from oxidation of foodstuffs is immediately stored in the phosphoanhydride bonds of ATP. This energy will later be used to power cellular processes; it may also be used to synthesize glucose or fats, which are longer-term energy storage molecules. This applies to *all* living organisms, from bacteria to humans. Even some viruses carry ATP with them outside the host cell, though viruses cannot make their own ATP.

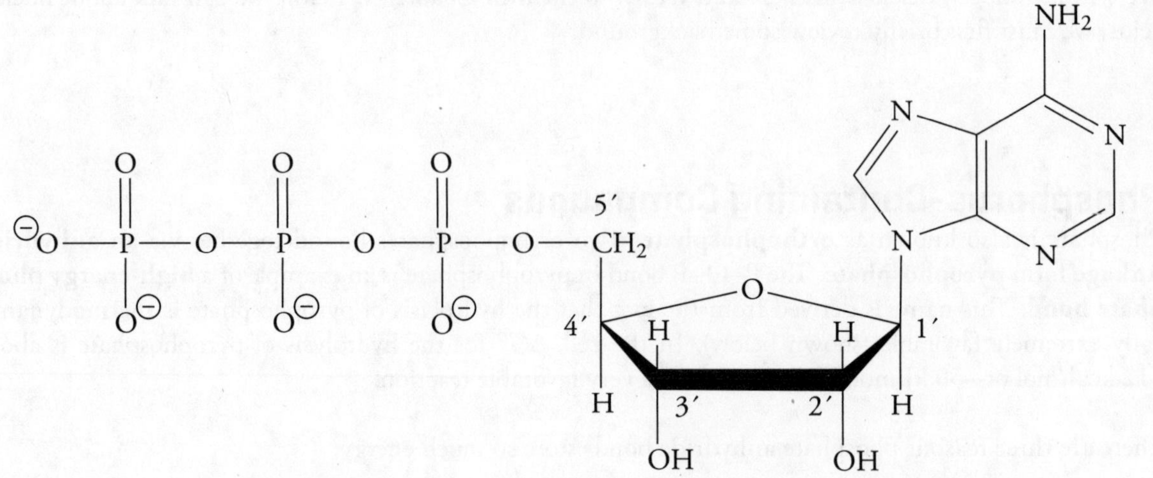

Figure 19 Adenosine Triphosphate (ATP)

Want More Practice?
Scan the QR code below to register your book for online chapter summaries, drills, practice tests, and more!

Chapter 3
Biochemistry

The notion of life refers to both the activities and the physical structures of living organisms. Storing and using energy, and synthesizing structures depend on a large number of chemical reactions that occur within each cell. Fortunately, these reactions do not proceed on their own spontaneously, without regulation. If they did, each cell's energy would rapidly dissipate, and total disorder would result. Most reactions are slowed by a large barrier known as the activation energy (E_a). The E_a is a bottleneck in a reaction, like a nearly closed gate. The role of an enzyme is to open this chemical gate. In this sense, the enzyme is like a switch. When the enzyme is on, the gate is open (low E_a), and the reaction accelerates. When the enzyme is off, the gate closes and the reaction slows. Before we can see how enzymes work, let's review some basics of thermodynamics.

3.1 THERMODYNAMICS

Thermodynamics is the study of the energetics of chemical reactions. We'll do an overview here of thermodynamics relevant to biology, but will review again in the Gchem section of this book. There are two relevant forms of energy in chemistry: heat energy (movement of molecules) and potential energy (energy stored in chemical bonds). [What is the most important potential energy storage molecule in all cells?[1]] The **first law of thermodynamics,** also known as the **law of conservation of energy**, states that the energy of the universe is constant. It implies that when the energy of a system *decreases*, the energy of the rest of the universe (the **surroundings**) must *increase*, and vice versa. The **second law of thermodynamics** states that the disorder, or **entropy**, of the universe tends to increase. Another way to state the second law is as follows: spontaneous reactions tend to increase the disorder of the universe. The symbol for entropy is S, and "a change in entropy" is denoted ΔS, where $\Delta S = S_{after} - S_{before}$. [If the ΔS of a system is negative, has the disorder of that system increased or decreased?[2]]

A practical way to discuss thermodynamics is the mathematical notion of **free energy** (**Gibbs free energy**), defined by Josiah Gibbs as follows:[3]

$$\Delta G = \Delta H - T\Delta S$$

T denotes temperature and H denotes **enthalpy**, which is defined by another equation:

$$\Delta H = \Delta E - P\Delta V$$

Here E represents the bond energy of products or reactants in a system, P is pressure, and V is volume. [Given that cellular reactions take place in the liquid phase, how is H related to E in a cell?[4]] ΔG increases with increasing ΔH (bond energy) and decreases with increasing entropy.

- Given the second law of thermodynamics and the mathematical definition of **ΔG**, which reaction will be favorable: one with a decrease in free energy ($\Delta G < 0$) or one with an increase in free energy ($\Delta G > 0$)?[5]

The change in the Gibbs free energy of a reaction determines whether the reaction is favorable (**spontaneous**, ΔG negative) or unfavorable (**nonspontaneous**, ΔG positive). In terms of the generic reaction

$$A + B \rightarrow C + D$$

the Gibbs free energy change determines whether the reactants (A and B) will stay as they are or be converted to **products** (C and D).

---

[1] ATP, which stores energy in ester bonds between its phosphate groups.

[2] If ΔS is negative, then the system lost entropy, which means disorder decreased.

[3] As in ΔS, the Greek letter Δ (delta) indicates "the change in." For example, $\Delta G_{rxn} = G_{products} - G_{reactants}$.

[4] $H \approx E$, since the change in volume is negligible ($\Delta V \approx 0$).

[5] Favorable reactions have $\Delta G < 0$. We can deduce this from the second law because the second law states that increasing entropy is favorable, and the equation has ΔG directly related to $-T\Delta S$.

Spontaneous reactions, ones that occur without a net addition of energy, have $\Delta G < 0$. They occur with energy to spare. Reactions with a negative ΔG are **exergonic** (energy *exits* the system); reactions with a positive ΔG are **endergonic**. Endergonic reactions only occur if energy is added. In the lab, energy is added in the form of heat; in the body, endergonic reactions are driven by reaction coupling to exergonic reactions (more on this later). Reactions with a negative ΔH are called **exothermic** and liberate heat. Most metabolic reactions are exothermic (which is how homeothermic organisms such as mammals maintain a constant body temperature). Reactions with a positive ΔH require an input of heat and are referred to as **endothermic**.

The signs of thermodynamic quantities are assigned from the point of view of *the system*, not the surroundings or the universe. Thus, a negative ΔG means that the system goes to a lower free energy state, and a system will always move in the direction of the lowest free energy.

Thermodynamics vs. Reaction Rates

The term *spontaneous* is used to describe a reaction system with $\Delta G < 0$. This can be misleading, since the common usage of the word *spontaneous* has a connotation of *rapid rate*; this is not what spontaneous means in the context of chemical reactions. For example, many reactions have a negative ΔG, indicating that they are "spontaneous" from a thermodynamic point of view, but they do not necessarily occur at a significant rate. Spontaneous means that a reaction may proceed without additional energy input, *but it says nothing about the rate of reaction*.

Thermodynamics will tell you where a system starts and finishes but nothing about the path traveled to get there. The difference in free energy in a reaction is only a function of the nature of the reactants and products. Thus, ΔG does not depend on the pathway a reaction takes or the rate of reaction; it is only a measurement of the difference in free energy between reactants and products.

- How does the ΔG for a reaction burning (oxidizing) sugar in a furnace compare to the ΔG when sugar is broken down (oxidized) in a human?[6]

3.2 KINETICS AND ACTIVATION ENERGY (E_a)

The reason some spontaneous (i.e., *thermodynamically favorable*) reactions proceed very slowly or not at all is that a large amount of energy is required to get them going. For example, the burning of wood is spontaneous, but you can stare at a log all day and it won't burn. Some energy (heat) must be provided to kick-start the process.

The study of reaction rates is called **chemical kinetics**. All reactions proceed through a transient **intermediate** that is unstable and takes a great deal of energy to produce. The energy required to produce the transient intermediate is called the **activation energy** (E_a). This is the barrier that prevents many reactions from proceeding even though the ΔG for the reaction may be negative. The match you use to light

---

[6] The ΔG is the same in both cases. ΔG does not depend on the pathway, only on the different energies of the reactants and products.

your fireplace provides the activation energy for the reaction known as burning. It is the activation energy barrier that determines the kinetics of a reaction. [How would the rate of a spontaneous reaction be affected if the activation energy were lowered?[7]]

The concept of E_a is key to understanding the role of enzymes, so let's spend some time on it. To illustrate, take this reaction:

$$Bob_{without\ a\ job} + job \rightarrow Bob_{with\ a\ job}$$

Is this a favorable reaction, i.e., will the universe be better off, with less total (nervous) energy, if Bob gets the job? Will things settle down? Let's assume yes. However, between the two states (without/with) there is an intermediate state, namely, $Bob_{applying\ for\ job}$. So the reaction will look this way:

$$Bob_{without\ a\ job} + job \rightarrow [Bob_{applying\ for\ job}]^{\ddagger} \rightarrow Bob_{with\ a\ job}$$

The middle term is the **transition state** (TS), traditionally written in square brackets with a double-cross symbol: $[TS]^{\ddagger}$. It exists for a very, very short time, either moving forward to form product or breaking back down into reactants. The energy required for Bob to be job hunting is much higher than the energy of Bob with a job *or* Bob without a job. As a result, he may not go job hunting, even though he'd be happier in the long run if he did. In this model, we can describe the E_a as the energy necessary to get Bob to apply for a job.

A **catalyst** lowers the E_a of a reaction *without changing the* ΔG. The catalyst lowers the E_a by *stabilizing the transition state*, making its existence less thermodynamically unfavorable. The second important characteristic of a catalyst is that it is not consumed in the reaction; it is *regenerated* with each reaction cycle.

In our model, an example of a catalyst would be a career planning service (CPS). Adding a CPS won't make $Bob_{without\ a\ job}$ any happier or sadder, nor will it make $Bob_{with\ a\ job}$ happier or sadder. But it will make it much easier for Bob to move between the two states: without a job vs. with a job. The traditional way to represent a reaction system like this is using a **reaction coordinate graph**, as shown in Figure 1. This is just a way to look at the energy of the reaction system as compared to the three possible states of the system: (1) reactants, (2) $[TS]^{\ddagger}$, and (3) products. The *x*-axis plots the physical progress of the reaction system (the "reaction coordinate"), and the *y*-axis plots energy.

---

[7]   The rate would be increased, since lowering E_a is tantamount to reducing the energy required to achieve the transition state. The more transition state species formed, the greater the amount of product produced, i.e., the more rapid the rate of reaction.

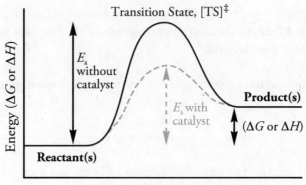

Figure 1 Reaction Coordinate Graph

- If the y-axis is ΔG, is this graph for an exergonic or endergonic reaction?[8]
- If the y-axis is ΔH, is this graph for an exothermic or endothermic reaction?[9]

Enzymes are catalysts. They increase the rate of a reaction by lowering the reaction's activation energy, but they *do not affect* ΔG between reactants and products. As catalysts, enzymes have a kinetic role, *not* a thermodynamic one. [Will an enzyme alter the concentration of reagents at equilibrium?[10]] Enzymes may alter the rate of a reaction enormously: a reaction that would take a hundred years to reach equilibrium without an enzyme may occur in just seconds with an enzyme.

ATP as an Energy Source: Reaction Coupling

Enzymes increase the rate of reactions that have a negative ΔG. These reactions would occur on their own without an enzyme (they are spontaneous) but far more slowly than with one. However, there are many reactions in the body that occur which have a positive ΔG. The biosynthesis of macromolecules such as DNA and protein is not spontaneous ($\Delta G > 0$), but clearly these reactions *do* take place (or we wouldn't be here). How can this be? Thermodynamically unfavorable reactions in the cell can be driven forward by **reaction coupling**. In reaction coupling, one very favorable reaction is used to drive an unfavorable one. This is possible because free energy changes are additive. [What is the favorable reaction that the cell can use to drive unfavorable reactions?[11]] In the lab, the $\Delta G°$ for the hydrolysis of one phosphate group from ATP is –7.3 kcal/mol, so it is a very favorable reaction. In the cell, ΔG is about –12 kcal/mol, so in the cell it is even more favorable. [What's the difference between the situation *in vitro* (lab) and *in vivo* (cell)?[12]]

---

[8] This would be an endergonic (non-spontaneous) reaction.

[9] This would be an endothermic (non-spontaneous) reaction.

[10] No. It will only affect the rate at which the reactants and products reach equilibrium.

[11] ATP hydrolysis!

[12] $Q_{cell} \neq K_{eq}$. This means that the relative concentrations of ATP and ADP + P_i are not at equilibrium levels in the cell. Actually, $Q_{cell} \ll K_{eq}$ because the cell keeps a high concentration of ATP around. For more information on K_{eq} and Q, see Chapter 19.

How does ATP hydrolysis drive unfavorable reactions? There are many ways. One example is by causing a conformational change in a protein; in this way ATP hydrolysis can be used to power energy-costly events like transmembrane transport. Another example is by transfer of a phosphate group from ATP to a substrate. Take the unfavorable reaction A + B → C. Let's say that Reactant A must proceed through an intermediate, APO_4^{2-} in order to participate. Let's say ΔG = +7 kcal/mol for the overall reaction. What if the two partial reactions have ΔGs as follows:

$$A + PO_4^{2-} \rightarrow APO_4^{2-} \qquad \Delta G = \quad +2 \text{ kcal/mol}$$

$$\underline{APO_4^{2-} + B \rightarrow C + PO_4^{2-} \qquad \Delta G = \quad +5 \text{ kcal/mol}}$$

$$Total \quad \Delta G = \quad +7 \text{ kcal/mol}$$

These reactions will not proceed, because the overall ΔG will be +7 kcal/mol. What will be the *overall* ΔG if we *couple* the reaction A + B → C to the hydrolysis of one ATP? All we have to do is add up all the ΔG values, as follows:

$$ATP \rightarrow ADP + PO_4^{2-} \qquad \Delta G = \quad -12 \text{ kcal/mol}$$

$$A + PO_4^{2-} \rightarrow APO_4^{2-} \qquad \Delta G = \quad +2 \text{ kcal/mol}$$

$$\underline{APO_4^{2-} + B \rightarrow C + PO_4^{2-} \qquad \Delta G = \quad +5 \text{ kcal/mol}}$$

$$Total \quad \Delta G = \quad -5 \text{ kcal/mol}$$

Now the overall reaction, shown below, is thermodynamically favorable. We have *coupled* the unfavorable reaction A + B → C to the highly favorable hydrolysis of ATP:

$$A + B + ATP \rightarrow C + ADP + PO_4^{2-} \qquad \Delta G = -5 \text{ kcal/mol}$$

Note that we first stated that the enzyme has only a kinetic role (influencing rate only), not a thermodynamic one (determining favorability). Then we went on to discuss reaction coupling, which allows enzymes to promote otherwise unfavorable reactions. There is no contradiction, however. The only difference is viewing reactions in an isolated manner or in the complex series of linked reactions more commonly found in the body. The same rule applies in either case: ΔG must be negative for either a single reaction or a series of linked reactions to occur spontaneously. In summary:

- One reaction in a test tube: the enzyme is a catalyst with a kinetic role only. It influences the rate of the reaction, but not the outcome.
- Many "real-life" reactions in the cell: enzyme controls outcomes by selectively promoting unfavorable reactions via reaction coupling.

3.3 ENZYME STRUCTURE AND FUNCTION

Most enzymes are proteins that must fold into specific three-dimensional structures to act as catalysts. (Some enzymes are RNA or contain RNA sequences with catalytic activity. Most catalyze their own splicing, and the rRNA in ribosomes helps in peptide-bond formation.) An enzyme may consist of a single polypeptide chain or several polypeptide subunits held together in a ___[13] (primary? secondary? etc.) structure. The reason for the importance of folding in enzyme function is the proper formation of the **active site**, the region in an enzyme's three-dimensional structure that is directly involved in catalysis. [What shape are enzymes more likely to have: fibrous/elongated or globular/spherical?[14]]

Reactants in an enzyme-catalyzed reaction are called **substrates**. Products have no special name; they're just "products." What is the role of the active site? That is, how do enzymes work? The enzyme is like a career-planning service (CPS), and the active site is like the room where Bob can sit and do his job hunting. The CPS has counselors, books, and job lists, all of which make job hunting easier. The **active site model**, commonly referred to as the "lock and key hypothesis," states that the substrate and active site are perfectly complementary. This differs from the **induced fit model**, which asserts that the substrate and active site differ slightly in structure and that the binding of the substrate induces a conformational change in the enzyme. The induced fit model has gained greater acceptance in recent years, but regardless of the model, enzymes accelerate the rate of a given reaction by helping to stabilize the transition state; the active site has amino acid residues that help with this. [For example, if a transition state intermediate possesses a transient negative charge, what amino acid residues might be found at the active site to stabilize the transition state?[15]] This lowers the activation energy barrier between reactants and products.

- Is it possible that amino acids located far apart from each other in the primary protein sequence may play a role in the formation of the same active site?[16]
- If, during an enzyme-catalyzed reaction, an intermediate forms in which the substrate is covalently linked to the enzyme via a serine residue, can this occur at any serine residue, or must it occur at a specific serine residue?[17]

The active site for enzymes is generally highly specific in its substrate recognition, including stereospecificity (the ability to distinguish between stereoisomers). For example, enzymes which catalyze reactions involving amino acids are specific for D or L amino acids, and enzymes catalyzing reactions involving monosaccharides may distinguish between stereoisomers as well.

---

[13] quaternary

[14] Globular. Structural proteins such as collagen tend to be fibrous, but proteins that act as catalysts tend to be roughly spherical to form an active site in a cleft in the sphere.

[15] A positive charge would stabilize the negative charge in the intermediate. Such a charge might be contributed by histidine, arginine, or lysine amino acids. Alternatively, the hydrogen of a $-NH_2$ group in glutamine or asparagine could hydrogen bond with the negative charge.

[16] Yes, amino acids at the active site may be distant from each other in a polypeptide's primary sequence but be near each other in the final folded protein. This is why protein folding is crucial for enzyme function.

[17] It must occur at a particular serine residue which sticks out into the active site.

What is a Cofactor?

Many enzymes require an additional small molecule, known as a **cofactor**, to aid with catalytic activity. Such an enzyme without its cofactor is referred to as an **apoenzyme**; the complete, catalytically active enzyme is called a **holoenzyme**. In other words:

$$\text{Apoenzyme} + \text{Cofactor} = \text{Holoenzyme}$$

Cofactors are small, non-protein molecules that function in reactions of enzymes. The exact role of the cofactor varies with each cofactor and its enzyme. Cofactors can be either inorganic molecules (such as metal ions) or small organic molecules (called coenzymes).

Inorganic Cofactors

A holoenzyme with a metal ion cofactor can also be called a **metalloenzyme**. While any enzyme containing a metal ion can be called a metalloenzyme, any protein containing a metal ion is called a **metalloprotein**.

Here are some examples of metalloenzymes:

- The enzyme carbonic anhydrase requires Zn^{2+} for its activity; it is a widely distributed metalloenzyme, which catalyzes the reversible hydration of CO_2 to carbonic acid (H_2CO_3).
- DNA polymerase is a holoenzyme with multiple protein subunits. It catalyzes the polymerization of deoxyribonucleotides during DNA replication. This synthesis reaction requires Mg^{2+} as a cofactor for catalysis, making DNA polymerase a metalloenzyme.
- RNA polymerase is also a metalloenzyme. It functions in transcription and contains zinc and magnesium cations as metal cofactors.

There are lots of examples of non-enzymatic metalloproteins. Ferritin is an intracellular protein found in almost all living organisms that stores iron. Transferrins are glycoproteins found in vertebrates that transport iron. These proteins do not have catalytic activity but still bind a metal ion.

Here is a trickier example: Ribozymes are RNA molecules with enzyme function, and many contain divalent metal ions such as Mg^{2+}. Ribozymes are therefore both holoenzymes and a metalloenzymes. However, because they are not made of protein, ribozymes are not metalloproteins.

Organic Cofactors

Cofactors that are small organic molecules are called **coenzymes**. Most coenzymes are derivatives of vitamins and are soluble in water. Some examples of common coenzymes are NADH, $FADH_2$, quinone, and coenzyme A (CoA).

Coenzymes can associate with enzymes in many ways. They can bind tightly or associate loosely. They can bind either covalently or noncovalently.

- Coenzymes that bind tightly to proteins or enzymes are called **prosthetic groups**; they are often attached to a protein by a covalent bond. Some prosthetic groups bind enzymes, but others bind proteins that have no enzymatic activity.
- Coenzymes that are loosely associated coenzymes are sometimes called **co-substrates** because they bind to and are released from the enzyme just as substrates and products are.

Here is an example:

Glycogen phosphorylase is an enzyme that mobilizes glycogen for energy. To do this, it requires the small organic molecule pyridoxal phosphate (PLP). PLP is the active form of vitamin B6 and is a coenzyme in a variety of enzymatic reactions.

Here is a more advanced example:

Cytochromes are small proteins that participate in electron transfer reactions. These enzymes contain both an inorganic cofactor (a metal ion) and an organic cofactor (heme). Cytochromes bind heme tightly and covalently. In this example, cytochrome bound to heme and a metal ion is a holoenzyme, metalloenzyme, and metalloprotein. The metal ion is the inorganic cofactor. Heme is a cofactor, a coenzyme, and a prosthetic group.

3.4 REGULATION OF ENZYME ACTIVITY

Metabolic pathways in the cell are not all continually on, but must be tightly regulated to maintain health. For example, if glycogen synthesis and breakdown occur in the same cell at the same time, a great deal of energy will be wasted without accomplishing anything. Therefore, the activity of key enzymes in metabolic pathways is usually regulated in one or more of the following ways:

1. **Covalent modification:** Proteins can have several different groups covalently attached to them, and this can regulate their activity, lifespan in the cell, and/or cellular location. The addition of a phosphoryl group from a molecule of ATP by a protein **kinase** to the hydroxyl of serine, threonine, or tyrosine residues is the most common example. Phosphorylation of these different sites on an enzyme can either activate or inactivate the enzyme. Protein **phosphorylases,** also phosphorylate proteins, use free-floating inorganic phosphate (P_i) in the cell instead of ATP. Protein phosphorylation can be reversed by protein **phosphatases**.

2. **Proteolytic cleavage:** Many enzymes (and other proteins) are synthesized in inactive forms (**zymogens**) that are activated by cleavage by a protease.

3. **Association with other polypeptides:** Some enzymes have catalytic activity in one polypeptide subunit that is regulated by association with a separate regulatory subunit. For example, there are some proteins that demonstrate continuous rapid catalysis if their regulatory subunit is removed; this is known as **constitutive activity** (*constitutive* means continuous or unregulated). There are other proteins that require association with another peptide in order to function. Still other proteins can bind many regulatory subunits. There are numerous examples of this in the cell, and many of them have diverse and complex regulatory mechanisms that all revolve around the theme of "associations with other polypeptides can affect enzyme activity."

4. **Allosteric regulation:** This is the modification of active-site activity through interactions of molecules with other specific sites on the enzyme (called **allosteric sites**). Let's look at this in a little more detail.

Allosteric Regulation

If the cell is to make use of the enzyme as a biochemical switch, there must be a way to turn the enzyme *on* or *off*. One mechanism of regulation is the binding of small molecules to particular sites on an enzyme that are distinct from the active site; this is allosteric regulation. This name comes from the fact that the particular spot on the enzyme which can bind the small molecule is *not* located close to the active site; *allo* means "other," and *steric* refers to a location in space (as in "steric hindrance"), so *allosteric* means "at another place." The binding of the allosteric regulator to the allosteric site is generally noncovalent and reversible. When bound, an allosteric regulator can alter the conformation of the enzyme to increase or decrease catalysis, even though it may be bound to the enzyme at a site distant from the active site or even on a separate polypeptide.

Feedback Inhibition

Enzymes usually act as part of pathways, not alone. Rather than regulate every enzyme in a pathway, usually there are one or two key enzymes that are regulated, such as the enzyme that catalyzes the first irreversible step in a pathway. The easiest way to explain this is with an example. Three enzymes (E1, E2, and E3) catalyze the three steps required to convert Substrate A to Product D. When plenty of D is around, it would be logical to shut off E1 so that excess B, C, and D are not made. This would conserve A and would also conserve energy. Commonly, an end-product such as D will shut off an enzyme early in the pathway, such as E1. This is called **negative feedback**, or **feedback inhibition**.

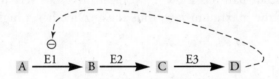

Figure 2   Feedback Inhibition

There are examples of **positive feedback** ("feedback *stimulation*")[18], but negative feedback is by far the most common example of feedback regulation. On the other hand, *feedforward stimulation* is common. This involves stimulation of an enzyme by its substrate, or by a molecule used in synthesis of the substrate. For example, in Figure 2, A might stimulate E1 or E3. This makes sense because when lots of A is around, we want the pathway for utilization of A to be active.

---

[18] There are two examples of positive feedback you need to be familiar with for the DAT: estrogen production by granulosa cells in the ovary and oxytocin levels during labor and delivery. We'll discuss both examples in the Reproduction and Development chapter.

3.5 ENZYME KINETICS

Enzyme kinetics is the study of the rate of formation of products from substrates in the presence of an enzyme.[19] The **reaction rate** (V, for velocity) is the amount of product formed per unit time, in moles per second (mol/s). It depends on the concentration of substrate, [S], and enzyme.[20] If there is only a little substrate, then the rate V is directly proportional to the amount of substrate added: double the amount of substrate and the reaction rate doubles, triple the substrate and the rate triples, and so forth. But eventually there is so much substrate that active sites of the enzymes are occupied much of the time, and adding more substrate doesn't increase the reaction rate as much, that is, the slope of the V vs. [S] curve decreases. Finally, there is so much substrate that every active site is continuously occupied, and adding more substrate doesn't increase the reaction rate at all. At this point the enzyme is said to be **saturated**. The reaction rate when the enzyme is saturated is denoted V_{max}; see Figure 3 below. This is a property of each enzyme at a particular concentration of enzyme. You can look it up in a book for the common ones. [If a small amount of enzyme in a solution is acting at V_{max}, and the substrate concentration is doubled, what is the new reaction rate?[21]]

Another commonly used parameter on these enzyme kinetics graphs is the Michaelis constant K_m. K_m is the substrate concentration at which the reaction velocity is half its maximum. To find K_m on the enzyme kinetics graph, mark the V_{max} on the y-axis; then divide this distance in half to find $V_{max}/2$. K_m is found by drawing a horizontal line from $V_{max}/2$ to the curve, and then a vertical line down to the x-axis. K_m is unique for each enzyme-substrate pair and gives information on the affinity of the enzyme for its substrate. If an enzyme-substrate pair has a low K_m, it means that not very much substrate is required to get the reaction rate to half the maximum rate; thus the enzyme has a high affinity for this particular substrate.

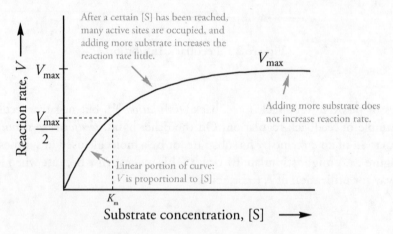

Figure 3   Saturation Kinetics

---

[19] It is not impossible for this content to be tested on the DAT, but this is pretty advanced biochemistry, and questions on this content are rare. Plan your study time accordingly.

[20] Usually the concentration of enzyme is kept fixed, and [S] is taken as the only independent variable (the one the rate depends on). This is applicable to biological systems, where substrate concentrations change much more than enzyme concentrations.

[21] If the enzyme is acting at V_{max}, it is saturated with substrate; adding more substrate will not increase the reaction rate; the rate is still V_{max}.

Inhibition of Enzyme Activity

Enzyme inhibitors can reduce enzyme activity by a few different mechanisms, including **competitive inhibition** and **noncompetitive inhibition**. **Competitive inhibitors** are molecules that *compete* with substrate for binding at the active site. [You can predict that structurally, competitive inhibitors resemble what?[22]] The key thing to remember about competitive inhibitors is that their inhibition can be overcome by adding more substrate; if the substrate concentration is high enough, the substrate can *outcompete* the inhibitor. Hence, V_{max} is not affected. You can get to the same V_{max}, but it takes more substrate (see Figure 4). Therefore, the K_m of the reaction to which a competitive inhibitor has been added is increased compared to the K_m of the uninhibited reaction. [If an enzyme has a reaction rate of 1 µmole/min at a substrate concentration of 50 µM and a rate of 10 µmole/min at a substrate concentration of 100 µM, does this indicate the presence of a competitive inhibitor?[23]]

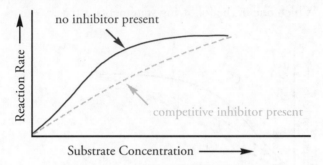

Figure 4   Competitive Inhibition

Noncompetitive inhibitors bind at an allosteric site, not at the active site. No matter how much substrate you add, the inhibitor will not be displaced from its site of action (see Figure 5). Hence, noncompetitive inhibition *does* diminish V_{max}. Remember that V_{max} is always calculated at the same enzyme concentration, since adding more enzyme will increase the measured V_{max}. Addition of a noncompetitive inhibitor changes the V_{max} and $V_{max}/2$ of the reaction, but typically does not alter K_m. This is because the substrate can still bind to the active site, but the inhibitor prevents the catalytic activity of the enzyme.

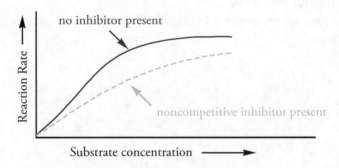

Figure 5   Noncompetitive Inhibition

---

[22] Structurally, competitive inhibitors must at least resemble the substrate; however, the most effective competitive inhibitors resemble the transition state which the active site normally stabilizes.

[23] No. The rate increase is greater than linear, indicating that the effect is caused by cooperativity. In positive cooperativity, the binding of a substrate to one subunit increases the affinity of the other subunits for substrate. This results in a sigmoidal (or "S-shaped") curve. A common example of cooperative binding is how hemoglobin binds O_2. See Figure 21 on page 291 for more information.

- Carbon dioxide is an allosteric inhibitor of hemoglobin. It dissociates easily when Hb passes through the lungs, where the CO_2 can be exhaled. Carbon monoxide, on the other hand, binds at the oxygen-binding site with an affinity 300 times greater than oxygen; it can be displaced by oxygen, but only when there is much more O_2 than CO in the environment. Which of the following is/are correct?[24]

    I. Carbon monoxide is an irreversible inhibitor.
    II. CO_2 is a reversible inhibitor.
    III. CO_2 is a noncompetitive inhibitor.

- In the figure below, the kinetics of an enzyme are plotted. In each case, an inhibitor may be present or absent. Which one of the following statements is true?[25]

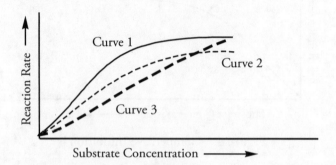

A. Curve 3 represents noncompetitive inhibition of the enzyme.
B. Curve 1 represents noncompetitive inhibition of the enzyme.
C. The V_{max} values of Curve 2 and Curve 3 are the same.
D. Curve 3 represents competitive inhibition of the enzyme, and the enzyme is uninhibited in Curve 1.
E. Curve 2 represents competitive inhibition of the enzyme, and the enzyme is uninhibited in Curve 1.

---

[24] **Statement I: False**. The question states that CO can be displaced by oxygen. **Statement II: True.** The question states that it dissociates easily. **Statement III: True**. The question states it binds allosterically, which means "at another site" (not the active site).

[25] Since Curve 3 and Curve 1 have the same V_{max}, but Curve 3 has a reduced rate of product formation, it suggests that Curve 3 represents competitive inhibition of the enzyme in Curve 1 (choice **D** is correct). If Curve 3 represented noncompetitive inhibition, its V_{max} would be reduced compared to Curve 1 (choice A is wrong). Note that this is what we see in Curve 2 (choice E is wrong). In no case would an inhibitor have a higher V_{max} than an uninhibited reaction (choice B is wrong). Lastly, it can be seen on the graph that Curve 2 has a reduced V_{max} compared to Curve 3 (choice C is wrong).

3.6 CELLULAR RESPIRATION

Energy Metabolism and Redox

Where does the energy in foods come from? How do we make use of this energy? Why do we breathe? The answers begin with **photosynthesis**, the process by which plants store energy from the sun in the bond energy of carbohydrates. Plants are **photoautotrophs** because they use energy from light ("photo") to make their own ("auto") food. We are **chemoheterotrophs**, because we use the energy of chemicals ("chemo") produced by other ("hetero") living things, namely plants and other animals. Plants and animals store chemical energy in reduced molecules such as carbohydrates and fats. These reduced molecules are oxidized to produce CO_2 and ATP. The energy of ATP is used in turn to drive the energetically unfavorable reactions of the cell. That's the basic energetics of life; all the rest is detail.

In essence, production and utilization of energy boil down to a series of **oxidation/reduction** reactions. **Oxidize** is a chemical term meaning just what it sounds like: "bind to oxygen." **Reduce** means the opposite: "remove oxygen." In fact, there are three ways to "oxidize" (and "reduce") an atom. *Memorize them.*

Three Meanings of Oxidize:
1. attach oxygen (or increase the number of bonds to oxygen)
2. remove hydrogen
3. remove electrons

Three Meanings of Reduce (just the opposite):
1. remove oxygen (or decrease the number of bonds to oxygen)
2. add hydrogen
3. add electrons

If you can answer questions like the following, you're set: Is changing CH_3CH_3 to $H_2C=CH_2$ an oxidation, a reduction, or neither?[26] What about changing Fe^{3+} to Fe^{2+}?[27] What about this: $O_2 \rightarrow H_2O$?[28]

When you reduce something, it's like compressing a spring; you store potential energy. The reduced substance "wants" to be oxidized back to where it started. Here is one other important fact about oxidation and reduction: when one atom gets reduced, another one *must* be oxidized; hence the term **redox pair**. As you study the process of glucose oxidation, you will see that each time an oxidation reaction occurs, a reduction reaction occurs too.

---

[26] It's an oxidation, because hydrogens have been removed.

[27] It's a reduction, because an electron has been added.

[28] It's a reduction, because bonds to oxygen have been replaced by bonds to hydrogen.

Catabolism is the process of breaking down molecules. The opposite is **anabolism**, which is "building-up" metabolism.[29] The way we extract energy from glucose is by **oxidative catabolism**. We break down glucose by oxidizing it. Oxidative catabolism of glucose involves four steps: glycolysis, pyruvate dehydrogenase complex (PDC), Krebs cycle, and electron transport/oxidative phosphorylation. The stoichiometry of glucose oxidation looks like this:

$$C_6H_{12}O_6 + 6\,O_2 \;\rightarrow\; 6\,CO_2 + 6\,H_2O$$

- What are the two members of the redox pair in this reaction?[30]

As we oxidize foods, we release the stored energy plants got from the sun. But we don't make use of that energy right away. Instead, we store it in the form of ATP. Thus, cellular respiration is theoretically very simple: *It's just a big coupled reaction* (described in Section 3.2). We make the unfavorable synthesis of ATP happen by coupling it to the very favorable oxidation of glucose. ATP can then be used to drive other cellular processes.

Introduction to Cellular Respiration

When glucose is oxidized to release energy, very little ATP is generated directly. Instead, oxidation of glucose is accompanied by the reduction of high-energy electron carriers, primarily reduction of **NAD⁺** (nicotinamide adenine dinucleotide) to **NADH**. The energy in reduced NADH is then used to pump protons out of the interior of mitochondria and create a proton gradient. The proton gradient energy is then used to finally drive the production of ATP.

Glucose is oxidized to produce CO_2 and ATP in a four-step process: glycolysis, pyruvate dehydrogenase complex (PDC), Krebs cycle, and electron transport/oxidative phosphorylation. The first stage is **glycolysis** ("glucose splitting"). Here glucose is partially oxidized while it is split in half, into two identical **pyruvic acid** molecules.[31] [How many carbon atoms does pyruvic acid have?[32]] Glycolysis produces a small quantity of ATP and a small quantity of NADH. Glycolysis occurs in the cytoplasm and does not require oxygen.

In the second stage (**pyruvate dehydrogenase complex**), pyruvate produced in glycolysis is decarboxylated to form an **acetyl group**. The acetyl group is then attached to **coenzyme A**, a carrier that can transfer the acetyl group into the Krebs cycle. A small amount of NADH is produced.

In the third stage, the **Krebs cycle** (also known as the **tricarboxylic acid cycle** or **citric acid cycle**), the acetyl group from PDC is added to **oxaloacetate** to form **citric acid**. The citric acid is then decarboxylated and isomerized to regenerate the original oxaloacetate. A modest amount of ATP, a large amount of NADH, and a small amount of **FADH₂** are produced. Note that although the PDC and Krebs cycle can

---

[29] The mnemonics are *cata* = breakdown, as in catastrophe, and *ana* = buildup, sounds like "add-a." (Think of anabolic steroids, which weightlifters use to bulk up.)

[30] The carbons in the sugar are oxidized (to CO_2), and oxygen is reduced (to H_2O).

[31] Pyruvate is formed when pyruvic acid loses a hydrogen atom; on the DAT, both terms are used interchangeably. At physiological pH (7.4), pyruvic acid is deprotonated and exists in the form of pyruvate. Pyruvate is an anion and pyruvic acid is neutral.

[32] The text states that glucose is split in half in the formation of pyruvate. Since glucose has six carbons, pyruvate must have three.

only occur when oxygen is available to the cell, *neither uses oxygen directly*. Rather, oxygen is necessary for stage four, in which NADH and $FADH_2$ generated throughout cellular respiration are reconverted into NAD^+ and **FAD**. The PDC and the Krebs cycle occur in the innermost compartment of the mitochondria: the **matrix**.

In stage four of energy harvesting, **electron transport/oxidative phosphorylation**, the high-energy electrons carried by NADH and $FADH_2$ are oxidized by the **electron transport chain** in the inner mitochondrial membrane. The reduced electron carriers dump their electrons at the beginning of the chain, and oxygen is reduced to H_2O at the end. (The word *oxidative* in "oxidative phosphorylation" refers to the use of oxygen to oxidize the reduced electron carriers NADH and $FADH_2$.) The electron energy liberated by the transport chain is used to pump protons out of the innermost compartment of the mitochondrion. The protons are allowed to flow back into the mitochondrion, and the energy of this proton flow is used to produce the high-energy triphosphate group in ATP.

Compartmentalization of Glucose Catabolism in Eukaryotes: Mitochondria

Of the four parts of cell respiration, only glycolysis occurs in the cytoplasm in eukaryotic cells. Thus, to understand cell respiration, you must know the structure of a **mitochondrion** (Figure 6). The mitochondrion contains two membranes, an **outer membrane** and an **inner membrane**, each composed of a lipid bilayer. The outer membrane is smooth and contains large pores formed by **porin** proteins. The inner membrane is impermeable, even to very small items like H^+, and is densely folded into structures termed **cristae**. The cristae extend into the **matrix**, which is the innermost space of the mitochondrion. The space between the two membranes, the **intermembrane space**, is continuous with the cytoplasm due to the large pores in the outer membrane. The enzymes of the Krebs cycle and the pyruvate dehydrogenase complex are located in the matrix, and those of the electron transport chain and ATP synthase involved in oxidative phosphorylation are bound to the inner mitochondrial membrane.

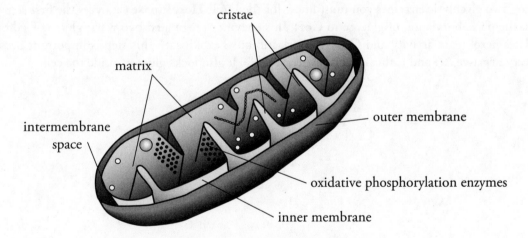

Figure 6 The Mitochondrion

Glycolysis

Glycolysis is an extremely old pathway, having evolved several billion years ago. It is the universal first step in glucose metabolism, extraction of energy from carbohydrates. All cells from *all domains* (a domain is the highest taxonomic category) possess the enzymes of this pathway. In glycolysis, a glucose molecule is oxidized and split into two **pyruvate** molecules, producing a net surplus of 2 ATP (from ADP + P_i) and producing 2 NADH (from NAD^+ + H^+):

$$\textbf{Glucose} + \textbf{2 ADP} + \textbf{2 P}_i + \textbf{2 NAD}^+ \rightarrow \textbf{2 Pyruvate} + \textbf{2 ATP} + \textbf{2 NADH} + \textbf{2 H}_2\textbf{O} + \textbf{2 H}^+$$

3.6

Of course it's not quite that simple. Glycolysis involves several reactions, each of which is catalyzed by a different enzyme (see Figure 7). The general strategy is to first phosphorylate glucose on both ends and then split it into two 3-carbon units which can go on to the PDC and Krebs cycle. In the first step of glycolysis, a phosphate is taken from ATP and used to phosphorylate glucose, producing glucose 6-phosphate (G6P). This is isomerized to fructose 6-phosphate (F6P), which is then phosphorylated on carbon #1 (with the phosphate again taken from ATP) to produce fructose 1,6-bisphosphate (F1,6bP). This is split into two 3-carbon units (called glyceraldehyde 3-phosphate, G3P, or GAP) that are eventually oxidized to pyruvate, producing 2 ATP and 1 NADH per pyruvate, or 4 ATP and 2 NADH per glucose (since we get two 3-carbon units from each glucose). Don't forget that *each* glucose gives rise to *two* 3-carbon G3Ps that pass through the second part of glycolysis and into the PDC. Make sure you understand glycolysis at the level we've described it here. You don't need to worry about details for the second half (e.g., G3P to pyruvate) for the DAT, as long as you know how many ATP and NADH are produced. You'll see a summary diagram of this on the next page.

- An extract of yeast contains all of the enzymes required for glycolysis, ADP, P_i, Mg^{2+}, NAD^+ and glucose, but when these are all combined, none of the glucose is consumed. Provided that there are no enzyme inhibitors present, why doesn't the reaction proceed?[33]

There are two glycolytic enzymes you must know for the DAT. **Hexokinase** catalyzes the first step in glycolysis, the phosphorylation of glucose to G6P. This enzyme is regulated two ways; glucose feedforward stimulates hexokinase activity and G6P feedback inhibits hexokinase. This step is important because it has a very negative ΔG and is thus effectively irreversible. It also locks glucose inside the cell.

---

[33] Although glycolysis results in a net ATP production, ATP is initially required to drive the reaction forward in the phosphorylation of glucose to glucose 6-phosphate and the phosphorylation of fructose 6-phosphate to fructose 1,6-bisphosphate. Without ATP to "prime the pump," there is no way to start the pathway. In case you're wondering about the Mg^{2+}, it's necessary for all reactions involving ATP.

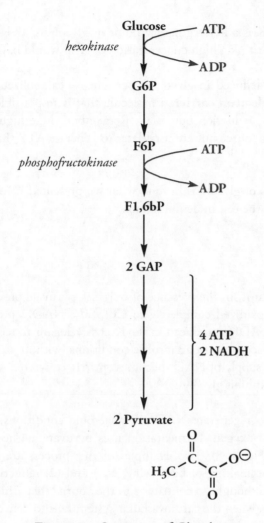

Figure 7   Summary of Glycolysis

Phosphofructokinase (**PFK**) catalyzes the third step: transfer of a phosphate group from ATP to fructose 6-phosphate to form fructose 1,6-bisphosphate (F1,6bP). This is an important step because the reaction catalyzed by PFK is thermodynamically very favorable (like burning wood: $\Delta G \ll 0$), so it's practically irreversible. Also, G6P can be shunted to various pathways, but F1,6bP can only react in glycolysis. So once you light the PFK fire, you're committed to glycolysis. Hence PFK is the key biochemical valve controlling the flow of substrate to product in glycolysis, and the conversion of F6P to F1,6bP is known as a **committed step**. In the remainder of glycolysis, F1,6bP is split into two 3-carbon molecules that are converted to pyruvate, with production of NADH and ATP. Very favorable steps in enzymatic pathways (those with a large negative ΔG) are practically irreversible (because the back-reaction is so unfavorable). These reactions are the ones that are usually subject to allosteric regulation. Another generalization about what steps get regulated is this: early steps in a long pathway tend to be regulated. This makes sense; if you're going from A to Z, it's more practical to regulate the A $\rightarrow$ B reaction than the W $\rightarrow$ X one.

For example, the enzyme PFK is a key regulatory point in glycolysis. PFK is allosterically regulated by ATP. [What effect would you think a high concentration of ATP would have on PFK activity?[34]]

Two molecules of NAD[+] are reduced in glycolysis per glucose catabolized, forming 2 NADH. As discussed above, NADH is an **electron carrier**, a molecule that is responsible for shuttling energy in the form of **reducing power** (i.e., reduction potential). Remember, these high energy electron carriers are not used directly as an energy source but are used later to generate ATP through electron transport and oxidative phosphorylation.

Don't worry about the details of glycolysis beyond what we presented here; this is DAT-level glycolysis. You can worry about learning the rest in dental school.

3.6

Fermentation

Under **aerobic** conditions (that is, in the presence of oxygen), pyruvate produced in glycolysis enters the PDC and Krebs cycle to be oxidized completely to CO_2. The NADH produced in glycolysis and the PDC, as well as NADH and $FADH_2$ produced in the Krebs cycle, are all reoxidized in electron transport, where O_2 is the final electron acceptor. In **anaerobic** conditions (without oxygen), electron transport cannot function, and the limited supply of NAD[+] becomes entirely converted to NADH. [Would a limiting supply of NAD[+] stimulate or inhibit glycolysis?[35]]

Fermentation has evolved to regenerate NAD[+] in anaerobic conditions, thereby allowing glycolysis to continue in the absence of oxygen. Fermentation uses pyruvate as the acceptor of the high energy electrons from NADH (see Figure 8). Two examples of this process are (1) reduction of pyruvate to **ethanol** (yeasts do this in the making of beer, wine, etc.) and (2) reduction of pyruvate to **lactate** in human muscle cells. Lactate is thought to contribute to the "burn" that athletes encounter during anaerobic exertion, such as sprinting, when the cardiovascular system fails to deliver enough oxygen to keep the electron transport chain running in muscle cells.

---

[34] When energy (ATP) is abundant, the cell should slow glycolysis. High concentrations of ATP inhibit PFK activity by binding to an allosteric regulatory site. It is interesting to note that since ATP is a reactant in the reaction catalyzed by PFK, you would expect a high concentration of ATP to increase the rate of the reaction (Le Châtelier's principle). However, the inhibitory allosteric effects of ATP on PFK outweigh this thermodynamic consideration. So lowering the concentration of ATP will increase the reaction rate, even though ATP is a reactant. Of course, if the ATP level went too low, the reaction could not proceed at all.

[35] If NAD[+] has all been converted to NADH, then the step in glycolysis that produces NADH (catalyzed by glyceraldehyde 3-phosphate dehydrogenase) cannot occur because it requires NAD[+] as a substrate. Thus, a lack of NAD[+] will *inhibit* glycolysis.

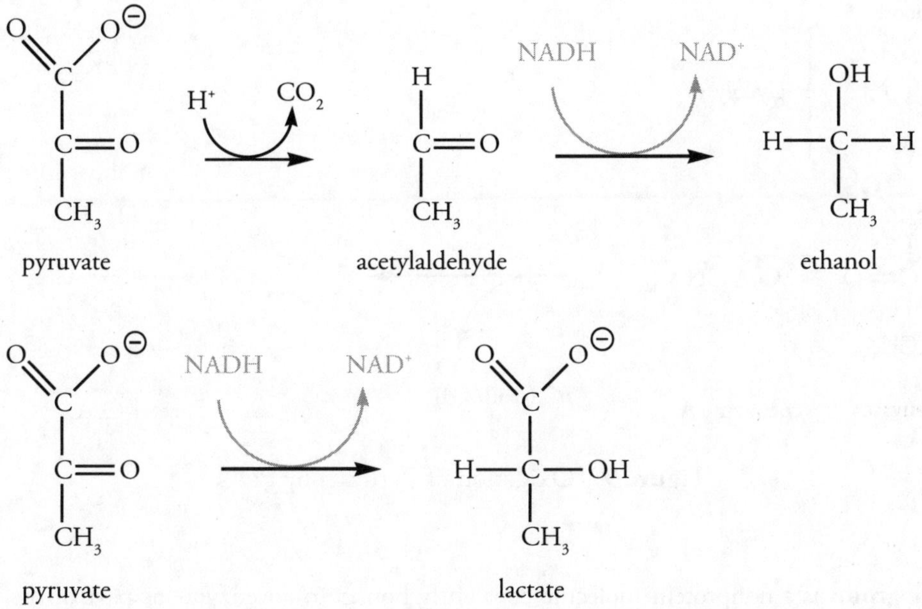

Figure 8 Anaerobic Pathways for Regeneration of NAD⁺ from NADH

NAD^+ produced by reducing pyruvate anaerobically is available for reuse in the glycolytic pathway, so more ATP can be produced. There is a limit to the use of anaerobic glycolysis as an energy source, however. The ethanol or lactate that is produced builds up, having no other use in the cell, and acts as a poison at high concentrations. Wine yeast die when the ethanol concentration reaches about 12 percent, and **lactic acid** is damaging at high concentrations in our tissues as well.

- What happens to the lactate in human muscle cells after a period of strenuous exercise?[36]

Pyruvate Dehydrogenase Complex (PDC)

Pyruvate produced in glycolysis in the cytoplasm is transported into the mitochondrial matrix, where it will be entirely oxidized to CO_2. Pyruvate does not enter the Krebs cycle directly, however. First it is oxidatively decarboxylated by the pyruvate dehydrogenase complex (PDC; Figure 9). **Oxidative decarboxylation** is a reaction repeated again in the Krebs cycle, in which a molecule is oxidized to release CO_2 and produce NADH. In oxidative decarboxylation, pyruvate is changed from a 3-carbon molecule to a 2-carbon molecule, while CO_2 is given off and NADH is produced. The PDC changes pyruvate into an activated acetyl unit. An acetyl unit is [(CH₃)(O=C–)], and *activated* means the acetyl is not floating around freely but rather is attached to a carrier, namely **coenzyme A.** This coenzyme is basically a long handle with a sulfur at the end, abbreviated CoA-SH. It is used in many reaction systems to pass acetyl units around (e.g., fatty acid and cholesterol synthesis and degradation). When loaded with an acetyl unit, CoA-SH is abbreviated acetyl-CoA.

---

[36] Lactate is exported from the muscle cell to the liver. When oxygen becomes available, the liver cell will convert the lactate back to pyruvate, while making NADH from NAD^+. Then the liver will use this excess NADH to make ATP in oxidative phosphorylation. This pyruvate can enter gluconeogenesis or the Krebs cycle in the liver, or it can be sent back to muscle. (This cycle, whereby the liver deals with lactate from muscle, is known as the **Cori Cycle**.)

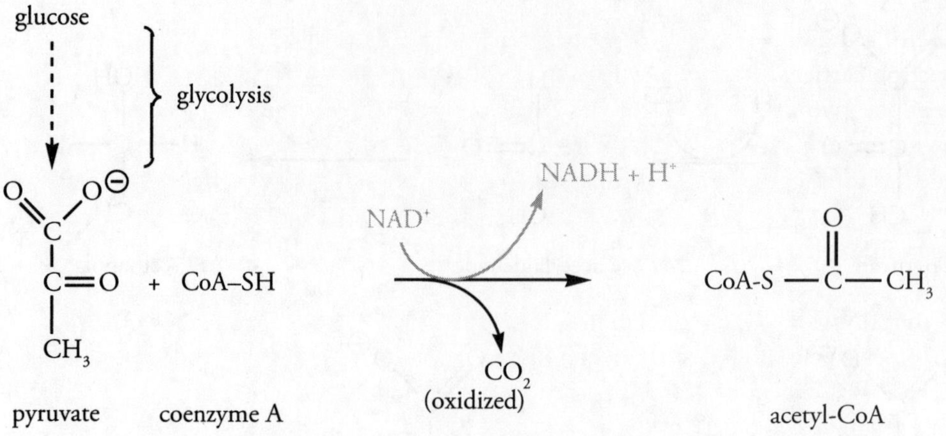

3.6

glucose

glycolysis

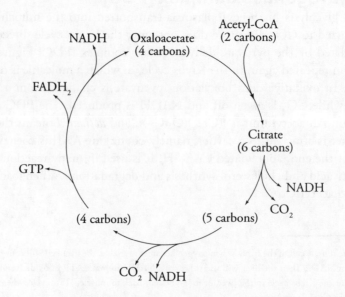

pyruvate   coenzyme A CO_2 (oxidized)   acetyl-CoA

Figure 9   Oxidation of Pyruvate by PDC

A **prosthetic group** is a nonprotein molecule covalently bound to an enzyme as part of the enzyme's active site. The PDC contains a thiamine pyrophosphate (TPP) prosthetic group at one of its active sites. The α-ketoglutarate dehydrogenase complex, which catalyzes the third step in the Krebs cycle, is very similar to the PDC; it has a TPP prosthetic group and catalyzes an oxidative decarboxylation. The **thiamine** in thiamine pyrophosphate is vitamin B_1. Vitamins often serve as prosthetic groups. Contrast this with NAD^+, which is a cofactor. **Cofactors** (which were discussed earlier) are various organic and inorganic substances necessary to the function of an enzyme but which never actually interact with the enzyme.

Krebs Cycle

Krebs cycle is a group of reactions that take the 2-carbon acetyl unit from acetyl-CoA, combine it with oxaloacetate (that contains four carbon atoms), and release two CO_2 molecules. NADH and $FADH_2$ are generated in the process. Figure 10 shows an overview of the process; note that many of the names are not necessary to know and have intentionally been left out.

Figure 10   Overview of the Krebs Cycle

Note that Figure 10 is drawn for one acetyl-CoA, so Krebs cycle as we've drawn it will run twice per glucose. The reduced electron carriers (NADH and $FADH_2$) go on to generate ATP in electron transport and oxidative phosphorylation. Two other names for the Krebs cycle are the **tricarboxylic acid cycle** (**TCA cycle**) and the **citric acid cycle**. Citrate is the first intermediate produced in the cycle, as soon as the acetyl unit is supplied. Citrate has three carboxylic acid functional groups, hence the term "tricarboxylic acid."

To review, oxidation of glucose has so far yielded:

1. 2 ATP and 2 NADH per glucose molecule in glycolysis
2. 2 NADH per glucose (one per pyruvate) via PDC
3. 6 NADH, 2 $FADH_2$, and 2 GTP per glucose in the Krebs cycle

3.6

Thus, most of the energy of glucose is not extracted directly as ATP (or GTP) but in high-energy electron carriers. We will now see how ATP is generated from NADH and $FADH_2$ in electron transport/oxidative phosphorylation.

3.6

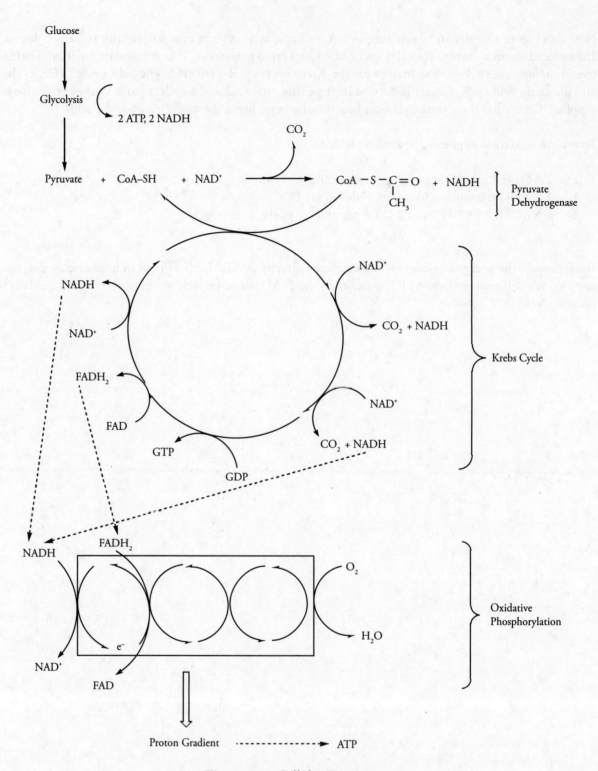

Figure 11 Cellular Respiration

The two goals of electron transport/oxidative phosphorylation are to:

1. reoxidize all electron carriers reduced in glycolysis, PDC, and Krebs cycle
2. store energy in the form of ATP in the process.

Where are all the reduced electron carriers located? Per each glucose catabolized, two NADH are created by glycolysis in the cytoplasm; the electrons from these NADH will have to be transported into the mitochondria before they can be passed along the electron transport chain. All the other NADHs and $FADH_2$s were produced inside the mitochondrial matrix, so they are in the right place to donate electrons to the electron transport chain.

The situation in prokaryotes is a bit different: all of the reduced electron carriers are located in the cytoplasm. In fact, everything is located in the cytoplasm, since there are *no membrane-bound organelles at all* in prokaryotes (no mitochondria, no nucleus, no lysosomes—everything just floats around in the cytoplasm). Since they have no mitochondria, can bacteria perform oxidative phosphorylation? *Yes, they can!* The way the process works is that a proton gradient must be created and then used to power ATP synthesis by the membrane-bound **ATP synthase**. So all that's required is a membrane impermeable to protons. Eukaryotes use the inner mitochondrial membrane; bacteria just use their cell membrane. The end result of this difference is that when eukaryotes perform aerobic respiration, they have to shuttle the electrons from cytosolic NADH into the mitochondrial matrix (at the cost of some energy), but bacteria do not. So, all things considered, prokaryotes get two more high-energy phosphate bonds from aerobic respiration than eukaryotes do (this will be discussed in more detail in just a bit). From this point forward, we will discuss the eukaryotic system. Remember that it's the same in prokaryotes except that they do it on the cell membrane instead of on the inner mitochondrial membrane (since they have no mitochondria!).

Electron Transport Chain and Oxidative Phosphorylation

Oxidative phosphorylation is oxidation of the high-energy electron carriers NADH and $FADH_2$ coupled to the phosphorylation of ADP to produce ATP. Energy released through oxidation of NADH and $FADH_2$ by the electron transport chain is used to pump protons out of the mitochondrial matrix. This proton gradient is the source of energy used to drive the phosphorylation of ADP to ATP. The **electron-transport chain** is a group of five electron carriers (Figure 12). Each member of the chain reduces the next member down the line. All five are named for their redox roles. Three of them are large protein complexes found embedded in the inner mitochondrial membrane. They contain heme prosthetic groups (as in hemoglobin) or iron-sulfur electron-transfer systems. The other two members of the electron transport chain are smaller electron carriers. The chain is organized so that the first large carrier receives electrons (reducing power) from NADH; the NADH is thus oxidized to NAD^+. Hence, the first large carrier in the e^- transport chain ("A" in the figure) is called **NADH dehydrogenase**. It passes its electrons to one of the small carriers in the transport chain, called **ubiquinone**, also known as **coenzyme Q**. NADH dehydrogenase is also known as **coenzyme Q reductase**.

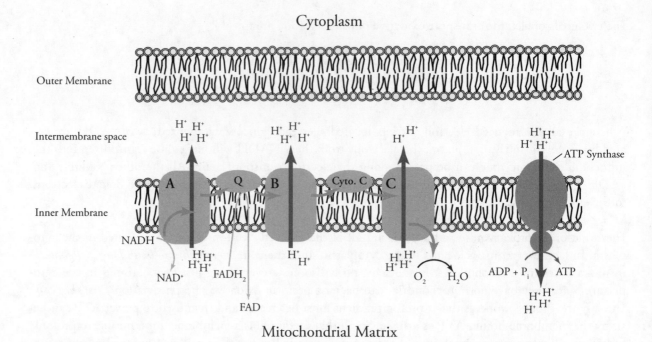

Figure 12 Electron Transport Chain

Ubiquinone then passes its electrons to the second large membrane-bound complex in the chain ("B"), known as **cytochrome C reductase**. From this name, you can guess what the next carrier in the chain is called; it is **cytochrome C**, a small hydrophilic protein bound loosely to the inner mitochondrial membrane. The last member of the electron transport chain ("C") is simply called **cytochrome C oxidase**. [Where does it pass its electrons to?[37]]

Each of the three large membrane-bound proteins in the electron transport chain pumps protons across the inner mitochondrial membrane every time electrons flow past. The first and second large protein pumps four protons each, and the third large protein pumps two protons. Protons are pumped out of the matrix, into the intermembrane space. The inner mitochondrial membrane is highly impermeable to protons. As a result, the electron transport chain creates a large proton gradient, with the pH being much ___ (higher/lower) inside the matrix than in the rest of the cell.[38]

What does this have to do with ATP synthesis? Well, there is one more very important protein embedded in the inner mitochondrial membrane: **ATP synthase**. It is a large protein complex which contains a proton channel that spans the inner membrane. The passage of protons from the intermembrane space through the ATP synthase channel causes it to synthesize ATP from ADP + P$_i$. Thus, ATP production is dependent on a **proton gradient**. The overall process of electron transport and ATP production is said to be *coupled* by the proton gradient. Together, electron transport and ATP production are known as **oxidative phosphorylation**. Make sure you understand these questions:

---

[37] If it's the last member of the chain, it must pass its reducing power to O_2, reducing it to H_2O, an end product of electron transport. This is the only reason we breathe and the only reason we evolved with lungs, RBCs, etc.

[38] higher (remember, high pH = low [H^+])

- Dinitrophenol (DNP) is an uncoupler: it destroys the proton gradient by allowing protons to flow into the matrix. Which one of the following processes does it inhibit first?[39]
  - A. Pyruvate decarboxylation by the PDC
  - B. The TCA cycle
  - C. Electron transport
  - D. Muscular contraction
  - E. Glycolysis

- The reason cyanide is a poison is that it inactivates cytochrome C oxidase by binding to its active site with high affinity. When a person is exposed to cyanide[40]
  - A. the difference in pH inside and outside the matrix is already as large as it can become, so no more electrons can be pumped against the gradient.
  - B. anaerobic glycolysis depletes pyruvate, thereby slowing the Krebs cycle and the electron transport chain and slowing the rate of proton pumping.
  - C. the electron transport chain ceases to transport electrons and therefore ceases to pump protons.
  - D. NADH becomes fully oxidized by the Krebs cycle and therefore cannot reduce NADH dehydrogenase, so no protons are pumped.
  - E. cytochrome C oxidase becomes reduced and therefore pumps more protons across the inner membrane.

Energetics of Glucose Catabolism

How is electron transport quantitatively connected to ATP synthesis? For every NADH that is oxidized to NAD^+, the three large electron transport proteins pump about 10 protons across the inner mitochondrial membrane, into the intermembrane space. The ATP synthase requires three protons to generate a molecule of ATP from ADP and P_i; however, an additional proton is required to bring P_i into the matrix. This brings the "cost" of ATP synthesis up to four protons per molecule of ATP. Since NADH is responsible for the pumping of 10 protons, each molecule of NADH provides the energy to produce approximately 2.5 ATP molecules.

Even though NADH and $FADH_2$ have similar functions, their fates are a little different. $FADH_2$ gives its electrons to ubiquinone instead of to NADH dehydrogenase. By bypassing the first proton pump, $FADH_2$ is only responsible for the pumping of six protons across the inner membrane.

- How many ATP are made every time an $FADH_2$ is reoxidized to FAD?[41]

---

[39] If the proton gradient is destroyed, the processes in A, B, C, and E will continue unabated, because NADH will be reoxidized to NAD^+ at a normal rate, or perhaps faster than normal. The problem will be that without a proton gradient no ATP will get made from all this glucose breakdown. The answer is **D** because this will be the first problem encountered from running out of ATP.

[40] If the active site of cytochrome C oxidase is occupied with cyanide, then oxygen cannot bind there to be reduced to water; in other words, cytochrome C oxidase will be unable to get rid of its electrons, will remain reduced, and will be unable to pump protons (choice E is wrong). It will also be unable to accept electrons from cytochrome C, which will be unable to accept electrons from cytochrome C reductase, which will be unable to accept electrons from coenzyme Q, etc., etc., all the way back up the electron transport chain. The end result will be a cessation of all electron transport chain activity (choice **C** is correct). Note that protons, not electrons, are pumped against their gradient (choice A is wrong), and this will stop completely, not just be slowed down (choice B is wrong). Also, NAD^+ is reduced to NADH in the Krebs cycle, not the other way around (choice D is wrong).

[41] Only 1.5 ATP are made as a result of the reoxidation of $FADH_2$. Six protons divided by four protons per ATP equals 1.5 ATP.

3.6

As mentioned earlier, PDC, Krebs cycle, and oxidative phosphorylation all occur in mitochondria in eukaryotes, while glycolysis occurs in the cytoplasm. Electrons from the NADH generated in glycolysis must be transported into the mitochondria before they can enter the electron transport chain. In most cells, they are transported by a pathway termed the **glycerol phosphate shuttle**. This shuttle delivers the electrons directly to ubiquinone (just like $FADH_2$), bypassing NADH dehydrogenase, and results in the production of only 1.5 molecules of ATP per cytosolic NADH, rather than the 2.5 normally formed from matrix NADH. Bacteria, because they lack cellular organelles, do not need to transport cytosolic electrons across any membranes. This explains the discrepancy in Table 1 in how much ATP is yielded from each NADH from glycolysis in eukaryotes compared to prokaryotes. All values in the following table are per glucose molecule catabolized.

Process	Molecules Formed/Used	ATP Equivalents
Glycolysis	−2 ATP 4 ATP 2 NADH	−2 ATP 4 ATP 3 ATP (eukaryotes) 5 ATP (prokaryotes)
PDC	2 NADH	5 ATP
Krebs Cycle	6 NADH 2 FADH₂ 2 GTP	15 ATP 3 ATP 2 ATP
Total		**30 ATP (eukaryotes)** **32 ATP (prokaryotes)**

Table 1 ATP Yield from Cellular Respiration

Notes:

1. These numbers are an estimate of the theoretical maximum amount of ATP that can be produced from a single molecule of glucose. As the proton gradient is used to transport other molecules into or out of the matrix, the actual yield may differ depending on the number of protons (i.e., the gradient) available for ATP synthesis.
2. These numbers reflect the most recent understanding of ATP synthesis, and as such, may not appear in some textbooks that still cling to the previously established counts of 36 ATP per glucose in eukaryotes and 38 ATP per glucose in prokaryotes.

3.7   OTHER METABOLIC PATHWAYS OF THE CELL

There are several other metabolic pathways that play important roles in maintaining sugar and energy levels.

Glycogenolysis vs. Gluconeogenesis

Glycogenolysis is the term for glycogen breakdown. Glycogen is a polymer of glucose that is found in muscle and liver cells in humans, and is the main form of carbohydrate storage in animals. The synthesis of glycogen (**glycogenesis**) and glycogenolysis are opposing processes, controlled by hormones that regulate blood sugar levels and energy (antagonistic peptide hormones insulin and glucagon, made in and released from the pancreas). Glycogenolysis occurs in response to glucagon, when blood sugar levels are low. It results in glucose being released into the blood.

Gluconeogenesis occurs when dietary sources of glucose are unavailable, and when the liver has depleted stores of glucose. This process occurs primarily in the liver (with a small amount occurring in the kidneys), and involves converting non-carbohydrate precursor molecules (such as lactate, pyruvate, Krebs cycle intermediates, and the carbon skeletons of most amino acids) into oxaloacetate and then glucose. There are some tissues that use glucose as their main energy fuel; your brain is a good example. Gluconeogenesis provides glucose when dietary intake is insufficient or absent.

β-Oxidation

Fatty acids are made in the cytoplasm of hepatocytes (liver cells) via fatty acid biosynthetic pathways, and are stored in adipocytes (fat cells) as triglycerides (triacylglycerol or TAG). Fatty acids can be broken down in the hepatocyte mitochondria via fatty acid β-oxidation in response to metabolic need. This process involves removing two carbons at a time from the fatty acid and converting these carbons to acetyl-CoA. β-oxidation generates one NADH and one $FADH_2$ for each 2-carbon group removed. Acetyl-CoA can then enter the Krebs cycle. The glycerol backbone of TAG can be converted into glucose and can enter cellular respiration at glycolysis.

Amino Acid Catabolism

Proteins in cells are constantly being made, kept for a certain period of time (minutes to weeks), and then degraded back into amino acids. In addition, humans absorb amino acids from dietary proteins. These free amino acids can be catabolized via several pathways. The amino group is removed and converted into urea for excretion. The remaining carbon skeleton (also called an α-keto acid) can either be broken down into water and CO_2, or can be converted to glucose or acetyl-CoA.

3.7

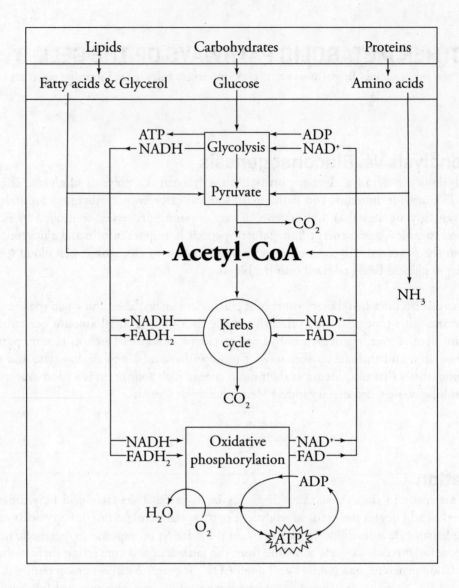

Figure 13 Summary of Metabolic Pathways

3.8 PHOTOSYNTHESIS

Overview

Photosynthesis is the process by which plants and other photoautotrophs use light energy to synthesize carbohydrates. [Besides plants, which other organisms can perform photosynthesis?[42]] It is an example of **carbon fixation**, a process in which carbon dioxide is incorporated into more complex organic molecules. Photosynthesis produces and maintains the oxygen content of the Earth's atmosphere. It also generates most of the energy necessary for life on Earth, and supplies all of the organic compounds. In plants, photosynthesis takes place in the **chloroplast**, a double-membrane organelle found in the cells of photosynthetic organisms (see Figure 14). A double membrane encloses the **stroma**, a dense fluid within the chloroplast. Inside the stroma are smaller membrane-bound compartments called thylakoids that are stacked into structures called **grana**.

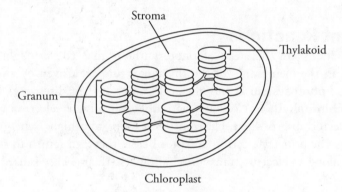

Figure 14   Chloroplast

The summarized chemical equation for photosynthesis is:

$$6\ CO_2 + 12\ H_2O + energy \rightarrow 6\ O_2 + C_6H_{12}O_6 + 6\ H_2O$$

Water appears on both sides of the equation because twelve molecules are split and six are newly formed. The reaction can be simplified by showing only net consumption of water:

$$6\ CO_2 + 6\ H_2O + energy \rightarrow 6\ O_2 + C_6H_{12}O_6$$

This net equation is essentially the chemical reverse of cellular respiration, although the actual metabolic processes that occur are not simply respiration in reverse. Although the carbohydrate in the equation is glucose, the actual product of photosynthesis is a three-carbon sugar called **glyceraldehyde 3-phosphate** (sometimes called G3P or GAP). Remember, we also saw this molecule in the middle of glycolysis. G3P can be used to produce glucose and other organic molecules.

---

[42] Photosynthesis is performed by all plants, as well as some bacteria (cyanobacteria) and some protists (algae). It is not performed by any fungi or animals.

Photosynthesis occurs in two steps, the **light-dependent reactions** and the **light-independent reactions**. The following table summarizes these two sets of reactions:

	Location	Energy Production/Use	Product
Light-dependent	thylakoid membrane	produces ATP and NADPH	oxygen
Light-independent	stroma	uses ATP and NADPH	carbohydrate

Table 2   Summary of Photosynthesis

The light-dependent reactions and the light-independent reactions are linked: the light-dependent reactions produce the chemical energy needed by the light-independent reactions to produce organic molecules.

3.8

Light-Dependent Reactions

The light-dependent reactions are the steps of photosynthesis that convert light energy to chemical energy. They occur within the membranes of the thylakoids and are driven by two light-absorbing systems: **photosystem I** and **photosystem II** (numbered in order of their discovery). Photosystems consist of pigment molecules (**chlorophyll**) in close association with a primary electron acceptor. In overview, when a chlorophyll molecule absorbs light, electrons are excited to a higher energy level. These excited electrons are captured by the primary electron acceptor before they can return to their ground state and are subsequently passed along an electron transport chain where their energy is used to produce ATP and **NADPH**.[43]

Let's look at the specific reactions more closely (see Figure 15 on the following page). When photosystem II absorbs light, electrons in chlorophyll are excited to a higher energy level and captured by the primary electron acceptor. This leaves "vacancies" for electrons in chlorophyll. These vacancies are filled by electrons gained from the splitting of a water molecule into two H^+ ions and an oxygen atom. The oxygen atom immediately combines with a second oxygen atom to produce O_2; this is the step in photosynthesis where oxygen is released. The release of protons from H_2O establishes a proton gradient across the **thylakoid** membrane.

The excited electrons then pass through an electron transport chain (very similar to the electron transport chain used in cellular respiration) on their way to photosystem I. The primary electron acceptor of photosystem II passes the electrons to plastoquinone (Pq), which passes them to a cytochrome complex, which passes them to plastocyanin (Pc), which passes them to photosystem I. Here they fill the vacancies produced when the electrons in chlorophyll of photosystem I were excited by light to a higher energy level.

---

[43] You need to be aware of three coenzymes for the DAT:

1. Nicotinamide adenine dinucleotide (NAD) is a coenzyme central to metabolism and is found in all living cells. It exists in two forms: oxidized NAD^+ and reduced NADH.

2. Flavin adenine dinucleotide (FAD) is also a coenzyme and is involved with several enzymatic reactions in metabolism. FAD is the fully oxidized form; it accepts two electrons and two protons to become $FADH_2$ (reduced form).

3. Nicotinamide adenine dinucleotide phosphate ($NADP^+$) is a coenzyme and reducing agent used in anabolic reactions, such as the Calvin cycle and lipid and nucleic acid syntheses. It is used by all forms of life. NADPH is the reduced form of $NADP^+$.

Note that $NADP^+$ differs from NAD^+ by the presence of an additional phosphate group on a ribose ring.

As electrons pass from Pq to the cytochrome complex, additional protons are pumped from the stroma into the thylakoid lumen. This is identical to the pumping of protons from the mitochondrial matrix into the intermembrane space during respiration. These H^+ ions, along with the H^+ ions released from the splitting of water, form a proton gradient that drives the production of ATP, again in a manner similar to that found in respiration. The protons diffuse down their concentration gradient to the stroma, through an ATP synthase that couples the movement of protons to the phosphorylation of ADP. ATP production in the light reactions is also called **photophosphorylation.**

Chlorophyll electrons excited by photosystem I are captured by its primary electron acceptor and are transferred to ferredoxin (Fd). An enzyme called **NADP⁺ reductase** then transfers a pair of electrons to $NADP^+$ (along with a pair of protons from the stroma), reducing it to NADPH. Note that both ATP and NADPH are made in the stroma.

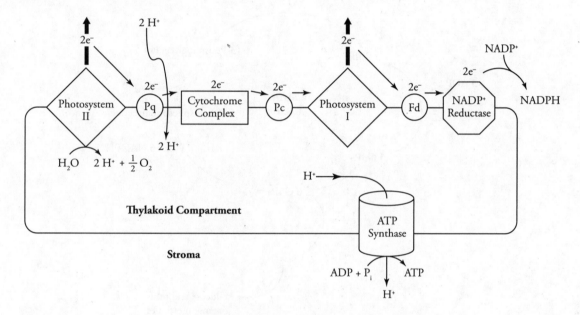

Figure 15   Light-Dependent Reactions

Most plants follow this electron flow, which is called linear, or noncyclic. However, some plants (such as C4 plants discussed below) perform cyclic electron flow instead. Cyclic photophosphorylation is similar to non-cyclic, but generates only ATP, and no NADPH. It takes place only at photosystem I: once the electron is displaced from the photosystem, it is passed down electron acceptor molecules (Fd, cytochromes and Pc) and returns to photosystem I, from where it was emitted.

Light–Independent Reactions

The light-independent reactions (**Calvin cycle**) use chemical energy produced during the light-dependent reactions to form carbohydrates. This cycle (Figure 16 on the following page) takes place in the stroma and is similar to the Krebs cycle in that the original carbon molecule is regenerated with each turn of the cycle.

The first step is the addition of three CO_2 molecules to three molecules of a 5-carbon sugar, **ribulose bisphosphate** (RuBP). This is the carbon fixation step, and the enzyme that catalyzes this reaction is **rubisco**. This forms three unstable 6-carbon intermediates that immediately split in half to form six 3-carbon sugars (3-phosphoglycerate). ATP is used to phosphorylate 3-phosphoglycerate, forming six molecules of 1,3-bisphosphoglycerate. By oxidizing NADPH to $NADP^+$, six molecules of 1,3-bisphosphoglycerate are reduced to six molecules of glyceraldehyde-3-phosphate which we've seen before, one of which leaves the cycle to be incorporated into glucose and other organic molecules. Finally, through a series of complex reactions involving ATP, the remaining five molecules of G3P are rearranged to regenerate the original three molecules of ribulose bisphosphate. Most plants perform carbon fixation in this way, and are thus called **C_3 plants**. C_3 photosynthesis is so named because the first organic product of carbon fixation is 3-phosphoglycerate, a 3-carbon molecule.

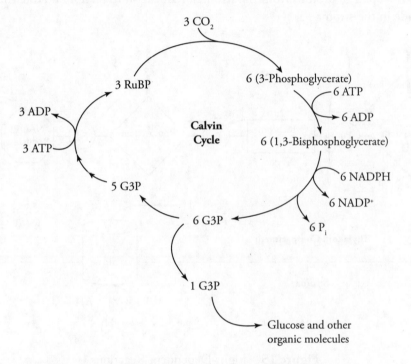

Figure 16   Light-Independent Reactions (Calvin Cycle)

Summary

The light-dependent and light-independent reactions are inexorably linked; neither set of reactions alone can produce carbohydrates from CO_2. The light-dependent reactions use water and light to produce ATP, NADPH, and O_2; light-independent reactions use CO_2, ATP, and NADPH to produce ADP, $NADP^+$, and carbohydrate.

The reactions share some similarities with respiration. In both cases, ATP production is driven by a proton gradient, and the proton gradient is created by an electron transport chain. In respiration, protons are pumped from the mitochondrial matrix to the intermembrane space, and they return to the matrix through an ATP synthase down their concentration gradient. In photosynthesis, protons are pumped from the stroma into the thylakoid's compartment, and they return to the stroma through an ATP synthase down their concentration gradient.

The Krebs cycle and the Calvin cycle are both series of reactions that ultimately regenerate their starting product. Both cycles have an indirect need for a particular substance; although they do not use it directly, without it they cease to run. For the Krebs cycle, that substance is oxygen; for the Calvin cycle, that "substance" is light.

Furthermore, the goals of the two cycles are opposite; the Krebs cycle seeks to oxidize carbohydrates to CO_2, while the Calvin cycle seeks to reduce CO_2 to carbohydrates. The figure below summarizes the main reactants and products of photosynthesis as it occurs in chloroplasts.

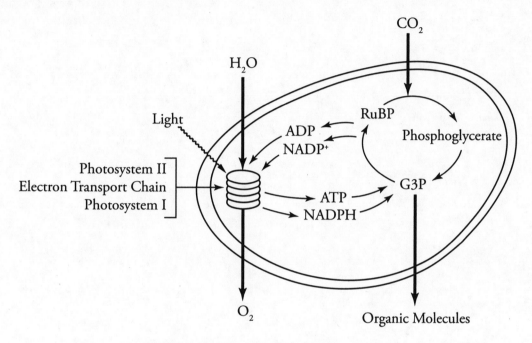

Figure 17   Summary of Photosynthesis

Alternate Mechanisms of Photosynthesis

Stomata are pores on the leaf surface that allow CO_2 to enter the leaf, and O_2 and water to exit. Most plants close their stomata on hot, dry days, to prevent water loss by transpiration (evaporative loss of water from leaves). While this conserves water, it also limits access to CO_2 and thus reduces photosynthetic yield. With less CO_2 available, O_2 accumulates, and plants start performing photorespiration instead of photosynthesis. **Photorespiration** is a wasteful process that uses ATP and O_2, produces more CO_2 and doesn't produce any sugars.

Plants that live in hot climates have evolved two different ways around this: **CAM plants** deal with this problem by temporally separating carbon fixation and the Calvin cycle. They open their stomata at night and incorporate CO_2 into organic acids. During the day, they close their stomata and release CO_2 from the organic acids while the light reactions run. In contrast, **C_4 plants** have slightly different leaf anatomy that allows them to perform CO_2 fixation in a different part of the leaf from the rest of the Calvin cycle. This prevents photorespiration. C_4 plants produce a 4-carbon molecule as the first product of carbon fixation and perform cyclic electron flow in the light reactions (discussed above).

Want More Practice?
Remember to register your book online for chapter summaries, drills, practice tests, and more!

Chapter 4
Molecular Biology

It was once thought that simple living organisms were generated spontaneously from nonliving matter. When a steak went bad and became infested with larvae, it was because the decomposing meat actually became squirming worms. Most religions have traditional explanations for the origin of human life, too. Children are derived from adults due to the will of a deity; the original adults were placed on the earth by that deity. But as empiricism developed during the Enlightenment, rigorous experiments were used to explain life, resulting in "scientific" models that are gradually replacing more traditional explanations.

One early conclusion was that simple organisms were derived not from decomposing matter but from parental organisms. Subsequently, it was found that some organisms are too small to be seen with the naked eye. These "germs" were eventually implicated as the cause of most major diseases. Gradually the scientific community came to the conclusion that all life was derived from other life. The patterns of inheritance and evolution were elucidated by a chain of scientists, from Mendel through Darwin. But the mechanism remained a mystery. Finally, cellular biology advanced to the point that scientists were aware of two substances found in cells which seemed appropriate vehicles for the transmission of inherited information: DNA and protein. The extreme length and orderly arrangement of repeating units in DNA and protein made it seem very likely that they could contain information. Researchers had waded through a chemical ocean of alphabet soup and suddenly come upon long strings of what looked like letters.

This is where biology stood in the early 1940s. In the 1940s and 1950s, two monumental achievements in microbiology finally clarified the gears in the clock of evolution and how they turn. One was the elucidation of the structure of DNA by Wilkins, Franklin, Watson, and Crick. The other was the proof by Avery, McCarty, MacLeod, Hershey, and Chase that DNA was the fundamental unit of genetic inheritance in microorganisms. In the following discussion, we will summarize the wealth of information that has been built upon these two prescient cornerstones.

4.1 DNA STRUCTURE

Nucleic acids were first introduced in Chapter 2. We will build on that introduction here.

Nucleotides

Understanding the structure of DNA provides great insight into its function, so let's start at the smallest level and work our way up. DNA is short for deoxyribonucleic acid. DNA and RNA (ribonucleic acid) are called **nucleic acids** because they are found in the nucleus and possess many acidic phosphate groups. The building block of DNA is the deoxyribonucleoside 5' triphosphate (dNTP, where N represents one of the four basic nucleosides). Deoxyadenosine 5' triphosphate (dATP) is shown in Figure 1 on the following page. Deoxyribonucleotides are built from three components. The first is a simple monosaccharide, ribose. In a dNTP, carbons on the ribose are referred to as 1', 2', etc. The next component of the dNTP is an aromatic nitrogenous base, namely **adenine** (A), **guanine** (G), **cytosine** (C), or **thymine** (T). (Don't mix up the DNA base thymine with vitamin B_1, thiamine.) These aromatic molecules are bases because they contain several nitrogens which have free electron pairs capable of accepting protons. G and A are derived from a precursor called purine, so they are referred to as the **purines**. C and T are the **pyrimidines**.[1] A **nucleo*side*** is ribose with a purine or pyrimidine linked to the 1' carbon and are named as follows: A-ribose = adenosine, G-ribose = guanosine, C-ribose = cytidine, T-ribose = thymidine, and U-ribose = uridine. Both purines and pyrimidines have abundant hydrogen bonding potential.

The final component of the deoxyribonucleotide building block of DNA is a phosphate group. **Nucleotides** are phosphate esters of nucleosides, with one, two, or three phosphate groups joined to the ribose ring by the 5' hydroxy group. When nucleotides contain three phosphate residues, they may also be referred to as **deoxynucleoside triphosphates**; they are abbreviated as **dNTP**, where d is for deoxy and N is for nucleoside. In individual nucleotides, N is replaced by A, G, C, T, or U.

---

[1] Some mnemonics for this are "pure As Gold" to remind you the purines are A and G, and "CUT the Py," meaning the pyrimidines are C, U, and T. Note that U stands for **uracil**, which is a pyrimidine found in RNA instead of T. This will be discussed more shortly.

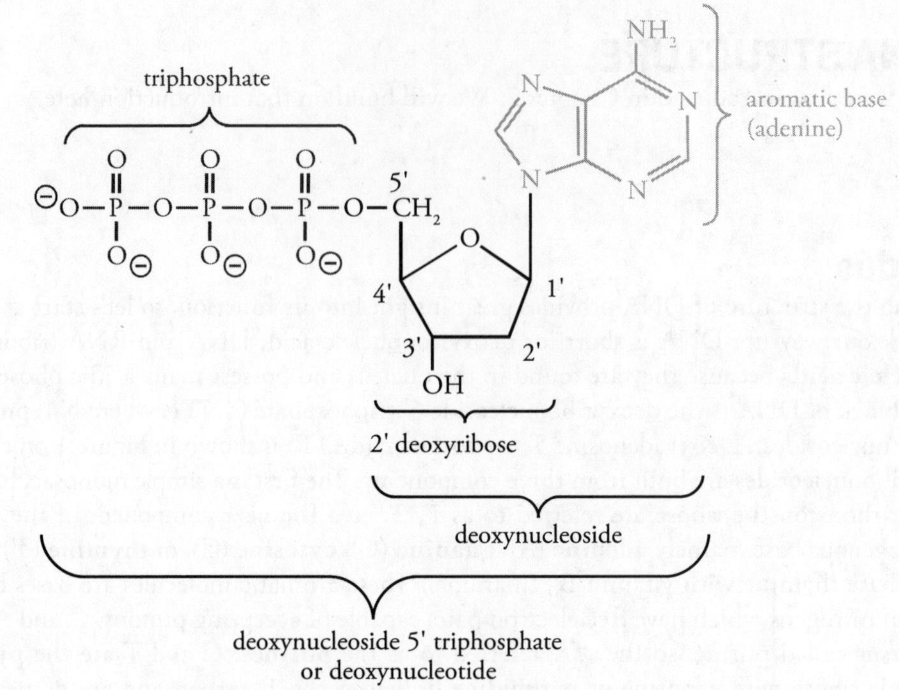

Figure 1   Deoxyadenosine Triphosphate (dATP)

The ribose + phosphate portion of the nucleotide is referred to as the **backbone** of DNA, because it is invariant. The nitrogenous base is the variable portion of the building block. Hence, there are four different dNTPs, and they differ only in the aromatic base. [What is the backbone in protein, and what is the variable portion of the amino acid?[2] If an enzyme binds to a specific sequence of nucleotides in DNA, will the binding specificity be derived from interactions of portions of the polypeptide enzyme with the ribose and phosphate groups or with the purine and pyrimidine bases?[3]]

Polynucleotides

Nucleotides in the DNA chain are covalently linked by **phosphodiester bonds** between the 3' hydroxy group of one deoxyribose and the 5' phosphate group of the next deoxyribose (Figure 2 on the following page). A polymer of several nucleotides linked together is termed an *oligo*nucleotide, and a polymer of many nucleotides is a *poly*nucleotide. Since the only unique part of the nucleotide is the base, the sequence of a polynucleotide can be abbreviated by simply listing the bases attached to each nucleotide in the chain. The end of the chain with a free 5' phosphate group is written first in a polynucleotide, with other nucleotides in the chain indicated in the 5' to 3' direction. [Which of the nucleotides in the oligonucleotide ACGT has a free 3' hydroxy group?[4]]

---

[2] Peptide bonds with a carbon between them are the backbone, and the R group attached to the α carbon is the variable portion.

[3] Since the backbone is the same regardless of the nucleotide sequence, the specificity in binding must be derived from interactions with bases.

[4] The T is written last and is therefore the 3' nucleotide, or the nucleotide with the free 3' hydroxy group.

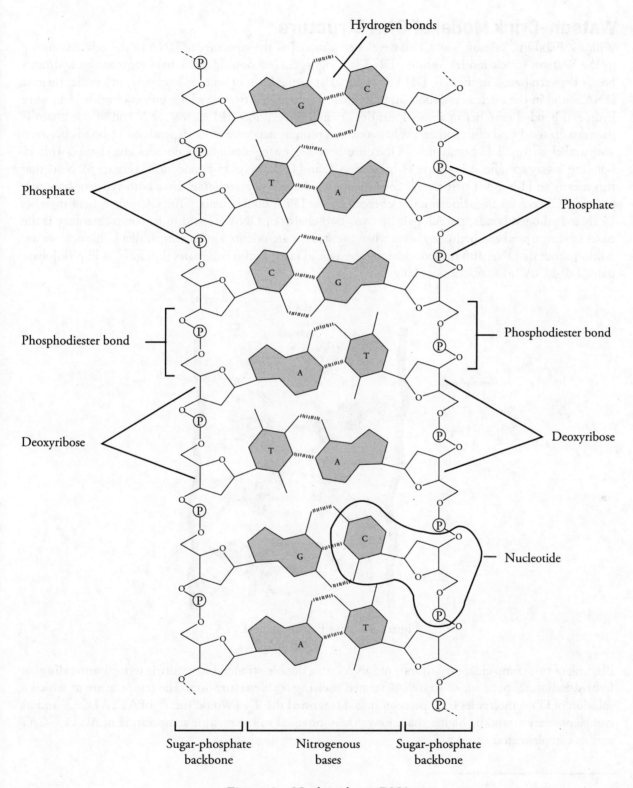

Hydrogen bonds

Phosphate

Phosphate

Phosphodiester bond

Phosphodiester bond

Deoxyribose

Deoxyribose

Nucleotide

Sugar-phosphate backbone

Nitrogenous bases

Sugar-phosphate backbone

Figure 2   Nucleotides in DNA

Watson-Crick Model of DNA Structure

Wilkins, Franklin, Watson, and Crick developed a model of the structure of DNA in the cell. According to the **Watson-Crick model**, cellular DNA is a right-handed **double helix** held together by hydrogen bonds between bases. In the cell, DNA does not exist in the form of a single long polynucleotide. Instead, DNA found in the nucleus is double-stranded (**ds**). In ds-DNA, two very long polynucleotide chains are hydrogen-bonded together in an **antiparallel** orientation. Antiparallel means the 5' end of one chain is paired with the 3' end of the other. [What common protein structure often depends on H-bonds between antiparallel chains?[5]] H-bonds in ds-DNA are between nitrogenous bases on adjacent chains. This H-bonding is very specific: A is always H-bonded to T, and G is always H-bonded to C (Figure 3). Note that this means an H-bonded pair always consists of a *purine plus a pyrimidine*. Thus both types of base pair (AT or GC) take up the same amount of room in the DNA double helix.[6] The GC pair is held together by three hydrogen bonds, the AT pair by two. Two chains of DNA are said to be complementary if the bases in each strand can hydrogen bond when the strands are oriented in an antiparallel fashion. If we are talking about ds-DNA 100 nucleotides long, we would say it is 100 base pairs (bp) long. A kbp (kilobase pair) is ds-DNA 1,000 nucleotides long.

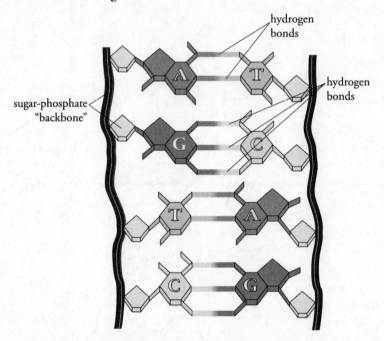

Figure 3   Base Pairing in ds-DNA

Binding of two complementary strands of DNA into a double-stranded structure is termed **annealing**, or **hybridization**. Separation of strands is termed **melting**, or **denaturation**. The temperature at which a solution of DNA molecules is 50 percent melted is termed the T_m. [Would the T_m of ATTATCAT and its complementary strand be higher than, lower than, or equal to the melting temperature of AGTCGCAT and its complementary strand?[7]]

---

[5]   Antiparallel H-bonding is reminiscent of a β-pleated sheet, which is a common secondary structure; it can also be part of quaternary protein structure, when two separate chains come together to form a sheet.

[6]   This fact has another benefit: we can calculate the number of purines if we know the number of pyrimidines. We can actually calculate several variables. Chargoff's rule states that [A] = [T] and [G] = [C]; and [A] + [G] = [T] + [C].

[7]   The T_m of the first oligonucleotide pair would be lower because it contains more AT pairs. A and T only form two hydrogen bonds while G and C form three. Thus, it takes less kinetic energy to disrupt A-T rich ds-DNA than G-C rich ds-DNA.

- Which of the following is/are true about ds-DNA?
  I. If the amount of G in a double helix is known, the amount of C can be calculated.
  II. If the fraction of purine nucleotides and the total molecular weight of a double helix are known, the amount of cytosine can be calculated.
  III. The two chains in a piece of ds-DNA containing mostly purines will be bonded together more tightly than the two chains in a piece of ds-DNA containing mostly pyrimidines.
  IV. The oligonucleotide ATGTAT is complementary to the oligonucleotide ATACAT.[8]

There is another important detail about DNA structure: not only is it double stranded, it is also *coiled*. In ds-DNA, the two hydrogen-bonded antiparallel DNA strands form a **right-handed double helix** with the bases on the interior and the ribose/phosphate backbone on the exterior. The bases lie in a plane, perpendicular to the length of the DNA molecule.

The sum total of an organism's genetic information is called its **genome**. Eukaryotic genomes are composed of several large pieces of linear ds-DNA; each piece of ds-DNA is called a **chromosome**. Humans have 46 chromosomes, 23 of which are inherited from each parent. Prokaryotic (bacterial) genomes are composed of a **single circular chromosome**. Viral genomes may be linear or circular DNA or RNA. The human genome consists of over 10^9 base pairs while bacterial genomes contain only 10^6 base pairs. But there is no direct correlation between genome size and evolutionary sophistication, since the organisms with the largest known genomes are amphibians. Much of the size difference in higher eukaryotic genomes is the result of repetitive DNA that has no known function.

One final point: if the DNA remained as a simple double helix floating free in the cell, it would be very bulky and fragile. Prokaryotes have a distinctive mechanism for making their single circular chromosome more compact and sturdy. An enzyme called **DNA gyrase** uses the energy of ATP to twist the gigantic circular molecule. Gyrase functions by breaking the DNA and twisting the two sides of the circle around each other. The resulting structure is a twisted circle that is composed of ds-DNA. As discussed above, the two strands are already coiled, forming a helix. The twists created by DNA gyrase are called **supercoils**, since they are coils of a structure that is already coiled.

Since eukaryotes have even more DNA in their genome than prokaryotes, the eukaryotic genome requires denser packaging to fit within the cell (Figure 4). To accomplish this, eukaryotic DNA is wrapped around globular proteins called **histones**. After being wrapped around histones, but before being completely packed away, DNA has the microscopic appearance of beads on a string. The beads are called **nucleosomes**; they are composed of DNA wrapped around an octamer (a group of 8) of histones. The string between the beads is a length of double-helical DNA called linker DNA and is bound by a single linker histone. Fully packed DNA is called **chromatin**; it is composed of closely stacked nucleosomes. [Based on your knowledge of the interactions of macromolecules and the chemical composition of DNA, do you suppose that histones are mostly basic or mostly acidic?[9]]

---

[8] **Statement I: True.** For every G, there is a C; and for every A there is a T. **Statement II: False.** The ratio of purines to pyrimidines is always the same (50:50) since each purine is paired with a pyrimidine. In order to calculate the amount of any one base, you have to know the ratio of AT to GC pairs. **Statement III: False.** Again, the ratio of purines to pyrimidines is always the same; (50:50). However, two chains containing mostly GC pairs will bond more tightly than two chains containing mostly AT pairs, since GC pairs are held together by 3 H-bonds while AT pairs have only 2. **Statement IV: True.** Remember: the strands are antiparallel, A and T pair, G and C pair, and the 5' end is always written first.

[9] They're mostly basic, since they must be attracted to the acidic exterior of the DNA double helix. This basicity is supplied by the amino acids arginine and lysine, which are unusually abundant in histones.

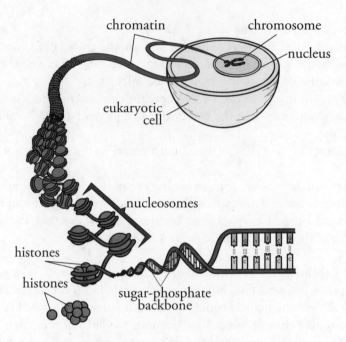

Figure 4 DNA Packaging

The **karyotype** is a display of an organism's genome (see Figure 5). A cell is frozen during metaphase, its chromosomes are stained, and a photograph is taken. The micrograph is enlarged, and each chromosome is cut out of the picture with an artist's blade. Then all homologues are paired, and the entire genome is examined for abnormalities.

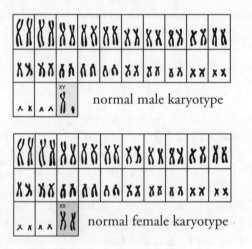

Figure 5 A Genetic Karyotype

The following flow equation summarizes the structure of DNA in the nucleus: **deoxyribose** → *add base* → **nucleoside** → *add three phosphates* → **nucleotide** → *polymerize with loss of two phosphates* → **oligo-nucleotide** → *continue polymerization* → **single-stranded polynucleotide** → *two complete chains H-bond in antiparallel orientation* → **ds DNA chain** → *coiling occurs* → **ds helix** → *wrap around histones* → **nucleosomes** → *complete packaging* → **chromatin**. Remember, each individual double-stranded piece of chromatin is condensed into a chromosome during mitosis and meiosis (see Chapters 5 and 6).

The Role of DNA

DNA encodes and transmits the genetic information passed down from parents to offspring. Before 1944 it was generally believed that protein, rather than DNA, carried genetic information, since proteins have an "alphabet" of 20 letters (the amino acids), while DNA's "alphabet" has only 4 letters (the four nucleotides). But in that year, Avery, McCarty, and MacLeod showed that DNA was the active agent in bacterial transformation. In short, this means they proved that pure DNA from one type of *E. coli* bacteria could transform *E. coli* of another type, causing it to acquire the genetic nature of the first type. Later, Hershey and Chase proved that DNA was the active chemical in the infection of *E. coli* bacteria by bacteriophage T2.

4.2   DNA REPLICATION

The DNA genome is the control center of the cell. When mitosis produces two identical daughter cells from one parental cell, each daughter must have the same genome as the parent. Hence, cell division requires duplication of the DNA, known as **replication**. This is an enzymatic process, just as the Krebs cycle and glycolysis are enzymatic processes. It occurs during **S** (synthesis) **phase** in interphase of the cell cycle (Chapter 5). But before we get bogged down with details, let's look at the big picture.

There is only one logical way to make a new piece of DNA that is identical to the old one: copy it. The old DNA is called **parental** DNA, and the new is called **daughter** DNA. The way it works is that the individual strands of the double-stranded parent are pulled apart. Then a new daughter strand is synthesized using the parental DNA as a template to copy from.[10] [Each new daughter chain is perfectly ___[11] to its template or parent.] After replication, one strand of the new double helix is parental (old), and one strand is newly synthesized daughter DNA, making DNA replication **semiconservative**.

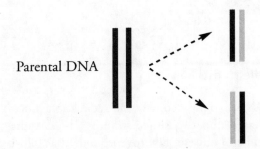

Parental DNA

Figure 6   Semiconservative Replication

---

[10]   A template is something that is copied. The metal plates used in printing presses are an example.

[11]   complementary

Steps of DNA Replication

Now we'll look at replication at the molecular level. Daughter DNA is created as a growing polymer. The enzyme that catalyzes the elongation of the daughter strand using the parental template is called **DNA polymerase** (**DNA pol**). DNA polymerase checks each new nucleotide to make sure it forms a correct base-pair before it is incorporated in the growing polymer. Here are some important replication rules you should know:

1. **Polymerization occurs in the 5' to 3' direction, without exception.**
   This means the existing chain is always lengthened by the addition of a nucleotide to the 3' end of the chain. [The template strand is read in what direction?[12]]

2. **DNA pol requires a *template*.**
   It cannot make a DNA chain from scratch but must copy an old chain. This makes sense because it would be pretty useless if DNA pol just made a strand of DNA randomly, without copying a template.

3. **DNA pol requires a *primer*.**
   It cannot start a DNA chain but can only add nucleotides to an existing chain. If DNA pol is responsible for making new daughter DNA by copying parental DNA, but is incapable of synthesizing DNA without a primer, where does the primer come from? A special RNA polymerase called **primase** begins DNA replication by creating a small RNA primer that DNA pol can elongate by adding deoxyribonucleotides to the existing ribonucleotide primer. The RNA primer is later replaced by DNA.

Can DNA polymerase make the following partially double-stranded structure completely double stranded in the presence of excess nucleotides, using the top strand as a primer?[13]

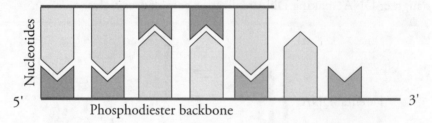

When it is not being replicated, DNA is tightly coiled. The replication process cannot begin unless the double helix is uncoiled and separated into two single strands. The enzyme that unwinds the double helix and separates the strands is called **helicase**. Hydrogen bonds that join base pairs rupture, and the molecule's two strands are separated. The two deoxyribose-phosphate strands do not fully separate before daughter strands begin to form. Rather, they partially diverge at what is called a replication bubble, which has two **replication forks**. [Would you expect helicase to use the energy of ATP hydrolysis to do its job?[14]] The place where the helicase begins to unwind is not random. It is a specific location on the chromosome called the **origin of replication** (or ORI). When helicase unwinds the helix at the origin, the helix gets wound more tightly upstream and downstream from this point.[15] The chromosome would

---

[12] If the daughter is made 5' to 3', and the two strands have to end up antiparallel, *the template must be read 3' to 5'.*

[13] No. The DNA strands are antiparallel, meaning that the upper strand would have to be extended in a 3' to 5' direction, which is impossible. Note that the phrase "in the presence of excess nucleotides" is extraneous. It just means there are plenty of building blocks around; typical DAT smokescreen.

[14] Yes. Separating the strands requires the breaking of many H-bonds.

[15] This is similar to what would happen if you had two long ropes wound around each other. If you pulled them apart in the middle, the ends of the rope would have to wind more tightly.

get tangled and eventually break except that enzymes called **topoisomerases** cut one or both of the strands and unwrap the helix, releasing the excess tension created by the helicases. Note that this is just the opposite of what DNA gyrase does; in fact, gyrase is considered a type of topoisomerase. Another potential problem is that single-stranded DNA is much less stable than ds-DNA. **Single-strand binding proteins** (or SSBPs) protect DNA which has been unpackaged in preparation for replication and help keep the strands separated. Replication may now begin.

The first step is the synthesis of an RNA primer on each template strand. Then DNA pol elongates the primer by adding dNTPs to its 3' end. Rapid elongation of the daughter strands follows. Since the two template strands are antiparallel, the two primers will elongate toward opposite ends of the chromosome. Replication proceeds along in both directions away from the origin. Both template strands are read 3' to 5' while daughter strands are elongated 5' to 3'.

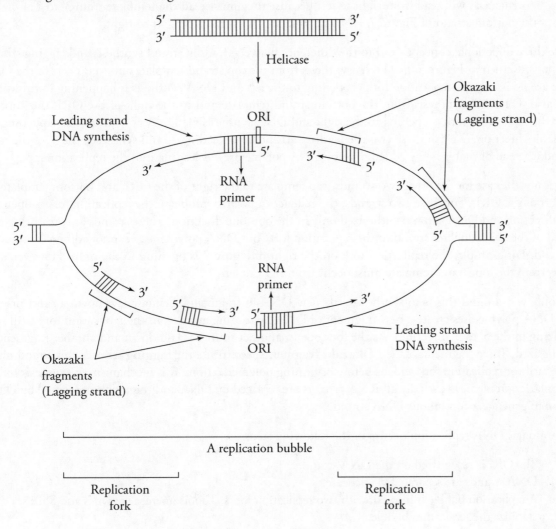

Figure 7 DNA Replication

The Polarity Problem and Its Solution

There are three directional concepts to keep in mind when going through DNA replication:

1. Recall that a DNA molecule's two deoxyribose-phosphate strands lie in antiparallel orientation. As depicted in Figure 7, the top strand runs in the 5' to 3' direction from left to right, and the bottom strand runs in the 5' to 3' direction from right to left; this is the convention when drawing double-stranded DNA.
2. Replication forks at either end of the replication bubble open in opposite directions; the fork on the left will continue opening to the left and the fork on the right will continue opening to the right.
3. DNA polymerases synthesize DNA in one direction only: 5' to 3'. A newly growing nucleotide chain does NOT take on new nucleotide units at its 5' end; DNA polymerases will add nucleotide units only to the 3' end of the growing chain. On the top strand in Figure 7, DNA polymerases will read from right to left because they must read the template from 3' to 5'. On the bottom strand of Figure 7, DNA polymerases will read from left to right.

These three directional concepts lead to the difference between leading strand synthesis and lagging strand synthesis. Return to Figure 7: For DNA synthesis from the top strand template and to the left of the ORI, there are no issues; the replication fork is opening to the left and DNA synthesis is happening in this direction also. For DNA synthesis from the bottom strand template and to the right of the ORI, the same is true; the replication fork is opening to the right and DNA synthesis via DNA polymerases is happening in the same direction. We call these two the **leading strands**. For leading strand synthesis, the 3' of the new strand (the end of that is being added onto by DNA polymerases) is leading into the replication fork.

This is not the case for the other two strands (top template to the right of the ORI, and bottom template to the left of the ORI). For these two strands, the cell faces a polarity problem: the replication fork is opening one direction and DNA can be synthesized only in the opposite direction. These strands are presenting the 5' end of the new daughter strand to the replication fork, but DNA polymerases cannot add nucleotides to this end. For example, the replication fork on the right of Figure 7 is opening to the right. However, synthesis from the top strand template must occur from right to left.

The only way around this is to synthesize the new DNA in fragments. Primase lays down a short primer and DNA polymerases create a new fragment of DNA by reading away from the replication fork (still synthesizing in the 5' to 3' direction). As the fork opens, another primer is laid down and another fragment is synthesized. These fragments, called **Okazaki fragments**, constitute the **lagging strand**; this strand must wait until the replication fork widens before beginning polymerization. This mechanism of synthesis solves the polarity problem. Eventually all RNA primers are replaced by DNA and fragments are joined by **DNA ligase** to generate a continuous DNA strand.

In summary, DNA replication occurs in the following steps:

1. The ORI is recognized on the DNA strand.
2. DNA strands are separated via helicase.
3. A replication bubble is formed, with two replication forks. Topoisomerase enzymes and SSBPs stabilize the replication bubble.
4. RNA primers are laid down by primase, an RNA polymerase.
5. DNA polymerases read the template strand (in the 3' to 5' direction) and synthesize a new complementary strand (in the 5' to 3' direction). This can occur in a continuous way (as in the leading strand) or discontinuously (as in the lagging strand). Replication forks grow away from the origin in both directions. Each replication fork contains a leading strand and a lagging strand. Each replication bubble contains two leading strands and two lagging strands.
6. The leading strand and Okazaki fragments of the lagging strand are joined by DNA ligase.
7. RNA primers are removed and replaced with DNA (this is done by DNA polymerases).

Eukaryotic vs. Prokaryotic Replication

In eukaryotic replication, each linear chromosome has several origins. This is necessary because eukaryotic chromosomes are so huge that replicating them from a single origin would be too slow. As the many replication forks continue to widen, they create an appearance of bubbles along the DNA strand, so they are referred to as "**replication bubbles**." Eventually the replication forks meet, and the many daughter strands are ligated together (Figure 8).

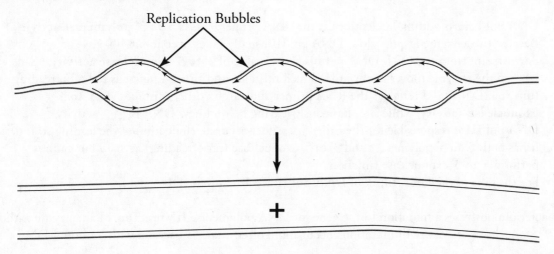

Figure 8   Eukaryotic Replication

Prokaryotes have only one chromosome, and this one chromosome has only one origin. Because the chromosome is circular, as replication proceeds the partially duplicated genome begins to look like the Greek letter θ (theta). Hence the replication of prokaryotes is said to proceed by the **theta mechanism** and is referred to as **theta replication** (see Figure 9).

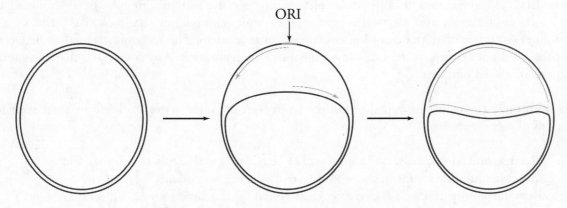

Figure 9   Theta (θ) Replication in Prokaryotes

DNA Polymerase

Eukaryotes have several different DNA polymerase enzymes, and their mechanisms of action are complex. You do not need to worry about this complexity for the DAT.

Prokaryotes on the other hand have at least three types of DNA polymerase. They are called DNA polymerase I, II, and III. You should know the basic purpose of each one:

- **DNA pol I** starts adding nucleotides at the RNA primer; this is **5' to 3' polymerase activity**. Because this enzyme is quite slow, DNA pol III usually takes over about 400 base pairs downstream from the ORI. DNA pol I is also capable of **3' to 5' exonuclease activity**.[16] This is when the enzyme moves backwards to fix a mistake, and this is known as the proofreading function. DNA pol I removes the RNA primer and can fix other mistakes via **5' to 3' exonuclease activity**, while simultaneously leaving behind new DNA in ___ activity.[17]
- **DNA pol III** is responsible for the super-fast, super-accurate elongation of the leading strand. It has both 5' to 3' polymerase and 3' to 5' exonuclease (proofreading) activity but cannot perform 5' to 3' exonuclease function.
- For the sake of the DAT, think of **DNA pol II** as a backup for DNA pol III.

[If a bacterium possesses a mutation in the gene for DNA polymerase III, resulting in an enzyme without 3' to 5' exonuclease activity, will mutations occur more often than in bacteria with a normal DNA polymerase gene?[18]]

Genetic Mutation

Genetic mutation refers to any alteration of the DNA sequence of an organism's genome. The causes of mutation include mistakes in replication of the genome during cell division, chance chemical malformations (such as spontaneous deamination, which means loss of a nitrogen group), and environmental agents such as chemicals and ultraviolet light. For example, compounds that look like purines and pyrimidines (with large flat aromatic ring structures) cause mutations by inserting themselves between base pairs, or **intercalating**, thereby causing errors in DNA replication. Any compound that can cause mutations is called a **mutagen**.

Point mutations are single base pair substitutions (A in place of G, for example). There are three subclassifications of point mutations:

1. **missense mutations**: cause one amino acid to be replaced with a different amino acid
2. **nonsense mutations**: cause a stop codon to replace a regular codon
3. **silent mutations**: change a codon into a new codon for the same amino acid (no change in protein amino acid sequence)

---

[16] Exonuclease means "cutting a nucleic acid chain at the end." An endonuclease will cut a polynucleotide acid chain in the middle of the chain, usually at a particular sequence. Two important types of endonucleases are repair enzymes that remove chemically damaged DNA from the chain, and restriction enzymes, which are endonucleases found in bacteria. Their role is to destroy the DNA of infecting viruses, thus restricting the host range of the virus.

[17] 5' to 3' polymerase; remember, all polymerization is 5' to 3'.

[18] Yes. 3' to 5' exonuclease activity is the polymerase's way of editing its work. Without this editing function, many more point mutations would occur due to the incorporation of wrong nucleotides. The normal polymerase is remarkably adept at sensing correct base pairing and removing bases that don't belong.

If a missense mutation leads to little change in the structure and function of the gene product (protein), it is referred to as a **conservative mutation**.

There are five kinds of gene rearrangement mutations. **Insertion** refers to the addition of one or more extra nucleotides into the DNA sequence. **Deletion** is the removal of nucleotides from the sequence. Both of these mutations can cause a shift in the **reading frame**. For example, AAACCCACC can be read as AAA, CCC, ACC. It would code for Lys-Pro-Thr. Inserting an extra G into the first codon could produce this: AGAACCCACC. This would be read AGA, ACC, CAC, C. It now codes for Arg-Thr-His (plus there's an extra C). Not only has the first codon changed; the whole piece of DNA will be read differently. Mutations causing a change in the reading frame are called **frameshift mutations**. Generally speaking, frameshift mutations are very serious. Note that a frameshift can lead to premature termination of translation (yielding an incomplete polypeptide) if it results in the presence of an abnormal stop codon. [Are all insertions and deletions frameshift mutations?[19] If the following oligonucleotide is mutated by inserting a G between the fifth and sixth codons, what effect will this have on the oligopeptide it encodes: AUG AAG GGG CCC UUU AAA UGA CCC?[20] For each type of mutation, does it involve a change in the genotype, the phenotype, or both?[21]]

- Sickle-cell anemia is a genetic disease caused by alteration of a single amino acid in the hemoglobin polypeptide. Which one of the following could cause such a mutation?[22]
  - A. An error in the translation of hemoglobin
  - B. Insertion of a single nucleotide into the DNA sequence of the gene encoding hemoglobin
  - C. A frameshift mutation
  - D. Alteration of a purine to a pyrimidine base
  - E. Deletion of three nucleotides from the DNA sequence of the gene encoding hemoglobin

---

[19] No. If you insert or delete one whole codon or several whole codons, you add or remove amino acids to the polypeptide without changing the reading frame.

[20] The original RNA codes for Met-Lys-Gly-Pro-Phe-Lys. After the insertion, the oligonucleotide will code for Met-Lys-Gly-Pro-Phe-Glu-Met-Thr. Note this contains different amino acids and is longer. The extra length is due to the fact that a stop codon, UGA, was changed to an amino acid by the frameshift.

[21] By definition, all mutations involve a change in the genotype. Most mutations also cause a change in the phenotype, but in the case of conservative mutations it is a very subtle change that would be hard to detect.

[22] Alteration of a purine to a pyrimidine base is described in the text as a transversion mutation, which is classified as a point mutation. Point mutations could result in a single amino acid change (choice **D** is correct). An error in translation would temporarily result in defective hemoglobin, but the defect would not be genetic (it wouldn't be passed from parents to offspring; A is wrong). Insertion of a single nucleotide into the DNA sequence would cause a frameshift mutation. Frameshift mutations lead to massive changes in amino acid sequence and protein structure, since every codon after the mutation is changed. This could not produce the single amino acid change described in the question (choices B and C are wrong). Deletion of three nucleotides would remove one entire codon from the sequence, and thus one entire amino acid from the protein, it would not alter an amino acid (choice E is wrong).

In addition to insertions and deletions (sometimes called "indels"), there are three other types of gene rearrangement mutations:

Mutation	Definition	Example
Inversion	Chromosome section is flipped	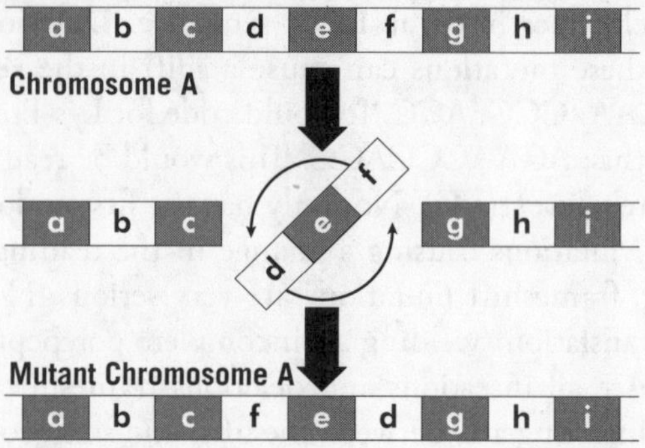
Amplification or Duplication	Chromosome section is duplicated	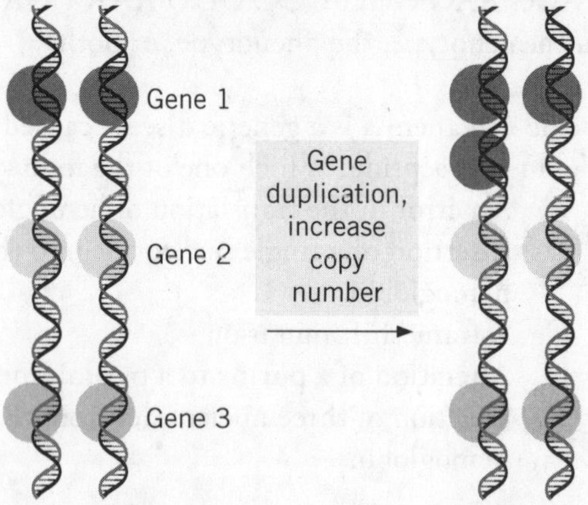
Translocation	Chromosome segment is swapped with another (nonhomologous) chromosome	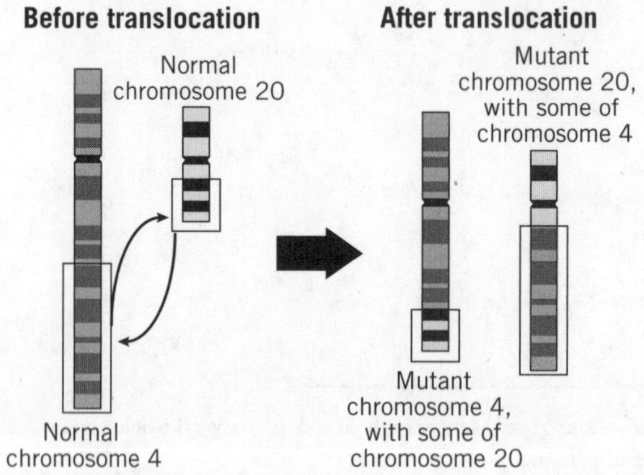

Table 1 Gene Rearrangement Mutations

4.3 TRANSCRIPTION: FROM DNA TO RNA

RNA Versus DNA

Chromosomes serve their critical function within the cell (and the organism) by mediating the synthesis of **ribonucleic acid (RNA)**. Both DNA and RNA are nucleic acids, polymers composed of nucleotide monomers. However, there are some differences between them:

Characteristic	DNA	RNA
Sugar in the backbone	Deoxyribose (no OH on the 2' carbon of ribose)	Ribose (has an OH on the 2' carbon of ribose)
Pyrimidines	Cytosine and thymine	Cytosine and uracil
Strandedness	Usually double-stranded (except in some viruses)	Usually single-stranded
Stability	More stable	Less stable
Lifespan in the cell	Permanent	Transient

Table 2 DNA vs. RNA

RNA, therefore, is a nucleic acid composed of a sugar-phosphate backbone in which the sugar component is ribose. Bound to each ribose unit of the backbone is one of the four nitrogenous bases:

1. adenine (A)   —a purine
2. cytosine (C)   —a pyrimidine
3. guanine (G)   —a purine
4. uracil (U)   —a pyrimidine

There are three common forms of RNA, each differing from the other in their function(s). Beyond the three well-recognized types, there are additional forms of RNA that serve enzymatic roles. The three predominant types of RNA are:

1. ribosomal RNA (rRNA)
2. transfer RNA (tRNA)
3. messenger RNA (mRNA)

[Why is the stability of RNA relatively unimportant?[23]]

---

[23] This is because a cell's DNA is necessary for the cell's entire life. RNA is a transient molecule which is transcribed, translated, and destroyed. As a matter of fact, the reason RNA contains uracil also has to do with the reduced need for fidelity in transcription as compared to replication. Without getting into the details, thymine is easier for DNA repair systems to work with, while uracil is much less energy-costly to make. So RNA has uracil, DNA has thymine.

Messenger RNA (mRNA) is the molecule that *carries genetic information from the nucleus to the cytoplasm* where it can be translated into protein. Each unique polypeptide is created according to the sequence of codons on a particular piece of mRNA, which was transcribed from a particular gene. Eukaryotic mRNA is **monocistronic** and obeys the "one gene, one protein" principle; this means that each piece of mRNA encodes one and only one polypeptide. Hence, *there are as many different mRNAs as there are proteins.* Messenger RNA is constantly produced and degraded, according to the cell's need for the protein encoded by each piece of mRNA; in fact, this is the principal means whereby cells regulate the amount of each particular protein they synthesize; this is an important point which will be emphasized later. Note that prokaryotic mRNA often codes for *more* than one polypeptide and is termed **polycistronic**. The different genes on the same polycistronic mRNA are generally related in function.[24]

There are only a few different types of **ribosomal RNA** (rRNA). They all have the same function: they serve as components of the ribosome, along with many polypeptide chains. rRNAs provide catalytic function of the ribosome. Take note: this is a little odd. In general, cellular machines (enzymes) are made only from polypeptides.

The last type of RNA is **transfer RNA** (tRNA); tRNA is responsible for translating the genetic code. Transfer RNA carries amino acids from the cytoplasm to the ribosome to be added to a growing protein.

The Genetic Code

DNA does not directly exert its influence on cells, but merely contains sequences of nucleotides known as **genes** that serve as **templates** for the production of another nucleic acid known as RNA. The process of reading DNA and writing the information as RNA is termed **transcription**. The RNA serves as a messenger from the nucleus to the cytoplasm. In the cytoplasm, the RNA is read, and the information is written down as protein. The production of proteins from RNA is termed **translation**.[25]

The overall process looks like this: DNA → RNA → protein. This unidirectional flow equation represents the **Central Dogma** (fundamental law) of molecular biology. This is the mechanism whereby inherited *information* is used to create actual *objects*, namely enzymes and structural proteins. An exception to the Central Dogma is that certain viruses (retroviruses) make DNA from RNA using the enzyme reverse transcriptase. Here we will examine the language DNA uses to orchestrate protein synthesis. The process goes like this:

1. Information contained in DNA is copied into a messenger, **messenger RNA (mRNA)**.
2. The mRNA travels to the cytoplasm, where it encounters the **ribosome** and other components of protein synthesis. The ribosome is a massive enzyme composed of many proteins and pieces of RNA (known as **ribosomal RNA** or **rRNA**).
3. The ribosome synthesizes polypeptides according to the DNA's original orders.

---

[24] For instance, if five enzymes are necessary for the synthesis of a particular molecule, then all five enzymes might be encoded on a single piece of mRNA.

[25] To *transcribe* a letter is to listen to spoken words and write them down as printed text. The message doesn't change, and the language, English, doesn't change. To *translate* a letter is to change it from one language to another. Cellular transcription is the process whereby a code is read from a nucleic acid (DNA) and written in the language of another nucleic acid (RNA), so the language is the same. In cellular translation, nucleic acids are read and polypeptides are written, so here the language does change.

The language used by DNA and mRNA to specify the building blocks of proteins is the **Genetic Code**. The alphabet of the genetic code contains only four letters (A, T, G, C). How can four letters specify the ingredients of the multitude of proteins in every cell? [What is the smallest "word" size that would allow this four-letter alphabet to encode 20 different amino acids?[26]] A number of experiments confirmed that the genetic code is written in three-letter words, each of which codes for a particular amino acid. A nucleic acid word (3 nucleotide letters) is referred to as a **codon**.

The genetic code is shown in Figure 10. The first nucleotide in a codon is given at the left, the second on top, and the third on the right. At the intersection of these three nucleotides is the amino acid called for by that codon. [Why is uracil (U) shown in the chart, and why is thymine (T) absent?[27] The codon GTG in DNA is transcribed in RNA as ___, which the ribosome translates into what amino acid?[28]]

1st Position (5' End)	2nd Position				3rd Position (3' End)
	U	**C**	**A**	**G**	
U	Phe	Ser	Tyr	Cys	U
	Phe	Ser	Tyr	Cys	C
	Leu	Ser	**Stop**	**Stop**	A
	Leu	Ser	**Stop**	Trp	G
C	Leu	Pro	His	Arg	U
	Leu	Pro	His	Arg	C
	Leu	Pro	Gln	Arg	A
	Leu	Pro	Gln	Arg	G
A	Ile	Thr	Asn	Ser	U
	Ile	Thr	Asn	Ser	C
	Ile	Thr	Lys	Arg	A
	Met	Thr	Lys	Arg	G
G	Val	Ala	Asp	Gly	U
	Val	Ala	Asp	Gly	C
	Val	Ala	Glu	Gly	A
	Val	Ala	Glu	Gly	G

Figure 10 The Genetic Code

There are 64 codons. Sixty-one of them specify amino acids; the remaining three are called **stop codons**. Their function is to notify the ribosome that the protein is complete and cause it to stop reading the mRNA. Stop codons are also called **nonsense codons**, since they don't code for any amino acid. Note that most of the 20 amino acids can be coded for by more than one codon. Often, all four of the codons

---

[26] With four nucleotides, if a "word" (codon) is two nucleotides long, there are 4^2 = 16 possible codons; too few to specify 20 unique amino acids. However, there are 4^3 = 64 possible 3-letter "words," and 64 is more than enough different codons to specify 20 unique amino acids. Thus, three nucleotides is the minimum codon size.

[27] RNA is the nucleic acid that actually encodes protein during translation. RNA has U instead of T.

[28] The RNA codon transcribed from the DNA will be CAC, coding for histidine.

with the same first two nucleotides (e.g., CU_) encode the same amino acid. [If the last nucleotide in the codon CUU is changed in a gene that codes for a protein, will the protein be affected?[29]] Two or more co-dons coding for the same amino acid are known as synonyms. Because it has such synonyms, the genetic code is said to be degenerate. However, it is very important to realize that though an amino acid may be specified by several codons, each codon specifies only a single amino acid. This means that each piece of DNA can be interpreted only one way: the code has no **ambiguity**.

While you do need to be able to read and interpret the genetic code for the DAT, you do not need to memorize the whole thing. You should know the start codon and the three stop codons only.

Steps of Transcription

In the synthesis of any of the three types of RNA, DNA serves as a template, and the process is termed **transcription**. Transcription is similar (but not identical) to DNA replication. Both DNA replication and transcription begin with separating the DNA molecule's two strands. In DNA replication, *both* strands serve as templates for the synthesis of a new DNA strand. In transcription, *one* of the strands serves as a template for the synthesis of an RNA molecule. The same base-pairing rules apply to DNA replication and transcription, except in DNA replication thymine is used, and in transcription, uracil is used. For example, if some portion of a DNA template carries the nucleotide sequence:

$$(5') - \quad T \quad G \quad A \quad C \quad A \quad - (3')$$

then the complementary sequence of the newly formed RNA molecule would be:

$$(3') - \quad A \quad C \quad U \quad G \quad U \quad - (5')$$

or, expressed in conventional 5' to 3' direction:

$$(5') - \quad U \quad G \quad U \quad C \quad A \quad - (3')$$

Because RNA is a single-stranded molecule, it results from the reading of only one DNA strand; between the two strands of DNA, only one serves as a template for RNA synthesis. The other one is complementary to the template, just like the RNA will be complementary to the template. Because of this, the DNA strands are given names: the one that serves as a template and is actually read and transcribed is called the template, the **non-coding strand** or the **anti-sense strand**. The other strand that does *not* serve as template is called the **coding strand** or **sense strand**. This is because RNA and the coding strand are both complementary to the template, and thus have the same sequence or code as each other (except for the T/U switch of course).

Recall that DNA polymerases generated the new daughter strands in DNA replication. In transcription, formation of an RNA polymer is catalyzed by enzymes called **RNA polymerases**. These two enzymes are similar in their mechanism of action; both DNA polymerases and RNA polymerases add nucleotides to the 3' end of the growing chain. Therefore, the template DNA is read in the 3' to 5' direction and the new nucleic acid molecule is synthesized in the 5' to 3' direction. Another important difference between transcription and DNA replication is that RNA polymerase has not been shown to possess the ability to remove mismatched nucleotides (it lacks exonuclease activity); in other words, it cannot correct its errors. Thus, transcription is a lower fidelity process than replication.

---

[29] No, since CUN codes for leucine, regardless of what N is. Notice that switching the 3rd nucleotide in the majority of codons will have no effect.

- Because both replication and transcription involve template-driven polymerization, the RNA transcript produced in transcription is ___[30] to the DNA template, just as the daughter strand produced in replication was.
- Transcription, like replication, can occur only in the ___[31] direction.
- Do the polymerase enzymes in both replication and transcription require a primer?[32]

Transcription occurs in three steps:

1. initiation
2. elongation
3. termination

During **initiation,** RNA polymerase binds the DNA template at a region called the **promoter.** The promoter is a particular sequence of DNA; it determines which DNA strand is the template, where transcription starts, and the direction of transcription. One common example of a promoter is called a **TATA box.** Next, RNA polymerase unwinds the template strand (there is no need for helicase here) and starts reading it in the 3' to 5' direction. Once it reaches a region called the **start site,** RNA polymerase starts creating an RNA transcript by reading the template DNA.

- DNA replication starts at the ___; transcription starts at ___ but RNA pol binds at ___.[33]

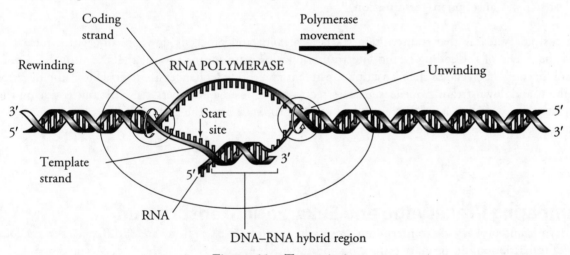

Figure 11   Transcription

It is customary to say that transcription starts at a point and proceeds **downstream,** which means toward the 3' end of the coding strand and transcript. **Upstream** means toward the 5' end of the coding strand, beyond the 5' end of the transcript. Upstream nucleotide sequences are referred to with negative numbers, and downstream sequences are referred to with positive numbers. The first nucleotide that is actually transcribed is given the number +1.

---

[30]   complementary

[31]   5' to 3'

[32]   No, RNA pol does not require a primer. Remember, the primer in replication is a piece of RNA, made by an RNA polymerase.

[33]   ORI, start site, promoter

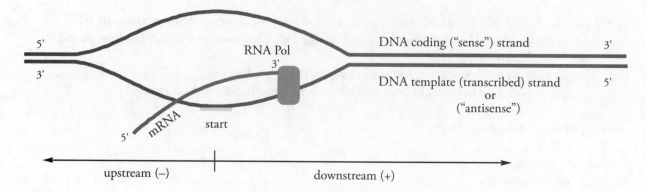

Figure 12 Reference Points in Transcription

During **elongation,** RNA polymerase builds RNA by adding nucleotides onto the 3' end of the new molecule, as in DNA replication. RNA polymerase catalyzes the creation of a phosphodiester bond between the 5' end of the one nucleotide and the 3' end of the next, releasing pyrophosphate (PP₁). RNA polymerase moves along the template, adding additional nucleotides to the growing chain of RNA. This continues until the enzyme reaches a sequence called the **terminator,** or **termination signal.** Here, RNA polymerase and the newly synthesized RNA transcript dissociate, and transcription is complete. This is the last step of transcription, **termination.**

It is customary to say that transcription starts at a point and proceeds downstream, which means toward the 3' end of the coding strand and transcript. Upstream means toward the 5' end of the coding strand, beyond the 5' end of the transcript. Upstream nucleotide sequences are referred to using negative numbers, and downstream sequences are referred to using positive numbers. The first nucleotide on the template strand which is actually transcribed is called the start site. The corresponding nucleotide on the coding strand is given the number +1.

Comparing Prokaryotic and Eukaryotic Transcription

Eukaryotic and prokaryotic transcription are similar, but you need to be aware of differences in the location of transcription, the primary transcript, and the mRNA.

Eukaryotic means "true-kerneled." Prokaryotic means "before-the-kernel." The **karyon** (kernel) is the nucleus. The fact that prokaryotes have no nucleus means transcription occurs freely in the cytoplasm, in the same compartment where translation occurs, and transcription and translation can occur *simultaneously.* Eukaryotes must transcribe their mRNA in the nucleus, modify it, then transport it across the nuclear membrane to the cytoplasm where it can be translated. Transcription and translation in eukaryotes *does not* occur simultaneously.

An important difference between prokaryotic and eukaryotic gene expression is that the primary transcript in prokaryotes is mRNA. In other words, the product of transcription by prokaryotic RNA polymerase is ready to be translated. In fact, translation of prokaryotic mRNA begins before transcription is completed!

In contrast, the eukaryotic primary transcript is modified extensively before translation. Immature RNA made in the nucleus (called heterogeneous nuclear RNA or hnRNA) must be spliced, stabilized by a cap and tail, and exported to the cytoplasm before it is considered mature mRNA (Figure 13). Let's talk about **splicing** first. Eukaryotic DNA has non-coding sequences intervening between the segments that actually code for proteins. Sometimes these intervening sequences contain enhancers or other regulatory sequences. As a result, eukaryotic mRNA is made with sequences intervening between those that actually code for proteins. The _int_ervening sequences in the RNA are called **introns**. Protein-coding regions of the RNA are termed _ex_ons because they actually get _ex_pressed. Before the RNA can be translated, introns must be removed and exons joined together; this process is called splicing and is mediated by the **spliceo-some**, a large ribonucleoprotein (RNP) complex.

The other example of the modification of eukaryotic RNA before translation is the addition of two tags to the mRNA which "customize" and stabilize it. The tags are called the **5' cap** and the **3' poly-A tail**. The 5' cap is a methylated guanine nucleotide stuck on the 5' end [which is the end made ___ (first or last?)[34]]. The poly-A tail is a string of several hundred adenine nucleotides. The cap is essential for translation, while both the cap and the poly-A tail are important in preventing digestion of the mRNA by exonucleases that are free in the cell. Finally, the eukaryotic transcript is exported to the cytoplasm where it can interact with a ribosome and act as a template for protein synthesis.

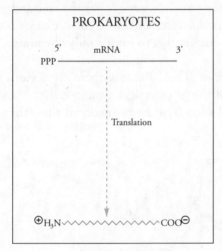 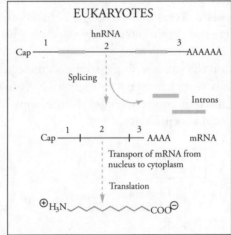

Figure 13 Prokaryotic vs. Eukaryotic Gene Expression

4.4   TRANSLATION: FROM RNA TO PROTEIN

Generally speaking, translation is a process in which mRNA issues orders that are read by a ribosome and carried out by molecules of tRNA coupled to amino acids. Translation is generally a process in which:

1.   The ribosome recognizes some portion of an mRNA molecule and binds it.
2.   The ribosome reads the mRNA molecule, three nucleotides at a time (these three nucleotides are called a **codon**).

---

[34] It is made first, since transcription proceeds from 5' to 3'.

3. When read by the ribosome, each codon on the mRNA orders that some particular amino acid be brought to the ribosome.
4. Molecules of tRNA within the cytosol bring amino acids to the ribosome, as instructed by mRNA.
5. Amino acids brought to the ribosome, one by one, in a sequence ordered by the mRNA molecule, are connected via peptide bonds to form a polypeptide.

Ribosome, tRNA, and Amino Acid Activation

Because translation involves ribosomes and tRNA, we first look at the nature of these complexes, and then at the thermodynamics tied to the bonding of tRNA with amino acid, a process called amino acid activation.

A prokaryotic ribosome contains two subunits, a large one and a small one, called the **50S** and **30S** subunits, respectively. The total ribosome is **70S**. In eukaryotes, the small subunit is **40S**, the large subunit is **60S**, and the total ribosome is **80S**. The "S" represents the unit "Svedberg" and denotes sedimentation rate; a higher value indicates a higher sedimentation rate and larger mass.[35] Each subunit is a complex of rRNA and proteins. The ribosome also features three tRNA binding sites called the **A site** (or aminoacyl-tRNA site), the **P site** (or peptidyl-tRNA site), and the **E site** (or exit-tRNA site). [During translation, the next codon to be translated is exposed in the ___.[36]] In both prokaryotes and eukaryotes, many ribosomes synthesizing the same protein simultaneously associate with one another to form a **polyribosome**.

Transfer RNA, or tRNA, is a single-stranded molecule of RNA. Because there are regions where the tRNA molecule is complementary to itself, tRNAs fold into a cloverleaf structure that is composed of stems (areas of internal complementarity) and loops. tRNAs have two functional sites, the **anticodon** and the **amino acid acceptor site**.

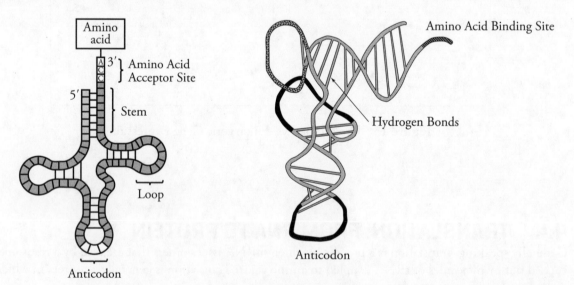

Figure 14 Cloverleaf (Two-Dimensional) Structure of tRNA

Figure 15 Three-Dimensional Structure of tRNA

---

[35] If you noticed that 50S + 30S ≠ 70S, you are correct, but it's not an error. Sedimentation rates are not arithmetically additive.

[36] The A site, since this is where the next amino acid to be added must bind.

The tRNA anticodon is a sequence of three nucleotides. Since the anticodon is three nucleotides in length and since there are four nucleotide options for each site (A, C, G, or U), there are 64 different anticodons (this comes from $4 \times 4 \times 4$). Like any set of nucleotides, those of the tRNA anticodon have complements according to the base-pairing rules described in earlier sections. The anticodon on tRNA is complementary to the codon on the mRNA transcript.

The tRNA molecule's amino acid acceptor site is a site at which the molecule binds (accepts) an amino acid. A given tRNA molecule with its particular anticodon has a binding site for one particular amino acid. However, since there are 64 anticodons and only 20 amino acids, there might be more than one tRNA molecule specific to a given amino acid. For example, the anticodon (3') - C G G - (5') is specific to alanine; it binds alanine and only alanine. On the other hand, the anticodons (3') - C G A - (5'), (3') - C G U - (5'), and (3') - C G C - (5') are also specific to alanine. They, too, bind alanine and only alanine.

The amino acid acceptor site of any tRNA molecule is the same as that of any other, which raises this question: on what basis does tRNA recognize the amino acid to which it is specific? For each amino acid, there exists (at least) one enzyme called an **aminoacyl-tRNA synthetase**. The synthetase enzyme recognizes both the tRNA carrier and the amino acid to which it is specific. Recognition between tRNA and amino acid, therefore, is mediated not by tRNA, but by the relevant aminoacyl-tRNA synthetase.

The binding of an amino acid to its tRNA to produce the corresponding aminoacyl-tRNA is called **amino acid activation**. The word "activation" comes from the thermodynamics of this process. The reaction in which an amino acid is bound to its tRNA is endergonic (meaning ΔG is positive). It involves the cleavage of two high-energy phosphate bonds (ATP $\rightarrow$ AMP + 2P$_i$), and the reaction looks like this:

$$\text{Amino Acid} + \text{ATP} + \text{tRNA} \rightarrow \text{Aminoacyl-tRNA} + \text{AMP} + \text{PP}_i$$

Subsequent cleavage of the pyrophosphate (PP$_i$) by pyrophosphatase drives the equilibrium forcefully to the right. The ester linkage between the amino acid and the tRNA is a relatively high-energy bond, and for that reason, the amino acid is said to be activated; the energy stored within this bond is later used to drive peptide bond formation. Each tRNA can be named according to the amino acid it's specific for. For example, a tRNA for valine would be written tRNA$_{Val}$. When the amino acid is attached, the tRNA is written this way: Val-tRNA$_{Val}$.

The principal functions of tRNA are to bind amino acids, bring them to the ribosome, line them up according to an order dictated by the mRNA codons, and facilitate the formation of peptide bonds to form proteins. Transfer RNA, therefore, mediates the process of translation.

Steps of Translation

Like transcription, translation proceeds in three steps:

1. initiation
2. elongation
3. termination

During **initiation,** the small ribosomal subunit (30S in prokaryotes and 40S in eukaryotes) binds near the 5' end of an mRNA. It scans the transcript sequence until it finds the AUG **start codon**. Next, a tRNA molecule (with the anticodon UAC and bound to the amino acid methionine) interacts with the AUG codon on the mRNA. These three molecules together (small ribosomal subunit, Met-tRNA, and a molecule of mRNA) are called the initiation complex. Finally, the large ribosomal subunit (50S in prokaryotes and 60S in eukaryotes) is recruited. The first amino acid added will be the N-terminus of the peptide chain.

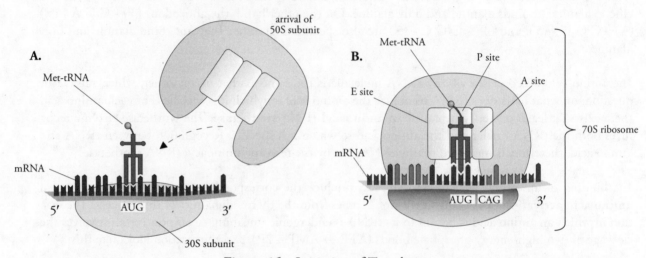

Figure 16 Initiation of Translation

During **elongation**, the ribosome reads the mRNA codons, tRNA molecules bearing appropriate anticodons bring amino acids to the ribosome, and peptide bonds form between the adjacent amino acids to form a polypeptide. The amino acid sequence of the polypeptide is dictated by the mRNA codons.

In more detailed terms, elongation involves this series of events:

1. An mRNA codon is exposed at the A site of the ribosome.
2. An aminoacyl-tRNA, whose anticodon is complementary to the codon, arrives at the A site and forms hydrogen bonds with the codon. This step requires the hydrolysis of one phosphate from GTP.
3. A peptide bond is formed between the two amino acids. The bond between the amino acid and the tRNA in the P site is broken.
4. The ribosome moves, or translocates, a distance of three nucleotides along the mRNA molecule in the 5' to 3' direction. Translocation moves the growing polypeptide anchored to a tRNA molecule to the P site of the ribosome, moves the old tRNA to the E site, and exposes the next mRNA codon at the A site. This step requires the hydrolysis of one GTP.

These steps repeat and the polypeptide chain grows, one amino acid at a time. The E site always contains a tRNA that has lost its amino acid to the growing peptide chain. This tRNA exits the ribosome and is recycled to the cytoplasm where it can be joined with another amino acid. The P site always contains a tRNA hydrogen bonded to the mRNA transcript, and this anchors the peptide chain to the ribosome.

The A site is always where the next aminoacyl-tRNA arrives.

Overall, it costs four high-energy phosphate bonds to add an amino acid. Two high energy bonds are required by aminoacyl-tRNA synthetase to join the tRNA with its amino acid, one phosphate bond is required to bring the aminoacyl-tRNA into the A site of the ribosome, and a final phosphate bond is required to translocate the ribosome so the next codon can be read. This means that for a cell to translate a short 250 amino acid peptide chain, it would require 1,000 molecules of ATP! Making proteins is highly expensive for the cell.

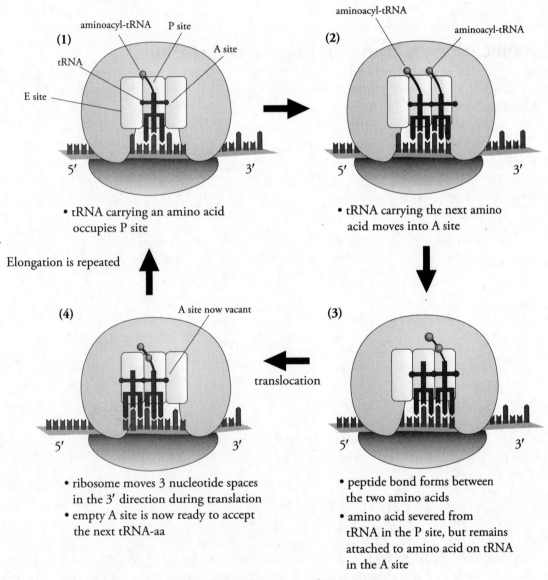

Figure 17 Elongation of Translation

The last amino acid added will be the C-terminus of the peptide chain. **Termination** occurs when a stop codon appears in the ribosomal A site. There are three stop codons (UAG, UGA, UAA), which can be remembered using the three phrases "You (U) Are Gone, U Go Away, U Are Away." Stop codons do not code for tRNA molecules. Rather, their arrival at the A site causes **release factors** (proteins) to stop the elongation process and to release the newly formed polypeptide from the ribosome. The ribosome dissociates into large and small subunits ready to begin the process of translation anew.

Not all of the mRNA transcript codes for a protein. The region of the transcript before the start codon is called the **5' untranslated region** (or 5' UTR). There is also some extra sequence on the other end of the RNA called the **3' untranslated region** (or 3' UTR). The 5' UTR contains upstream regulatory sequences that help with initiation; the 3' UTR contains downstream regulatory sequences that help with termination.

DNA Replication vs. Transcription vs. Translation

Now that we have covered all of molecular biology, let's review. Recall that transcription involved a small portion of DNA from promoter to terminator. The relationship between DNA, RNA, and a peptide chain might look like this:

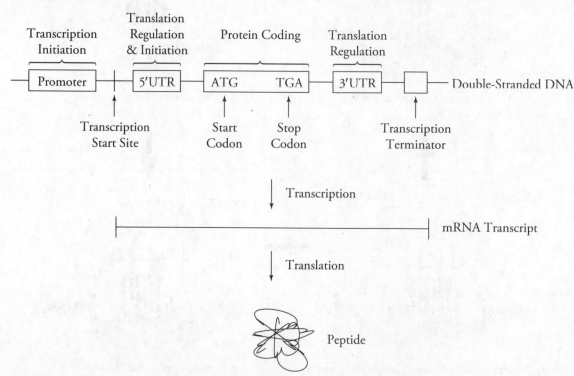

Figure 18   Central Dogma of Molecular Biology

Notice that transcription is initiated at the promoter, starts at the start site (downstream from the promoter), and ends at the terminator. The protein coding region is within the mRNA transcript, but is not the entire mRNA transcript; mRNA also contains regulatory regions at the 5' and 3' ends (the 5'UTR and 3'UTR). Translation is initiated at the 5'UTR, starts at the start codon (ATG on the DNA coding strand or AUG on the mRNA transcript), and ends at one of the stop codons (UAG, UGA, UAA).

It is important to remember the similarities and differences between DNA replication, transcription, and translation. In summary:

	DNA Replication	Transcription	Translation
Signal to get ready	ORI	Promoter	5' UTR
Signal to start	ORI	Start site	AUG start codon
Key enzyme	DNA polymerase	RNA polymerase	Ribosome (made of rRNA and peptides)
Other enzymes	Helicase Primase Ligase	Spliceosome (eukaryotes only)	Aminoacyl tRNA synthetases
Template molecule	DNA	DNA	mRNA
Read direction	3' to 5' on the DNA template	3' to 5' on the DNA template	5' to 3' on the RNA template
Molecule synthesized	DNA	RNA	Peptides
Build direction	5' to 3'	5' to 3'	N-terminus to C-terminus
Prokaryotic location	Cytoplasm	Cytoplasm	Cytoplasm
Eukaryotic location	Nucleus	Nucleus	Cytoplasm
Signal to stop	When the replication bubbles or newly synthesized strands meet and are ligated together	Terminator	Stop codon (UAG, UGA, UAA)

Table 3   Summary of Molecular Biology Processes

4.5   CONTROLLING GENE EXPRESSION

The body of an adult human is composed of four types of tissues (connective tissue, muscle, nervous tissue, and epithelial tissue), but over 220 different types of cells. These cells all have the same genome, but can have different attributes such as morphology, lifespan, function, ability to secrete, response to signaling molecules, and mobility. These changes are due to differences in gene expression and subsequent protein function. In each cell type, some genes are expressed, and others are silenced. Genes that are expressed can have different levels of expression, where in one cell type the gene is expressed at a high level (to produce lots of RNA or protein), and in a different cell, the same gene is expressed at a low level. Proteins can also have varying activity, stability, and half-life. These variations in gene expression can be altered using seven different mechanisms (Figure 19).

4.5

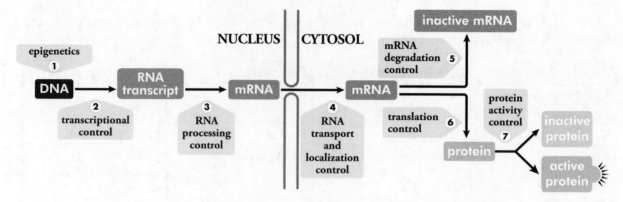

Figure 19 Mechanisms of Controlling Gene Expression in Eukaryotes

In the sections that follow, we'll look at regulation of gene expression, starting with DNA and working toward a mature and active protein.

Epigenetics

Broadly speaking, epigenetics is the study of how behavior and the environment (e.g., diet and exercise) can cause changes that affect the way genes work. Epigenetics focuses on changes in gene expression that are not due to changes in DNA sequences, but rather are either heritable or have a long-term effect. There are three types of epigenetic control:

1. DNA methylation
2. Histone modification
3. RNA interference

Unlike genetic changes, epigenetic changes are reversible and do not change the DNA sequence. However, they can affect how a DNA sequence is read. For example, epigenetic changes can turn gene expression on and off.

DNA Methylation

Both prokaryotic and eukaryotic DNA can be covalently modified by adding a **methyl group**. Bacteria methylate adenine nucleotides, via the enzyme **DNA adenine methylase**. Newly synthesized DNA is methylated shortly after synthesis. In contrast, eukaryotes methylate cytosine nucleotides that are on the 5' side of a guanine nucleotide. This motif is called "CpG," which stands for cytosine-phosphate-guanine (where the phosphate is in the backbone, linking together C and G nucleosides). A family of enzymes called **DNA methyltransferases** catalyze CpG methylation.

DNA methylation has been found in every vertebrate genome studied so far, and about 75% of CpG sites are methylated in a typical mammalian genome. Broadly speaking, methylation plays an important role in controlling gene expression (especially during embryonic development) and has also been implicated in several diseases. Methyl groups can be removed through a process called **demethylation**. Typically, methylation turns genes off and demethylation turns genes on.

Histone Modification

Eukaryotic DNA is wound around histone proteins, and these proteins can be **acetylated**, or have acetyl groups added to lysine amino acids. Histone modification via acetylation affects how tightly DNA is wound around histones and thus causes chromatin remodeling:

- Acetyl groups are added by enzymes called **histone acetyltransferases**; this causes DNA to be loosely wrapped around histones and makes the DNA more accessible to transcriptional machinery.
- In contrast, **histone deacetylases** are a family of enzymes that remove acetyl groups from lysine amino acids on histone proteins. When histones are deacetylated, they wrap DNA more tightly, forming **heterochromatin** (compact and inactive chromatin). This chromatin remodeling inhibits transcription.[37]

RNA Interference

DNA is used as a template to make both coding and **non-coding RNA (ncRNA)**. Coding RNA (or mRNA) is used to make proteins. [What are the two types of ncRNA you have already learned about in this chapter?[38]] There are additional non-coding RNA molecules: miRNA and siRNA, which are discussed later in this section. Long ncRNA can bind to DNA and block gene expression; this is a type of epigenetic control of gene expression. Non-coding RNA can also recruit proteins to modify histones acetylation. RNA interference is discussed more later in this section.

Examples of Epigenetics

Genomic **imprinting** is when only one allele of a gene is expressed. In some situations, the maternal allele is expressed, and in others the paternal allele is expressed. Imprinted genes tend to be clustered together on chromosomes. Imprinting is a dynamic process and can change from generation to generation. In other words, a gene that is imprinted in an adult may still be expressed in that adult's offspring. Imprinting is an epigenetic process; silencing of a certain gene involves DNA methylation, histone modification, and binding of long ncRNAs.

Female mammals have two X chromosomes in every cell, but one X chromosome is silenced, or inactive, while the other is active. In humans, **X-inactivation** occurs early in development, at the blastocyst stage (see Chapter 11 for more information on development). Each cell in the inner cell mass randomly inactivates an X chromosome, and this decision is irreversible. Because each cell makes its own decision, an adult can have different X chromosomes inactivated in different tissues and cells. Because of X-inactivation, all humans have the same number of gene products for the X chromosome; males have only one X chromosome, and females have only one *active* X chromosome. X chromosome inactivation is an epigenetic process; the inactive X chromosome binds a long ncRNA, is very condensed and packaged as heterochromatin, and has high levels of DNA methylation and low levels of histone acetylation.

---

[37] Be careful with DNA methylation and histone acetylation. DNA methylation usually turns gene expression off, while histone acetylation usually turns gene expression on.

[38] Both tRNA and rRNA are non-coding RNA because they are not used to make proteins.

Transcriptional Control

Transcription is the principal site of the regulation of gene expression in both eukaryotes and prokaryotes. This means that the amount of each protein made in every cell is affected by the amount of mRNA that gets transcribed.

Regulation of Transcription: Prokaryotes

In prokaryotes, the primary method of regulation of gene expression is regulation of transcription. One simple mechanism of transcriptional regulation in bacteria is that some promoters are simply stronger than others. However, this mechanism of regulation is "pre-set"; it does not respond to changing conditions within the cell. Bacteria also possess far more complex regulatory mechanisms, which activate or suppress transcription depending on current needs for specific gene products. For example, bacteria only produce the enzyme β-galactosidase and other proteins required for lactose catabolism when lactose is present.

- Assuming these protein products do not have a harmful effect on the cell, what advantage might there be in turning off the genes when the protein products are not required?[39]
- Are the terms *polypeptide enzyme* and *gene product* synonymous? Are there gene products that are not polypeptide enzymes? Are there polypeptides that are not enzymes?[40]

Enzymes involved in anabolism (biosynthesis) should be produced when the item they help make (their product) is scarce. Enzymes involved in catabolism (degradative metabolism) should be produced when the item they help break down (their substrate) is abundant, such as food. Hence there are two basic ways we can imagine how transcription is regulated. Transcription of enzymes involved in biosynthetic pathways should be inhibited by their product. Transcription of enzymes involved in catabolic pathways should be automatically inhibited whenever the substrate is not around and activated when it is. That is in fact exactly what happens. Anabolic enzymes whose transcription is inhibited in the presence of excess amounts of product are **repressible**. Catabolic enzymes whose transcription can be stimulated by the abundance of a substrate are called **inducible enzymes**.[41]

There are two common examples of this:

1. The lac operon is inducible since the enzymes it codes for are part of lactose catabolism.
2. The trp operon is repressible since the enzymes it codes for mediate tryptophan biosynthesis or anabolism.

An operon has two components: a coding sequence for enzymes, and upstream regulatory sequences or control sites. Operons may also include genes for regulatory proteins, such as repressors or activators, but don't have to. These genes can be located elsewhere in the genome and typically have their own promoters.

---

[39] It takes a great deal of ATP to synthesize RNA and protein, so it's more energy-efficient to transcribe and translate only the proteins that are needed.

[40] The terms "polypeptide enzyme" and "gene product" are not synonymous. All polypeptides are gene products, but some gene products are not polypeptides, and some polypeptides are not enzymes. tRNA and rRNA are gene products, but not polypeptides. Microfilaments and other elements of the cytoskeleton, as well as collagen and many other polypeptides, are not enzymes.

[41] Note: the default for repressible systems is "ON"; for inducible systems the default is "OFF."

Lac Operon

The **lac operon** contains several components, two of which are at distant sites:

1. *crp* gene: located at a distant site, this gene codes for catabolite activator protein (CAP) and helps couple the lac operon to glucose levels in the cell
2. *I* gene: located at a distant site, this gene codes for the lac repressor protein
3. P region: the promoter site on DNA to which RNA polymerase binds to initiate transcription of *Y*, *Z*, and *A* genes
4. O region: the operator site to which the lac repressor protein binds
5. *Z* gene: codes for the enzyme β-galactosidase, which cleaves lactose into glucose and galactose
6. *Y* gene: codes for permease, a protein which transports lactose into the cell
7. *A* gene: codes for transacetylase, an enzyme which transfers an acetyl group from acetyl-CoA to β-galactosides (note this function is not required for lactose metabolism)

Overall, there are five protein coding genes, and two regulatory sequences. Both *crp* and *I* have their own promoters. The protein products of these two genes control gene expression of *Z*, *Y*, and *A*.

Bacterial cells preferentially use glucose as an energy source. This means that in the presence of glucose, the lac operon will be off (Figure 20). Regulation of the lac operon is mediated by CAP and the lac repressor protein. When glucose levels are high, the CAP protein cannot bind the lac operon promoter and the lac repressor protein binds the operator of the lac operon. This prevents RNA pol from binding the promoter and transcribing *Z*, *Y*, and *A* genes. Overall, transcription of the operon is blocked when glucose levels are high and lactose is absent (Figure 20).

When glucose levels are low, bacterial cells will use lactose as an energy source. In these conditions, the lac operon will be on. When glucose is absent, the CAP protein binds the lac operon promoter and helps activate RNA polymerase activity. The lac repressor protein binds lactose, which changes the tertiary structure of the repressor protein. This conformational change means the lac repressor protein is no longer capable of binding the operator and thus falls off the DNA (Figure 21).

With CAP bound to the promoter and without the lac repressor protein bound to the operator, RNA pol binds the promoter. High transcription of *Z*, *Y*, and *A* genes occurs and produces a polycistronic mRNA that is translated to produce β-galactosidase, permease, and transacetylase.

4.5

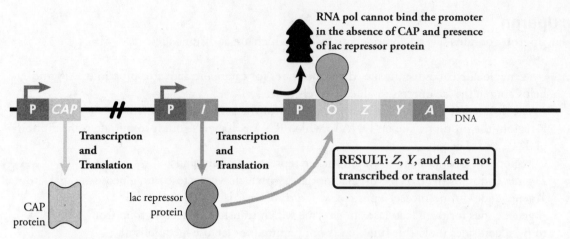

RNA pol cannot bind the promoter in the absence of CAP and presence of lac repressor protein

Transcription and Translation

Transcription and Translation

RESULT: *Z*, *Y*, and *A* are not transcribed or translated

CAP protein

lac repressor protein

Figure 20 Lac Operon in the Presence of Glucose (Glu⁺) and Absence of Lactose (Lac⁻)

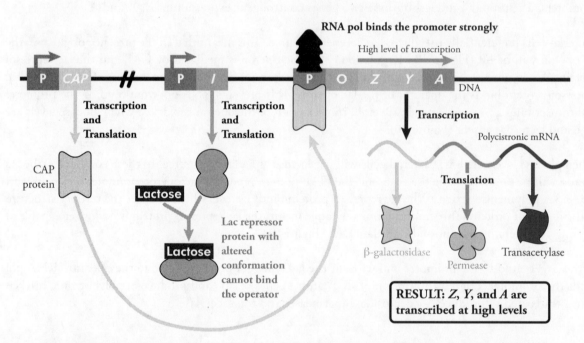

RNA pol binds the promoter strongly

High level of transcription

Transcription and Translation

Transcription and Translation

Transcription

Polycistronic mRNA

CAP protein

Lactose

Lactose

Lac repressor protein with altered conformation cannot bind the operator

Translation

β-galactosidase

Permease

Transacetylase

RESULT: *Z*, *Y*, and *A* are transcribed at high levels

Figure 21 Lac Operon in the Absence of Glucose (Glu⁻) and Presence of Lactose (Lac⁺)

- If the operator is mutated so the lac repressor can no longer bind, what effect will this have on transcription?[42]
  - A. Transcription of gene *Z* will be activated, and genes *Y* and *A* will not be affected.
  - B. None of the genes will be transcribed, regardless of the presence or absence of lac repressor.
  - C. Transcription will still be activated by lactose.
  - D. All three genes will be expressed constitutively, regardless of the presence of lactose.

---

[42] If the repressor cannot bind to the operator, nothing will prevent RNA polymerase from transcribing all the genes on the operon in an unregulated, constitutive (or continuous) fashion (choice **D** is correct, eliminate B). All genes on the operon are expressed or repressed together (eliminate A), and lactose will no longer have any effect. In other words, expression of the genes is unregulated (eliminate C).

Trp Operon

Bacteria use a five-enzyme synthetic pathway to make the amino acid tryptophan from chorismic acid. In the presence of tryptophan, there is little point in making these enzymes, which are found together in the trp operon.

The repressor protein is coded by the *trpR* gene (Figure 22). The repressor binds tryptophan when it is present, and the two together then bind the operator, to turn off transcription of the other five *trp* genes. In the absence of tryptophan, the bacterial cell must make its own. With no tryptophan present, the repressor protein cannot bind the operator. Without this block, RNA polymerase transcribes the five genes in the trp operon, and the five gene products allow the cell to make tryptophan. This is an example of anabolic repressible transcription.

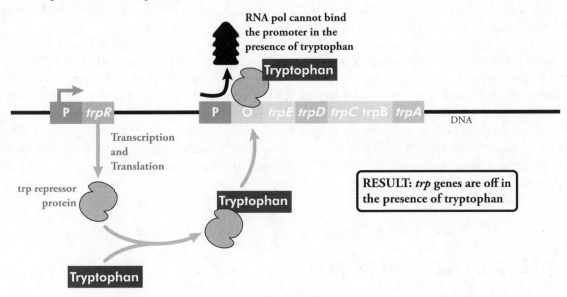

Figure 22   Trp Operon in the Presence of Tryptophan (Trp⁺)

Regulation of Transcription: Eukaryotes

Given the complexity of eukaryotes compared to prokaryotes, it is not surprising that regulation of eukaryotic transcription is also more complex. Most of this regulation happens at initiation.

- The DNA sequence contains several regulation regions (e.g., upstream control elements, promoter, TATA box). These affect transcription complex assembly and initiation.
- Enhancer sequences in DNA can bind activator proteins to promote transcription and make genes more accessible.
- Gene repressor proteins inhibit transcription.
- Transcription factors have DNA-binding domains and are crucial in transcription regulation. They can bind promoters or other regulatory sequences.

If a mutation in a eukaryotic fat cell reduces the level of several proteins related to fat metabolism, does this mean the proteins are encoded by the same mRNA?[43]

---

[43]   No, it does not. Eukaryotic mRNA is monocistronic. A more likely explanation is that a number of different genes located throughout the genome have related regulatory sequences that bind the same sequence-specific transcription factors. This is how eukaryotes achieve coordinated expression of genes. Related proteins are clumped together on the same piece of mRNA in prokaryotes only.

RNA Processing Control

We have already talked about how eukaryotes process hnRNA to make mRNA. [What are the three things that must happen after transcription finishes and before translocation?[44]] These processes are tightly regulated and affect RNA stability and lifespan. This means they also affect the types of levels of protein a cell can make.

RNA Transport and Localization Control

After processing, mRNA transcripts must be exported from the nucleus to the cytoplasm. Nuclear export of RNA is mediated by a family of transport proteins that bind RNA molecules and interact with nuclear pore proteins to help get the transcript to the cytoplasm.

Once outside the nucleus, RNA location is controlled by different proteins that bind to the RNA and control its localization to the cytoplasm. This system is especially important in cells that have a high level of polarity, where one area or end of the cell is distinctly different from the other (in terms of shape, structure and/or function). Neurons have polarity; some transcripts are transported to the dendrites, while others stay in the soma. Many embryonic and developing cells also have polarity. While protein trafficking is well known, RNA trafficking is a newer field. Nonetheless, eukaryotes control RNA location as a way of controlling gene expression: mRNA transcripts aren't translated into proteins until they are localized properly in the cell.

mRNA Degradation and Control

mRNA Surveillance

Cells closely monitor mRNA molecules. Three mechanisms of mRNA surveillance have been discovered, and these function to ensure that only high-quality mRNA transcripts are read by the ribosome.

1. Transcripts that contain premature termination codons are targeted for destruction. These transcripts code for truncated proteins, which may be harmful to a cell.
2. Transcripts without a stop codon are also targeted for destruction. Without a stop codon, ribosomes keep reading the transcript through the poly-A tail, and then stall. The ribosome cannot dissociate from the transcript and gets stuck.
3. Another pathway rescues ribosomes that have stalled in translation and are stuck on a transcript. This mechanism results in the ribosome being released, and the transcript being degraded.

Each of these pathways is mediated by protein complexes and ends with the defective transcript being broken down. mRNA surveillance is part gene expression control because it removes defective transcripts from the library of mRNA in a cell. Since prokaryotes perform transcription and translation at the same time, they don't have the opportunity to assess mRNAs before translation. However, they can rescue stalled ribosomes.

---

[44] After an hnRNA is made, it must be spliced, a 5' cap must be added, and a 3' poly-A tail must be added.

RNA Interference

RNA interference (RNAi) is a way to silence gene expression after a transcript has been made. It is mediated by microRNA (miRNA) and small interfering RNA (siRNA). Both can bind specific mRNA molecules. Once a double-stranded RNA is made (transcript and miRNA, or transcript and siRNA), it is degraded. This decreases translation.

Translation Control

Almost all control of translation occurs at initiation. [Why might this be the case?[45]] This requires coordination of many regulatory proteins into complexes, which are themselves regulated by cell signaling pathways. This allows the cell to control translation rates. In both prokaryotes and eukaryotes, this is a highly regulated process, and links protein synthesis with upstream signaling pathways.

Protein Activity Control

Newly synthesized proteins released from the ribosome are rarely able to function. They need to be correctly folded, modified and/or processed, and transported to where they function in the cell. These modifications are called **post-translational modifications** since they occur after protein synthesis.

Protein Folding

First, the newly synthesized protein is folded into its correct three-dimensional shape. This is accomplished by a family of proteins called **chaperones**. Chaperone proteins are found across all types of organisms (from bacteria to plants to mammals), and function in assembly or folding of other macromolecular structures. For example, chaperone proteins assist in nucleosome assembly from folded histones and DNA.

Covalent Modification

Next, many proteins are covalently modified. Some proteins have hydrophobic groups added to facilitate membrane localization. Smaller chemical groups can also be added. For example, proteins can be **glycosylated**, when a glycosyl group is added to certain amino acids, or **phosphorylated**, when a phosphate group (PO_4^{3-}) is added to a serine, threonine, or tyrosine amino acid. Overall, protein covalent modifications can have many effects on a protein and its function. They can change protein subcellular localization, target a protein for degradation, change interactions between proteins and other molecules, activate or inhibit enzyme activity, or change enzyme affinity for substrates. These modifications are typically studied in the lab using mass spectrometry (see Chapter 29) or western blotting.

---

[45] Regulating a process near the start is generally more efficient that regulating a process later.

Processing

Many proteins require cleavage of some sort to become mature or functional. Cleavage can occur at either end of a peptide chain, or in the middle. Protein precursors are often used when the mature protein may be dangerous to an organism. Because the precursor is already made, cleavage allows large quantities of mature protein to be available on short notice.

Enzyme precursors were already discussed in Chapter 3 and are called zymogens or proenzymes. You'll see more examples in Chapter 9 because many digestion enzymes are made as zymogens. Another example is the hormone insulin, which is made from a proenzyme (Figure 23). Preproinsulin is the primary translational product of the human *INS* gene. This peptide is 110 amino acids in length. To form proinsulin, an N-terminus signal peptide is removed and disulfide bonds form, in the endoplasmic reticulum. Three cleavage events are necessary to process proinsulin: the C peptide is removed by a family of enzymes called proprotein convertases, and a dipeptide fragment is removed from the C-terminus of the B chain peptide by a carboxypeptidase. These cleavage events occur in a secretory vesicle. The biological effects of insulin are well known, but it's recently been shown that peptide C also has signaling properties.

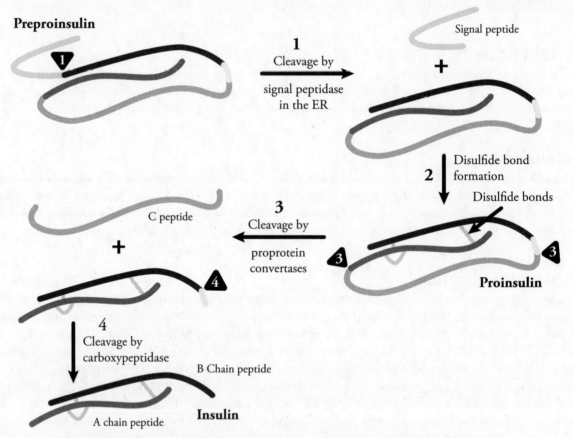

Figure 23 Insulin Processing: An Example of Post-Translational Modification

Translocation and Trafficking

Especially in complex eukaryotic cells, protein translocation is crucial for proper protein function. Each subcellular compartment contains many proteins, most of which are made by cytoplasmic or ER-associated ribosomes. Protein trafficking, how newly synthesized proteins are transported around the cell to their final destination, will be discussed more in Chapter 5.

4.6 MOLECULAR BIOLOGY LAB TECHNIQUES

You should be familiar with some basic molecular biology techniques for the DAT. We will review some here and introduce cell biology lab techniques in the next chapter. **Plasmids** are often used to transfer and replicate DNA. They are double-stranded and circular DNA molecules that are smaller than a chromosome. Plasmids are self-replicating and extra-chromosomal (non-essential). They can be added to eukaryotic cells by **transfection,** and added to prokaryotic cells by **transformation.**

One important characteristic of the plasmids used in molecular biology labs is that they give a transformed cell selective advantage. For example, most plasmids contain an antibiotic resistance gene such as Amp^R, which allows bacteria with the plasmid to survive when ampicillin is added to the growth culture. Bacterial cells without the plasmid will die in the presence of ampicillin. This is a clever way scientists can find out which bacteria have taken up a plasmid.

Restriction enzymes are used to make plasmids and other types of recombinant DNA. They cut double-stranded DNA at specific sites (called **recognition sites**) and can generate compatible "sticky ends" on the DNA. These ends can be ligated back together by **DNA ligase,** thus creating unique DNA that is not found in nature.

Complementary DNA (cDNA) is double-stranded DNA synthesized from a single-stranded RNA. It is made by the enzyme **reverse transcriptase.** This process is often used to clone eukaryotic genes in prokaryotes because the cDNA of a gene has no introns, so is shorter than the genomic DNA sequence of the same gene. cDNAs are often used to study gene expression.

The **polymerase chain reaction (PCR)** is a quick and inexpensive way to duplicate DNA. It makes millions of copies of a certain DNA template, and occurs in three steps, repeated about 30 times. First, the template DNA is "melted" using heat (hydrogen bonds that hold double-stranded DNA together are broken), turning the template into two single-stranded pieces of DNA. Next, primers that bind to either end of the template anneal. Finally, a heat-stable DNA polymerase elongates each primer and synthesizes new DNA that is complementary to the template.

Gel electrophoresis is a technique used to separate biological macromolecules (DNA, RNA, proteins) by size and charge, using an electric current. Samples of a certain molecule are applied to a gel and the molecules migrate through the gel based on their size. Small molecules migrate quickly and move farthest. Larger molecules move slowly and stay closer to the start position.

Techniques in molecular biology and genetic engineering have been used to sequence whole genomes, and to make cloned and transgenic organisms. For example, **cloned animals** are genetically identical to each other. These animals are made using reproductive cloning: a nucleus from a donor adult cell (somatic cell) is transferred to an egg that has no nucleus. Dolly the sheep was formed from a nucleus of an udder cell of her 6-year-old biological mother (a Finn-Dorset ewe). **Transgenic animals** have one or more gene(s) deliberately inserted into their genome, so they are genetically altered. Transgenic mice, rats, fish and flies are commonly used in biology labs to model human diseases (such as cancer and Parkinson's) and biological processes (such as development and aging).

Want More Practice?
Scan the QR code below to register your book for online chapter summaries, drills, practice tests, and more!

Chapter 5
Cell Biology

The first cells were prokaryotes. They consisted of a cell membrane and a cell wall surrounding the cytoplasm or cell fluid. All the structures necessary for survival and reproduction floated in the cytoplasm, including the double-stranded circular DNA genome, ribosomes, enzymes of aerobic and anaerobic metabolism, etc. As evolution proceeded, cell complexity increased. The greatest landmark in the evolution of the cell was the development of membrane-bound compartments within the cytoplasm known as organelles. These served to organize the cytoplasm, with each membrane acting to seal its compartment. The most important organelle is the control center of the cell: the nucleus. In fact, "eukaryotic" is from the Greek "karyon," meaning "kernel" or "nucleus," plus the prefix "eu," meaning "true." "Prokaryotic" means "before the nucleus" and also implies "before organelles." All true living organisms are either prokaryotes or eukaryotes. As we'll see in Chapter 7, there are four Kingdoms of eukaryotes (protists, fungi, plants, and animals), and two Domains of prokaryotes (Eubacteria and Archaea). In this chapter we'll review the eukaryotic and prokaryotic cell biology you need to be familiar with for the DAT.

5.1 INTRODUCTION

In this chapter we will examine each of the principal organelles, beginning with the nucleus. Next we will focus on the plasma membrane, then the cytoskeleton, and finally we will finish with a discussion of the cell cycle. You should be able to explain the function of each item labeled in Figure 1 below.

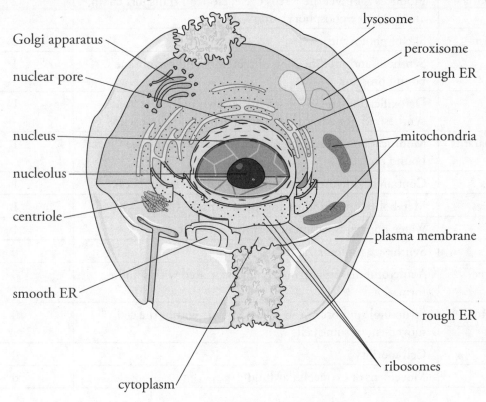

Figure 1 A Typical Eukaryotic Cell

5.2 EUKARYOTIC ORGANELLES

An **organelle** is a small structure within a cell that carries out specific cellular functions. Most organelles are bound by their own lipid bilayer membrane. The membrane acts like a plastic bag to seal off the contents of the organelle from the rest of the **cytoplasm** and control what enters and exits. A summary of the major animal cell organelles is given in the table on the next page.

Organelle	Function	Number of Membranes
Nucleus	Contains and protects the DNA genome, transcription, partial assembly of ribosomes	2
Mitochondria	Produces ATP via the Krebs cycle, electron transport chain, and oxidative phosphorylation	2
Chloroplast[1]	Site of photosynthesis	2
RER	Synthesis and modification of secretory and membrane-bound proteins	1
SER	Detoxification and glycogen breakdown in liver, steroid synthesis in gonads, calcium storage in skeletal muscle	1
Golgi apparatus	Modification and sorting of secretory and membrane-bound proteins	1
Lysosomes	Contain acid hydrolases that digest various substances	1
Peroxisomes	Metabolize lipids and toxins, producing H_2O_2	1
Vacuole	Water storage, isolation of harmful substances	1
Ribosomes	Synthesize proteins via translation	0
Centrosome	A microtubule-organizing center associated with spindle formation	0
Cytoskeleton	Structural support of the cell, transport within the cell, movement of some cells	0
Flagella	Cell motility	0
Cilia	Movement of extracellular fluid	0

Table 1   Eukaryotic Organelles

The Nucleus

One of the primary features of eukaryotic cells distinguishing them from prokaryotic cells is the **nucleus**. The nucleus contains the genome surrounded by the **nuclear envelope** that separates the contents of the nucleus into a distinct compartment, isolated from other organelles and from the cytoplasm.

The Genome

Eukaryotic genomes are organized into linear molecules of double-stranded DNA, while the genome of prokaryotes is a single circular DNA molecule. The large size of the typical eukaryotic genome appears to make it necessary to split the genome into pieces, each a separate linear DNA molecule, termed a **chromosome**. Yeast have four different chromosomes, while there are 23 different human chromosomes. Since humans and most adult animals are **diploid**, they have two copies of each chromosome (except for the sex chromosomes; see Chapter 6). Chromosomes have a **centromere** near the middle to ensure

---

[1] Plastids are found almost solely in plant cells, contain pigment, and function in photosynthesis as well as in other cellular processes. The most abundant of the plastids are chloroplasts, which contain the green pigment chlorophyll.

that newly replicated chromosomes are sorted properly during cell division, one copy to each daughter cell; we'll see more on this when we review mitosis later in this chapter and meiosis in Chapter 6. Each eukaryotic chromosome also has special structures at both ends termed **telomeres**. Telomeres have large numbers of repeats of a specific DNA sequence and, with the help of a special DNA polymerase termed **telomerase**, maintain the ends of the linear chromosomes during DNA replication. Some regions of a chromosome are folded into densely packed chromatin, termed **heterochromatin**, within which genes tend to be inaccessible and turned off. Other regions known as **euchromatin** are more loosely packed (although still packaged into chromatin) and allow genes to be activated. We'll see more on chromosome structure later in this chapter.

The Nucleolus

The **nucleolus** ("little nucleus") is a region within the nucleus which functions as a ribosome factory. There is no membrane separating the nucleolus from the rest of the nucleus. It consists of loops of DNA, RNA polymerases, rRNA, and the protein components of the ribosome. [Would you expect the nucleolus to be larger in cells that are actively synthesizing protein, or in quiescent cells?[2]]

The nucleolus is the site of transcription of rRNA by RNA pol I. Transcription of mRNA and tRNA is performed by other polymerases (RNA pol II and RNA pol III, respectively) in other areas of the nucleus. The ribosome is partially assembled while still in the nucleolus. Protein components of the ribosome are not produced in the nucleolus; they are transported into the nucleus from the cytoplasm (remember that *all* translation takes place in the cytoplasm). After partial assembly, the ribosome is exported from the nucleus, remaining inactive until assembly is completed in the cytoplasm.

The Nuclear Envelope

Surrounding the nucleus and separating it from the cytoplasm is the **nuclear envelope**, composed of two **lipid bilayer** membranes. The inner nuclear membrane is the surface of the envelope facing the nuclear interior, and the outer nuclear membrane faces the cytoplasm. The membrane of the endoplasmic reticulum is at points continuous with the outer nuclear membrane, making the interior of the ER (the **lumen** of the ER) contiguous with the space between the two nuclear membranes. [Is the space between the inner and outer membranes contiguous with the cytoplasm?[3]]

The nuclear envelope is punctuated with large **nuclear pores** that allow the passage of material into and out of the nucleus (see Figures 2 and 3 on the following page). Molecules that are smaller than 60 kilodaltons, including small proteins, can freely diffuse from the cytoplasm into the nucleus through the nuclear pores. Larger proteins cannot pass freely through nuclear pores and are excluded from the nuclear interior unless they contain a sequence of basic amino acids called a **nuclear localization sequence**. Proteins with a nuclear localization sequence are translated on cytoplasmic ribosomes and then imported into the nucleus by specific transport mechanisms. RNA is transported out of the nucleus by a specific transport system rather than freely diffusing into the cytoplasm. [If a 15 kD protein has a nuclear localization sequence that is then deleted from its gene, will the mutated protein still be found in the nucleus?[4]]

---

[2] The nucleolus is largest in cells that are producing large amounts of protein. The increased size reflects increased synthesis of ribosomes. More on quiescence later in this chapter.

[3] No, it is not. The space between the nuclear membranes is contiguous with the ER lumen, which is isolated from the cytoplasm.

[4] Yes. The protein is small enough that it can still pass through the nuclear pores by diffusion even without a nuclear localization sequence.

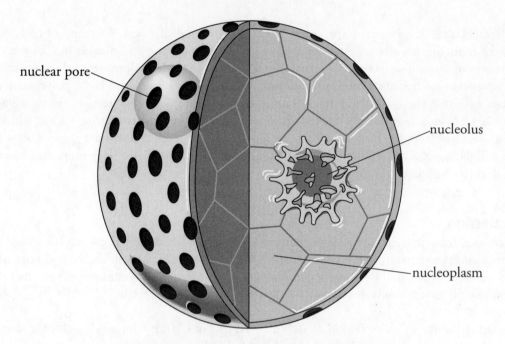

Figure 2 The Nucleus, Showing Pores

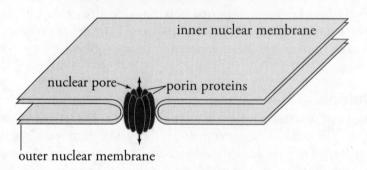

Figure 3 A Nuclear Pore Close-Up

- A researcher injects tiny gold beads into a cell and waits an hour. Then she examines the cell and finds gold beads in the cytoplasm and in the nucleus. When she injects larger gold beads, they are not found in the nucleus. However, when she binds the larger beads to a nuclear localization sequence, she finds that they end up in the nucleus. One can conclude that[5]
  A. the nuclear localization sequence is lysine-rich.
  B. gold beads have an inherent import signal.
  C. the nuclear localization mechanism is nonspecific enough to confer nuclear import on gold beads.
  D. nuclear import relies primarily on simple diffusion.

---

[5] Gold beads are not normally found in cells, so there cannot be an existing mechanism for moving them. However, since the cell is capable of moving them when the localization signal is attached, the localization signal must be somewhat non-specific (choice **C** is correct). It is true that the nuclear localization signal is lysine-rich, but this cannot be concluded based on the given information (true, but doesn't answer the question; A is wrong). If gold beads had an inherent import signal, then they would be transported into the nucleus on their own, without the researcher having to bind them to the localization sequence (choice B is wrong). If simple diffusion were the primary means of moving things into the nucleus, no import signal would be needed (choice D is wrong).

Mitochondria

As we saw in Chapter 3, **mitochondria** are the site of oxidative phosphorylation. We'll quickly review mitochondrial structure again here because this is important for you to know for the DAT. The interior of mitochondria, the **matrix**, is bound by the inner and outer mitochondrial membranes (see Figure 4). The matrix contains pyruvate dehydrogenase and the enzymes of the Krebs cycle. The inner membrane is the location of the electron transport chain and ATP synthase and is the site of the proton gradient used to drive ATP synthesis by ATP synthase. The inner membrane is impermeable to the free diffusion of polar substances, like protons, and is folded into the matrix in projections called **cristae**. The outer membrane is smooth and contains large pores that allow free passage of small molecules. The space between the membranes is called the intermembrane space. ATP produced within mitochondria is transported out into the cytoplasm to drive a great variety of cellular processes. [Why is the inner membrane folded into cristae?[6]]

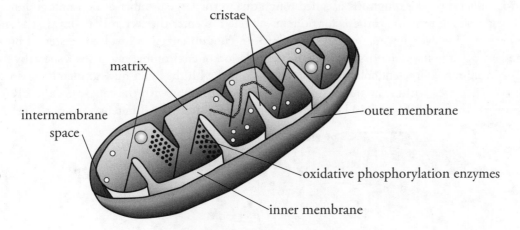

Figure 4   The Mitochondrion

Mitochondria possess their own genome which is far smaller than the cellular genome and consists of a single circular DNA molecule. (Sound familiar?) It encodes rRNA, tRNA, and several proteins, including some components of the electron transport chain and parts of the ATP synthase complex although most mitochondrial proteins are encoded by nuclear genes. Even more curious, mitochondria use a different system of transcription and translation than nuclear genes do. This includes a unique genetic code and unique RNA polymerases, DNA replication machinery, ribosomes, and aminoacyl-tRNA synthetases. In order to explain the fact that mitochondria possess a second system of inheritance, investigators have postulated that mitochondria originated as independent unicellular organisms living within larger cells. This is known as **symbiogenesis** or the **endosymbiotic theory** of mitochondrial evolution (*endo* = within; *symbiotic* = living together). In fact, if you compare a mitochondrion to a Gram-negative bacterium, you'll note that they look pretty similar. Pay attention to where the enzymes of electron transport are located and the genome shape.[7]

---

[6]   The folding of the membrane increases its surface area and allows for increased electron transport and ATP synthesis per mitochondrion. (Folding is used elsewhere to increase surface area, such as in the kidney tubules and the lining of the small intestine.)

[7]   Remember that bacterial electron transport depends on a proton gradient across the cell membrane. In a Gram-negative bacterium, this membrane would correspond to the mitochondrial inner membrane. We'll discuss Gram staining soon!

Mitochondria exhibit **maternal inheritance**. This means that mitochondria are inherited only from the mother, since the cytoplasm of the egg becomes the cytoplasm of the zygote; sperm contribute only genomic (or nuclear) DNA. Maternal inheritance departs from the rules of Mendelian genetics, which state traits are inherited from both parents (more on this in Chapter 6). [If a woman has a disease caused by an abnormality in her mitochondrial genome, what are the chances that her children will have the disease, assuming her mate does not have the disease?[8]]

Endoplasmic Reticulum (ER)

The **endoplasmic reticulum** (**ER**) is a large system of folded membrane accounting for over half of the membrane of some cells. There are two types of ER (see Figure 5): **rough ER** and **smooth ER**, each with distinct functions. The rough ER is called rough due to the large number of ribosomes bound to its surface; it is the site of protein synthesis for proteins targeted to enter the secretory pathway. The smooth ER is not actively involved in protein processing but can contain enzymes involved in steroid hormone biosynthesis (especially in gonad tissue) or in the degradation of environmental toxins (especially in liver tissue). The membrane of the endoplasmic reticulum is joined with the outer nuclear membrane in places, meaning that the space within the nuclear membranes is continuous with the interior of the ER (called the ER **lumen**). The rough ER plays a key role directing protein traffic to different parts of the cell.

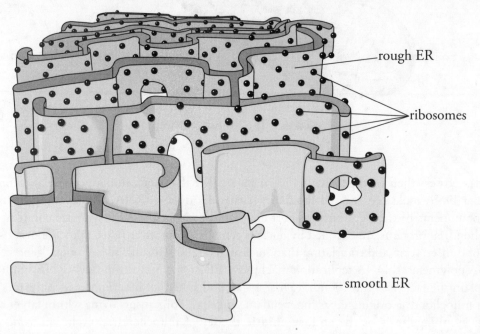

rough ER

ribosomes

smooth ER

Figure 5   The ER

---

[8]   All her children will have the disease since they will inherit mitochondria exclusively from her. For a maternally inherited trait, it doesn't matter whether the father has it or not; this is in fact the essence of maternal inheritance.

RER and the Secretory Pathway

Protein trafficking (as we'll review here) is a pretty advanced DAT topic. It is possible you'll see a question on this stuff on test day, but it is not very likely. Plan your study time accordingly. There are two sites of protein synthesis in the eukaryotic cell: either on ribosomes free in the cytoplasm or on ribosomes bound to the surface of the rough ER. Proteins translated on free cytoplasmic ribosomes are headed toward peroxisomes, mitochondria, the nucleus, or will remain in the cytoplasm. Proteins synthesized on the rough ER will end up either 1) secreted into the extracellular environment, 2) as plasma membrane proteins, or 3) in the membrane or interior of the ER, Golgi apparatus, or lysosomes. Membrane-bound vesicles pass between these cellular compartments. Since the membranes of these organelles communicate through the traffic of vesicles, the interior of the ER, the Golgi apparatus, lysosomes, and the extracellular environment are in a sense contiguous. Proteins synthesized on the rough ER are transported in vesicles that bud from the ER to the Golgi apparatus, then to the plasma membrane or lysosome. A secreted protein that enters the ER lumen is separated by a membrane from the cytoplasm until the protein leaves the cell.

Whether a protein is translated on the rough ER is determined by the sequence of the protein itself. All proteins start translation in the cytoplasm; however, some proteins (secreted proteins and lysosomal proteins) have an amino acid sequence at their N-terminus called a **signal sequence.** The signal sequence of a nascent polypeptide is recognized by the **signal recognition particle** (**SRP**), which binds to the ribosome. The rough ER has SRP receptors that dock the ribosome-SRP complex on the cytoplasmic surface (along with the nascent polypeptide and mRNA). Translation then pushes the polypeptide, signal peptide first, into the ER lumen. After translation is complete, the signal peptide is removed from the polypeptide by a signal peptidase in the ER lumen. For secreted proteins, once the signal sequence is removed, the protein is transported in the interior of vesicles through the Golgi apparatus to the plasma membrane, where it is released by exocytosis into the extracellular environment.

- The mRNA for a secreted protein encodes a longer protein than is actually observed in the cellular exterior. Why?[9]
  - A. The protein was cleaved by a cytoplasmic protease.
  - B. The mRNA was not spliced properly.
  - C. The gene encoding the protein contained a nonsense mutation.
  - D. The signal sequence of the protein was removed in the rough ER.

Plasma membrane proteins are processed slightly differently. Integral membrane proteins have sections of hydrophobic amino acid residues called **transmembrane domains** that pass through lipid bilayer membranes. The transmembrane domains (TMD) also act as signal sequences, but are found in the interior of the protein (instead of at the N-terminus). TMD are *not* removed after translation. A single polypeptide can have several transmembrane domains passing back and forth through a membrane. During translation, transmembrane domains are threaded through the ER membrane. The protein is then transported in vesicles to the Golgi apparatus and plasma membrane in the same manner as a secreted protein (see Figure 6 on the following page). [For a protein in the plasma membrane, does the portion of the protein in the ER lumen end up facing the cytoplasm or the cellular exterior?[10]]

Additional functions of the rough ER include post-translational modification of proteins. Although glycosylation (the addition of saccharides to proteins) is usually associated with the Golgi apparatus, some glycosylation occurs in the lumen of the ER. Disulfide bond formation also occurs in the ER lumen.

---

[9] The only way a protein can be smaller than would be expected from its mRNA would be if some post-translational modification were to occur (**D** is correct). Choices B and C are pre-translational modifications and would not account for a size difference between mRNA and protein, and since secreted proteins are synthesized on the rough ER, they are inaccessible to cytoplasmic proteases (so A is wrong).

[10] The cellular exterior

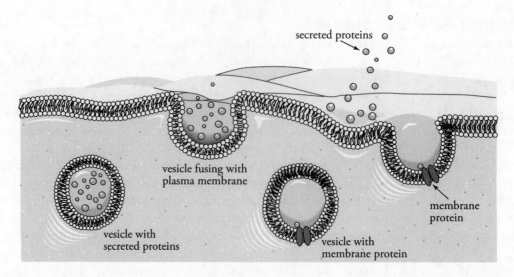

secreted proteins

vesicle fusing with
plasma membrane

membrane
protein

vesicle with
secreted proteins

vesicle with
membrane protein

Figure 6   Protein Trafficking of Secreted and Membrane Proteins

The Golgi Apparatus

The **Golgi apparatus** is a group of membranous sacs stacked together like collapsed basketballs (see Figure 7). It has the following functions:

1. Modification of proteins made in the RER; especially important is the modification of oligosaccharide chains
2. Sorting and sending proteins to their correct destinations
3. Synthesis of certain macromolecules, such as polysaccharides to be secreted

Vesicle traffic to and from the Golgi apparatus is mostly unidirectional; membrane-bound or secreted proteins which are to be sorted and modified enter at one defined region and exit at another. (Traffic is said to be *mostly* unidirectional because on occasion, proteins that are supposed to reside in the ER accidentally escape, and must be returned to the ER from the Golgi. This is called "retrograde traffic.") Each region of the Golgi has different enzymes and a different microscopic appearance. The portion of the Golgi nearest the rough ER is called the *cis* stack, and the part farthest from the rough ER is the *trans* stack. The *medial* stack is in the middle.[11] Vesicles from the ER fuse with the *cis* stack. The proteins in these vesicles are then modified and transferred to the *medial* stack, where they are further modified before passing to the *trans* stack. Proteins leave the Golgi at the *trans* face in transport vesicles. [If vesicle fusion with the *cis* Golgi was inhibited, could plasma membrane proteins still reach the cell surface?[12]] The route taken by a protein is determined by signals within the protein that determine which vesicle a protein is sorted into in the *trans* Golgi.

---

[11] Note that *cis* means "near," as in a *cis* double bond. *Trans* means "far." *Medial* means "in the middle." Also note that the order is alphabetical: *cis-medial-trans*.

[12] No. Secretory proteins must proceed via a specific path: from the ER to the *cis* Golgi to the medial and *trans* Golgi and from there to the cell surface.

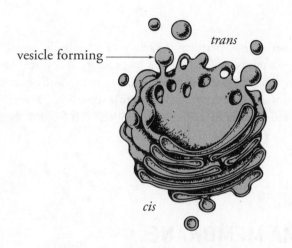

vesicle forming

trans

cis

Figure 7 The Golgi Apparatus

When a vesicle moves from the *trans* Golgi toward the cell surface, it fuses with the cell membrane. As a result, contents of the vesicle are released into the extracellular environment in a process termed **exocytosis**. Alternatively, if the vesicle contains proteins anchored to its membrane, these proteins will remain attached to the cell as cell-surface proteins. Some proteins are sent in vesicles from the Golgi immediately to the cell surface, in the **constitutive secretory pathway**. *Constitutive* connotes *continuous* or *unregulated*. In contrast, specialized secretory cells (such as pancreatic cells, B cells of the immune system, etc.) store secretory proteins in **secretory vesicles** and release them only at certain times, usually in response to a change in (or signal from) the extracellular environment. This is a **regulated secretory pathway**.

Lysosomes

Lyse means cut. The **lysosome** is a membrane-bound organelle that is responsible for degradation of biological macromolecules by hydrolysis. Lysosome proteins are made in the RER, modified in the Golgi, and released in their final form from the *trans* face of the Golgi. Organelles such as mitochondria that have been damaged or are no longer functional may be degraded in lysosomes in a process termed **autophagy** (self-eating). Lysosomes also degrade large particulate matter engulfed by the cell by **phagocytosis** (cell eating). For example, **macrophages** of the immune system engulf bacteria and viruses. The particle or microorganism ends up in a **phagocytic vesicle**, which will fuse with a lysosome. Finally, **crinophagy** refers to lysosomal digestion of unneeded (excess) secretory products. After hydrolysis, the lysosome will release molecular building blocks into the cytoplasm for reuse.

The enzymes responsible for degradation in lysosomes are called **acid hydrolases**. This name reflects the fact that these enzymes only hydrolyze substrates when they are in an acidic environment; this is a safety mechanism. The pH of the lysosome is around 5, so the acid hydrolases are active. But the pH of the cytoplasm is 7.4. If a lysosome ruptures, its enzymes will not damage the cell because the acidic fluid will be diluted, and the acid hydrolases will be inactivated. However, if many lysosomes rupture at once, the cell may be destroyed.

Peroxisomes

Peroxisomes are small organelles that perform a variety of metabolic tasks. The peroxisome contains enzymes that produce hydrogen peroxide (H_2O_2) as a by-product. They are essential for lipid breakdown in many cell types. In the liver they assist in detoxification of drugs and chemicals. H_2O_2 is a dangerous chemical, but peroxisomes contain an enzyme called **catalase** which converts it to $H_2O + O_2$. Separating these activities into the peroxisomes protects the rest of the cell from damage by peroxides or oxygen radicals.

5.3   THE PLASMA MEMBRANE

Evolution of life most likely began with a separation of "inside" from "outside." Once this had occurred, processes in the cell could increase their orderliness despite the entropic chaos of the surroundings. An alternate hypothesis is that life began with self-replicating RNA floating free in the ocean. As it grew more complex, this early genome would require protection. In any case, separation of the cytoplasm from the extracellular environment was a major milestone in evolution. Bacteria, plants, and fungi accomplish this by forming a **cell membrane** and a cell wall (made of peptidoglycan, **cellulose**, and **chitin**, respectively). Eukaryotic animal cells have no cell wall and thus rely on the cell membrane as the only boundary between inside and outside. And they must devise another means of structural support: just as chordates have a bony endoskeleton instead of the primitive exoskeleton arthropods have, animal cells rely on an internal cytoskeleton instead of an external cell wall. Further problems arise in multicellular eukaryotes. Not only must each cell maintain its structural integrity, but it must also interact with its neighbors in an organized fashion. In the following discussion, we will study how each of these goals is accomplished.

Membrane Structure

All membranes of the cell are composed of **lipid bilayer** membranes.[13] The three most common lipids in eukaryotic membranes are **phospholipids**, **glycolipids**, and **cholesterol**, of which phospholipids are the most abundant. An example of a phospholipid is *phosphatidyl choline* (see Figure 8 on the following page) with two long hydrophobic fatty acids esterified to glycerol, along with a charged phosphoryl choline group. Thus, phospholipids have portions that are distinctly hydrophilic and hydrophobic. Glycolipids, with fatty acid groups and carbohydrate side chains, also have hydrophilic and hydrophobic regions. As we saw in Chapter 2, when fatty acids or phospholipids are mixed with water, they spontaneously arrange themselves with the hydrophobic tails facing the interior to avoid contact with water and the hydrophilic regions facing outward toward water (see Figure 9 on the following page). Fatty acids form small micelles, but, due to steric hindrance, phospholipids arrange themselves spontaneously into **lipid bilayer membranes**. Since the lipid bilayer is the lowest energy state for these molecules, the bilayer membrane can reseal and repair itself if a small portion of membrane is removed.

The interior of the lipid bilayer membrane is very hydrophobic, with water largely excluded. Hydrophilic molecules such as water, ions, carbohydrates, and amino acids are not soluble in this environment, making the membrane a barrier to the passage of these molecules. These molecules can pass through the

---

[13] On the DAT, the terms cell membrane and plasma membrane are often used interchangeably. Technically, the cell membrane is the boundary of the cell whereas plasma membrane is a more generic term for the boundary of a cell or an organelle. All plasma membranes are selectively permeable to molecules.

membrane; they just need the help of specialized protein channels, which we'll discuss shortly. Small, nonpolar molecules such as CO_2, O_2, and steroid hormones can cross the membrane easily and without the help of a protein.

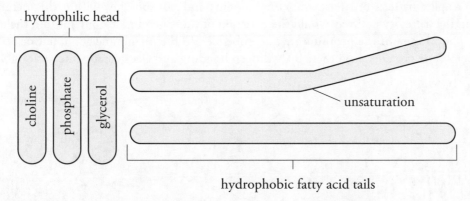

Figure 8   Phosphatidyl Choline, a Phospholipid

- Which one of the following statements best describes the physical characteristics of phospholipids?[14]
  - A.   Negatively charged at pH 7 and therefore entirely hydrophilic
  - B.   Hydrophobic
  - C.   Partially hydrophilic and partially hydrophobic
  - D.   Positively charged at pH 7 and therefore entirely hydrophilic

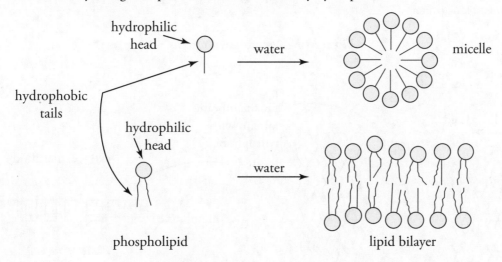

Figure 9   Lipid Behavior in an Aqueous Solvent

In addition to lipids, proteins are a major component of membranes. Some proteins act to mediate interactions of the cell with other cells. Other proteins called **cell-surface receptors** bind extracellular signaling molecules such as hormones and relay these signals into the cell so that it can respond accordingly. **Channel proteins** selectively allow ions or molecules to cross the membrane. Each of these types of membrane protein is discussed on the next page.

---

[14] Choice **C**. Phospholipids have hydrophobic components (fatty acid acyl chains) and hydrophilic components (phosphate and choline, for example, in phosphatidyl choline).

5.3

In general, membrane proteins are classified as peripheral or integral (see Figure 10). **Integral membrane proteins** are actually embedded in the membrane, held there by hydrophobic interactions. Membrane-crossing regions are called **transmembrane domains** (see Figure 11). Integral membrane proteins may have a complex pattern of transmembrane domains and portions not within the membrane. [At which point in the secretory pathway would the insertion of transmembrane domains into the membrane occur?[15]] **Peripheral membrane proteins** are not embedded in the membrane at all, but rather are stuck to integral membrane proteins, held there by hydrogen bonding and electrostatic interactions.

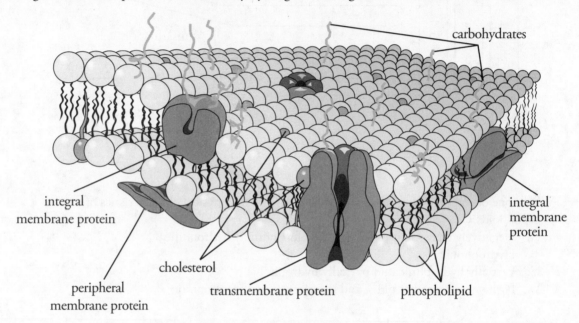

Figure 10 Membrane Proteins

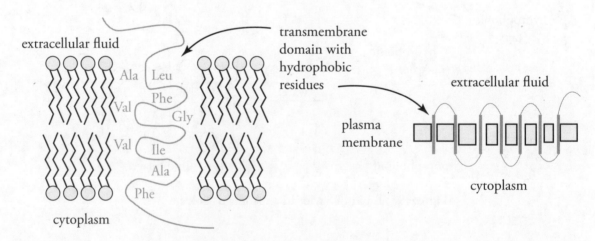

Figure 11 Transmembrane Domains

---

[15] It occurs in the rough ER as the protein is translated and threaded across the ER membrane.

The current understanding of membrane dynamics is termed the **fluid mosaic model**, because the membrane is seen as a mosaic of lipids and proteins that are free to move back and forth fluidly. According to this model, lipids and proteins are free to diffuse laterally, in two-dimensions, but are not free to flip-flop. Phospholipid head groups and hydrophilic protein domains are restricted from entering the hydrophobic membrane interior just as hydrophilic molecules in the extracellular space are. Hence the membrane is said to have **polarity**. This just means that the inside face and the outside face remain different. We have already discussed one such difference: all glycosylations are found on the extracellular face. So the "fluid" in "fluid mosaic" means that things are free to move back and forth, but in two dimensions only. One exception is that some proteins are anchored to the cytoskeleton and thus cannot move in any direction.

- Phospholipids can be covalently attached to a fluorescent tag and then integrated into a lipid bilayer. If one cell has a red fluorescent tagged lipid in its plasma membrane and another cell has a green fluorescent tagged lipid in its membrane, what will happen if the two cells are fused together?[16]

Fluidity of a membrane is affected by composition of lipids in the membrane (see Figure 12). Hydrophobic van der Waals interactions between fatty acid side chains are a major determinant of membrane fluidity. Saturated fatty acids, lacking any double bonds, have a very straight structure and pack tightly in the membrane, with strong van der Waals forces between side chains. Unsaturated fatty acids, with one or more double bonds, have a kinked structure and pack in the membrane interior more loosely. As we discussed in Chapter 2, cholesterol also plays a key role in maintaining optimal membrane fluidity by fitting into the membrane interior. [If the percentage of unsaturated fatty acids in a membrane is increased, will membrane fluidity increase or decrease at body temperature?[17]]

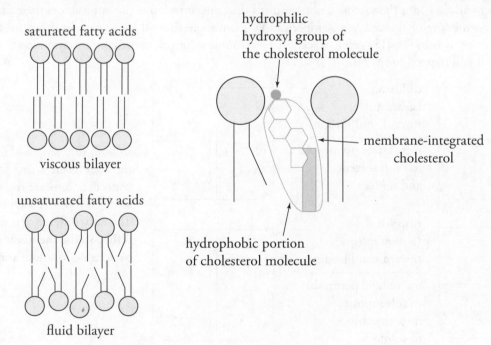

Figure 12 Factors Affecting Membrane Fluidity

---

[16] After a short period of time, the red and green tagged lipids will diffuse laterally and mix. An even distribution of the tags will be seen across the surface of the new hybrid cell.

[17] Unsaturated fatty acids, with a kinked structure, have fewer van der Waals interactions, and therefore allow a more fluid membrane structure. Increasing the unsaturated fatty acids will increase membrane fluidity.

5.3

Transmembrane Transport

The cell requires membranes to act as barriers to diffusion but also requires the transport of many different substances across membranes. Integral membrane proteins transport material through membranes that cannot diffuse on their own across membranes. Transport across a membrane can be either **passive** (does not require cellular energy) or **active** (requires cellular energy).

Review of Diffusion and Osmosis

Passive transport involves diffusion across a membrane. **Diffusion** is the tendency for liquids and gases to fully occupy the available volume (Figure 13). Particles in the liquid or gas phase are in constant motion, depending on temperature. If all particles are concentrated in one portion of a container, we have an orderly situation, which is unfavorable according to the second law of thermodynamics (law of entropy, see Chapter 3). The constant thermal motion of particles in the cell leads to their spreading out to occupy all available space, which maximizes entropy. A solute will always diffuse *down its* **concentration gradient**, which means *from high to low concentration*. Diffusion continues until a solute is evenly distributed throughout the available volume. At this point, movement of solute back and forth continues, but no net movement occurs.

Osmosis is a special type of diffusion in which solvent diffuses rather than solute (Figure 13). For example, if a chamber containing water and a chamber containing a solution of sucrose are connected directly, sucrose will diffuse throughout the entire volume until a uniform concentration is reached. However, if the two chambers are separated by a **semipermeable membrane** that allows water but not sucrose to cross, then diffusion of sucrose between the chambers cannot occur. In this case, osmosis draws water into the sucrose chamber to reduce the sucrose concentration as well as the volume in the water chamber. Ignoring gravity, water will flow into the sucrose chamber until the concentration is the same across the membrane. The plasma membrane of the cell is a semipermeable membrane that allows water—but not most polar solutes—to cross by osmosis. [If a cell is placed in a hypotonic solution (solute concentration lower than in the cell), what will happen to the cell?[18]]

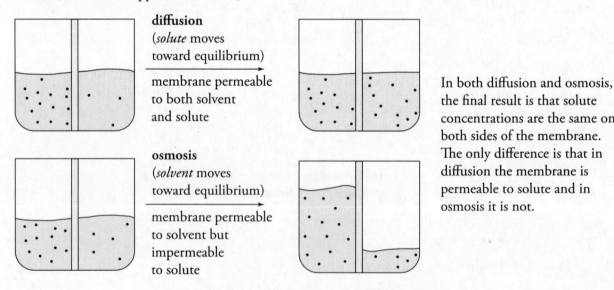

diffusion
(*solute* moves toward equilibrium)

membrane permeable to both solvent and solute

osmosis
(*solvent* moves toward equilibrium)

membrane permeable to solvent but impermeable to solute

In both diffusion and osmosis, the final result is that solute concentrations are the same on both sides of the membrane. The only difference is that in diffusion the membrane is permeable to solute and in osmosis it is not.

Figure 13   Diffusion and Osmosis

---

[18] Water will flow into the cell through the plasma membrane until the cell volume increases to the point that the cell bursts.

The term **tonicity** is used to describe osmotic gradients. If the environment is **isotonic** to the cell, the solute concentration is the same inside and outside. A **hypertonic** solution has more total dissolved solutes than the cell, a **hypotonic** solution has less. You may also hear the terms **isosmotic**, **hyperosmotic**, and **hypoosmotic**. The tendency of water to move down its concentration gradient can be a powerful force, able to cause cells to explode. This force is known as **osmotic pressure**. The greater the difference in tonicity across a semipermeable membrane, the greater the osmotic pressure. This is what accounts for the difference in fluid levels in the beaker at the bottom right-hand corner of Figure 13. The large difference in fluid levels may be a rather extreme example, but it is conceptually accurate: just as osmotic forces can cause a cell to rupture, they can overcome gravity, as shown.

Passive Transport

Passive transport is a biochemical term that means diffusion. It refers to any thermodynamically favorable movement of solute across a membrane. Another way to phrase this is to say that passive transport is any movement of solute down a gradient. No energy is required since the concentration gradient drives movement of the solute. There are two types of passive transport: simple diffusion and facilitated diffusion.

Simple Diffusion

Simple diffusion is diffusion of a solute through a membrane without help from a protein. For example, steroid hormones are free to move back and forth across the membrane by simple diffusion as pushed by concentration gradients, thanks to their ___.[19] Small and hydrophobic molecules can simply diffuse across the plasma membrane; these include O_2, CO_2, steroids, cholesterol, and fatty acids.

However, lipid bilayer membranes are impermeable to most solutes; that is one of the main functions of membranes. The plasma membrane is a barrier to the free movement of all large and/or hydrophilic solutes. **Facilitated diffusion** is the movement of a solute across a membrane, down a gradient, when the membrane itself (the pure lipid bilayer) is intrinsically impermeable to that solute. Specific integral membrane proteins allow material to cross the plasma membrane down a gradient in facilitated diffusion. For example, red blood cells require glucose, which they get from the bloodstream. However, glucose is a bulky hydrophilic molecule that cannot cross the RBC lipid bilayer. Instead, it must be shuttled across by a particular protein in the RBC plasma membrane. There are two well-characterized types of proteins which serve this sort of function: **channel proteins** and **carrier proteins**. Channels and carriers give the membrane its essential feature of **selective permeability**; permeability to *some* things despite impermeability to *most* things.

Facilitated Diffusion: Channels

Channel proteins in the plasma membrane allow material that cannot pass through the membrane by simple diffusion to flow through the plasma membrane down a concentration gradient. Channels do this by forming a narrow opening in the membrane surrounded by the protein. Channels are very selective in what passes through the opening in the membrane. There are many kinds of channels, each of which allows the passage of only one type of molecule (usually an ion) through the channel down a gradient (see Figure 14 on the following page). All cells have potassium ion leak channels, for example, that allow

---

[19] hydrophobicity

only potassium (and not sodium) to flow through the plasma membrane down a gradient. **Aquaporins**, also called water channels, are channel proteins that form pores in the membrane of biological cells, facilitating transport of water. Cell membranes of most bacteria, fungi, animal, and plant cells contain aquaporins. Ion channels are said to be **gated** if the channel is open in response to specific environmental stimuli. A channel that opens in response to a change in the electrical potential across the membrane is called a **voltage-gated** ion channel. One that opens in response to binding of a specific molecule like a neurotransmitter is called a **ligand-gated** ion channel. The regulation of membrane potential by gated ion channels plays a key role in the nervous system, which we'll discuss in Chapter 8. [Can ion channels move ions against an electrochemical gradient?[20]]

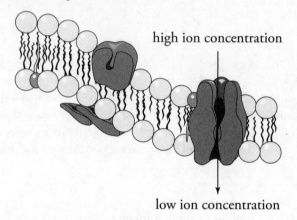

high ion concentration

low ion concentration

Figure 14   An Ion Channel

Facilitated Diffusion: Carriers

Carrier proteins also can transport molecules through membranes by facilitated diffusion, but they do so by a mechanism different from that of ion channels. Carrier proteins do not form a tunnel through membranes like ion channels do. Instead, carriers appear to bind the molecule to be transported at one side of the membrane and then undergo a conformational change to move the molecule to the other side of the membrane. Some carriers, called **uniports**, transport only one molecule across the membrane at a time (see Figure 15). Other carriers termed **symports** carry two substances across a membrane in the same direction. **Antiports**, on the other hand, carry two substances in opposite directions.

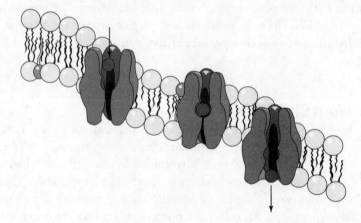

Figure 15   A Uniport

---

[20] No. Ion channels are only involved in facilitated diffusion, the movement of molecules down an electrochemical gradient with the help of a protein.

Pores and Porins

A **pore** is a tube through the membrane that is so large, it is *not selective* for any particular molecule. Rather, all molecules below a certain size may pass. Also, a molecule that is just barely small enough to cross may not cross if it has the wrong charge on its surface. Pores are formed by polypeptides known as **porins**. You are already familiar with several examples of pores. We have studied pores in the double nuclear membrane and the outer mitochondrial membrane. The eukaryotic plasma membrane does not have pores, because pores destroy the barrier function of the membrane, allowing solutes in the cytoplasm to freely diffuse out of the cell. [Are porins and ion channels found in the same membranes?[21]]

Active Transport

Active transport is the movement of molecules through the plasma membrane against a gradient. Active transport requires energy input, since it is working against a gradient, and always involves a protein. Another way of saying that active transport requires energy input is to say that the thermodynamically unfavorable transport process ($\Delta G > 0$) is coupled to a process which is thermodynamically favorable ($\Delta G < 0$). The gradient being pumped against is not necessarily just a concentration gradient, but for charged molecules, like ions, it can also involve electric potentials that form a combined electrochemical gradient that must be pumped against. The form of energy input used to drive movement of molecules against an electrochemical gradient varies. In **primary active transport**, the transport of a molecule is coupled to ATP hydrolysis. In **secondary active transport**, the transport process is not coupled *directly* to ATP hydrolysis. Instead, ATP is first used to create a gradient; then the potential energy in that gradient is used to drive the transport of some other molecule across the membrane. Since ATP is not used in the actual transport of the "other" molecule, the ATP use is described as *indirect*. For example, the transport of glucose into some cells is driven *against the glucose* concentration gradient by the cotransport of sodium ions *down the sodium* electrochemical gradient, previously established by an ATPase pump. A common mechanism driving secondary active transport of many different molecules involves coupling transport to the flow of sodium ions down a gradient.

- If a protein moves sodium ions across the plasma membrane down an electrochemical gradient, what form of transport is this?[22]
  - A. Simple diffusion
  - B. Facilitated diffusion
  - C. Primary active transport
  - D. Secondary active transport

---

[21] No. Porins are large holes, and ion channels are small, usually regulated channels. If porins and ion channels were found in the same membrane, the ion channels would be useless, because ions would flow in an unregulated manner through the pores.

[22] Facilitated diffusion is the movement of molecules down a gradient with the help of a protein (choice **B** is correct). Membrane proteins are not required for simple diffusion (choice A is wrong), and active transport involves moving things *against* their gradients (choices C and D are wrong). Note also that in secondary active transport, the ion movement down its gradient must be coupled to the movement of some other molecule against *its* gradient.

Na⁺/K⁺ ATPase and the Resting Membrane Potential

Na⁺/K⁺ ATPase is a transmembrane protein in the plasma membrane of pretty much all animal cells. This protein can also be called the sodium/potassium pump. It pumps 3 Na⁺ out of the cell, 2 K⁺ into the cell, and hydrolyzes one ATP to drive the pumping of these ions against their gradients (see Figure 16 on the following page). [The pumping of sodium and potassium by the Na⁺/K⁺ ATPase is an example of what form of transport?[23]] The sodium that is pumped out of the cell stays outside, since the plasma membrane is impermeable to sodium ions. Some of the potassium ions are able to leak back out, however, through **potassium leak channels**. Potassium flows down its concentration gradient out of the cell through leak channels. The movement of ions out of the cell helps the cell to maintain osmotic balance with its surroundings. As potassium leaves the cell through the leak channels, movement of positive charge out of the cell creates an electric potential across the plasma membrane with a net negative charge on the interior of the cell. This potential created by the Na⁺/K⁺ ATPase is known as the **resting membrane potential**. (The resting membrane potential will be examined again in Chapter 8 in relation to action potentials in neurons.) The concentration gradient of high sodium outside of the cell established by the Na⁺/K⁺ ATPase is the driving force behind secondary active transport of many different molecules, including sugars and amino acids. To summarize, the activity of the Na⁺/K⁺ ATPase is important in three ways. It:

1. maintains osmotic balance between the cellular interior and exterior
2. establishes the resting membrane potential
3. provides the sodium concentration gradient used to drive secondary active transport

- If an inhibitor of Na⁺/K⁺ ATPase is added to cells, which of the following may occur?[24]
   A. The cell will shrink and lose water.
   B. The interior of the cell will become less negatively charged.
   C. Secondary active transport processes will compensate for the loss of primary active transport.
   D. The cell will begin to proliferate.

---

[23] The pumping of ions against a gradient that is coupled to ATP hydrolysis is primary active transport.

[24] The Na⁺/K⁺ ATPase is required to establish the resting membrane potential in which the cellular interior has a negative charge. It pumps out one net positive ion. If this net positive ion stays inside the cell, the resting potential becomes less negative (choice **B** is correct). Since the interior of the cell is now more charged, the cell will have a tendency to take on water by osmosis, and will swell (choice A is wrong). Secondary active transport depends on the gradient established by primary active transport (the Na⁺/K⁺ pump). If the pump is shut down, the gradient won't be established, and secondary active transport will also stop (choice C is wrong). The Na⁺/K⁺ ATPase has nothing to do with cellular proliferation (choice D is wrong).

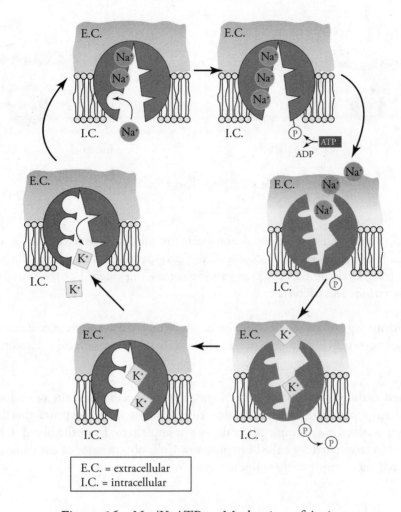

Figure 16 Na$^+$/K$^+$ ATPase Mechanism of Action

E.C. = extracellular
I.C. = intracellular

Endocytosis and Exocytosis

Another mechanism used to transport material through the plasma membrane is within membrane-bound vesicles that fuse with the membrane (see Figure 17 on the following page). This section is a pretty advanced DAT topic. It is possible you'll see a question on this stuff on test day, but it is not very likely. Focus on knowing a basic definition for key terms (which we've bolded for you) and plan your study time accordingly. **Exocytosis** is a process to transport material outside of the cell in which a vesicle in the cytoplasm fuses with the plasma membrane, and the contents of the vesicle are expelled into the extracellular space. The materials released are products secreted by the cell, such as hormones and digestive enzymes.

Endocytosis is the opposite of exocytosis: generally, materials are taken into the cell by an invagination of a piece of the cell membrane to form a vesicle. Again, the cytoplasm is not allowed to mix with the extracellular environment. The new vesicle which is formed is called an **endosome**. There are three types of endocytosis:

1. phagocytosis
2. pinocytosis
3. receptor-mediated endocytosis

5.3

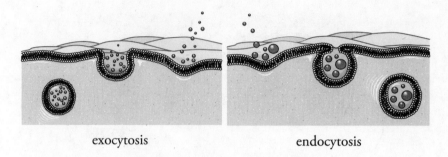

exocytosis   endocytosis

Figure 17   Endo- and Exocytosis

Phagocytosis means "cell eating." It refers to nonspecific uptake of large particulate matter into a phago-cytic vesicle, which later merges with a lysosome. Thus, phagocytosed material will be broken down. The prime example of phagocytic human cells are macrophages ("big eaters") of the immune system, which engulf and destroy viruses and bacteria.

Pinocytosis (cell drinking) is nonspecific uptake of small molecules and extracellular fluid via invagination. Primitive eukaryotic cells obtain nutrition in this manner, but virtually all eukaryotic cells participate in pinocytosis.

Receptor-mediated endocytosis, on the other hand, is very specific. The site of endocytosis is marked by pits coated with the molecule **clathrin** (inside the cell) and with **receptors** that bind to a specific molecule (outside the cell). One example is the uptake of cholesterol from the blood. Cholesterol is transported in the blood in large particles called lipoproteins. Cells obtain some of the cholesterol they require by receptor-mediated endocytosis of these lipoproteins.

Cell-Surface Receptors

Receptors form an important class of integral membrane proteins that transmit signals from the extracellular space into the cytoplasm. Each receptor binds a particular molecule in a highly specific lock-and-key interaction. The molecule that serves as the key for a given receptor is termed the **ligand** and is usually a hormone or a neurotransmitter. Binding of a ligand to its receptor on the extracellular surface of the plasma membrane triggers a response within the cell, a process termed **signal transduction**. Many cancers result from mutant cell-surface receptors that constitutively relay their signal to the cytoplasm, whether ligand is present or absent. For example, a growth factor exerts its effects by binding to a cell-surface receptor, and constitutive activity of a receptor for the growth factor causes uncontrolled growth of the cell. There are three main types of signal-transducing cell-surface receptors: ligand-gated ion channels, G-protein-linked receptors, and catalytic receptors.

Ligand-gated ion channels in the plasma membrane open an ion channel upon binding a particular neurotransmitter. An example is the ligand-gated sodium channel on the surface of the muscle cell at the neuromuscular junction. When the neurotransmitter acetylcholine binds to this receptor, the receptor undergoes a conformational change and becomes an open Na^+ channel. The result is a massive influx of sodium down its electrochemical gradient, which depolarizes the muscle cell and causes it to contract. We'll explore these channels more in the physiology chapters of this book.

A **G-protein-linked receptor** does not directly transduce its signal, but transmits it into the cell with the aid of a **second messenger**. This is a chemical signal that relays instructions from the cell surface to enzymes in the cytoplasm. The most important second messenger is **cyclic AMP (cAMP)**. It is known as a "universal hunger signal" because it is the second messenger of the hormones epinephrine and glucagon, which cause energy mobilization (glycogen and fat breakdown). Second messengers such as cAMP allow a much greater signal than a receptor alone produces (see Figure 18 on the following page). Let's look at an example: an epinephrine molecule activates one G-protein-linked receptor which activates many G-proteins, each G-protein activates many adenylyl cyclase enzymes, each adenylyl cyclase makes lots of cAMP from ATP, each cAMP activates many kinases, and each kinase phosphorylates many enzymes. Some of these enzymes will be activated, and others inactivated by phosphorylation, with the end result that the entire cell harmoniously works toward the same goal: energy mobilization.

Catalytic receptors have an enzymatic active site on the cytoplasmic side of the membrane. Enzyme activity (often kinase activity) is initiated by ligand binding at the extracellular surface. This initiates a signaling cascade, often using a small second messenger [What was the first messenger?[25]]. The message amplifies as it is propagated through the cell. Kinases phosphorylate macromolecules and phosphatases dephosphorylate them. Remember, phosphates act as molecular switches, turning biological macromolecules on and off. This can affect cell growth, transcription and gene expression, protein translation, and lots of their core cellular processes. The insulin receptor is an example of a tyrosine kinase. Modification of proteins with phosphates regulates their activity.

Catalytic and G-protein linked receptors are advanced DAT topics. It is possible you'll see a question on this content on the DAT, but it is not very likely. Plan your study time accordingly.

5.4 OTHER STRUCTURAL ELEMENTS OF THE CELL

Cytoskeleton

The animal cell **cytoskeleton** provides the structural support supplied by the cell wall in bacteria, plants, and fungi. It also allows movement of the cell and its appendages (such as cilia and flagella) and transport of substances within the cell. Animal cells have an internal cytoskeleton composed of three types of proteins: **microtubules**, **intermediate filaments**, and **microfilaments** (see Figure 18). Microtubules are the thickest; microfilaments the thinnest. All three are composed of noncovalently polymerized proteins; in other words, they are a massive example of quaternary protein structure.

---

[25] The primary (or first) messenger was the ligand binding a receptor on the cell surface. This is what initiates signal transduction.

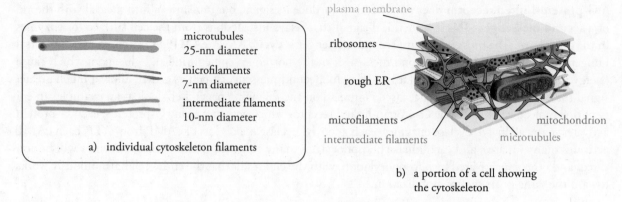

a) individual cytoskeleton filaments

b) a portion of a cell showing the cytoskeleton

Figure 18   Cytoskeleton

Microtubules

The **microtubule** is a hollow rod composed of two globular proteins: **α-tubulin** and **β-tubulin**, polymerized noncovalently. First, α-tubulin and β-tubulin form an αβ-tubulin dimer. Then many dimers stick to each other noncovalently to form a sheet, which rolls into a tube. Microtubules are dynamic and can get longer or shorter by adding or removing tubulin monomers from one end. The other end cannot elongate, because it is anchored to the **microtubule-organizing center** (**MTOC**), located near the nucleus.

The microtubule-organizing center is a structure found in eukaryotic cells from which microtubules emerge. There are two types of MTOCs in animal cells that you should be familiar with: centrosomes and basal bodies, associated with cilia and flagella.

Centrosomes are the major MTOC within a cell and play a key role in forming the spindle apparatus required to accurately separate and divide genetic material (chromosomes) between daughter cells during cell division (mitosis or meiosis). The majority of cells in our body contain either one or two centrosomes. Centrosomes are composed of two **centrioles** arranged at right angles to each other (Figure 19), and surrounded by a cloud of protein termed the pericentriolar material (PCM).

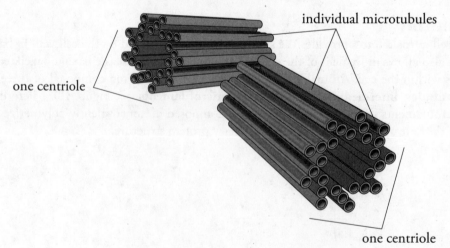

individual microtubules

one centriole

one centriole

Figure 19   A Pair of Centrioles

Each centriole is composed of a ring of nine microtubule triplets. When cell division occurs, centrioles duplicate, and one pair moves to each end of the cell. During mitosis, microtubules radiating out from the centrosomes attach to replicated chromosomes and pull them apart so that one copy of each chromosome (one chromatid) moves to each end of the cell. The resulting daughter cells each get a full copy of the genome plus a centriole pair. Things happen a little differently in meiosis but we'll discuss that in the next chapter.

The other type of MTOCs you should know are basal bodies that anchor and organize microtubules that make up cilia and flagella, which we'll discuss shortly.

Microtubules also mediate transport of substances within the cell. For example, in nerve cells, materials are transported from the cell body to the axon terminus on a microtubule railroad. Transport is driven by proteins that hydrolyze ATP and act as molecular motors along the microtubule.

Eukaryotic Cilia and Flagella

Cilia are small hairs on the cell surface that move fluids past the cell surface. For example, cilia on lining cells of the human respiratory tract continually sweep mucus toward the mouth in a mechanism termed the **mucociliary escalator**. A **flagellum** is a large tail which moves the cell by wiggling. The only human cell which has a flagellum is the ___.[26] Cilia are small and flagella are long, but they have the same structure, with a "**9 + 2**" arrangement of microtubules (see Figure 20). Nine pairs of microtubules form a ring around two lone microtubules in the center. Each microtubule is bound to its neighbor by a contractile protein called **dynein** which causes movement of the filaments past one another. The cilium or flagellum is anchored to the plasma membrane by a **basal body**, which has the same structure as a centriole (a ring of nine triplets of microtubules). The prokaryotic flagellum will be discussed later in this chapter; it is different in structure, and its motion is driven by a different mechanism.

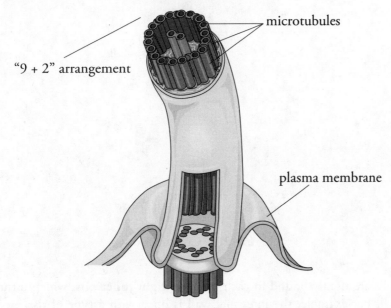

microtubules

"9 + 2" arrangement

plasma membrane

Figure 20 The Base of a Cilium or Flagellum

---

[26] sperm

Microfilaments

Microfilaments are rods formed in the cytoplasm from polymerization of the globular protein **actin**. Actin monomers form a chain, and then two chains wrap around each other to form an actin filament. Microfilaments are dynamic and are responsible for gross movements of the entire cell, such as pinching the dividing parent cell into two daughters during cell division, and **amoeboid movement**. Amoeboid movement involves changes in the cytoplasmic structure that cause a cell to move in one direction. As we'll see in Chapter 7, some protists (amoebae) use pseudopodia to perform amoeboid movement. In humans, some leukocytes (or white blood cells) can do this, too.

Intermediate Filaments

Intermediate filaments are named for their thickness, which is between that of microtubules and microfilaments. Unlike microtubules and microfilaments, intermediate filaments are heterogeneous, composed of a wide range of polypeptides, such as keratins. Another difference is that intermediate filaments are more permanent, whereas microfilaments and microtubules are often disassembled and reassembled as needed by the cell. Intermediate filaments are involved in providing strong cell structure, such as in resisting mechanical stress.

Cell Adhesion and Cell Junctions

There are three types of cell junctions you should recognize for the DAT: tight junctions, desmosomes, and gap junctions (Figure 21).

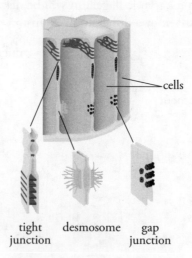

cells

tight junction   desmosome   gap junction

Figure 21   Cell Junctions

In some tissues, cells are tightly bound to each other by **tight junctions**, which form a band and tight seal around the cell. For example, the intestinal wall is lined with a type of tissue called epithelium.[27] These epithelial cells are connected by tight junctions to prevent items from moving freely between the intestinal lumen and the body.

---

[27] An epithelial cell layer is a layer of cells which lies "upon nipples" of a type of extracellular connective tissue called *basement membrane* (*epi-* means "upon," and *-thele* means "nipple," in the sense of a small bump). The basement membrane is a strong molecular sheet made of collagen. Under the microscope the basement membrane under epithelial cells has "bumps" which make epithelial cell layers easy to recognize.

5.4

Epithelial cells in the skin are held together tightly but do not form a complete seal; this is accomplished by **desmosomes**. Desmosomes do not form a band around the cell, but rather hold cells together at specific spots or concise points. These cell junctions are composed of a cytoplasmic plaque in the cell (which is anchored by intermediate filaments) and cadherin proteins.

Some specialized cell types are connected by holes called **gap junctions** that allow ions to flow back and forth between them. Gap junctions form pore-like connections (or tunnels) between adjacent cells, allowing their cytoplasms to mix. The connection is large enough to permit exchange of solutes such as ions, amino acids, and carbohydrates, but not polypeptides and organelles. Gap junctions in smooth muscle and cardiac muscle allow membrane depolarization of an action potential to pass directly from one cell to another.

5.5 THE CELL CYCLE AND MITOSIS

Cell Cycle

Our cells must reproduce themselves in order to replace lost or damaged cells and so that tissues can grow. Cells reproduce themselves by first doubling everything in the cytoplasm and the genome and then splitting in half. Some cells continually go through a cycle of growth and division, which is traditionally discussed in four phases (see Figure 22 on the following page). M phase includes mitosis and cytokinesis. Mitosis is the partitioning of cellular components (genes, organelles, etc.) into two halves. Cytokinesis is the physical process of cell division. The period of the cell's life cycle between mitotic divisions is called **interphase**. Interphase has three subphases: (1) G_1 **phase**, also called **gap phase 1**; (2) **S phase**, also called the **synthesis phase**; and (3) G_2 **phase**, also called **gap phase 2**.

- During G_1, the cell grows, runs metabolic pathways such as cell respiration, and builds proteins and organelles.
- During the S phase the cell reproduces its genome in preparation for division. This is done via DNA replication, which we reviewed earlier.
- During G_2, the cell continues to grow and synthesize proteins and organelles. It also prepares for mitosis.

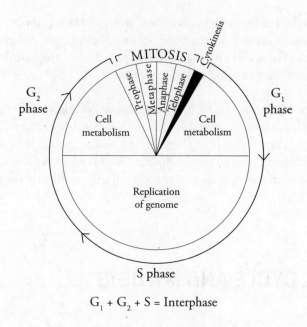

$$G_1 + G_2 + S = \text{Interphase}$$

Figure 22 The Cell Cycle

Replication of the Genome

We introduced chromosome structure in the last chapter. Let's return to it now, so you can understand how chromosomes move around during cell division. Centromeres divide a chromosome into arms; the p chromosome arm is the short one (p stands for petit, the French word for small) and the q chromosome arm is the larger one. Centromeres are also the part of a chromosome where identical sister **chromatids** are connected. Kinetochores are complexes of proteins associated with the centromere. This is where spindle fibers attach to move chromosomes around. Finally, telomeres are the ends of a chromosome. They vary in length and affect chromosome stability and cell aging or lifespan (which we'll talk about more later).

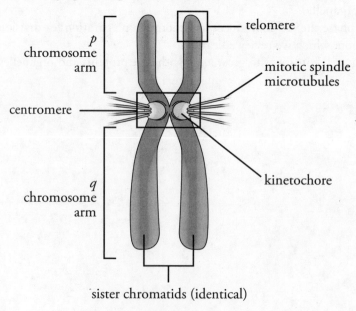

Figure 23 Chromosome Structure

During interphase, the genome is spread out in a form that is only visible using special stains under a light microscope, and DNA is accessible to the enzymes of replication. By the end of S phase, the nucleus contains two complete copies of the genome and the cell now has twice the normal amount of DNA. Let's look at how this happens. During the S phase of interphase, all 23 pairs of the cell's chromosomes replicate. When replication is complete, each chromosome has a duplicate. Each pair of duplicates is joined at a **centromere**. These duplicates are called sister chromatids and because they are the product of DNA replication, sister chromatids are identical to each other.

Before a chromosome duplicates itself, it is, of course, one chromosome. Even after it duplicates itself (and the DNA quantity is doubled), the duplicated unit is still considered one chromosome. Here is another way to think about this: before DNA replication, each of your 46 chromosomes is present in a single copy. This means there is one chromatid per chromosome. Each chromosome has a centromere that divides it into two arms, and each chromosome is made of one long piece of double-stranded DNA. After DNA replication, each chromosome is made of two identical chromatids, connected together at the centromere. Now there are two identical pieces of DNA and four arms coming out of the centromere, so each chromosome looks like the letter X (once it is condensed).

This section is pretty confusing for most people, so let's look at this another way:

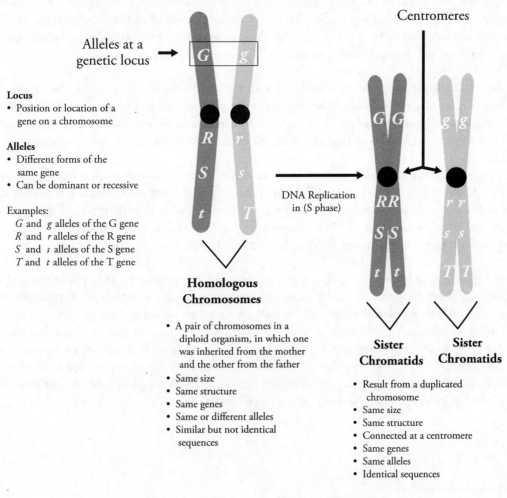

Figure 24 Chromosomes and Chromatids

Before DNA replication, a human cell has 23 pairs of chromosomes. Even after replication, for as long as duplicated pairs are joined at their centromeres, the cell still has only 23 pairs of chromosomes, each chromosome comprising a pair of sister chromatids. Each pair of sister chromatids (joined at a centromere) represents what *will* become two separate chromosomes. It is very important that you're clear on all this terminology before getting into mitosis, so you may want to go back and read that section again.

Mitosis is divided into four phases: **prophase**, **metaphase, anaphase**, and **telophase**.[28] The first sign of prophase is that the genome becomes visible upon condensing into densely packed chromosomes, instead of diffuse chromatin. [Why do the chromosomes condense?[29]] Observing a human cell under the light microscope at the beginning of prophase, one can see 46 X-shaped chromosomes; each contains two identical sister chromatids. Spending a little more time staring at the nucleus, you might notice that the jumble of 46 chromatid pairs actually consists of 23 **homologous pairs** of identical-appearing sister chromatid pairs (23 pairs of pairs). Homologous chromosomes are different copies of the same chromosome, one from your mother and the other from your father. To repeat:

Sister chromatids are identical copies of a chromosome, attached to each other at the centromere. Homologous chromosomes are equivalent but nonidentical and do not come anywhere near each other during mitosis.

Other important events occur during prophase. The nucleolus disappears, the spindle and kinetochore fibers appear, and the centriole pairs begin to move to opposite ends of the cell. So now the cell has two MTOCs, called **asters** (stars) because of the star-like appearance of microtubules radiating out. Also at the end of prophase, the nuclear envelope converts itself into many tiny vesicles.

During metaphase, kinetochore fibers associated with the centromeres interact with the mitotic spindle, allowing movement of chromosomes. Chromosomes are pushed and pulled by the mitotic spindle and eventually align on the **metaphase plate** so that centromeres lie in a plane along an axis at the cell's midpoint. Kinetochore fibers help to align and maintain the chromosomes on the metaphase plate.

During anaphase, the spindle fibers shorten, and the centromeres of each sister chromatid pair are pulled apart. Sister chromatids separate as a result of the splitting of the centromere and move toward opposite poles of the cell along the path marked by the spindle apparatus. With the separation of sister chromatids, each chromatid is called a **daughter chromosome**. The cell elongates, and **cytokinesis** begins with the formation of a **cleavage furrow** along the equator of the cell, which is accomplished by ___.[30]

In telophase (*telos* is Greek for "end"), daughter chromosomes are positioned at opposite poles of the cell, and kinetochore fibers disappear. A nuclear membrane forms around the bunch of chromosomes at each end of the cell, and the chromosomes decondense and are no longer visible by light microscopy. A nucleolus becomes visible within each new daughter nucleus. Each daughter nucleus has $2n$ chromosomes; mitosis and nuclear division are now complete. Meanwhile, the cleavage furrow continues to deepen until it ultimately divides the cell, forming two daughter cells. Cytokinesis is complete, and the cell is split in two (see Figure 25 on the following page). Each daughter cell possesses a diploid number of chromosomes. The daughter cells then enter the interphase period of the cell cycle.

---

[28] A mnemonic is "I Pee on the MAT," where I is for interphase.

[29] Presumably so that they can be separated without tangling.

[30] A ring of microfilaments encircling the cell and contracting

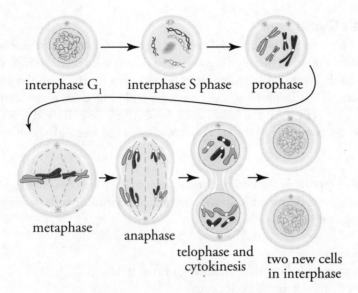

interphase G_1 interphase S phase   prophase

metaphase   anaphase   telophase and cytokinesis   two new cells in interphase

Figure 25   Phases of Mitosis

The above diagram is worth considering for a moment before you move on. In the prophase and metaphase diagrams, we were looking at a cell with four X-shaped chromosomes. In anaphase, the cell has eight linear chromosomes. When sister chromatids separate from each other, each becomes a chromosome; the number of chromosomes doubles. This means that during anaphase, the cell goes from being $2n$ with duplicated chromosomes, to being $4n$ (**tetraploid**) with single copy chromosomes. For example, human cells at this point contain 96 chromosomes.

Inappropriate cell division can have disastrous consequences. A mutation in a protein that is normally involved in regulating progression through the cell cycle can result in unregulated cell division and cancer. Cancer means "**crab**," as in the zodiac sign. The name derives from the observation that malignant tumors grow into the surrounding tissue, embedding themselves like clawed crabs. Mutated genes that induce cancer are termed **oncogenes.** ("*Onco-*" is a prefix denoting cancer.) Normally, these genes are required for proper growth of the cell.

- In normal eukaryotic cells, mitosis will not begin until the entire genome is replicated. If this inhibition is removed so that mitosis begins during S-phase, which one of the following would occur?[31]
  - A.   The cells would grow more quickly.
  - B.   The genome would become fragmented and incomplete.
  - C.   The cells would display unregulated, cancerous growth.
  - D.   The genome would be temporarily incomplete in each daughter cell, but DNA repair will fill in missing gaps.

---

[31] If the genome is not completely replicated and condensed prior to mitosis, it will be torn during cell division. Each daughter cell will receive only pieces of the genome rather than the complete genome and will not be able to survive (choice **B** is correct and A and C are wrong). DNA repair systems can only repair sequence errors or minor structural problems; this problem would be too large to fix (choice D is wrong).

Some Cells Don't Cycle

Eukaryotic cells don't have to always actively cycle and grow. Cells can exit the cell cycle to become a more specialized (or differentiated) non-cycling cell or to die via apoptosis. In fact, the more specialized a cell becomes, the less likely it is to remain capable of reproducing itself. Examples are neurons, blood cells, and cells on the surface of the skin. These cells must be replenished by reproduction of less specialized precursor cells called stem cells.[32] All the blood cells, for example, are derived from a single type of stem cell found in the bone marrow. One of things that can cause a cell to exit the cell cycle is the length of its telomeres.

Telomeres are disposable repeats at the end of chromosomes. They are consumed and shorten during each cell division. When telomeres become too short, they reach a critical length where a chromosome can no longer replicate. In response to this, cells can:

1. Activate DNA repair pathways
2. Enter a senescent state (where they are alive but not dividing)
3. Activate apoptosis (programmed cell death)

The **Hayflick limit** is the number of times a normal human cell type can divide until telomere length stops cell division. Many age-related diseases are linked to telomere shortening.

Senescence and Quiescence

Cells can stay alive without actively growing and progressing through the cell cycle. For example, senescent cells are alive and metabolically active but do not actively divide. Entering **senescence** is irreversible; the cell cannot re-enter the cell cycle. Some examples of senescent cells in your body are your red blood cells and the cells on the surface of your skin.

In contrast, some cells can exit the cell during G_1, enter a state called **quiescence**, and then go back into the cell cycle and continue dividing and growing. Quiescence can also be called G_0, and cells can usually only get into G_0 from G_1. Like senescent cells, quiescent cells are alive and metabolically active, but not actively dividing. However, unlike senescent cells, quiescent cells can re-enter the cell cycle. Many types of nerve cells and cardiac muscle cells are typically quiescent.

Apoptosis

Apoptosis, or programed cell death, allows a cell to shrink and die while simultaneously minimizing damage to neighboring cells and limiting the exposure of other cells to its cytosolic contents. Death of a cell is triggered by a stressor which may be external (such as nitric oxide, a toxin, or cytokines) or internal (such as when the level of the p53 tumor suppressor protein reaches a critical level). This activates a signaling pathway that increases the permeability of the mitochondria. As a result, **cytochrome c** is released from mitochondria. You may remember cytochrome c from cell respiration. This small hemeprotein is normally found loosely associated with the inner membrane of the mitochondrion. It is a component of the electron transport chain in mitochondria, where it performs a redox reaction but does not transfer any protons across the inner mitochondrial membrane. However, cytochrome c is also involved in initiation of apoptosis.

---

[32] Stem cells are undifferentiated cells from which all other cells with specialized functions are derived. Under the right conditions, stem cells divide to form either new stem cells or more specialized and differentiated cells. No other cell in the body has the natural ability to generate new cell types. In Chapter 11, we'll review two types of stem cells: embryonic stem cells and adult stem cells.

The process of apoptosis involves dismantling the cell from the inside. This is mainly done by a family of proteases, referred to as **caspases**. Because these enzymes damage cellular material, they are produced in their inactive (or zymogen) form as procaspases. Twelve different caspases have been identified in humans, and they are generally grouped into two categories, initiators and effectors. Initiator caspases respond to extra- or intracellular death signals by clustering together. This clustering allows them to activate each other. Activation of the initiators leads to activation of effector caspases in a cascade of activation. Effector caspases then cleave a variety of cellular proteins to trigger apoptosis.

Consequently, the cell begins shrinking. The cytoskeleton is disassembled. While the cellular infrastructure is taken apart, the nuclear envelope breaks down and the genome is broken into pieces. The ER, Golgi, and mitochondria are fragmented, and hundreds of proteins are degraded. A different profile of cell surface proteins emerges, thus signaling various phagocytic cells, including macrophages, to finish deconstructing and clearing away the dead cell.

While cell death sounds like it is a bad thing, apoptosis is a normal part of development and health in multicellular organisms. It protects us against pre-cancerous cells and cells that have been infected by a virus and contributes to normal cell turnover.

5.6 CELL BIOLOGY LAB TECHNIQUES

Several types of microscopes are used in biology labs. **Light microscopes** use visible light and a system of lenses to magnify images of small samples. Many models are available with varying resolution and sample contrast. **Electron microscopes** use a beam of accelerated electrons as a source of illumination. Since the wavelength of an electron is much shorter than that of a visible light photon, electron microscopes have a higher resolving power than light microscopes. **Transmission electron microscopes (TEMs)** produce 2D images that have very high magnification and great resolution, whereas **scanning electron microscopes (SEMs)** produce 3D images.

Centrifugation

Centrifugation is the process of spinning a sample at high speed. This pellets cells and precipitates molecules at the bottom of the tube, and leaves everything else in the liquid layer above (called the **supernatant**). Here is an example:

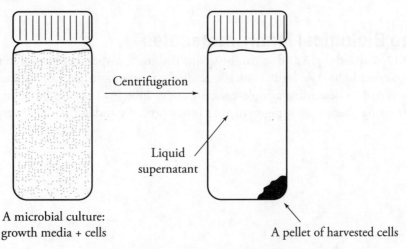

Centrifugation

Liquid supernatant

A microbial culture: growth media + cells

A pellet of harvested cells

Figure 26   Centrifugation

Cell Lysis

Protein biochemistry often requires lysates to be collected. A **cell lysate** is a solution that contains hundreds of different proteins from a certain cell population. Here is a summary of the steps used to collect a lysate sample:

1. If a tissue is being used, it must be **homogenized** in a buffer solution first. Homogenization breaks up the tissue structure and cell-to-cell connections to release individual cells into solution. Mechanisms for homogenization include grinding, mincing, and chopping.
2. Cells are collected as a soft pellet at the bottom of a tube via centrifugation.
3. Cells are resuspended in a **lysis buffer**, which contains buffers and detergents. The detergent solubilizes the plasma membrane to release cytoplasmic contents. If the cell contains a cell wall, mechanical disruption can be used in this step to help break the cell wall open. For example, yeast cells are shaken at high speeds with small glass beads to help break open their thick chitin cell wall.
4. The solution is centrifuged again. Insoluble proteins, broken membranes, unlysed cells, organelles and other cell debris from a pellet at the bottom of the tube (which is thrown out). The solution above the pellet (or supernatant) is the lysate sample.

Cell Fractionation

Cell fractionation separates subcellular components into different samples, while preserving individual functions of each component. A lysate is centrifuged in several steps, starting with low speeds, and gradually increasing the speed; this is called differential centrifugation and allows the separation and collection of cell components and organelles according to their density and size. After each centrifugation, the pellet is removed, and the centrifugal force is increased. Here is the general order that cell components are collected, from low speeds and short intervals (a) to more force and longer durations (d):

a. Whole cells, nuclei, cytoskeleton
b. Mitochondria, chloroplasts, lysosomes, peroxisomes
c. Endoplasmic reticulum, Golgi, vesicles, plasma membrane; these components usually fragment into small membrane-bound structures called **microsomes**
d. Ribosomes, centrosomes, centrioles, cytosol, proteins, viruses

Quantifying Biological Macromolecules

Both DNA and RNA absorb light and so can be quantified using a **spectrophotometer**. DNA (or RNA) is exposed to ultraviolet light (UV light). Nucleic acids absorb the light, and this is quantified as optical density, then converted to determine sample concentration. Proteins can also be quantified in a spectrophotometer by reacting them with a pigment that binds proteins and shifts the absorption peak of the sample.

Blots

Western blotting allows you to detect the presence of certain proteins within a sample (usually a cell lysate) and serves as a diagnostic tool. Proteins are separated by electrophoresis; then a primary antibody is used to detect a specific protein. An enzyme-linked secondary antibody is added to amplify and detect the signal of the target protein.

Southern blotting allows you to detect the presence of specific sequences within a heterogeneous sample of DNA. The method is named after Edwin Southern (a British biologist) who first published it in 1975. First, DNA fragments are separated via gel electrophoresis. Hybridization probes complementary to the target DNA are generated (often with radiolabeled nucleotides) and detected to identify a particular DNA sequence. **Northern blots** work the same way but study RNA (which is much less stable than DNA. This makes Northern blots typically more difficult to perform than Southern blots).

5.7

5.7 PROKARYOTES (DOMAIN BACTERIA)

The primary feature of prokaryotes that distinguishes them from eukaryotes is that they do not contain **membrane-bound organelles** (nucleus, mitochondria, lysosomes, etc.). *Prokaryote* means "before the nucleus," and the lack of a nucleus indicates that prokaryotes are evolutionarily the oldest kingdom. Unlike viruses however, prokaryotes possess all of the machinery required for life. They are true cells, true living organisms. The prokaryotes include **Eubacteria**, **Archaea** (extremophiles), and **blue-green algae** (cyanobacteria).

Classification of living organisms, **taxonomy**, is an important part of biology because it is used to determine the evolutionary relationship of organisms to one another. The largest taxonomic division is the **Domain**. There are three recognized domains: Bacteria, Archaea, and Eukarya. Domains Bacteria and Archaea include prokaryotic organisms, and Domain Eukarya includes eukaryotic organisms. Each domain can be further subdivided into **Kingdoms**. Currently there are three well-recognized eukaryotic kingdoms (Animalia, Plantae, and Fungi), and great debate over the number of kingdoms that should be present in the other prokaryotic domains and in the single-celled eukaryotes (protists).

Bacterial Structure and Classification

Contents of the Cytoplasm

In this section we will tour the bacterial cell from the inside out. Unlike a eukaryotic cell, there are *no membrane-bound organelles* in prokaryotic cells (note that ribosomes, which are *not* membrane-bound, *are* found in bacteria). The prokaryotic genome is a single double-stranded circular DNA chromosome.[33] It is not located in a nucleus and is not associated with histone proteins, as the eukaryotic genome is. In prokaryotes the genome is localized in the cell, but without a nuclear envelope to form a separate compartment, the genome remains accessible to the cytoplasm. In prokaryotes, replication, transcription and

---

[33] There are a few exceptions to this (e.g., bacteria with more than one chromosome and/or linear chromosomes), but you do not have to know them for the DAT.

translation, and everything else all happen in the same compartment (the cytoplasm). Remember, in eukaryotes, replication, transcription, and splicing occur in the nucleus, while translation occurs in the cytoplasm.

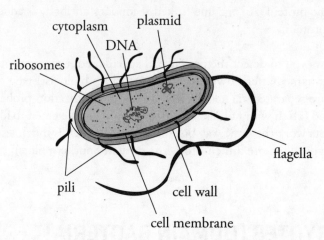

Figure 27   A Prokaryote

In bacteria, transcription and translation occur not only in the same place, but at the same time. Ribosomes begin to translate mRNA before it is completely transcribed. Many ribosomes translating a single piece of mRNA form a structure known as a polyribosome.

[In Figure 28 below, is the free end of the mRNA the 3' or the 5' end? Which end of the nascent polypeptides is the free end?[34]] Remember that the bacterial ribosome is structurally different from the eukaryotic ribosome, though both function the same way. The differences allow us to prescribe various antibiotics which interfere with bacterial translation without disrupting our own. (Examples are streptomycin and tetracycline, which only bind to bacterial ribosomes.)

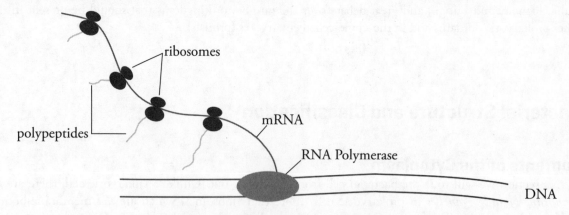

Figure 28   A Prokaryotic Polyribosome

---

[34] The 5' end of the mRNA polymer is free, since elongation of mRNA proceeds 5' to 3'. Proteins are made N to C, so the free end of the polypeptides is the N terminus.

One last genetic element that can be found in prokaryotic cells is the **plasmid**. This is a circular piece of double-stranded DNA which is much smaller than the genome. Plasmids are referred to as **extrachromosomal genetic elements**. They often encode gene products which may confer an advantage upon a bacterium carrying the plasmid. For example, plasmids frequently carry antibiotic-resistance genes (genes that encode proteins which can break down antibiotics). Many plasmids are capable of autonomous replication, which means that a single plasmid molecule within a bacterial cell may cause itself to be replicated into many copies. Plasmids are important not only because they may encode advantageous gene products, but also because they orchestrate bacterial exchange of genetic information, or **conjugation.**

Bacterial Shape

Bacteria are often classified according to their shape. The three shapes and their proper names are organized in the following table:

Shape	Proper name (plural)	Proper name (singular)
round	cocci	coccus
rod-shaped	bacilli	bacillus
spiral-shaped	spirochetes or spirilla	spirochete, spirillum

Table 2   Bacterial Classification by Shape

Cell Membrane and Cell Wall

The bacterial cytoplasm is bound by a lipid bilayer which is similar to our own plasma membrane. Outside the lipid bilayer is a rigid **cell wall**. It provides support for the cell, preventing lysis due to osmotic pressure. (As we have discussed, animal cells lack a cell wall. They deal with the problem of osmotic pressure by continuously pumping ions across the cell membrane.) The bacterial cell wall is composed of **peptidoglycan**, a complex polymer unique to prokaryotes. It contains cross-linked chains made of sugars and amino acids, including D-alanine, which is not found in animal cells (our amino acids have the L configuration). The bacterial cell wall is the target of many antibiotics, such as penicillin. The enzyme **lysozyme**, which is found in tears and saliva and made by lytic viruses, destroys the peptidoglycan in the bacterial cell wall, resulting in an osmotically fragile structure called a **protoplast**. [Would a protoplast moved from salt water to fresh water shrivel or burst?[35]]

Gram Staining of the Cell Wall

As part of our tour of the bacterial cell, we will say a word about classification of bacteria according to two different types of cell wall. The method of classification is derived from the extent to which bacteria turn color in a procedure termed **Gram staining**. The two groupings are **Gram-positive**, which stain strongly (a dark purple color), and **Gram-negative** bacteria, which stain weakly (a light pink color).

Gram-positive bacteria have a thick peptidoglycan layer outside of the cell membrane and no other layer beyond this. Gram-negative bacteria have a thinner layer of peptidoglycan in the cell wall but have an additional outer layer containing lipopolysaccharide. The intermediate space in Gram-negative bacteria between the cell membrane and the outer layer is termed the **periplasmic space**, in which are sometimes found enzymes that degrade antibiotics (see Figure 29). The increased protection of Gram-negative

---

[35]   It would burst, since water would flow into the cell by osmosis.

bacteria from the environment is reflected in their weak staining, as well as in their increased resistance to antibiotics. [Which bacteria would be more susceptible to lysis when treated with lysozyme: Gram-positive or Gram-negative?[36]]

5.7

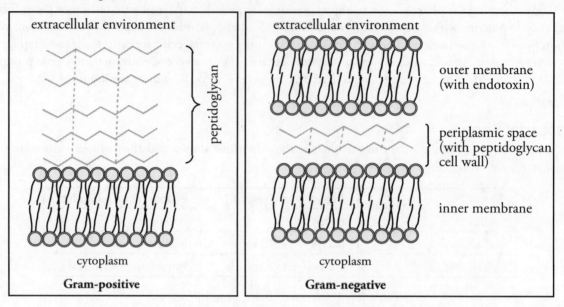

Figure 29 Gram-positive vs. Gram-negative Bacteria

The Capsule

Another attribute that only some bacteria have is the **capsule** or **glycocalyx**. This is a sticky layer of polysaccharide "goo" surrounding the bacterial cell and often surrounding an entire colony of bacteria. It makes bacteria more difficult for immune system cells to eradicate. It also enables bacteria to adhere to smooth surfaces such as rocks in a stream or the lining of the human respiratory tract.

Flagella

Another item only some bacteria have are long, whip-like filaments known as **flagella**, which are involved in bacterial motility. A bacterium which possesses one or more flagella is said to be **motile**, because flagella are the only means of bacterial locomotion. Bacteria may be **monotrichous** (meaning they have a flagellum located at only one end), **amphitrichous** (meaning they have a flagellum located at both ends), or **peritrichous** (meaning that they have multiple flagella). The following is which?[37]

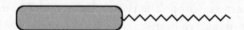

The structure of the flagellum is fairly complicated, with components encoded by over 35 genes, but it can be broken down into a few major components: the **filament**, the **hook**, and the **basal structure** (Figure 30). The basal structure contains a number of rings that anchor the flagellum to the inner and

---

[36] Lysozyme hydrolyzes linkages in peptidoglycan to weaken the cell wall. The peptidoglycan in Gram-positive cells is more accessible, since these cells do not possess an additional outer layer; therefore, Gram-positive cells will lyse more easily when treated with lysozyme.

[37] Monotrichous

outer membrane (for a Gram-negative bacterium) and serve to rotate the **rod** and the rest of the attached flagellum in either a clockwise or counterclockwise manner. The most important thing to remember about the prokaryotic flagellum is that its structure is different from the eukaryotic one (which contains a "9 + 2" arrangement of microtubules, discussed earlier in this chapter). In addition, the prokaryotic flagellum spins in a circle while the eukaryotic flagella waves from side to side.

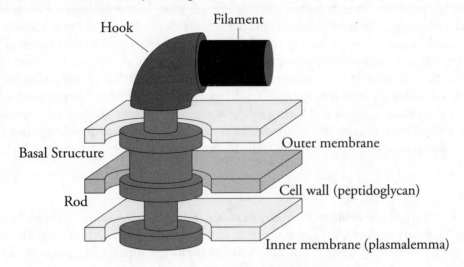

Figure 30   The Prokaryotic Flagellum

Rotation of the rod requires a large amount of energy (that is, ATP), which is supplied by diffusion of H^+ down a proton gradient generated across the inner membrane by electron transport. Bacterial motion can be directed toward attractants, such as food, or away from toxins, such as acid, in a process termed **chemotaxis**. The connection between chemotaxis and flagellar propulsion is dependent upon **chemoreceptors** on the cell surface that bind attractants or repellents and transmit a signal which influences the direction of flagellar rotation. A good analogy would be the blind man's bluff game played by children, in which a person is blindfolded and moves randomly but selects among favorable or unfavorable movements toward the goal based on the responses "warmer" or "colder" (like chemoreceptors binding attractant or repellent and sending a signal to the bacteria to tumble or not to tumble). The response of flagellar rotation to chemical attractants (or repellents) is not dependent on an *absolute* concentration, but to a *change* in the concentration over time. Thus, as the bacterium moves through the solution, it is able to detect whether it is moving toward or away from the highest concentration and respond accordingly.

Pili

Pili are long projections or protein bristles on the bacterial surface involved in attaching to different surfaces. They can also be called **fimbriae**. The **sex pilus** is a special pilus attaching F^+ (male) and F^- (female) bacteria that facilitates the formation of **conjugation bridges**. Other pili are smaller and function in adhering to surfaces. [What other bacterial structure is involved in adhering to surfaces? Is it possible that pili play a role in infection by pathogenic organisms?[38]]

---

[38] The capsule, or glycocalyx is also involved in adherence. Yes, short fimbriae do play a role in infection, by facilitating adhesion to cells so that the bacteria can colonize a tissue.

Bacterial Growth Requirements and Classification

Temperature

Another characteristic of bacteria used to categorize them is their ability to tolerate environmental variables, such as temperature. Though bacteria as a group can grow at a wide range of temperatures, each species has an optimal growth temperature. If the temperature is too high or too low, bacteria fail to grow and may be killed, hence the use of boiling to kill bacteria and refrigeration to slow bacterial growth and prevent food spoilage. Most bacteria favor mild temperatures similar to the ones that humans and other organisms favor; this is usually in the range of room temperature (20°C) to body temperature (37°C). These bacteria are called **mesophiles**. They are moderate temperature lovers. **Thermophiles** (heat lovers) can survive at temperatures up to 100°C in boiling hot springs or near geothermal vents in the ocean floor. Bacteria that thrive at very low temperatures (near 0°C) are termed **psychrophiles** (cold lovers). [How might a decrease in temperature increase the bacterial growth rate of a psychrophile?[39]]

Nutrition

Bacteria can be classified according to their *carbon source* and their *energy source*. "Troph" is a Latin root meaning "eat." **Autotrophs** use CO_2 as their carbon source. **Heterotrophs** rely on organic nutrients (glucose, for example) created by other organisms. **Chemotrophs** get their energy from chemicals. **Phototrophs** get their energy from light; not only plants but also some bacteria and some protists do this. Each bacterium is either a chemotroph or a phototroph and is either an autotroph or a heterotroph. There are thus four types of bacteria:

1. **Chemoautotrophs** build organic macromolecules from CO_2 using the energy of chemicals. They obtain energy by oxidizing inorganic molecules like H_2S.
2. **Chemoheterotrophs** require organic molecules such as glucose made by other organisms as their carbon source and for energy. We are chemoheterotrophs.
3. **Photoautotrophs** use only CO_2 as a carbon source and obtain their energy from the Sun. Plants are photoautotrophs.
4. **Photoheterotrophs** are odd in that they get their energy from the Sun, like plants, but require an organic molecule made by another organism as their carbon source.

* A bacterium that causes an infection in the bloodstream of humans is most likely to be classified as which one of the following?[40]
    A. Chemoautotroph
    B. Photoautotroph
    C. Chemoheterotroph
    D. Photoheterotroph

---

[39] Normally you expect decreasing temperature to decrease the rate of all chemical, biochemical, and biological processes, since reactions accelerate when kinetic energy increases. However, bacteria which have evolved to live at low temperatures (psychrophiles) possess enzymes which may be optimally active at low temperatures, leading to better growth.

[40] Since there's no sunlight in the bloodstream, B and D are out. If it's a parasite, it most likely uses some of our chemicals, so it must be a heterotroph, which eliminates A. The answer is **C**.

5.7

- Which one of the following categories best describes an organism which uses sunlight to drive ATP production but cannot incorporate carbon dioxide into sugars?[41]
  A. Chemoautotroph
  B. Photoautotroph
  C. Chemoheterotroph
  D. Photoheterotroph

Growth Media

The environment in which bacteria grow is the **medium** (plural: **media**). In the lab, the most common solid medium is agar, a firm transparent gel made from seaweed. Bacteria live in the agar but do not metabolize it. The agar is usually kept in a clear plastic plate called a **Petri dish**, and the process of putting bacteria on such a plate is called **plating**. When one bacterium is plated onto a dish, if it grows, it will eventually give rise to many progeny in an isolated spot called a **colony. Minimal medium** contains nothing but glucose (in addition to the agar). More key terms: a **wild-type** bacterium (or a wild-type strain) is one which possesses all the characteristics normal to that particular species. The dense growth of bacteria seen in laboratory Petri dishes is known as a bacterial **lawn**. A **plaque** is a clear area in the lawn. Plaques result from death of bacteria and are caused by lytic viruses or toxins.

Bacteria can reproduce very rapidly, provided that the conditions of their environment are favorable and nutrients are abundant. The **doubling time** is the amount of time required for a population of bacteria to double its number. It ranges from a minimum of 20 minutes for *E. coli* to a day or more for slow growers, such as the bacteria responsible for tuberculosis and leprosy. The doubling time of a bacterial species will vary, depending upon the availability of nutrients and other environmental factors.

One other important term in bacterial nutrition is **auxotroph** (don't confuse this term with *auto*troph; you must read carefully enough on the DAT to ensure you notice differences like this). This is a bacterium which cannot survive on minimal medium because it can't synthesize a molecule it needs to live. Hence, it requires an *aux*iliary *troph*ic substance to live. For instance, a bacterium which is auxotrophic for arginine won't form a colony when plated onto minimal medium, but if the medium is supplemented with arginine, a colony will form. This arginine auxotrophy is denoted Arg⁻. Auxotrophy results from a mutation in a gene coding for an enzyme in a synthetic pathway.

Bacteria can be differentiated not only by what substances they require, but also by what substances they are capable of metabolizing for energy. For instance, a strain of bacteria may be capable of surviving on minimal medium that has the disaccharide lactose as the only carbon source (no glucose). This would be denoted lac⁺. Mutation in a gene for the enzyme lactase would impair the bacterium's ability to survive on lactose-only medium. A bacterial strain incapable of growing with lactose as its only carbon source would be denoted lac⁻. Now is a good time to go back and review the lac operon (which we reviewed in the last chapter) if you need a refresher. Genetic exchange between bacteria by means of conjugation, transduction, or transformation (discussed later in this section) can remedy these disadvantages.

---

[41] The ability to use sunlight indicates that the organism is a phototroph, and the inability to use carbon dioxide as a carbon source indicates that it is a heterotroph—it must use organic molecules as a carbon source. The answer is **D**.

5.7

Oxygen Use and Tolerance

Oxygen metabolism is *aerobic* metabolism. Bacteria that require oxygen are called **obligate aerobes**. Bacteria that do not require oxygen are called **anaerobes**. There are three subcategories: **facultative anaerobes** will use oxygen when it's around, but don't need it. [How much more ATP can they make per glucose molecule when O_2 is present?[42]] **Tolerant anaerobes** can grow in the presence or absence of oxygen but do not use it in their metabolism. **Obligate anaerobes** are poisoned by oxygen. This is because they lack certain enzymes necessary for the detoxification of free radicals which form spontaneously whenever oxygen is around.[43] Obligate anaerobes commonly infect wounds.

- If a bacterium cannot use oxygen as an electron acceptor, is it an obligate anaerobe, a tolerant anaerobe, a facultative anaerobe, or is it not possible to distinguish based on the information given?[44]

- A sample of bacteria is evenly mixed into a cool liquid agar nutrient mix in the absence of oxygen and then poured into a glass-walled tube that is open to the atmosphere on top. When the agar mix cools, it solidifies, and bacterial growth is observed as shown in Figure 31. How would you classify the bacteria in terms of oxygen utilization and tolerance? (*Note*: Agar is practically impermeable to oxygen.)[45]

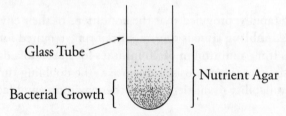

Glass Tube

Bacterial Growth

Nutrient Agar

Figure 31 Bacterial Reproduction

Fermentation vs. Respiration

This was covered in Chapter 3. To review briefly, respiration is glucose catabolism with use of an inorganic electron acceptor such as oxygen. In contrast, fermentation is glucose catabolism which does not use an electron acceptor such as O_2; instead, a reduced by-product of glucose catabolism such as lactate or ethanol is given off as waste. [Why is fermentation necessary whenever an external electron acceptor is not used?[46]]

---

[42] Sixteen times as much.

[43] The enzymes include superoxide dismutase (converts O_2^- to H_2O_2) and catalase (converts H_2O_2 to $H_2O + O_2$). An example of a harmful O_2 by-product is superoxide anion, O_2^-.

[44] The bacterium cannot be a facultative anaerobe, since the question states it cannot use O_2. It could be either an obligate or a tolerant anaerobe depending on its ability to neutralize harmful oxygen free radicals.

[45] Since the bacteria grew only at the bottom of the tube, farthest away from any oxygen, this indicates that they could only grow in the absence of oxygen. Thus, they are obligate anaerobes.

[46] Because NAD^+ must be regenerated from NADH for glycolysis to continue. In fermentation, the electrons are passed from NADH to a molecule other than O_2, such as pyruvic acid.

Anaerobic Respiration

This is not a contradiction in terms! It refers to glucose metabolism with electron transport and oxidative phosphorylation relying on an external electron acceptor *other than* O_2. For example, instead of reducing O_2 to H_2O, some anaerobic bacteria reduce SO_4^{2-} to H_2S, or CO_2 to CH_4. Nitrate (NO_3^-) is another possible electron acceptor.

- In an experiment, facultative anaerobic bacteria that are growing on glucose in air are shifted to anaerobic conditions. If they continue to grow at the same rate while producing lactic acid, then the rate of glucose consumption will[47]
    - A. increase 16 fold.
    - B. decrease 16 fold.
    - C. decrease 2 fold.
    - D. not change.

5.7

Bacterial Life Cycle

Bacteria reproduce asexually but do not perform mitosis. In asexual reproduction, there is no meiosis, no meiotic generation of **haploid** gametes, and no fusion of gametes to form a new individual organism. Instead, each bacterium grows in size until it has synthesized enough cellular components for two cells rather than one, replicates its genome, then divides in two. This process in bacteria is also known as **binary fission** (fission means "to split"). [In prokaryotes, does reproduction increase genetic diversity?[48] If a eukaryote reproduces strictly by asexual reproduction, how will this affect the genetic diversity of a population?[49] How is asexual reproduction in a eukaryote different from asexual reproduction in a prokaryote?[50]] Although bacteria do not reproduce sexually, they do possess three mechanisms for exchanging genetic information (more on this later).

Growth of bacterial populations is described in stages (see Figure 32). Under ideal conditions, bacterial population growth is exponential, meaning that the number of bacterial cells increases exponentially with time. This also means the log of the population size grows linearly with time, hence the name **log phase.** [If 10 bacteria in log phase are placed in ideal growth conditions and the doubling time is 20 minutes, how many bacteria will there be after four hours?[51]]

---

[47] Aerobic respiration produces 32 ATP per glucose in prokaryotes compared to only 2 ATP per glucose in fermentation. If the rate of growth is to remain the same, the rate of ATP production must remain the same to drive biosynthetic pathways forward. Since fermentation produces 1/16 the amount of ATP per glucose, the rate of glucose consumption must increase 16 fold to maintain the rate of growth at the same level. The answer is **A**. (In reality the growth rate would probably decrease.)

[48] No. Each daughter cell is identical to the parent cell (assuming no mutation took place).

[49] Many eukaryotes reproduce asexually. Sexual reproduction allows for a generation of new allelic combinations through meiotic recombination and random union of gametes. Without this, diversity will decrease over time.

[50] In eukaryotes, asexual reproduction occurs through mitosis. Prokaryotes do not go through mitosis.

[51] Since four hours is equal to 240 minutes, the bacteria will divide twelve times. Therefore, one bacterium will produce $2^{12} = 4,096$ bacteria after 12 divisions. Since there are 10 bacteria initially, the total after four hours will be $10 \times 2^{12} = 40,960$.

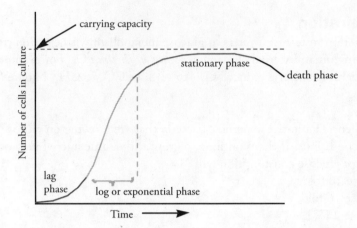

Figure 32 Growth of Bacterial Populations

Prior to achieving exponential growth, bacteria that were not previously growing undergo a **lag phase**, during which cell division does not occur even if the growth conditions are ideal.

- If growth conditions are ideal, why wouldn't cell division occur immediately?[52]
- Will bacteria that are transferred from a culture that is in log phase to a fresh new culture show a lag phase?[53]

As metabolites in the growth medium are depleted, and metabolic waste products accumulate, the bacterial population passes from log phase to **stationary phase**, in which cells cease to divide for lack of nutrients. The maximum population at the stationary phase is referred to as the **carrying capacity** for that environment. In the last stages of the stationary phase, cell death may occur as a result of the medium's inability to support growth. [If bacteria are grown in a medium with glucose as the main source of energy, when will the glycolytic pathway be more active: during the lag phase or during the stationary phase?[54]]

Endospore Formation

Some types of Gram-positive bacteria, such as the bacteria responsible for botulism, form **endospores** under unfavorable growth conditions. Endospores have tough, thick external shells comprised of peptidoglycan. Within the endospore are the genome, ribosomes, and RNA, which are required for the spore to become metabolically active when conditions become favorable. Endospores are able to survive temperatures above 100°C, which is why autoclaves or pressure cookers are required to completely sterilize liquids and substances that cannot be heated sufficiently in a dry oven. The metabolic reactivation of an endospore is termed **germination**. A single bacterium is able to form only one spore per cell. Thus, bacteria cannot increase their population through spore formation. [When are bacteria most likely to form endospores: during lag phase, log phase, or stationary phase? Is endospore formation a means for bacteria to reproduce?[55]]

---

[52] Cells that are not growing are not actively producing components that are needed for cell division, such as dNTPs. The lag period is a time when biosynthetic pathways are very actively producing new cellular components so that cells can then begin to divide.

[53] No, since they will have all the gear necessary for population growth at the ready.

[54] The bacteria will use glucose during the lag phase to produce ATP and cellular machinery. During this period, glucose is abundant, and the cell is actively performing biosynthesis, so glycolysis is very active. During the stationary phase, however, the glucose will be depleted, and the rate of metabolism will have slowed dramatically, so the rate of glycolysis will decrease as well.

[55] Stationary. Forming an endospore is like hibernating, not reproducing. Bacteria do it in order to sleep through the bad times.

Genetic Exchange Between Bacteria

Bacteria reproduce asexually, but genetic exchange is evolutionarily favorable because it fosters genetic diversity. Bacteria have three mechanisms of acquiring new genetic material: **transduction**, **transformation**, and **conjugation**. Note that none of these has anything to do with reproduction! Transduction is the transfer of genomic DNA from one bacterium to another via a lysogenic phage; we'll talk about this more in Chapter 7, when we review virology. Transformation is when a bacterial cell takes DNA from the external environment into the cell; the DNA can be a fragment of genomic DNA (or chromosome) or a plasmid. Once inside the bacteria, a plasmid will be exposed to the host's DNA replication and protein synthesis machinery. Genomic DNA fragments must be recombined into the genome to be maintained by the bacterial cell; otherwise, chromosome fragments will be degraded and lost over time.

While transformation is a naturally occurring process, only a small percentage of bacteria are naturally willing to accept pieces of DNA floating around in their environment. These "competent" bacteria express special machinery that translocate hydrophilic DNA across the lipid membrane. In the lab, bacteria must be coaxed (via heat shock or electroporation) to take up a plasmid. A high temperature for a short period of time (e.g., 42°C for 30 sec) or applying an electric field increases permeability of the plasma membrane, allowing DNA to enter the cell.

Conjugation

Although bacteria reproduce asexually, they have developed conjugation to exchange genetic information. In conjugation, bacteria make physical contact and form a bridge between the cells. One cell copies DNA, and this copy is transferred through the bridge to the other cell. A key to bacterial conjugation is an extrachromosomal element known as the **F (fertility) factor**. Bacteria that have the F factor in a plasmid are **male**, or **F⁺**, and will transfer the F factor to female cells. Bacteria that do not contain the F factor are **female**, **F⁻**, and will receive the F factor from male cells to become male. [If all cells in a population are F⁺, will conjugation occur?[56]]

The F factor is often found in a plasmid and contains several genes, many of which are involved in conjugation itself. [Which cell will produce sex pili: the male cell or the female cell?[57]] After the male cell produces sex pili and the pili contact a female cell, a **conjugation bridge** forms. The F factor is replicated and transferred from the F⁺ to the F⁻ cell. DNA transfer between F⁺ and F⁻ cells is unidirectional; it occurs in one direction only (see Figure 33 on the next page).

Although the F factor is an extrachromosomal element, it does sometimes become integrated into the bacterial chromosome through recombination. A cell with the F factor integrated into its genome is called an **Hfr (high frequency of recombination) cell**. [Will an Hfr cell undergo conjugation with an F⁻ cell?[58]] When an Hfr cell performs conjugation, the chromosome is replicated and the entire genome is gradually donated to the female cell. How much genetic information is shared depends on how long the Hfr and female cells remain attached. In Figure 33b, the cells remained attached long enough for the A and b loci to transfer, but not long enough for the C and D loci or the F factor to be shared. As with transformation, genomic DNA fragments must be recombined into the genome to be maintained by a bacterial cell; otherwise, chromosome fragments will be degraded and lost over time.

---

[56] No. Conjugation occurs only between F⁺ (male) and F⁻ (female).

[57] The male cell contains the F factor that encodes the genes for pili production and will produce pili.

[58] Yes. All of the genes of the F factor are still present and expressed normally in the Hfr cell.

- If bacteria contain only one copy of the bacterial genome, how can recombination occur?[59]

- If the F factor in an Hfr strain integrates near a gene required for lactose metabolism, is it likely that other genes involved in lactose metabolism will be transferred during conjugation at the same time?[60]

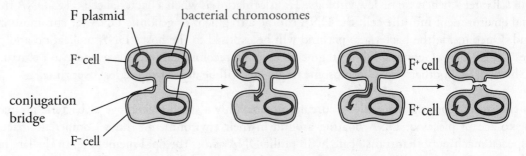

a) Conjugation and transfer of an F plasmid from an F⁺ donor to an F⁻ recipient

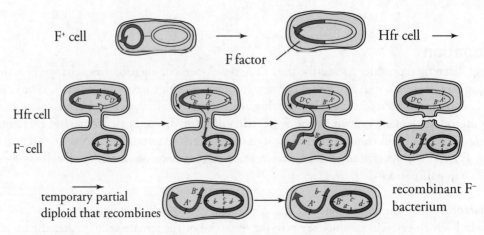

b) Conjugation and transfer of part of the bacterial chromosome from an Hfr donor to an F⁻ recipient, resulting in recombination

Figure 33   Conjugation

Conjugation Mapping

Hfr bacteria provide a mechanism of mapping the bacterial genome. By allowing Hfr cells to conjugate in the lab and stopping the conjugation process after different time intervals, researchers can figure out the order of the genes on the bacterial chromosome by analyzing recipient cells to see what genes were transferred.

---

[59] When an Hfr cell conjugates with an F⁻ cell and transfers a portion of the bacterial chromosomes, the F⁻ cell will have two copies of some genes, and recombination can occur between the two copies.

[60] Yes. Genes for proteins of related functions are often adjacent to each other in prokaryotes (in operons) and so will transfer to an F⁻ cell together.

For example, you have two strains of *E. coli*. One is a normal Hfr bacterium. The other is F$^-$ and auxotrophic for arginine, leucine, and histidine (F$^-$ Arg$^-$ Leu$^-$ His$^-$). You allow conjugation to begin and stop it after 2 minutes. You find that all the recipients are now F$^-$ Arg$^-$ Leu$^-$ His$^+$. Then you take another bunch of bacteria and allow conjugation to proceed for 5 minutes. Now all the recipients are F$^-$ Arg$^+$ Leu$^-$ His$^+$. You do the experiment a third and final time, allowing 8 minutes of conjugation, and find the recipients to be F$^-$ Arg$^+$ Leu$^+$ His$^+$.

- What is the arrangement on the genome of the enzymes responsible for synthesis of each amino acid, relative to the site of F plasmid integration?[61]

5.7

Want More Practice?
Scan the QR code below to register your book for online chapter summaries, drills, practice tests, and more!

---

[61] The experiments showed that the ability to make histidine was transferred in a short time. After a slightly longer time, the ability to make both histidine and arginine was transferred. Lastly, the ability to make leucine was transferred. So the arrangement on the genome (the map) must be: His-Arg-Leu-plasmid integration site.

Chapter 6
Genetics

The nature of the fundamental unit of inheritance, the gene, has been agreed upon by scientists only since the mid-19th century. Aristotle believed traits were passed on in the form of "pangenes," particles derived from all parts of the body and distilled into eggs and sperm. In the 17th century, different theorists believed that all genetic information was passed by either the father or the mother. Finally, early in the 19th century, people began to see that characteristics are passed from both parents; this led to the idea that parental characteristics were evenly mixed in offspring, in a process termed "blending." The notion that some characteristics were inherited in an either-or fashion, while others were in fact blended, remained unconceived.

The proponents of these early theories cannot be faulted for their lack of electron microscopes and other modern tools and techniques. But one is tempted to criticize their ideas for their obvious irrelevance to reality. One didn't need a supercomputer to figure out that both parents contributed to a child's genetic makeup. Why did researchers fail to arrive at this seemingly obvious hypothesis? Probably for two reasons: methods and dogma.

Their approach to discovery was not empirical, but rather *a priori*. They believed knowledge could be derived by speculation alone, and that to perform experiments in the physical world was to dirty one's hands. Prevailing religious dogma strongly censored empirical exploration, since it threatened the metaphysical tenets of the church.

What is different today is the approach to discovery known as the scientific method. Modern scientists know that only through careful, sober consideration of a question, formulation of a tentative answer, and testing of that hypothesis can new knowledge be uncovered. In this chapter we will examine what is now considered to be the truth about genetics.

We challenge you to attack this knowledge in the way its discoverers did. This is difficult material. Spend time thinking about the in-text questions before reading the answers. If you have trouble with a topic, stop and take out a fresh piece of paper. Write down all the facets of your current understanding, and look for internal inconsistencies and fallacies. Make your own sketches of chromosomes during meiosis and write out your own calculations. Finally, as you review, ask yourself which modern "truths" will one day be looked back on as preposterous ponderings of blindfolded pseudo-scientists.

6.1 MEIOSIS

As we saw in the last chapter, mitotic cell division produces two daughter cells that are identical to the parent; it is a form of asexual cell replication. However, the production of **haploid** cells such as **gametes** from a **diploid** cell requires a type of cell division that reduces the number of copies of each chromosome from two to one; this method of cell division is called **meiosis**. In males, meiosis occurs in the testes with haploid spermatozoa as the end result; in females, meiosis in the ovaries produces ova. (*Note*: this is not always the case, and while meiosis begins in the ovaries, it is completed only after fertilization; see Chapter 11 for a further discussion on oogenesis.) Specialized cells termed **spermatogonia** in males and **oogonia** in females undergo meiosis. Spermatogenesis and oogenesis share the same basic features of meiosis but differ in many of the specific features of gamete production. Meiosis itself will be discussed in this chapter, while the specifics of spermatogenesis and oogenesis will be discussed in Chapter 11.

Mitosis and meiosis are similar in many respects. Both are preceded by one round of DNA synthesis or replication of the genome (S phase). As in mitosis, DNA replication turns single copy linear chromosomes with one chromatid (sometimes called 1x chromosomes) into duplicated X-shaped chromosomes with two **sister chromatids** joined at the centromere (sometimes called 2x chromosomes).[1] In other words, before starting prophase of mitosis or meiosis, the cell is diploid with four copies of the genome (Figure 1). The different phases in cell division are referred to by the same names (prophase, metaphase, anaphase, and telophase) in both meiosis and mitosis and are mechanistically very similar. The primary difference between meiosis and mitosis is that replication of the genome is followed by one round of cell division in mitosis and two rounds of cell division in meiosis, **meiosis I** and **meiosis II** (Figure 2). Another important difference is that in meiosis, recombination occurs between homologous chromosomes.

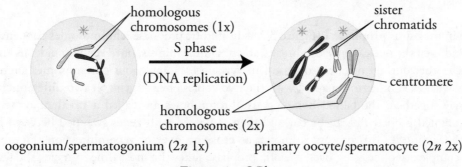

Figure 1   S Phase

---

[1]   It is worth spending time reading that sentence again and thinking about what it means. If you want to know the ploidy of a cell (e.g., haploid, diploid, tetraploid), you need to count the chromosomes. Counting centromeres works too. If you see a human cell with 23 chromosomes, it is haploid. A human cell with 46 chromosomes is diploid and contains two of each chromosome (one set inherited from the father and the other set inherited from the mother). A human cell with 96 chromosomes is tetraploid and is in anaphase of mitosis, as we saw in the last chapter. 1x and 2x tell you whether the chromosomes have been replicated, or whether S phase has happened, or whether there is one or two chromatids per chromosome; these are all different ways of saying the same thing. If chromosomes are linear (as on the left of Figure 1 above), the cell is 1x and before DNA replication/S phase. If chromosomes are X-shaped (as on the right of Figure 1 above), the cell is 2x and DNA replication/S phase has occurred.

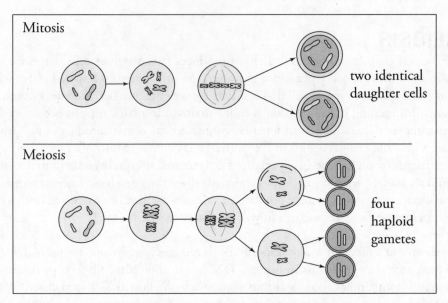

Figure 2   Mitosis vs. Meiosis

To depict meiosis, we will use a hypothetical model organism with a diploid genome and two different (nonhomologous) chromosomes.

- How many chromosomes are present in a cell from this organism at the very beginning of meiosis?[2]

The first step in meiosis is **prophase I** (Figure 3). As in mitotic prophase, chromosomes condense in meiotic prophase I, and then the nuclear envelope breaks down. Unlike mitosis, however, homologous chromosomes pair with each other during meiotic prophase I in **synapsis**. Homologous chromosomes align themselves very precisely with each other in synapsis, with the two copies of each gene on two different chromosomes brought closely together. The paired homologous chromosomes are called a **bivalent** or **tetrad**. When the DNA is aligned properly, it can be cut and then re-ligated with genes swapped between homologous chromosomes (Figure 5). This process is known as **crossing over** or **recombination** (Figure 4). Due to the extreme complexity of crossing over, meiotic prophase takes the most time in meiosis, days sometimes. Recombination during meiosis is an important source of genetic variation during sexual reproduction.

- Does crossing over change the number of genes on a chromosome?[3]
- Does recombination create combinations of alleles on a chromosome that are not found in the parent?[4]

---

[2] The organism is diploid and has two different chromosomes. This means it must have two of each chromosome, so four chromosomes in total. After DNA synthesis, and at the beginning of meiosis, the cell still has four chromosomes; however, the chromosomes are replicated and held together at each centromere. Thus each chromosome consists of two sister chromatids, and the cell has a total of eight sister chromatids.

[3] Not if it is done correctly. Error-free recombination involves a one-for-one swap of DNA between homologous chromosomes.

[4] Yes. Although each chromosome contains the same genes after crossing over, it may contain different alleles of some genes that were not present on the same chromosome previously.

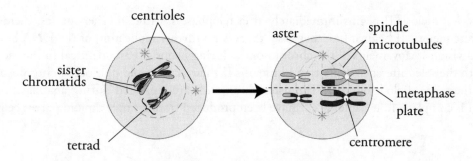

Figure 3 Prophase I and Metaphase I

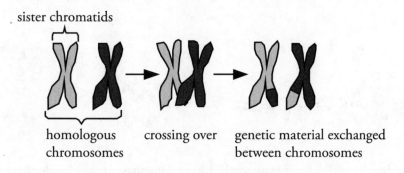

Figure 4 Crossing Over (Recombination)

After prophase I is **metaphase I**. In meiotic metaphase I, alignment along the metaphase plate occurs, as in mitosis. The difference is that in meiotic metaphase I, the *tetrads* are aligned at the center of the cell (the metaphase plate), whereas in mitosis, *sister chromatids* are aligned on the metaphase plate. In **anaphase I**, homologous chromosomes separate, and sister chromatids remain together (Figure 5). The cell then divides into two cells during **telophase I** (Figure 5). *It is important to note that at this point the cells are considered to be haploid.* Each cell has a single set of chromosomes. The chromosomes, however, are still replicated (still exist as a pair of sister chromatids, or are 2x). The whole point to the second set of meiotic divisions is to separate sister chromatids so that each cell has a single set of unreplicated chromosomes.[5]

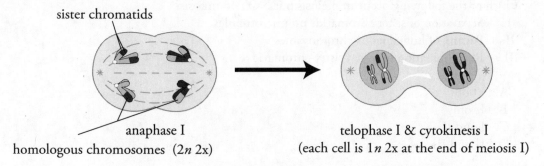

Figure 5 Anaphase I, Telophase I, and Cytokinesis I

---

[5] Another way to think about this is that meiosis I decreases ploidy ($2n \rightarrow 1n$), while both mitosis and meiosis II decrease the DNA content of the cell ($2x \rightarrow 1x$). You might be wondering what can increase n and x. The only way to increase ploidy (n) is to join two cells together (e.g., haploid sperm fuses with haploid egg to form a diploid zygote) or rip apart double copy ($2x$) chromosomes into single copy linear ($1x$) chromosomes (as we saw in mitosis and will see again shortly in anaphase II). The only way to increase x is to perform DNA replication ($1x \rightarrow 2x$ chromosomes).

In some species, meiosis II begins immediately after telophase I, while in other species, there is a period of time before meiosis II begins. In either case, there is no further replication of the DNA before the second set of divisions. Movements of the chromosomes during meiosis II are identical to the movements in mitosis, with the sole difference being that in meiosis II there is a haploid number of chromosomes, while in mitosis there is a diploid number. The sister chromatids are separated during anaphase II, and after telophase II is complete, four haploid cells have been produced from a single diploid parent cell (Figure 6).

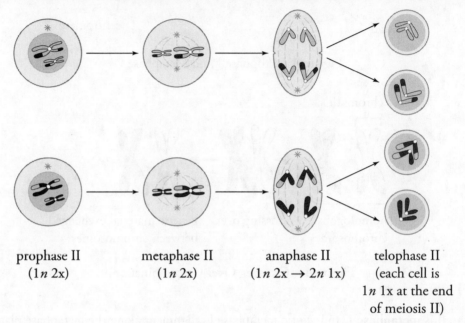

prophase II   metaphase II   anaphase II   telophase II
($1n$ 2x)   ($1n$ 2x)   ($1n$ 2x $\rightarrow$ 2n 1x)   (each cell is
                                                                 $1n$ 1x at the end
                                                                 of meiosis II)

Figure 6   Meiosis II

• When homologous chromosomes separate, do all paternal and maternal chromosomes stay together in the daughter cells?[6]

• Are the sister chromatids that separate during meiotic anaphase II identical in their DNA sequence?[7]

• Which of the following occur in meiosis but NOT in mitosis?[8]
  I.   Separation of sister chromatids on microtubules
  II.   Pairing of homologous chromosomes
  III. Recombination between sister chromatids

  A. I only
  B. II only
  C. I and II
  D. II and III

---

[6] No. Homologous chromosomes separate (segregate) randomly. This is one aspect of meiosis that increases genetic variation during sexual reproduction.

[7] The sister chromatids *would* be identical, except that recombination with homologous chromosomes occurred earlier in meiosis, during prophase I, altering the sister chromatids.

[8] **Statement I is false**: The spindle separates sister chromatids during both (eliminate A and C). Note both remaining answer choices include Statement II, so **Statement II must be true**. **Statement II is true**: Only meiosis involves pairing and recombination between homologous chromosomes. **Statement III is false**: Meiotic recombination occurs between homologous chromosomes, not sister chromatids (eliminate D, and **B** is correct).

- If cells are blocked in meiotic metaphase II and prevented from moving on in meiosis, which one of the following will be prevented?[9]
    - A. Crossing over
    - B. Separation of homologous chromosomes
    - C. Separation of sister chromatids
    - D. Breakdown of the nuclear envelope
    - E. Production of haploid cells

Nondisjunction

Sometimes during meiosis I homologous chromosomes fail to separate, and sometimes during meiosis II sister chromatids fail to separate. Such a failure of chromosomes to separate correctly during meiosis is called **nondisjunction**. [A human gamete normally contains how many copies of each chromosome?[10] If two homologous chromosomes of chromosome 12 fail to separate during meiosis I, how many copies of chromosome #12 will the resulting gametes have?[11]] Gametes resulting from nondisjunction will have two copies or no copies of a given chromosome. In other words, nondisjunction results in daughter cells with abnormal chromosome numbers (**aneuploidy**). Such a gamete can fuse with a normal gamete to create a zygote with either three copies of a chromosome (**trisomy**) or one copy of a chromosome (**monosomy**).

The genetic defect caused when an entire chromosome is either added or removed is usually so great that a zygote with either trisomy or monosomy cannot develop into a normal individual. The clinical significance is high, as nondisjunction is the leading cause of pregnancy loss and birth defects. There are examples in which nondisjunction is not lethal in humans, although it usually results in significant developmental abnormalities. Trisomy of chromosome 21 results in Down syndrome, which is usually associated with physical growth delays and mild to moderate intellectual disability.[12] Nondisjunction of the sex chromosomes is also generally not lethal during development. Individuals who have only one X chromosome and no Y, for example, have Turner syndrome, with external female appearance but underdeveloped ovaries and sterility. Klinefelter syndrome is the most common sex chromosome aneuploidy in humans; most individuals with this syndrome have one extra X chromosome resulting in the karyotype XXY. Individuals with nondisjunction of the sex chromosomes will develop to have male appearance if they have at least one Y, no matter how many X chromosomes are present, and will have female genitalia if only X chromosomes are present. Most will be sterile, however, and many will have intellectual disability. [In an individual with Down syndrome, are the defects in development caused by an absence of genetic information?[13] If not, why does trisomy of this chromosome or other chromosomes have such dramatic effects?[14]]

---

[9] Crossing over occurs during prophase I, separation of homologous chromosomes occurs during anaphase I, and nuclear envelope breakdown occurs during prophase I and sometimes prophase II (eliminate A, B, and D). Remember that cells are haploid after telophase I (eliminate E). Only separation of sister chromatids occurs after metaphase II, in anaphase II (choice **C** is correct).

[10] Normal gametes have one copy of each chromosome; this is the definition of haploid.

[11] If homologous chromosomes do not separate in meiosis I, then one daughter cell from this division will have four copies of this chromosome and the other cell will have none. In meiosis II, sister chromatids will separate, leaving two gametes with two copies of the chromosome and two gametes with no copies of the chromosome.

[12] Human somatic trisomies compatible with live birth, other than Down syndrome (trisomy 21), are Edwards syndrome (trisomy 18) and Patau syndrome (trisomy 13). Complete trisomies of other somatic chromosomes are usually not viable and represent a relatively frequent cause of miscarriage.

[13] There is no information missing in a person with trisomy. All chromosomes are present, and there is no reason to believe that any of the genes on these chromosomes are deleted or mutated to render them inactive.

[14] The issue with trisomy is not to be that genetic information is missing, but that there is *too much* present. A mechanism involved might be gene dosage. Genes are regulated to produce a certain amount of each gene product. In trisomy, many genes are present in one more copy than usual, resulting in greater quantities of gene products encoded on this chromosome. Extra quantities of so many gene products, even if they are wild type in sequence, can have dramatic consequences.

6.2 GENETICS DEFINITIONS

Genes, Allele, and Locus

Genetics is the science that describes the inheritance of traits from one generation to another. At the origin of genetics, patterns of inheritance were observed to follow certain predictable patterns, as described by Mendel's laws. The reasons for these patterns of inheritance were to remain a mystery until the nature of DNA as the genetic material was known. Today we can use our knowledge of DNA and the cell to understand Mendel's laws at the molecular level.

One of the basic tenets of genetics is that children inherit traits from both parents. As we saw in the previous section, humans have a life cycle which begins with a diploid cell, the **zygote**. Diploid organisms (or cells) have two copies of the genome in each cell, while haploid cells have one copy of the genome. In sexual reproduction, the diploid zygote is produced by fusion of two haploid gametes: a haploid ovum from the mother and a haploid spermatozoon from the father. The zygote then goes through many mitotic divisions to develop into an adult, with half of the genetic material in each cell from each parent. The adult, male or female, produces haploid gametes by meiotic cell division to repeat the life cycle once again.

Development of a zygote into an adult and maintenance of adult cells and tissues requires many thousands of different gene products. All of these gene products are encoded in the genome and inherited from mother and father. The **gene**, a length of DNA coding for a particular gene product, is the fundamental unit of inheritance. [Are gene products always proteins?[15]] Genes are distributed among the chromosomes that compose the genome, and every gene can be pinpointed to a specific location called the **locus** (plural: **loci**) on a specific chromosome. [Can all physical traits of an organism be mapped to a single locus?[16]]

Chromosomes

The human genome is split into 23 different chromosomes, of which every cell has two different copies. In other words, our genome is made of 23 pairs of chromosomes, 46 chromosomes in total. Twenty-two of these pairs, called **autosomes**, look the same in both males and females. The 23rd pair, the **sex chromosomes**, differ between males and females. Females have two copies of the X chromosome, while males have one X and one Y chromosome. The 22 autosomes are numbered by size, as we saw in Chapter 4 when we discussed karyotypes. Humans inherit one copy of each chromosome from the mother and one from the father. The two nonidentical copies of a chromosome are called **homologous chromosomes**. Although these two copies look the same when examined at the crudest level under a microscope, and although they contain the same genes, the copies of the genes in the two homologous chromosomes may differ in their DNA sequence. Different versions of a gene, called **alleles**, may carry out the gene's function differently. Since a person carries two copies of every gene, one on each homologous chromosome, a person can carry two different alleles. [Is it possible for there to be more than two different alleles of a specific gene?[17]]

---

[15] No. tRNA and rRNA genes, as well as other small nuclear RNA genes, do not encode polypeptides.

[16] No. Every gene is located at a specific locus, but physical traits, particularly complex traits, like weight or height, can be controlled by many different genes and therefore do not map to a single locus, but to many.

[17] Yes, there can be many versions (alleles) of a particular gene in a population or species. Under normal circumstances, however, one individual cannot have more than two of those different alleles, since they have only two copies of a gene (one on each homologous chromosome). An exception is when an individual is polyploid for a certain -chromosome (i.e., they have more than two homologous chromosomes, for example in Down syndrome and Klinefelter syndrome).

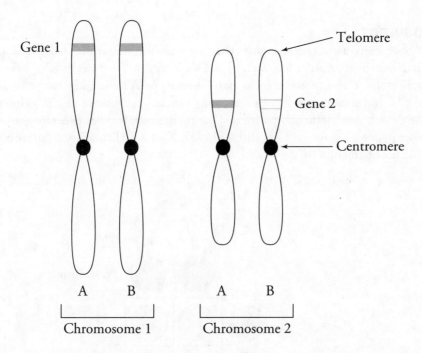

Figure 7 Two Genes, Located at Two Different Loci on Two Different Chromosomes

Figure 7 shows two chromosomes, 1 and 2. For each chromosome, two copies are shown (A and B), as would be present in a diploid organism. The individual that has these chromosomes in their genome would have received or inherited one Chromosome 1 and one Chromosome 2 from their mother and one Chromosome 1 and one Chromosome 2 from their father. The two homologous pairs of Chromosome 1 are the same size and code for the same genes in the same location. The same is true of Chromosome 2.

At any given genetic locus, the two chromosomes of a given homologous pair might be:

- identical in DNA sequence and code for the same form of the gene (shown on Chromosome 1 in Figure 7)
- different in DNA sequence and code for different versions of the same gene (shown on Chromosome 2 in Figure 7)

Alleles have different DNA sequences and a given gene can have numerous alleles. (For example, more than 400 alleles of the *GLA* gene have been published! Many of these can cause a rare genetic disorder called Fabry disease.) However, since humans are diploid, our genome can at most contain two alleles of a given single-copy gene. Some humans contain only one allele of some genes, if both their homologous chromosomes contain the same allele.

Sex Chromosomes

Female humans have 23 pairs of chromosomes that are homologous, while males have only 22 pairs of chromosomes that match in appearance; males have an X and a Y, while females have two X chromosomes. The presence of a Y chromosome in humans (**genotype XY**) is a key factor in determination of the sex of an embryo, and subsequent development into a male. The absence of a Y (**genotype XX**) results in a female as the default developmental pathway. During meiosis, females generate gametes that contain an X chromosome; males generate gametes with either an X or a Y chromosome, meaning the male gamete determines the sex of an embryo.

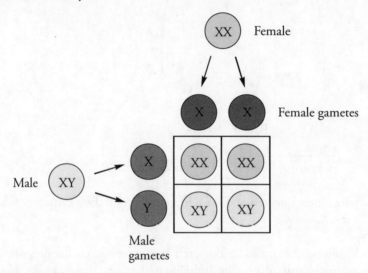

Figure 8   Determination of the Zygote's Sexual Genotype

The sex chromosomes also function in inheritance of other traits that are not directly involved in sexual development. Much of what has been discussed about inheritance was dependent on the assumption that there are two copies of every chromosome and therefore two copies of every gene in each cell. This is true for genes found on every pair of chromosomes except for one pair: the sex chromosomes. Genes that lie on the X chromosome will be present in two copies in females but only in one copy in males. [What pattern of expression will a recessive allele on the X chromosome display in males?[18]] Traits that are determined by genes on the X or Y chromosome are called sex-linked traits because of their unique patterns of expression and inheritance. We'll discuss this more later in this chapter.

Genotype and Phenotype

The full complement of alleles possessed by an organism represents its **genotype**. The ultimate significance of a genotype lies in the **traits** it produces, meaning the features, attributes, or characteristics it imparts to an organism. Height, color-blindness, and lactose intolerance all constitute "traits." When we discuss an organism's traits, we refer to its **phenotype**. For example, we might say that one individual's phenotype is blue eye color and that another's phenotype is green eye color; eye color is a trait and blue and green are phenotypes that would be associated with different alleles in the genotype. An organism's phenotype is governed by its genotype—by its overall inventory of alleles. More specifically, phenotype comes about according to the way in which combined alleles interact to produce traits.

---

[18] In males, recessive alleles on the X chromosome are always expressed, since no other allele is present to mask the recessive allele.

Consider hypothetical Trait X and two parents—a father who is positive for Trait X and a mother who is negative for Trait X. Depending on the nature of the two inherited alleles and the way in which they interact, the offspring might manifest:

a. Trait X fully
b. Trait X not at all
c. Trait X in some intermediate, attenuated, or hybrid form

The dynamics through which an individual's genotype creates its phenotype are intimately tied to the phenomena of homozygous and heterozygous genotypic states.

Homozygous and Heterozygous Genotypes

With respect to a given genetic locus, an individual's two alleles might be identical, meaning that the two alleles inherited from its two parental gametes were identical. Such an individual is **homozygous** with reference to that genetic locus. The essence of the word homozygous refers to an organism whose two alleles for a given locus, or gene, are identical.

On the other hand, if, for some genetic locus, an organism carries two different alleles on corresponding sites of homologous chromosomes, it is said to be **heterozygous**. The phenomena of homozygous and heterozygous genotypes give phenotypic effect to dominant and recessive alleles.

Look back at Figure 7. For Gene 1 on Chromosome 1, the same form of the gene is shown (gray). The DNA sequences of these two copies of Gene 1 are identical and the gene codes for the same gene product. The individual would be called homozygous at this locus. In contrast, this individual contains two different alleles of Gene 2 on Chromosome 2 (one grey and one white). These two forms of Gene 2 code for different versions of the gene product and have different DNA sequences. Since this individual has two different alleles at this locus, they would be called heterozygous for Gene 2.

Dominant and Recessive Alleles

Consider a hypothetical trait T. Assume that trait T appears when the organism manufactures protein T and does not appear when the organism fails to manufacture protein T. Finally, suppose that the production or failure to produce protein T is governed by a particular allele that exists in two forms:

1. allele *T* codes for protein T
2. allele *t* does not code for protein T

Imagine that a particular individual is homozygous for the allele that produces protein T. We designate her genotype as *TT,* meaning that at the relevant homologous pair, both chromosomes code for the production of protein T. The cells of this individual will manufacture protein T and she will, therefore, manifest trait T; her genotype is *TT,* and her phenotype for trait T is positive.

Imagine another individual who is homozygous for the allele that does not code for protein T. We designate his genotype as *tt,* meaning that at the relevant homologous pair, both chromosomes fail to code for protein T. This individual will fail to produce protein T and fail to manifest trait T. Their genotype is *tt* and their phenotype for trait T is negative.

Now, imagine an individual who is heterozygous for the allele under discussion. We designate the genotype as *Tt*, meaning that at the relevant chromosomal pair, one chromosome carries the allele that codes for protein T and the other carries the allele that does not code for protein T. Since one of the two alleles codes for protein T, this individual will produce protein T and will consequently manifest trait T. Their genotype is *Tt* and their phenotype for trait T is positive.

In the example of trait T, if the individual carries one allele that codes for Protein T (*T*) and one that does not (*t*), that individual will manifest trait T. This means the *T* allele is **dominant** over the *t* allele. In the heterozygous individual (*Tt*), the *T* allele (positive for the trait) expresses itself over the phenotype of the *t* allele (negative for the trait). The *t* allele expresses itself only when present on both alleles, or when the individual is homozygous for that allele (*tt*).

- Which one of the following is true if an individual has two different alleles at a given locus?[19]
  A. The individual has two phenotypes, e.g., one brown eye and one blue.
  B. There are two alleles in one place on one particular chromosome.
  C. Two siblings have different appearances.
  D. There is a different allele on each of the two members of a homologous pair.
  E. The individual's parents must have two different alleles at that locus.

When two alleles interact in the way just described, we say that they exhibit **classical dominance**. This is based on Mendel's Law of Dominance (that one trait can mask the effects of another trait), and so can also be called Mendelian inheritance. The essential features and phenomena associated with classical dominance are:

1. Dominant alleles are denoted by a capital letter and recessive traits are denoted by a lowercase letter.
2. When an individual is either homozygous for the dominant allele (such as *TT*) or heterozygous (such as *Tt*), that individual expresses the dominant phenotype (such as T positive).
3. When an individual is homozygous for the recessive allele (such as *tt*), that individual expresses the recessive trait (such as T negative).

- If the dominant allele for curly (*C*) results in curly hair and the recessive allele (*c*) causes straight hair, what are the phenotypes of *CC*, *Cc*, and *cc* individuals?[20]

---

[19] An individual with two different alleles at a given locus has one allele on one chromosome and the other allele on its homologous partner (eliminate B, and **D** is correct). While A may be possible, it is an exceedingly complex phenomenon and not discernible from the information given. The question discusses a single individual, not a pair of siblings (eliminate C), and the fact that this individual has two different alleles does not provide much information on the alleles of the parents (eliminate E).

[20] *CC* and *Cc* individuals have curly hair, while *cc* individuals have straight hair. Only homozygous recessive individuals express recessive traits. In heterozygotes, the presence of a recessive allele is masked by the dominant allele, so there are only two different phenotypes, although there are three different genotypes. This type of interaction between alleles is called classical dominance.

6.3 MENDELIAN GENETICS

Gregor Mendel described the statistical behavior of the inheritance of traits in pea plants long before the nature of DNA and chromosomes was known. Unlike Mendel, however, we are now familiar with the molecular basis of genetics in meiosis and genes, and the laws of genetics that Mendel formulated can now be presented with insight based on this knowledge. Although Mendelian genetics generally only involves the simplest patterns of inheritance, it forms the foundation for understanding more complicated situations.

Mendel observed that traits were governed by pairs of hereditary material (alleles). The first of Mendel's laws, the **law of segregation**, states that the two alleles of an individual are separated and passed on to the next generation singly. [At what stage during meiosis are different alleles of a gene separated?[21]] Mendel's second law, the **law of independent assortment**, states that the alleles of one gene will separate into gametes independently of alleles for another gene. We will illustrate these principles using the garden pea plant, but the principles apply equally well to humans and many other organisms.

A trait that can be studied in the pea plant is the color of the pea. We can call *G* the allele for green color, while *g* is the allele for yellow pea color. Mating between plants, a **cross**, is used as a tool in genetics to discern genotypes by looking at the phenotypes of progeny from a cross. A **pure-breeding strain** of yellow or green peas consistently yields progeny of the same color when mated within the strain. For example, if mating yellow plants with yellow plants always produces yellow progeny, yellow is a pure-breeding strain. [Can anything be deduced about the genotype of the pure-breeding strain of yellow peas?[22] If a pure-breeding yellow and pure-breeding green strain are crossed, and all of the progeny are green, what does this indicate about the expression of the yellow and green alleles?[23]] Let's assume that *G* is the dominant allele of the color gene, and *g* is the recessive allele. [Is it possible to deduce the genotype of a pea plant at the color gene if it is green?[24]] If a green plant is encountered, to deduce the genotype of the plant one can do a **testcross**; this is when an individual is crossed with another that is homozygous recessive for all loci under study. [For example, to testcross an individual with an *AABbccDdEEff* genotype, the other individual would have genotype ___.[25]] The results of a testcross are dependent on statistics and follow Mendel's laws.

The principle of segregation can be illustrated with the color gene described above for the pea. If a pea is heterozygous *Gg*, its gametes will contain either the *G* allele or the *g* allele, but never both. [If a gamete contained both *G* and *g*, what occurred during meiosis?[26]] The probability that a gamete in the heterozygote will contain one allele or the other is 50%, completely random. [Would the principle of segregation apply to a gene on the X chromosome in a female human?[27]] To illustrate the law of independent assortment, we need to introduce a second gene, one that controls the shape of the pea. *W* is the dominant allele, resulting in wrinkled peas, while *w* is the recessive allele, resulting in smooth peas in homozygous

---

[21] During meiosis I, when homologous chromosomes separate.

[22] If a strain always produces the same trait when mated with itself, it is likely to be homozygous for the trait. The pure-breeding yellow pea is homozygous for the yellow allele *g* of the color gene.

[23] The two strains were both pure-breeding and could only produce gametes containing one type of allele. All of the progeny would be the *Gg* genotype. If all progeny are green, then the green allele is dominant and the yellow allele is recessive.

[24] No. A green plant could either be heterozygous *Gg* or homozygous *GG*.

[25] A testcross with *AABbccDdEEff* would be *aabbccddeeff*, all homozygous recessive.

[26] The gamete must be the result of nondisjunction.

[27] Yes. The principles are the same for human genes as for pea genes, as long as an organism is diploid and goes through sexual reproduction.

6.3

ww plants. According to the law of independent assortment, genes for the color of peas and the shape of peas are passed from one generation to another independently. [If the color gene and the shape gene are right next to each other on a chromosome, will they display independent assortment?[28]] The nature of the shape gene in a given gamete does not depend on and is not influenced by the color gene, if independent assortment is true. [If an individual is heterozygous at the color gene, *Gg*, and heterozygous at the shape gene, *Ww*, what are the chances that a gamete containing the *G* allele will also contain the *W* allele?[29]]

Here is a summary of Mendel's principles of genetics:

Law of Dominance	One trait can mask the effects of another trait	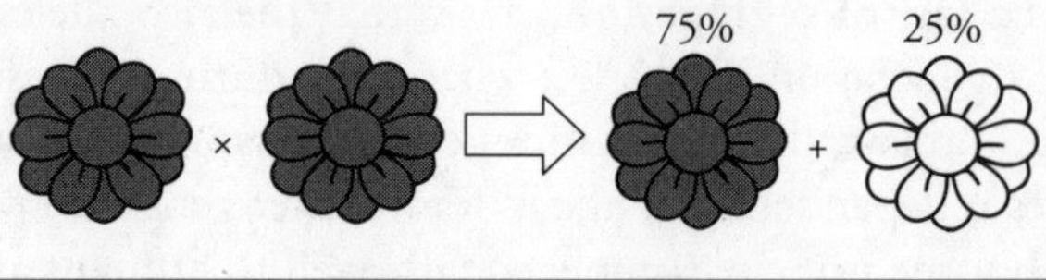
Law of Segregation	Alleles of a gene are distributed randomly but equally in gametes	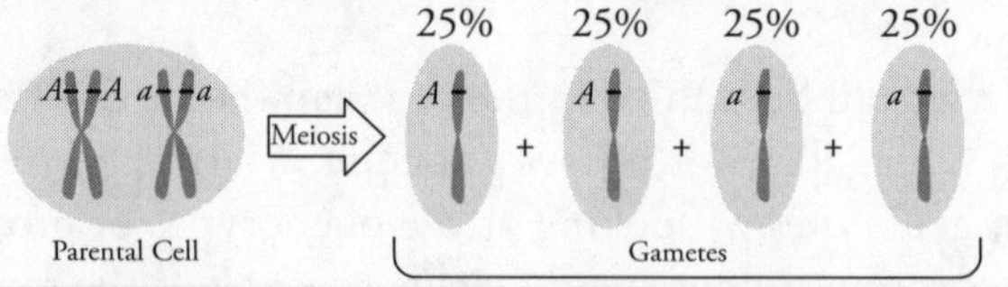
Law of Independent Assortment	Traits can segregate and recombine independently of other traits	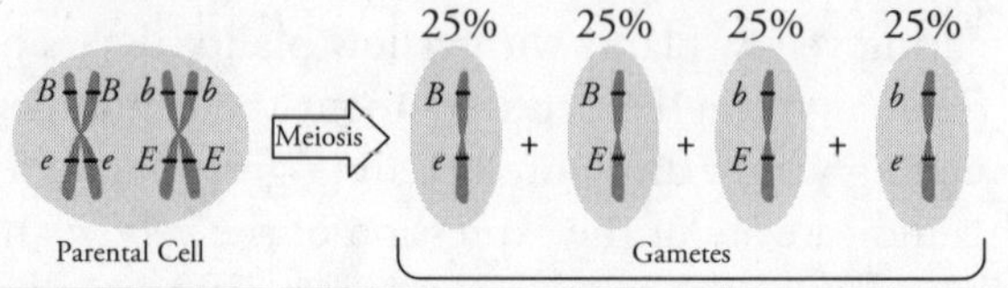

Table 1 Mendel's Principles of Genetics

Generations in genetic crosses are given specific names. The first generation in an experiment is called the parental or **P generation**. Their offspring, the second generation in an experiment, are called the first filial or **F$_1$ generation**. In other words, progeny of the P generation are F$_1$. The progeny of F$_1$ are called **F$_2$**, and so on. [If a green plant is testcrossed with a pure-breeding yellow strain, and some of the F$_1$ generation are yellow while others are green, what is the genotype of the original green plant?[30]]

The Punnett Square

It is possible to predict the results of a cross between two individuals using the laws of segregation and independent assortment. Determining the result can be complex, however, so a visual tool called the **Punnett square** is often employed to make the process simpler. Let's use a simple square first, with only one trait involved (see Figure 9):

---

[28] No, they would not. They would display an important exception to independent assortment, **linkage**, which is discussed later.

[29] According to independent assortment, segregation of one gene does not depend on segregation of another. The chances of a gamete containing the *W* allele are 50%, regardless of the identity of the color allele.

[30] The original pea is heterozygous *Gg*.

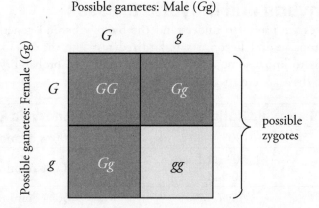

Figure 9 A Punnett Square Involving One Gene

In Figure 9, a Punnett square depicts a cross between two pea plants that are heterozygous for the color gene, with *G* being the dominant green allele and *g* the recessive yellow allele. To draw a Punnett square, the following steps are involved:

Step 1: Determine the gametes that are possible from each parent in the cross.
Step 2: Draw a square with the possible gametes from each parent on two sides.
Step 3: Fill in the square with the zygote genotypes that would result from each possible combination of gamete.
Step 4: Determine the phenotype of each genotype.
Step 5: Find the probability of each genotype and each phenotype.

- In the situation shown in Figure 9, which one of the following will be true?[31]
  - A. 25% of the offspring will be green, and 75% will be yellow.
  - B. 50% of the offspring will be green, and 50% will be yellow.
  - C. 75% of the offspring will be green, and 25% will be yellow.
  - D. 100% of the offspring will be green.

If you have to work a probability question more complicated than this on the DAT (for example, one that involves two different genes), you are better off using some basic rules of probability and doing a small amount of math. Let's look at how to do this quickly and accurately.

---

[31] If *G* (green allele) is dominant, then both *GG* homozygotes and *Gg* heterozygotes will be green, while only *gg* homozygotes will be yellow. 25% of the offspring in Figure 9 will be *GG* homozygotes, and 50% will be *Gg* heterozygotes, so a total of 75% of the offspring will be green (choice **C** is correct).

Common Monohybrid and Dihybrid Crosses

Although Punnett squares are useful to understand the biology behind genetic crosses, they are time-consuming and error prone, especially on a standardized test like the DAT. Another way to answer genetic cross questions is to know some common crosses and two probability rules. Let's look at the monohybrid crosses first; these are crosses that involve only one gene:

Parental Cross	Genotypic Ratio of Offspring	Phenotypic Ratio of Offspring
$AA \times aa$	100% Aa	100% dominant A phenotype
$AA \times Aa$	50% AA 50% Aa	100% dominant A phenotype
$Aa \times aa$	50% Aa 50% aa	50% dominant A phenotype 50% recessive a phenotype
$Aa \times Aa$	25% AA 50% Aa 25% aa This is also called a 1:2:1 ratio	75% dominant A phenotype 25% recessive a phenotype

Table 2 Common Monohybrid Crosses

It is also useful to know some probability rules for two common dihybrid genetic crosses (those that involve two genes). They are:

Parental Cross	Genotypic Ratio of Offspring	Phenotypic Ratio of Offspring
$AaBb \times aabb$[32]	25% $AaBb$ 25% $Aabb$ 25% $aaBb$ 25% $aabb$	25% A and B phenotypes 25% A and b phenotypes 25% a and B phenotypes 25% a and b phenotypes
$AaBb \times AaBb$	n/a[33]	A 9:3:3:1 ratio of: 9 offspring have A and B phenotypes 3 offspring have A and b phenotypes 3 offspring have a and B phenotypes 1 offspring has a and b phenotypes

Table 3 Common Dihybrid Crosses

---

[32] This cross can also be called a **testcross**, because one of the individuals is homozygous recessive.

[33] Notice the table above has an n/a in the genotypic column of the second cross. It is quite complicated to predict genotypic ratios in a heterozygous dihybrid cross. Instead, you would break the cross down into two separate genes, calculate the probabilities associated with each, and then multiply these two numbers, since you want to include the results from gene 1 *and* gene 2 in your final answer. Let's look at how to do this.

Rules of Multiplication and Addition

The **Rule of Multiplication** states that the probability of both of two independent events happening can be found by multiplying the odds of either event alone. For example, if the probability of being struck by lightning is 1 in a million (10^{-6}) and the probability of winning the lottery is 10^{-7}, then the probability of both happening is the product: $10^{-6} \times 10^{-7} = 10^{-13}$.

The **Rule of Addition** can be used to calculate the chances of either of two events happening. The chance of either A or B happening is equal to the probability of A added to the probability of B, minus the probability of A and B occurring together. For example, the chance of either getting hit by lightning *or* winning the lottery is $10^{-6} + 10^{-7} = 1.1 \times 10^{-6}$. (*Note*: the product of 10^{-6} and 10^{-7} is so small that it can be neglected from the equation.)

These rules can be a shortcut to using a Punnett square in many genetics problems. Let's look at some examples.

Assume G is the allele for green pea color, while g is the allele for yellow pea color. A cross is performed between Plant 1, heterozygous at the color gene, and Plant 2, also heterozygous at the color gene. Plant 1 is also homozygous for the dominant allele of the shape gene (wrinkled peas, W) while Plant 2 is homozygous for the recessive allele (smooth peas). Based on this:

- What are the phenotypes and genotypes of the plants being crossed?[34]
- What percentage of the F_1 generation will have smooth peas?[35]
- What percentage of peas will be green and wrinkled?[36]
- What percentage of peas will be yellow and wrinkled?[37]
- Assume this cross was performed and produced 77 green wrinkled plants and 20 yellow wrinkled plants; why do these results not agree exactly with the ratios predicted?[38]
- In this cross, how does the shape gene affect inheritance of the alleles for the color gene?[39]
  - A. The percentage of green peas is increased by the shape gene.
  - B. The shape gene has no effect on the inheritance of the alleles for the color gene.
  - C. The percentage of green peas is decreased by the shape gene.
  - D. The shape gene prevents segregation of the alleles for the color gene.
  - E. The percentage of yellow peas is increased by the shape gene.

---

[34] Plant 1 has green wrinkled peas ($GgWW$), while Plant 2 has green smooth peas ($Ggww$).

[35] All peas receive one w allele and one W allele, so all are wrinkled Ww heterozygotes. This means 0% of the F_1 plants will be smooth.

[36] All F_1 peas are wrinkled (Ww) and 75% are green (GG or Gg), so 75% are green and wrinkled.

[37] All F_1 peas are wrinkled (Ww) and 25% are yellow (gg), so 25% are yellow and wrinkled.

[38] The results obtained in reality rarely agree exactly with the predicted result. If the results differ slightly from the prediction, the most likely explanation is statistical variability. The more progeny from the cross, the closer the result should be to the prediction.

[39] Independent assortment and the principle of segregation are inherent in Mendelian genetics and classical dominance. There is no reason to believe these rules are not followed (choice **B** is correct). All other choices assume either independent assortment or segregation did not occur.

A green wrinkled plant from the F1 generation is crossed with a pure-breeding yellow smooth pea plant.

- What phenotypes and genotypes are possible?[40]
- If any yellow smooth progeny are observed in this testcross, what does this indicate about the genotype of the F_1 plant?[41]

A man homozygous for eye color, *bb*, mates with a woman who is heterozygous at the same gene. What are the chances that a child will have the *Bb* genotype and be male?[42]

6.4 NON-MENDELIAN GENETICS

Incomplete Dominance

Alternative alleles do not always (or even usually) interact to exhibit classic dominance. For some traits, alleles interact to produce an intermediate phenotype or a blended phenotype. In this case, we say that the trait exhibits **incomplete dominance**. For example, suppose flower color in plants exhibits incomplete dominance, plants with an *RR* genotype have red flowers, and plants with a *WW* genotype have white flowers. In this case, plants with an *RW* genotype would have pink flowers. For alleles that display incomplete dominance, different capital letters are used for alleles of a gene (e.g., *R* and *W* instead of *R* and *r*).

- If a gene for flower color has two alleles, *R* (red) and *r* (white), what is the phenotype of *Rr* heterozygotes? [43]
- A different flowering plant has a gene with two alleles, *P* (dark purple) and *W* (white). What is the phenotype of *PW* heterozygotes?[44]
- How many phenotypes are possible if *P* and *W* display incomplete dominance?[45]
- If two heterozygous plants are crossed, what are the expected phenotypic and genotypic ratios in the F_1 generation?[46]

---

[40] A pure-breeding yellow smooth pea plant has the genotype *ggww*; this plant acts as a testcross. There are two different genotypes possible for the green wrinkled phenotype in the F_1 generation: *GGWw* or *GgWw*. Let's work through each option separately. If the F_1 plant is *GGWw*, the cross is *GGWw × ggww*. Every plant will be *Gg* and green. 50% of the plants will be *Ww* (wrinkled) and 50% will be *ww* (smooth). Overall then, half the F_2 will be green and wrinkled (*GgWw*) and half will be green and smooth (*Ggww*). The other possible cross is *GgWw × ggww*. Because one parent is a dihybrid heterozygote, this testcross will give four different genotypes and phenotypes in a 1:1:1:1 ratio. The F_2 offspring will be 25% green wrinkled (*GgWw*), 25% yellow wrinkled (*ggWw*), 25% green smooth (*Ggww*), and 25% yellow smooth (*ggww*).

[41] If yellow smooth progeny are observed, the F_1 plant must be *GgWw*.

[42] All children must receive at least one *b* allele from the father. 50% of children will receive a *B* allele from the mother; thus, 50% of the children will be *Bb*. The odds of a male offspring (XY) are 50%. Therefore, the odds a child is both male and has a *Bb* genotype are (by the rule of multiplication) 0.5 × 0.5 = 0.25, or 25%.

[43] *Rr* heterozygotes will have the phenotype of the dominant allele: red.

[44] In this case, *PW* heterozygote plants will have flowers that are neither dark purple nor white, but a blend of the two: lavender or light purple.

[45] Three phenotypes and three genotypes: *PP* (dark purple flowers), *PW* (lavender or light purple flowers, the blended phenotype), and *WW* (white).

[46] This cross is *PW × PW* and will yield 25% *PP* (plants with dark purple flowers), 50% *PW* (lavender flowers), and 25% *WW* (white flowers). Notice this is three phenotypes for three genotypes, something we didn't see when working with Mendelian inheritance (dominant/recessive alleles).

Codominance

In other cases, two different alleles for the same locus might express themselves not as an intermediate phenotype, but as two distinct phenotypes both present in a single individual. Alleles for the human blood groups (which determine your blood type) exhibit this form of interaction, known as **codominance.**

Human blood is commonly typed as A, B, or O, and either positive or negative. Blood type is determined by the expression of antigens on the surface of red blood cells (also called **erythrocytes**). An antigen is a molecule that is recognized by an antibody. We'll introduce the genetics of human blood type here, and will return to this concept again in Chapter 8.

The blood group (A, B, AB, or O) is governed by three alleles designated I^A, I^B, and i at one locus:

- The I^A allele codes for an enzyme that adds the sugar galactosamine to the lipids on the surface of red blood cells. People with this allele express antigen A on their erythrocytes.
- The I^B allele codes for an enzyme that adds the sugar galactose to the lipids on the surface of red blood cells. People with this allele express antigen B on their erythrocytes.
- The i allele does not add any sugar to the surface of red blood cells.

An individual of genotype:

1. $I^A I^A$ or $I^A i$ shows the addition of galactosamine to the surface lipids of the red blood cells (or expresses **antigen A**); this person has blood type A.
2. $I^B I^B$ or $I^B i$ shows the addition of galactose to the surface lipids of the red blood cells (or expresses **antigen B**); this person has blood type B.
3. $I^A I^B$ shows the addition of *both* galactose and galactosamine to the surface lipids of the red blood cells (or expresses both antigens A and B); this person has blood type AB.
4. ii shows the addition of no sugar to the surface lipids of the red blood cells (expresses neither antigen A nor antigen B); this person has type O blood.

Note the alleles I^A and I^B exhibit codominance. The individual who carries both alleles exhibits the trait tied to each. Neither allele is recessive in relation to the other. At the same time, however, the i allele, which does not code for the addition of any sugar on the red blood cell surface, *is* recessive in relation to both the I^A and I^B alleles. Only the genotype ii produces the blood type O phenotype.

Positive or negative blood type is determined by a separate gene called the Rh factor or **antigen D**, which exhibits classical dominance. Individuals who express antigen D have positive blood (genotype DD or Dd). If they do not express antigen D, they have negative blood (genotype dd).

- What is the phenotype of an individual heterozygous for I^A and I^B alleles?[47]
- What is the phenotype of an individual heterozygous for I^B and i?[48]
- If a woman heterozygous for type A blood mates with a man who is heterozygous for type B blood, what are the possible genotypes and blood types of their children?[49]

---

[47] This individual's RBC will express both A and B antigens, so they will have type AB blood.

[48] This individual's RBC will express B antigen only, and they will have type B blood.

[49] Because they are both heterozygous, the woman's genotype is $I^A i$ and the man's genotype is $I^B i$. Their children could be $I^A I^B$ (type AB blood, 25% probability), $I^A i$ (type A, 25% probability), $I^B i$ (type B, 25% probability), or ii (type O, 25% probability).

Linkage

The traits that Mendel studied and based the law of independent assortment on were located on separate chromosomes. Genes that are located on the *same* chromosome may not display independent assortment, however. The failure of genes to display independent assortment is called **linkage**.

Linkage and Recombination

Linkage is an exception to the law of independent assortment. When genes are located close to each other on the same chromosome, they will display linkage and may not assort independently. Meiotic recombination provides the exception to linkage. During formation of gametes, meiotic recombination between homologous chromosomes can separate alleles that were located on the same chromosome. In the example in Figure 10, three genes are located on the same chromosome. Prior to recombination, *ABC* were found on one chromosome and *abc* were found on the homologous chromosome. [What combinations of alleles will be found in gametes in the absence of recombination?[50]] Recombination produces new combinations of alleles not found in the parent and also allows genes located on the same chromosome to assort independently.

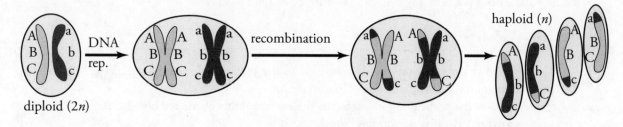

Figure 10   Recombination

Recombination Example

Let's look at an example of linkage using a pea gene for height. There are two alleles of the height gene, tall (*T*) and short (*t*). If the height gene and the green/yellow color gene we were discussing earlier are very near each other on the same chromosome, then the alleles of these genes on a specific chromosome will probably assort together into gametes during meiosis (Figure 11). This can limit the possible combinations of alleles in gametes or change their relative probabilities.

---

[50] *ABC* or *abc* genotypes

1. *TtGg* individual with independent assortment between the two genes

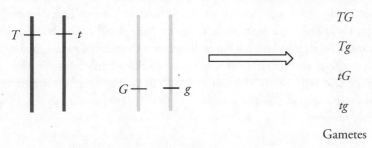

2. *TtGg* individual with complete linkage of the two genes

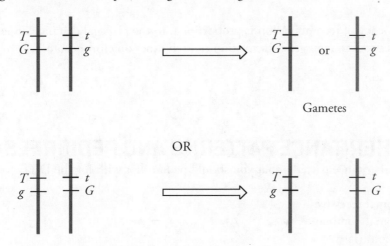

Figure 11   Linkage of Alleles during Meiosis

In the first example, although the genes are on the same chromosome, they are far apart. Recombination can occur between them and each of the resultant gametes will be present 25% of the time. This example follows Mendel's rules.

In the second example, the two genes are right beside each other with no space in between; they are 0 map units apart. They are completely **linked** and will be inherited as a unit. To know how linked alleles will assort during meiosis, it is necessary to know which alleles are on a chromosome together. As seen in Figure 11, there are two possible ways the height and color genes could be linked. The dominant alleles of two different genes can be linked together on the same chromosome (*TG*); the recessive alleles of two different genes can be linked (*tg*) on the other chromosomes. The other option is that one dominant and one recessive allele can be linked (*Tg* and *tG*). In either case, the genes are inherited as a unit, in the same allele combinations as in the parental cell.

There is also an intermediate option, in which genes are on the same chromosome as each other and more than 0 but less than 50 map units apart. In this case, some recombination can occur between the genes, but not as much as if the genes were far apart and unlinked. In this instance, parental combinations of alleles occur at a higher frequency and the products of recombination occur at a lower frequency.

The frequency of recombination between two genes on a chromosome is proportional to the physical distance between the genes along the linear length of the DNA molecule. [Does recombination occur between genes more frequently if they are near each other or far apart?[51]] The farther apart two genes are on a chromosome, the more likely recombination will occur between the genes during meiosis. If the genes are located far enough apart, recombination will occur so frequently between the genes that they will no longer display linkage and will assort as independently as if they were on separate chromosomes. The **frequency of recombination** is given as the *number of recombinant phenotypes* resulting from a cross *divided by the total number of progeny.*

$$RF = \text{recombination frequency} = \frac{\text{number of recombinants}}{\text{total number of offspring}}$$

Since the frequency of recombination is proportional to the physical distance of genes from each other, it can be used as a tool to map genes in relation to each other on chromosomes.

6.5 INHERITANCE PATTERNS AND PEDIGREES

There are six inheritance patterns that you should be familiar with for the DAT:

1. Autosomal recessive
2. Autosomal dominant
3. Mitochondrial
4. Y-linked
5. X-linked recessive
6. X-linked dominant

Autosomal Traits

Autosomal traits are caused by genetic variation on the autosomes (the 22 pairs of non-sex chromosomes in humans). These traits can be **autosomal dominant** (in which case a single copy of the allele will confer the trait or disease phenotype) or **autosomal recessive** (in which case two copies of the allele are required for the affected phenotype). Both tend to affect males and females equally; in other words, there is no sex bias for these traits.

Sex-Linked Traits

Traits that are determined by genes located on the X or Y chromosome are called **sex-linked traits** and display unusual patterns of inheritance. Traits encoded by genes on the Y chromosome (Y-linked traits) would only be passed from male parents to male children. [Would it be possible for a father to pass a

---

[51] The farther two genes are away from each other, the greater the odds that recombination will occur between them.

Y-linked trait to female children?[52] Can males be carriers of recessive Y-linked traits without expressing them?[53] Y-linked traits are quite rare, because the Y chromosome is small and contains a relatively small number of genes. Many of the genes on the Y-chromosome function in sex determination.

X-linked traits are observed quite frequently, and most are X-linked recessive. There are several well-studied examples of X-linked recessive traits that are common in the human population; hemophilia is an example. Women are often **carriers** of X-linked recessive alleles but only express recessive X-linked traits when they are homozygous. Men are **hemizygous** for X-linked traits; they have only one copy of genes on the X chromosome. As a result, males *always* express recessive X-linked alleles. [From which parent do males receive X-linked traits?[54]] These traits tend to affect males more than females.

Red-green colorblindness, an X-linked trait, is caused by a defect in a visual pigment gene on the X chromosome. The allele that is responsible for colorblindness is a pigment gene that does not produce functional protein. [Is the colorblindness allele recessive or dominant?[55]] The color blindness allele, like many recessive traits carried in the population, is not expressed in heterozygotes. Colorblindness is unusual in women but fairly common in men. Females have two copies of the gene, so will not express the trait if they are heterozygotes, while males have only one X chromosome and so will always express the allele whenever they receive it. [A man is colorblind, and his wife is homozygous normal for genes encoding visual pigment proteins. What will be the phenotypes and genotypes of sons and of daughters of this couple?[56]]

X-linked dominant traits can be tricky to identify. A female will display an X-linked dominant phenotype if she has one or two copies of the allele on her X chromosomes. A male will express the phenotype if he inherited the affected allele from his mother. From a population point of view, many of these traits affect males more than females; however this is not always the case.

Mitochondrial Inheritance

There is a small, haploid DNA genome inside the mitochondria and humans inherit this genome from their mothers. This is because sperm contribute only nuclear chromosomes to the zygote; the ova contributes nuclear chromosomes and the rest of the cellular material including the organelles. There are some traits that are inherited via the mitochondrial genome, although these **mitochondrial traits** are rare. Luckily, they are easy to spot because affected females have all affected offspring (sons and daughters). Affected individuals must have an affected mother. Individuals cannot inherit this trait from their father.

---

[52] No. Females never have a Y chromosome and so can never carry or express a Y-linked trait.

[53] No. Y-linked traits are carried in only one copy, since there is only one Y chromosome per cell. If a male carries a recessive Y-linked trait, he will express it.

[54] Since males receive their X chromosome from their mother (and their Y chromosome from their father), they receive X-linked traits from their mother.

[55] An allele that encodes inactive protein or no protein is generally recessive, since the gene's function can be compensated for by the remaining normal copy of the gene.

[56] Sons will have a normal phenotype and carry one copy of the normal gene. Daughters will carry one normal gene and one recessive colorblindness allele and will have the normal phenotype.

Table 4 summarizes the inheritance patterns you should be familiar with, and lists some strategies you can use to distinguish between them.

6.5

Inheritance Pattern	Identification Techniques	Unaffected Genotypes	Affected Genotypes
Autosomal recessive	• can skip generations (affected individuals can have unaffected parents) • number of affected males is usually equal to the number of affected females • unaffected parents can have affected offspring	AA Aa	aa
Autosomal dominant	• usually doesn't skip generations (affected individuals must have an affected parent) • number of affected males is usually equal to the number of affected females • an affected parent passes the trait to either all or half of offspring	aa	AA Aa
Mitochondrial	• maternal inheritance • affected female has all affected children • affected male cannot pass the trait onto his children • unaffected female cannot have affected children	a	A
Y-linked	• affects males only; females never have the trait • affected male has all affected sons • unaffected father cannot have an affected son	XY^a	XY^A
X-linked recessive	• can skip generations (affected individuals can have unaffected parents) • tends to affect males more than females • unaffected females can have affected sons • affected female has all affected sons, but can have both affected and unaffected daughters	X^AX^A X^AX^a X^AY	X^aX^a X^aY
X-linked dominant	• hardest to identify • does not skip generations (affected individuals must have an affected parent) • usually affects males more than females • affected males have all affected daughters • affected females can have unaffected sons, and give the trait equally to sons and daughters	X^aX^a X^aY	X^AX^A X^AX^a X^AY

Table 4 Summary of Inheritance Patterns

- Two mouse genes located on the X chromosome are being studied. The alleles of the genes are:
Fuzzy hair: *F*, dominant (normal hair) and *f*, recessive (fuzzy hair)
Extra toes: *E*, dominant (extra toes), and *e*, recessive (normal toes)
A female with normal hair and extra toes is crossed with a male with normal hair and extra toes. The progeny have the following phenotypes:

Phenotype	Male	Female
Normal hair, extra toes	51	100
Fuzzy hair, normal toes	49	0

- Which one of the following is true concerning this experiment?[57]
  A. Males have a higher rate of recombination than females do.
  B. In the absence of recombination, all males would have normal hair and extra toes.
  C. Since all female offspring have normal hair and extra toes, the female parent must be homozygous for these alleles.
  D. Fuzzy hair and normal toes are lethal in females.
  E. The female parent is heterozygous for the genes being studied.

Often it is not possible to perform controlled genetic crosses to ascertain the nature of inheritance of a trait, particularly when people are involved. In these cases, families can be studied to determine the pattern of inheritance. Researchers organize the information learned from families into **pedigrees**, which are charts depicting inheritance of a trait (See Figure 12 on the next page). By studying the pedigree of families, researchers can determine the pattern of inheritance of a gene, whether it is linked to other genes, and whether an individual is likely to pass on a trait to their offspring. Pedigrees follow certain conventions in how they are drawn:

1. Males are represented by squares and females by circles.
2. A cross (mating) between a male and female is represented by a horizontal line connecting them.
3. Offspring from a cross are connected to their parents by a vertical line, and to each other by a horizontal line with vertical branches for each sibling.
4. Offspring of unknown gender (unborn children) are represented by a diamond shape.
5. Individuals afflicted with a trait being studied are shaded in; unaffected or normal individuals are not shaded in.

Many pedigrees make a common assumption: individuals mating into the family (i.e., individuals for which you have no information on their parents or grandparents) are assumed to be homozygous normal unless their phenotype tells you differently. The basis of this assumption is that the traits being studied are usually relatively rare in the human population and therefore it is most likely that a non-family member is homozygous for the wild type allele.

---

[57] The genotype of the male parent must be $X^{FE}Y$. The presence of both the normal hair-extra toes and fuzzy hair-normal toes phenotypes in the males of the F_1 generation indicates that the female parent must have one X chromosome with both dominant alleles together, and one X chromosome with both recessive alleles together, in other words, her genotype must be $X^{FE}X^{fe}$ (eliminate C, and **E** is correct). There is no reason to assume a higher rate of recombination in males than in females, and in any case, the phenotypes of the offspring do not indicate recombination. They are simply the result of the random distribution of the mother's X chromosomes in the male offspring (eliminate A and B). Fuzzy hair and normal toes are not lethal in females; they just aren't present in the offspring because all the male parent had to donate was an X^{FE} chromosome to his daughters (eliminate D).

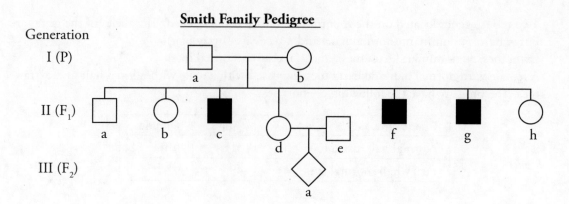

Figure 12 A Pedigree

Once drawn, a pedigree can be analyzed as follows:

1. Figure out the mode of inheritance for the trait:
    A. Check for mitochondrial inheritance. Affected females will have all affected children but affected males cannot pass the trait on.
    B. Check for Y-linked inheritance. Diseases linked to the Y chromosome affect only males and will show father-to-son transmission.
    C. Is the allele that causes the trait dominant or recessive? Recessive traits commonly skip generations, but dominant traits do not.
    D. Is the gene involved carried on a sex chromosome? If so, there tends to be an unequal distribution of affected males (more) vs. affected females (fewer). If the numbers of affected males and females are approximately equal, the gene is most likely autosomal.
2. Assign alleles and write down on your noteboard which letters stand for which alleles. For example, D = normal, d = affected.
3. You may want to also write down genotypes. For example, DD and Dd = normal, dd = affected.
4. Start with the individual you're being asked about and work backwards up the pedigree. Figure out genotypes as you go.
5. Calculate probabilities of inheritance where necessary.
6. It is highly unlikely you will have to look at two different traits on one pedigree, but if you do, repeat the steps above for the other trait.

*   In the pedigree in Figure 12, the darkened squares represent individuals afflicted with a certain genetic disease. This disease is most likely caused by:[58]
    A. a dominant allele.
    B. an autosomal recessive allele.
    C. an X-linked recessive allele.
    D. a Y-linked allele.

---

[58] Since the affected individuals have unaffected parents, the disease is most likely recessive (eliminate A), and since the affected individuals are all male, it is most likely sex-linked (eliminate B). There is no father-to-son transmission (all affected males have an unaffected father), so the disease is most likely X-linked (eliminate D; **C** is correct).

6.5

- In the pedigree in Figure 12, what is the probability that IIIa will have the disease?[59]
  - A. If male, IIIa will have the disease.
  - B. Overall, there is a 1/8 chance that IIIa will have the disease.
  - C. Overall, there is a 1/4 chance that IIIa will have the disease.
  - D. IIIa will not have the disease.

Below are example pedigrees for six modes of inheritance (X-linked recessive, X-linked dominant, autosomal recessive, autosomal dominant, mitochondrial, and Y-linked). For each pedigree, determine which mode of inheritance is displayed. The explanation is on the next page.

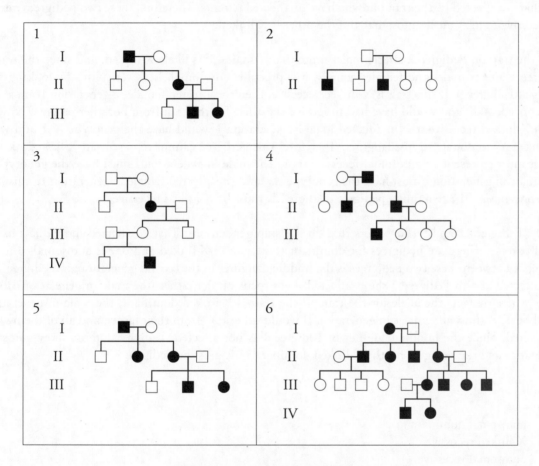

Figure 13 Example Pedigrees

---

[59] The disease is X-linked recessive, and IIe (IIIa's father) is not affected, so IIe cannot pass the allele on. Thus the probability of IIIa getting the disease depends on the genotype of IId (she would have to be a carrier) and what she passes on to IIIa. It also depends on the sex of IIIa; females would not be affected because they would have to receive the allele from both IId and IIe, and IIe does not carry the disease allele. Bottom line, in order for IIIa to get the disease, IId would have to be a carrier, would have to pass the disease allele on, and IIIa would have to be male. The probability of IId being a carrier is 1/2; we know she received a wild type X chromosome from her father Ia (all he has is a wild type X chromosome), and the probability she received the affected X chromosome from her mother (Ib) is 1/2. The probability she passes the affected X chromosome on to IIIa is 1/2; she has one wild type X and one affected X. The probability that IIIa is male is 1/2. Finally, we can use the rule of multiplication to determine the overall probability: $1/2 \times 1/2 \times 1/2 = 1/8$ overall probability (choice **B** is correct; eliminate C and D). Note that A is wrong because being male does not guarantee the disease; IIIa could be male (get the Y chromosome from IIe) and still be unaffected (get the wild type X chromosome from IId).

6.5

Explanation

The easiest inheritance patterns to spot are mitochondrial (passed from mothers to all offspring) and Y-linked (passed from fathers to sons, and females are never affected). Let's start by finding these two. Since Pedigree 6 shows a trait with maternal inheritance, this must be mitochondrial inheritance. The affected father in generation II does not pass the trait to any of his children, but the affected mothers in generations I, II and III pass the trait onto all their offspring. Pedigree 4 shows a trait with Y-linked inheritance. The trait is passed from father to all sons and does not affect females.

Next, Pedigrees 2 and 3 both show traits that skip generations. That is, there are individuals on the pedigree that are affected by the trait but who have unaffected parents. Therefore, these two pedigrees must be for recessive traits. One is autosomal and the other is X-linked.

Since the trait on Pedigree 2 affects males more than females, it is likely X-linked, and since the trait on Pedigree 3 affects males and females equally, it is probably autosomal. Let's verify this by looking more closely at Pedigree 3. If this trait is X-linked recessive, then the affected female in generation II must have the genotype X^aX^a and would have had to receive the allele for the trait from both her parents. However, for an X-linked recessive, the unaffected male in generation I would have the genotype X^AY and would only have X^A to donate to his daughter. Therefore, this pedigree cannot represent an X-linked recessive trait; it must represent an autosomal recessive trait. The male in generation I must have the genotype Aa, the female in generation I must have the genotype Aa, and the affected female in generation II must have the genotype aa. The remaining pedigree, Pedigree 2, must be X-linked recessive.

Finally, Pedigrees 1 and 5 show traits that do not skip generations. That is, affected individuals have affected parents. These are pedigrees for dominant traits; one is X-linked and one is autosomal. The only difference between these two pedigrees is the middle daughter in the second generation; in Pedigree 1 she is unaffected and in Pedigree 5 she is affected. Let's focus on her father (the male in generation I) since this is where she gets the allele for the trait. If the trait is X-linked dominant, the male in generation I would be X^AY; thus, all females in generation II would inherit X^A from their father, and all of them would be affected. Since the middle daughter in Pedigree 1 is not affected, Pedigree 1 must show autosomal dominance and the pedigree for the X-linked dominant trait must be Pedigree 5.

Overall:

1. autosomal dominant
2. X-linked recessive
3. autosomal recessive
4. Y-linked
5. X-linked dominant
6. mitochondrial inheritance

6.6 POPULATION GENETICS

Mendelian genetics describes the inheritance of traits in progeny of specific individuals. For the purposes of large topics such as natural selection and evolution, however, the more relevant issue is not inheritance of traits from individuals but in a whole population from one generation to another. **Population genetics** describes the inheritance of traits in populations over time. The word *population* has a specific meaning in this setting: *a population consists of members of a species that mate and reproduce with each other*; we'll talk about this more in the next chapter. [If a group of sea turtles lives most of the year dispersed over a large area of ocean without contact with each other but congregate once a year to reproduce, is this group a population?[60]] To a population geneticist, each individual is merely a temporary carrier of the alleles in a population.

In population genetics, the units of genetic inheritance are alleles of genes, just as in Mendelian genetics. However, in population genetics alleles are examined across the entire population rather than in individuals. The sum total of all genetic information in a population is called the **gene pool**. [For an autosomal gene in a population of 2,000 individuals, how many copies of the gene are present in the gene pool?[61]] The frequency of an allele in a population is a key variable used to describe the gene pool. [If there are 5,000 hippos in a population, out of which there are 100 homozygotes of an autosomal allele h and 400 heterozygotes, what is the frequency of the h allele in the population?[62] If 20% of the population is heterozygous for an allele Q and 10% is homozygous, what will be the frequency of the allele in the population?[63]]

Hardy-Weinberg in Population Genetics

Population genetics does not simply describe the gene pool of a population but attempts to predict the gene pool of a population in the future. The **Hardy-Weinberg law** states that the *frequencies of alleles in the gene pool of a population will not change over time*, provided five assumptions are true:

1. There is no mutation.
2. There is no migration.
3. There is no natural selection.
4. There is random mating.
5. The population is sufficiently large to prevent random drift in allele frequencies.

At the molecular level, this means segregation of alleles, independent assortment, and recombination during meiosis can alter the combinations of alleles in gametes. However, these processes will not change the frequency of an allele in the population as a whole.

---

[60] Yes. A population does not need to live with each other, only to reproduce sexually with each other.

[61] There are two copies of the gene in each of the 2,000 individuals, for a total of 4,000 copies in the gene pool.

[62] Allele frequency is the number of copies of a specific allele divided by the total number of copies of the gene in the population. If there are 5,000 hippos, and each has 2 copies of the gene, there are 10,000 copies of the gene in the population. There are 100 homozygotes of the h allele, each with 2 copies of it, and 400 heterozygotes with one h allele, for a total of 600 h alleles in the population. Thus, the frequency of the h allele is 600/10,000 = 0.06.

[63] In this case, the number of individuals in the population is not provided, but it is not needed. The total number of alleles is 100%. The frequency of the allele is 0.5 × (20% heterozygotes) + 10% homozygotes = 20%.

- If 100 homozygous green pea plants and 100 homozygous yellow pea plants are crossed, 1,000 green pea plants are produced. Does this mean that the yellow alleles disappeared from the population?[64]
- What is the frequency of the yellow allele in the gene pool of the progeny?[65]
- If the green peas from the F_1 generation are allowed to mate randomly within the population, and there is no mutation, migration, natural selection, or random drift, what will be the frequency of the yellow allele in the population after four generations?[66]
- If two genes are closely linked on the same chromosome, will Hardy-Weinberg still apply to these genes?[67]
- According to Hardy-Weinberg, what will happen to the frequency of the yellow allele if predation occurs on yellow plants, but yellow plants attract bees more successfully?[68]

The Hardy-Weinberg law has also been translated into mathematical terms. Assuming that there are two alleles of a gene in a population, the letter p is used to represent the frequency of the dominant allele, and the letter q is used to represent the frequency of the recessive allele. Since there are only two alleles, the following fundamental equation must be true:

$$p + q = 1$$

Based on allele frequency, it is possible to calculate the proportion of genotypes in a population. Take a situation where frequency of a dominant allele (G) equals p and frequency of a recessive allele (g) equals q. If the equation above is squared on both sides, it becomes:

$$(p + q)^2 = 1$$

$$p^2 + 2pq + q^2 = 1$$

where

$$p^2 = \text{frequency of the } GG \text{ genotype}$$
$$2pq = \text{frequency of the } Gg \text{ genotype}$$
$$q^2 = \text{frequency of the } gg \text{ genotype}$$

- If frequency of the G allele is 0.25 in a population of 1,000 mice, determine the number of individuals who are Gg heterozygotes if there is random mating but no migration, mutation, random drift, or natural selection.[69]

---

[64] The yellow alleles are still there (but in the heterozygous state) so they do not appear in the phenotype.

[65] The frequency of the yellow allele will be 50%, just as it was in the parents. None of the alleles in a population were destroyed, so the frequency is the same as in the parental generation.

[66] According to Hardy-Weinberg, there will be no change in the frequency of the allele. The frequency of the yellow allele will still be 50% after four generations.

[67] Yes. Independent assortment is not a requirement of Hardy-Weinberg. Allele frequencies for the genes will still remain constant, regardless of the extent of recombination between the genes, as long as the assumptions of Hardy-Weinberg hold true.

[68] Hardy-Weinberg says nothing about this situation. Once the assumptions no longer hold true, Hardy-Weinberg no longer applies.

[69] If frequency of the G allele (p) is 0.25, then frequency of the g allele (q) must be 0.75, since $p + q = 1$. Frequency of the heterozygotes in the population will be $2pq = 2(0.25)(0.75) = 0.375$. Therefore, the number of individuals in this population who are heterozygotes will be $0.375 \times 1,000 = 375$.

- If allele frequencies in a population are constant, and genotype frequencies can be calculated from allele frequencies, how will genotype frequencies vary over time?[70]

After one generation, a population will reach **Hardy-Weinberg equilibrium**, in which allele frequencies no longer change. Since allele frequencies do not change, and genotype frequencies can be calculated from allele frequencies, it follows that genotype frequencies also do not change over time. [If 100 green peas (*GG*) and 100 yellow peas (*gg*) are allowed to mate randomly, will the genotype frequencies in the next generation (F_1) be the same?[71] If not, why not?[72] If the plants are allowed to mate randomly for another generation (F_2), will the genotype frequencies in the F_1 and F_2 generations be the same?[73]]

6.6

Hardy-Weinberg in the Real World

Hardy-Weinberg requires a number of assumptions in order to be true. The assumptions, as presented earlier, are that in a population there is random mating and no mutation, migration, natural selection, or random drift. Thus, Hardy-Weinberg describes a highly idealized set of conditions required to prevent alleles from being added or removed from a population. In reality, it is not possible for a population to meet all of the conditions required by Hardy-Weinberg.

1. **Mutation**: Mutation is inevitable in a population. Even if there are no chemical mutagens or radiation, inherent errors by DNA polymerase would over time cause mutations and introduce new alleles in a population.
2. **Migration**: If migration occurs, animals leaving or entering the population will carry alleles with them and disturb the Hardy-Weinberg equilibrium. In ecological systems, it is hard to prevent at least some migration.
3. **Natural Selection**: For there to be no natural selection, there would have to be unlimited resources, no predation, no disease, and so on. This is not a set of conditions encountered in the real world.
4. **Non-random Mating**: If individuals pick their mates preferentially based on one or more traits, alleles that cause those traits will be passed on preferentially from one generation to another. For a lot of organisms (including us) truly random mating is rare.
5. **Random Drift**: If a population becomes small, it cannot contain as great a variety of alleles. In a very small population, random events can alter allele frequencies significantly and have a large influence on future generations.

Want More Practice?
Scan the QR code below to register your book for online chapter summaries, drills, practice tests, and more!

---

[70] Genotype frequencies, as well as allele frequencies, will remain constant according to Hardy-Weinberg.

[71] No. The next generation will include *GG, Gg,* and *gg* genotypes.

[72] The population was not at Hardy-Weinberg equilibrium to start out.

[73] Yes. A population reaches Hardy-Weinberg equilibrium after one generation. The F_2 generation (and all generations after that) will have the same genotype frequencies as the F_1 generation.

Chapter 7
Evolution, Diversity of Life, Ecology, and Animal Behavior

7.1 ORIGIN OF LIFE

Based on radioisotope dating, the earth is thought to be 4.5 billion years old. All life evolved from pro-karyotes. The oldest fossils are 3.5-billion-year-old outlines of primitive prokaryotic cell walls found in stromatolites (layered mats formed by colonies of prokaryotes). Even older life-forms certainly existed but lacked cell walls and thus left no fossil record (at least none have yet been discovered). Hence, life on Earth is older than 3.5 billion years, nearly as old as the planet itself.

The atmosphere of the young Earth was different from today's atmosphere. The predominant gases then were probably H_2O, CO, CO_2, and N_2. The most important thing to note here is the absence of O_2. It is thought that the early atmosphere was a **reducing environment**, where electron donors were prevalent. Oxygen is an electron acceptor and thus tends to break organic bonds. In this early world, simple organic molecules, or monomers ("single units") could form spontaneously. The energy for this synthesis was provided by lightning, radioactive decay, volcanic activity, or the Sun's radiation, which was more intense than it is today due to the thinner atmosphere. Laboratory recreations of the early environment result in the spontaneous formation of amino acids, carbohydrates, lipids, and ribonucleotides, as well as other organic compounds.

Spontaneous polymerization of these monomers can also be observed in the lab (including spontaneous polymerization of ribonucleotides). No enzymes were present when this was occurring for the first time in nature, but it is thought that metal ions on the surface of rocks and especially clay acted as catalysts. This is known as **abiotic synthesis**. Polypeptides made in this way are called **proteinoids**.

Proteinoids in water spontaneously form droplets called **microspheres**. When lipids are added to the solution, **liposomes** form, with lipids forming a layer on the surface of proteins. A more complex particle known as a **coacervate** includes polypeptides, nucleic acids, and polysaccharides. Coacervates made with pre-existing enzymes are capable of catalyzing reactions. Microspheres, liposomes, and coacervates are collectively referred to as **protobionts**.

Protobionts resemble cells in that they contain a protected inner environment and perform chemical re-actions. They can also reproduce to a certain extent: when they grow too large, they split in half. What is lacking, however, is an organized mechanism of heredity. This was first provided by RNA. As noted above, RNA chains form spontaneously in the appropriate solution. Even more interesting is the observa-tion that single-stranded RNA chains can be self-replicating. A daughter chain lines up on the parent by base pairing and then spontaneously polymerizes with a surprisingly low error rate. A nonspecific catalyst such as a metal ion can further increase the efficiency of RNA self-replication. Furthermore, it is now known that RNA has catalytic activity in modern cells. For example, in primitive eukaryotes, introns are spliced out of the mRNA by **ribozymes**, which are RNA enzymes.

Somehow, a mechanism evolved for polypeptides to be copied from early RNA genes. You already know about the inherent tendency for phospholipids to form lipid bilayers. Given all this information, it's not too hard to imagine true cells evolving from a primordial soup at the dawn of time. The last step in the evolution of the earliest cells would have been the switch from RNA to DNA as the genetic material. DNA is more stable due to its 2'-deoxy structure and because it spontaneously forms a compact double-stranded helix.

7.2 EVOLUTION

At one time, life on Earth was generally viewed as static and unchanging, but we now know that this is not the case. Over the geologic span of Earth's history, many species have arisen, changed over millions of years, given rise to new species, and died out. These changes in life on Earth are called **evolution**. Although he did not arrive at his theory alone, Charles Darwin played an important role in shaping modern thought by proposing natural selection as the mechanism that drives evolution. **Natural selection** is an interaction between organisms and their environment that causes differential reproduction of different phenotypes and thereby alters the gene pool of a **population**. In essence the theory of evolution by natural selection is this:

1. In a population, there are heritable differences between individuals.
2. Heritable traits (alleles of genes) produce traits (phenotypes) that affect the ability of an organism to survive and have offspring.
3. Some individuals have phenotypes that allow them to survive longer, be healthier, and have more offspring than others.
4. Individuals with phenotypes that allow them to have more offspring will pass on their alleles more frequently than those with phenotypes that have fewer offspring.
5. Over time, those alleles that lead to more offspring are passed on more frequently and become more abundant, while other alleles become less abundant in the gene pool.
6. Changes in allele frequency are the basis of evolution in species and populations.

To put it simply, evolution occurs when natural selection acts on genetic variation to drive changes in the genetic composition of a population. A key term in evolution is **fitness**. In evolutionary terms, fitness is not how well an animal is physically adapted to a niche in the environment, or how well it can feed itself, but how successful it is in passing on its alleles to future generations. The way to have greater fitness is by having more offspring that pass on their alleles to future generations of the population. Some species achieve greater fitness through sheer numbers of progeny produced, who are then left to fend for themselves. Other species have fewer progeny, but protect and nurture the young to maturity.

- If an allele of a gene causes cancer in elderly polar bears after their reproductive years have passed, how will it affect the fitness of bears carrying the allele?[1]
- If a recessive allele causes sterility in homozygotes, how will it affect the fitness of heterozygotes?[2]
- Which of the following will have greater fitness: a fish that has two offspring and protects and nurtures its young to maturity, or a fish that has 10 offspring and abandons them, resulting in the death of 8 young fish before maturity?[3]
- The recessive allele that causes cystic fibrosis is strongly selected against in modern society, since individuals with this disease often die before sexual maturity. However, the frequency of the allele takes many generations to decrease in the population. Why?[4]

---

[1] The allele will not affect fitness. The bears will only be affected at a time when they can no longer have offspring, so it will not affect the ability of bears to transmit their alleles to future generations.

[2] If the allele is truly recessive, it will not affect fitness at all. Natural selection can act only on phenotypes, not genotypes.

[3] The fish will technically have the same fitness, since both will contribute to the gene pool of future generations equally.

[4] Natural selection acts on phenotypes, not genotypes. Even if the allele is lethal in homozygotes, heterozygotes will not be selected against if the allele is not expressed. It takes many generations for deleterious recessive alleles to decrease in frequency in a population.

- A certain genetic disease is caused by a recessive allele. In the absence of effective therapy, homozygous individuals with this allele generally die before reaching sexual maturity. The allele also protects heterozygous individuals against several life-threatening viral diseases. If a medicine is found that provides a complete remedy for the disease, allowing individuals with the disease to live an entirely normal life, which of the following statements describes what will happen to the frequency of the allele in the population after that time?[5]
    - A. The frequency of the allele will decrease.
    - B. The frequency of the allele will remain constant.
    - C. The frequency of the allele will increase.
    - D. It is not possible to predict the future frequency of the allele.

Sources of Genetic Diversity

Natural selection acts on the genetic diversity in a population to alter allele frequencies, causing evolution. Genetic diversity in a population is a requirement for natural selection to occur. [If a population of sea otters contains only one allele of a gene that protects against cold, can natural selection drive evolution of this trait?[6] Can natural selection cause new alleles to appear in the population?[7]] Natural selection does not introduce genetic diversity, however; it can act only on existing diversity to alter allele frequencies.

There are two sources of genetic variation in a population: *new alleles* and *new combinations of existing alleles*. New alleles are the result of mutations in the genome. New combinations of alleles are generated during sexual reproduction as a result of independent assortment, recombination and segregation during meiosis. By increasing and maintaining genetic variation in a population, sexual reproduction allows for greater capacity for adaptation of a population to changing environmental conditions.

- Do new alleles in a population generally confer greater or lesser fitness on an individual carrying them?[8]
- If a mutation occurs in a muscle cell of an individual who then has many progeny, does this mutation increase genetic variation in the population?[9]
- Does mitosis contribute to the genetic variation in a population?[10]

---

[5] The correct answer is **C**. Homozygotes have low fitness in the absence of medicine, while heterozygotes have increased fitness due to their resistance to viral disease. In the absence of the medicine, natural selection tends to reduce the frequency of the allele by removing individuals who are homozygous but tends to increase the frequency of the allele through the higher fitness of heterozygotes. Over time these opposing selection pressures can be balanced to keep the allele at a relatively constant frequency. If medicine removes the selection against homozygotes, then the heterozygotes with the increased fitness cause allele frequency to increase over time.

[6] If there is only one allele, there is no variability for natural selection to act on, and no way allele frequencies can change to cause evolution.

[7] No. Natural selection can only alter the frequency of existing alleles, not create new alleles.

[8] This is a tricky question to answer because our understanding of molecular and evolutionary biology is constantly changing. Ten years ago, we thought new alleles caused by mutation generally rendered gene products less active or even inactive. Animals adapted over long periods of time to have most gene products function in an optimal manner, so most genetic changes were thought to be harmful rather than beneficial. However, in research and clinical practice, mutations are usually called "genetic variants" now because we are starting to understand that not all mutations are bad. In fact, many genetic variants have little or no effect on the protein, cell, tissue, and organism. Several gain-of-function mutations have also been studied, and while these usually confer less fitness to an organism, some can offer an evolutionary advantage.

[9] No. Mutation must occur in the germ line to introduce a new allele into a population. A mutation in a somatic cell cannot be passed on to the next generation.

[10] No. Mitosis can only copy a cell into an identical cell; it is not involved in creating new combinations of alleles in the same manner as meiosis.

- If a population of flowers loses the ability to reproduce sexually and reproduces only asexually, how will this affect natural selection in the population?[11]
- Plants that are pollinated by insects sometimes have physical features of the flower that prevent self-pollination. What is the advantage to the plant of preventing self-pollination?[12]
- Which one of the following can create new alleles in a population?[13]
    A. Non-random mating
    B. Random drift
    C. Recombination
    D. Deletion
    E. Natural selection

Modes of Natural Selection

Natural selection can occur in many different manners and have different effects in a population. The following are a few examples:

1. **Directional Selection:** Polygenic traits often follow a bell-shaped curve of expression, with most individuals clustered around the average and some members of a population trailing off in either direction away from the average. If natural selection removes those at one extreme, the population average over time will move in the other direction. Example: giraffes get taller as all short giraffes die for lack of food.

2. **Divergent Selection:** This can also be called **disruptive selection.** Rather than removing extreme members in the distribution of a trait in a population, this type of natural selection removes members near the average, leaving those at either end. Over time divergent selection will split the population in two and perhaps lead to a new species. Example: small deer are selected because they can hide, and large deer are selected because they can fight, but mid-sized deer are too big to hide and too small to fight.

3. **Stabilizing Selection:** Both extremes of a trait are selected against, driving the population closer to the average. Example: birds that are too large or too small are eliminated from a population because they cannot mate.

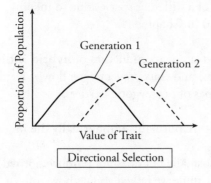
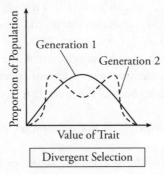
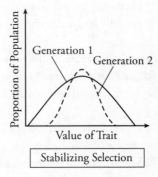

Figure 1

---

[11] If the flowers can only reproduce asexually, they have lost the ability of meiosis to generate new combinations of alleles and new genetic variation for natural selection to act on.

[12] Self-pollination reduces genetic variability. More variability is maintained in the population if different individuals mate, making new combinations of alleles.

[13] Nonrandom mating, random drift, and natural selection will alter allele frequencies but do not create new alleles (eliminate A, B, and E). Recombination will not alter allele frequencies or create new alleles, but create new combinations of alleles (eliminate C). The correct answer is **D.** Only mutation of the genome can create new alleles. A deletion can create a new allele, even if the new allele is a truncated gene product or does not express any gene product at all.

7.3

4. **Artificial Selection:** Humans intervene in the mating of many animals and plants, using artificial selection to achieve desired traits through controlled mating. Example: the pets and crop plants we have are the result of many generations of artificial selection.

5. **Sexual Selection:** Animals often do not choose mates randomly, but have evolved elaborate rituals and physical displays that play a key role in attracting and choosing a mate. Example: some birds have bright plumage to attract a mate, even at the cost of increased predation.

6. **Kin Selection:** Natural selection does not always act on individuals. Animals that live socially often share alleles with other individuals and will sacrifice themselves for the sake of the alleles they share with another individual. Example: a female lion sacrifices herself to save her sister's children.

7.3 THE SPECIES CONCEPT AND SPECIATION

A **species** is a group of organisms that are capable of reproducing with each other sexually. Other criteria, such as morphology, are used to classify species that only reproduce asexually. [What's the difference between a population and a species?[14]] Two individuals are not members of the same biological species if they cannot mate and produce fit offspring. [When a horse mates with a donkey a mule is born. Mules are healthy animals with long life spans, but they are sterile. Are horses and donkeys members of the same species?[15]] **Reproductive isolation** keeps existing species separate. There are two types of reproductive isolation: prezygotic and postzygotic.

Prezygotic barriers prevent formation of a hybrid zygote. Such barriers may be:

- Ecological: individuals who could otherwise mate live in different habitats and thus cannot access each other.
- Temporal: individuals mate at different times of the day, season, or year.
- Behavioral: some species require special rituals or courtship behaviors before mating can occur.
- Mechanical: reproductive structures or genital organs of two individuals are not compatible (even if they court and attempt copulation).
- Gametic: sperm from one species cannot fertilize the egg of a different species due to incompatibilities in the sperm–egg recognition system, discussed in Chapter 11.

Postzygotic barriers to hybridization prevent development, survival, or reproduction of **hybrid individuals** (those that arise from a mating between two different species) and thus prevent gene flow if fertilization between two different species does occur. There are three types of postzygotic barriers:

- Hybrid inviability: hybrid offspring do not develop or mature normally and normally die in the embryonic stage.
- Hybrid sterility: a hybrid individual is born and develops normally but does not produce normal gametes and thus is incapable of breeding. For example, the mule we talked about above (offspring of a mating between a horse and a donkey) is sterile and an example of a hybrid animal.[16]

---

[14] Members of a species *can* mate and produce fit offspring. Members of a population *do*. Remember it this way: a population is a subset of a species.

[15] No, since their offspring are unfit (unable to reproduce).

[16] Several hybrid animals have been reported or observed. Some examples (with their parent species in parentheses) are cama (camel/lama), coywolf (coyote/wolf), grolar bear or pizzly bear (grizzly bear/polar bear), liger or tion (lion/tiger), wholphin (killer whale/bottlenose dolphin), zorse (zebra/horse). Most of these hybrids are the result of artificial breeding programs, but a few have been observed in the wild.

- Hybrid breakdown: two hybrids mate successfully to produce a hybrid offspring, but this second-generation hybrid is somehow biologically defective.

The creation of new species is known as **speciation**. An important premise in modern biology is that all species come from preexisting species. **Cladogenesis** is branching speciation (*clado* is from the Greek for branch), where one species diversifies and becomes two or more new species. **Anagenesis** is when one biological species simply becomes another by changing so much that if an individual were to go back in time, it would be unable to reproduce sexually with its ancestors. One type of cladogenesis, **allopatric isolation**, is initiated by geographical isolation. Over time, geographical isolation leads to reproductive isolation. **Sympatric speciation** occurs when a species gives rise to a new species in the same geographical area, such as through divergent selection.

Cladogenesis has left traces which taxonomists use to classify organisms. **Homologous structures** are physical features shared by two different species as a result of a common ancestor. For example, bird wings have five bony supports which resemble distorted human fingers, and dog paws also resemble distorted human hands. The explanation is that dogs, birds, and people all have a common ancestor which had five-toed feet. **Analogous structures** serve the same function in two different species, but *not* due to common ancestry. The flagellum of the human sperm and bacterial flagella are an example; they have entirely different structures from different organisms yet play the same role in motility. **Convergent evolution** is when two different species come to possess many analogous structures due to similar selective pressures. For example, bats and birds appear very similar even though bats are mammals. The opposite of convergent evolution is **divergent evolution**, in which divergent selection causes cladogenesis. **Parallel evolution** describes the situation in which two species go through similar evolutionary changes due to similar selective pressures. For example, in an ice age, all organisms would be selected for their ability to tolerate cold.

A **cladogram** is a diagram used in cladistics to show how organisms are related. They are based on phylogeny, or the study of evolutionary relationships. Lines branch off in different directions and end in a clade, or a group of organisms with a common ancestor. The lengths of the lines in cladograms are not important, but the order of the splitting is important. The branch point represents a hypothetical ancestor and the organisms that stem from the branch point share features, traits or characteristics. Cladograms are made based on morphological characteristics, DNA and RNA sequencing, and statistics.

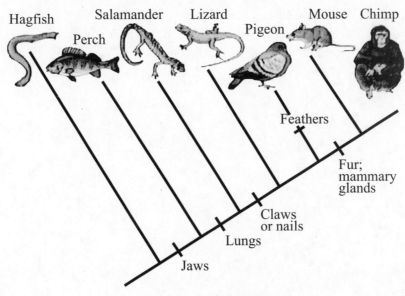

Figure 2   A Cladogram

7.4

In Figure 2:

- Jaws, lungs, claws or nails, feathers, and fur were used to create the cladogram.
- The original ancestor is represented by the beginning of the line on the lower left.
- The first node (just to the left of jaws) splits the animals into things without jaws and things with jaws. The only thing without jaws is the hagfish.
- The next node splits the jawed animals into those with jaws and no lungs, and those with jaws and lungs. This splits off the perch.
- In other words, hagfish have no jaws and no lungs, perch have jaws but not lungs, and salamanders have jaws and lungs but not claws.

Cladograms can misrepresent relationships if species have traits in common but not ancestors in common; sometimes the same traits evolve independently. For example, if a cladogram used the trait of wings, then birds and bats would get lumped together. In reality, bats are mammals; they are not birds. Their wings evolved differently than birds' wings.

7.4 INTRODUCTION TO DIVERSITY OF LIFE

Binomial Classification System

Taxonomy is the science of biological classification, originated by Carolus Linnaeus in the 18th century. He devised the **binomial classification** system we use today, in which each organism is given two names: genus and species. The binomial name of an organism is written in italics (or is underlined) with the genus capitalized and the species not, as in *Homo sapiens* (man the wise). There are eight principal taxonomic categories: **Domain**, **Kingdom**, **Phylum**, **Class**, **Order**, **Family**, **Genus**, and **Species**.

Overview

Below is a chart summarizing domains and kingdoms. Each will be discussed in greater detail in the sections that follow.

7.4

Domain	Bacteria	Archaea	Eukarya			
Kingdom	**Formerly Monera**		**Protista**	**Fungi**	**Plantae**	**Animalia**
Cell Wall	Peptidoglycan	Chain mail proteins	Optional and varied	Chitin	Cellulose	None
Membrane-Bound Organelles	None	None	Typical eukaryotic organelles such as nucleus, RER, SER, Golgi, peroxisome, lysosomes, chloroplasts, vacuoles, mitochondria, etc.			
Chromosomes	1 circular ds DNA	1 circular ds DNA	Several linear ds DNA chromosomes			
Life cycle and Reproduction	Asexual repro. (binary fission)	Asexual repro. (binary fission)	Varied (sexual and asexual)	Varied (sexual and asexual)	Mostly sexual repro.	Mostly sexual repro.
Cellularity	Unicellular	Unicellular	Mostly unicellular	Mostly multicellular	Multicellular	Multicellular
Ploidy	Haploid	Haploid	Haploid or diploid	Mostly haploid	Alternate between haploid and diploid	Diploid
Cellular motility	Flagella	Flagella	Amoeboid or flagellar	Non-motile	Some flagellated sperm	Amoeboid or flagellar
Cilia	None	None	Characteristic 9 + 2 arrangement of microtubules			
Flagella	Bacterial flagellin proteins	Archaeal flagellin proteins				
Nutrition	Varied, absorptive	Varied, absorptive	Varied	Chemotroph Heterotroph Absorptive	Autotroph via photosynth.	Chemotroph Heterotroph Ingestive
Glycolysis/ ATP	All living organisms perform glycolysis & use ATP. All kingdoms contain at least some members which perform oxidative phosphorylation.					
Examples	Bacteria *E. coli* Blue-green algae	Extremophiles	Euglena Paramecium Plasmodium Seaweed	Yeasts Molds Mushrooms	Trees Flowers Mosses Ferns	Sponges Worms Mollusks Insects Reptiles Mammals

Table 1 Taxonomic Characteristics

7.5   DOMAIN EUBACTERIA

Most prokaryotes fall into this category. They are ubiquitous organisms that are small, and have simple circular genomes (made of double-stranded DNA) and no membrane-bound organelles. Eubacteria have a cell wall made of **peptidoglycan**. Under the previous five kingdom classification system of taxonomy, these organisms were grouped with Archaebacteria in Kingdom Monera.

The cell biology of this domain was discussed in Chapter 5. These organisms divide asexually via binary fission but can undergo genetic exchange via **lateral gene transfer**. **Conjugation** allows for genetic exchange between two bacterial cells via sex pili, **transduction** is genetic exchange via a lysogenic phage, and **transformation** occurs when bacteria take up nucleic acid material from the environment. Some use flagella for motility, and they are scored as Gram positive or Gram negative depending on their cell wall and membrane composition. Some species in this domain live in mutualistic relationships, such as the *E. coli* in your large intestine. Others are pathogenic, and some are **decomposers**. Cyanobacteria—plant-like prokaryotes that have chlorophyll and perform photosynthesis—are also Eubacteria. Cyanobacteria are sometimes called blue-green algae and they live primarily in fresh water.

7.6   DOMAIN ARCHAEBACTERIA

Most of these unicellular organisms live in extreme conditions, such as hot springs or extremely salty ponds. Archaea are extremophiles and prokaryotic. They are relatively small, have simple circular genomes and no membrane-bound organelles. The Archaea flagella functions like bacterial flagella, but is synthesized differently. Most Archaea possess a cell wall, made of surface-layer proteins, that covers the outside of the cell like chain mail. This provides both chemical and physical protection, and can prevent macromolecules from contacting the cell membrane. Archaea perform some basic pathways differently than Eubacteria, including membrane synthesis, some metabolic pathways and protein synthesis.

7.7   DOMAIN EUKARYA

Four Kingdoms are included in this eukaryotic domain: Protista, Fungi, Plantae and Animalia.

Kingdom Protista

Protists are extremely varied unicellular eukaryotes (note that a small few are multicellular and many of the unicellular species can form colonies). Most protists live in aquatic or damp environments such as damp soil, leaf litter, oceans, ponds and lakes. They make up most of the slimes and scums you see around you and are divided into animal-like, fungal-like, or plant-like categories, mostly depending on how they obtain food and nutrients.

Animal-Like Protists (Protozoa)

Protozoa are unicellular, animal-like, ingestive protists; **ingestive feeders** are organisms that ingest food and then digest it inside the body or cell (similar to animals). This group includes the following phyla:

- Amoebas move via **pseudopodia**, which are temporary extensions of the plasma membrane created by actin filaments; pseudopodia can also help amoebas engulf food particles.
- Zooflagellates move using flagella. An example is Euglena, an algae that lives in murky ponds.
- Ciliophores (or ciliates) move via cilia. A well characterized example is the Paramecium.
- Protists in the Apicomplexa phyla are non-motile. Many are parasites and a common example is the animal parasite Plasmodium (which causes malaria).

Fungus-Like Protists (Molds and Mildews)

This category includes many slime molds, water molds, and mildews. These species are **absorptive feeders**, which means they digest molecules outside the cell then transport them in (similar to fungi). Many species are decomposers and live in damp terrestrial areas. This group includes slime molds (which reproduce via spores) as well as mildews and water molds (which reproduce using an egg cell and a sperm cell).

Plant-Like Protists (Algae)

Algae are photosynthetic **autotrophs** (similar to plants) and generally have multiple chlorophyll pigments. Almost all algae contain **chlorophyll a** (the same pigment found in plants) but there is great diversity in accessory pigments that give them their characteristic colors. Most of these organisms live in aquatic biomes[17]. Some are unicellular and others are multicellular.

- Brown Algae (or Phaeophyta) contain the brownish pigment **fucoxanthin**. Most are multicellular algae, including seaweeds of colder northern hemisphere waters; kelp is an example.
- Golden Algae (or Chrysophyta) contain chlorophyll a, **chlorophyll c**, and fucoxanthin, giving them a golden-brown color. This group includes unicellular **diatoms**, which are major constituents of sediment; their glasslike cell walls made of silica remain behind after the cell dies, and function in water filtration.
- Red Algae (or Rhodophyta) contain chlorophyll a and **phycobiliproteins**. Most species are multicellular and macroscopic. They are used to make agar in microbiology laboratories.
- Green Algae (or Chlorophyta) contain chlorophyll a and **chlorophyll b**. Some species of green algae can be found in terrestrial biomes and in symbiotic associations with fungi to form lichens.

---

[17] Remember that this includes both marine (salt water) and freshwater environments.

KINGDOM FUNGI

Cell Biology

Fungi are eukaryotic and possess all of the features that distinguish eukaryotes from prokaryotes, like nuclei and mitochondria (see Chapter 5). Fungi possess a rigid cell wall composed of **chitin**, which is different from plant and bacterial cell walls[18], but is found in the exoskeleton of insects. Fungi can be haploid, diploid or **heterokaryotic**, where one cell has more than one nucleus. For example, **dikaryotes** have two nuclei per cell. [What is the benefit of a haploid organism being heterokaryotic?][19]

7.7

Organism Structure

Most fungi are non-motile, multicellular eukaryotes. One exception is yeasts, which are unicellular. Multicellular fungi have two main structures: a vegetative mycelium and a reproductive fruiting body.

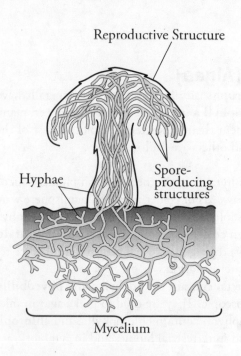

Reproductive Structure

Hyphae

Spore-producing structures

Mycelium

Figure 3   Fungal Structure

---

[18]   Remember that the plant cell wall is made of cellulose and the bacterial cell wall is made of peptidoglycan.

[19]   One benefit of having more than one haploid nucleus per cell is that one genome can compensate for mutations in the other. This is one reason many fungi undergo sexual reproduction (which generates heterokaryotes) when living conditions are not ideal.

A **mycelium** is the undifferentiated vegetative tissue of fungi. Mycelia are non-reproductive and usually microscopic; they function in obtaining nutrients for the fungus. They are rarely seen because they are buried in the fungal food source (such as rotting matter in soil, leaf litter or feces). The **fruiting body** is a reproductive structure and supports spore-producing structures (such as sporangia, asci or basidia; see below). It is usually macroscopic and above ground. Mushrooms are fruiting bodies. Both the mycelium and the fruiting body are made out of hyphae. **Hyphae** (singular: hypha) are long filaments, made of many cells joined end-to-end. They can be mononucleate or multinucleate (depending on how the cells join) and grow at their tips via mitosis.

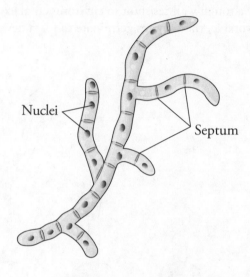

Figure 4   Fungal Hyphae

Nutrition and Symbiosis

All fungi are non-photosynthetic decomposers that acquire their nutrition through absorptive feeding; this means digestion of nutrients takes place outside fungal cells, and simple organic molecules are then absorbed across the fungal cell wall. To facilitate this, fungi excrete digestive enzymes, and hyphae generally have a large surface area to accomplish sufficient absorption for the organism.

Most fungi are obligate aerobes, although yeasts are facultative anaerobes. All fungi are chemoheterotrophs. Most are either **saprophytes** (feed off dead plants and animals) or parasites (feed off living organisms, doing harm to the host). Some are mutualists (they live in a symbiotic relationship where both organisms benefit). For example, **lichen** consist of a fungus and an algae living in mutualistic **symbiosis**.

Reproduction

Fungi reproduce by releasing sexual or asexual spores. The spores of fungi are distinct from bacterial endospores.[20]

---

[20] For example, each fungus can produce a great number of spores, while a bacterial cell can produce only a single endospore.

Fungal Asexual Reproduction

Asexual reproduction of fungi can occur either by budding, fragmentation, or spore production.[21] A very small number of fungi divide using **fission**.

- **Budding**: a new smaller hypha (or single cell) grows outward from an existing one. Most unicellular yeasts perform budding.
- Fragmentation: the mycelium can be broken into small pieces, each of which develops itself into separate mycelia.
- Asexual spores form through mitosis, to generate many spores from one cell. Some fungal spores are surrounded by a tough wall resistant to environmental extremes. When environmental conditions are favorable, these spores germinate to form new hyphae.

7.7

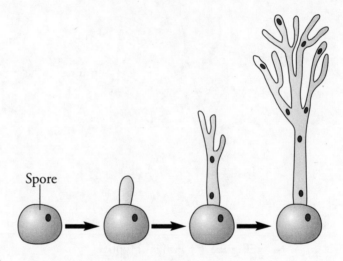

Figure 5   Spore Germination

Fungal Sexual Reproduction

Fungi use spores for sexual reproduction, and there are typically three phases in the sexual reproduction of fungi: plasmogamy, karyogamy and meiosis. First, the cytoplasms of two spores fuse (**plasmogamy**). This produces a cell with two different nuclei and one cytoplasm (a **dikaryote**). Nuclear fusion occurs next (**karyogamy**), and this turns the dikaryote into a diploid cell. Next, the cell enters meiosis to produce haploid cells. These cells divide repeatedly via mitosis, to produce a new haploid adult.

Fungal Phyla

Three common phyla in Kingdom Fungi (Zygomycota, Ascomycota and Basidiomycota) are discussed on the next page.

---

21   Remember that in asexual reproduction, the result is multiple identical genetic clones of the original fungi.

Phylum Zygomycota

This phylum includes bread and other common molds. These organisms live on decaying plant and animal matter. Zygomycota reproduce asexually unless food is scarce, in which case they will reproduce sexually. The resulting cells are called **zygosporangia** and exhibit resistance to unfavorable or harsh conditions. When conditions are again favorable, germination results in **sporangia** development on the fruiting body. Haploid spores (called **zygospores**) are released and grow into a new fungal organism.

Phylum Ascomycota (Sac Fungi)

This phylum includes a range of organisms from unicellular yeast to multicellular truffles. These fungi get their name from the production of sexual spores (called **ascospores**) in sac-like structures called **asci** (singular: ascus).

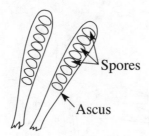

Figure 6   Ascospores in an Ascus

These organisms can also reproduce asexually through the production of "naked" spores called **conidia**.

Phylum Basidiomycota (Club Fungi)

This group includes mushrooms and shelf fungi. They are important decomposers of wood and other plant material. Many are edible and asexual reproduction is uncommon. Most species in this phylum produce sexual spores (called **basidiospores**) on **basidiocarp** (or **basidia**) structures located on the fruiting body.

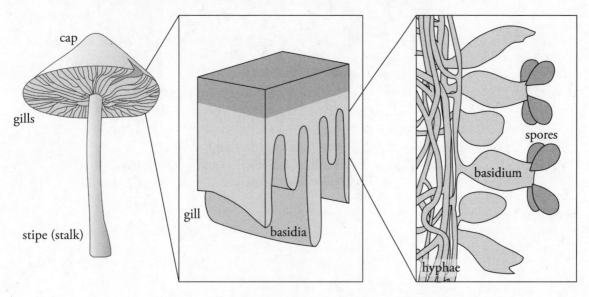

Figure 7   Basidiocarps on a Common Mushroom

KINGDOM PLANTAE

Plant Structure

Most plants have three main vegetative organs: roots, stems and leaves.

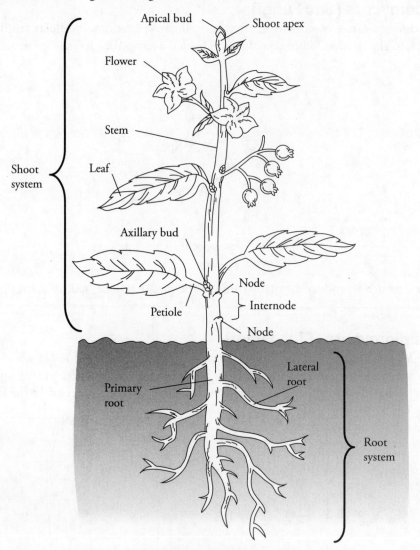

Figure 8 Plant Structure

Roots

Roots are typically below ground and have two primary functions. They anchor the immobile plant to the ground, and help with water and nutrient absorption from the soil. The end of each root is called a **root cap**, and helps push developing and growing roots into the soil. The **apical meristem** is where cell division occurs to push the root cap forward.

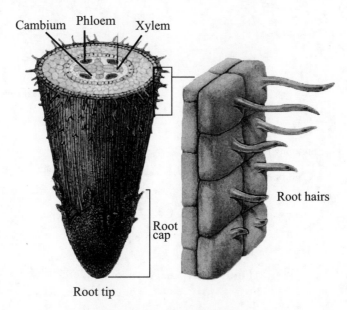

Figure 9   Root Structure

Stems

Leaves attach to stems at structures called **nodes**. Internodes are areas of stem between nodes (or between leaf attachments). A bud is an area of new stem growth.

Leaves

The outermost layer of leaves is the epidermis. This layer of cells is covered in a waxy **cuticle** to prevent water loss. Guard cells surround and control **stomata**, which are holes or pores in the leaves that allow exchange with air. Inside the leaf there are three tissue types (Figure 10): veins contain vascular tissue (**xylem** and **phloem**), palisade mesophyll tissue contains high amounts of chlorophyll and has high photosynthetic rates, and spongy mesophyll functions in gas exchange.[22]

---

[22] Palisade mesophyll can also be called palisade parenchyma, and spongy mesophyll can also be called spongy parenchyma.

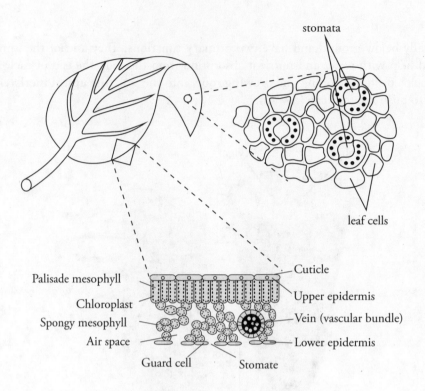

Figure 10   Leaf Structure

Vascular System

Plants do not have blood vessels like humans do. Instead, they have vascular tissue to transport water, minerals, and sugars. The main components are xylem and phloem.

- Xylem moves water and is made of tracheids and vessel elements.
- Phloem moves sugars and is made of sieve tubes and companion cells.

Both xylem and phloem are found within vascular bundles. If a plant has xylem and phloem, it is said to be vascular. Plants that don't have these systems are called nonvascular.

Xylem

Xylem is made of three cell types. **Parenchyma cells** are alive and do not transport water, but are associated with the other xylem cell types. They typically do not have chloroplasts. **Tracheids** and **vessel elements** are dead and hollow. They connect to form a column for water transport and give structural support to the plant.

Water transport in xylem is unidirectional, and always flows from roots to leaves. Water is transported due to two main forces. First, water evaporates from cells within leaves, creating a negative pressure which pulls water upwards. This only works if the vessels transporting the water are very narrow. This is known as **transpiration**, or pull force. Second, root hairs actively transport ions into the root creating a gradient which draws water in through osmosis. Continuous influx of water pushes more water upward.

This is called **root pressure**, or **push force**. **Guttation** is the process of water being forced out of the plant due to unusually high root pressure.

Phloem

Phloem vascular tissue transports organic nutrients (especially sucrose and other carbohydrates) throughout the plant, and is composed of **sieve cells** and **companion cells**. Companion cells carry out metabolism and other essential cell processes, and are attached to sieve cells by **plasmodesmata**; sieve cells transport nutrients while companion cells support them.

Sugar movement through the phloem is not unidirectional, although the majority of phloem flow goes from leaves down. Generally, sugar flow goes from source (where carbohydrates are made) to sink (the location in the plant where carbohydrates are deposited). This is done via **bulk flow** or **translocation**: sugars are actively transported into sieve cells at the source, to create a gradient. Water follows via osmosis, which drives sugars through sieve cells. Sugars are actively removed at the sink.

7.7

Photosynthesis

Plants are autotrophs because they use carbon dioxide as their sole source of carbon, and inorganic sources of nitrogen (such as nitrates and ammonium salts) and other elements as their sole starting materials for biosynthesis. Photosynthesis was discussed in Chapter 3.

Alternation of Generations

The plant life cycle alternates between two different forms. One generation of the plant is haploid (called a **gametophyte**) and generates gametes. Two gametes (originating from different organisms of the same species or from the same organism) fuse during fertilization, to produce a diploid zygote. Rounds of mitosis generate a mature diploid plant called a **sporophyte**. Haploid spores are generated via meiosis, and when a spore germinates, mitosis again generates a haploid mature gametophyte. All plants alternate between diploid and haploid life forms, although one of the two forms is usually dominant in both size and generation length. It is important to remember that both sporophytes and gametophytes are separate, multicellular, independent organisms, which may or may not have a similar appearance. Some protists and some fungi also undergo **alternation of generations**.

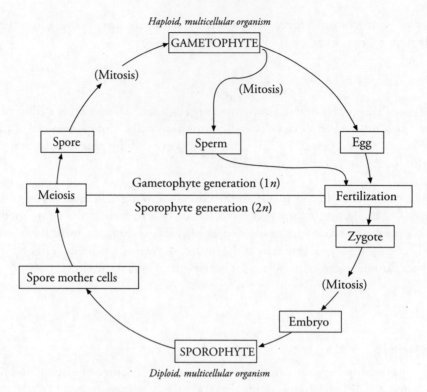

Figure 11 Alternation of Generations

Kingdom Plantae is divided into 12 common divisions.[23] They are:

- Three nonvascular divisions: Bryophyta, Hepatophyta, Anthocerophyta
- Four vascular seedless divisions: Pterophyta, Psilophyta, Lycophyta, Sphenophyta
- Five vascular seeded divisions, which are divided into:
  - Gymnosperms: Pinophyta, Cycadophyta, Ginkgophyta and Gnetophyta
  - Angiosperms: Anthophyta

Nonvascular Plants (Bryophytes)

The main feature of non-vascular plants is that they lack xylem and phloem. They tend to live in damp or humid conditions because they use motile sperm in fertilization. Many bryophytes lack specialized tissues and structures. They have a gametophyte-dominant life cycle. For example, Figure 12 shows the moss life cycle.

---

[23] In biology, a phylum is a level of classification or taxonomic rank below kingdom and above class. Traditionally, the term "phylum" was used in zoology, and the term "division" was used in botany. These days, most scientists agree that for algae, fungi, and plants, the terms "phylum" and "division" are equivalent, and both can be used. The DAT usually uses the term "division" when referring to plants, so that is what we'll do here too.

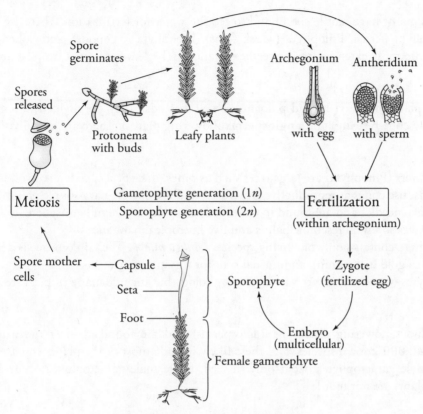

Figure 12   Life Cycle of Moss

There are 3 divisions of bryophytes:

- Mosses (Bryophyta) grow in tight packs known as mats. They do not have formal roots but do have multicellular root-like filaments called **rhizoids**, which help with anchoring and absorption.
- Liverworts (Hepatophyta) resemble a lobed liver. They use **gemmae** to reproduce asexually via fragmentation[24], but can also reproduce sexually.
- Hornworts (Anthocerophyta) are rather unremarkable and are found in most habitats.

Vascular Plants (Tracheophytes)

These plants have xylem and phloem, and are further divided into seedless and seeded plants. They typically have a sporophyte-dominant life cycle; gametophytes tend to be reduced in size and different in morphology.

---

[24] Small bundles of cells form a modified bud on the plant, which detaches and develops into a new plant.

Vascular seedless plants have motile sperm and so require water for fertilization. There are four common divisions: Pterophyta (ferns), Psilophyta (whisk ferns), Lycophyta (lycopods), and Sphenophyta (horsetails). Ferns are the most extensive of the seedless plants.[25] The leaves of ferns (fronds) are divided into several leaflets.

Vascular seeded plants have xylem and phloem, as well as seeds. They are divided into **gymnosperms** (flowerless, mostly cone-bearing) and **angiosperms** (flowering plants). There are four divisions of gymnosperms:

- Most conifers (Pinophyta) are large trees such as pines, firs, spruce, cedar, redwoods. They are evergreens, use cones as reproductive structures, and are our primary source of lumber. Most species have needles and are found in cool climates in the northern hemisphere.
- Cycads (Cycadophyta) resemble palms and live in tropical habitats.
- Ginkgophyta contains only one living species, *Ginkgo biloba*. The Ginkgo tree is deciduous (leaves turn gold in autumn), an unusual trait for a gymnosperm.
- Gnetophytes (Gnetophyta) are varied in morphology but include many tropical trees and vines.

Anthophyta includes flowering plants (or angiosperms) and are found all over the world. There are approximately 240,000 known species, and these likely include most of the plants you are familiar with, see and eat. Female gametophytes occur only in seed, while male gametophytes occur only in pollen. Sperm of these plants are not motile.

Flowers are the sexual organs of flowering plants. The **stamen** is the plant's male component. It consists of the anther and the filament. The filament supports the anther, which makes pollen. Pollen is made from little cells called microspores, and mature pollen grains contain a cell that can divide to form two sperm cells.

The **pistil** is the plant's female component. It consists of the stigma, style, ovule and ovary. Inside the ovary is the ovule, which forms cells called megaspores. Megaspores can divide to form eggs and polar bodies.

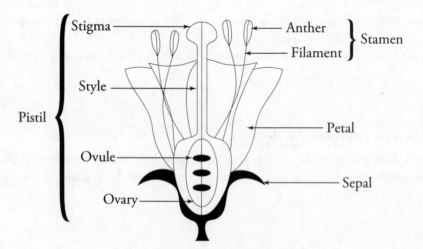

Figure 13 Parts of a Flower

---

[25] There are over 12,000 species of ferns.

Here is how a flowering plant reproduces:

1. Pollen grains fall onto the stigma, which is sticky. There are many ways this can happen: they can be blown there, fall there or be placed there by insects.
2. Once on the stigma, pollen grains germinate.
3. During germination, the pollen tube grows down through the style and connects to the ovary.
4. Two sperm (from the pollen) travel down the pollen tube and enter the ovule inside the ovary.
5. Double fertilization occurs, where one sperm fertilizes the egg and the other combines with polar bodies.
6. The fertilized egg becomes the plant embryo and the polar bodies become **endosperm**, a food-storing tissue that surrounds the plant embryo.
7. The entire ovule, which contains the embryo and the endosperm, develops into a seed. The ovary develops into a fruit. The fruit protects the seed and helps it disperse by wind or animals.
8. The seed is released (the fruit drops, the plant is eaten, etc.) and when it finds a suitable environment, it develops into a new plant.

Anthophyta are divided into two classes: monocotyledons (or **monocots**) and dicotyledons (or **dicots**).[26] A **cotyledon** is a seed leaf, or the first leaf to form from a developing seed. Monocots form one leaf during seed development, and dicots form two. There are several other differences between these two classes, as shown in Figure 14 on the following page. Parallel leaf venation is common in monocots, whereas dicots have net-like veins in their leaves. Monocots have multiples of three floral parts in flowers and fibrous roots. Dicots have multiples of four or five in floral parts, and taproots. Finally, vascular bundles in stems are also characteristically different, where monocots have a complex, usually scattered arrangement, and dicots have vascular bundles arranged in a ring. Common examples of monocots are grasses, corn and wheat. Dicots include legumes (peas and beans) and most flowering trees (oaks and maples).[27]

---

[26] Recently, some new categories of angiosperms have been defined (you don't need to worry about these for the DAT) and dicots are now called eudicots.

[27] About 1/3 of angiosperms are monocots (70,000 species) and about 2/3 of angiosperms are dicots (170,000 species).

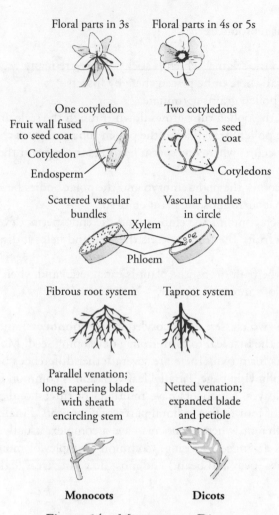

Figure 14   Monocots vs. Dicots

KINGDOM ANIMALIA

Animals are eukaryotic, multicellular, heterotrophic, and the most diverse of the six types of organisms. All animals evolved from one common ancestor organism, which is no longer alive. This organism had no tissues, symmetry, body cavity, or segmentation. Each of these characteristics evolved as Kingdom Animalia developed over millions of years.

Terms and Concepts

Tissues

Parazoa refers to animals without tissues, and **metazoa** includes animals with tissues. Only metazoans evolved symmetry, body cavities and segmentation.

Symmetry

Metazoans evolved two different types of symmetry. Animals with **radial symmetry** resemble a pie, where each cross-section of a pie piece looks the same. An example is a jellyfish (Cnidaria). Most animals with radial symmetry are **diploblastic** (see Chapter 11). They also have less efficient locomotion and did not evolve body cavities or segmentation. **Bilateral symmetry** is the same as plane symmetry, where the organism has an internal line of symmetry and two halves that are mirror images. Humans, cats and butterflies are all examples. Bilateral symmetry is associated with cephalization (see the next page) and more efficient locomotion. These organisms tend to be **triploblastic** (see Chapter 11).

Anatomical Axes

Anatomists describe bodies with reference to axes such as the dorsal-ventral axis and the anterior-posterior axis (Figure 15). These are imaginary planes through the body. **Anterior** means "front-facing"; **posterior** is the opposite. **Dorsal** means "on top." A shark has a "dorsal fin," and the spines of dogs and humans are considered dorsal as well. **Ventral** is the opposite of dorsal. The bellybutton is a ventral structure in dogs and humans. In humans, **superior** is used to indicate "toward the head." **Inferior** means "toward the feet." Another way to say "toward the head" is cephalad; *cephalus* is Latin for head. The opposite is caudad, meaning "toward the tail."

7.7

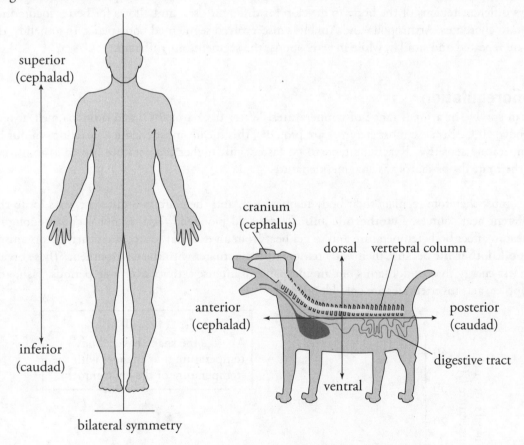

Figure 15 Bilateral Symmetry and the Anatomical Axes

Body Cavity

Some organisms with bilateral symmetry evolved a body cavity. This is important because a body cavity allows better storage of food, and increased storage of eggs and sperm. **Acoelomates** do not have a body cavity and instead have a solid body (this includes parazoans and metazoans with radial symmetry). **Pseudocoelomates** have a body cavity that develops between the endoderm and mesoderm, while **coelomates** have a body cavity that forms within the mesoderm. This allows for more specialized organs and structures. The body cavity of coelomates is fluid-filled, and separates the digestive tract from the body wall.

Cephalization

This is an evolutionary trend, where nervous system tissue becomes concentrated at one end of the organism, and can eventually become a head with sensory organs. Most animals with bilateral symmetry have some level of **cephalization**, while Chordata have a high degree of cephalization.

Segmentation

This refers to the division of some animal body plans into a series of repetitive segments. For example, vertebrates have a segmented vertebral column. **Segmentation** of the body plan is important because it allows different regions of the body to develop for different uses, and allows for better locomotion. In addition to chordates, Arthropoda and Annelida also evolved segmented body plans. In annelids, the segments are repeated and similar, while in arthropods, the segments are different.

Thermoregulation

Cells can survive in a small range of temperatures. Water freezes at 0°C, and proteins melt at temperatures above 40°C. Because most enzymes are proteins, this means most chemical reactions in our bodies are temperature sensitive. Reactions tend to go faster with higher temperature, up to a point, beyond which their rate drops sharply as enzymes denature.

Animals must therefore regulate their body temperature, and there are two different ways to do this, using different heat sources. **Ectothermic** animals are cold blooded. They do not produce enough metabolic heat to affect body temperature and so get heat from an external source. Ectothermic organisms are called **poikilothermic** because their body temperature fluctuates with the environment. These organisms require less energy than endotherms but are incapable of intense activity over long periods. Fish, amphibians, reptiles, and invertebrates are cold blooded.

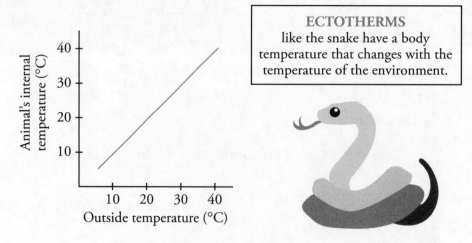

ECTOTHERMS
like the snake have a body temperature that changes with the temperature of the environment.

Figure 16 Ectotherms

Like all living things, ectotherms generate some metabolic heat. However, they cannot use this heat production to maintain a specific internal temperature.

Endothermic organisms are warm blooded in that their bodies are warmed by internal metabolic heat independent of the environment. In other words, they internally generate the heat required. These animals are **homeothermic** as their body temperature is constant and must be maintained at a certain level to maintain life. Birds and mammals are warm blooded. Generally, endotherms have a higher metabolic rate than ectotherms. This higher metabolic rate means more chemical fuel is being burned, and more heat is produced.

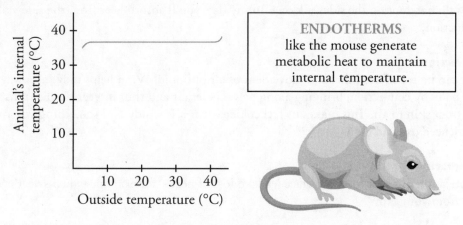

Figure 17 Endotherms

For both endotherms and ectotherms, body temperature depends on the balance between heat generated by the organism and heat exchanged with the environment. Organisms lose or gain heat from the environment via four different mechanisms:

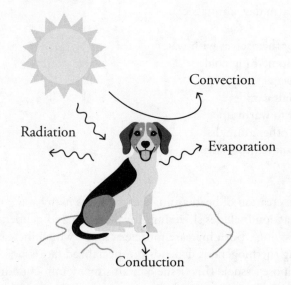

Figure 18 Heat Transfer in Living Organisms

1. **Radiation**
   Radiation is the transfer of heat from a warmer object to a cooler one by infrared radiation. This type of heat transfer occurs without direct contact. For example, animals warm themselves using heat from the sun. You may have warmed your hands by placing them near a fire or a radiator in a building.

2. **Conduction**
   Heat can be transferred between two objects in direct contact by means of conduction. For example, if you pick up an ice cube, you'll lose heat to the ice by means of conduction. If you walk barefoot on the sidewalk on a sunny day, you'll absorb heat from the sidewalk by conduction.

3. **Convection**
   Heat can be transferred through movement of air or liquid. Wind helps move air away from your body by convection, bringing along new, cooler air and thus increasing the transfer of heat from skin to air. This makes us feel colder when it is windy out, something you may have experienced as wind chill.

4. **Evaporation**
   Vaporization of water from a surface leads to loss of heat—for example, when sweat evaporates from your skin.

Animals can use behavior, anatomy, and physiology to help regulate body temperature. These adaptations arose by natural selection and help animals stay warm in cool temperatures and stay cool enough in the heat. Here are some examples:

1. **Behavioral Strategies**
   Animals can change their behavior to help control body temperature.
   For example, on a warm day, animals can:
   - Seek shade
   - Swim or spray themselves with water
   - Eat or drink something cold
   - Drink more water
   On a cool day, animals can:
   - Sit in the sun to warm up
   - Huddle with other animals
   - Eat or drink something warm

2. **Thermogenesis**
   Thermogenesis is the creation of heat; animals can do this many ways:
   - Muscle contraction includes shivering (involuntary) and deliberate movements (such as rubbing or moving). Both increase muscle activity, which increases heat production.
   - Non-shivering thermogenesis depends on specialized fat tissue known as brown fat (or brown adipose tissue). This tissue contains many mitochondria and specialized proteins. As a consequence, metabolic pathways are used to release energy from fuel molecules directly as heat instead of using it to build ATP. Brown fat is plentiful in some mammals, especially hibernators and baby animals.

3. **Circulatory Mechanisms**

Controlling blood flow to the skin is an important way to control heat exchange with the environment. For example:

- Small blood vessels near the surface of the skin can be constricted to reduce blood flow and retain heat; this is called vasoconstriction and decreases the diameter of blood vessels. For example, iguanas reduce blood flow to the skin when they go swimming in cold water. This helps them retain heat.
- In some animals, blood can be sent through an alternative "shunt" blood vessel, allowing it to bypass the skin surface completely. This is another way to conserve heat.
- Expanding blood vessels (vasodilation) in the skin leads to increased blood flow and heat loss to the environment.
- Some furry mammals have specialized networks of blood vessels located in areas of bare skin. Because there is no fur in these regions, these blood vessels are great heat exchangers. For example, jackrabbits have large ears with many blood vessels. This allows quick heat loss and aids their survival in the **hot desert**.
- Some birds and mammals have countercurrent heat exchangers. These structures allow heat transfer from blood vessels containing warmer blood to those containing cooler blood. For example, if a bird is standing in cool water but warm air, the blood in the body will be warmer than the blood in the foot of the bird. In the leg, the artery carrying warm blood down is located beside a vein carrying cool blood up from the foot. Heat exchange between these two vessels keeps the body warm and reduces heat loss in the foot.

4. **Insulation**

Animals can minimize the heat they lose to the environment via insulation. Common examples are fat, fur, and feathers. For example, marine mammals (such as whales) use blubber, a thick layer of fat, as insulation. Fur and feathers trap a layer of air beside the skin and reduce heat transfer to the environment. In cold weather, birds fluff their feathers and animals raise their fur to thicken the insulating layer. The same response in people—goosebumps or "chicken skin"—is not so effective because of our limited body hair.

5. **Evaporative Mechanisms**

Land animals often lose water from their skin, mouth, and nose by evaporation into the air. Evaporation removes heat and can act as a cooling mechanism. For example, many mammals sweat to increase evaporative cooling in response to high body temperature. In addition, both birds and mammals can pant to increase evaporation.

Circulation

Some animals (Annelida, Mollusca, Arthropoda, Echinoderms, and Chordata) evolved a circulatory system. In an **open circulatory system**, there is no difference between blood and interstitial fluid. This fluid is called **hemolymph**, and it bathes organs and tissues. Hemolymph is composed of water, inorganic salts (such as Na^+ and K^+), and organic compounds (mostly carbohydrates, proteins, and lipids). The primary oxygen transporter molecule is **hemocyanin**, and free-floating cells (**hemocytes**) function in immune protection. In a **closed circulatory system**, blood is contained within vessels and is distinct from the fluid in the body cavity. A pumping heart is required for either system; two-, three-, and four-chambered-hearts are common in the animal kingdom.

7.7

Digestive Systems

An **incomplete digestive system** (found in cnidarians and Platyhelminthes) is where a single opening to a pouch-like cavity serves as both mouth and anus. A **complete digestive system** (found in Nematoda, Annelida, Mollusca, Arthropoda, Echinodermata, and Chordata) means that food processing occurs within a tube-like enclosure (the alimentary canal), running lengthwise through the body from mouth to anus.

Structural Support

Many animals have some sort of skeleton to support their body and help with movement. An **exoskeleton** is found near the exterior, whereas an **endoskeleton** is found inside. Arthropoda have a hard exoskeleton made of chitin.[28] Some chordates (such as Chondrichthyes) have a flexible endoskeleton made of cartilage, while others (such as Osteichthyes, amphibians, reptiles, birds and mammals) have stronger endoskeletons made of bone.

Reproduction and Development

Many animals perform sexual reproduction, and fertilization can occur internally or externally. Vertebrates evolved two different developmental pathways: that of protostomes and deuterostomes. This will be discussed more in Chapter 11.

Animalia Phyla

Phylum Porifera (Sponges)

These parazoans have no tissues, organs, symmetry, body cavity (they are acoelomates) or segmentation. They are sessile and resemble multicellular blobs and perforated sacs. Most sponges are **hermaphroditic** (they possess both male and female reproductive parts), though some can do asexual budding. Most species in this phyla live in marine environments. If these animals are chopped or blended, they can reform. Sponges are **filter-feeders** (also called suspension feeders) because they feed by straining suspended matter and food particles from water, using a filter. This plays an important role in water clarification. Many other animals are filter feeders, including bivalves (mollusks), some fish, sharks, whales and birds (such as flamingos).

Phylum Cnidaria

Members of this phylum are metazoans and have radial symmetry. They are diploblastic, acoelomates and do not have segmentation. Most cnidarians live in marine environments. Cnidarians have no circulatory or respiratory systems, but they do have an incomplete digestive system. Most cnidarians are carnivores and use **nematocysts** on tentacle ends to capture prey and push food into their mouths. These venomous cells release toxin when they have anchored into prey and are responsible for jellyfish stings, which you may have been unfortunate enough to have felt.

Cnidarians have two body forms. The **medusa** form is free-floating and usually undergoes sexual reproduction. It consists of an umbrella-shaped body (called a bell), a fringe of tentacles that hang from the edge of the bell, a mouth opening located on the underside of the bell, and a gastrovascular cavity. The

---

28 Remember, this is the same substance that makes up the fungal cell wall.

polyp form is sessile and attaches to the sea floor. Polyps often form large colonies and undergo budding, a form of asexual reproduction.

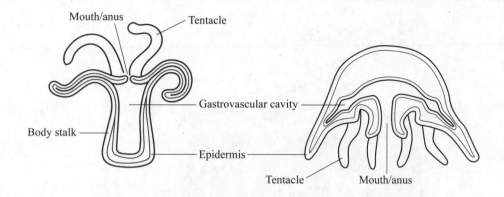

Figure 19   Body Forms of Cnidarians (Polyp vs. Medusa)

Some cnidarians (such as the hydra) alternate between polyp and medusa forms. Others are predominantly medusa (such as jellyfish) and some (such as sea anemones and corals) occur only as polyps.

Phylum Platyhelminthes (Flatworms)

These metazoans have bilateral symmetry, are triploblastic and are acoelomates. They are flattened dorso-ventrally and exhibit some cephalization. Many flatworms are parasites. They have no respiratory system but do gas exchange via diffusion through skin (**cutaneous respiration**), and have an incomplete digestive tract, similar to cnidarians. They can eliminate waste via diffusion across outer cells or using **flame cells** (specialized excretory cells that serve a function similar to mammalian kidneys). Flatworms reproduce either sexually (most are hermaphroditic) or asexually (via fragmentation). Planarians and tapeworms are common examples.

Phylum Nematoda (Roundworms)

Members of this phylum are pseudocoelomate worms that inhabit bodies of water, soil, plants, and the tissues of other animals. Nematodes usually reproduce sexually. Many species are parasites of plants or animals. These worms are metazoans with bilateral symmetry. They develop from three primary germ layers (are triploblastic) and are protostomes. They have a complete digestive tract, but no circulatory or respiratory systems. Instead, nutrients are transported via diffusion, and cutaneous respiration occurs via diffusion through skin. Excretion function is performed by flame cells, similar to flatworms. Some common examples of roundworms are *C. elegans* (a model organism commonly used in molecular and developmental biology labs), and organisms in the genus *Trichinella* (parasites that causes trichinosis).

Phylum Annelida (Segmented Worms)

Segmented worms are metazoans with bilateral symmetry; they are triploblastic. They have a body cavity (are coelomates) and are segmented protostomes. In fact, annelids represent the first phyla to evolve body segmentation. Segmented worms have multiple hearts and a closed circulatory system. They have well developed and complete digestive systems, with several specialized regions (such as the pharynx, esophagus,

7.7

crop, gizzard, intestine). Waste removal in annelids is carried out by **metanephridia**, excretory tubes found in each segment. Metanephridia have ciliated funnels that remove waste from the blood and interstitial fluid. Funnels lead to exterior pores where wastes are discharged.

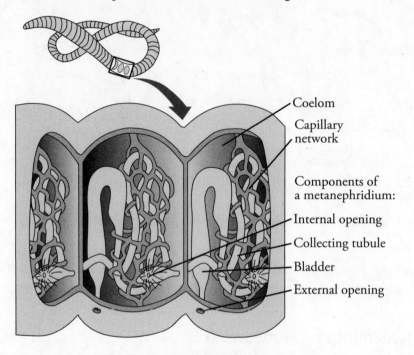

Coelom

Capillary network

Components of a metanephridium:

Internal opening

Collecting tubule

Bladder

External opening

Figure 20 Metanephridium

Segmented worms have a brain, eyes and other sensory organs, and nerve cords. They have no formal respiratory system, as they perform cutaneous respiration. They can perform sexual or asexual reproduction via fragmentation. Some species are also capable of **regeneration**. Earthworms and leeches are common annelids.

Phylum Mollusca

Mollusks are metazoans with bilateral symmetry. They are triploblastic, coelomates and protostomes. The soft bodies of mollusks are usually protected by a tough **calcium carbonate** shell, and are made up of three main parts: the **muscular foot** (for movement), the **visceral mass** (contains most of the internal organs), and the **mantle** (this is responsible for the secretion of the shell). Mollusks do not demonstrate true segmentation. Metanephridia are used for waste removal, and most mollusks have a three-chambered heart and an open circulatory system. Gills or lungs are used for respiratory function and these animals have complete digestive tracts. Reproduction is usually sexual, and some species are hermaphroditic. Most mollusks live in marine or fresh water, and some live on land.

There are three classes of Phylum Mollusca you should be familiar with: gastropods (such as snails and slugs), bivalves (such as clams and oysters) and cephalopods (such as squids and octopuses). Bivalves are divided into two halves and most are suspension-feeders, using their gills for the filtering of food particles. Cephalopods have some differences from the rest of the mollusks. Almost all members of this class have a reduced or missing shell. Cephalopods are carnivores that move much faster than the other mollusks. They are also the only members of this phylum that possess a closed circulatory system.

Phylum Arthropoda

There are close to one million known species in this phylum. Arthropods are considered to be the most successful phylum of animals. They have tissues (metazoans) and a body cavity (coelomates). Their symmetry pattern is bilateral, they develop from three primary germ layers (triploblastic), and are protostomes. Arthropods are segmented (with distinct head, thorax, and abdomen), with a hard exoskeleton (made of chitin) and jointed appendages. When they grow in size, they must shed their exoskeleton and synthesize a new one (this process is known as **molting**). Arthropods have well-developed sensory organs, a brain, and specialized organs (tracheoles, **book lungs** or **gills**) for gas exchange. The circulatory system in arthropods is open and is filled with hemolymph. A complete digestive system is present, and the crop stores food for digestion. A **crop** is a thin-walled expanded portion of the alimentary tract used for the storage of food prior to digestion; many other animals, including gastropods, earthworms, leeches, and birds also use a crop. Waste removal is accomplished via **malpighian tubules** in most arthropods; these tubules are outpocketings of the gut. They absorb water and waste from the circulating hemolymph, and dump it into the alimentary canal. Wastes are then secreted as solid from the hindgut.

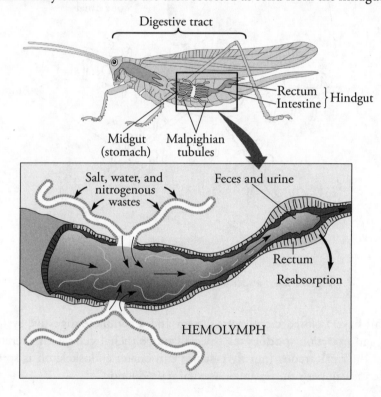

Figure 21   Malpighian Tubules

However, some arthropods use metanephridia instead (similar to mollusks and annelids discussed above). Arthropods typically perform sexual reproduction. This phylum includes arachnids (such as scorpions and spiders), millipedes (which eat decaying leaves and plant matter), centipedes (which are carnivores), insects and crustaceans (such as crabs and lobster).

Insects have three pairs of legs and undergo **metamorphosis**, a biological process by which an animal physically develops after birth or hatching. Many other animals undergo metamorphosis, including some amphibians, mollusks, crustaceans, cnidarians, echinoderms, and tunicates. Some common examples of insects are wasps, earwigs, beetles, ants, flies, and moths.

7.7

Phylum Echinodermata

Echinoderms are metazoans, coelomates, triploblastic and deuterostomes. Starfish, sea urchins and sea cucumbers are some common examples of echinoderms. They have secondary radial symmetry, which means adults have radial symmetry, but larvae have bilateral symmetry. Members of this phylum are sessile or slow moving (although the larvae are mobile) and have a **water vascular system** that ends in **tube feet**. The water vascular system is a hydraulic or fluid system, where internal canals connect numerous tube feet. This system is used for movement: muscles are alternatively contracted to force water into the tube feet (causing them to extend and push against the ground), then relaxed (to allow the feet to retract). This type of movement is powerful but very slow. In addition to locomotion, the water vascular system also functions in food and waste transportation, feeding, respiration and gas exchange.

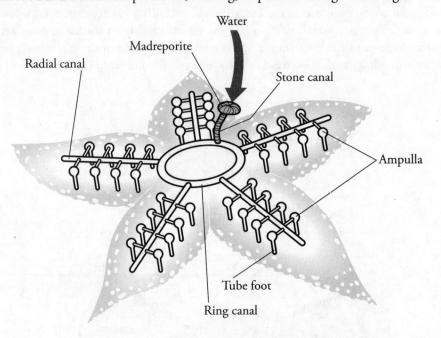

Figure 22   Echinoderm Water Vascular System

These marine animals have a closed circulatory system and a complete digestive system. They use skin gills for respiration and excretion; **podocytes** (specialized epithelial cells with excretory function) also help with excretion. Their calcareous (mostly calcium carbonate) endoskeleton is spiny and covered by thick skin. Echinoderms can perform sexual or asexual reproduction.

Phylum Chordata

The chordates are varied, but have major evolutionary features in common. These metazoans have bilateral symmetry, segmentation, and a body cavity. They are deuterostomes which develop from three primary germ layers (therefore are triploblastic). In addition, there are four main characteristics that define chordates and separate them from all other animals. All chordates possess the following four structures at some point in their lifetime:

1.   Neural tube: embryonic precursor to the central nervous system, which becomes the brain and spinal cord in vertebrates. It is sometimes called the **dorsal hollow nerve cord**.

2. **Notochord**: embryonic precursor to the spine. It is a flexible, rod-shaped structure found in embryos of all chordates and is composed of cells derived from the mesoderm. The notochord defines the primitive axis of the embryo. It persists as the main axial support in lower vertebrates, and is replaced by the vertebral column in higher vertebrates.

3. **Pharyngeal slits**: openings through which water is taken into the pharynx, or throat. They are used in primitive chordates to strain water and filter out food particles, and are modified in fish for respiration. Most terrestrial vertebrates have these structures only during the embryonic stage.

4. A muscular **post-anal tail**.

In many chordates these structures are present only in the embryonic stage.

Chordate Evolution

Generally speaking, chordates evolved in the order "FARBM," or fish, amphibians, reptiles, birds, mammals. However, it's important to keep in mind that evolution is not linear, it is branched. Organisms evolved from common ancestors (many of which are now extinct) and not from each other. The evolution tree below summarizes when common chordate branches evolved, and which characteristics (vertebrae, jaws, lungs, limbs, etc.) are common to each.

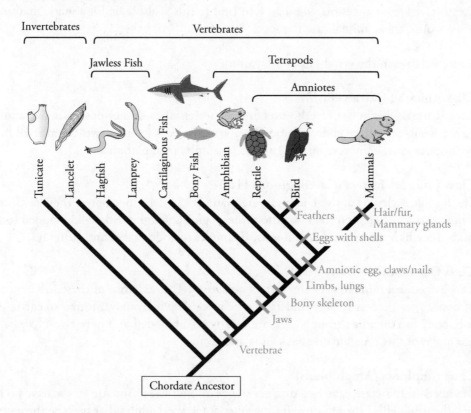

Figure 23   Cladogram of Chordate Evolution

Not all chordates are vertebrates. For example, both tunicates (also called sea squirts) and lancelets are marine chordates that are **invertebrates**.

Subphylum Vertebrata

There are several additional characteristics common to all **vertebrates**; the first 6 of these help differentiate vertebrates from other chordates:

1. The presence of a vertebral column, which replaces the notochord.
2. Vertebrates are highly cephalized, in that the anterior part of the nerve cord is enlarged. This distinct head also includes a well-formed cranium to protect the brain. The cranium and vertebral column are the main axis of the body.
3. The presence of neural crest cells. These unique embryonic cells are transient, multipotent, and migratory.
4. The presence of specialized internal organs, such as liver, kidneys, and endocrine glands.
5. Physiological adaptations that support their increased demand for energy.
6. An endoskeleton, made of bone or cartilage, for support.
7. Closed circulatory system.
8. Complete digestive tract, where food processing occurs in a tube-like enclosure (alimentary canal), which connects the mouth and the anus.
9. Many vertebrates (including amphibians, reptiles, birds, and mammals) are **tetrapods**, meaning they have four limbs. Note that snakes and other legless reptiles are tetrapods because they evolved from ancestors who had four limbs. This is also true for aquatic mammals. In other words, these animals are tetrapods by descent.

There are seven classes in the vertebrate subphylum:

1. **Class Agnatha (Jawless Fish)**
   These animals live in both fresh water and sea water. They do not possess a jaw, and they have a flexible cartilage endoskeleton. They are ectothermic, have two-chambered hearts and breathe via gills. Lampreys and hagfish are examples of agnathans.

2. **Class Chondrichthyes (Cartilaginous Fish)**
   The flexible skeletons of these animals are made of cartilage, not bone. They have jaws and paired fins. Cartilaginous fish breathe through gills and are mostly cold blooded (ectothermic). They have two-chambered hearts. Examples include sharks and stingrays.

3. **Class Osteichthyes (Bony Fish)**
   This is the most numerous of the vertebrate classes. The skeletons of these fish are composed of bone. They possess swim bladders that help regulate buoyancy. Similar to cartilaginous fish, bony fish breathe through gills, are mostly cold blooded and have two-chambered hearts. Examples of this class include bass, tuna and trout.

4. **Class Amphibia (Amphibians)**
   Members of this class have two distinct stages in their lives. Aquatic larvae have no legs and breathe using gills. They mature into terrestrial tetrapod adults that breathe through lungs or their skin. Most amphibians therefore live close to the water. They have three-chambered hearts, and are mostly ectothermic. Amphibians have an endoskeleton made of bone. Some representative amphibians include frogs, toads, and salamanders.

5. **Class Reptilia (Reptiles)**
   These terrestrial animals are ectotherms. Most breathe through lungs, but some can perform cutaneous respiration. Reptiles have an endoskeleton made of bone and thick, scaly skin to

7.7

prevent water loss. Most species in this class have three-chambered hearts. Representatives of this class include lizards, snakes, crocodiles, and turtles. Many (but not all) dinosaurs were reptiles.

6. **Class Aves (Birds)**
Birds share many characteristics with reptiles, including amniotic eggs (with shells) and scales (on their legs). Birds are tetrapods: they have four limbs, where the two forelimbs are wings. The bodies of birds have been modified to improve flight; they possess feathered wings and a lightweight honeycomb skeleton. Birds have a four-chambered heart, breathe through lungs, are endothermic, and have high metabolic and heart rates. Birds also have a gizzard, a digestive organ responsible for grinding food (since they don't have teeth). Members of this class include owls, eagles and penguins.

7. **Class Mammalia (Mammals)**
Mammals are endothermic animals with hair and teeth. The heart of a mammal has four chambers and respiration occurs via lungs. All female members of this class use mammary glands to provide milk to nourish their offspring. Fertilization is internal, and most young are born (not hatched). Mammals have proportionately larger brains. Some examples of mammals are rodents (like mice and rats), kangaroo, antelope, monkeys and humans.

Human Taxonomy

You should know how humans are classified and the defining characteristics of each taxonomy category.

Category	Human	Characteristics
Domain	Eukarya	The presence of membrane-bound organelles such as a nucleus and mitochondria.
Kingdom	Animalia	Multicellular, diploid, eukaryotic organisms; chemoheterotrophs that perform ingestive digestion.
Phylum	Chordata	Possess notochord, neural tube, pharyngeal gill slits and a post-anal tail at some time in embryonic development.
Subphylum	Vertebrata	Have bilateral symmetry, cephalization, an endoskeleton with a vertebral column, four limbs (or fins), a closed circulatory system, a respiratory system, and an excretory system with kidneys.
Class	Mammalia	Have hair, 4 limbs, a 4-chambered heart, a diaphragm for respiration, mammary glands which produce milk to feed young offspring, internal fertilization.
Order	Primates	Well-developed cerebral cortex, opposable thumbs, omnivorous, forward-facing eyes.
Family	Hominidae	Erect posture, intelligence, long period of parental care, cooperation.
Genus	Homo	Includes modern humans and species closely related to them (which are now extinct); this genus is approximately 2.4 million years old and is differentiated from ancestors by an increase in cranial capacity.
Species	Sapiens	Originated in Africa about 200,000 years ago; highly developed brain and capable of abstract reasoning, language, introspection, problem solving, self-awareness and rationality; unique in their abilities to communicate and share ideas; ability to organize; advanced and complex social structures.

Table 2   Human Taxonomy

Additional Animalia Phyla

In addition to the 9 phyla discussed above, there are many others that are part of Kingdom Animalia, such as:

- Phylum Ctenophora—comb jellies
- Phylum Nemertea—proboscis worms
- Phylum Phoronida—horseshoe worms
- Phylum Onychophora—walking worms
- Phylum Rotifera—wheel animals
- Phylum Bryozoa—moss animals
- Phylum Brachiopoda—lamp shells

7.8   VIRUSES

What Is a Virus?

With the identification of bacteria as the cause of anthrax and other diseases, medical science appeared in the late 1800s to be headed toward an explanation of all infectious disease. Researchers soon found, however, that some infectious agents could not be trapped by passage through filters in the same manner as bacteria. These agents also proved invisible to the light microscope, unlike bacteria. With the advent of electron microscopy, the tiny infectious agents known as **viruses** were finally visualized. Today, molecular biology has shed great light onto viruses, down to the nucleotide sequence of entire viral genomes. However, viruses remain one of the most serious threats to health, indicating there is still much to learn.

Viruses infect all life-forms on earth, including plants, animals, protists, and bacteria. A virus is an **obligate intracellular parasite**. As such, they are only able (obligated) to reproduce within (intra) cells. While within a host cell, viruses have some attributes of living organisms, such as the ability to reproduce; outside cells, viruses are without activity. Viruses on their own are unable to perform any of the chemical reactions characteristic of life, such as synthesis of ATP and macromolecules.[29] Viruses are not cells or even living organisms. To reproduce, they commandeer the cellular machinery of the host they infect and use it to manufacture copies of themselves. In the final analysis, a virus is nothing more than a package of nucleic acid that says, "Pick me up and reproduce me." Remember this crucial definition: a virus is an obligate intracellular parasite that relies on host machinery whenever possible. In the following sections, we will look at some of the variations on this basic theme.

---

[29]   Note, however, that some viruses store some ATP in their capsids. They acquired this ATP from the previous host and typically use it to power penetration.

- Cyanide (an inhibitor of the electron transport chain) is added to a culture of virus-infected mammalian cells. The virus has none of the components of electron transport or any other proteins that are inhibited by cyanide. Which one of the following best describes the effect of cyanide?[30]
    - A. The mammalian cells will die, and all viruses will be destroyed as well, regardless of their stage of development.
    - B. Mammalian cells are killed, and viral replication halted, but the culture remains infectious.
    - C. Mammalian cells stop growing, and viral replication is unaffected.
    - D. Mammalian cells continue to grow, but viral replication is halted.
    - E. There will be no effect on either the mammalian cells or the viruses.

Viruses have a major impact on human health. For example:

- Rabies, hepatitis, measles, mumps, smallpox, rubella, polio, and yellow fever are all caused by viruses.
- HIV (human immunodeficiency virus) is a virus that attacks the body's immune system. If HIV is not treated, it can lead to AIDS (acquired immunodeficiency syndrome).
- There are over 100 varieties of human papillomavirus (HPV), more than 40 of which are passed through sexual contact. Some types of HPV infection cause warts, and some can cause different types of cancer.
- Herpes simplex is a viral infection caused by the herpes simplex virus; about 67% of the world population under the age of 50 has HSV-1.
- Chickenpox is an infection caused by the varicella-zoster virus.
- Flu is caused by influenza viruses, whereas the common cold can be caused by several different viruses, including rhinoviruses, parainfluenza, and seasonal coronaviruses. Seasonal coronaviruses are not the same as SARS-COV-2, the virus that causes COVID-19.

Safe and effective vaccines have been developed for many of these viruses.

Viral Structure and Function

The structure of viruses reflects their life cycle. In general, all viruses possess a nucleic acid genome packaged in a protein shell. The exterior protein packaging helps to convey the genome from one cell to infect other cells. Once in a cell, the viral genome directs the production of new copies of the genome and of the protein packaging needed to produce more virus. However, the nature of the genome, the protein packaging, and the viral life cycle vary tremendously between different viruses.

---

[30] Mammalian cells are directly dependent on the ATP generated by the electron transport chain, so if cyanide inhibits the electron transport chain, mammalian cells will die (eliminate choices D and E). Viruses are dependent on the mammalian cells for the ATP and enzymes needed for replication, so if the mammalian cells die, viral replication will stop (eliminate choice C). However, any viruses that had already completed the replication process when the cyanide was added will not be affected and will remain infectious (eliminate choice A, and option **B** is correct).

A viral genome may consist of either DNA *or* RNA that is either single- *or* double-stranded and is either linear *or* circular. Viruses use virtually every conceivable form of nucleic acid as their genome. However, a given type of virus can have only one type of nucleic acid as its genome, and a mature virus does not contain nucleic acid other than its genome.[31]

- If the ratio of adenine to thymine in a DNA virus is not one to one, what can be said about the genome of this virus?[32]
- A disease agent that is isolated from a human cannot reproduce on its own in cell-free broth but can reproduce in a culture of human cells. In its pure form, it possesses both RNA and DNA. Is it possible that the disease agent is a virus?[33]

A factor that influences all viral genomes, regardless of the form of the nucleic acid used as genome, is size as a limiting factor. Viruses are much smaller than the hosts they infect, both prokaryotic and eukaryotic. The following figure depicts the relative size of a **bacteriophage** (a virus that infects bacteria) and its host:

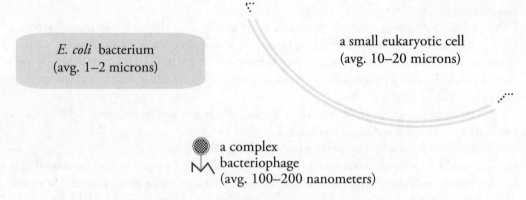

Figure 24   Relative Size of a Virus

Not only are viruses small, but the exterior protein shell of a virus is typically a rigid structure of fixed size that cannot expand to accommodate a larger genome. [What is the likely result if a viral genome is tripled in size?[34]] To adapt to this size constraint, viral genomes have evolved to be extremely economical. One adaptation is for the viral genome to carry very few genes and for the virus to rely on host-encoded proteins for transcription, translation, and replication. [How do ribosomes used to translate viral proteins compare to host ribosomes?[35]] Another adaptation found in viral genomes is the ability to encode more than one protein in a given length of genome. A virus can accomplish this feat by using more than one reading frame within a piece of DNA so that genes may overlap with each other.

---

[31]   There are exceptions. For example, the hepatitis B virus has a circular DNA genome that is part single stranded and part double stranded. The take-home point here is that when a virus is not inside a host cell, it contains only its genome, which is always the same (except in special situations such as when a piece of host genome accidentally becomes incorporated in the viral genome). In contrast, a true cell contains not only its genome but also mRNA, rRNA, and tRNA.

[32]   Adenine base pairs with thymine in double-stranded DNA. Thus, for every A there should be one T for a one-to-one ratio of A to T. If the ratio differs from this, the genome must be single-stranded DNA, or RNA, which has no T.

[33]   No, it cannot be a virus. Viruses possess only one kind of nucleic acid. The disease agent is another kind of obligate intracellular parasite (certain bacteria can only reproduce inside host cells, e.g., chlamydia).

[34]   The viral genome will probably no longer fit within the normal viral structure, and the genome will therefore not be packaged into infectious viral particles.

[35]   Viruses use host ribosomes. Viral and host proteins are translated by the same ribosomes.

- A 1,000 base pair region of viral genome is found to encode two polypeptides unrelated in amino acid sequence during infection of eukaryotic cells. If one of these polypeptides is 250 amino acids in length and the other is 300, what is the best explanation for this?[36]
  - A. A missense mutation occurred.
  - B. Viruses use a different genetic code than eukaryotes do.
  - C. The virus uses overlapping multiple reading frames.
  - D. The polypeptides are splicing variants.
  - E. A silent mutation is present.

Surrounding the viral nucleic acid genome is a protein coat called the **capsid**. The capsid provides the external morphology that is used to classify viruses. It is made from a repeating pattern of only a few protein building blocks. Helical capsids are rod shaped, while polyhedral capsids are multiple-sided geometric figures with regular surfaces. Complex viruses may contain a mixture of shapes. For example, the T4 bacteriophage has a helical sheath and a polyhedral head (Figure 25). This virus is commonly used in research; its host is the bacterium *E. coli*. The genome is located within the capsid head. Other parts of the capsid are used during infection of the host. Tail fibers attach to the surface of the host cell, as does the base plate. The sheath contracts using the energy of stored ATP, injecting the genome into the host. [Why might a bacteriophage inject its DNA, while animal viruses do not?[37]]

7.8

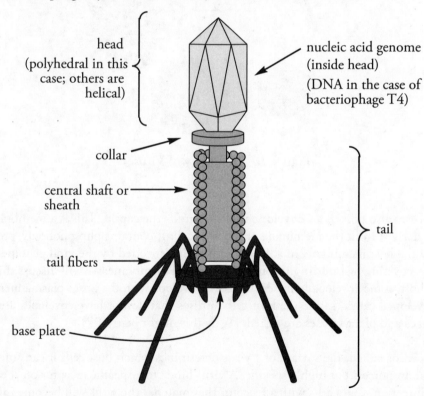

head
(polyhedral in this case; others are helical)

nucleic acid genome
(inside head)
(DNA in the case of bacteriophage T4)

collar

central shaft or sheath

tail

tail fibers

base plate

Figure 25   Bacteriophage T4

---

[36] The problem is that the virus must contain at least 750 bp (250 amino acids) and 900 bp (300 amino acids) of genetic information for unrelated polypeptides in 1,000 bp of DNA. The only way to do this is overlapping multiple reading frames (choice **C** is correct).

[37] Phages must puncture the bacterial cell wall, while animal viruses can be internalized whole into animal cells (since they do not have a cell wall).

The most important thing to understand is that the entire viral capsid is composed of protein, while the viral genome is composed of nucleic acid (DNA or RNA). Most viruses are not as structurally complex as the bacteriophage shown above. Here are more examples of viruses:

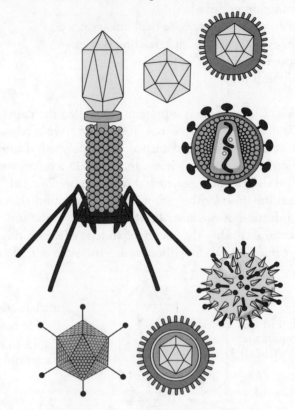

Figure 26   A Variety of Viruses

Many animal viruses also possess an **envelope** that surrounds the capsid. This is a membrane on the exterior of the virus derived from the membrane of the host cell. It contains phospholipids, proteins, and carbohydrates from the host membrane, in addition to proteins encoded by the viral genome. Enveloped viruses acquire this covering by **budding** through the host cell membrane; we will discuss this more shortly. To infect a new host, some enveloped viruses fuse their envelope with the host's plasma membrane, which leaves the de-enveloped capsid inside the host cell. Viruses that do not have envelopes are called **naked viruses**. All phages and plant viruses are naked. [Why this might be true?[38]]

Whether enveloped or naked, the surface of a virus determines which host cells it can infect. Viral infection is not a random process but highly specific. A virus binds to a specific receptor on the cell surface as the first step in infection. Only cells with a receptor that matches the virus will become infected, explaining why only specific species or specific cell types are susceptible to infection. The viral surface is also important for recognition by our immune system. [If antibodies to a viral capsid protein are ineffective in blocking infection, what might this indicate about the virus?[39]]

---

[38]   Remember: viruses acquire envelopes by budding through host membranes. Phages and plant viruses infect hosts that possess cell walls. When viruses begin to exit the cell, the cell wall is destroyed, and host membranes rupture. Thus, there is no membrane through which the remaining viruses must bud; they simply escape in a lytic explosion.

[39]   It suggests that the virus is enveloped, so the antibody cannot reach its epitope on the capsid surface in infectious virus.

Bacteriophage Reproduction

Since viruses lack the ability to produce energy and replicate on their own, they use machinery of the host cell to carry out these processes. The first step in viral reproduction is binding to the exterior of a bacterial cell in a process termed **attachment** or **adsorption**. The next step is injection of the viral genome into the host cell in a process termed **penetration** or **eclipse**; this is called "eclipse" because the capsid remains on the outer surface of the bacterium while the genome disappears into the cell, removing infectious virus from the media. From this point forward, a phage follows one of two different paths: it enters either the **lytic cycle** or the **lysogenic** cycle.

Lytic Cycle

As soon as the phage genome has entered the host cell, host polymerases and/or ribosomes begin to rapidly transcribe and translate it. This is because the viral genome contains genes that redirect the infected cell to produce viral products. One of the first viral gene products made is sometimes an enzyme called **hydrolase**, a hydrolytic enzyme that degrades the entire host genome. Hydrolase is an example of an **early gene**, one of a group of genes that are expressed immediately after infection, and which include any special enzymes required to express viral genes. Next, multiple copies of the phage genome are produced, using the dNTPs resulting from degradation of the host genome, as well as an abundance of capsid proteins. Next, each new capsid automatically assembles itself around a new genome. Finally, an enzyme called **lysozyme** is produced. An example of a **late gene**, lysozyme is also present in human tears and saliva. It destroys the bacterial cell wall. [What is the bacterial cell wall made of? Is this the same or different from fungal and plant cell walls?[40]] Because osmotic pressure is no longer counteracted by protection of the cell wall, the host bacterium bursts ("lyses," hence the name lytic), releasing hundreds of progeny viruses, which can begin another round of the cycle (Figure 27). [If lysozyme were an early gene, would this be advantageous to the virus?[41]]

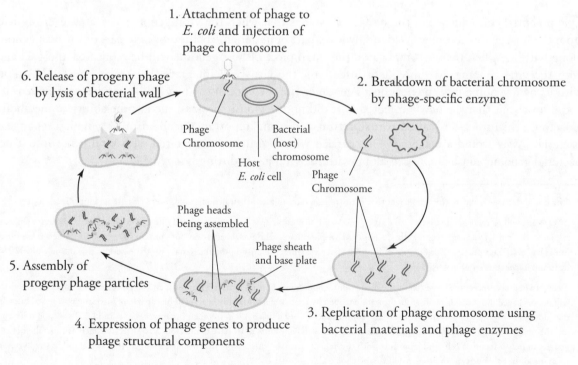

1. Attachment of phage to *E. coli* and injection of phage chromosome

6. Release of progeny phage by lysis of bacterial wall

2. Breakdown of bacterial chromosome by phage-specific enzyme

Phage Chromosome

Bacterial (host) chromosome

Host *E. coli* cell

Phage Chromosome

Phage heads being assembled

Phage sheath and base plate

5. Assembly of progeny phage particles

4. Expression of phage genes to produce phage structural components

3. Replication of phage chromosome using bacterial materials and phage enzymes

Figure 27 Lytic Cycle

---

[40] The bacterial cell wall is made of peptidoglycan; the fungal cell wall is made of chitin, and the plant cell wall is made of cellulose.

[41] No. The host cell would lyse before the phage had time to replicate and assemble.

- When phages are first added to a bacterial culture, the number of infective viruses initially decreases before it later increases. Why does this occur?[42]
- Bacteria cultured in the presence of ^{35}S-labeled cysteine and ^{32}P-labeled phosphates are infected with phage T4. When phages from this culture are used to infect a new non-radiolabeled bacterial culture, which of the isotopes will be found in the interior of the newly infected bacteria?[43]
- A bacteriophage with an important capsid gene deleted infects the same cell as another virus with a normal copy of the same gene. At the time of host-cell lysis[44]:
    - A. All released viruses will be capable of infecting new hosts, but only some of these new infections will give rise to phage capable of infecting new hosts.
    - B. No infective viruses will be released.
    - C. Each individual virus that is released will produce a mixture of infective and noninfective viruses in subsequent infections.
    - D. Only normal viruses will be released.

Lysogenic Cycle

The lytic cycle is an efficient way for a virus to rapidly increase its numbers. It presents a problem though: all host cells are destroyed. This is an evolutionary disadvantage. Some viruses are cleverer: they enter the **lysogenic cycle**. Upon infection, the phage genome is incorporated into the bacterial genome and is now referred to as a **prophage**; the host is now called a **lysogen** (Figure 28). The prophage is silent; its genes are not expressed, and viral progeny are not produced. This dormancy is because transcription of phage genes is blocked by a phage-encoded repressor protein that binds to specific DNA elements in phage promoters (operators). The cleverness of the lysogenic cycle lies in the fact that every time the host cell reproduces itself, the prophage is reproduced too. Eventually, the prophage becomes activated. It now removes itself from the host genome (in a process called **excision**) and enters the lytic cycle.

One potential consequence of the lysogenic cycle is that when the viral genome activates, excising itself from the host genome, it may accidentally leave part of its genome behind or take part of the host genome along with it. When the virus replicates, the small piece of host genome will be replicated and packaged with the viral genome. In subsequent infections, the virus will integrate the "stolen" host DNA along with its own genome into the new host's genome. The presence of the new DNA will become evident if it codes for a trait that the newly infected host did not previously possess, such as the ability to metabolize galactose. This process is called **transduction** and is an important mechanism of genetic exchange in bacteria. [Why would a bacterial gene, carried with a virus and integrated with viral genes into a new bacterial genome, not be repressed along with the viral genes during lysogeny?[45]]

---

[42] The initial decrease is due to the simple fact that many phages have injected their genomes into hosts and are no longer infectious.

[43] ^{35}S cysteine will be incorporated into viral coat proteins and ^{32}P phosphate will be incorporated into the viral nucleic acid genome in newly released viral particles; proteins generally do not contain phosphate, and nucleic acids do not contain sulfur atoms. When these viruses infect bacteria, their nucleic acids are injected into the bacteria while the capsid proteins remain on the exterior. This means only 32P will be found in the interior of newly infected cells.

[44] When two viruses infect the same cell, it is called co-infection. Some normal viruses will result, and some genomes from defective viruses will get packaged into capsids made from proteins encoded by the normal virus. The latter will be capable of infecting new hosts, but when they do, their progeny will not survive due to the capsid abnormality (choice **A** is correct; eliminate choices B and D). Think about it: where did the phage with the deleted capsid gene come from? The deficient virus must have come from a co-infection such as this. The deficient phage can only infect host cells and reproduce with the help of normal viruses. Note that because a single virus carries only a single genome, it can produce only one type of progeny (eliminate choice C).

[45] Prophage latency results from a viral repressor protein binding to viral DNA in a sequence-specific manner. The specific DNA sequence to which the repressor binds is present in the viral genes but not in the bacterial genes, so the bacterial gene can be expressed while the viral genes are repressed.

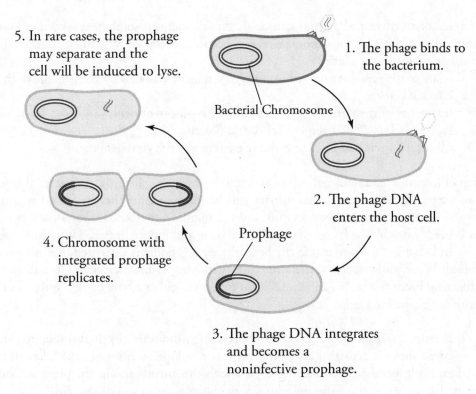

5. In rare cases, the prophage may separate and the cell will be induced to lyse.

1. The phage binds to the bacterium.

Bacterial Chromosome

4. Chromosome with integrated prophage replicates.

Prophage

2. The phage DNA enters the host cell.

3. The phage DNA integrates and becomes a noninfective prophage.

Figure 28   Lysogenic Cycle

Animal Virus Reproduction

There are several differences between phages and viruses that infect animal cells; animal viruses don't have a special name like "phage." The general outline of the viral life cycle, however, remains the same. The virus must specifically bind to a proper host cell, release its genetic material into the host, take over host machinery, replicate its genome, synthesize capsid components, assemble itself, and finally escape to infect a new cell.

Animal cells have proteins on the surface of their plasma membranes that serve as specific receptors for viruses. These receptors play a role in normal cellular function; they do not exist simply for the benefit of the virus. Part of the tissue specificity of animal viruses is due to the distribution of receptors necessary for adsorption. For example, binding of the HIV virus protein gp120 to a T-cell membrane protein termed CD4 is one of the first steps in HIV infection.

- Would treatment of an HIV-infected person with a soluble form of CD4 protein affect the infectivity of the virus?[46]
- Mutation of the cell surface receptor that viruses attach to would be a means for an organism to become resistant to viral infection. Why is this mechanism not common?[47]

---

[46]   Yes, it would. The soluble CD4 protein would bind to the virus's CD4 receptor (gp120) and block attachment of the virus to the T cells.

[47]   Two reasons: 1) the receptor has a specific role in the normal physiology of the host, which a mutation might compromise. 2) Viruses generally evolve so rapidly that they can keep up with any changes in the host, but this is not an absolute rule. Cells of our immune system keep us alive by keeping up with most microorganisms' tricks.

7.8

- Treatment of an enveloped animal virus with a mild detergent solubilizes several proteins from the virus, although the genome does not become accessible. Which one of the following is consistent with this scenario?[48]
  - A. Some of the proteins released by detergent may be encoded by the genome of the infected cell.
  - B. Infectivity of the virus is not affected by detergent treatment.
  - C. Proteins released by detergent are capsid proteins.
  - D. All proteins released by detergent are encoded by the viral genome.

The next step of infection of an animal cell is penetration into the cell just as in bacterial infection by a phage. After receptor binding, enveloped viruses will be internalized either by fusion with the plasma membrane or by receptor-mediated endocytosis; indeed, many animal viruses enter their host cell by endocytosis, a process whereby the host cell engulfs the virus and internalizes it. [Why don't phages enter their hosts by endocytosis?[49]] Once inside the host, the viral genome is uncoated, meaning it is released from the capsid. When fusion occurs, the virus fuses with the plasma membrane to release its contents into the cytoplasm. From this point, an animal virus may enter either a lytic cycle, a lytic-like cycle called the productive cycle, or a lysogenic cycle.

The lytic cycle in animal viruses is the same as in phages. The **productive cycle** is similar to the lytic cycle but does not destroy the host cell. This is possible because enveloped viruses exit the host cell by budding through the host's cell membrane, becoming coated with this membrane in the process. Budding does not necessarily destroy a cell since the lipid bilayer membrane can reseal as the virus leaves. Finally, in the animal virus lysogenic cycle, the dormant form of the viral genome is called a **provirus** (analogous to a prophage). For example, herpes simplex I is the virus that causes oral herpes. After infection, it may remain dormant as a provirus for an indefinite period. Then one day, usually when the host encounters stress (e.g., lack of sleep, upcoming professional school entrance exams), the virus reactivates.

Overall, many factors determine the uniqueness of each virus. The type of genome, possession or lack of an envelope, nature of cell-surface proteins, and type of life cycle are examples. All these parameters are used in the classification of viruses, and all are potential targets for therapeutic intervention.

---

[48] The detergent solubilized the viral envelope (eliminate choice C). Some envelope proteins are encoded by the virus, and some are derived from the host's membranes during budding (choice **A** is correct; eliminate choice D). Removal of envelope proteins will impair viral adsorption and reduce infectivity (eliminate choice B).

[49] Bacteria do not perform endocytosis, in part because they have a rigid cell wall.

7.8

Retroviruses

HIV, the virus that causes AIDS, and HTLV (human T-cell leukemia virus) are examples of retroviruses. These are (+) RNA viruses that undergo lysogeny. Let's look at what this means.

- A (+) RNA virus has a single-stranded RNA genome; this is the simplest imaginable type of viral genome. The (+) notation means the viral RNA functions as mRNA and is a template for translation.
- Because retroviruses undergo lysogeny, they integrate into the host genome as proviruses. To integrate into a double-stranded DNA genome, a viral genome must also be composed of double-stranded DNA. Since these viral genomes enter the cell in an RNA form, they must undergo reverse transcription to make DNA from an RNA template. This snubbing of the central dogma is accomplished by an **RNA-dependent DNA polymerase (reverse transcriptase)** encoded by the viral genome. Retroviruses are theoretically not required to carry this enzyme, only to encode it. [Why is this the case?[50]] The three main retroviral genes are gag (codes for viral capsid proteins), pol (polymerase codes for reverse transcriptase) and env (envelope codes for viral envelope proteins). [After integration of a retrovirus into the cellular genome, a reverse transcriptase inhibitor is added to the cell. Will the production of new viruses be blocked?[51]]

7.8

---

[50] Retroviruses are not required to carry the reverse transcriptase enzyme, only to encode it, because the viral RNA genome can be translated by host ribosomes; this means that reverse transcriptase may be made after the viral genome enters the host. That said, some retroviruses encode and also carry this enzyme. For example, HIV carries its reverse transcriptase within its capsid. You should understand why this is not a theoretical necessity.

[51] No, it will not. Reverse transcriptase is required for only one phase of the retrovirus life cycle: the copying of the viral RNA genome into DNA so that it can integrate into the host genome and be transcribed. Once the viral genome has integrated, transcription to produce viral mRNA and new viral RNA genomes does not involve reverse transcriptase. It can proceed with the normal host-cell enzymes.

7.9 ECOLOGY

Ecology is the study of organisms and their interactions with their environments.

Biomes

Biomes are **ecosystems** and communities that are typical of major geographical regions. They are characterized by different vegetation and animal types, depending on differences in climate and other factors, including water availability, sunlight, soil type, wind, and temperature. There are eight major terrestrial biomes:

1. **Tropical forests** are found near the equator, where the average amount of sunlight and the average temperature vary very little. They can be divided into **tropical dry forests** (little rainfall), **tropical deciduous forests** (moderate rainfall), and **tropical rain forests** (heavy rainfall). Tropical rain forests have the greatest diversity of plant and animal life of all the biomes.

2. **Savanna** biomes are located north and south of tropical forest biomes. They have less rainfall and a longer dry season. The vegetation is predominately grasses with some scattered trees; they are sometimes referred to as tropical grasslands. This biome is home to some of the largest herbivores in the world (such as giraffes and elephants).

3. **Deserts** are extremely dry biomes, characterized by extremely low rainfall. Although we typically think of deserts as being very hot, the average temperature of a desert can be very hot or very cold, depending on the location. The vegetation is drought resistant (succulents and cacti), and animals must be heat tolerant. Most animals are seed eaters, with reptiles such as snakes and lizards preying on them.

4. **Temperate deciduous forests** receive a fairly large amount of precipitation and thus support a dense environment of deciduous trees. There is a wide diversity of plant and animal life. They usually have cool winters and warm summers.

5. **Grassland** biomes are mostly found in the interiors of continents. They have large seasonal temperature variations (cold winters and hot summers), and moderate precipitation. Vegetation is mostly grasses with few trees or shrubs. This biome houses many large terrestrial animals that graze (kangaroos, horses, bison). It is sometimes referred to as the **prairies** and has some of the most fertile soils in the world. Grasslands are used primarily for farming and grazing.

6. **Chaparral** (or the Mediterranean climate biome) is found near coastal regions and is characterized by short, shrubby vegetation. It has hot, long, dry summers and mildly rainy winters. Animal life is similar to the desert, but includes deer, birds, and coyote.

7. **Taiga** is the largest biome, consisting of coniferous forest. It is sometimes called the Northern **coniferous forest biome** or the **Boreal forest**. Most precipitation falls as snow, and long, cold winters characterize this area. Animal populations include squirrels, birds, deer, moose, rabbits, bears, wolves, and lynx. The most common tree is the conifer.

8. **Tundra** is characterized by an extremely cold climate and permanently frozen subsoil (permafrost). There is very little precipitation, and very few plants. Most animals are insects, although there are a fair number of mammals as well, including caribou, wolves, polar bears, foxes and reindeer.

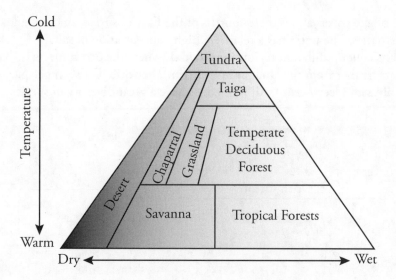

Figure 29   Terrestrial Biomes

There are two aquatic biomes:

1.   Freshwater biomes have low salt concentration. They include ponds and lakes, streams and rivers, and wetlands.
     •   Lakes and ponds are divided into three different zones, determined by distance from the shoreline and depth of the water. The **littoral zone** is close to the shore and near the top of the lake. It is usually shallow and thus the warmest part of the lake. Farther from the shore and near the top is the **limnetic zone,** home of plankton and fish. The **profundal zone** is the deepest part of the lake. It is typically colder and darker, and home to **heterotrophs** instead of autotrophs.

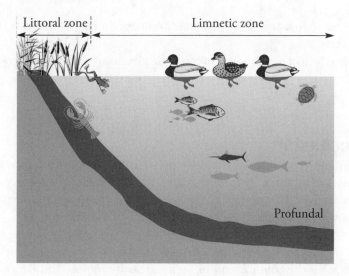

Figure 30   Lake Zones

     •   Streams and rivers flow in one direction, from the source to the mouth.
     •   Wetlands include marshes, swamps, and bogs, all areas of standing water that support aquatic plants. They tend to have high species diversity.

2. The Marine biome covers about three-fourths of the Earth's surface and includes oceans, coral reefs, and estuaries. The water has a relatively high concentration of salt.
   - Oceans contain different regions: **intertidal** (where the ocean meets the land), **pelagic** (waters further from the land, or open ocean), **benthic** (between pelagic and abyssal), and **abyssal** (deep ocean). All four zones have a great diversity of species.

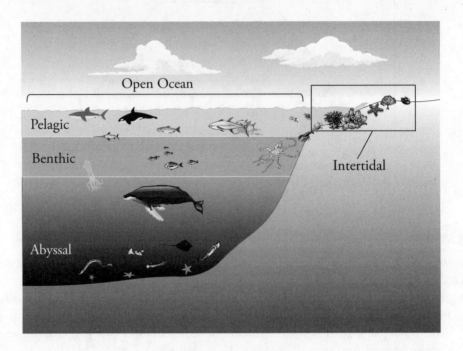

Figure 31 Ocean Zones

- Coral reefs are found in warm shallow waters and contain corals, fishes, sea urchins, octopuses, and sea stars.
- Estuaries are areas where ocean water merges with freshwater streams or rivers.

Ecological Succession

Changes in ecosystems and communities typically occur after some disturbance to the system, such as a fire, flood or other natural disaster. This may change the availability of resources and could allow new species to establish themselves. Communities typically pass through a series of predictable stages. This transition period is known as **ecological succession.**

If this process begins in an as yet lifeless area (a new lava flow, for example), it is known as **primary succession** and begins with the colonization of rocky areas by mosses and lichen. These organisms are known as **pioneer organisms.** The community then passes through stages of colonization by shrubs, conifers, and deciduous trees. The entire process takes about two centuries to complete, and the final stage community is known as the **climax community.**

If succession occurs in an area previously supporting life (a hillside devastated by fire, for example), the process is known as **secondary succession.**

7.9

Population and Community Ecology

A **population** can be defined as a group of individuals of a single species that live in the same general area and are thus subject to the same environmental factors and resources. Two characteristics that help to define a population are its **density** (number of individuals per unit area) and its **dispersion** (the spacing among individuals within the population). Resources, being limited, often define the **carrying capacity** of an area, that is the maximum stable population size that can be supported by that particular environment. Other factors that can play a role are defined as **density-dependent** or **density-independent.**

Density-dependent factors are those that increase in intensity as the population grows. For example, food availability and territory (space) availability can both be density-dependent factors affecting the size of a population. Density-independent factors are not related to population size; the most common are related to climate and weather.

- Which of the following are **not** density-independent factors affecting a bird population?[52]
    - I. The number of earthworms available as food
    - II. The average temperature in the area
    - III. The number of trees available for nesting

7.10 SYMBIOTIC RELATIONS

Many different populations existing together make up a community, and community interactions can have different effects on a population's density. The interaction between predator and prey can affect both populations' densities.

Other common interactions are those that involve two species in a symbiotic relationship. There are three common symbiotic relationships: commensalism, mutualism, and parasitism.

Commensalism is defined as a symbiotic relationship between two species in which one member of the pair is helped by the association and the other member is unaffected. Examples include the relationship between egrets and buffalo, and the relationship between humans and skin bacteria. In the egret-buffalo relationship, the egret benefit by eating the bugs flushed from the grass as the buffalo graze. The buffalo do not care one way or the other about the egrets. Likewise, skin bacteria benefit from their symbiotic relationship with humans by being provided with food (dead, sloughed-off skin), while the humans are unaffected.

In a **mutualistic relationship**, both partners benefit from the association. Probably the best known example is the relationship between legumes and nitrogen-fixing bacteria. The plants benefit by the additional nitrogen provided by bacteria, and the bacteria benefit from the nutrients provided by the plant.

---

[52] I is density-dependent: as the population size increases, competition for resources (such as food) will become more intense, and not all birds will survive. II is density-independent: temperature and other climate-related factors affect all populations similarly, regardless of size. III is density-dependent: space availability will also become an issue as the population size increases.

Parasitic relationships are those in which one partner benefits and the other is harmed. An example is the relationship between an intestinal tapeworm and its human host. The tapeworm receives nutrients at the expense of the host, who develops nutritional deficiencies.

- Humans have a large population of normal intestinal bacteria that provide us with a good source of vitamin K. This relationship is best described as ___.[53]
- The relationship between a virus and the animal cell it infects can be described as ___.[54]

Within each community different organisms have different roles. Overall, the roles can be divided into producers and consumers. **Producers** are those organisms that can produce their own food, and as such, provide a source of food for organisms that cannot make their own food. Examples of producers are plants and photosynthetic microorganisms. [Are fungi producers?[55]] **Consumers** are those organisms that rely on the food made by the producers (either directly or indirectly) for their nutrition. Consumers can be further subdivided into three categories: **primary consumers** (who eat the producers), **secondary consumers** (who eat both primary consumers and producers), and **tertiary consumers** (who eat both primary and secondary consumers). Primary consumers are also known as **herbivores** (plant eaters), secondary consumers as **omnivores** (plant and meat eaters), and tertiary consumers as **carnivores** (meat eaters). [How would a hawk be classified?[56] How about a sparrow?[57]] Since each level of the **food chain** is supported by the previous level, the actual numbers of organisms at each level tend to decrease the further up the chain we progress. Thus there are very few top carnivores, and the world's largest animals (elephants, rhinos, etc.) tend to be herbivores (primary consumers). There just physically aren't enough organisms at the higher levels to support their great body size.

7.11 ANIMAL BEHAVIOR

The study of animal behavior is the study of *how* an animal acts and *why* it acts in that manner. Behaviors can generally be classified into two main groups: innate behavior and learned behavior (see Figure 32).

Innate Behaviors

Innate behaviors (also called **instinctive patterns**) are present at birth or are preprogrammed to occur; they do not have to be taught or learned. They include innate predispositions for certain associations and include kinesis, taxis and fixed action patterns. In **kinesis**, movement or activity of a cell or organism occurs in response to a stimulus. The response is non-directional. During **taxis**, an organism responds to a stimulus directionally. Guided movement occurs toward the stimulus (positive taxis) or away from the

---

[53] mutualistic. The bacteria benefit from the nutrients received in the material the human host could not digest, and the human host benefits from the vitamin K produced by the bacteria.

[54] parasitic. The virus benefits (it is able to reproduce using the host cell's machinery), but the host cell is harmed (and often killed) in the process.

[55] No. Fungi rely on absorption of nutrients from other (usually dead) organisms. Only photosynthetic organisms can be producers. Fungi have no chloroplasts and are not photosynthetic. They are classified as decomposers.

[56] Hawks are strict meat eaters (birds of prey) and are thus classified as carnivores and tertiary consumers.

[57] Sparrows consume insects as well as seeds and berries and are thus classified as omnivores and secondary consumers.

stimulus (negative taxis). There are many types of taxis behaviors, and they are named using prefixes to specify the stimulus. For example, **chemotaxis** is a response to chemicals, **geotaxis** is a response to gravity, and **thermotaxis** is a response to temperature changes. **Fixed action patterns** are stereotypical behaviors that are triggered by specific stimuli. Examples include the feeding of baby birds by their parents, displays of territoriality, and sexual or mating behaviors. These are instinctive behavioral sequences that run to completion once started. They are invariant and are produced in response to an external sensory stimulus.

Learned Behaviors

Learning is the process of either acquiring new, or modifying existing, knowledge, behaviors, skills, values, or preferences. It often involves synthesizing different types of information and requires interaction with other organisms or the environment. The ability to learn occurs in animals (including humans). There are two types of learned behaviors: simple non-associative and associative, and each has different subtypes.

Simple non-associative learning occurs when an organism changes its response to a stimuli without associating it with positive or negative reinforcement. Habituation and sensitization are both examples. **Habituation** is a progressive *decrease* in the probability of a behavioral response, in response to a repeated stimulus. In other words, an organism responds to a stimulus at first; however, if it is neither rewarding nor harmful, the organism reduces subsequent responses. For example, if a certain hallway always smells weird, you will notice at first but eventually learn not to notice it. The basic response (smell) has not been lost, merely modified by learning. For example, if you walk down a new hallway and it has the same weird smell, you will notice it. In contrast, **sensitization** leads to a progressive *increase* in the probability of a behavioral response, in response to a repeated stimulus. In other words, repeated administrations of a stimulus lead to progressive amplification of the response that follows.

Associative learning is also called **conditioning**, and occurs when a response is taught through association with a separate, pre-occurring reinforcement or stimulus (either positive or negative). There are two types. **Classical or Pavlovian conditioning** is named after Pavlov and his dog experiments.[58] It is characterized as an involuntary reaction (or reflex) that has been linked to a stimulus, and involves strengthening of the stimulus-outcome association with exposure. The stimulus may be totally unrelated to the actual behavior. For example, a dog that runs to the kitchen when it hears the can opener is exhibiting classical conditioning, as is a fish that swims to the top of the bowl when a tap is heard, because it has associated the tap with food at the surface. These behaviors will occur even if the true stimulus (food) is not present.

Operant conditioning is a voluntary reaction in response to a stimulus, in anticipation of a reward or punishment. In other words, it uses consequences, reinforcement or punishment to modify the occurrence or form of behavior. For example, a rat that learns to press a lever because every time it does so it receives a food pellet is exhibiting operant conditioning. Operant conditioning is also known as trial-and-error learning.

7.11

---

[58] Ivan Pavlov was a Russian physiologist who researched salivation in dogs in response to being fed. He noticed that his dogs began to salivate when they heard the footsteps of his assistant who was delivering the food, not when food was placed in front of the dogs. In fact, Pavlov discovered that any object or event which the dogs learned to associate with food would trigger the same response.

Imprinting is a combination of instinctive behavior and learned behavior. It is a type of phase-sensitive learning, in that it occurs at a particular age or stage of life. For example, in filial imprinting, a young animal acquires several of its behavioral characteristics from its parent. This is most obvious in birds such as geese, which imprint on their parents and then follow them around. In this example, the identity of the goose's mother was learned, but the goose's behavior toward the mother was instinctive. In some cases, behaviors occur even if the stimulus is not the actual stimulus encountered in nature. For example, certain fish display aggressive behavior toward any object with a particular coloring, even if that object is not real. Baby goslings will recognize any object (a balloon, a ticking clock, a human) seen during a critical time period shortly after birth as "mother."

7.11

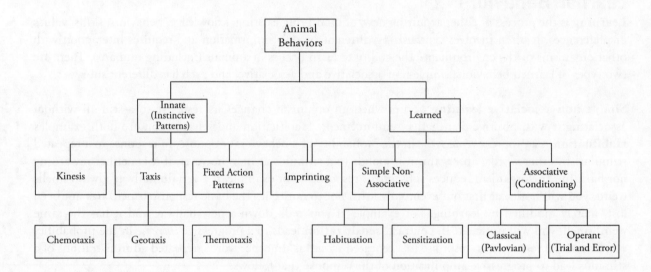

Figure 32   Animal Behavior

Want More Practice?
Scan the QR code below to register your book for online chapter summaries, drills, practice tests, and more!

Chapter 8
Structure and Function of Systems:
Body Control and Communication

The nervous and endocrine systems are presented in the same chapter since their functions are related: they both provide communication, integrating and coordinating activities of the tissues and organs of the body. The means of communication by the two systems are quite different (although complementary) in many ways. The nervous system communicates through electrochemical signals (action potentials), while the endocrine system uses chemical messengers carried in the blood (hormones). The nervous system in general regulates rapid responses such as those of skeletal muscle or smooth muscle, while the endocrine system takes longer to have an effect and regulates longer-term responses such as metabolism and homeostasis. The two systems are interconnected, with two of the primary endocrine glands—the pituitary and the adrenals—regulated by the nervous system, and with the endocrine system feeding back to modulate the nervous system.

8.1   NEURONAL STRUCTURE AND FUNCTION

Neurons are specialized cells that transmit and process information from one part of the body to another. This information takes the form of electrochemical impulses known as **action potentials**. The action potential is a localized area of depolarization of the plasma membrane that travels in a wave-like manner along an axon. When an action potential reaches the end of an axon at a synapse, the signal is transformed into a chemical signal with the release of neurotransmitter into the synaptic cleft, a process called **synaptic transmission** (Section 8.1). The information of many synapses feeding into a neuron is integrated to determine whether that neuron will in turn fire an action potential. In this way the action of many individual neurons is integrated to work together in the nervous system as a whole.

Structure of the Neuron

The basic functional and structural unit of the nervous system is the **neuron** (see Figure 1 on the following page); nerves, ganglia, and the brain are composed of clusters of neurons. The structure of these cells is highly specialized to transmit and process action potentials, the electrochemical signals of the nervous system. Neurons have a central cell body, the **soma**, which contains the nucleus and is where most of the biosynthetic activity of the cell takes place. Slender projections, termed **axons** and **dendrites**, extend from the cell body. Neurons have only one axon (as long as a meter in some cases), but most possess many dendrites. Neurons with one dendrite are termed **bipolar**; those with many dendrites are **multipolar**. Neurons generally carry action potentials in one direction, with dendrites receiving signals and axons carrying action potentials away from the cell body. Axons can branch multiple times and terminate in **synaptic knobs** that form connections with target cells. When action potentials travel down an axon and reach the synaptic knob, chemical messengers are released and travel across a very small gap called the **synaptic cleft** to the target cell. The nature of the action potential and the transmission of signals across the synaptic cleft are key aspects of nervous system function. [In Figure 1, in what direction does an action potential travel in the axon shown?[1] What's the difference between a neuron and a nerve?[2]]

---

[1] Action potentials travel from the cell body down the axon, or from left to right in Figure 1.

[2] A neuron is a single cell. A nerve is a large bundle of many different axons from different neurons.

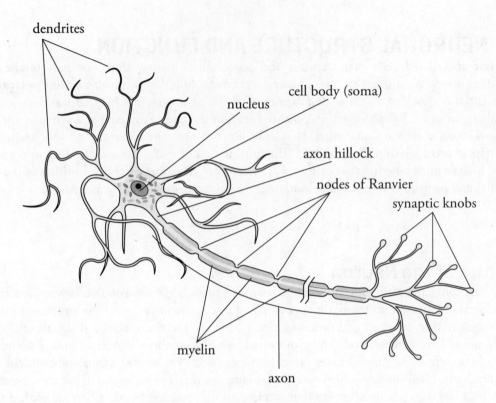

Figure 1 A Multipolar Neuron

The Action Potential

Resting Membrane Potential

The **resting membrane potential** (or RMP) is an electric potential across the plasma membrane of approximately −70 millivolts (mV), with the interior of the cell negatively charged with respect to the exterior of the cell. Two primary membrane proteins are required to establish the resting membrane potential: the Na^+/K^+ ATPase and the **potassium leak channels**. The **Na^+/K^+ ATPase** pumps three sodium ions out of the cell and two potassium ions into the cell with the hydrolysis of one ATP molecule. [What form of transport is carried out by the Na^+/K^+ ATPase?[3]] The result is a sodium gradient with high sodium outside of the cell and a potassium gradient with high potassium inside the cell. **Leak channels** are open all the time and allow ions to "leak" across the membrane according to their gradient. Potassium leak channels allow potassium, but no other ions, to flow down their gradient out of the cell. The combined loss of many positive ions through Na^+/K^+ ATPases and potassium leak channels leaves the interior of the cell with a net negative charge, approximately 70 mV more negative than the exterior of the cell; this difference is the resting membrane potential. Note that there are very few **sodium leak channels** in the membrane (the ratio of K^+ leak channels to Na^+ leak channels is about 100:1), so the cell membrane is virtually impermeable to sodium.

---

[3] The Na^+/K^+ ATPase uses ATP to drive transport against a gradient; this is primary active transport.

- Are neurons the only cells with a resting membrane potential?[4]
- If the potassium leak channels are blocked, what will happen to the membrane potential?[5]
- What would happen to the membrane potential if sodium ions were allowed to flow down their concentration gradient?[6]

The resting membrane potential establishes a negative charge along the interior of axons (along with the rest of the neuronal interior). Thus, the cells can be described as **polarized**—negative on the inside and positive on the outside. An action potential is a disturbance in this membrane potential, a wave of **depolarization** of the plasma membrane that travels along an axon. Depolarization is a change in the membrane potential from the resting membrane potential of approximately –70 mV to a less negative, or even positive, potential. After depolarization, **repolarization** returns the membrane potential to normal. The change in membrane potential during passage of an action potential is caused by movement of ions into and out of the neuron through ion channels. The action potential is therefore not strictly an electrical impulse, like electrons moving in a copper telephone wire, but an electro*chemical* impulse.

Depolarization

Key proteins in the propagation of action potentials are the **voltage-gated sodium channels** located in the plasma membrane of the axon. In response to a change in the membrane potential, these ion channels open to allow sodium ions to flow down their gradient into the cell and depolarize that section of membrane. [What is the effect of opening the voltage-gated sodium channels on the membrane potential?[7]] These channels are opened by depolarization of the membrane from the resting potential of –70 mV to a **threshold potential** of approximately –50 mV.[8] Once this threshold is reached, the channels are opened fully, but below the threshold they are closed and do not allow the passage of any ions through the channel. When the channels open, sodium flows into the cell, down its concentration gradient, depolarizing that section of the membrane to about +35 mV before inactivating. Some sodium ions flow down the interior of the axon, slightly depolarizing the neighboring section of membrane. When the depolarization in the next section of membrane reaches threshold, those voltage-gated sodium channels open as well, passing the depolarization down the axon (see Figure 2 on the following page). [If an action potential starts at one end of an axon, can it run out of energy and not reach the other end?[9]]

---

[4] No. All cells have a resting membrane potential. Neurons and muscle tissue are unique in using the resting membrane potential to generate action potentials.

[5] The flow of potassium out of the cell makes the interior of the cell more negatively charged. Blocking potassium leak channels would reduce the resting membrane potential, making the interior of the cell less negative.

[6] Sodium ions would flow into the cell and reduce the potential across the plasma membrane, making the interior of the cell less negative and even relatively positive if enough ions flow into the cell.

[7] Sodium (positively charged) flows into the cell, down its concentration gradient, making the interior of the cell less negatively charged, or even positively charged.

[8] In the next section, we'll discuss summation and how action potentials start.

[9] No, it cannot. Action potentials are continually renewed at each point in the axon as they travel. Once an action potential starts, it will propagate without a change in amplitude (size) until it reaches a synapse.

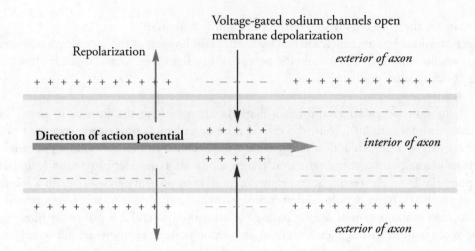

Figure 2 The Action Potential is a Wave of Membrane Depolarization

- Which one of the following can cause the interior of the neuron to have a momentary positive charge?[10]
    A. Opening of potassium leak channels
    B. Activity of the Na^+/K^+ ATPase
    C. Opening of voltage-gated sodium channels
    D. Opening of voltage-gated potassium channels

- Which of the following best describes the response of voltage-gated sodium channels to a membrane depolarization from –70 mV to –60 mV?[11]
    A. All the channels open fully
    B. 50% of the channels open fully
    C. All the channels open 50%
    D. 50% of the channels open 50%
    E. None of the channels open

Voltage-gated sodium channels have three conformations (Figure 3):

1. Closed: in this conformation, the channel does not allow sodium into the cell.
2. Open: in this conformation, the channel is activated and open wide, which allows sodium into the cell. The channel opens when the plasma membrane reaches the threshold potential of –50 mV.
3. Inactivated: when the cell has depolarized to +35 mV, voltage-gated sodium channels inactivate. In this conformation, they do not allow sodium into the cell, but they are also unable to open. The channel must be reset to the closed conformation before they can open again, which occurs during the absolute refractory period; we'll talk more about this shortly.

---

[10] Choices A, B, and D all make the interior of the cell more negative. Choice **C** is the correct answer. Voltage-gated sodium channels can make the interior of the cell momentarily positive during passage of an action potential.

[11] Voltage-gated sodium channels require a threshold depolarization to open. A depolarization below the threshold will produce essentially no response, while a depolarization greater than or equal to the threshold will cause all of the channels to open fully. This is called an **all-or-none** response. The correct answer is **E**. The depolarization is less than the threshold, so there is no response.

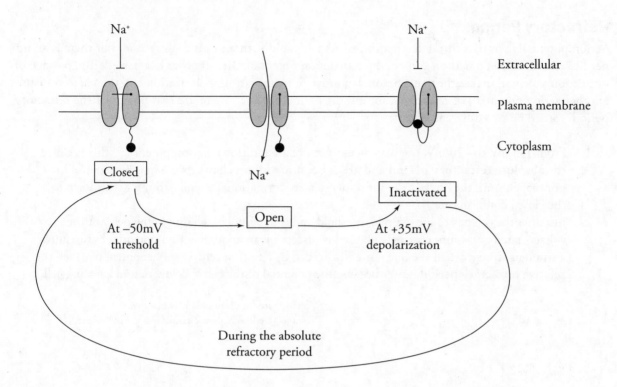

Figure 3 Conformations of Voltage-Gated Sodium Channels

Repolarization

At the peak of an action potential (when the cell potential is +35mV), voltage-gated sodium channels become inactivated. At just about the same time, **voltage-gated potassium channels** have finished opening up; they actually start doing this around –50mV but take awhile to complete the process. With the potassium channels open, potassium ions rush out of the cell along their concentration gradient (created initially by the sodium-potassium ATPase pump).

By moving outward across the neuronal cell membrane, positively charged potassium ions reduce electrical potential within the cell. The cell's interior once again becomes negative and is then said to be **repolarized.** During this time, the voltage-gated sodium channels are resetting from the inactivated state back to closed. When the potential of the cell reaches –70mV once again, the voltage-gated potassium channels close. However, there is a delay between when these channels should close and when they actually close; voltage-gated potassium channels are effectively slow to open and slow to close. Because the voltage-gated potassium channels stay open a little too long, too many potassium ions flow out of the cell and the potential drops to approximately –90mV. During this time, the cell is said to be **hyperpolarized.** After the voltage-gated potassium channels close, the sodium-potassium ATPase and the potassium leak channels steadily bring the membrane back to the resting potential of –70mV.

The phrase "action potential" is therefore used to describe a combination of two sequential events:

1. depolarization (–70mV to +35mV) due to sodium inflow
2. repolarization (+35mV to –70mV) due to potassium outflow

Refractory Periods

Action potentials can pass through a neuron extremely rapidly, thousands each second, but there is an upper limit to how soon a neuron can conduct an action potential after another has passed. The passage of one action potential makes the neuron nonresponsive to membrane depolarization and unable to transmit another action potential, or refractory, for a short period of time. There are two phases of the refractory period, caused by two different factors:

1. From +35 mV to –70 mV, the neuron cannot fire an additional action potential. This is called the **absolute refractory period** and arises because sodium channels are inactivated and cannot reopen until they have reset (or undergo a conformational switch from inactive form to the closed conformation).

2. Just after the cell passes the –70mV threshold and is hyperpolarized due to the delay of the voltage-gated potassium channels, the cell is susceptible to another action potential but requires a stimulus stronger than the one normally needed by a resting cell. This phenomenon, called the **relative refractory period,** arises because the potential of the cell is below that of a resting cell.

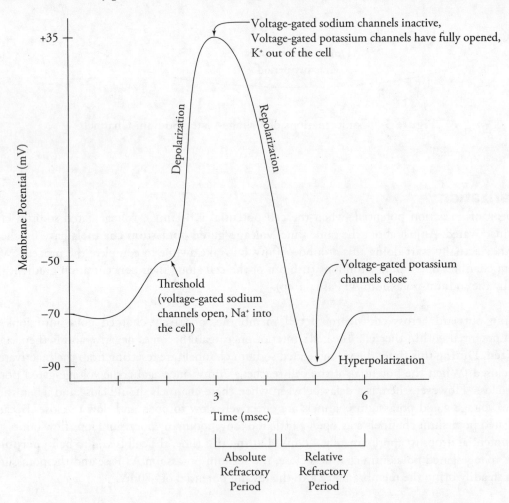

Figure 4 Principal Stages and Ion Flows Associated with an Action Potential

- If a toxin prevents voltage-gated sodium channels from closing, which of the following will occur?[12]
  I. Voltage-gated potassium channels will open but not close.
  II. The membrane will not repolarize to the normal resting membrane potential.
  III. Na$^+$/K$^+$ ATPases will be inactivated.

  A. I only
  B. II only
  C. I and II only
  D. II and III only
  E. I, II, and III

Saltatory Conduction

The axons of many neurons are wrapped in an insulating sheath called **myelin** (Figure 5). The myelin sheath is not created by the neuron itself, but by cells called glial cells, specialized, non-neuronal cells that provide structural and metabolic support to neurons. Glia maintain a resting membrane potential but do not generate action potentials. There are two types of glial cells you should be familiar with for the DAT: **Schwann cells** that form the myelin sheath in the peripheral nervous system (PNS) and **oligodendrocytes** that form the myelin sheath in the central nervous system (CNS). These cells exist in conjunction with neurons, wrapping layers of specialized membrane around the axons. No ions can enter or exit a neuron where the axonal membrane is covered with myelin. [Would an axon be able to conduct action potentials if its entire length were wrapped in myelin?[13]] There is no membrane depolarization and no voltage-gated sodium channels in regions of the axonal plasma membrane that are wrapped in myelin. There are periodic gaps in the myelin sheath however, called **nodes of Ranvier**. Voltage-gated sodium and potassium channels are concentrated in the nodes of Ranvier in myelinated axons. Rather than impeding action potentials, the myelin sheath dramatically speeds the movement of action potentials by forcing the action potential to jump from node to node. This rapid jumping conduction in myelinated axons is termed **saltatory conduction**.

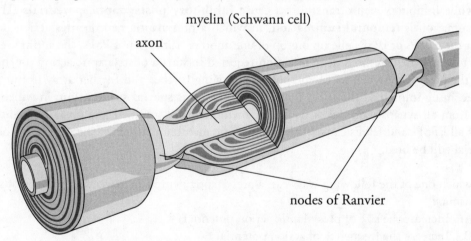

myelin (Schwann cell)

axon

nodes of Ranvier

Figure 5 A Schwann Cell Wrapping an Axon with Myelin

---

[12] **Statement I is true:** Voltage-gated potassium channels are normally closed by the repolarization of the membrane, so if the membrane is not repolarized, they will not close. **Statement II is true:** Sodium ions will continue to flow into the cell, even as the Na$^+$/K$^+$ ATPase works to pump them out. This will prevent the repolarization of the membrane. **Statement III is false:** The Na$^+$/K$^+$ ATPase will work harder than ever. The answer is **C**.

[13] No. The action potential requires the movement of ions across the plasma membrane to create a wave of depolarization.

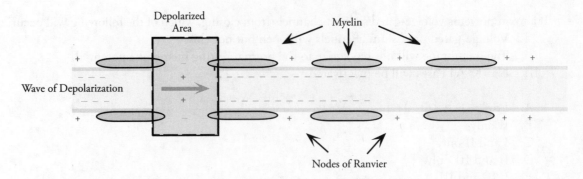

Figure 6   Propagation of the AP in a Myelinated Axon (cross-section)

Summation

Once an action potential is initiated in a neuron, it will propagate to the end of the axon at a speed and magnitude of depolarization that do not vary from one action potential to another. The action potential is an "all-or-nothing" event. The key regulated step in the nervous system is whether or not a neuron will fire an action potential; this will be decided at the **axon hillock**, a region that sums incoming signals and determines if threshold (–50 mV) has been reached or not. A postsynaptic neuron has many different neurons with synapses leading to it, and each of these synapses can release neurotransmitters many times per second. The "decision" by a postsynaptic neuron of whether to fire an action potential is determined by adding the effect of all synapses impinging on a neuron, both **excitatory** and **inhibitory**. This addition of stimuli is termed **summation**.

Excitatory neurotransmitters cause postsynaptic depolarization, or **excitatory postsynaptic potentials (EPSPs)**, while inhibitory neurotransmitters cause **inhibitory postsynaptic potentials (IPSPs)**. One form of summation is **temporal summation**, in which a presynaptic neuron fires action potentials so rapidly that the EPSPs or IPSPs pile up on top of one another. If they are EPSPs, the additive effect might be enough to reach the threshold depolarization required to start a postsynaptic action potential. If they are IPSPs, the postsynaptic cell will hyperpolarize, moving further and further away from threshold, effectively becoming inhibited. The other form of summation is **spatial summation**, in which the EPSPs and IPSPs from all synapses on the postsynaptic membrane are summed at a given moment in time. If the total of all EPSPs and IPSPs causes the postsynaptic membrane to reach the threshold voltage, an action potential will be fired.

- In which one of the following ways can a presynaptic neuron increase the intensity of signal it transmits?[14]
    - A. Increase the size of presynaptic action potentials
    - B. Increase the frequency of action potentials
    - C. Change the type of neurotransmitter it releases
    - D. Change the speed of action potential propagation

---

[14] A neuron cannot change the size of action potentials it transmits, but it can increase the number of action potentials it transmits in a given amount of time (frequency of action potentials). Increased frequency of action potentials will add up through temporal summation in the postsynaptic cell to produce an increased response (choice **B** is correct). Action potentials are all-or-nothing once they are started. The magnitude of membrane depolarization during propagation of an action potential does not change (eliminate A). A neuron does not change the neurotransmitter it releases (eliminate C), and speed of propagation cannot be varied from one action potential to the next (eliminate D).

Synaptic Transmission

A **synapse** is a junction between the axon terminus of a neuron and the dendrites, soma, or axon of a second neuron. It can also be a junction between the axon terminus of a neuron and an organ. There are two types of synapses: electrical and chemical. **Electrical synapses** occur when cytoplasms of two cells are joined by gap junctions. If two cells are joined by an electrical synapse, an action potential will spread directly from one cell to the other. Electrical synapses are not common in the nervous system although they are quite important in propagating action potentials in smooth muscle and cardiac muscle. In the nervous system, **chemical synapses** are found at the ends of axons where they meet their target cell; here, an action potential is converted into a chemical signal. The following steps are involved in the transmission of a signal across a chemical synapse in the nervous system (see Figure 7), as well as at the junctions of neurons with other cell types, such as skeletal muscle cells:

1. An action potential reaches the end of an axon, the synaptic knob.
2. Depolarization of the presynaptic membrane opens **voltage-gated calcium channels**.
3. Calcium influx into the presynaptic cell causes exocytosis of neurotransmitter stored in secretory vesicles.
4. **Neurotransmitter molecules** diffuse across the narrow synaptic cleft (small space between cells).
5. Neurotransmitter binds to receptor proteins in the postsynaptic membrane. These receptors are **ligand-gated ion channels**.
6. Opening of these ion channels in the postsynaptic cell alters membrane polarization.
7. If membrane depolarization of the postsynaptic cell reaches the threshold of voltage-gated sodium channels, an action potential is initiated.
8. Neurotransmitter in the synaptic cleft is degraded and/or removed to terminate the signal.

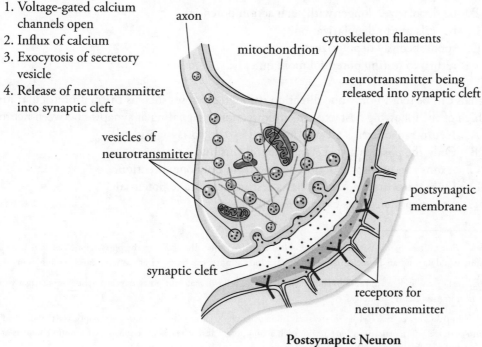

1. Voltage-gated calcium channels open
2. Influx of calcium
3. Exocytosis of secretory vesicle
4. Release of neurotransmitter into synaptic cleft

axon

mitochondrion

cytoskeleton filaments

neurotransmitter being released into synaptic cleft

vesicles of neurotransmitter

postsynaptic membrane

synaptic cleft

receptors for neurotransmitter

Postsynaptic Neuron
1. Neurotransmitter binds to ligand-gated ion channel
2. Ions enter or exit postsynaptic cell
3. Membrane polarization is increased or decreased

Figure 7   Synaptic Function

An example of a chemical synapse that is commonly used is the **neuromuscular junction** between neurons and skeletal muscle. The neurotransmitter that is released at the neuromuscular junction is **acetylcholine (ACh)**. When an action potential reaches such a synapse, acetylcholine is released into the synaptic cleft. Acetylcholine binds to an acetylcholine receptor on the surface of the postsynaptic cell membrane. When acetylcholine binds to its receptor, the receptor opens its associated sodium channel, allowing sodium to flow down a gradient into the cell, depolarizing the postsynaptic cell membrane. Meanwhile, acetylcholine in the synaptic cleft is degraded by the enzyme **acetylcholinesterase (AChE)**.

There are several different neurotransmitters and neurotransmitter receptors. Acetylcholine and **norepinephrine** are important neurotransmitters to recognize for the DAT. Other examples of neurotransmitters are gamma-aminobutyric acid (GABA), serotonin, and dopamine. If a neurotransmitter, such as acetylcholine, opens a channel that depolarizes the postsynaptic membrane, the neurotransmitter is termed **excitatory**. Other neurotransmitters, however, have the opposite effect, making the postsynaptic membrane potential more negative than the resting potential, or hyperpolarized. Neurotransmitters that induce hyperpolarization of the postsynaptic membrane are termed **inhibitory**.[15] Each presynaptic neuron can release only one type of neurotransmitter, although a postsynaptic neuron may respond to many different neurotransmitters.

- If a neurotransmitter causes the entry of chloride into the postsynaptic cell, is the neurotransmitter excitatory or inhibitory?[16]

- If an inhibitor of acetylcholinesterase is added to a neuromuscular junction, then the postsynaptic membrane will:[17]
  A. be depolarized by action potentials more frequently.
  B. be depolarized longer with each action potential.
  C. be resistant to depolarization.
  D. spontaneously depolarize.
  E. return to resting potential more quickly.

- Signals can be sent in only one direction through synapses such as the neuromuscular junction. Which of the following best explains unidirectional signaling at synapses between neurons?[18]
  A. Neurotransmitter is always degraded by the postsynaptic cell.
  B. Only the postsynaptic cell has neurotransmitter receptors.
  C. Axons can propagate action potentials in only one direction.
  D. Only the postsynaptic cell has a resting membrane potential.
  E. Presynaptic neurons cannot be depolarized.

---

[15] Note, however, that ultimately it is not the *neurotransmitter* that determines the effect on the postsynaptic cell, it is the *receptor* for that neurotransmitter and its associated ion channel. The same neurotransmitter can be excitatory in some cases and inhibitory in others.

[16] Chloride ions are negatively charged. Entry of chloride ions into the cell will make the postsynaptic potential more negative, or hyperpolarized, so the neurotransmitter is inhibitory.

[17] Choice **B** is the correct answer. If acetylcholinesterase is inhibited, acetylcholine will remain in the synaptic cleft longer, and acetylcholine-gated sodium channels will remain open longer with each action potential that reaches the synapse. If sodium channels are open longer, depolarization of the postsynaptic membrane will last longer.

[18] Signaling is unidirectional because only the presynaptic cell has vesicles of neurotransmitter that are released in response to action potentials, and only the postsynaptic neuron has receptors that bind neurotransmitter (choice **B** is correct). Degradation of neurotransmitter is irrelevant to the direction of signal propagation (eliminate A), axons are capable of propagating action potentials in both directions (even though this is not what they normally do; eliminate C), all cells have a resting membrane potential (eliminate D), and all neurons can be depolarized (eliminate E).

8.2 NERVOUS SYSTEM

Functional Organization of the Human Nervous System

The nervous system must receive information, decide what to do with it, and cause muscles or glands to act upon that decision. Receiving information is the **sensory** function of the nervous system (carried out by the **peripheral nervous system**, or PNS), processing the information is the **integrative** function (carried out by the **central nervous system**, or CNS), and acting on it is the **motor** function (also carried out by the PNS). **Motor neurons** carry information from the nervous system toward organs which can act upon that information, known as **effectors**. [What are the two types of effectors?[19]] Notice that "motor" neurons do not lead only "to muscle." Motor neurons, which carry information away from the central nervous system and innervate effectors, are called **efferent** neurons (remember, efferents go to effectors). **Sensory neurons**, which carry information toward the central nervous system, are called **afferent** neurons.

The main anatomical division of the nervous system is between the central nervous system and the peripheral nervous system. The CNS is the brain and spinal cord. The PNS includes all other axons, dendrites, and cell bodies. The great majority of neuronal cell bodies are found within the central nervous system. Sometimes they are bunched together to form structures called **nuclei.** (Don't confuse this with the nucleic-acid-containing nuclei of cells.) Somas located outside the central nervous system are found in bunches known as **ganglia.** Finally, it is worth noting that most axons in the CNS and PNS are myelinated.

The peripheral nervous system can be subdivided into several functional divisions (Figure 8). The portion of this system concerned with conscious sensation and deliberate, voluntary movement of skeletal muscle is the **somatic** division. The portion concerned with digestion, metabolism, circulation, perspiration, and other involuntary processes is the **autonomic** division. Both the somatic and autonomic divisions include afferent and efferent functions. The efferent portion of the autonomic division is further split into two subdivisions: sympathetic and parasympathetic. When the **sympathetic** system is activated, the body is prepared for "fight or flight." When the **parasympathetic** system is activated, the body is prepared to "rest and digest."

---

[19] Muscles and glands

8.2

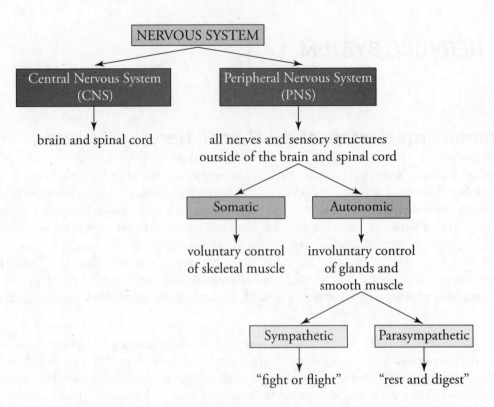

Figure 8   Overall Organization of the Nervous System

CNS

The CNS includes the **spinal cord** and the **brain**. The brain has three subdivisions: the **hindbrain** (or the rhombencephalon), the **midbrain** (or the mesencephalon), and the **forebrain** (or the prosencephalon). These four regions of the CNS perform increasingly complex functions. The entire CNS (brain and spinal cord) floats in **cerebrospinal fluid** (**CSF**), a clear liquid that serves various functions such as shock absorption and exchange of nutrients and waste with the CNS.

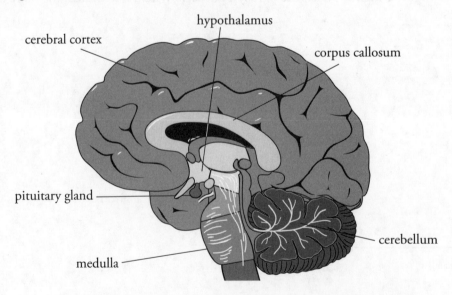

Figure 9   Organization of the CNS (cross-section of the brain)

The following table summarizes major regions of the brain you should be familiar with, along with their functions.

Structure	General Function	Specific Functions
Spinal cord	Simple reflexes	• controls simple stretch and tendon reflexes • controls primitive processes such as walking, urination, and sex organ function
Pons	Relay station and balance	• controls antigravity posture and balance • connects the spinal cord and medulla with upper regions of the brain • relays information to the cerebellum and thalamus
Cerebellum	Movement coordination	• integrating center • coordination of complex movement, balance and posture, muscle tone, spatial equilibrium
Hypothalamus	Homeostasis and behavior	• controls homeostatic functions (such as temperature regulation, fluid balance, appetite) through both neural and hormonal regulation • controls primitive emotions such as anger, rage, and sex drive • controls the pituitary gland
Limbic system	Emotion, memory, and learning	• controls emotional states • links conscious and unconscious portions of the brain • helps with memory storage and retrieval
Cerebral cortex	Perception, skeletal muscle movement, integration center	• divided into four lobes (frontal, parietal, temporal, and occipital) with specialized subfunctions • conscious through processes and planning, awareness, and sensation • intellectual function (intelligence, learning, reading, communication) • abstract thought and reasoning • memory storage and retrieval • initiation and coordination of voluntary movement • complex motor patterns
Corpus callosum	Connection	• connects the left and right cerebral hemispheres

Table 1 Summary of Brain Functions

PNS

Remember, there are two divisions of the PNS: the somatic system and the autonomic nervous system (ANS). All somatic motor neurons innervate skeletal muscle cells and use acetylcholine as their neurotransmitter. They mediate voluntary control of skeletal muscle.

The ANS controls all involuntary processes that regulate and maintain our systems and processes. The ANS innervates cardiac muscle, smooth muscle, and glands:

- Cardiac muscle is found in your heart.
- Smooth muscle is found in the walls of hollow tubes (e.g., blood vessels, respiratory tract, digestive tract) and hollow organs (e.g., bladder).
- There are several types of glands controlled by the ANS; some examples are sweat glands, glands that release hormones, or glands that release digestive secretions.

The sympathetic system primarily uses the neurotransmitter norepinephrine as it drives the fight or flight response. The parasympathetic system primarily uses acetylcholine as it maintains your rest and digest state. Remember that these two branches of the ANS generally act in opposition to one another; at any given moment, one or the other is active.

The following table summarizes the main effects of the ANS.

Organ or System	Parasympathetic: rest and digest	Sympathetic: fight or flight
digestive system: glands	stimulation	inhibition
motility	stimulation (stimulates digestion)	inhibition (inhibits digestion)
sphincters	relaxation	contraction
urinary system: bladder	contraction (stimulates urination)	relaxation (inhibits urination)
urethral sphincter	relaxation (stimulates urination)	contraction (inhibits urination)
bronchial smooth muscle	constriction (closes airways)	relaxation (opens airways)
cardiovascular system		
heart rate and contractility	decreased	increased
blood flow to skeletal muscle	—	increased
skin	—	sweating and ↑ blood flow (flushing)
eye: pupil	constriction	dilation
muscles controlling lens	near vision accommodation	accommodation for far vision
adrenal medulla	—	release of epinephrine
genitals	erection / lubrication	ejaculation / orgasm

Table 2 Effects of the Autonomic Nervous System

Adrenal Medulla

The adrenal gland is named for its location: "Ad-" connotes "above," and "renal" refers to the kidney. There are two adrenal glands, one above each kidney. The adrenal has an inner portion known as the medulla and an outer portion known as the cortex. The cortex is an important endocrine gland, secreting **glucocorticoids** (the main one is cortisol), **mineralocorticoids** (the main one is **aldosterone**), and some sex hormones.

The adrenal medulla, however, is part of the sympathetic nervous system. It is embryologically derived from sympathetic postganglionic neurons and is directly innervated by sympathetic preganglionic neurons. Upon activation of the sympathetic system, the adrenal gland is stimulated to release **epinephrine**, also known as **adrenaline**.[20] Epinephrine is a slightly modified version of norepinephrine, the neurotransmitter released by sympathetic postganglionic neurons. Epinephrine is a hormone because it is released into the bloodstream by a ductless gland, but in many ways it behaves like a neurotransmitter. It elicits its effects very rapidly, and the effects are quite short-lived. Epinephrine released from the adrenal medulla is what causes the sudden flushing and sweating one experiences when severely startled. In general, epinephrine's effects are those listed in Table 2 for the sympathetic system. Stimulation of the heart is an especially important effect.

8.3   SENSATION

Types of Sensory Receptors

Sensory receptors provide an organism with crucial information about its environment. They are designed to detect stimulus from either the interior of the body or the external environment and convey information in the form of action potentials to the central nervous system. Each sensory receptor receives only one kind of information and transmits that information via sensory neurons. There are several types of sensory receptors, based on the stimuli they detect:

1. **Mechanoreceptors** respond to mechanical disturbances. These include stretch receptors, tactile receptors, **proprioceptors** (which provide cues to changes in pressure or tension in muscles), and auditory receptors. For example, Pacinian corpuscles are pressure sensors located deep in the skin. A Pacinian corpuscle is shaped like an onion and is composed of concentric layers of specialized membranes. When they are distorted by firm pressure on the skin, the nerve ending becomes depolarized and the signal travels up the dendrite. Another important mechanoreceptor is the **auditory hair cell**; this is a specialized cell found in the cochlea of the inner ear. It detects vibrations caused by sound waves.
2. **Chemoreceptors** respond to specific chemicals and register taste and smell. For example, the hairlike projections of the **taste receptors**, located in the taste buds, are sensitive to molecules in the mouth. The four basic types of **gustatory receptors** register sourness, sweetness, saltiness, and bitterness. **Olfactory receptors** are also chemoreceptors. They are located in the olfactory epithelium of the nasal cavity and detect airborne chemicals. Olfactory receptors allow us to smell things. Finally, autonomic chemoreceptors in the walls of carotid and aortic arteries respond to changes in arterial pH, P_{CO_2}, and P_{O_2} levels.
3. **Thermoreceptors** are stimulated by changes in temperature.

---

[20] In Greek, "epi" means upon or on top of, and "nephr" refers to the kidney (as in nephron, the microscopic functional unit of the kidney); hence, epinephrine is "the hormone secreted by the gland on top of the kidney." Another name for epinephrine is adrenaline. In Latin, "ad" also means upon, and "renal" likewise refers to the kidney.

4. **Electromagnetic** receptors are stimulated by electromagnetic waves. In humans, the only examples are **photoreceptors**: rods and cones in the eye. **Rods** are more sensitive to dim light and are responsible for night vision. **Cones** require abundant light and are responsible for color and high-acuity vision. Other animals can sense infrared radiation, and some creatures (e.g., certain whales) can even sense the earth's magnetic field.

5. **Nociceptors** are pain receptors. They are stimulated by tissue injury. Nociceptors are the simplest type of sensory receptor, generally consisting of a free nerve ending that detects chemical signs of tissue damage; in that sense, the nociceptor is a simple chemoreceptor.

Using sensory receptors, humans can respond to five types of stimuli: tactile (touch), olfactory (smell), gustatory (taste), auditory (hearing), and visual. This is summarized in the following table.

Modality	Receptor	Receptor type	Organ	Stimulus
Vision	rods and cones	electromagnetic	retina	light
Hearing	auditory hair cells	mechanoreceptor	organ of Corti	vibration
Olfaction	olfactory nerve endings	chemoreceptor	individual neurons	airborne chemicals
Taste	taste cells	chemoreceptor	taste bud	food chemicals
Touch (a few examples)	Pacinian corpuscles free nerve endings temperature receptors	mechanoreceptor nociceptor thermoreceptor	skin	pressure pain temperature
Interoception (two examples)	aortic arch baroreceptors pH receptors	baroreceptor chemoreceptor	aortic arch aortic arch / medulla oblongata	blood pressure pH

Table 3   Summary of Sensation

8.4   ENDOCRINE SYSTEM

Endocrine vs. Exocrine Glands

The endocrine system controls body homeostasis over hours and days by promoting communication among various tissues and organs through the secretion of hormones. Hormones are secreted by endocrine organs, more commonly called **endocrine glands**. Hormones usually act at considerable distances from the sites of their release. They are released from an endocrine gland into the bloodstream, by which they are carried to their target cells. In contrast, **exocrine organs** secrete their products into the external environment (including the lumen of the gut) via ducts. These secretions can be mucus-based or serous (watery secretions that usually contain enzymes). Some examples of exocrine organs are the salivary glands, mammary glands, pancreatic acinar cells, or sweat glands.

Most endocrine hormones act slowly and for a long period of time (i.e., minutes to years) to maintain homeostasis. Their secretion is modulated by changes in bodily needs and conditions. Because they are secreted directly into the bloodstream, endocrine hormones come into contact with nearly every cell of the body. Despite that fact, a given hormone may not have any effect on a given cell type. Most hormones affect a cell only if the cell has a receptor that binds them, either on the surface of the cell or inside the cell. A hormone's target cells, then, are those cells that have receptors for it. A given cell type might be the target of one hormone, many hormones, or no hormones, depending on the number and kind of receptors it expresses.

Types of Hormones

Hormones can be generally grouped into one of three classes: peptide hormones, steroid hormones, or amino acid derivatives. These chemical classes of hormones are made differently, travel in the blood differently, function at the target cell differently, and affect the target cell differently. Below is a summary table of the key features of peptide and steroid hormones. Most amino acid derivatives act like peptide hormones (for example, epinephrine), but some can act like steroid hormones (for example, thyroid hormone).

	Peptide Hormones	**Steroid Hormones**
Chemical Class	Hydrophilic	Hydrophobic
Synthesis	Made in RER, Golgi apparatus	Made from cholesterol in SER
Storage	Stored in vesicles	Secreted right away; no storage
Blood travel	Dissolve in the plasma (because they are hydrophilic)	Travel in the blood bound to proteins (because they are hydrophobic)
Receptor binding	Bind to receptors on surface of the target cell; because they are hydrophilic, they cannot diffuse across the plasma membrane	Diffuse across the plasma membrane and bind to receptors in the cytoplasm of the target cell
Effect on target	Induce second messenger cascades that result in modifying the existing enzymes and proteins	Go to nucleus and alter transcription; change amount and types of proteins in the target cell
Length of effect	Rapid but short-lived	Slow but long-lasting

Table 4   Key Features of Peptides vs. Steroid Hormones

Organization and Regulation of the Endocrine System

The endocrine system has many different roles. Hormones are essential for gamete synthesis, ovulation, pregnancy, growth, sexual development, and overall level of metabolic activity. Despite this diversity of function, endocrine activity is harmoniously orchestrated. Regulation of the endocrine system is generally automatic and relies on feedback regulation.

An example of feedback regulation is the interaction between the hormone **calcitonin** and serum $[Ca^{2+}]$. The function of calcitonin is to prevent serum $[Ca^{2+}]$ from peaking above normal levels, and the amount of calcitonin secreted is directly proportional to increases in serum $[Ca^{2+}]$ above normal. When serum $[Ca^{2+}]$

becomes elevated, calcitonin is secreted. Then when serum $[Ca^{2+}]$ levels fall, calcitonin secretion stops. The falling serum $[Ca^{2+}]$ level (*that which is regulated*) feeds back to the cells which secrete calcitonin (*regulators*). The serum $[Ca^{2+}]$ level is a physiological endpoint which must be maintained at constant levels. This demonstrates the role of the endocrine system in maintaining homeostasis, or physiological consistency.

An advantage of the endocrine system and its feedback regulation is that very complex arrays of variables can be controlled automatically. It's as if the variables controlled themselves. However, some integration (a central control mechanism) is necessary. Superimposed upon the hormonal regulation of physiological endpoints is another layer of regulation: hormones that regulate hormones. Such meta-regulators are known as **tropic hormones**.

For example, **adrenocorticotropic hormone** (**ACTH**) is secreted by the anterior pituitary. The role of ACTH is to stimulate increased activity of the portion of the adrenal gland called the **adrenal cortex**, which is responsible for secreting cortisol (among other steroid hormones). ACTH is a tropic hormone because it does not directly affect physiological endpoints, but merely regulates another regulator (cortisol). Cortisol regulates physiological endpoints, including cellular responses to stress and serum [glucose]. Feedback regulation applies to tropic hormones as well as to direct regulators of physiological endpoints; the level of ACTH is influenced by the level of cortisol. When cortisol is needed, ACTH is secreted, and when the serum [cortisol] increases sufficiently, ACTH secretion slows.

You may have noticed that in both of our examples, the effect of feedback was inhibitory: the result of hormone secretion inhibits further secretion. Inhibitory feedback is called **negative feedback** or **feedback inhibition**. Most feedback in the endocrine system (and if you remember, most biochemical feedback) is negative. There are few exceptions (examples of **positive feedback**), which will be reviewed in Chapter 11.

There is a final layer of control. Many functions of the endocrine system depend on instructions from the brain. The portion of the brain which controls much of the endocrine system is the **hypothalamus**, located at the center of the brain. The hypothalamus controls the endocrine system by releasing tropic hormones that regulate other tropic hormones, called **releasing and inhibiting factors** or **releasing and inhibiting hormones**.

For example (Figure 10), the hypothalamus secretes corticotropin releasing hormone (CRH, also known as CRF, where "F" stands for factor). The role of CRH is to cause increased secretion of ACTH. Just as ACTH secretion is regulated by feedback inhibition from cortisol, CRH secretion, too, is inhibited by cortisol. You begin to see that regulatory pathways in the endocrine system can get pretty complex.

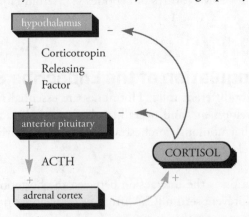

Figure 10 Feedback Regulation of Cortisol Secretion

Understanding that the hypothalamus controls the anterior pituitary and that the anterior pituitary controls most of the endocrine system is important. Damage to the connection between the hypothalamus and the pituitary is fatal, unless daily hormone replacement therapy is given. This endocrine control center is given a special name: **hypothalamic-pituitary control axis** (Figure 11). The hypothalamus exerts its control of the pituitary by secreting its hormones into the bloodstream, just like any other endocrine gland; what's unique is that a special miniature circulatory system is provided for efficient transport of **hypothalamic releasing and inhibiting factors** to the anterior pituitary. This blood supply is known as the **hypothalamic-pituitary portal system**.[21]

One more bit of background information is necessary before we can delve into specific hormones. The pituitary gland has two halves: front (anterior) and back (posterior); see Figure 11. The **anterior pituitary** is also called the **adenohypophysis** and the **posterior pituitary** is also known as the **neurohypophysis**. It is important to understand the difference. The anterior pituitary is a normal endocrine gland, and it is controlled by hypothalamic releasing and inhibiting factors (essentially tropic hormones). The posterior pituitary is composed of axons which descend from the hypothalamus. These hypothalamic neurons that send axons down to the posterior pituitary are an example of **neuroendocrine cells**, neurons which secrete hormones into the bloodstream.

All hormones released from the hypothalamus and pituitary glands are peptides. The anterior pituitary synthesizes and secretes six hormones you need to know about for the DAT. You can remember these using the mnemonic FLAT PiG.[22]]

The two hormones of the posterior pituitary are ADH (antidiuretic hormone or vasopressin), which causes the kidney to retain water during times of thirst, and **oxytocin**, which causes milk letdown for nursing as well as uterine contractions during labor. [Are these hormones made by axon termini in the posterior pituitary or by somas in the hypothalamus?[23]]

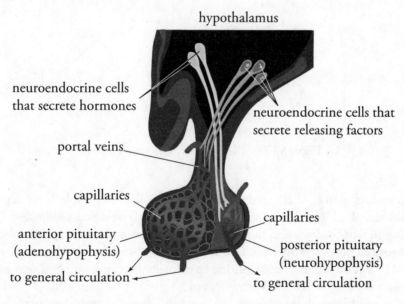

Figure 11   The Hypothalamic-Pituitary Control Axis

---

[21] This can also be called the hypothalamic-hypophysial portal system; hypophysis is another name for the pituitary gland.

[22] This stands for FSH, LH, ACTH, TSH, prolactin, ignore (no hormone here, we just needed a vowel!), GH.

[23] All hypothalamic and pituitary hormones are peptides, and there is no protein synthesis at axon termini. Hence, ADH and oxytocin must be made in nerve cell bodies in the hypothalamus and transported down the axons to the posterior pituitary.

Principal Endocrine Organs

There are eight major endocrine glands in humans: pancreas, adrenal glands, thyroid gland, parathyroid glands, hypothalamus, pituitary, ovaries, and testes. This is not an exhaustive list; there are other organs (such as the thymus, heart, and kidney) that can also be classified as endocrine glands, but these will not be focused on here.

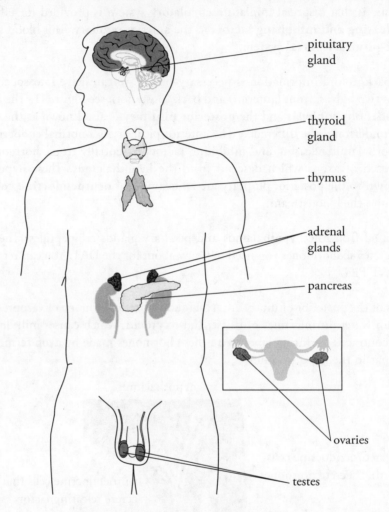

Figure 12 The Major Endocrine Glands

The major hormones and glands of the endocrine system are listed in Table 5 on page 276; make sure you know this table for the DAT! Many of these hormones will be discussed in detail in later chapters. **Insulin** and **glucagon** will be discussed in the chapter on digestion and energy metabolism (Chapter 9). **Testosterone, estrogen, progesterone,** FSH and LH will be presented in the chapter on reproductive biology (Chapter 11). The function of epinephrine has already been presented as part of the sympathetic nervous system response. In general, the hormones are involved in development of the body and in maintenance of constant conditions, homeostasis, in the adult. [Is epinephrine secreted by a duct into the bloodstream?[24]]

---

[24] No. Endocrine hormones are not secreted through ducts.

Thyroid hormone and **cortisol** have broad effects on metabolism and energy usage. Thyroid hormone is produced from the hydrophobic amino acid tyrosine in the thyroid gland, and comes in two forms (with three or four iodine atoms per molecule). Production of thyroid hormone is increased by thyroid stimulating hormone (TSH) from the anterior pituitary, which is regulated by the hypothalamus and the central nervous system in turn. The mechanism of action of thyroid hormone is to bind to a receptor in the cytoplasm of cells that then regulates transcription in the nucleus; thyroid hormone is an amino acid derivative that acts like a steroid because it is derived from a hydrophobic amino acid. The effect of this regulation is to increase the overall metabolic rate and body temperature, and, in children, to stimulate growth. Exposure to cold can increase the production of thyroid hormone. Cortisol is secreted by the adrenal cortex in response to ACTH from the pituitary. In general, the effects of cortisol tend to help the body deal with stress. Cortisol helps to mobilize glycogen and fat stores to provide energy during stress and also increases the consumption of proteins for energy. These effects are essential, since removal of the adrenal cortex can result in the death of animals exposed to even a small stress. Long-term high levels of cortisol tend to have negative effects, however, including suppression of the immune system.

- Would an inhibitor of protein synthesis block the action of thyroid hormone?[25]
- Would the production of ATP by mitochondria be stimulated or repressed by thyroid hormone?[26]
- Would thyroid hormone affect isolated mitochondria directly?[27]

---

[25] Yes. Thyroid hormone binds to a receptor that regulates transcription. mRNA stimulated by thyroid hormone receptor in the nucleus must be processed and translated before the effects of thyroid hormone can become evident.

[26] Thyroid hormone stimulates the basal metabolic rate throughout the body. More ATP will be consumed, so mitochondria are stimulated to make more ATP.

[27] No. Thyroid hormone affects mitochondria *indirectly*, through the regulation of nuclear genes.

8.4

Gland	Hormone [class]	Target/effect
Hypothalamus	releasing and inhibiting factors (peptides)	anterior pituitary/modify activity
Anterior pituitary	growth hormone (GH) (peptide)	↑ bone & muscle growth, ↑ cell turnover rate
	prolactin (peptide)	mammary gland/milk production
tropic	thyroid stimulating hormone (TSH) (peptide)	thyroid/↑ synthesis & release of TH
	adrenocorticotropic hormone (ACTH) (peptide)	↑ growth & secretory activity of adrenal cortex
gonadotropic	luteinizing hormone (LH) (peptide)	ovary/ovulation, testes/testosterone synth.
	follicle stimulating hormone (FSH) (peptide)	ovary/follicle development, testes/ spermatogenesis
Posterior pituitary	antidiuretic hormone (ADH, vasopres-sin) (peptide)	kidney/water retention
	oxytocin (peptide)	breast/milk letdown, uterus/contraction
Thyroid	thyroid hormone (TH, thyroxine) (modified amino acid)	child: necessary for physical & mental development; adult: ↑ metabolic rate & temp.
thyroid C cells	calcitonin (peptide)	bone, kidney; lowers serum [Ca^{2+}]
Parathyroids	parathyroid hormone (PTH) (peptide)	bone, kidney, small intestine/raises serum [Ca^{2+}]
Thymus	thymosin (children only) (peptide)	T cell development during childhood
Adrenal medulla	epinephrine (modified amino acid)	sympathetic stress response (rapid)
Adrenal cortex	cortisol ("glucocorticoid") (steroid)	longer-term stress response; ↑ blood [glucose]; ↑ protein catabolism; ↓ inflammation and immunity
	aldosterone ("mineralocorticoid") (steroid)	kidney/↑ Na^+ reabsorption to ↑ blood pressure
	sex steroids	not normally important
Endocrine pancreas (islets of Langerhans)	insulin (β cells secrete) (peptide) —absent or ineffective in diabetes mellitus	↓ blood [glucose]/↑ glycogen & fat storage
	glucagon (α cells secrete) (peptide)	↑ blood [glucose]/↓ glycogen & fat storage
	somatostatin (SS—δ cells secrete) (peptide)	inhibits many digestive processes
Testes	testosterone (steroid)	male characteristics, spermatogenesis
Ovaries/placenta	estrogen (steroid)	female characteristics, endometrial growth
	progesterone (steroid)	endometrial secretion, pregnancy
Heart	atrial natriuretic factor (ANF) (peptide)	kidney/↑ urination to ↓ blood pressure
Kidney	erythropoietin (peptide)	bone marrow/↑ RBC synthesis

Table 5   Summary of Hormones of the Endocrine System

8.5 CARDIOVASCULAR AND CIRCULATORY SYSTEMS

The cells of a multicellular organism have the same basic requirements as unicellular organisms. Living so close to billions of other cells has many advantages, but there are drawbacks too. Each cell must compete with its neighbors for nutrients and **oxygen** and must also cope with the waste products that are inevitable in so dense a civilization. Other requirements of community living are efficient communication and homeostasis. The circulatory system addresses these problems by accomplishing the following goals:

1. Distributes nutrients from the digestive tract, liver, and adipose (fat) tissue
2. Transports oxygen from the lungs to the entire body and **carbon dioxide** from the tissues to the lungs
3. Transports metabolic waste products from tissues to the excretory system (i.e., the kidneys)
4. Transports hormones from endocrine glands to targets and provides feedback
5. Maintains homeostasis of body temperature
6. Hemostasis (blood clotting). This does not address a need of a multicellular organism *per se*, but rather is necessitated by the presence of the circulatory system itself

Flow of blood through a tissue is known as **perfusion**. Inadequate blood flow, known as **ischemia**, results in tissue damage due to shortages of O_2 and nutrients, and buildup of metabolic wastes. When adequate circulation is present but the supply of oxygen is reduced, a tissue is said to suffer from **hypoxia**. [What's the difference between ischemia and hypoxia?[28]]

Components of the Circulatory System

Functions of the circulatory system involve transport of blood throughout the body and exchange of material between the blood and tissues. The **heart** is a muscular pump that forces blood through a branching series of vessels to the lungs and the rest of the body. Vessels that carry blood away from the heart at high pressure are **arteries**, and vessels that carry blood back toward the heart at low pressure are **veins**. As arteries pass farther from the heart, the pressure of blood decreases, and they branch into increasingly smaller arteries called **arterioles**. The arterioles then pass into the **capillaries**, very small vessels, often just wide enough for a single blood cell to pass. Arterioles have smooth muscle in their walls that can act as a control valve to restrict or increase the flow of blood into the capillaries of tissues. The capillaries have thin walls made of a single layer of cells, and are designed to allow the exchange of material between the blood and tissues. After passing through capillaries, blood collects in small veins called **venules**, and then into the veins leading back to the heart. From the heart, the blood can be pumped out once again through the arteries to the capillaries in the tissues.

- If the arterioles constrict in a tissue, will material diffuse through the wall of the arterioles into the tissue?[29]

---

[28] In hypoxia, wastes are adequately removed, but in ischemia they build up. Ischemia is worse.

[29] No. All exchange of material between the blood and tissues must occur in capillaries. The walls of arterioles are too thick and muscular for exchange to occur.

To achieve both efficient oxygenation of blood in the lungs and transport of oxygenated blood to the tissues, the heart has evolved in humans to have two sides separated by a thick wall to pump blood in two separate circuits.[30] The right side of the heart pumps blood to the lungs, and the left side of the heart pumps blood to the rest of the body. The flow of blood from the heart to the lungs and back to the heart is the **pulmonary circulation**, and the flow of blood from the heart to the rest of the body and back again is the **systemic circulation** (Figure 13).

By having two separate circulations, most blood passes through only one set of capillaries before returning to the heart. There are exceptions to this, however: **portal systems**. In the hepatic portal system, blood passes first through capillaries in the intestine, then collects in veins to travel to the liver, where the vessels branch and the blood passes again through capillaries. Another example is the hypothalamic-hypophysial portal system, in which blood passes through capillaries in the hypothalamus to the portal veins, then to capillaries in the pituitary. The portal systems evolved as direct transport systems, to transport nutrients directly from the intestine to the liver, or hormones from the hypothalamus to the pituitary without passing through the whole body.

- If the hypothalamic-hypophysial portal circulation is severed, how does this affect the function of the pituitary?[31]

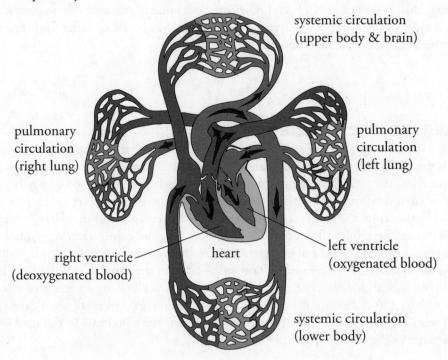

Figure 13 Pulmonary and Systemic Circuits

---

[30] Remember from the previous chapter that fish have two-chambered hearts, amphibians and reptiles have three-chambered hearts, and birds and mammals have four-chambered hearts.

[31] Normally, the pituitary receives hormones directly from the hypothalamus. If the portal system is severed, hormones must take a longer route and will be diluted and degraded before they reach the pituitary. As a result, secretion by the pituitary will not be effectively regulated by the hypothalamus.

The Heart

The heart has two kinds of chambers involved in pumping blood, **atria** and **ventricles** (Figure 14). The atria are reservoirs, or "waiting rooms," where blood can collect from the veins before getting pumped into the ventricles. The muscular ventricles pump blood out of the heart at high pressures into the arteries. The systemic circulation and the pulmonary circulation are separated within the heart, so the right and left sides of the heart each have one atrium and one ventricle. The **right atrium** receives deoxygenated blood from the systemic circulation (from the large veins: the **inferior vena cava** and the **superior vena cava**) and pumps it into the **right ventricle**. From the right ventricle, blood passes through the **pulmonary artery** to the lungs. Oxygenated blood from the lungs returns through the **pulmonary veins** to the **left atrium** and is pumped into the **left ventricle** before being pumped out of the heart in a single large artery, the **aorta**, to the systemic circulation.

- Do all of the arteries of the body carry oxygenated blood?[32]

- Based on the above, you can conclude that blood flows[33]
    A. from the lungs into the right atrium, since the right side of the heart deals with deoxygenated blood.
    B. from the right ventricle to the right atrium, since the atrium is a low-pressure chamber.
    C. from the right atrium to the left ventricle, since the right side of the heart deals with deoxygenated blood and the left side must pump blood to the body.
    D. from the lungs into the left atrium and from there to the left ventricle, since the left side of the heart deals with oxygenated blood.
    E. from the pulmonary arteries to the left side of the heart, since all arteries carry oxygenated blood and the left side of the heart deals with oxygenated blood.

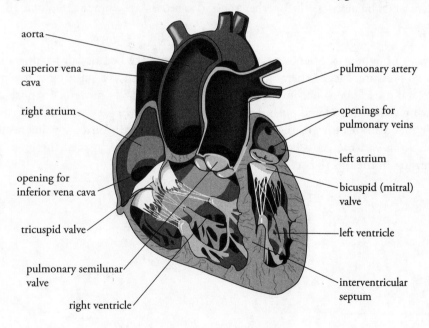

Figure 14   The Heart

---

[32] No. The pulmonary artery carries deoxygenated blood from the heart to the lungs.

[33] Oxygenated blood flows from the lungs to the left atrium (eliminate A), then to the left ventricle (eliminate C, and **D** is correct). The atrium is a low-pressure chamber; however blood flow from the ventricles to the atria is prevented by the atrioventricular valves (eliminate B). Not all arteries carry oxygenated blood; the pulmonary arteries carry deoxygenated blood from the heart to the lungs (eliminate E). All arteries carry blood away from heart chambers.

8.5

The heart is a large muscular organ which requires a blood supply of its own. The very first branches from the aorta are **coronary arteries** which branch to supply blood to the wall of the heart. They are called "coronary" because they encircle the heart forming a crown shape. Deoxygenated blood from the heart collects in **coronary veins**, which merge to form the **coronary sinus**, located beneath a layer of fat on the outer wall of the heart.[34] Blood in the coronary sinus is the only deoxygenated blood which does not end up in the inferior vena cava or superior vena cava. Instead, the coronary sinus drains directly into the right atrium.

8.5

Valves

Valves are necessary to ensure one-way flow through the circulatory system. Valves in the heart are especially important, since the pressure differentials there are so extreme. In particular, ventricular pressure is very high and atrial pressure is lower. Hence, an **atrioventricular valve** (**AV valve**) between each ventricle and its atrium is necessary to prevent backflow.

The AV valve between the left atrium and the left ventricle is the **bicuspid** (or **mitral**) **valve**. [The mitral valve must withstand enormous pressures. What would happen if it ruptured?[35]] The AV valve between the right atrium and the right ventricle is the **tricuspid valve**. [What valve prevents blood flow between the left ventricle and the right ventricle?[36]]

Another set of valves is needed between the large arteries and the ventricles; these are the **pulmonary** and **aortic semilunar valves**. [Since the ventricles are ultra high-pressure chambers, why is it necessary to put valves between them and the arteries?[37]] Together these two valves are known simply as the **semilunar valves**.

There are also valves throughout the venous system. This is necessary because in passing through capillaries, blood loses its pressure. Hence there is not much of a driving force pushing it toward the heart. Contraction of skeletal muscle becomes important, because normal body movements push and squeeze the veins, pressurizing venous blood and pushing it along. Venous valves prevent backflow; as long as the valves hold up, the blood moves toward the heart. When the valves fail, varicose veins result. Pregnant women often suffer from varicose veins because the growing fetus presses against the inferior vena cava, causing venous pressure in the legs to rise.

---

[34] A sinus is an open space; in the case of the cardiovascular system, it is a pool of low-pressure blood.

[35] The left ventricle would pump blood in both directions, out the aorta and back into the left atrium. The result would be elevated pulmonary blood pressure and pulmonary edema.

[36] None! The two ventricles are separated by a thick muscular wall. Remember: the left and right halves are separate.

[37] The ventricles are only pressurized while contracting. When they are not contracting, they must have a very low pressure so that blood can flow into them from the atria.

Cardiac Cycle

The heart contracts, then relaxes, in a cycle which ends only in death. The left and right sides of the heart proceed through the same cycle at the same time. The cardiac cycle is divided into two periods, **diastole** and **systole**.[38] During diastole, the ventricles are relaxed, and blood is able to flow into them from the atria. In fact, the atria contract during diastole to propel blood into the ventricles more rapidly. [How strong is atrial compared to ventricular contraction?[39]] At the end of diastole, the ventricles contract, initiating systole. The ensuing buildup of pressure causes the AV valves to slam shut. Over the next few milliseconds, the pressure in the ventricles increases rapidly, until the semilunar valves fly open and blood rushes into the aorta and pulmonary artery. Systole is the period of time during which the ventricles are contracting, beginning at the "lub" sound and ending at the "dup." At the end of systole, the ventricles are nearly empty[40] and stop contracting. As a result, the pressure inside falls rapidly, and blood begins to flow backward, from the pulmonary artery into the right ventricle, and from the aorta into the left ventricle. But very little backflow actually occurs, because the semilunar valves slam shut when the pressure in the ventricles becomes lower than the pressure in the great arteries. At this point, the heart has completed a full cardiac cycle and is back in diastole.

- Which one of the following is true during systole?[41]
  A. The bicuspid valve is open.
  B. The tricuspid valve is open.
  C. Blood does not flow through the aortic valve.
  D. Both semilunar valves are closed.
  E. Pressure in the atria is low, and thus the atria fill with blood from the vena cava and pulmonary veins.

Heart Sounds, Heart Rate, and Cardiac Output

The "lub-dup" of the heartbeat is produced by valves slamming shut. The "lub" results from the closure of the AV valves at the beginning of systole, and the "dup" is the sound of the semilunar valves closing at the end of systole. [Based on this, which is longer: systole or diastole?[42]]

The **heart rate** (HR) or **pulse** is the number of times the "lub-dup" cardiac cycle is repeated per minute. The normal pulse rate is about one beat per second, ranging from 45 beats per minute (b.p.m.) in athletes to 80 or more beats per minute in the elderly and in children. The explanation for this variation is that a stronger heart pumps more blood each time it contracts, and thus may beat fewer times per minute and

---

[38] Pronounced dy-AS-toe-lee and SIS-toe-lee

[39] Much weaker. The atria really only contract to ensure that most of the blood they contain passes into the ventricles. In contrast, the ventricles must propel blood through arteries, capillary beds, and veins. Hence, the muscular walls of the atria are much thinner than those of the ventricles.

[40] Actually, only about 2/3 of the blood is normally ejected from the ventricle; this is called ejection fraction.

[41] During systole the ventricles are contracting. The bicuspid valve separates the left atrium from the left ventricle, and the tricuspid valve separates the right atrium from the right ventricle; both valves must be closed to prevent backflow into the atria (eliminate A and B). The high pressures generated during systole force blood out of the ventricles through the aortic and pulmonary semilunar valves (eliminate C and D). While the ventricles are contracting, the atria are resting, and blood can flow into them from the vena cava and pulmonary veins. This flow would be prevented if there were any pressure in the atria (**E** is correct). Note that closure of the AV valves ensures that the super-high ventricular pressure does not spread to the atria.

[42] Diastole is longer, since it occupies the space between *lub-dup* and *lub-dup*. Systole is shorter, since it occupies the space between *lub* and *dup*.

still provide adequate circulation. Athletes have strong hearts, while children and the elderly have weaker hearts. The amount of blood pumped with each systole is known as the **stroke volume** (SV). The total amount of blood pumped per minute is termed the **cardiac output** (CO), defined by the equation

$$\text{cardiac output (L/min)} = \text{stroke volume (L/beat)} \times \text{heart rate (beats/min)}$$
$$CO = SV \times HR$$

- An overweight child weighing 110 pounds, a female athlete weighing 110 pounds, and an elderly man weighing 110 pounds all require a cardiac output of about 5 L/min. But the child and the old man have a stroke volume of 1/16 L, while the athlete's stroke volume is 1/9 L. How can the child and the old man supply enough blood to their bodies?[43]

- Which is larger: the cardiac output of the right ventricle or of the left ventricle?[44]

Rhythmic Excitation of the Heart

Interestingly, the heart is *not* stimulated to contract by neuronal or hormonal influences, although these can change the rate and strength of contraction (the **contractility** of the heart). Instead, initiation of each action potential that starts each cardiac cycle occurs automatically from within the heart itself, in a special region of the right atrium called the **sinoatrial (SA) node**. Under normal circumstances, the cells of the SA node act as the **pacemaker of the heart**. SA node cells transmit their action potential to cardiac muscle cells (or **myocytes**) of the atrium, and to the rest of the conduction cells in the heart. We will discuss each of these routes.

The signal from the SA node causes both atria to contract simultaneously and fill the ventricles with blood. An action potential (and thus contraction) spreads throughout the cardiac muscle because cardiac muscle is a **functional syncytium.** A **syncytium** is a tissue in which the cytoplasm of different cells can communicate via gap junctions. In cardiac muscle, gap junctions are found in intercalated disks, the connections between cardiac muscle cells. Depolarization of a cardiac muscle cell can be communicated directly through the cytoplasm to neighboring cardiac muscle cells through these gap junctions. As a result, once an action potential starts, it spreads in a wave of depolarization throughout the cardiac muscle tissue in the atria or the ventricles. The atria and the ventricles are separate syncytia.

The action potential also spreads down the special conduction pathway, which transmits action potentials very rapidly without contracting. The pathway connects the SA node to the **atrioventricular (AV) node.** Since this pathway connects two nodes, it is referred to as the **internodal tract**. Note that while the impulse travels to the AV node almost instantaneously, it spreads through the atria more slowly, because contracting heart muscle cells pass the impulse more slowly than specialized conduction fibers. At the AV node, the impulse is delayed slightly; it then passes from the node to the ventricles via the conduction pathway again. This part of the conduction pathway is known as the **AV bundle (bundle of His)**. The AV bundle divides into the **right** and **left bundle branches**, and then into the **Purkinje fibers**, which allow the impulse to spread rapidly and evenly over both ventricles. As the ventricles contract, blood is pushed up and out of the heart.

---

[43] The athlete's heart can provide the necessary cardiac output by pumping at a leisurely rate of 45 beats per minute. But the hearts of the child and old man will have to work hard to pump enough blood; their pulses will be 80 beats per minute.

[44] Neither, they are equal. The same amount of blood must pass through both sides of the heart or blood would back up in either the pulmonary or systemic circulatory system.

8.5

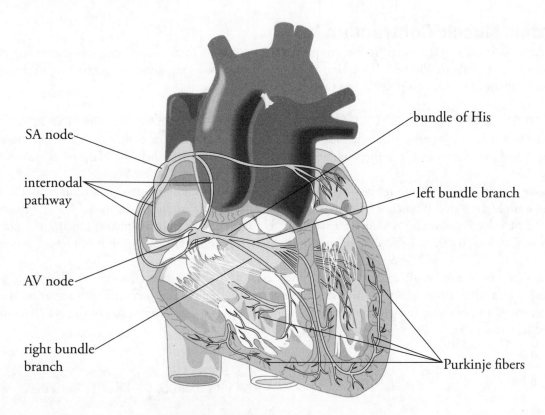

SA node

internodal
pathway

AV node

right bundle
branch

bundle of His

left bundle branch

Purkinje fibers

Figure 15   Cardiac Conduction System

Regulation of the Heart by the Autonomic Nervous System

The autonomic nervous system regulates the rate of contraction. The intrinsic firing rate of the SA node is about 120 beats per minute, but the normal heart rate is only about 60–80 beats per minute because the parasympathetic nervous system continually inhibits depolarization of the SA node. In particular, the **vagus nerve** causes the release of ACh onto the SA node. ACh inhibits depolarization by binding to receptors on cells of the SA node. This constant level of inhibition provided by the vagus nerve is known as **vagal tone**.

The sympathetic system can also influence the heart. It kicks in when increased cardiac output is needed during a "fight or flight" response. First, sympathetic postganglionic neurons directly innervate the heart, releasing norepinephrine. Second, epinephrine secreted by the adrenal medulla binds to receptors on cardiac muscle cells. The effect of sympathetic activation is stimulatory: heart rate increases, and so does the force of contraction.

Cardiac Muscle Contraction

Cardiac muscle cells of the heart have a unique action potential. These muscle cells have a resting membrane potential of about –90 mV. The action potentials here have a long duration, up to 300 milliseconds normally. Phases of an action potential in these cells are:

Phase 0 (depolarization) is caused by the transient increase in Na^+ conductance (just like in neurons). Action potentials propagating through the intercalated discs stimulate myocytes to reach threshold for voltage-gated Na^+ channels. Once threshold is reached, the Na^+ channels open and Na^+ rushes into the cell.

In **Phase 1** (initial repolarization) Na^+ channels inactivate and K^+ channels open. This leads to an efflux of K^+ and a slight drop in cell potential. Furthermore, increased potential due to the initial Na^+ influx causes opening of voltage-gated Ca^{2+} channels; this leads to **Phase 2**, the **plateau** phase. During the plateau, influx of Ca^{2+} ions balance the K^+ efflux from Phase 1, leading to a transient equilibrium in cell potential.

Phase 3 (repolarization) occurs when Ca^{2+} channels close and K^+ channels continue to allow K^+ to leave the cell (again, this is just like in neurons). **Phase 4** (resting membrane potential) is the period during which inward and outward current are equal. Remember, this is dictated by action of the Na^+/K^+ ATPase and K^+ leak channels.

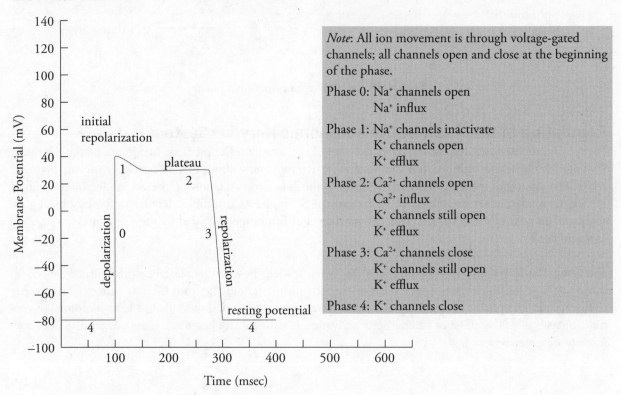

Figure 16   Phases of the Membrane Potential in a Cardiac Muscle Cell

8.6 BLOOD AND HEMODYNAMICS

Blood Pressure

When physicians measure blood pressure, they measure **systemic arterial pressure**. This is the force per unit area exerted by blood upon the walls of arteries. You may recall that a typical blood pressure reading looks like this: 120/80, pronounced "120 over 80." What do the two numbers mean? 120 mm Hg is the **systolic pressure**, and 80 mm Hg is the **diastolic pressure**. In other words, 120 mm Hg is the highest pressure that ever occurs in the circulatory system of this particular patient during the time the blood pressure is being measured. This level is attained as the ventricles contract (that is, during systole). 80 mm Hg is as low as the pressure gets between heartbeats (that is, during diastole) during the measurement.

Blood pressure denotes *arterial* pressure; throughout the cardiac cycle, pressure in the vena cava is about *zero* mm Hg! The highest pressures in the circulatory system are in the left ventricle, aorta, and other large arteries. But every large artery branches, giving rise to many arterioles, and every arteriole gives rise to many capillaries. The result of all this branching is that the pressure generated by the heart is dissipated (Figure 17). By the time blood reaches the vena cava, it depends on valves to prevent backflow because the driving pressure is negligible.

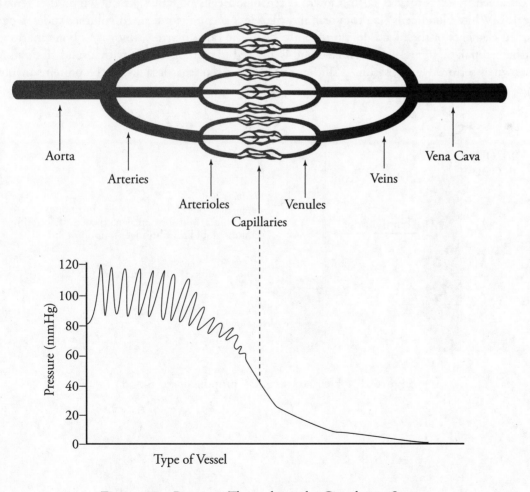

Figure 17 Pressures Throughout the Circulatory System

Components of Blood

Blood has a liquid portion called **plasma**, and a portion which is composed of cells. The cellular elements of blood are known as **formed elements**. Plasma accounts for 55 percent of the blood volume and consists of the following items dissolved in water:

- **Electrolytes**, such as Na^+, K^+, Cl^-, Ca^{2+}, and Mg^{2+} ions
- Buffers, such as bicarbonate (HCO_3^-), to maintain a constant pH of 7.4
- Sugars, mainly glucose
- **Blood proteins**, most of which are made by the liver
- **Lipoproteins**, which transport lipids in the bloodstream
- CO_2 and O_2
- Metabolic waste products, such as urea and bilirubin

Some examples of blood proteins include:

- **albumin**: essential for maintaining osmotic pressure in the capillaries
- **immunoglobulins** (or antibodies): a key part of the immune system
- **fibrinogen**: essential for blood clotting (or hemostasis)

Centrifuging whole blood separates plasma from formed elements, as shown below. The volume of blood occupied by erythrocytes (also known as red blood cells or RBCs) is known as the **hematocrit** (Figure 18). White blood cells (**leukocytes**) and **platelets** account for a small volume (about 1 percent). All formed elements of the blood develop from cells in the bone marrow, known as bone marrow stem cells or hematopoietic stem cells. If whole blood is allowed to clot, one is left with a solid clot plus a clear fluid known as serum. Hence, serum is similar to plasma except that it lacks all the proteins involved in clotting.

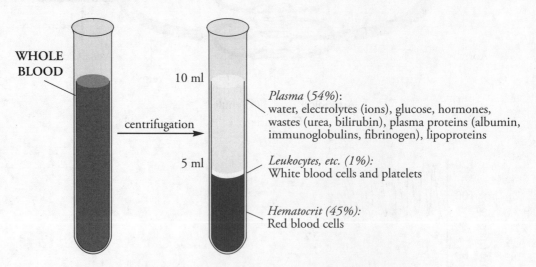

Figure 18   Hematocrit and Components of Blood

Erythrocytes

Erythrocytes are also known as **red blood cells** or RBCs. An erythrocyte is a cell but has no nucleus or other organelles such as mitochondria. However, it does require the energy of ATP for processes such as ion pumping and basic maintenance of cell structure during its 120-day lifetime in the bloodstream. Lacking mitochondria, the RBC relies on glycolysis for ATP synthesis. The purpose of the RBC is to transport O_2 to the tissues from the lungs and CO_2 from the tissues to the lungs. Hence it requires a large surface area for gas exchange. A high surface-to-volume ratio is achieved by the RBC's flat, **biconcave** shape (like a deflated basketball or a throat lozenge; see Figure 19). The RBC is able to carry oxygen because it contains millions of molecules of **hemoglobin**, which we will talk about shortly.

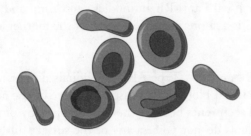

Figure 19   Red Blood Cells (Erythrocytes)

The hormone **erythropoietin** (made in the **kidney**) stimulates RBC production in the bone marrow. Aged RBCs are eaten by phagocytes in the spleen and liver.

Blood Typing

Blood typing is the classification of a person's blood based on the presence or absence of certain surface antigens on their red blood cells. The two most important blood group antigens are the **ABO blood group** and the **Rh blood group**. The ABO blood group consists of glycoproteins that are coded for by three different alleles: I^A, I^B, and i. These alleles and their genotypes and phenotypes were discussed in more detail in Chapter 6.

The other main antigen used in blood typing is the **Rh (rhesus) factor**. Expression of this antigen follows a classically dominant pattern: *RR* and *Rr* genotypes lead to protein expression on the surface of red blood cells (Rh positive), and the *rr* genotype leads to absence of protein expression (Rh negative). Combinations of ABO and Rh alleles determine overall blood type of an individual. Table 6 summarizes these blood types.

	$I^A I^A$ or $I^A i$	$I^B I^B$ or $I^B i$	$I^A I^B$	ii
RR or *Rr*	A+	B+	AB+	O+
rr	A–	B–	AB–	O–

Table 6   Blood Group Genotypes and Phenotypes

Determining blood type is critical when performing blood transfusions. Antibodies to A and B antigens are produced early in infancy and can cause clumping and destruction of red blood cells bearing the incorrect antigen (called a **transfusion reaction**). For example, a person with A+ blood produces anti-B antibodies; if transfused with type B blood, these antibodies will clump and destroy the donated type B cells, possibly leading to the death of the recipient. Note this early production of antibodies without prior exposure to the antigen is unusual; typically the immune system must be exposed to a foreign protein before it produces antibodies against it.

Antibodies to the Rh antigen do not develop unless a person with Rh– blood is exposed to Rh+ blood, an event called "sensitization"; note that this is the typical response of the immune system to a foreign protein (antigen). Subsequent exposure to Rh+ blood can then result in a transfusion reaction. This is particularly dangerous in the case of an Rh– mother carrying an Rh+ baby. Typically, if it is the first baby, there are no complications (unless the mother had been previously sensitized); the mother's blood and the baby's blood do not mix during pregnancy. However, on delivery, some Rh+ cells from the child can mix with the mother's Rh– blood and lead to her sensitization. Future Rh+ babies are then at risk, since the anti-Rh antibodies can cross the placental barrier to clump and/or destroy the Rh+ baby's red blood cells. This is known as hemolytic disease of the newborn, or erythroblastosis fetalis, and can be fatal. Injection of the mother at the time of birth with anti-Rh antibodies can clump and lead to the destruction of any stray Rh+ cells from the baby; this can prevent sensitization of the mother and protect any future unborn Rh+ children.

Two special blood types are AB+ and O–. Type AB+ individuals do not make antibodies to any of the blood group antigens, since their red blood cells possess all three of the antigens. Thus, type AB+ individuals are known as **universal recipients** because they can receive any of the other blood types without complication. Type O– individuals do not possess any of the surface antigens that could trigger a reaction in an individual with a different blood type. Thus, O– individuals are known as **universal donors** because they can donate blood to any of the other blood types, typically without complication.[45]

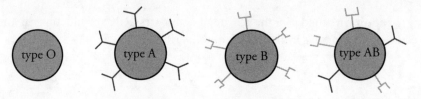

Figure 20   RBC Surface Antigens

Leukocytes

Leukocytes are also known as white blood cells or WBCs. They are all derived from **hematopoietic stem cells** (HSCs), which reside in your bone marrow. Their role is to fight infection and dispose of debris. All WBCs are large, complex cells with all the normal eukaryotic cell structures (nucleus, mitochondria, etc.). Some white blood cells (such as macrophages and **neutrophils**) move by amoeboid motility (crawling). This is important because they are able to squeeze out of capillary intercellular junctions (spaces between capillary endothelial cells) and can therefore roam free in the tissues, hunting for foreign particles and pathogens. Some WBCs exhibit chemotaxis, which means movement directed by chemical stimuli. The chemical stimuli can be toxins or waste products released by pathogens or can be chemical signals released from other white blood cells.

Basophils, neutrophils, and eosinophils are types of granulocytes. These white blood cells are important in the innate immune system and are characterized by the presence of specific granules in their cytoplasm. These cells are attracted to injury sites via chemotaxis and phagocytize antigens to neutralize them. Phagocytosis is a type of endocytosis in which a cell uses its plasma membrane to engulf a large particle. Once inside the cell, the engulfed material is neutralized, killed, or degraded.

---

[45]   Note that type O– individuals do make anti-A and anti-B antibodies, and these can sometimes cause issues in recipients. It is always best to match blood types between donors and recipients when possible.

Cell	Class	Role
Macrophage	Monocyte	• phagocytose debris, dead cells, microorganisms, pathogens • amoeboid motility • exhibit chemotaxis
Neutrophil	Granulocyte	• phagocytose bacteria • amoeboid motility • exhibit chemotaxis
Basophil	Granulocyte	• store and release histamine • destroy parasites such as bacteria, fungi, viruses • function in allergic response and inflammation
Eosinophil	Granulocyte	• destroy parasites such as bacteria, fungi, viruses • function in allergic response and inflammation
CD8$^+$ cyto-toxic T cell	Lymphocyte	• kill cells marked for destruction, e.g., virus-infected cell or tumor cell, tissue graft
CD4$^+$ helper T cell	Lymphocyte	• activate other immune cells • control and coordinate the immune response, e.g., cross talk between humoral and cell-mediated immune responses
Memory T cell	Lymphocyte	• can survive for decades • repeatedly generate an accelerated and robust immune response when an antigen is seen a second time • responsible for the fast secondary immune response and long-term immunity • created in response to vaccination
Plasma cell	Lymphocyte	• mature B cell • produce antibodies
Memory B cell	Lymphocyte	• can survive for decades • repeatedly generate an accelerated and robust antibody-mediated immune response when an antigen is seen a second time • responsible for the fast secondary immune response and long-term immunity • created in response to vaccination
NK cell	Lymphocyte	• kill cells marked for destruction, e.g., virus-infected cell or tumor cell, tissue graft
Dendritic cell	Monocyte or lymphocyte	• antigen-presenting cells • activate other immune cells • cross talk between innate and adaptive immune responses

Table 7　Roles of Leukocytes

8.6

Platelets and Hemostasis

Like red blood cells, platelets have no nuclei and a limited lifespan. They are derived from the fragmentation of large bone marrow cells called **megakaryocytes**, which are derived from the same stem cells that give rise to red blood cells and white blood cells. The function of platelets is to aggregate at the site of damage to a blood vessel wall, forming a **platelet plug**. This immediately helps stop bleeding. **Hemostasis** is a term for the body's mechanism of preventing bleeding.

The other component of the hemostatic response is **fibrin**. This is a threadlike protein which forms a mesh that holds the platelet plug together. When the fibrin mesh dries, it becomes a scab, which seals and protects the wound. The plasma protein **fibrinogen** is converted into fibrin by a protein called **thrombin** when bleeding occurs. A blood clot, or **thrombus**, is a scab circulating in the bloodstream. Calcium as well as many accessory proteins are necessary for the activation of thrombin and fibrinogen. Several of the proteins depend on **vitamin K** for their function. Defects in these proteins result in **hemophilia** ("loving to bleed"), an X-linked recessive group of diseases involving excessive bleeding.

Transport of Gases

Oxygen

Oxygen is too hydrophobic to dissolve in the plasma in significant quantities. Hence, RBCs are used to bind and carry O_2. RBCs are able to carry oxygen because they contain millions of molecules of **hemoglobin** (Hb). This is a complex protein composed of four polypeptide subunits. Each subunit contains one molecule of **heme**, which is a large multi-ring structure that has a single **iron** atom bound at its center. The role of heme with its iron atom is to bind O_2. Since each hemoglobin has four subunits and each subunit has one heme, each molecule of hemoglobin can carry four molecules of oxygen. Hemoglobin is more saturated with oxygen in areas where oxygen partial pressure is high than in areas where O_2 partial pressure is low.

- Does hemoglobin have higher affinity for oxygen in the tissues or in the lungs?[46]

This has monumental significance for the ability of the blood to transport oxygen efficiently. The level of O_2 in active tissues is very low, because they use it in oxidative phosphorylation. Hence, in the tissues, hemoglobin has low affinity for oxygen and tends to release any oxygen that it carries. The level of O_2 in the lungs is of course very high. Hence, when a red blood cell is passing through a capillary in the lungs, the hemoglobin it contains will have higher affinity due to cooperative binding and will tend to bind oxygen very strongly. The result is that a lot of oxygen is picked up by RBCs in the lungs, and most of it is released as they pass through active tissues that need oxygen. This is an amazing example of how structural biochemistry determines physiology (or vice versa).

---

[46] At higher partial pressure of oxygen, more of the hemoglobin protein will have at least one of the subunits occupied with oxygen. Since binding is cooperative, the more oxygen that is bound, the higher the affinity for oxygen. The partial pressure of oxygen is higher in the lungs than in the tissues, so hemoglobin will have higher affinity for oxygen in the lungs.

There is even more complexity to the hemoglobin story. It turns out that certain factors stabilize the low O_2 affinity state of hemoglobin. These factors are:

1. decreased pH
2. increased P_{CO_2} (level of CO_2 in the blood)
3. increased temperature

The fact that these factors stabilize tense hemoglobin and thus reduce its oxygen affinity is known as the **Bohr effect**. This system is truly incredible when you realize that these three factors perfectly characterize the environment within active tissues. [What is the significance of this?[47]]

This information can be depicted graphically, using an **O_2-Hemoglobin Dissociation Curve**, which plots % sat. vs. P_{O_2} (Figure 21).

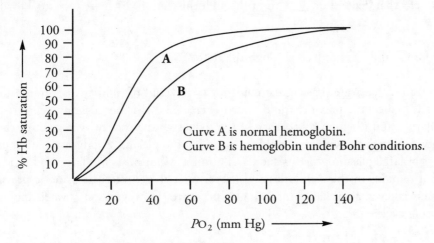

Curve A is normal hemoglobin.
Curve B is hemoglobin under Bohr conditions.

Figure 21 O_2-Hemoglobin Dissociation Curves

Carbon Dioxide

Carbon dioxide is transported in the blood in three ways:

1. 73% of CO_2 transport is accomplished by the conversion of CO_2 to **carbonic acid**, which can dissociate into **bicarbonate** and a **proton** according to this reaction:
    $CO_2 + H_2O \rightleftharpoons H_2CO_3 \rightleftharpoons HCO_3^- + H^+$. These compounds are extremely water-soluble and are thus easily carried in the blood. Conversion of CO_2 into carbonic acid is catalyzed by an RBC enzyme called **carbonic anhydrase**. This reaction is also important as the principal plasma pH buffer.
2. Some CO_2 (~20%) is transported by simply being stuck onto hemoglobin. It does *not* bind to the oxygen-binding sites, but rather to other sites on the protein. Binding of CO_2 to hemoglobin is important in the Bohr effect because it stabilizes tense Hb.
3. CO_2 is somewhat more water-soluble than O_2, so a fair amount (~7%) can be dissolved in the blood and carried from the tissues to the lungs. Virtually no oxygen can be dissolved in the blood.

---

[47] When a tissue is active, its cells metabolize a lot of glucose, and this results in an elevated P_{CO_2}. Soon the cells run low on oxygen and begin to perform lactic acid fermentation. The result is a drop in pH. Finally, whenever there is a lot of metabolic activity, the temperature increases. So, due to the Bohr effect, hemoglobin is most ready to release its load of oxygen in regions of the body where oxygen is most needed!

Exchange of Substances Across the Capillary Wall

Capillaries are the site of exchange between the blood and tissues. To facilitate exchange, capillaries have walls of only a single layer of flattened endothelial cells, and there are spaces (**intercellular clefts**) between the cells.

Three types of substances must be able to pass through the clefts:

1. Nutrients such as amino acids, glucose, and fatty acids pass through capillary clefts, usually from the bloodstream into the tissues.
2. Metabolic wastes go in the opposite direction, from the tissues that produce them, across a cleft, and into the blood.
3. White blood cells must be able to pass out of capillaries in order to patrol the tissues for invading microorganisms. Two types of WBCs can squeeze through the clefts: ____ and ____. These are large cells that depend on ____ to fit through the clefts, which are too small to allow RBCs to pass.[48]

- Is it necessary for O_2 and CO_2 to pass through the clefts?[49]

It is also important to realize that water has a great tendency to flow out of capillaries, through the clefts. There are two reasons: (1) hydrostatic pressure (fluid pressure) created by the heart simply tends to squeeze water out of the capillaries, and (2) high osmolarity of the tissues tends to draw water out of the bloodstream. The circulatory system deals with this problem by giving the plasma a high osmolarity, provided by high concentrations of large plasma proteins such as albumin. Albumin is too large and rigid to pass through the clefts, so it remains in the capillaries and keeps water there, too. The osmotic pressure provided by plasma proteins is given a special name: **oncotic pressure**. However, some water does leak out, resulting in an interesting cycle.

1. At the beginning of the capillary, hydrostatic pressure is high. The result is that water squeezes out into the tissues.
2. As water continues to leave the capillary, the relative concentration of plasma proteins increases.
3. At the end of the capillary hydrostatic pressure is quite low, but since the blood is now very concentrated, oncotic pressure is very high. As a result, water flows back into the capillary from the tissues.

Thus, some water is lost into the tissues, but due to the oncotic pressure of the plasma proteins, the net loss is normally low.

- What would occur if capillaries throughout the circulatory system were made more permeable?[50]
- Albumin is made in the liver. Alcoholics with diseased livers make insufficient amounts of albumin, and thus have insufficient plasma oncotic pressure. What result would you predict?[51]

---

[48] Macrophages and neutrophils can squeeze through the clefts, even though they are larger than RBCs, because they are capable of amoeboid motility. RBCs are not capable of independent motility.

[49] No, they can pass straight through any cell by simple diffusion.

[50] A significant volume of fluid would be lost from the plasma into tissues, decreasing the blood volume and cardiac output. Circulatory shock can result.

[51] This would result in water in the tissues, or swelling, a condition called edema. This could affect the limbs, abdomen, and/or lungs.

8.7   LYMPHATIC SYSTEM

The **lymphatic system** (Figure 22) is a one-way flow system which begins with tiny lymphatic capillaries in all the tissues of the body that merge to form larger lymphatic vessels. These merge to form large lymphatic ducts. Lymphatic vessels have valves, and the larger lymphatic ducts have smooth muscles in their walls. As a result, the lymphatic system acts like a suction pump to retrieve water, proteins, and white blood cells from the tissues. The fluid in lymphatic vessels is called **lymph**. Lymph is filtered by numerous **lymph nodes**. Large lymphatic ducts merge to form the **thoracic duct**, which is the largest lymphatic vessel, located in the chest. The thoracic duct empties into a large vein near the neck. Also, lymphatic vessels from the intestines dump dietary fats into the thoracic duct.

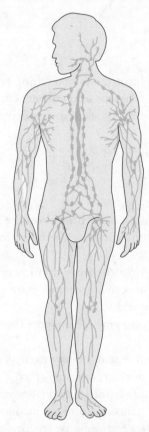

Figure 22   The Lymphatic System: Vessels and Lymph Nodes

Lymph Nodes

Numerous lymph nodes are found along each lymph vessel. They are an important part of the immune system because they contain millions of white blood cells that can initiate an immune response against anything foreign that may have been picked up in the lymph. Infection in one part of the body causes swelling of regional lymph nodes as lymphocytes in the nodes multiply to combat the infection.

Other Lymphatic Organs

The spleen and thymus are also components of the lymphatic system. The spleen, located under the stomach, functions much like a large lymph node except that the spleen acts as a lymphatic filter for blood while lymph nodes filter the lymph fluid. In addition, the spleen destroys old erythrocytes.

Found in the middle of the upper chest, the thymus is a small lymphoid organ that is especially active between birth and puberty. T lymphocytes mature in the thymus, which degenerates during adolescence and adulthood, becoming largely non-functional.

8.8   IMMUNE SYSTEM

The interior of the body provides a warm, protective, nourishing environment where microorganisms can flourish. We could not survive without a versatile and efficient immune system to destroy invaders without destroying the body itself. There are three types of immunity: innate, humoral, and cell-mediated.

Innate Immunity

Innate immunity refers to the general, nonspecific protection the body provides against various invaders. The principal components of innate immunity include the following:

1.   The skin is an excellent barrier against the entry of microorganisms. It prevents many types of pathogens from infecting us and is the most important part of our innate immune system; skin is our barrier to the outside world.
2.   Tears, saliva, and blood contain **lysozyme**, an enzyme that kills some bacteria by destroying their cell walls.
3.   The extreme acidity of the stomach destroys many pathogens which are ingested with food or swallowed after being passed out of the respiratory tract.
4.   **Macrophages** and **neutrophils** indiscriminately phagocytize microorganisms.[52]
5.   **Basophils** and **eosinophils** fight parasites and help mediate the allergic response.
6.   **Natural killer (NK) cells** provide a fast response to virus-infected cells and tumor formation. They quickly recognize and kill stressed cells (usually within 3 days), acting as a first line of defense while the adaptive immune system is preparing for attack.
7.   **Inflammation,** which occurs when cells or tissues have been injured, is triggered by **histamine** release. This results in dilation and increased permeability of blood vessels, which causes increased blood flow to the site of damage.
8.   The **complement system** is a group of about 20 blood proteins that can nonspecifically bind to the surface of foreign cells, leading to their destruction.

The innate immune system is preprogrammed to react to common broad categories of pathogens. It is not specific and has no immunological memory.

---

[52] Do not confuse this portion of innate immunity with cell-mediated immunity. Cells are involved, but this activity is placed in the "innate" category because we are referring to non-specific phagocytosis. As we'll see shortly, humoral and cell-mediated immunity are highly specific. One other subtlety: when a macrophage eats an antigen that has been coated with specific antibodies, we are dealing with humoral immunity; this is different from indiscriminate, nonspecific pathogen phagocytosis discussed here.

Humoral Immunity, Antibodies, and B Cells

Humoral immunity refers to specific protection by proteins in the plasma called **antibodies** (**Ab**) or **immunoglobulins** (**Ig**). Antibodies specifically recognize and bind to microorganisms (or other foreign particles), leading to their destruction and removal from the body. Each antibody molecule is composed of two copies of two different polypeptides, **light chains** and **heavy chains**, joined by disulfide bonds (see Figure 23). In addition, each antibody molecule has two regions, the **constant region** and the **variable (antigen binding) region**. There are several different classes of immunoglobulins: IgG, IgA, IgM, IgD, and IgE. Each class of immunoglobulins has slightly different functions, with most of the antibodies circulating in plasma in the IgG class. The variable regions are responsible for specificity of antibodies in recognizing foreign particles.

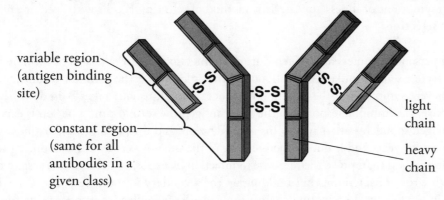

variable region (antigen binding site)

constant region (same for all antibodies in a given class)

light chain

heavy chain

Figure 23   Antibody Structure

Each antibody forms a unique variable region that has a different binding specificity. The molecule that an antibody binds to is known as an **antigen** (**Ag**). Examples of antigens are viral capsid proteins, bacterial surface proteins, and toxins in the bloodstream (such as tetanus toxin). Specificity of antigen binding is determined by the fit of antigen in a small three-dimensional cleft formed by the variable region of the antibody molecule. Antigens are often large molecules which have many different recognition sites for different antibodies. (This is similar to the specific binding of a substrate to the three-dimensional active site of an enzyme.) The small site that an antibody recognizes within a larger molecule is called an **epitope**. Very small molecules often do not elicit the production of antibodies on their own but will when bound to an antigenic large molecule like a protein. The protein in this case is called a **carrier**, and the small molecule that becomes antigenic is known as a **hapten**. When an antibody binds to an antigen, the following can contribute to removal of the antigen from the body:

1. Binding of an antibody may directly inactivate the antigen. For example, binding of an antibody to a viral coat protein may prevent the virus from binding to cells.
2. Binding of an antibody can induce phagocytosis of a particle by macrophages and neutrophils.
3. The presence of antibodies on the surface of a cell can activate the complement system to form holes in the cell membrane and lyse the cell.

Antibodies are produced by a type of lymphocyte called **B cells**. Antibodies produced by an individual B cell can recognize only one specific antigen, but B cells in general produce antibodies that recognize an immense array of antigens. How do B cells produce such a broad array of antibodies? Does the genome encode a gene for every possible antibody molecule, a million genes for a million different potential antibodies? No. Immature B cells are derived from precursor stem cells in the bone marrow. The genes that encode antibody proteins are assembled by recombination from many small segments during B cell

8.8

development. Thus, there are many different B cell clones, each with a different variable region. Immature B cells express **B cell receptors** (BCRs) on their surface. A BCR is a transmembrane protein on the surface of a B cell and is composed of a membrane-bound immunoglobulin molecule and a signal transduction subpart. When an antigen binds to the antibody on the surface of a specific immature B cell, that cell is stimulated to proliferate and differentiate into two kinds of cells: **plasma cells** and **memory cells**. Plasma cells actively produce and secrete antibody protein into the plasma. Memory cells are produced from the same clone and have the same variable regions, but do not secrete antibodies; they are like pre-activated, dormant B cells. Memory cells remain dormant, sometimes for years, waiting for the same antigen to reappear. If it does, the memory cells *then* become activated, and start producing antibodies very quickly, so quickly that no symptoms of illness appear. This method of selecting B cells with specific antigen binding is called **clonal selection**.

The first time a person encounters an antigen during an infection, it can take a week or more for B cells to proliferate and secrete significant levels of antibodies. This is known as the **primary immune response** and is too slow to prevent symptoms of the infection from occurring. It usually takes 7–14 days. The **secondary immune response**, the immune response to the same antigen the second time a person is exposed is much swifter and stronger, so much so that symptoms never develop, and the person is said to "be immune." This immunity can last for years and is due to the presence of the memory cells produced during the first infection. **Vaccination** is used to improve the response to infection by exposing the immune system to an antigen associated with a virus or bacterium, thus building up the secondary immune response if the live pathogen is encountered in the future. [Vaccination against some viruses is ineffective in preventing future infection, while it is highly effective against other viruses. Does the failure of vaccination to protect against some viruses indicate a failure in the ability to produce memory cells?[53]]

Cell-Mediated Immunity and T Cells

There are two main types of **T cells: Helper T cells** can also be called T helpers or **CD4⁺ cells. Killer T cells** are also known as T killers, **cytotoxic T cells**, or **CD8⁺ cells**.[54] Helper T cells activate B cells, killer T cells, and other cells of the immune system. Hence, helper T cells are the central controller of the whole immune response. These cells communicate with other cells by releasing special hormones called **lymphokines** and **interleukins**.[55] Helper T cells are the host of HIV, the virus that causes AIDS.

Killer T cells destroy abnormal host cells such as:
1. virus-infected host cells
2. cancer cells
3. foreign (but still human) cells such as the cells of a skin graft or donor liver tissue from an incompatible donor

---

[53] No. It is probably the result of mutation by the virus. Vaccination against one form of virus and production of memory cells will not protect against a virus if the viral antigen mutates so that it is no longer recognized by the immune system.

[54] "CD" stands for "Cell Differentiation marker."

[55] *Lympho-* is short for lymphocytes, and *-kine* means move or activate. *Inter-* means between, and *-leukin* is for leukocytes or white blood cells.

The "T" in "T cell" stands for **thymus**. T cells are named after this gland because this is where they develop during childhood. Trillions of different T cells are produced in the bone marrow during childhood. Each of these is specific for a particular antigen, just as with B cells. [If a T cell is specific for an antigen, does that mean it releases antibodies that bind to the antigen?[56]] The protein on the T cell surface that can bind antigen is the **T cell receptor** (TCR).

Production of these trillions of different T cells with different T cell receptors is random. As a result, many of them will be specific for normal molecules found in the human body, or self antigens. It is very important to get rid of all T cells specific for self antigen, because such T cells can cause an **autoimmune reaction**, in which the immune system attacks the host. The role of the thymus in T cell development is to destroy all self-specific T cells. The result of this is that billions of T cells survive, but billions of others do not. The ones that survive go on to proliferate if stimulated by antigen in the proper context, each producing a group of identical T cells, all specific for a particular antigen. Such a group is known as a **T cell clone.** Clonal selection in response to antigen recognition is similar in B and T cells.

The function of T cells is exceedingly complex. As a brief introduction, the way a T cell recognizes a bad cell is by "examining" (binding to) proteins on its surface. One important group of cell-surface proteins is known as the **major histocompatibility complex** (**MHC**). Our cells are all programmed to have MHC proteins on their surfaces so the immune system can keep an eye on what is going on inside every cell. There are two kinds of MHCs, known as MHC class I and MHC class II, or simply **MHC I** and **MHC II**. MHC I proteins are found on the surface of every nucleated cell in the body. Their role is to randomly pick up peptides from the inside of the cell and display them on the cell surface. This allows T cells to monitor cellular contents. For example, if a cell is infected with a virus, one of its class I MHC complexes will display a piece of a virus-specific protein. When a T killer cell detects the viral protein (by binding to it) displayed on the cell's MHC I, it becomes activated and will proliferate.

The role of MHC II is more complex. Only certain special cells have MHC II. These cells are known as **antigen-presenting cells** (**APCs**). The antigen-presenting cells include macrophages and B cells. Their role is to phagocytize particles or cells, chop them up, and display fragments using the MHC II display system, which T helpers then recognize and bind to. After a T helper is activated by antigen displayed in MHC II, it will activate B cells (and stimulate proliferation of T killer cells) specific for that antigen. Activated B cells mature into plasma cells and secrete antibodies specific for the antigen. The complexity of this process helps explain why the primary immune response takes a week or more.

- Can a T helper cell become activated after encountering a foreign particle floating in the blood? If so, how? If not, why not, and what else is required?[57]

---

[56] No, only B cells make antibodies. If a T helper is specific for an antigen, it will activate B cells or T killers to destroy it.

[57] No, T helpers are only activated by antigen presented on MHC II. For a foreign particle to activate a helper T cell, the particle must first be displayed by an antigen-presenting cell (macrophage or B cell). The antigen-presenting cell must phagocytize the particle, hydrolyze it into fragments in a lysosome, and allow it to bind to an MHC II which will be displayed on the cell surface.

Other Tissues Involved in the Immune Response

There are several additional tissues and organs that contribute to our immunity:

- **Bone marrow** is where all blood cells are synthesized from a common progenitor. The cell that gives rise to all other blood cells is the bone marrow stem cell (also called the hematopoietic stem cell).
- The **spleen** filters blood and is a site of immune cell interactions, just like **lymph nodes.** The spleen also destroys aged red blood cells (RBCs).
- The thymus is the site of T cell maturation. The thymus shrinks in size in adults since maturation of the immune system and creation of T cells happen mostly in children.
- **Tonsils** are masses of lymphatic tissue in the back of the throat that help "catch" pathogens entering the body through respiration or ingestion. Tonsils are not required for survival and are sometimes removed if they become infected, especially in children.
- The **appendix,** which is found near the beginning of the large intestine, is very similar to the tonsils, both in structure and function. Like tonsils, the appendix is not required for survival and is often removed if it becomes infected.

Want More Practice?
Scan the QR code below to register your book for online chapter summaries, drills, practice tests, and more!

8.8

Chapter 9
Structure and
Function of Systems:
Nutrients and Waste

9.1 RESPIRATORY SYSTEM

Functions of the Respiratory System

Single-cell eukaryotes that require oxygen to perform oxidative phosphorylation can acquire it by simple diffusion of oxygen from the surrounding medium. Larger organisms, such as the vertebrates, evolved a respiratory system to exchange O_2 and CO_2 between the atmosphere and the blood, and a circulatory system to transport those gases between the respiratory system and the rest of the tissues of the body. [What parts of glucose metabolism produce CO_2, and what point in glucose metabolism uses oxygen?[1]]

Additional tasks performed by the respiratory system include the following:

1. pH regulation: In the blood, CO_2 is converted to carbonic acid by the RBC enzyme carbonic anhydrase. When CO_2 is exhaled by the lungs, the amount of carbonic acid in the blood is decreased, and as a result the pH of the blood increases (becomes more alkaline). Hence, minute-to-minute variations in respiration affect blood pH. **Hyperventilation** (too much breathing) causes alkalinization of the blood, known as **respiratory alkalosis**. **Hypoventilation** (too little breathing) causes acidification of the blood, or **respiratory acidosis**. [Which organ regulates pH over a period of hours to days?[2]]
2. Thermoregulation: Breathing results in significant heat loss. Dogs depend on panting for dissipation of excess heat because they cannot sweat.
3. Protection from disease and particulate matter: The lungs provide a large moist surface where chemicals and pathogens can do harm. There are two protection mechanisms. First, specialized cells secrete mucus, which traps pathogens and inhaled particles. Other cells have **cilia** that constantly sweep the layer of mucus up so it is swallowed or coughed out; this is called the **mucociliary escalator.** Second, alveolar macrophages patrol alveoli and engulf foreign particles.

Anatomy of the Respiratory System

Simple movement of air into and out of the lungs is called **ventilation,** whereas the actual exchange of gases (between either lungs and blood, or blood and other tissues of the body) is called **respiration.**[3] Inhaled air follows this pathway:

nose → nasal cavity → pharynx → larynx → trachea → bronchi → terminal bronchioles → respiratory bronchioles → alveolar ducts → alveoli

---

[1] Pyruvate dehydrogenase and the Krebs cycle produce CO_2 during oxidative respiration, and oxygen is reduced to water by the last electron carrier in electron transport, cytochrome c oxidase.

[2] Kidneys

[3] Sometimes these terms are used interchangeably. For example, we refer to "respiratory rate" when we really mean "ventilation rate."

Parts of the respiratory system that participate only in ventilation are referred to as the **conduction zone;** this starts at the nose and ends at the respiratory bronchioles. The parts that participate in actual gas exchange are referred to as the **respiratory zone;** this starts at respiratory bronchioles and ends at alveoli.

Conduction Zone

The **nose** is important for warming, humidifying, and filtering inhaled air; nasal hairs and sticky mucus act as filters. The **nasal cavity** is an open space within the nose. The **pharynx** is another word for the throat, a common pathway for air and food. The **larynx** has three functions:

1. It is made entirely of cartilage and thus keeps the airway open.
2. It contains the **epiglottis**, which seals the trachea during swallowing to prevent the entry of food.
3. It contains the **vocal cords**, which are folds of tissue positioned to partially block the flow of air and vibrate, thereby producing sound.

The **trachea** is a passageway which must remain open to permit air flow. Rings of cartilage prevent its collapse. The trachea branches into two **primary bronchi**, each of which supplies one lung. Each bronchus branches repeatedly to supply the entire lung. Collapse of bronchi is prevented by small plates of cartilage. Very small bronchi are called **bronchioles**. They are about 1 mm wide and contain no cartilage. Their walls are made of smooth muscle, which allows their diameters to be regulated to adjust airflow into the system. The smallest (and final) branches of the conduction zone are aptly called the **terminal bronchioles**.

The smooth muscle of the walls of the terminal bronchioles is too thick to allow adequate diffusion of gases; this is why no gas exchange occurs in this region. The conduction zone is strictly for ventilation.

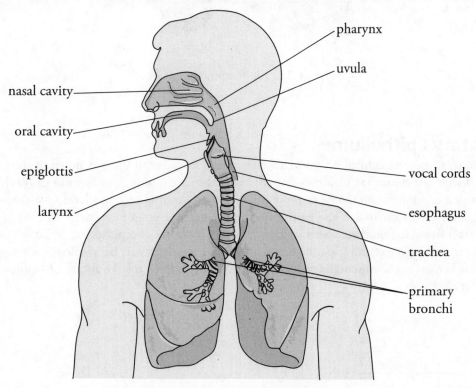

Figure 1   The Conduction Zone

Respiratory Zone

The region of the system where gas exchange occurs is the respiratory zone (Figure 2). The actual structure across which gases diffuse is called the **alveolus** (plural: **alveoli**). Alveoli are tiny sacs with very thin walls; they're so thin that they're transparent. The wall of the alveolus is only one cell thick, except where capillaries pass across its outer surface. The duct leading to the alveoli is called an **alveolar duct**, and its walls are entirely made of alveoli. The alveolar duct branches off a **respiratory bronchiole**. This is a tube made of smooth muscle, just like the terminal bronchioles, but with one important difference: the respiratory bronchiole has a few alveoli scattered in its walls. This allows it to perform gas exchange, so it is part of the respiratory zone.

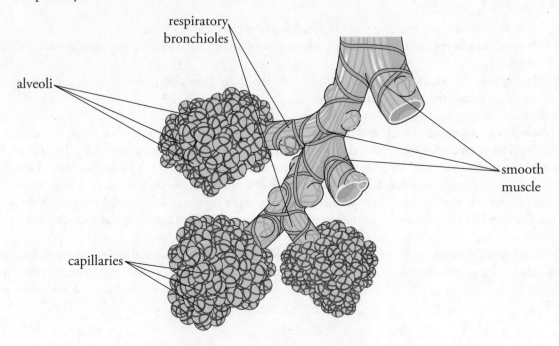

Figure 2   The Respiratory Zone

Respiratory Epithelium

The entire respiratory tract is lined by epithelial cells. From the nose all the way down to the bronchioles, epithelial cells are tall **columnar** (column-shaped) cells. They are too thick to assist in gas exchange; they merely provide a conduit for air. Some of these cells are specialized to secrete a layer of sticky mucus and are called **goblet cells** (just like in the gastrointestinal tract). The columnar epithelial cells of the upper respiratory tract have cilia on their apical surfaces which constantly sweep the layer of mucus toward the pharynx, where mucus containing pathogens and inhaled particles can be swallowed or coughed out. This system is known as the **mucociliary escalator**. [What would be the advantage of swallowing pathogens and particles?[4]]

---

[4]   Gastric acidity destroys many pathogens. Also, particles that would likely harm the delicate alveoli are unlikely to harm the tough lining of the GI tract.

Alveoli, alveolar ducts, and the smallest bronchioles (respiratory bronchioles) are involved in gas exchange. Oxygen and CO_2 must be able to diffuse across the layer of epithelial cells in order to pass freely between the bloodstream and the air in the lungs. Tall columnar cells with cilia would be too large to permit rapid diffusion. Hence, gas-exchanging surfaces are lined with a single layer of thin, delicate squamous epithelial cells.[5] A single layer of squamous epithelial cells is called **simple squamous epithelium**. It would also be unacceptable to have a layer of mucus covering the gas exchange surface, so another method of protection from disease and inhaled particles is necessary. **Alveolar macrophages** fill this role by patrolling the alveoli, engulfing foreign particles.

Surfactant

Imagine a beehive made of tissue paper. If you put it in a steamy bathroom, what would happen? Would all the small air spaces remain filled with air? No, the hive would collapse into a wet ball, because the mutual attraction of water molecules would overcome the flimsy support structure provided by the fine paper fibers. The tendency of water molecules to clump together creates **surface tension**, which is the force that causes wet hydrophilic surfaces (e.g., tissue paper) to stick together in the presence of air. Think of it this way: air is hydrophobic, so hydrophilic substances in the presence of air tend to clump together. Now imagine a beehive made of thin wax paper. If you put it into a steamy room, does it collapse? No, because the wax on the surface of the paper prevents adjacent pieces of paper from being strongly attracted. In other words, the wax destroys surface tension.

Alveoli are as fine and delicate as tissue paper, and they too tend to collapse due to surface tension. This problem is solved by a soapy substance called **surfactant** (*surf*ace *acti*ve substance), which coats the alveoli (Figure 3). Just like the wax in our example above, surfactant reduces surface tension. Surfactant is a complex mixture of phospholipids, proteins, and ions secreted by cells in the alveolar wall. [Is it likely that these are the principal lining cells of the alveolar wall?[6]]

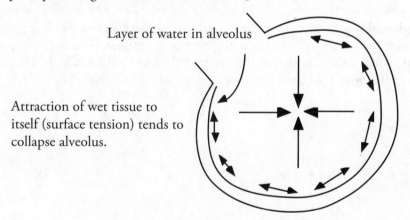

Layer of water in alveolus

Attraction of wet tissue to itself (surface tension) tends to collapse alveolus.

Figure 3   Surface Tension in an Alveolus

---

[5]   Squamous means flat.

[6]   No, the principal cells of the alveolar wall are thin squamous cells designed to allow diffusion of gases. Cells which actively secrete substances (i.e., surfactant) are large, metabolically active cells with many mitochondria. The basic alveolar lining cells (simple squamous epithelium) are called Type 1 alveolar cells. The fat (cuboidal) epithelial cells that secrete surfactant are called Type 2 alveolar cells.

- There is not sufficient surfactant within a fetus's lungs until about the eighth month of gestation, so some premature infants lack the protective effects of surfactant when they are born. Which of the following statements best describes resulting effects upon respiration in babies born prematurely?[7]
    - A. Surface tension would be abnormally low.
    - B. Alveoli would collapse.
    - C. Oxygen would be unable to diffuse through water.
    - D. Respiration is unnecessary, since the infant is dependent on the mother.

Pulmonary Ventilation

Pulmonary ventilation is the circulation of air into and out of the lungs to continually replace the gases in the alveoli with those in the atmosphere. Drawing air into the lungs is termed **inspiration**, and movement of air out of the lungs is termed **expiration**. Inspiration is an active process driven by the contraction of the diaphragm, which enlarges the chest cavity (and the lungs along with the chest cavity), drawing air in. Passive expiration is driven by the elastic recoil of the lungs and does not require active muscle contraction. These processes will be described in more detail in the following pages.

Pleural Space and Lung Elasticity

The lungs are large elastic bags that tend to collapse in upon themselves if removed from the chest cavity. Structures of the chest prevent this collapse and allow the lungs to remain inflated during inspiration and expiration. The lungs are not directly connected to the chest wall, however. Each lung is surrounded by two membranes, or **pleura**: the **parietal pleura**, which lines the inside of the chest cavity, and the **visceral pleura**, which lines the surface of the lungs (Figure 4). Between the two pleura is a very narrow space called the **pleural space**. Pressure in the pleural space (**pleural pressure**) is negative, meaning that the two pleural membranes are drawn tightly together by a vacuum. This negative pressure keeps the outer surface of the lungs drawn up against the inside of the chest wall. Additionally, a thin layer of fluid between the two pleura helps hold them together through surface tension.

---

[7] In the absence of surfactant, surface tension would be high (eliminate A), and alveoli would collapse on every exhalation like tissue-paper beehives (choice **B** is correct). It would take an enormous exertion to reopen the collapsed alveoli to get any air (oxygen) into them; the result is poor oxygen delivery to the alveoli and thus to the blood. For this reason, babies born prematurely are typically kept on ventilators until their surfactant levels are higher and they are stronger in general. Note that oxygen has some ability to diffuse through water, but choice C is wrong mostly due to irrelevance. It's not as though in the absence of surfactant the lungs suddenly fill with water. Respiration is always necessary once a baby is born; this question specifically refers to infants born prematurely (eliminate D).

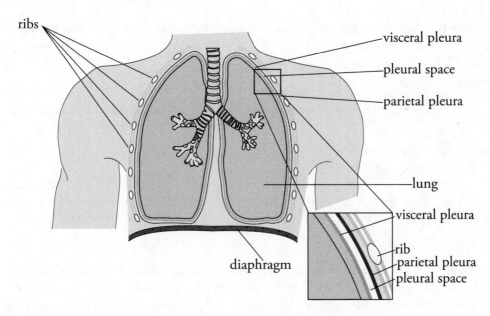

Figure 4 Lungs and Pleura

- If the pleural space is punctured, opening it to the external atmosphere, which one of the following will occur?[8]
    - A. Fluid will leak out of the pleural space.
    - B. Air will leak out of the pleural space.
    - C. Air will leak into the pleural space.
    - D. Since the pressure within the pleural space is equal to atmospheric pressure during expiration, nothing will happen.
    - E. Respiration could occur normally through the puncture site.

Inspiration is caused by muscular expansion of the chest wall, which draws the lungs outward (expands them), and causes air to enter the system. The lungs expand along with the chest due to the negative pressure in the pleural space. The expansion of the chest during inspiration is driven primarily by contraction of the **diaphragm**, a large skeletal muscle that is stretched below the ribs between the abdomen and the chest cavity. When resting, the diaphragm is shaped like a dome, bulging upward into the chest cavity. When it contracts, the diaphragm flattens and draws the chest cavity downward, forcing it and the lungs (which are stuck to the inside wall of the chest cavity) to expand. The external **intercostal muscles** between the ribs also contract during inspiration, pulling the ribs upward and further expanding the chest cavity. Inspiration is an *active* process, requiring contraction of muscles to occur.

Resting expiration, by contrast, is a *passive* process (no muscle contraction required). When the diaphragm and rib muscles relax, elastic recoil of the lungs draws the chest cavity inward, reducing the volume of the lungs and pushing air out of the system into the atmosphere. During exertion (or at other times when a more forcible exhalation is required), contraction of abdominal muscles helps the expiration process by pressing upward on the diaphragm, further shrinking the size of the lungs and forcing more air out. This is called a **forced expiration** and is an active process.

---

[8] The pleural space is always at negative pressure, or the lungs would collapse. If the pleural pressure is negative, and an opening to the atmosphere is made, then air will rush into the pleural space and the lungs will collapse. This prevents normal respiration. The correct answer is **C**. Note that A will probably also occur, but the amount of fluid is so minimal as to be insignificant; C is the better answer.)

The pressure of air in the alveoli and the pleural pressure vary during inspiration and expiration. During inspiration, the following steps occur:

1. The diaphragm contracts and flattens (moves downward).
2. The volume of the chest cavity expands.
3. Pleural pressure decreases, becoming more negative.
4. The lungs expand outward.
5. Pressure in the alveoli becomes negative.
6. Air enters the lungs and the alveoli.

The opposite steps occur during expiration. Typically inspiration and expiration are not consciously controlled although they are mediated by voluntary muscle, which means we *can* control the processes if we want to.

The **tidal volume** (**TV**) is the amount of air that moves into and out of the lungs with normal light breathing and is equal to about 10 percent of the total volume of the lungs (0.5 liters out of 5–6 liters). **Residual volume** (**RV**) is the amount of air that remains in the lungs after the strongest possible expiration. The **vital capacity** (**VC**) is the maximum amount of air that can be forced out of the lungs after first taking the deepest possible breath. The **total lung capacity** (**TLC**) is the vital capacity plus the residual volume (TLC = VC + RV).

- Is the total volume of the lungs exchanged with each breath?[9]

Gas Exchange

Pulmonary Circulation

Deoxygenated blood is carried toward the lungs by the pulmonary artery, which has left and right branches. These large arteries branch many times, eventually giving rise to a huge network of **pulmonary capillaries**, also called **alveolar capillaries**. Each alveolus is surrounded by a few tiny capillaries, which are just wide enough to permit passage of RBCs, and have extremely thin walls to permit diffusion of gases between blood and alveolus. The capillaries drain into venules, which drain into pulmonary veins. The lungs are supplied with lymphatic vessels as well.

The lungs are "designed" to expose a large amount of blood to a large amount of air. Hence the primary property of the lung is its enormous surface area, close to that of a tennis court. The goal is to allow O_2 from the atmosphere to diffuse into pulmonary capillaries, where it is bound by hemoglobin in RBCs. Simultaneously, CO_2 diffuses from the blood to the alveolar gas.

In the lungs, oxygen and carbon dioxide diffuse between the alveolar air and blood in the alveolar capillaries (Figure 5). The driving force for the exchange of gases in the lungs is the difference in partial pressures between the alveolar air and the blood. For diffusion to occur (from the air to the blood), gases must

---

[9] No, some air always remains in the lungs; this is called the functional residual capacity (FRC) during relaxed breathing or RV during deep breathing.

first pass across the alveolar epithelium, then through the interstitial liquid, and finally across the capillary endothelium. These three barriers to diffusion together form the **respiratory membrane**. Note that the pathway is reversed for diffusion from the blood to the air.

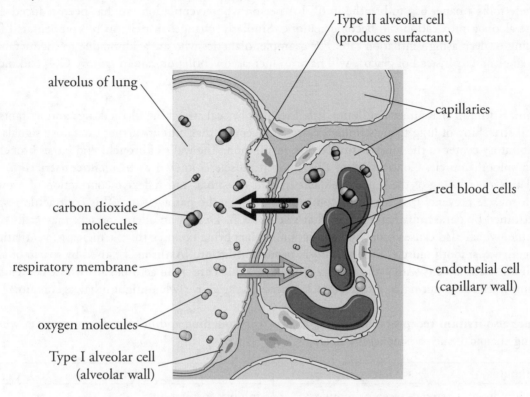

Figure 5   Diffusion of Gases Between an Alveolus and a Capillary

Regulation of Ventilation Rate

Proper regulation of the rate and depth of breathing is essential. Although breathing can be voluntarily controlled for short periods of time, it is normally an involuntary process directed by the **respiratory control center** in the medulla of the brain stem. The stimuli that affect ventilation rate are both mechanical and chemical (see Table 1 on the following page).

The principal chemical stimuli that affect ventilation rate are increased P_{CO_2}, decreased pH, and decreased P_{O_2} (with CO_2 and pH being the primary regulators and O_2 secondary). These variables are monitored by special autonomic sensory receptors. **Peripheral chemoreceptors** are located in the aorta and the carotid arteries and monitor the P_{CO_2}, pH, and P_{O_2} of the blood, while **central chemoreceptors** are found in the medullary respiratory control center, and monitor P_{CO_2} and pH of the cerebrospinal fluid (CSF). pH and P_{CO_2} are connected through the carbonic acid buffer system of the blood.

$$CO_2 + H_2O \rightleftharpoons H_2CO_3 \rightleftharpoons H^+ + HCO_3^-$$

Respiration eliminates CO_2 from the body. Thus, changes in ventilation rate can have rapid effects on pH due to the decrease or increase in P_{CO_2} and the resulting shift to maintain the above equilibrium. For example, a person hyperventilating during an anxiety attack can have an elevated pH. [Why do we give these folks a paper bag to breathe into?[10]] A person whose ventilation rate has been reduced due to extreme alcohol intoxication can become acidic. Similarly, changes in pH can be compensated for by increasing or decreasing ventilation rate. For example, diabetics who are acidic due to the metabolism of proteins and fats instead of glucose will have an increased ventilation rate to remove CO_2 and increase pH.

Mechanical stimuli that affect ventilation rate include physical stretching of the lungs and irritants. Mechanical stretching of lung tissue stimulates stretch receptors that inhibit further excitatory signals from the respiratory center to the muscles involved in inspiration. The walls of bronchi and larger bronchioles contain smooth muscle. Contraction of this smooth muscle is known as **bronchoconstriction**. Irritation of the inner lining of the lung stimulates irritant receptors, and reflexive contraction of bronchial smooth muscle prevents irritants from continuing to enter the passageways. This contractile response is determined by parasympathetic nerves that release ACh. During an allergy attack, mast cells release histamine, which also causes bronchoconstriction. Epinephrine opposes this; it increases ventilation by causing airway smooth muscles to relax; this is **bronchodilation**. [**Asthma** is caused by spasm of airway smooth muscles. Patients with asthma carry "inhalers," which are small aerosol cans whose contents they spray into their lungs during an asthma attack. Based on the above, what might inhalers contain?[11]]

There are also **irritant receptors** in the lung that trigger coughing and/or bronchoconstriction when an irritating chemical (such as smoke) is detected.

Stimulus	Receptor	Effect
stretch of lung	stretch receptor in lung	inhibits inspiration
$\uparrow P_{CO_2}$	peripheral chemoreceptors and medullary respiratory center	increased P_{CO_2} causes $\downarrow$pH via carbonic anhydrase; $\downarrow$pH is what is actually sensed (see below)
$\downarrow$pH	as above	increases respiratory rate
$\downarrow P_{O_2}$	peripheral chemoreceptors	increases respiratory rate
chemical irritation	irritant receptor in lung	coughing and/or bronchoconstriction

Table 1 Factors that Regulate Ventilation Rate

---

[10] Breathing into a paper bag forces them to rebreathe their exhaled CO_2. This pushes the equilibrium of the equation to the right and brings pH back down to normal.

[11] They contain epinephrine, antihistamines (drugs that block histamine receptors on smooth muscle cells), and anticholinergics (drugs that block acetylcholine receptors on smooth muscle cells).

9.2 DIGESTIVE SYSTEM

Food contains molecules that are substrates in **catabolic reactions** (reactions that break down molecules to supply energy) and **anabolic reactions** (synthesis of macromolecules). **Digestion** is the breakdown of polymers (polypeptides, fats, starch) into their building blocks. There are two types of digestion: mechanical and chemical. **Mechanical digestion** begins with the shredding and grinding of food into small pieces by chewing (mastication). It continues with vigorous churning in the stomach. **Chemical digestion** occurs via **enzymatic hydrolysis**; digestive enzymes are produced by several different organs associated with the alimentary canal. Enzymes break down food into absorbable molecules. Food also contains vitamins, which are not substrates, but rather serve a catalytic role as enzyme cofactors or prosthetic groups. Digestion and absorption of foodstuffs is the primary function of the digestive system. A secondary function, which we will touch on only briefly, is protection from disease.

Over the course of this section, we'll see how and where each of the following reactions take place.[12]

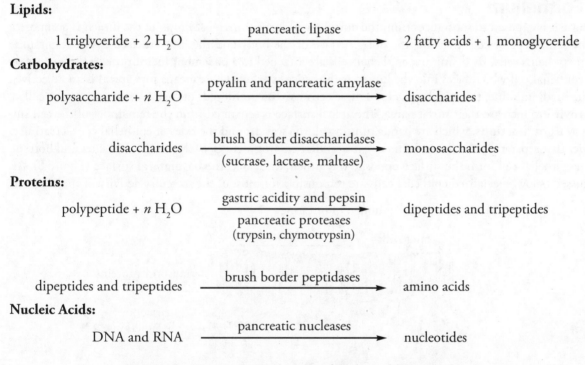

Lipids:

$$1 \text{ triglyceride} + 2 \text{ H}_2\text{O} \xrightarrow{\text{pancreatic lipase}} 2 \text{ fatty acids} + 1 \text{ monoglyceride}$$

Carbohydrates:

$$\text{polysaccharide} + n \text{ H}_2\text{O} \xrightarrow{\text{ptyalin and pancreatic amylase}} \text{disaccharides}$$

$$\text{disaccharides} \xrightarrow[\text{(sucrase, lactase, maltase)}]{\text{brush border disaccharidases}} \text{monosaccharides}$$

Proteins:

$$\text{polypeptide} + n \text{ H}_2\text{O} \xrightarrow[\substack{\text{pancreatic proteases}\\\text{(trypsin, chymotrypsin)}}]{\text{gastric acidity and pepsin}} \text{dipeptides and tripeptides}$$

$$\text{dipeptides and tripeptides} \xrightarrow{\text{brush border peptidases}} \text{amino acids}$$

Nucleic Acids:

$$\text{DNA and RNA} \xrightarrow{\text{pancreatic nucleases}} \text{nucleotides}$$

Figure 6 Enzymatic Hydrolysis of Biological Macromolecules

Digestion is accomplished along the **gastrointestinal (GI) tract**, also known as the **digestive tract**, **alimentary canal**, or simply the **gut**. The GI tract is a long, muscular tube extending from the mouth to the anus. This tube is derived from the cavity produced by **gastrulation** during embryogenesis; the anus is derived from the **blastopore** (discussed in Chapter 11). The inside of the gut is the **GI lumen**. The lumen is continuous with the space outside the body. Food could go from the plate into the lumen and from there into the toilet bowl without ever contacting the bloodstream, the muscles, the bones, etc. The GI lumen is a compartment where the usable components of foodstuffs are extracted, while wastes are left to be excreted as feces. The entire GI tract is composed of specific tissue layers which surround the lumen (Figure 7).

---

[12] We suggest you review this whole section and then come back and go through these reactions again.

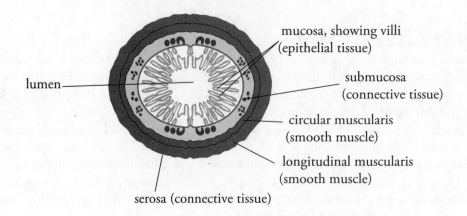

Figure 7 Cross-section and Layers of the GI Tract

GI Epithelium

Because it is exposed to substances from the outside world, the innermost lining of the lumen is composed of the same type of cells that line the outer surface of the body and the inner surface of the respiratory tract: epithelial cells. By definition, epithelial cells are attached to a **basement membrane**.[13] The surface of the epithelial cell which faces into the lumen is the **apical surface** (apex means top; apical is an adjective). In the small intestine, the apical surfaces of these cells have outward folds of their plasma membrane called **microvilli** to increase their surface area. The apical surface is separated from the remainder of the cell surface by **tight junctions**, which are bands running all the way around the sides of epithelial cells, creating a barrier that separates body fluids from the extracellular environment (see Chapter 5). The sides and bottom of an epithelial cell form the surface opposite the lumen, known as the **basolateral** surface (Figure 8). As discussed below, specialized epithelial cells are responsible for most of the secretory activity of the GI tract.

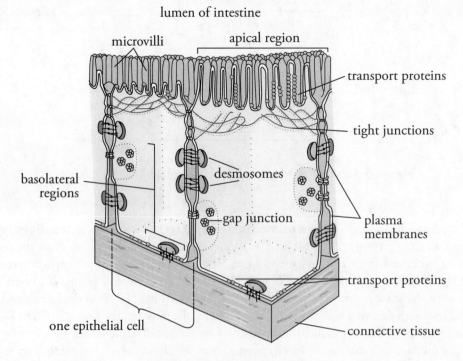

Figure 8 Epithelial Cells

---

[13] *Epi-* means "upon," and *-thelial* refers to the bumpy microscopic appearance of the basement membrane (it means "nippley").

GI Smooth Muscle

The walls of the alimentary canal contain **smooth muscle**.[14] In most regions of the alimentary canal, there are two layers of smooth muscle lining the gut. The **longitudinal layer** runs along the gut lengthwise, while the **circular layer** encircles it. The stomach has a third layer of smooth muscle, the oblique layer, which allows it to churn.

GI motility refers to the rhythmic contraction of GI smooth muscle. It is determined by a complex interplay between five factors:

1. Like cardiac muscle (Chapter 8), GI smooth muscle exhibits *automaticity*. In other words, it contracts periodically without external stimulation, due to spontaneous depolarization.
2. Like cardiac muscle, GI smooth muscle is a **functional syncytium**, meaning that when one cell has an action potential and contracts, the impulse spreads to neighboring cells.
3. The GI tract contains its own massive nervous system, known as the **enteric nervous system**. The enteric nervous system plays a major role in controlling GI motility.
4. GI motility may be increased or decreased by hormonal input.
5. The parasympathetic nervous system stimulates motility and causes sphincters to relax (allowing the passage of food through the gut), while sympathetic stimulation does the opposite.

GI motility serves two purposes: mixing of food and movement of food down the gut. Mixing is accomplished by disordered contractions of GI smooth muscles, which result in churning motions. Movement of food down the GI tract is accomplished by an orderly form of contraction known as **peristalsis** (Figure 9). During peristalsis, contraction of **circular smooth muscles** at point A prevents food located at point B from moving backward. Then **longitudinal muscles** at point B contract, with the result being shortening of the gut so that it is pulled up over the food like a sock. As a result, food moves toward point C. Then circular smooth muscles at point B contract to prevent the food from moving backward, and longitudinal muscles at point C contract, with the result being movement of food past point C, and so on. A ball of food moving through the GI tract is called a **bolus**.

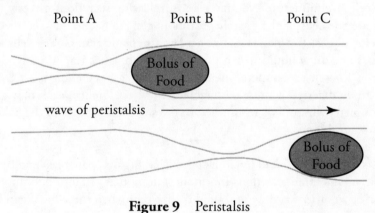

Figure 9 Peristalsis

---

[14] Smooth muscle is so named because of its smooth microscopic appearance. This contrasts with striated muscle, which appears striped under magnification. Skeletal (voluntary) muscle and cardiac (heart) muscle are striated. We'll review the three types of muscle you need to know for the DAT in the next chapter.

GI Secretions

Generally speaking, GI secretion (release of enzymes, acid, bile, etc.) is stimulated by food in the gut and by the parasympathetic nervous system, and is inhibited by sympathetic stimulation. There are two types of secretion: **endocrine** and **exocrine**. [What's the difference?[15]] Exocrine glands are composed of specialized epithelial cells, organized into sacs called **acini** (singular: **acinus**). Acinar cells secrete products that pass into ducts. It is important to keep the contrast between endocrine and exocrine in mind. Figure 10 below shows the microscopic structure of an exocrine gland.

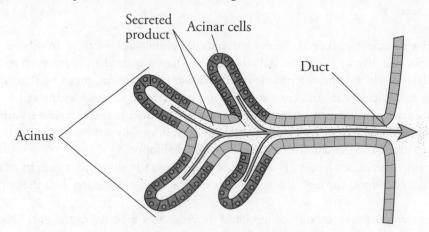

Figure 10   Exocrine Gland Structure

Most exocrine secretion in the GI tract is performed by exocrine glands within special digestive organs. These glands release enzymes into ducts (see Figure 10) that ultimately empty into the GI lumen. The digestive organs primarily involved in exocrine secretion include the liver, gallbladder, and pancreas. However, some exocrine secretion is performed by specialized individual epithelial cells in the wall of the gut itself. These cells are miniature exocrine glands, releasing secretions directly into the gut lumen. Important examples are the cells of the **gastric glands** in the stomach and specialized mucus-secreting cells called **goblet cells**. The gastric glands secrete acid and **pepsinogen**. Goblet cells are found along the entire GI tract. Mucus is a slimy liquid which protects and lubricates the gut; any physiological surface covered with mucus is known as a **mucus membrane**. One last secretion must be mentioned: water. Whenever a meal is to be digested it must be dissolved in water. Hence, each day, gallons of water are secreted into the GI lumen. Most of it is reabsorbed in the small intestine, and the colon is responsible for reclaiming whatever water is left.

Endocrine secretion is also accomplished by both specialized organs (pancreas) and by cells in the wall of the gut. Remember that endocrine secretions (hormones) do not empty into ducts but instead are picked up by nearby capillaries. In other words, you should realize that when the same organ has both endocrine and exocrine activities, these functions are accomplished by separate cells, which are usually grouped in such a way as to be microscopically distinguishable. We'll see an example of this in the pancreas shortly.

---

[15] Exocrine glands secrete their products (digestive enzymes, etc.) into *ducts* that drain into the GI lumen. *Endocrine* glands are ductless glands; their secretions (hormones) are picked up by capillaries and thus enter the bloodstream.

Alimentary Canal

The alimentary canal is a continuous tube from mouth to anus, and each portion is seen as a separate organ. It includes the following:

1. mouth or oral cavity
2. throat or pharynx
3. esophagus
4. stomach
5. small intestine
6. large intestine

We will review each of these in turn. Later in this chapter, we will review the accessory organs.

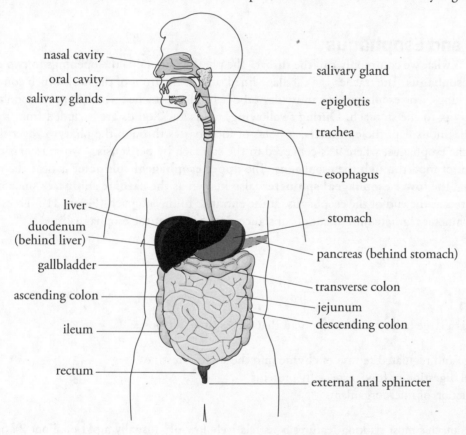

Figure 11 Organs of the Digestive System

Mouth

The mouth has three roles in the digestion of food: **mechanical digestion** (or fragmentation), lubrication, and some chemical digestion. Fragmentation is accomplished by **mastication** (**chewing**). The **incisors** (front teeth) are for cutting, the **cuspids** (canine teeth) are for tearing, and the **molars** are for grinding.

Lubrication and some digestion are accomplished by **saliva**, a viscous fluid secreted by **salivary glands**. Saliva contains **salivary amylase** (**ptyalin**), which hydrolyzes starch, breaking it into disaccharides and trisaccharides. Saliva also contains a small amount of **lingual lipase** for fat digestion. No digestion of proteins occurs in the mouth. Lastly, saliva also contains **lysozyme**, which attacks ___.[16] Hence the mouth also participates in innate immunity.

The muscles of the mouth and the muscular tongue are important for compacting chewed food into a smooth lump (**bolus**) which can be swallowed.

- When carbohydrates are broken down by ptyalin, can they be absorbed in the mouth?[17]

Pharynx and Esophagus

The **pharynx** is what we commonly call the throat. The pharynx contains the openings to two tubes: the **trachea** and **esophagus**. The trachea is a cartilage-lined tube at the front of the neck which conveys air to and from the lungs. The esophagus is a muscular tube behind the trachea which conveys food and drink from the pharynx to the stomach. During swallowing, solids and liquids are excluded from the trachea by a flat cartilaginous flap, the **epiglottis**. A bolus of food passes through the pharynx, over the epiglottis, and into the esophagus, where it is conveyed to the stomach by peristalsis. Two muscular rings regulate movement of food through the esophagus. The **upper esophageal sphincter** is near the top of the esophagus, and the **lower esophageal sphincter** (also known as the **cardiac sphincter** since it is found near the heart) is at the end of the esophagus, at the entrance to the stomach (Figure 11). [Does the lower esophageal sphincter regulate movement of substances into or out of the esophagus?[18]]

Stomach

The stomach is a large hollow muscular organ that serves three purposes:

1. storage and regulated release of **chyme** into the small intestine
2. partial digestion of food, especially proteins
3. destruction of microorganisms

Among the stomach's most striking features is its relatively low pH (usually a pH of about 2). Specialized cells, called **parietal cells**, in the lining of the stomach secrete **hydrochloric acid** (**HCl**) into the stomach's lumen. The acidity of the stomach is part of innate immunity, as it kills microorganisms in the food we eat. It is also essential to the functioning of the gastric enzyme **pepsin**. Secreted by **chief cells** in the stomach wall, pepsin initiates the chemical breakdown of proteins. Once food has been churned and digested by pepsin, it passes through the **pyloric sphincter** into the first section of the small intestine, the **duodenum**. One way to think about this is that the pyloric sphincter releases chyme (from the stomach) a squirt at a time.

---

[16] bacterial cell walls, which are made of peptidoglycan. Remember, lytic phages make lysozyme too.

[17] No. Sugars are not broken down into monosaccharides until they reach the intestinal brush border as we'll see shortly. Only monosaccharides can be absorbed into the body. Absorption requires special transmembrane transporters located on the intestinal brush border; each transporter is specific for a particular monosaccharide.

[18] It is there to prevent reflux from the stomach into the esophagus. There is no reason to regulate movement of substances out of the esophagus into the stomach, since nothing is stored in the esophagus; it's just a conduit.

- Pepsinogen is unique because it is activated by ___ instead of ___.[19]

Gastrin is a hormone secreted by cells in the stomach wall known as **G cells**. It stimulates acid, pepsin secretion, and gastric motility. Gastrin secretion is stimulated by food in the stomach and by parasympathetic stimulation. [Is this hormone secreted into the lumen of the duodenum or into the lumen of the stomach?[20]]

Small Intestine

Food leaving the stomach enters the small intestine, a tube which is about an inch wide and 10 feet long. (After death, it measures about 25 feet due to relaxation of longitudinal muscles.) The small intestine is divided into three segments: the **duodenum**, **jejunum**, and **ileum**. Digestion begins in the mouth, continues in the stomach, and is completed in the duodenum and jejunum. Absorption begins in the duodenum and continues throughout the small intestine.

Surface Area

The key feature that allows the small intestine to accomplish absorption is its large surface area; this results from (1) length, (2) plicae or folds, (3) villi, and (4) microvilli. **Villi** (singular: **villus**) are macroscopic (multicellular) projections in the wall of the small intestine. **Microvilli** are microscopic foldings of the cell membranes of individual intestinal epithelial cells. The lumenal surface of the small intestine is known as the **brush border** due to the brush-like appearance of microvilli. Let's look more closely at a villus (Figure 12).

These finger-like projections protrude into the lumen and have three important structures:

1. The villus contains capillaries, which absorb dietary monosaccharides and amino acids into the bloodstream.
2. The villus also contains small lymphatic vessels called **lacteals**, which absorb dietary fats. Lacteals merge to form large lymphatic vessels, which transport dietary fats to the thoracic duct, which empties into the bloodstream.

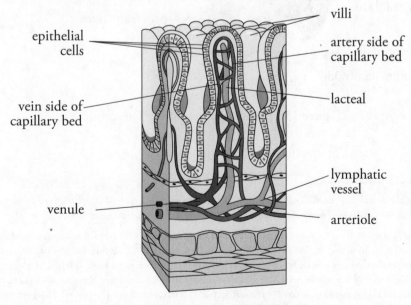

Figure 12   An Intestinal Villus

---

[19] Pepsinogen is unusual in that it is activated to pepsin by acidic proteolysis (autocleavage) instead of proteolytic cleavage by another enzyme.

[20] Neither! It's a hormone; by definition, it is secreted into the bloodstream.

9.2

Bile and Pancreatic Secretions in the Duodenum

A key anatomical feature of the duodenum is that two ducts empty into it (see Figure 13). One is the **pancreatic duct**, which delivers the exocrine secretions of the pancreas (digestive enzymes and bicarbonate, as we'll review shortly). The other is the **common bile duct**, which delivers **bile**. This is a green fluid containing **bile acids**, which are made from **cholesterol** in the liver and are normally absorbed and recycled. Bile is stored in the **gallbladder** until it is needed. Bile has two functions: it is a vehicle for the disposal (excretion) of waste products by the liver, and it is essential for digestion of fats, as discussed below. The bile duct and the pancreatic duct empty into the duodenum via the same orifice, known as the **sphincter of Oddi** (Figure 13).

- If a gallstone became lodged in the sphincter of Oddi, what would happen?[21]
- Bile acids secreted into the duodenum are normally reabsorbed in the ileum. Bile acid sequestrants are drugs which bind bile acids in the small intestine, causing them to remain in the GI lumen and eventually be excreted as feces. Each of the following is most likely true about such drugs EXCEPT:[22]
    - A. they are stable at low pH levels.
    - B. they result in a decrease in the level of cholesterol in the bloodstream.
    - C. it would be reasonable to be concerned that they might disrupt fat absorption.
    - D. they would be administered intravenously (injected into a vein).

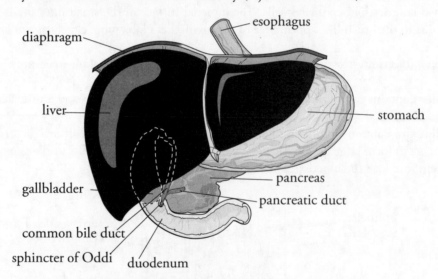

Figure 13 Anatomy Around the Duodenum

---

[21] Both bile and pancreatic ducts would be blocked, and digestion would be severely impaired (especially fat digestion, but also protein and carbohydrate digestion due to failure of pancreatic zymogens and amylase to reach the intestinal lumen).

[22] Since the drugs must pass through the stomach, they should be stable at low pH levels (choice A is true and can be eliminated). The text states that bile acids are made from cholesterol and normally recycled. It is reasonable to assume that blocking this recycling would require the conversion of more cholesterol into bile acids, which would lower the serum cholesterol level. This is in fact what bile acid sequestrants are used for (choice B is true and can be eliminated). It would be reasonable to be concerned about fat absorption, based on the fact that bile acids are necessary for this absorption, as stated in the text (choice C is true and can be eliminated). However, the drugs would have to be *swallowed* to end up within the GI lumen, not injected (choice **D** is false and is the correct answer).

Duodenal Secretions

Some duodenal epithelial cells secrete enzymes. Duodenal **enterokinase** activates the pancreatic zymogen **trypsinogen** to trypsin. Other duodenal enzymes are peculiar in that they are not truly secreted, but rather do their work inside or on the surface of the brush border epithelial cell. **Brush border peptidases** hydrolyze di- and tripeptides into amino acids. **Brush border disaccharidases** (such as **sucrase**, **maltase**, and **lactase**) hydrolyze disaccharides into monosaccharides.

Other duodenal epithelial cells secrete hormones. The three main duodenal hormones are **cholecysto-kinin (CCK)**, **secretin**, and **enterogastrone**. CCK is secreted in response to fats in the duodenum. It causes the pancreas to secrete digestive enzymes, stimulates gallbladder contraction (bile release), and decreases gastric motility; these processes cooperate to deal with fats in the duodenum, by digesting them and preventing further stomach emptying. Secretin is released in response to acid in the duodenum. It causes the pancreas to release large amounts of a high-pH aqueous buffer, namely HCO_3^- in water. This neutralizes HCl released by the stomach. Duodenal pH must be kept neutral or even slightly basic for pancreatic digestive enzymes to function. Enterogastrone decreases stomach emptying.

Jejunum and Ileum

Most substances are absorbed in the jejunum and ileum. Amino acids and glucose are absorbed into villi capillaries. These small blood vessels merge to form veins, which merge to form the large **hepatic portal vein**, which transports blood containing amino acid and carbohydrate nutrients from the gut to the liver. It is called a portal vein because it connects two capillary beds: the one in the intestinal wall and the one inside the liver. The liver stores amino acids and glucose and releases them into the bloodstream as needed.

Fats are absorbed from the intestine and packaged into **chylomicrons**, which are a type of **lipoprotein**. Chylomicrons enter lacteals, tiny lymphatic vessels in intestinal villi. Lacteals empty into larger lymphatics, which eventually drain into a large vein near the neck.[23] Chylomicrons are taken up by the liver, repackaged, and then released again into the bloodstream. Fats are taken up by **adipocytes** (fat cells) for storage. When fats are to be used for energy, adipocyte triglycerides are hydrolyzed, and free fatty acids are released into the bloodstream. A valve called the **ileocecal valve** separates the ileum from the cecum, which is the first part of the large intestine.

Large Intestine

The large intestine is the last part of the alimentary canal. The sections are:

- cecum and appendix
- ascending colon
- transverse colon
- descending colon
- sigmoid colon
- rectum
- anus

---

[23] This means that dietary fats bypass the hepatic vein.

The colon is the largest portion of the large intestine. Like the rest of the intestine, the large intestine is a muscular tube. It is 3 or 4 feet long and several inches wide. Its role is to absorb water and minerals, and to form and store feces until the time of **defecation**. Abnormalities of colon function result in poor fluid absorption and diarrhea, which can cause dehydration and death.

The first part of the colon is the **cecum**. Entrance of chyme into the cecum is controlled by the ileocecal valve. The **appendix** is a finger-like appendage of the cecum. It is composed primarily of lymphatic tissue.

The colon contains billions of bacteria of various species.[24] Many are facultative or obligate anaerobes. Undigested materials are metabolized by colonic bacteria. This often results in gas, which is given off as a waste product of bacterial metabolism. **Colonic bacteria** are important for two reasons:

1. The presence of large numbers of normal bacteria helps keep dangerous bacteria from proliferating, due to competition for space and nutrients.
2. Colonic bacteria supply us with **vitamin K,** which is essential for blood clotting.

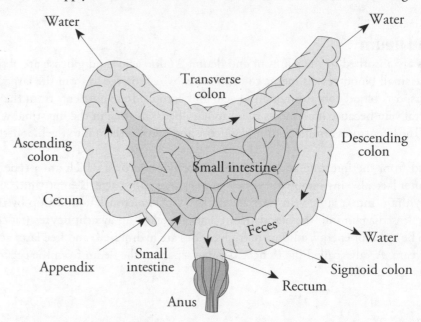

Figure 14 Large Intestine

The last portion of the colon is called the **rectum**. Exit of feces (defecation) from the rectum occurs through the **anus**. Defecation is controlled by the **anal sphincter**, which has an internal portion and an external portion. The internal anal sphincter consists of smooth muscle, which is under autonomic control. The external anal sphincter consists of skeletal muscle and is under voluntary control.[25] Most of the wastes from a meal are defecated about a day after it is eaten. However, the wastes from a meal are first present in stool after just a few hours and some residue of a meal is typically still present in the colon after several days.

---

[24] This is called your gut microbiome and is an active area of research.

[25] Note this is the same arrangement as seen in the urinary sphincters.

Digestive Accessory Organs

There are four **digestive accessory organs** that play a role in digestion but are not actually part of the alimentary canal. They are:

1. salivary glands
2. pancreas
3. liver
4. gallbladder

Salivary glands make and release saliva, which we have already discussed. The **pancreas** and liver are essential for GI function; the gallbladder is not essential.

Exocrine Pancreas

There are two principal cell types in the pancreas. Exocrine cells, referred to simply as **pancreatic acinar cells**, are organized into acini that drain into ducts. These cells secrete digestive enzymes and **bicarbonate**. Endocrine cells are clumped together in groups known as **islets of Langerhans**; we'll talk about these in the next section. Pancreatic enzymes are made by acinar cells and released into the duodenum; they are essential for digestion. **Pancreatic amylase** hydrolyzes polysaccharides to disaccharides. **Pancreatic lipase** hydrolyzes triglycerides at the surface of a **micelle**. **Nucleases** hydrolyze dietary DNA and RNA. Several different **pancreatic proteases** are responsible for hydrolyzing polypeptides to di- and tripeptides. Pancreatic proteases are secreted in their inactive **zymogen** forms. [Why do you suppose digestive enzymes are stored and released in an inactive form?[26]] Zymogens must be activated by removal of a portion of the polypeptide chain. **Trypsinogen** is a zymogen which is converted to the active form, **trypsin**, by **enterokinase**, a duodenal enzyme. Other pancreatic enzymes are then activated by trypsin. These include **chymotrypsinogen** (active form: **chymotrypsin**), **procarboxypeptidase** (active form: **carboxypeptidase**), and **procollagenase** (active form: **collagenase**).

The pancreas also makes and releases bicarbonate to neutralize acid entering the small intestine from the stomach. The stomach has protective measures that allow it to survive a pH of 2. The duodenum has no such protection, so the low pH needs to be neutralized once in the small intestine.

Two hormones discussed previously help to control pancreatic secretion. Cholecystokinin (CCK) secreted into the bloodstream by the duodenum causes the pancreas to secrete enzymes. Secretin, also released by the duodenum, causes the pancreas to secrete water and bicarbonate. Parasympathetic nervous system activation increases pancreatic secretion; sympathetic activation reduces it.

---

[26] It is a safety mechanism. Active digestive enzymes could be dangerous to the pancreatic cells themselves.

Endocrine Pancreas

The endocrine pancreas consists of small regions within the pancreas known as **islets of Langerhans**. There are three types of cells in the islets, and each secretes a particular hormone into the bloodstream.

1. α cells secrete **glucagon** in response to low blood sugar. Glucagon mobilizes stored fuels by stimulating the liver to hydrolyze glycogen and release glucose into the bloodstream, and by stimulating adipocytes to release fats into the bloodstream.
2. β cells secrete **insulin** in response to elevated blood sugar (e.g., after a meal). Its effects are opposite those of glucagon: insulin stimulates removal of glucose from the blood for storage as glycogen and fat.
3. δ cells secrete **somatostatin**. This hormone inhibits many digestive processes.

Focus on Blood Glucose

1. **Lowering blood glucose:** Insulin is essential for life because it causes sugar to be removed from the bloodstream and stored. Diabetics lack insulin or have dysfunctional insulin receptors. Their blood sugar levels are extraordinarily high. Excess glucose directly destroys many physiological systems at the cellular level, including neurons, blood vessels, and the kidneys.

2. **Raising blood glucose:** Three hormones can raise the blood glucose level: glucagon (a polypeptide hormone from the pancreas), epinephrine (an amino acid derivative from the adrenal medulla), and cortisol (a steroid or glucocorticoid from the adrenal cortex). Note that of these three hormones, one is a steroid, one is a polypeptide, and one is an amino acid derivative. Also note that there is only one hormone that can lower blood glucose, while three different hormones can raise blood glucose. It makes sense to have many ways to raise blood glucose, and for it to be less easy to lower blood glucose, since low blood glucose levels are immediately fatal, while elevated blood glucose is harmless in the short term. (Over several years, however, it is harmful.)

- Which one of the following statements is true?[27]
    - A. Insulin stimulates release of glucose into blood and also stimulates peristalsis in the small intestine.
    - B. Gastrin stimulates stomach emptying and inhibits secretion of gastric acid.
    - C. Cholecystokinin stimulates peristalsis in the intestine and inhibits stomach emptying.
    - D. Glucagon stimulates the storage of glucose and stimulates small intestinal peristalsis.
    - E. Trypsin hydrolyzes polysaccharides to disaccharides.

Liver and Gallbladder

The exocrine secretory activity of the liver is simple: it secretes bile. The liver actually produces about 1 liter of bile a day. The principal ingredients of bile include bile acids (known as **bile salts** in the deprotonated—anionic—form), cholesterol, and **bilirubin** (from RBC breakdown). Bile emulsifies large fat particles in the duodenum, creating smaller clusters of fat particles called **micelles**. These smaller particles have a greater collective surface area than the large particles, and thus are more easily digested by hydrophilic lipases (from the pancreas). Also, bile helps fatty particles to diffuse across the intestinal mucosal membrane.

---

[27] Insulin stimulates *removal* of glucose from the blood (eliminate A), gastrin *causes* acid secretion (eliminate B), glucagon functions to *raise* blood glucose (eliminate D), and trypsin hydrolyzes polypeptides (proteins) not polysaccharides (eliminate E). Only **C** is a true statement.

Bile made in the liver can go to one of two places: it is either directly secreted into the duodenum or it is stored for later use in the **gallbladder**. Bile stored in the gallbladder is concentrated, and released when a fatty meal is eaten. The gallbladder itself has no secretory activity. Bile release from this organ is dictated by both the endocrine system and the nervous system. Both CCK (released by the duodenal cells) and the parasympathetic nervous system stimulate contraction of the gallbladder wall.

The liver has many other functions. It assists in lipid metabolism and stores iron, vitamins, and as we saw earlier, glucose in the form of glycogen. Hepatocytes (liver cells) monitor blood and make changes to the body's physiology based on what is and is not present (much as the hypothalamus does in the hypothalamic–pituitary portal system). For example, if blood glucose is low, the liver will initiate a cascade that leads to glycogen breakdown as well as new glucose production (gluconeogenesis); free glucose can be released to raise blood glucose levels.

Waste products from protein catabolism (breakdown) are also regulated through the liver. When proteins are broken down into amino acids, and amino acids are broken down even further (e.g., to enter the Krebs cycle to generate ATP during starvation), nitrogenous by-products are released in the form of NH_3 (ammonia). Ammonia in high levels is toxic to the body, so it is transported to the liver where it is converted into urea. Urea is then absorbed into the bloodstream and excreted by the kidney in urine.

Many important plasma proteins (such as albumin, globulins, fibrinogens, and other clotting factors necessary to stop bleeding) are made in the liver and secreted into the plasma. People with liver disease often have problems with sealing wounds due to a lack of clotting factors. They also have a tendency to swell up; the lack of albumin allows fluid to leave the bloodstream and enter the tissues.

Finally, the liver is the major center for drug and toxin detoxification in the body. The smooth ER in hepatocytes contains enzyme pathways that break down drugs and toxins into forms that are less toxic and more readily excreted by the renal and gastrointestinal systems.

Vitamins

Vitamins are nutrients which must be included in the diet because they cannot be synthesized in the body. They are divided into **fat-soluble** and **water-soluble** categories. Fat-soluble vitamins require bile acids for solubilization and absorption. Excess fat-soluble vitamins are stored in adipose tissue. Some fat-soluble vitamins are:

- vitamin A (retinol): a visual pigment that changes conformation in response to light
- vitamin D: stimulates Ca^{2+} absorption from the gut; helps control Ca^{2+} deposition in bones
- vitamin K: necessary for formation of blood coagulation factors

Excess water-soluble vitamins are excreted in urine by the kidneys. Vitamin B (of which there are many subtypes), vitamin C, and folate are water-soluble vitamins.

9.3 EXCRETORY SYSTEM

Overview

Excretion is the disposal of waste products. "The excretory system" generally refers to the kidneys, even though the liver, large intestine, and skin are involved in excretion too. Let's begin by summarizing the excretory roles of these organs to see where the kidneys fit into the picture.

The **liver** is responsible for excreting many wastes by chemically modifying them and releasing them into bile. In particular, the liver deals with hydrophobic or large waste products, which cannot be filtered out by the kidney. The liver also synthesizes **urea** and releases it into the bloodstream. Urea is a carrier of excess nitrogen and is excreted in urine.

The large intestine processes wastes destined for excretion; these are molecules we ingest but do not absorb into our blood. The colon is also capable of excreting excess ions (e.g., sodium, chloride, calcium) into the feces, using active transport.

Skin produces sweat, which contains water, ions, and urea. In other words, sweat is similar to urine.[28] In this sense, the skin is an excretory organ. However, sweating is not primarily controlled by the amount of waste that needs to be excreted, but rather by temperature and level of sympathetic nervous system activity. Therefore, the excretory role of the skin is secondary.

Most humans have two kidneys, which are responsible for several important functions:

1. excreting hydrophilic wastes
2. maintaining constant solute concentration
3. maintaining constant pH
4. maintaining constant fluid volume, which is important for blood pressure and cardiac output

Gross Anatomy of the Urinary System

Each kidney is a filtration system that removes unwanted materials from the blood and passes them to the bladder for storage and eventual elimination. Blood enters the kidney from a large **renal artery**, which is a direct branch of the lower portion of the aorta (Figure 15). Purified blood is returned to the circulatory system by the large **renal vein**, which empties into the inferior vena cava. Urine leaves each kidney through a **ureter**, which empties into the **urinary bladder**. The bladder is a muscular organ which stretches as it fills with urine. There are two sphincters controlling release of urine from the bladder: an **internal sphincter** made of smooth (involuntary) muscle and an **external sphincter** made of skeletal (voluntary) muscle.

---

[28] In Chapter 7, we learned about metanephridia, excretory tubes used by annelids, mollusks, and some arthropods. Metanephridia have ciliated funnels that remove waste from the blood and interstitial fluid; funnels lead to exterior pores where wastes are discharged. Given these animals essentially urinate via their skin, it shouldn't be a surprise that sweat and urine share many characteristics.

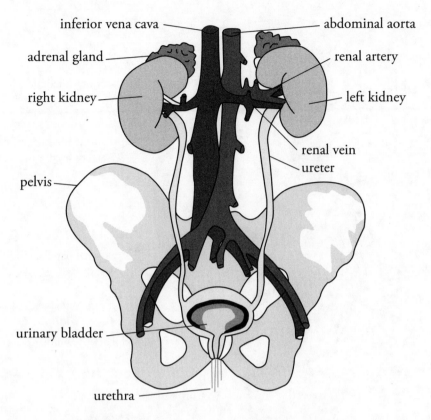

inferior vena cava

abdominal aorta

adrenal gland

renal artery

right kidney

left kidney

renal vein

ureter

pelvis

urinary bladder

urethra

Figure 15   Gross Anatomy of the Urinary System

A frontal section (separating front from back) through the kidney demonstrates its internal anatomy. The outer region is known as the **cortex**, and the inner region is the **medulla**. It is important to note that there is an osmolarity gradient in the interstitium of the kidney: the cortex has a low osmolarity and the medulla has a high osmolarity. This will be important later because it drives reabsorption and urine concentration in the renal tubules. Let's add two nomenclature reminders here:

- **Osmolarity** is the measure of solute concentration, usually compared to the plasma. In the renal system, the main solutes are ions like Na^+, Cl^-, and K^+. Saying the cortex has a low osmolarity just means it is not very salty. Saying the renal medulla has a high osmolarity means it is quite salty.
- **Interstitium** is a generic word for "tissue." It literally means "an in-between region"; in this case it refers to the kidney tissue in between the renal tubules.

Let's return to kidney anatomy (see Figure 16). The **medullary pyramids** are pyramid-shaped striations within the medulla. This appearance is due to the presence of many collecting ducts. Urine empties from the collecting ducts and leaves the medulla at the tip of a pyramid, known as a **papilla** (plural: **papillae**). Each papilla empties into a space called a **calyx** (plural: **calyces**). The calyces converge to form the **renal pelvis**, which is a large space where urine collects. The renal pelvis empties into the ureter.

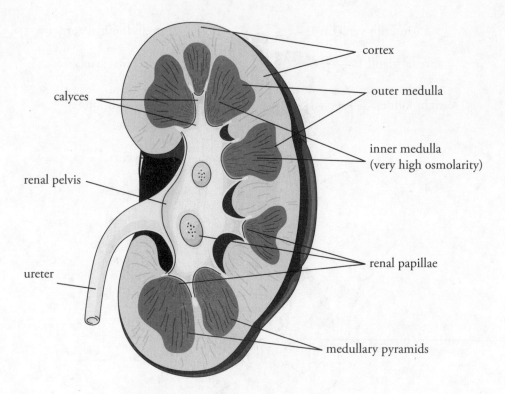

Figure 16 Internal Anatomy of the Kidney

The Nephron

The functional unit of the kidney is the **nephron**. It consists of two components:

1. **capsule**: a rounded region surrounding the capillaries where filtration takes place
2. **renal tubule**: a coiled tube that receives filtrate from the capillaries in the capsule at one end and empties into a **collecting duct** at the other end

Capsule and Filtration

Blood from the renal artery flows into an **afferent arteriole**, which branches into a ball of capillaries known as the **glomerulus** (Figure 17). Blood pressure causes fluid (essentially blood plasma) to leak out of the glomerular capillaries. The fluid passes through a filter known as the **glomerular basement membrane (GBM)** and enters **Bowman's capsule**. The lumen of Bowman's capsule is continuous with the lumen of the rest of the tubule. **Filtrate,** the fluid in the tubule, will eventually be made into urine.

The glomerular basement membrane acts like a colander.[29] Small molecules are squeezed into the renal tubule during filtration; these molecules include water, ions, glucose, amino acids, and urea. Substances which are too large to pass through the glomerular basement membrane are not filtered; they remain in the glomerular capillary blood and drain into an **efferent arteriole**. These substances include blood cells (both RBC and WBC) and plasma proteins.

---

[29] The glomerular basement membrane is actually a layer lining each capillary of the glomerulus.

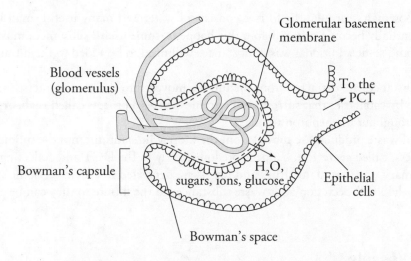

Figure 17   Filtration of Blood at the Glomerulus

Filtration occurs in the renal cortex, the outer layer of the kidney. The **glomerular filtration rate (GFR)** depends directly on blood pressure:

- Constriction of the efferent arteriole increases blood pressure in the glomerulus and increases GFR.
- Dilation of the afferent arteriole increases blood flow to the glomerulus; this increases blood pressure and GFR.

- Which of the following are present in the filtrate in Bowman's capsule in concentrations similar to those seen in blood?[30]
    - I.   Albumin (a plasma protein)
    - II. Glucose
    - III. Sodium

    - A. I and II
    - B. II only
    - C. I and III
    - D. II and III
    - E. I, II, and III

Reabsorption and Secretion

The tubule of the nephron contains five different regions. In order, they are:

1. Proximal convoluted tubule (PCT)
2. Descending loop of Henle
3. Ascending loop of Henle
4. Distal convoluted tubule (DCT)
5. Collecting duct

---

[30] **Statement I: False**. Plasma proteins are too large to pass through the filter (eliminate A, C, and E). **Statement II: True**. Glucose passes through into the filtrate and must be reclaimed during selective reabsorption (eliminate C). **Statement III: True**. Sodium also passes into the filtrate. It will be reclaimed or left in the filtrate to be urinated out, depending on physiological needs (eliminate B, and **D** is correct).

Coming out of Bowman's capsule, the filtrate consists of water and many useful small hydrophilic molecules; it will eventually become urine. Before this happens, some useful substances must be returned to the bloodstream and some additional waste substances will need to be added to the filtrate.

- Useful substances are extracted from the tubule, moved into the kidney interstitium, and picked up by capillaries that surround the tubule. This is a process called **reabsorption**, and it occurs throughout the nephron tubule.
- Additional waste products are moved from the kidney interstitium into the tubule filtrate. This process, called **secretion**, happens predominantly in the DCT and collecting duct; this is the primary way that many drugs and toxins are deposited in the urine. Some secretion also occurs in the PCT. Secretion adds waste substances to the filtrate so they can be eliminated in urine.

Renal Blood Vessels

Many blood vessels surround the nephron. They carry arterial blood toward the capsule for filtration, and then surround the tubule to carry filtered blood and reabsorbed substances away from the tubule:

- **Peritubular capillaries** surround the proximal and distal tubules in the cortex.
- **Vasa recta** go into the medulla to surround the loop of Henle.

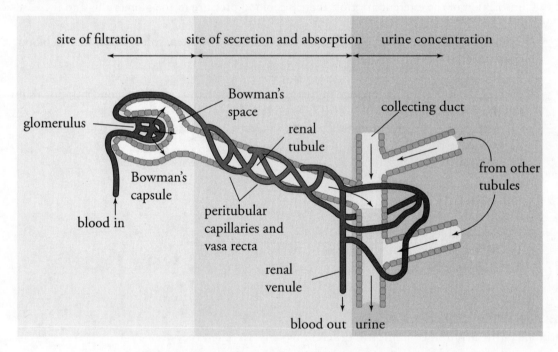

Figure 18   Blood Vessels and the Renal Tubule

These blood vessels return reabsorbed substances to the bloodstream; they drain into venules that lead to the renal vein.

Renal Tubule

Bowman's capsule empties into the first part of the tubule, the PCT. Here, most of the reabsorption occurs. All solute movement in the PCT is accompanied by water movement, so a lot of water reabsorption occurs in this region also; roughly 70 percent of the volume of the filtrate is reabsorbed in the PCT. For useful substances, the PCT reabsorbs as much as possible. Like Bowman's capsule, the PCT is located in the renal cortex, the outer layer of the kidney.

The PCT empties into the next region of the nephron, the **loop of Henle**. This is a long loop that dips down into the renal medulla. The loop of Henle has two parts:

- The descending loop of Henle starts in the cortex and goes down into the renal medulla. It is permeable to water, but not to ions. Because the renal interstitium has a high osmolarity, water is reabsorbed. This makes the filtrate more concentrated.
- The ascending loop of Henle starts in the medulla and heads back up toward the cortex. It is permeable to ions but not water. Because the filtrate is highly concentrated at the bottom of the loop of Henle, ions are reabsorbed as the filtrate moves up. These ions (mostly Na^+ and Cl^-) make the medullary interstitium salty.

As we continue through the tubule, the loop of Henle becomes the DCT, which is located in the renal cortex. The filtrate composition is optimized and fine-tuned in the DCT. Reabsorption here is more regulated than in the PCT, usually via hormones. Some secretion also happens here. The DCT dumps into a collecting duct and by the end of the collecting duct, whatever remains in the renal tubule gets excreted as urine. Many collecting ducts merge to form larger tributaries which empty into renal calyces and then the renal pelvis. Urine is sent to the bladder for storage, via the ureter.

The DCT and the collecting duct are together known as the distal nephron and cooperate in the last step of urine formation: concentration or dilution. This involves the selective reabsorption of water and is where we decide whether to make dilute urine or concentrated urine. Before filtrate is discarded into the ureter as urine, adjustments are made so urine volume and osmolarity are appropriate. This is controlled by two hormones: antidiuretic hormone (ADH) and **aldosterone**. Remember that ADH is also known as **vasopressin**.

- Which one of the following best describes selective reabsorption?[31]
    - A. In normal individuals, only a small portion of the serum glucose is filtered into the tubule. Of this amount, about 50% is reabsorbed by the epithelial cells of the tubule.
    - B. In normal individuals, the concentration of glucose which is filtered into the tubule is identical to the serum [glucose]. Of the filtered glucose, 100% is reabsorbed by the epithelial cells of the tubule.
    - C. Epithelial cells of the renal tubule actively transport glucose into the filtrate.
    - D. Glucose is kept in the bloodstream by the filtering action of the glomerular basement membrane.
    - E. Whether glucose is reabsorbed or excreted depends on the body's glucose levels.

---

[31] As stated in the section on filtration, glucose is small enough that all of it freely passes through the glomerular basement membrane (eliminate D), as are ions, amino acids, and water. However, even though glucose is filtered into the tubule, it must be reclaimed into the bloodstream, or we would constantly lose glucose into the urine. 100 percent of filtered glucose is normally reclaimed (choice **B** is correct, eliminate A and E), and in no instance is glucose ever transported *into* the filtrate (eliminate C). Note that in diabetes, the blood glucose level is so high that the cotransporters responsible for glucose reabsorption become saturated, and large amounts of glucose are left in the urine.

Endocrine Role of the Kidney

When you are dehydrated, the volume of fluid in your bloodstream is low and the solute concentration in the blood is high. Hence, you need to make small amounts of highly concentrated urine. Under these conditions (low blood volume and high blood osmolarity), ADH is released by the posterior pituitary. ADH prevents water loss in the urine by increasing water reabsorption in the distal nephron. This is accomplished by making the distal nephron permeable to water; without ADH, the distal tubule is impermeable to water.[32] In response to ADH, water flows out of the filtrate into the tissue of the kidney, where it is picked up by the peritubular capillaries. [Why would water tend to flow out of the tubule into the tissue of the kidney?[33]]

In contrast, after drinking a lot of water, plasma volume is too high, and a large volume of dilute urine is necessary. In this case, no ADH is secreted. The result is that the distal tubule is not permeable to water. This means that any water in the filtrate remains in the tubule and is lost in the urine. The reason that drinking alcohol causes many bathroom runs is that it inhibits ADH secretion by the posterior pituitary.

When blood pressure is low, aldosterone is released by the adrenal cortex. It increases reabsorption of Na^+ by the distal nephron. The result is increased plasma osmolarity, which leads to increased thirst and water retention, which raises the blood pressure. When the blood pressure is high, aldosterone is not released. As a result, sodium is lost in the urine; plasma osmolarity (and eventually blood pressure) fall.

ADH and aldosterone work together to increase blood pressure. First, aldosterone causes sodium reabsorption, which results in increased plasma osmolarity. This causes ADH to be secreted, which results in increased water reabsorption and thus increased plasma volume.

There are a few other hormones that affect the kidney, and the kidney makes one as well. All are peptides except aldosterone, which is a steroid. You should know the basic role and source of each of the following hormones:

Hormone	Source	Target and effect
Aldosterone	Adrenal cortex	Increases sodium reabsorption and potassium secretion in the distal nephron; this increases blood volume through the action of ADH and thus increases blood pressure
Antidiuretic hormone (ADH) or vasopressin	Posterior pituitary	Increases water reabsorption in the distal nephron, to increase urine concentration, dilute the blood, increase plasma volume, and increase systemic blood pressure
Calcitonin	Thyroid	Decreases serum $[Ca^{2+}]$ by deposition in bone, reduced absorption in the gut, and excretion in urine
Parathyroid hormone (PTH)	Parathyroid	Increases serum $[Ca^{2+}]$ by breaking down bone, increased absorption in the gut, and reabsorption from the filtrate
Erythropoietin (EPO)	Kidney	Increases synthesis of red blood cells in the bone marrow

Table 2   Hormones Affecting or Secreted by the Kidney

---

[32] Note this is the first time we have encountered a layer in the body that is impermeable to water.

[33] Because the renal medulla has a very high osmolarity, which causes water to exit the tubule by osmosis.

Countercurrent Multiplier

A system called the **countercurrent multiplier** allows the kidney to reabsorb 99% of the filtrate in the tubule and to produce urine that has a much higher osmolarity than plasma. The basis of this system is a series of tubes running in opposite directions through the interstitial space of the kidney, and a combination of active and passive transport across the tubule wall:

- The descending loop of Henle runs down, from the cortex into the medulla. It is permeable to water, but not to ions, so water is reabsorbed.
- Like the loop of Henle, vasa recta blood vessels form a loop; the ascending portions of the vasa recta are near the descending limb of the loop of Henle and carry off water that leaves the descending limb.
- The ascending loop of Henle runs up, from the medulla to the cortex of the kidney. It is permeable to ions but not water, so ions are reabsorbed. These ions contribute to the high osmolarity in the medulla.
- The collecting duct runs down, from the cortex to the medulla. The high osmolarity of the interstitium sucks water out of the collecting duct in the presence of ADH.

The countercurrent multiplier makes the medulla very salty, and this facilitates water reabsorption from the descending loop of Henle and the collecting duct. This is how the kidney is capable of making urine with a much higher osmolarity than plasma.

9.3

Now that we have looked at all aspects of renal physiology, let's look at a full labeled diagram of the nephron:

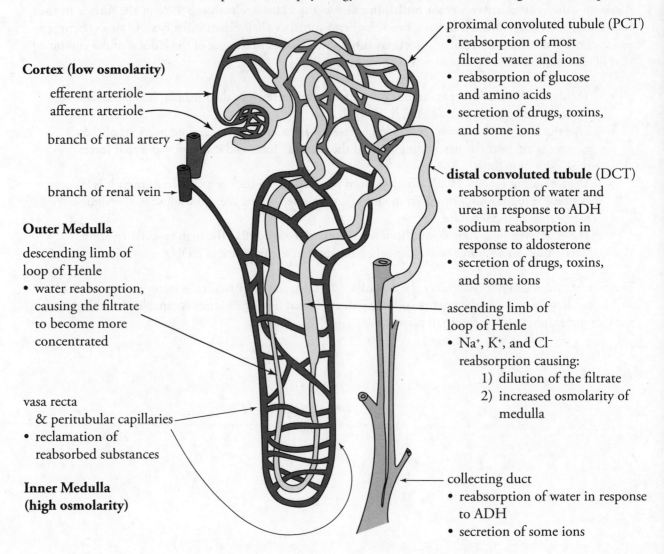

proximal convoluted tubule (PCT)
- reabsorption of most filtered water and ions
- reabsorption of glucose and amino acids
- secretion of drugs, toxins, and some ions

Cortex (low osmolarity)

efferent arteriole

afferent arteriole

branch of renal artery

branch of renal vein

distal convoluted tubule (DCT)
- reabsorption of water and urea in response to ADH
- sodium reabsorption in response to aldosterone
- secretion of drugs, toxins, and some ions

Outer Medulla

descending limb of loop of Henle
- water reabsorption, causing the filtrate to become more concentrated

ascending limb of loop of Henle
- Na^+, K^+, and Cl^- reabsorption causing:
  1) dilution of the filtrate
  2) increased osmolarity of medulla

vasa recta & peritubular capillaries
- reclamation of reabsorbed substances

Inner Medulla (high osmolarity)

collecting duct
- reabsorption of water in response to ADH
- secretion of some ions

Figure 19 Regions and Functions of the Nephron

Renal Regulation of Blood Pressure

Since GFR depends directly on pressure, the kidney has built-in mechanisms to help regulate systemic and local (glomerular) blood pressure. The **juxtaglomerular apparatus (JGA)** contains **baroreceptors** that monitor systemic blood pressure. When there is a decrease in blood pressure, juxtaglomerular (JG) cells secrete an enzyme called **renin** into the bloodstream. Renin catalyzes the conversion of **angiotensinogen** (a plasma protein made by the liver) into **angiotensin I**, which is further converted to **angiotensin II** by **angiotensin-converting enzyme (ACE)** in the lungs. Angiotensin II is a powerful vasoconstrictor that immediately raises the blood pressure. It also stimulates the release of aldosterone; see Figure 20.

The cells of the **macula densa** are chemoreceptors that monitor filtrate osmolarity in the distal tubule. A low filtrate osmolarity indicates a low filtration rate; the macula densa stimulates the JG cells to release renin. The macula densa also increases blood flow to the glomerulus, which increases filtration.

Let's look at a summary of how these two processes work together to increase systemic blood pressure:

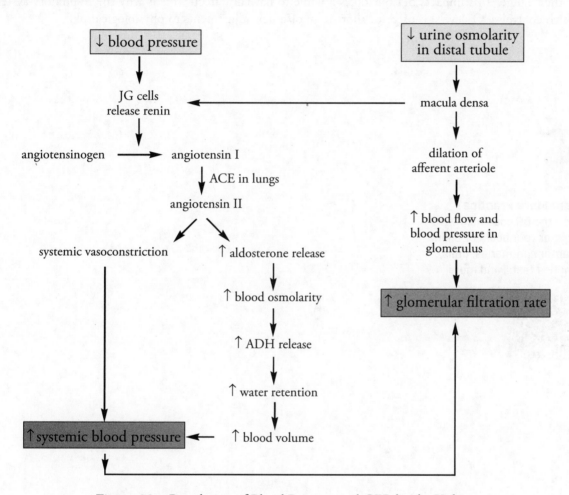

Figure 20 Regulation of Blood Pressure and GFR by the Kidney

Renal Regulation of pH

The kidney is essential for maintaining constant blood pH. It accomplishes this by a direct mechanism:

- When plasma pH is too high, HCO_3^- is excreted in the urine.
- When plasma pH is too low, H^+ is excreted in the urine.

9.3

These modifications affect the CO_2 equilibrium reaction we saw earlier in this chapter:

$$CO_2 + H_2O \rightleftharpoons H_2CO_3 \rightleftharpoons HCO_3^- + H^+$$

By excreting molecules in the urine, they are lost from the body and the equilibrium shifts to compensate for the change. This impacts pH but takes a while to have an effect. This is why the respiratory system (which controls CO_2 levels) is used for short-term or quick adjustments to physiological pH.

Want More Practice?
Scan the QR code below to register your book for online chapter summaries, drills, practice tests, and more!

Chapter 10
Structure and Function of Systems: Support and Structure

10.1 CELLS, TISSUES, AND ORGANS

Organization in living things exists in a hierarchical structure. Arranged from the simplest to most complex, they are: atoms, molecules, organelles, cells, tissues, organs, organ systems, organisms, populations, communities, ecosystem, biome, and biosphere. In other words, cells make up tissues, tissues make up organs, organs make up organ systems, organ systems make up an organism, and so on.

The human body consists of approximately 100 trillion cells, of which there are about 220 different types. Cells are generally grouped together to form **tissues**, groups of cells that function together as a unit and usually have similar structures. The space between cells is filled by a nonliving material, called the extracellular matrix, intercellular matrix, or interstitium.

There are four major types of tissues in the human body: epithelial tissue, muscle tissue, nervous tissue, and connective tissue. **Epithelial tissue** is located at the body's surface and where the body meets the external environment, such as the lining of the digestive tract. There are three common shapes of epithelial cells: **squamous** (flat), **columnar** (tall and thin), and **cuboidal** (shaped like a cube). Here are some examples of each:

- Epithelial tissue of the skin is made of many layers of (or stratified) squamous cells lying on a basement membrane.
- **Endothelial cells** are squamous epithelial cells that make up blood vessels.
- Alveoli of the lung are made of many squamous epithelial cells and a smaller number of cuboidal cells that make and secrete surfactant.
- Columnar cells line most of the digestive tract.
- Ciliated columnar cells make up the upper respiratory tract, such as the trachea and bronchi.
- Cuboidal cells make up the epithelia of kidney tubules and many glands.

Not all cells in your body are these shapes. For example, hepatocytes (liver cells) are polygonal in shape, the acinar cells of the pancreas are shaped like pyramids.

There are three types of **muscle tissue**. Skeletal muscle allows gross motor movement and is made of myofibers. Cardiac muscle tissue is found in the heart and smooth muscle tissue lines hollow organs and tubes. Cardiac and smooth muscle cells are both called myocytes.

Nerve tissue is made of neurons (or nerve cells) and glial cells, both of which were discussed earlier in this chapter.

There are six types of **connective tissue**:

1. cartilage, made of chondrocytes
2. bone tissue, containing osteoblasts, osteoclasts, and osteocytes
3. tendons
4. ligaments
5. fat (**adipose**), made of adipocytes
6. blood, containing red blood cells (erythrocytes) and white blood cells (leukocytes)

All together there are 78 main organs within the human body, many of which we've explored in this chapter. Of the 78 organs, only five organs are vital for survival: the heart, brain, kidneys, liver, and lungs. If you think about what each of these organs does for us, you will appreciate why they are important enough to make this list. Organs coordinate and work together in organ systems, and organ systems also work together. This coordination and cooperation are essential to maintain homeostasis and facilitate survival of the organism.

10.2   OVERVIEW OF MUSCLE TISSUE

There are three types of muscle which differ in cellular physiology, anatomy, and function. **Skeletal muscle** is also known as voluntary muscle, because its role is to contract in response to conscious intent. The next muscle type is called **cardiac muscle** because it is found only in the wall of the heart. Skeletal and cardiac muscle are said to be **striated** because of their appearance under a microscope. The third type of muscle is **smooth muscle**, which is found in the walls of all hollow organs such as the GI tract, urinary system, uterus, etc. It is responsible for GI motility, constriction of blood vessels, uterine contractions, and so on. We have no conscious control over cardiac or smooth muscle because they are innervated only by the autonomic nervous system. The three types of muscle share some characteristics and differ in others. We'll start with skeletal muscle because it is the most important type you should know for the DAT. Cardiac and smooth muscle will be discussed later in this chapter.

10.3   SKELETAL MUSCLE

Skeletal Muscle Function: Movement of Joints

Skeletal muscle provides voluntary movement of the body in response to stimulation by somatic motor neurons, but skeletal muscle alone cannot move the body. Skeletal muscle requires the framework of the bones of the skeleton for movement to occur. Skeletal muscles are attached at each end to two different bones. Muscles are often attached to bones by **tendons**, strong connective tissue formed primarily of collagen. By contracting, skeletal muscle can draw the points of attachment on the two bones closer together. One of the two bones joined by a skeletal muscle is generally closer to the center of the body and tends to stay in place when the muscle contracts. The point on this bone where the muscle attaches is called the **origin** of that skeletal muscle, and the point where the muscle attaches on the bone more distant from the center of the body is referred to as the muscle's **insertion**. When a muscle contracts, its insertion point is brought closer to its origin.

An example of a skeletal muscle and its action is the **flexion** of the elbow joint by the biceps brachii (see Figure 1 on the following page). The origin of this muscle lies in the shoulder joint, and the insertion lies in the bones of the forearm. Contraction of the biceps brachii brings its insertion (the forearm) closer to its origin (the shoulder). Since muscles can only *contract* to move a joint, different muscles are necessary for flexion and **extension** (opposite movements) of a joint. For the elbow, the triceps brachii (the muscle on the back of the upper arm) is responsible for extension. [Where is the origin of the triceps brachii?[1]] The origin and the insertion for the triceps brachii are on the opposite side of the arm as for the biceps brachii, so that contraction of the triceps has the opposite effect on the lower arm as contraction of the biceps. Muscles that are responsible for movement in opposite directions are termed **antagonistic**, while muscles that move a joint in the same direction are **synergistic**. Usually, contraction of antagonistic muscles is coordinated by the nervous system so that one muscle relaxes while the other contracts.

---

[1]   The origin of the triceps is the point of attachment nearer the center of the body, or the shoulder, on the opposite side of the biceps attachment.

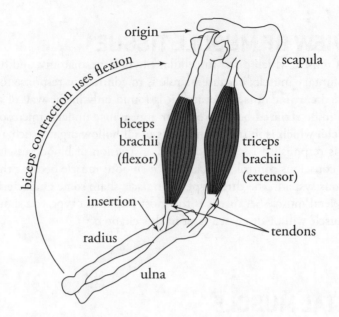

origin

scapula

biceps contraction uses flexion

biceps
brachii
(flexor)

triceps
brachii
(extensor)

insertion

radius

tendons

ulna

Figure 1   Skeletal Muscle

Structure of Skeletal Muscle

Each skeletal muscle is composed not only of muscle tissue, but also of connective tissue that holds the contractile tissue together in bundles called **fascicles** to allow flexibility within the muscle (Figure 2). Looking within each bundle, it is possible to see many fine **muscle fibers** (also called **myofibers**). Each muscle fiber is a single skeletal muscle cell. Skeletal muscle cells are **multinucleate syncytia** formed by the fusion of individual cells during development. They are innervated by a single nerve ending, and stretch the entire length of the muscle. The myofiber has a cell membrane, called the **sarcolemma**, that is made of the plasma membrane and an additional layer of polysaccharide and collagen. This additional layer helps the cell to fuse with tendon fibers. Within each skeletal muscle cell (myofiber) there are many smaller units called **myofibrils**. The myofibril in the muscle cell is like a specialized organelle; it is responsible for the striated appearance of skeletal muscle and generates the contractile force of skeletal muscle.

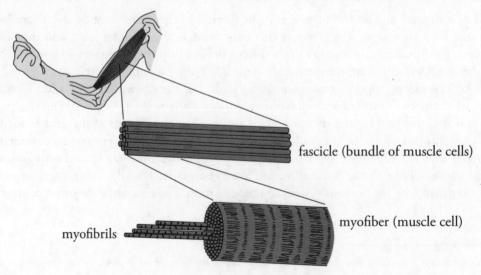

fascicle (bundle of muscle cells)

myofibrils

myofiber (muscle cell)

Figure 2   Levels of Skeletal Muscle Organization

The proteins in the myofibril that generate contraction are polymerized **actin** and **myosin**. Actin polymerizes to form **thin filaments** visible under the microscope, and myosin forms **thick filaments** (Figure 3). The striated appearance of skeletal muscle is due to the overlapping arrangement of bands of thick and thin filaments in **sarcomeres**. A myofibril is composed of many sarcomeres aligned end-to-end. Each sarcomere is bound by two **Z lines**. Thin filaments (actin) attach to each Z line and overlap with thick filaments (myosin) in the middle of each sarcomere; the thick filaments are not attached to the Z lines. The regions of the sarcomere composed only of thin filaments are referred to as the **I bands**. The full length of the thick filament represents the **A band** within each sarcomere; this includes both the overlapping regions of thick and thin filaments (where contraction is generated), as well as the region composed of only thick filaments (this is seen in resting sarcomeres only and is referred to as the **H zone**). See Figure 3.

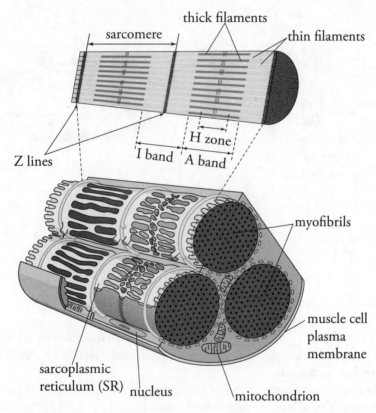

Figure 3 The Sarcomere and a Cross-Section of a Myofiber

Sliding Filament Model of Muscle Contraction

Within each sarcomere, actin and myosin filaments overlap with each other (Figures 3 and 4). Contraction of muscle is achieved by sliding actin and myosin filaments, bringing Z lines of each sarcomere closer together, and shortening the length of the muscle cell. Filament sliding is powered by ATP hydrolysis; myosin is an enzyme that uses ATP energy to create movement. Each myosin monomer contains a head and a tail, and contraction occurs when the angle between the head and tail decreases. Before contraction starts, actin is hidden from myosin by the troponin/tropomyosin complex (which we'll discuss in the next section), and myosin is in a high energy state, ready to contact. Each myosin head is bound to ADP and P_i.

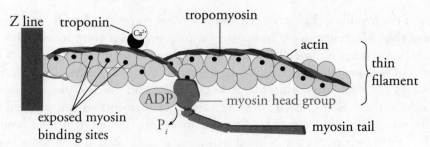

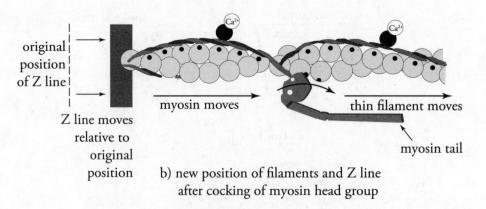

a) original position of filaments and Z line
prior to cocking of myosin head group

b) new position of filaments and Z line
after cocking of myosin head group

Figure 4 Filament Sliding

Filament sliding occurs in four steps:

1. Tropomyosin is shifted off actin by troponin, exposing **myosin-binding sites** on actin. The myosin head attaches to these specific sites on an actin molecule[2] and P_i dissociates. This is called **crossbridge formation**.
2. Myosin heads rotate towards the center of the sarcomere. This is called the **power stroke**. In doing so, the myosin head uses its stored energy and moves to a low-energy conformation. ADP is released. If enough myosin heads do this, Z lines come closer together and the sarcomere shortens; this step effectively completes what we think of as "muscle contraction."[3] Now it is time to reset and get ready for the next round.
3. A new ATP molecule enters. As the myosin head binds ATP, the crossbridge detaches from actin.[4]
4. The myosin head performs ATP hydrolysis immediately and the myosin head is cocked (set in a high-energy conformation, like the hammer of a gun). Myosin is now back to a high energy state (bound to ADP and P_i) and ready for the next round of contraction. The next cycle begins when the myosin head binds to a new binding site on the thin filament.

---

[2] In order for a muscle to contract, its thin and thick filaments must physically interact.

[3] Shortening of a sarcomere means the myofiber to which it belongs shortens as well. Shortening of many sarcomeres within a myofiber means the myofiber undergoes significant reduction in length; this amounts to contraction.

[4] It is very important to remember that binding of a new ATP molecule is necessary for release of actin by the myosin head, not for crossbridge formation or the power stroke.

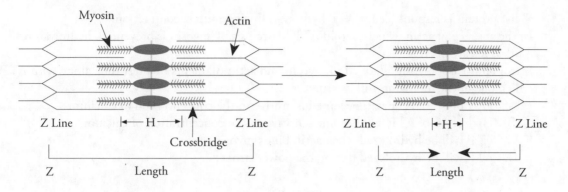

Figure 5 Shortening of Sarcomeres During Contraction

Excitation-Contraction Coupling in Skeletal Muscle

The above four steps in the contractile cycle occur spontaneously. In other words, if you put actin and myosin into a beaker and add ATP and Mg^{2+} (necessary for all reactions involving ATP), ATP will be hydrolyzed, and the filaments will slide past one another. But in the myofiber, contraction occurs only when cytoplasmic $[Ca^{2+}]$ increases. This is because in addition to polymerized actin, the thin filament contains the **troponin-tropomyosin complex** (see Figure 6 below) that prevents contraction when Ca^{2+} is not present. **Tropomyosin** is a long fibrous protein that winds around the actin polymer, blocking all the myosin-binding sites. **Troponin** is a globular protein bound to the tropomyosin that can bind Ca^{2+}. When troponin binds Ca^{2+}, troponin undergoes a conformational change that moves tropomyosin out of the way, so that myosin heads can attach to actin and filament sliding can occur.

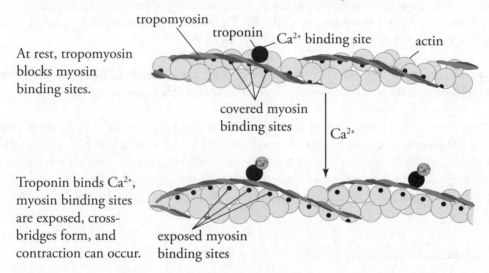

Figure 6 Troponin-Tropomyosin Complex

- What protein is responsible for ATP hydrolysis during muscle contraction?[5]
- In the absence of actin, which step in ATP hydrolysis by myosin is prevented, hydrolysis of ATP or release of ADP?[6]
- If troponin-tropomyosin is added to myosin and actin filaments in a test tube along with ATP, which one of the following will be true?[7]
    A. Hydrolysis of ATP will become insensitive to the concentration of calcium.
    B. Hydrolysis of ATP will become sensitive to the concentration of calcium.
    C. ATP will be hydrolyzed when actin binds myosin.
    D. ATP will be hydrolyzed during the power stroke.

The Neuromuscular Junction and Impulse Transmission

The **neuromuscular junction** (**NMJ**) is the synapse between an axon terminus (synaptic knob) and a myofiber. The NMJ is not a single point, but rather a long trough or invagination (infolding) of the cell membrane; the axon terminus is elongated to fill the long synaptic cleft. The purpose of this arrangement is to allow the neuron to depolarize a large region of the postsynaptic membrane at once. The postsynaptic membrane (the myofiber cell membrane) is known as the **motor end plate**. ACh is the neurotransmitter at the NMJ.

Impulse transmission at the NMJ is typical of chemical synaptic transmission: An action potential (AP) arrives at the axon terminus, triggering the opening of ___ channels; the resulting increase in ___ triggers the ___ of acetylcholine.[8] The postsynaptic membrane contains ACh receptors, which are ligand-gated Na^+ channels. ACh must reach its receptor by diffusing across the synaptic cleft. Binding of ACh to its receptor results in a postsynaptic sodium influx, which depolarizes the postsynaptic membrane. This depolarization is known as an **end-plate potential** (**EPP**). The smallest measurable EPP, caused by exocytosis of a single ACh vesicle, is known as a **miniature EPP** (**MEPP**).

ACh will continue to stimulate postsynaptic receptors until it is destroyed. This is accomplished by the enzyme **acetylcholinesterase**, which hydrolyzes ACh to choline plus an acetyl unit.

As in neurons, summation is required to initiate an AP in the postsynaptic cell. In other words, a single MEPP is insufficient to cause the myofiber to contract. When a sufficient EPP occurs, threshold is reached, and ___ channels open in the postsynaptic membrane.[9] This initiates an AP in the myofiber. The AP is propagated as in neurons, by a continuing wave of voltage-gated sodium channel opening. The shape of this AP on a graph is similar to the shape of the neuronal AP (see Chapter 8).

---

[5] Myosin is the protein with the ATPase activity.

[6] In the absence of actin, myosin can still hydrolyze ATP, but it cannot release ADP after hydrolysis.

[7] Choice **B is correct.** Without troponin-tropomyosin, ATP hydrolysis will begin as soon as ATP, actin, and myosin are mixed. In the presence of troponin-tropomyosin, myosin cannot bind actin, but if calcium is added, the troponin-tropomyosin complex allows binding and ATP hydrolysis can occur once again.

[8] An action potential arrives at the axon terminus, triggering opening of **voltage-gated Ca^{2+} channels**; the resulting increase in **intracellular Ca^{2+}** triggers **release of vesicles** of acetylcholine.

[9] voltage-gated sodium channels

This AP must depolarize the entire myofiber if contraction is to occur. But there is a problem: action potentials occur only at the cell surface, because they are by nature a depolarization of the cell membrane. The myofiber is so thick that an AP on its surface will not depolarize its interior. The solution is to have deep invaginations of the cell membrane, which allow the AP to travel into the thick cell. These deep infoldings are called **transverse tubules** (**T-tubules**).

Another specialized membrane in the myofiber is the **sarcoplasmic reticulum** (**SR**). This is a huge, specialized smooth endoplasmic reticulum, which enfolds each myofibril in the cell (see Figure 3 on page 337). The SR is specialized to sequester and release Ca^{2+}. Active transporters in the SR rapidly remove calcium from the **sarcoplasm** (myofiber cytoplasm). Then, when an AP travels down the T-tubular network, it depolarizes the cell, and with it, the SR. The SR contains voltage-gated Ca^{2+} channels, which allow Ca^{2+} to rush out of the SR into the sarcoplasm upon depolarization. The increase in sarcoplasmic $[Ca^{2+}]$ causes troponin-tropomyosin to change conformation, allowing myosin to bind actin. Actin and myosin fibers slide across each other, and the muscle fiber contracts. When the cell repolarizes, calcium is actively sequestered by the SR, and contraction is ended.

Mechanics of Contraction

The smallest measurable muscle contraction is known as a muscle **twitch**. The nervous system can increase the force of contraction in two ways.

1. **Motor unit recruitment**. A motor unit is a group of myofibers innervated by the branches of a single motor neuron's axon. A muscle twitch results from activation of one motor neuron, and a larger twitch can be obtained by activating ("recruiting") more motor neurons (and thus more myofibers).
2. **Frequency summation**. Each contraction ends when the SR returns the $[Ca^{2+}]$ to low resting levels. If a second contraction occurs rapidly enough, however, there is insufficient time for the Ca^{2+} to be sequestered by the SR, and the second contraction builds on the first.[10] The force of contraction increases. A rapidly repeating series of stimulations results in the strongest possible contraction, known as **tetanus**. This is a normal occurrence which the nervous system uses to obtain strong contractions.[11]

---

[10] A note of clarification: a skeletal muscle action potential has a refractory period as does the neural AP. For frequency summation to occur, the amount of time between successive stimulations must be greater than the duration of the refractory period, but brief enough so that the sarcoplasmic $[Ca^{2+}]$ has not been returned to its low resting level.

[11] Do not confuse this with the disease tetanus, caused by *tetanospasmin*, a bacterial toxin. The disease is an exaggerated, uncontrolled example of the normal process.

- The central nervous system can increase the strength of skeletal muscle contraction by:[12]
    A. increasing the size of action potentials in somatic motor neurons that innervate the muscle.
    B. increasing the number of neurons that innervate each skeletal muscle cell.
    C. increasing the number of motor neurons leading to a muscle that are firing action potentials.
    D. decreasing firing by inhibitory neurons that innervate the skeletal muscle.
    E. increasing firing of inhibitory neurons that innervate opposing muscles.

Energy Requirements for Muscle Contraction

Muscular function requires energy to maintain:

1. Resting potential that allows for depolarization and action potential.
2. Dynamic interaction of myosin and actin that underlies physical shortening of the sarcomere.
3. Return of calcium ions from the sarcoplasm to the SR after contraction is complete.

The myofiber, like most human cells under most conditions, derives its energy most directly by dephosphorylation of ATP into ADP and inorganic phosphate. The muscle cell stores only very small amounts of ATP. In order to sustain its activity, therefore, it must somehow regenerate ATP from ADP and inorganic phosphate, and for that, it needs other energy sources.

Myofibers store (relatively small) amounts of **phosphocreatine**, which, like ATP and GTP, embodies a high-energy phosphate bond. Dephosphorylation of phosphocreatine, therefore, releases energy, which the myofiber uses to regenerate ATP from ADP and inorganic phosphate. Yet, the total amount of ATP and phosphocreatine normally stored within a muscle cell is sufficient to maintain meaningful contraction for only 5 or 10 seconds. For contractile activity that lasts longer, the cell must resort to yet another source of ATP generation.

Muscle cells store glycogen, which is readily broken down into glucose. Glucose then undergoes glycolysis to produce ATP and pyruvate, which, in the presence of an adequate oxygen supply, enters the Krebs cycle, electron transport, and oxidative phosphorylation. Muscle is highly aerobic tissue, with abundant mitochondria. **Myoglobin** is a globular protein and is similar to one of the four subunits of hemoglobin. The role of myoglobin is to provide an oxygen reserve by taking O_2 from hemoglobin and then releasing it as needed.

Where oxygen supply is inadequate to sustain aerobic metabolism, muscle cells resort to anaerobic processes alone (glycolysis and fermentation). **Lactic acid** is produced and moves into the bloodstream, causing a drop in pH. Cramps may result from exhaustion of energy supplies (temporary lack of ATP) in muscle cells. The liver processes lactate and converts it into pyruvate, which can be used in various pathways.

---

[12] Each muscle cell is innervated by a single neuron (eliminate B), and if more neurons fire, more muscle cells will contract; more muscle cells will contract, the greater the total force of contraction (choice **C** is correct). Action potentials are all-or-none events; depolarization is the same size in a given neuron (eliminate A), and there are no inhibitory neurons that innervate the neuromuscular junction. Only acetylcholine, which is excitatory to muscle cells, is released at these synapses (eliminate D and E). (All motor neurons release a constant, small, baseline amount of ACh onto the muscle cell; this provides a baseline level of contraction that we commonly call "muscle tone." To inhibit a muscle, the amount of baseline ACh is reduced.)

Rigor mortis is rigidity of skeletal muscles which occurs soon after death. It results from complete ATP exhaustion; without ATP, myosin heads cannot release actin, and the muscle can neither contract nor relax.

10.4 CARDIAC MUSCLE

We discussed cardiac muscle in Chapter 8; it is found only in the wall of the heart. Cardiac muscle is similar to skeletal muscle in the following ways:

- Like skeletal muscle, cardiac muscle is striated under the microscope and thus contains actin and myosin proteins arranged into sarcomeres.
- T-tubules are present and serve the same function (transmission of APs into the interior of the large, thick cell).
- Sliding filaments and excitation-contraction occur as in skeletal muscle.
- Troponin-tropomyosin regulates contraction in the same way.

Cardiac muscle is different from skeletal muscle in some important ways:

- Cardiac muscle contraction does not depend on stimulation by motor neurons. [If neurons don't trigger cardiac contraction, what does?[13]]
- You have no conscious control over cardiac muscle because it is innervated by the autonomic nervous system. Cardiac muscle operates involuntarily, with the sinoatrial (SA) node acting as the initiator of its rhythmic contractions.
- Cardiac muscle cells are each connected to several neighbors by **intercalated disks**.
- Cardiac muscle cells have one nucleus per cell, but all the muscle cells of the heart are interconnected by gap junctions. This allows action potentials to propagate throughout the entire heart without allowing cells to share nuclei or cytoplasmic contents. Only small items like ions can pass through gap junctions. Heart muscle is thus called a **functional syncytium** because it acts like a syncytium (but isn't really).[14]
- While ACh induces skeletal muscle contraction, this neurotransmitter inhibits depolarization of the SA node and thus decreases the heart rate.

---

[13] Pacing by the sinoatrial node, as discussed in Chapter 8.

[14] Skeletal cells function as a real syncytium because each myofiber (cell) is a tube of cells that fuse during development, end to end. As a consequence, skeletal muscle cells are huge and multinucleate. An action potential will affect the whole cell.

10.5 SMOOTH MUSCLE

Smooth muscle is found in the walls of hollow tubes and hollow organs (such as the stomach, bladder, and uterus). It is responsible for gastrointestinal motility, constriction of blood vessels, uterine contractions, urination, and so on. You have no conscious control over smooth muscle because it is innervated by the autonomic nervous system.

Smooth muscle cells are mononucleate, elongated, and nonstriated. These cells still contain actin and myosin filaments, but they are scattered in a network instead of organized into sarcomeres. Like cardiac muscle, smooth muscle cells are connected by gap junctions so that the action potential is readily and rapidly transmitted from one cell to the next.

Smooth muscle contracts via a mechanism similar to skeletal and cardiac muscle; contraction is triggered by an action potential that releases calcium ions from the sarcoplasmic reticulum. However, smooth muscle cells do not use tropomyosin and troponin to control actin and myosin. Instead, they use a protein called **calmodulin**, which binds calcium.

Feature	Skeletal Muscle	Cardiac Muscle	Smooth Muscle
Location	Attached to skeletal system	Wall of the heart	Walls of all hollow organs
Function	Gross movement	Heart contraction	Tube contraction
Microscopic appearance	Striated with sarcomeres	Striated with sarcomeres	Smooth, no sarcomeres
Cell morphology	• large, cylindrical • multinucleate • not branched	• short • mononucleate • branching fibers	• narrow, short • mononucleate • not branched
T-tubules	Yes	Yes	No
Syncytium	Real syncytium	Functional syncytium; cells are connected via gap junctions	Functional syncytium; cells are connected via gap junctions
Somatic (voluntary) innervation	Stimulated via Ach	None	None
Autonomic (involuntary) innervation	None	Simulated by NE (sympathetic) Inhibited by Ach (parasympathetic, vagal tone)	Yes, via Ach, NE and many others
Hormone influence	None	Epinephrine	Many
Initiation of contraction	Requires input from motor neuron	Autorhythmic (SA node)	Can be autorhythmic
Contraction	↑ in cytoplasmic Ca^{2+} from SR	↑ in cytoplasmic Ca^{2+} from VG Ca^{2+} channels & SR	↑ in cytoplasmic Ca^{2+} from VG Ca^{2+} channels
Contraction regulation	Troponin-tropomyosin complex	Troponin-tropomyosin complex	Calmodulin

Table 1 Comparison of Skeletal, Cardiac, and Smooth Muscle

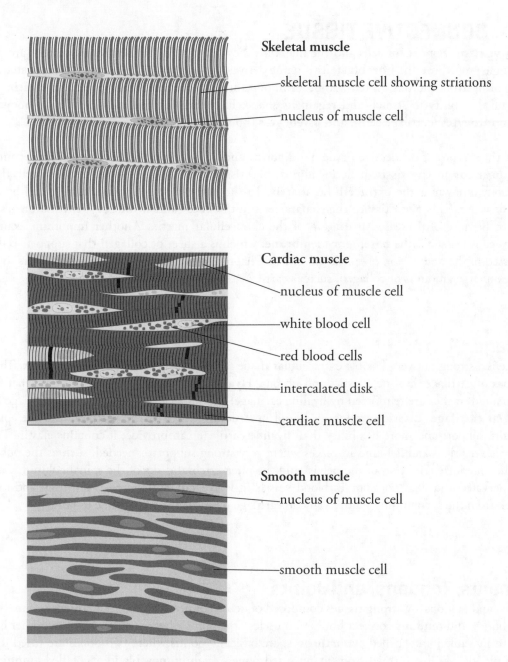

Figure 7 Three Types of Muscle Tissue

10.6   CONNECTIVE TISSUE

Connective tissue consists of cells and the materials they secrete. All connective tissue cells are derived from a single progenitor, the **fibroblast**. This name derives from its ability to secrete fibrous material such as **collagen**, a strong fibrous protein. Another important fibrous extracellular protein is **elastin**, which gives tissue the ability to stretch and regain its shape. Fibroblast-derived cells include **adipocytes** (fat cells), **chondrocytes** (cartilage cells), and **osteocytes** (bone cells).

There are three types of connective tissue: fluid, loose, and dense. Blood and lymph are fluid connective tissues. **Loose connective tissue** includes adipose (fat) tissue and material located between cells throughout the body, known as the **extracellular matrix**. In the body, they are always surrounded by a large amount of water. This gives tissues their characteristic thickness and firmness. Dehydration results in saggy skin because of decreased hydration of the extracellular matrix. Another important example of loose connective tissue is the **basement membrane**, which is a sheet of collagen that supports cell layers (as discussed in the description of epithelial cells in Chapter 9). **Dense connective tissue** refers to tissues that contain large amounts of collagen, such as cartilage tendons, ligaments, and bones.

Cartilage

Cartilage is a strong but very flexible extracellular tissue secreted by cells called **chondrocytes**. There are three types of cartilage: hyaline, elastic, and fibrous. **Hyaline cartilage** is strong and somewhat flexible. The larynx and trachea are reinforced by hyaline cartilage, and joints are lined by hyaline cartilage known as **articular cartilage**. **Elastic cartilage** is found in structures (such as the outer ear and the epiglottis) that require support and more flexibility than hyaline cartilage can provide; it contains elastin. **Fibrous cartilage** is very rigid and is found in places where very strong support is needed, such as the pubic symphysis (the anterior connection of the pelvis) and the intervertebral disks of the spinal column. Cartilage is not innervated and does not contain blood vessels (it is **avascular**). It receives nutrition and immune protection from the surrounding fluid. [Why do cartilage injuries take a long time to heal?[15]]

Ligaments, Tendons, and Joints

Ligaments and tendons are strong tissues composed of dense connective tissue. **Ligaments** connect bones to other bones, and **tendons** connect bones to muscles. The point where one bone meets another is called a **joint**. Immovable joints, called **synarthroses**, are basically points where two bones are fused together. For example, the skull is formed from many fused bones. Slightly movable joints, called **amphiarthroses**, provide both movability and a great deal of support (*amphi-* means "both"). The vertebral joints are an example. Freely movable joints (i.e., most of the joints in the body) are called **diarthroses**. There are several types, for example, ball and socket (hip, shoulder), and hinge (elbow). All movable joints are supported by ligaments.

Movable joints are lubricated by **synovial fluid**, which is kept within the joint by the **synovial capsule**. The surfaces of the two bones that contact each other are perfectly smooth because they are lined by special **articular cartilage** (composed of hyaline cartilage). Like all cartilage, articular cartilage lacks blood vessels. Hence, it is easily damaged by overuse or infection. Inflammation of joints (**arthritis**) leads to destruction of the articular cartilage, which causes pain and stiffness.

---

[15] Cells in cartilage are not directly supplied by blood and have a low rate of metabolism. Thus, they are slow to repair damage. Often damaged cartilage is simply removed or repaired surgically.

10.7 SKELETAL SYSTEM

As vertebrates, we have an **endoskeleton** made of bone[16]. This contrasts with the chitinous **exoskeleton** of arthropods. The vertebrate skeletal system serves five roles:

1. support the body and provide our framework
2. provide an anchor for muscular contraction
3. protect vital organs such as the brain, spinal cord, heart, and lungs
4. store calcium, phosphate, and other important ions
5. synthesize formed elements of the blood (red blood cells, white blood cells, platelets). This occurs in the marrow of flat bones and is called **hematopoiesis**.

The vertebrate endoskeleton is divided into **axial** and **appendicular** components. The axial skeleton consists of the skull, the vertebral column, and the rib cage. All other bones are part of the appendicular skeleton (see Figure 8).

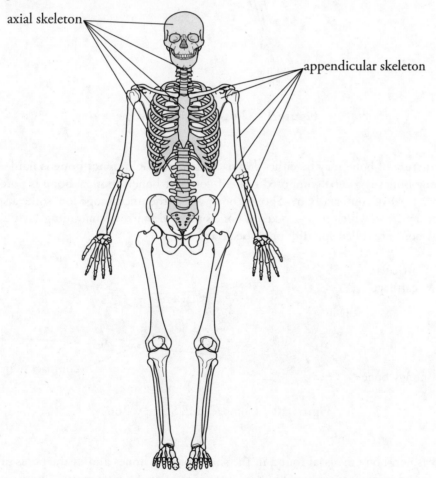

axial skeleton

appendicular skeleton

Figure 8   Axial and Appendicular Skeletons

---

[16] Not all vertebrates have an endoskeleton made of bone. Remember, *Agnatha* (jawless fish) and *Chondrichthyes* (cartilaginous fish) have skeletons primarily composed of cartilage.

Bone Structure

There are two primary bone shapes: **flat** and **long**. Flat bones, such as the scapula, ribs, and bones of the skull, are the location of hematopoiesis and are important for protection of organs. Bones of the limbs are long bones, important for support and movement. The main shaft of a long bone is called the **diaphysis**; the flared end is called the **epiphysis**.

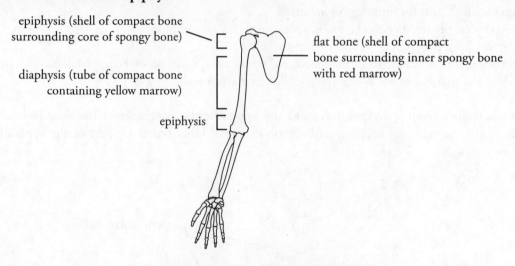

epiphysis (shell of compact bone surrounding core of spongy bone)

flat bone (shell of compact bone surrounding inner spongy bone with red marrow)

diaphysis (tube of compact bone containing yellow marrow)

epiphysis

Figure 9 Gross Anatomy of Bone

The general structure of bone may be either compact or spongy. **Compact bone** is hard and dense. The diaphysis of long bones is a tube composed only of compact bone. **Spongy bone** is porous and always surrounded by a layer of compact bone. Spongy bone under the microscope looks like a sponge. It has a disorganized structure in which many spikes of bone surround marrow-containing cavities. The spikes of bone in spongy bone are called **spicules** or **trabeculae**.

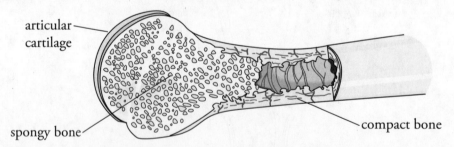

articular cartilage

spongy bone

compact bone

Figure 10 Compact and Spongy Bone

Bone marrow is non-bony material found in the shafts of long bones and in the pores of spongy bones. **Red marrow**, found in spongy bone within flat bones, is the site of hematopoiesis. Its activity increases in response to erythropoietin, a hormone made by the kidney. **Yellow marrow**, found in the shafts of long bones, is filled with fat and is inactive.

Compact bone has a specific organization (Figure 11). The basic unit of compact bone structure is the **osteon** (sometimes referred to as a **Haversian system**). In the center of the osteon is a hole called the **central** (or **Haversian**) **canal**, which contains blood, lymph vessels, and nerves. Surrounding the canal

10.7

are concentric rings of bone termed **lamellae** (which just means "sheets" or "layers"). Tiny channels, or **canaliculi**, branch out from the central canal to spaces called **lacunae** ("lakes"). In each lacuna is an **osteocyte**, or mature bone cell. Osteocytes have long processes which extend down the canaliculi to contact other osteocytes through gap junctions. This allows the cells to exchange nutrients and waste through an otherwise impermeable membrane. **Perforating** (or **Volkmann's**) **canals** are channels that run perpendicular to central canals to connect osteons.

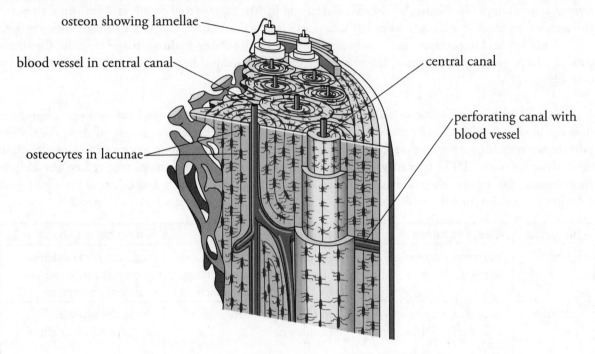

Figure 11   Microscopic Structure of Compact Bone

Bone Cells, Growth, and Remodeling

Bone is a dynamic connective tissue composed principally of matrix and cells. The matrix is made of **hydroxyapatite** (a crystalline compound of calcium and phosphorous), ions, collagen, and additional proteins. Bone contains three different cell types:

- **Osteoblasts** are located on the inner surfaces of bone tissue. They synthesize collagen and other organic components of the matrix.
- **Osteocytes** occupy minute spaces (**lacunae**) within the bony matrix and function to maintain the matrix.
- **Osteoclasts** promote ongoing breakdown, resorption, and remodeling of bone.

Overall, both osteoblasts and osteocytes build and nourish bone, while osteoclasts break bone down.

Growth of long bones proceeds as follows: During childhood, a structure called the **epiphyseal plate** is seen between the diaphysis and the epiphysis. The epiphyseal plate is a disk of hyaline cartilage that is actively being produced by chondrocytes. As the chondrocytes divide, the epiphysis and diaphysis are forced apart. Then the cartilage is replaced by bone (ossified). This process is stimulated by growth hormone, and the rate of ossification is slightly faster than the rate of chondrocyte cell division (cartilage growth). Thus, at about the age of 18, the diaphysis and epiphyses meet and fuse together, and lengthening can no longer occur. This "fusion of the epiphyses" is easily observed in X-rays and can be used to notify adolescents when they have stopped growing taller. In adults, the fusion point is referred to as the **epiphyseal line**.

During adulthood, bones do not elongate. However, bone is continually degraded and remade in a process termed **remodeling**. Osteoblasts lay down collagen and hydroxyapatite and synthesize bone until they are surrounded by bone. The space they're left inhabiting is called a lacuna, and the osteoblast differentiates into an **osteocyte**. **Osteoclasts** continually destroy bone by dissolving hydroxyapatite crystals. The osteoclast is a large phagocytic cousin of the macrophage. Bone destroyed by osteoclasts must be replaced by osteoblasts.

An increased ratio of osteoclast to osteoblast activity results in the liberation of calcium and phosphate into the bloodstream (and a decreased ratio has the opposite effect). Hence, activity of these cells is important not only for bone structure, but also for maintenance of proper blood levels of calcium and phosphate. The hormones **PTH (parathyroid hormone)**, **calcitonin**, and **calcitriol** (derived by the kidney from vitamin D) regulate their activity and thus blood calcium levels. PTH and calcitriol increase blood calcium, and calcitonin reduces it. The specific effects of these hormones are listed in Table 2.

Hormone	Effect on bones	Effect on kidneys	Effect on intestines
PTH	stimulates osteoclast activity	increases reabsorption of calcium, stimulates conversion of vitamin D into calcitriol	indirectly (via calcitriol) increases intestinal calcium absorption
calcitriol	may stimulate osteoclast activity, but minor effect	increases reabsorption of phosphorus	increases intestinal absorption of calcium
calcitonin	inhibits osteoclast activity	decreases reabsorption of calcium	n/a

Table 2   Hormonal Control of Calcium Homeostasis

10.8   INTEGUMENTARY SYSTEM

The integumentary system (or skin) is the largest organ in the body, by size and by weight (Figure 12). Its role is to protect us from pathogens, to prevent excessive evaporation of water, and to regulate body temperature. The outermost layer of the skin is called the **epidermis**; it lies upon the deeper **dermis**, which rests on **subcutaneous tissue** or **hypodermis**. The hypodermis is a protective, insulating layer of fat (adipose tissue).

The epidermis is composed of stratified (many layers of) squamous epithelial cells. These cells are constantly sloughed off and then replenished by mitosis of cells at the deepest part of the epidermis, the **stratum basale**. A cell in this layer divides, and one of the resulting daughter cells moves outward. Soon this cell will die and be pushed farther and farther outward by continued mitosis below, until it flakes away from the surface of the body. The significance of many layers of epithelial cells is that they provide a strong protective structure.

Another important facet of the stratified squamous cells of the epidermis is that they are **keratinized**. This means that as they die, they become filled with a thick coating of the tough, hydrophobic protein **keratin**. Keratin helps make the skin waterproof.

Epidermal epithelial cells also contain **melanin**. This is a brown pigment, produced by specialized cells in the epidermis termed **melanocytes**, that helps absorb the ultraviolet light of the sun to prevent damage to underlying tissues.

Beneath the epidermis lies the **dermis**. The dermis consists of various cell-types embedded in a connective tissue matrix. It contains blood vessels that nourish both the dermis and the epidermis (the epidermis has no blood vessels of its own). The dermis also contains **sensory receptors**, which convey information about touch, pressure, pain, and temperature to the central nervous system. Also found in the dermis are **sudoriferous** (sweat) glands, **sebaceous** (oil) glands, and **hair follicles**. Hairs consist of dead epithelial cells bound tightly together. Some specialized regions of skin contain **ceruminous** (wax) glands (e.g., the external ear canal).

10.8

The sudoriferous gland is composed of a tube-like structure that originates in the dermis and leads through the epidermis to a pore on the surface of the skin. The purpose of sweat is to allow loss of excess heat by evaporation. Sweat contains water, electrolytes, and urea. **Sweat glands** are responsive to aldosterone. People living in hot climates must sweat a lot. In order to conserve sodium, they have a high level of aldosterone, and thus their sweat does not waste salt.

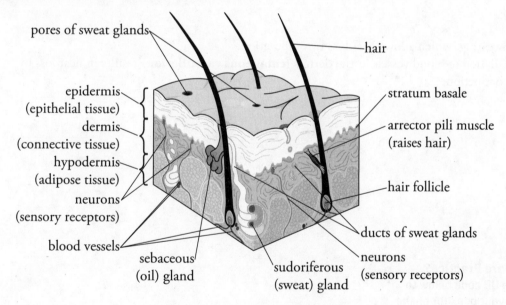

Figure 12 Skin Layers

Temperature Regulation by the Skin

Humans are **homeotherms**, meaning their body temperature is relatively constant. Heat is generated by metabolic processes and muscle contraction. Some homeotherms (e.g., bears) can increase their temperature by burning special fat called **brown adipose tissue**; this process is called **chemical thermogenesis** or **non-shivering thermogenesis**. But this is *not* an important mechanism of temperature regulation in adult humans. Also, while it is true that an increased level of thyroid hormone can increase the metabolic rate and thus increase body temperature, this mechanism takes several weeks to kick in and is not thought to be important in day-to-day temperature regulation. So, practically, only four strategies are available to cope with cold weather:

1. Contraction of skeletal muscles produces heat, whether it is involuntary (shivering) or voluntary (jumping up and down).
2. The skin insulates us so that we conserve heat generated by metabolism. Subcutaneous (beneath the skin) tissue contains a layer of insulating fat, which helps.
3. Heat loss by conduction is minimized by constriction of blood vessels in the dermis (**cutaneous vasoconstriction**). Cutaneous vasoconstriction occurs in response to cold weather or upon activation of the sympathetic nervous system. This is why the skin becomes cold and pale when one is frightened.
4. Contrivances such as clothing and blankets help us conserve heat.

A mechanism for dissipation of excess heat is also necessary. This is accomplished by two mechanisms in the skin:

1. Sweating, which allows heat loss by evaporation.
2. Dilation of blood vessels in the dermis (**cutaneous vasodilation**) results in heat loss by conduction.

Want More Practice?
Scan the QR code below to register your book for online chapter summaries, drills, practice tests, and more!

Chapter 11 Structure and Function of Systems: Reproduction and Development

11.1 METHODS OF REPRODUCTION

Organisms can either reproduce asexually or sexually. **Asexual reproduction** is a mode of reproduction where offspring arise from a single parent, and inherit the genes of that parent only. As a consequence, there is no variation in genetic material and the offspring are genetically identical to the parent. Asexual reproduction may have short-term benefits when rapid population growth is important, or in stable environments. Asexual reproduction is common in each of the major domains/kingdoms. For example, bacteria and Archaea domains reproduce asexually via **binary fission** (see Chapter 7). Many protists, plants and fungi reproduce asexually as well. Most multicellular organisms (fungi, plants and animals) can perform sexual reproduction.

There are six common modes of asexual reproduction:

- **Fission**: the parent organism is replaced by two daughter organisms by dividing in two. The two daughter cells are usually approximately equal in size. This is common in bacteria, Archaea, protists and some unicellular fungi (yeasts).
- **Budding**: a small daughter cell/organism buds off a larger mother cell/organism. The bud grows into a fully mature organism and breaks off from the parent. This can occur in unicellular organisms such as budding yeast (also called baker's yeast or *Saccharomyces cerevisiae*) and in multicellular organisms such as the *Hydra*.
- **Vegetative Reproduction**: when a new plant is formed without the production of seeds or spores. For example, a new strawberry plant can grow from a runner attached to a parent plant.
- **Spore Formation**: many organisms (all plants, most protists and most fungi) produce spores. Some spores are resistant to harsh conditions, and so are a survival mechanism for organisms when growing conditions are not ideal. When spores germinate, they grow into multicellular individuals without a fertilization event. **Sporogenesis** can involve **meiosis** (when the ploidy number is lower in the spore compared to the parent organism) or **mitosis** (where the parent and the spore have the same genetic content). Plants typically perform **meiotic sporogenesis** (where a diploid parent plant generates haploid spores) and fungi typically perform **mitotic sporogenesis** (where the parent and the spore are both haploid).
- **Fragmentation**: when a new organism grows from a fragment of the parent (note that this is different from regeneration, see below). Each fragment develops into a mature, fully grown individual. Fragmentation is seen in many organisms such as animals (some annelid worms and sea stars), fungi, and plants. Some plants have specialized structures for reproduction via fragmentation, such as gemmae in liverworts. Most lichens, which are a symbiotic union of a fungus and photosynthetic algae or bacteria, reproduce through fragmentation to ensure that new individuals contain both symbionts.
- **Parthenogenesis**: a type of **agamogenesis** (reproduction that does not involve a male gamete), where an unfertilized egg develops into a new individual. Parthenogenesis occurs naturally in many plants, invertebrates (such as rotifers and some insects), and vertebrates (including some reptiles, amphibians, fish, and very rarely birds).

Regeneration is commonly mistaken as asexual reproduction, but is not a mode of reproduction. This is a wound healing mechanism, where lost tissues, organs or limbs can be regrown in an organism. For example, sea stars can regrow lost arms, geckos can regenerate tails, humans can regenerate liver tissue, and the planarian flatworm can regenerate just about anything.

Sexual reproduction increases genetic variation in individuals, because each offspring inherits genetic information from two parents. Genetic diversity allows adaptation to changing environments. Plants use both spores and gametes in sexual reproduction, because they perform alternation of generations. Fungi typically use sexual spores. Animals reproduce sexually via gametes. Each of these will be discussed more below.

Sexual reproduction via gametes requires two processes:

1. Genetic ploidy is decreased via meiosis, and haploid (n) gametes are generated.
2. Gametes join during fertilization, restoring the ploidy of the organism to diploid ($2n$).

11.2 DEVELOPMENT OF REPRODUCTIVE SYSTEMS

What processes in a human being involve meiosis? Only one: **gametogenesis**. This is the process whereby **diploid germ cells** undergo **meiotic division** to produce **haploid gametes**. As discussed in Chapter 6, meiotic cell division fosters genetic diversity in the population (by independent assortment of genes and by recombination). The gametes produced by a male are known as **spermatozoa**, or **sperm**; females produce **ova**, or **eggs**. The role of the sperm is to swim through the female genital tract to reach the egg and fuse with it. This fusion is known as **syngamy**, and it results in a **zygote**. The gametes produced by males and females differ dramatically in structure but contribute equally to the genome of the zygote. [There are two exceptions to this.[1]] Although both gametes contribute equally to the nuclear genome, the egg provides *every other part of the zygote*, since the only part of the sperm which enters the egg is a haploid genome. This leads to **maternal inheritance** of certain traits, specifically for genes located in the mitochondrial genome.

The sex of a developing embryo is determined by its sex chromosomes, either **XX** in females or **XY** in males. During the early weeks of development, however, male and female embryos are indistinguishable. Early embryos, whether male or female, have undifferentiated gonads, and possess both **Wolffian ducts** that can develop into male internal genitalia (epididymis, seminal vesicles, and ductus deferens) and **Müllerian ducts** that can develop into female internal genitalia (uterine tubes, uterus, and vagina). In the absence of a Y chromosome, Müllerian duct development occurs by default, and female internal genitalia result. Female external genitalia (labia, clitoris) are also the default but are not derived from Müllerian ducts. Genetic information on the Y chromosome of XY embryos leads to the development of testes, which cause male internal and external genitalia to develop by producing testosterone and **Müllerian inhibiting factor** (**MIF**).

MIF is produced by the testes and causes regression of the Müllerian ducts; this prevents development of female internal genitalia. Testosterone secretion by cells, which will later give rise to the testes, begins around week 7 of gestation. By week 9, testes are formed, and their interstitial cells supply testosterone. The testosterone that is responsible for the development of male external genitalia enters the systemic circulation and must be converted to **dihydrotestosterone** in target tissues in order to exert its effect (Figure 1).

---

[1] One exception is that an egg always contributes an X chromosome, while a sperm can contribute an X or a Y chromosome. Remember, X and Y chromosomes are very different in size. The other exception is the mitochondrial genome. While sperm and egg contribute roughly equally to the *nuclear* genome, every human inherits their mitochondrial genome from their mother.

- If an XY genotype embryo fails to secrete testosterone, will it have testes or ovaries?[2]

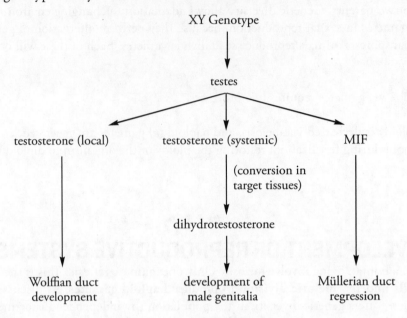

Figure 1   Reproductive System Development

- Which of the following would best characterize an embryo with an XY genotype that lacks the receptor for testosterone?[3]
  A.   Testes, ductus deferens, and seminal vesicles are present; external genitalia are female.
  B.   Ovaries, uterine tubes, and uterus are present; external genitalia are female.
  C   Testes are present; external genitalia are female; neither Müllerian nor Wolffian ducts develop.
  D.   Testes and male external genitalia are present.

The development of the male and female reproductive systems is closely related. As described above, the three main fetal precursors of the reproductive organs are the Wolffian ducts, the Müllerian ducts, and the gonads. While the Wolffian ducts are the precursors of internal male genitalia, they essentially disappear in the female reproductive system. For the Müllerian ducts, this process is reversed; they essentially disappear in the male reproductive system and form the internal genitalia of the female system. Structures arising from these ducts tend to have the same function (e.g., **ductus deferens** in males and the **uterine tubes** in females both carry gametes), but because they arise from different precursors, they are considered to be **analogous structures**.

In both sexes, the **gonads** go on to form either the testes or the ovaries; because they are derived from the same undeveloped structure, testes and ovaries are considered homologous organs. There are a number of other homologous structures in males and females due to their common origins within the fetus (see Table 1). We'll discuss these organs in more detail in the following sections.

---

[2]   Testosterone is *produced by* the embryonic testes. Their development does not depend on testosterone. Hence, an XY embryo which didn't secrete testosterone would most likely have testes nonetheless.

[3]   An XY genotype would lead to development of testes (eliminate B), and testes would produce MIF and testosterone. MIF would cause degeneration of the Müllerian ducts, and no female internal genitalia would develop. However, the inability to respond to testosterone (because of the missing receptor) would prevent development of the Wolffian ducts (eliminate A) as well as the male external genitalia (eliminate D). External genitalia would default to female (choice **C** is correct).

Male Organ	Female Organ	Function
Testis	Ovary	Gamete and hormone reproduction
Penis	Clitoris	Erectile tissue, sensation
Bulbourethral glands	Greater vestibular glands	Lubrication
Scrotum	Labia majora	External skin folds

Table 1 Homologous Reproductive Structures

11.3   ANDROGENS AND ESTROGENS

All hormones involved in development and maintenance of biologically male characteristics are termed **androgens**, while those involved in development and maintenance of biologically female characteristics are termed **estrogens**. The primary androgen produced in the testes is testosterone. It is converted into dihydrotestosterone within the cells of target tissues. The primary estrogen produced in the ovaries is estradiol.

Testosterone is required for embryonic development of male internal and external genitalia and spermatogenesis. After birth the level of testosterone falls to negligible levels until puberty, at which time it increases and remains high for the remainder of adult life. Elevated levels of testosterone are responsible for development and maintenance of biologically male **secondary sexual characteristics** (maturation of genitalia, male distribution of facial and body hair, deepening of the voice, increased muscle mass). The pubertal growth spurt and fusion of the epiphyses also result.

The roles of estrogen in females are analogous to the roles of testosterone in a male. Beginning at puberty, estrogen is required to regulate the uterine cycle and for development and maintenance of biologically female secondary sexual characteristics (maturation of genitalia, breast development, wider hips, pubic hair). Estrogen causes the fusion of the epiphyses in females.

During puberty and adult life, sex steroid production is controlled by the **hypothalamus** and the anterior pituitary. **Gonadotropin releasing hormone (GnRH)** from the hypothalamus stimulates the pituitary to release the gonadotropins, follicle-stimulating hormone (FSH) and luteinizing hormone (LH).[4] In men, LH acts on interstitial (or Leydig) cells to stimulate testosterone production, and FSH stimulates the sustentacular (or Sertoli) cells. In women, FSH stimulates the granulosa cells to secrete estrogen, and LH simulates formation of the corpus luteum and progesterone secretion.[5] Feedback inhibition by the steroids inhibits the production of GnRH and LH and FSH. Inhibin, produced by sustentacular cells and the granulosa cells, provides further feedback regulation of FSH production (see Figure 2 on the following page).

---

[4]   Remember, GnRH, FSH, and LH are all peptide hormones.

[5]   Don't worry! We'll be looking at all these structures and processes in this chapter. We suggest you review this whole chapter and then come back and read this section again.

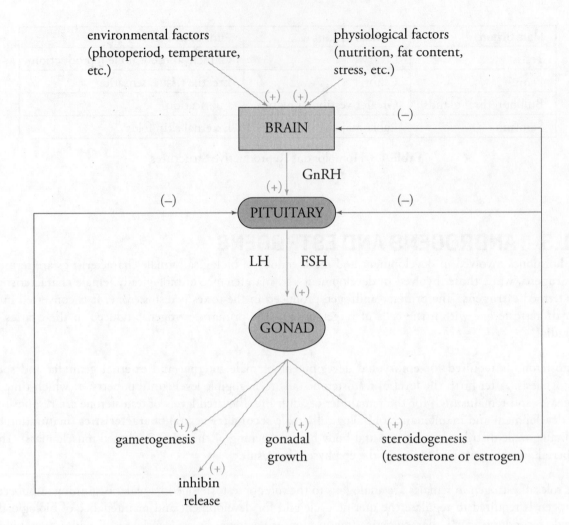

Figure 2 Regulation of Sex Steroid Production

11.4 HUMAN PHYSIOLOGY: MALE REPRODUCTIVE SYSTEM

Anatomy

The principal male reproductive structures visible on the outside of the body are the scrotum and the penis. The **scrotum** is essentially a bag of skin containing the male gonads, which are known as **testes** (testicles). [Does the scrotum have any active role, or is it merely a container?[6]] The testes have two roles: (1) synthesis of sperm (**spermatogenesis**), and (2) secretion of male sex hormones (**androgens**, e.g., testosterone) into the bloodstream. We're going to start our review of this system by tracing the path of a sperm from its origination to its final destination.

---

6 The scrotum is important for temperature regulation. Sperm synthesis in the testes must occur at a few degrees below normal body temperature. This is why the testes are located outside the body. Relaxation of the scrotum facilitates cooling of the testes. When the environment is cold, the scrotum contracts, pulling the testes up against the body, warming them.

The sites of spermatogenesis within the testes are the **seminiferous tubules**. The walls of seminiferous tubules are formed by cells called **sustentacular cells** (also known as **Sertoli cells**). Sustentacular cells protect and nurture developing sperm, both physically and chemically; their role will be discussed in more detail below. The tissue between the seminiferous tubules is referred to as testicular interstitium.[7] Important cells found in the testicular interstitium are **interstitial cells** (also known as **Leydig cells**). They are responsible for androgen (testosterone) synthesis.

Seminiferous tubules empty into the **epididymis**, a long coiled tube located on the posterior (back) of each testicle (see Figure 3). The epididymis from each testicle empties into a **vas deferens** (also call the **ductus deferens**), which in turn leads to the **urethra** (the tube inside the penis). To get to the urethra, the vas deferens leaves the scrotum and enters the **inguinal canal**, a tunnel that travels along the body wall toward the crest of the hip bone.[8] Next, the vas deferens enters the pelvic cavity. Near the back of the urinary bladder, it joins the duct of the seminal vesicle (discussed below) to form the **ejaculatory duct**. Ejaculatory ducts from both sides of the body then join the urethra.

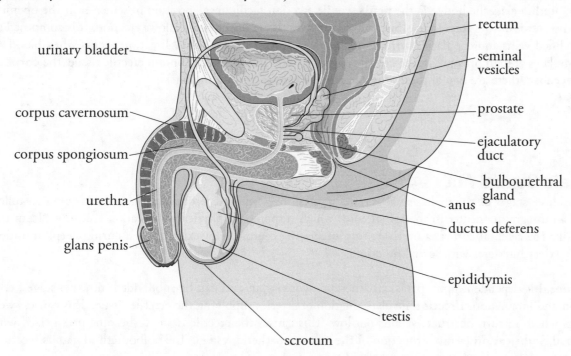

Figure 3   Male Reproductive System

A pair of glands known as **seminal vesicles** is located on the posterior surface of the bladder. They secrete about 60 percent of the total volume of the **semen** into the ejaculatory duct. Semen is a highly nourishing fluid for sperm and is produced by three separate glands: seminal vesicles, **prostate**, and **bulbourethral glands**. These are collectively referred to as the **accessory glands** (see Table 2). The ejaculatory duct empties into the **urethra** as it passes through the prostate gland. One final set of glands, the bulbourethral glands, contributes to the semen near the beginning of the urethra.

---

[7]   Interstitium is a term used to describe a thing or a region that is "between" other structures.

[8]   There are two inguinal canals: left and right.

11.4

Gland	Secretions	Function of secretions	% of total ejaculate volume
Seminal vesicles	Mostly fructose	Nourishment of sperm	60%
Prostate gland	Fructose and a coagulant	Nourishment, allows semen to coagulate after ejaculation	35%
Bulbourethral glands	Thick, alkaline mucus	Lubricate urethra, neutralize acids in male urethra and in female vagina	3%
Testes	Sperm	Male gamete	2%

Table 2 Accessory Glands

The urethra exits the body via the **penis**. Penile erection facilitates deposition of semen near the opening of the uterus during intercourse. Specialized **erectile tissue** in the penis allows erection. It is composed of modified veins and capillaries surrounded by a connective tissue sheath. Erection occurs when blood accumulates at high pressure in the erectile tissue. Three compartments contain erectile tissue: the **corpora cavernosa** (there are two of these) and the **corpus spongiosum** (only one).

Male Sexual Act

The three stages of the male sexual act are: arousal, orgasm, and resolution. These events are controlled by an integrating center in the spinal cord, which responds to physical stimulation and input from the brain. The cerebral cortex can activate this integrating center (as in sexual arousal during sleep) or inhibit it (anxiety interferes with sexual function).

Arousal is dependent upon parasympathetic nervous input and can be subdivided into two stages: erection and lubrication. **Erection** involves dilation of arteries supplying the erectile tissue. This causes swelling, which in turn obstructs venous outflow. This causes the erectile tissue to become pressurized with blood. **Lubrication** is also a function of the parasympathetic system. The bulbourethral glands secrete a viscous mucous which serves as a lubricant.

Stimulation by the sympathetic nervous system is required for **orgasm**, which can also be divided into two stages: emission and ejaculation. **Emission** refers to propulsion of sperm (from the vas deferens) and semen (from accessory glands) into the urethra by contractions of smooth muscle surrounding these organs. Emission is followed by **ejaculation**, in which semen is propelled out of the urethra by rhythmic contractions of muscles surrounding the base of the penis. Ejaculation is actually a reflex reaction caused by the presence of semen in the urethra. Emission and ejaculation together constitute the male orgasm.

Resolution, or a return to a normal, unstimulated state, is also controlled by the sympathetic nervous system. It is caused primarily by a constriction of the erectile arteries. This results in decreased blood flow to the erectile tissue and allows the veins to carry away the trapped blood, returning the penis to a flaccid state. This typically takes 2–3 minutes.

- Name four glands that contribute to semen.[9]
- Which components of the male sexual act can occur if all sympathetic activity is blocked?[10]
- What is the difference between emission and ejaculation?[11]

Spermatogenesis

Sperm synthesis is called **spermatogenesis** (Figure 4). It begins at puberty and occurs in the testes throughout adult life. [Do females also make gametes throughout adult life?[12]] Seminiferous tubules are the site of spermatogenesis. The entire process of spermatogenesis occurs with the aid of specialized sustentacular cells found in the wall of the seminiferous tubule. Immature sperm precursors are found near the outer wall of the tubule, and nearly-mature spermatozoa are deposited into the lumen; from there they are transported to the epididymis. The cells that give rise to **spermatogonia** (and to their female counterparts, oogonia) are known as **germ cells**; under the right conditions, they *germ*inate, and give rise to a complete organism.

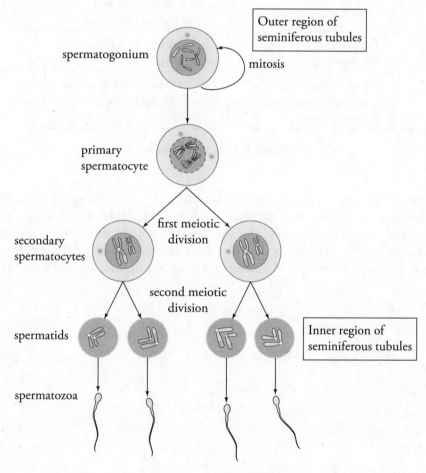

Figure 4   Spermatogenesis

---

[9] Seminal vesicles, prostate, testes, and bulbourethral glands

[10] Erection and lubrication (arousal only)

[11] Emission is the movement of sperm and semen components into the urethra; ejaculation is the movement of semen from the urethra out of the body.

[12] No. This is discussed in the next section.

Table 3 below gives the names of the sperm precursors, along with the meiotic role of each stage, and some mnemonic comments. Fill in the female version when you read that section.

Stage	Jobs	Mnemonic	Female version
spermatogonium	1. Mitotically reproduce prior to meiosis 2. Replicate DNA in S phase of meiosis	The spermatoGONium is GONNA become a sperm.	
primary spermatocyte	Meiosis I	Any gamete precursor (male or female) with "cyte" undergoes a meiotic division. The *primary* spermatoCYTE undergoes the *first* meiotic division.	
secondary spermatocyte	Meiosis II	The *secondary* spermatoCYTE undergoes the *second* meiotic division.	
spermatid	Turn into a spermatozoan	The spermatid's a kid, almost mature	
spermatozoan	Finish maturing in the 1. seminiferous tubule 2. epididymis	Remember a mature sperm is called a spermatozoan.	

Table 3 Gametogenesis

As noted in Table 3, the final stages of sperm maturation occur in the epididymis. When they first enter the epididymis, spermatozoa are incapable of motility. Many days later, when they reach the ductus deferens, they are fully capable of motility. But they remain inactive due to the presence of inhibitory substances secreted by the ductus deferens. This inactivity causes sperm to have a very low metabolic rate, which allows them to conserve energy and thus remain fertile during storage in the ductus deferens for as long as a month.

- Do spermatogonia divide by mitosis or by meiosis?[13]
- How many mature sperm result from a single spermatogonium after it becomes committed to meiosis?[14]
- Which of the following statements is/are true?[15]
   - I. During gametogenesis, sister chromatids remain paired with each other until anaphase of the second meiotic cell division.
   - II. A difference between mitosis and meiosis is that mitosis requires DNA replication prior to cell division but meiosis does not.
   - III. Recombination between sister chromatids during gametogenesis increases the genetic diversity of offspring.

Spermatids develop into spermatozoa in the seminiferous tubules with the aid of sustentacular cells. The DNA condenses, the cytoplasm shrinks, and the cell shape changes so that there is a **head**, containing the haploid nucleus and the acrosome, and a flagellum, which forms the **tail**. There is also a **neck** region at the base of the tail, which contains many mitochondria. The **acrosome** is a compartment on the head of the sperm that contains hydrolytic enzymes required for penetration of the ovum's protective layers. **Bindin** is a protein on the sperm's surface that attaches to receptors on the zona pellucida surrounding the ovum.

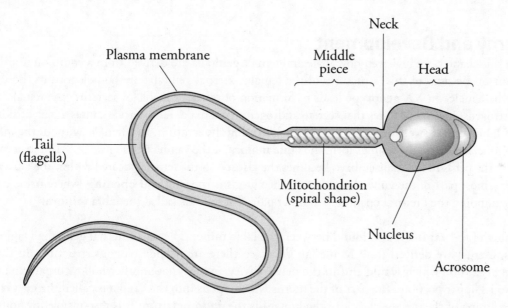

Figure 5   Spermatozoa

---

[13] Mitosis. Spermatogonia undergo the meiotic S phase (replicate the genome), but the stages which undergo the actual meiotic *divisions* are called spermatocytes. All gamete precursors with "cyte" in their names undergo a meiotic division.

[14] Four haploid cells result from the reductive division (meiosis) of one diploid spermatogonium. Compare this to oogenesis, which we're talking about soon.

[15] **Statement I is true.** Meiosis I involves the pairing, recombination, and separation of homologous chromosomes. Meiosis II is like mitosis, in which sister chromatids separate. **Statement II is false.** Both require DNA replication in a preceding S phase. **Statement III is false.** Sister chromatids don't recombine; homologous chromosomes do. Even if sister chromatids did recombine, it would make no difference since they are identical.

Hormonal Control of Spermatogenesis

Testosterone plays the essential role of stimulating division of spermatogonia. **Luteinizing hormone (LH)** stimulates the interstitial cells to secrete testosterone. **Follicle stimulating hormone (FSH)** stimulates the sustentacular cells. The hormone **inhibin** is secreted by sustentacular cells; its role is to inhibit FSH release.

11.5

- Which of the following is/are true?[16]
  I. Luteinizing hormone reaches its target tissue through the hypothalamic-hypophysial portal system.
  II. The absence of luteinizing hormone does not affect spermatogenesis.
  III. Increased testosterone levels in the blood decrease the production of follicle stimulating hormone.

11.5 HUMAN PHYSIOLOGY: FEMALE REPRODUCTIVE SYSTEM

Anatomy and Development

Earlier in this chapter, we reviewed how male and female genitalia are derived from a common undifferentiated precursor. Because of this, structures of the female external genitalia are homologous to those of the male. In the female, an **XX genotype** leads to formation of ovaries capable of secreting the female sex hormones (estrogens) instead of testes that secrete androgens. In a male, testosterone causes a pair of skin folds known as **labioscrotal swellings** to grow and fuse, forming the scrotum. In a female, without the influence of testosterone, labioscrotal swellings form the **labia majora** of the vagina (see Figure 6).[17] The structure that gave rise to the penis in the male embryo becomes the **clitoris** in the female, located within the labia majora in the uppermost part of the vulva. Just beneath the clitoris is the **urethral opening**, where urine exits the body. Surrounding the urethral opening is another pair of skin folds called the **labia minora**.

The opening of the **vagina** is also found between the labia minora. Female internal genitalia (vagina, uterine tubes, uterus) are derived from Müllerian ducts, so there are no homologous structures in the male. The vagina is a tube which would end in the pelvic cavity, except that another hollow organ, the **uterus**, opens into its upper portion. The part of the uterus which opens into the vagina is called the **cervix**[18]. The innermost lining of the uterus (closest to the lumen) is the **endometrium**. It is responsible for nourishing a developing embryo, and in the absence of **pregnancy** it is shed each month, producing menstrual bleeding. Surrounding the endometrium is the **myometrium**, which is a thick layer of smooth muscle comprising the wall of the uterus. The uterus ends in two **uterine tubes** (also called **fallopian tubes**), which extend into the pelvis on either side. Each uterine tube ends in a bunch of finger-like structures called **fimbriae**. The fimbriae brush up against the **ovary**, which is the female gonad. [At the time of ovulation, where does the oocyte come from and where does it go?[19]]

---

[16] **Statement I is false.** LH is secreted by the anterior pituitary and reaches its targets via systemic circulation. GnRH reaches its target via the portal system. **Statement II is false.** LH is necessary because it stimulates interstitial cells to secrete testosterone, which is necessary for germ cell stimulation. **Statement III is true.** Testosterone, estrogen, progesterone, and inhibin are all hormones, which exert feedback inhibition upon the anterior pituitary and hypothalamus.

[17] labia = lips, majora = larger

[18] "neck," as in "cervical"

[19] It emerges from the ovary (sometimes causing pain in the middle of the menstrual cycle) and must be swept into the uterine tube by a constant flow of fluid into the uterine tube caused by cilia.

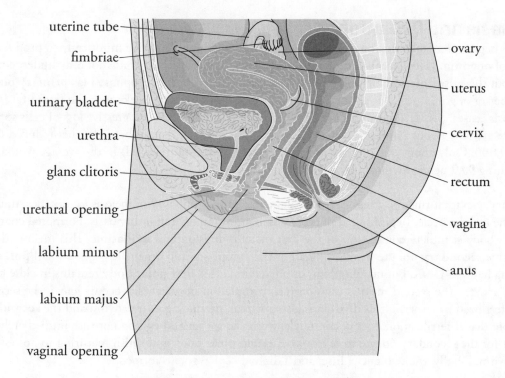

Figure 6   Female Reproductive System

- What is the fate of the Wolffian ducts and their derivatives in the female?[20]
- Is estrogen production by the ovaries required for the development of the uterine tubes and uterus?[21]

Female Sexual Act

The stages of the female sexual act are the same as in the male: **arousal**, **orgasm**, and **resolution**. The arousal stage, as in the male, is subdivided into erection and lubrication and is controlled by the parasympathetic nervous system. The clitoris and labia minora contain erectile tissue and become engorged with blood, just as in the male. Lubrication is provided by mucus secreted by **greater vestibular glands** (also called **Bartholin glands**) and by vaginal epithelium. Orgasm in the female is controlled by the sympathetic nervous system and involves muscle contractions, just as in the male, in addition to a widening of the cervix. These events are thought to facilitate the movement of sperm into the uterus. The female does not experience ejaculation. Resolution is also the same as in the male, controlled by the sympathetic system, but can take up to 20–30 minutes (compared to 2–3 minutes in the male).

---

[20] In the absence of testosterone, they atrophy.

[21] No, the Müllerian ducts develop into vagina, uterus, and uterine tubes by default as long as MIF is absent.

Oogenesis and Ovulation

Oogenesis begins prenatally. In the ovary of a female fetus, germ cells divide mitotically to produce large numbers of **oogonia**. [How is this different from the male scenario?[22]] Oogonia not only undergo mitosis *in utero*, but they also enter the first phase of meiosis and are arrested in prophase I (as **primary oocytes**). The number of oogonia peaks at about 7 million at mid-gestation (20 weeks into the fetal life). At this time mitosis ceases, conversion to primary oocytes begins, and there is a progressive loss of cells so that at birth there are only about 2 million primary oocytes. By puberty this number is further reduced to only about 400,000. Only about 400 oocytes are ever actually **ovulated** (released) in the average woman, and the remaining 99.9 percent will simply degenerate.

The primary oocytes formed in a female fetus can be frozen in prophase I of meiosis for decades, until they re-enter the meiotic cycle. Beginning at puberty and continuing on a monthly basis, hormonal changes in a woman's body stimulate completion of the first meiotic division and **ovulation**. This meiotic division yields a large **secondary oocyte** (containing all of the cytoplasm and organelles) and a small **polar body** (containing half the DNA, but no cytoplasm or organelles). This **first polar body** remains in close proximity to the oocyte. The second meiotic division (i.e., completion of oogenesis) occurs *only if* the secondary oocyte is fertilized by a sperm; this division is also unequal, producing a large ovum and the **second polar body**. Note that if fertilization does occur, nuclei from the sperm and egg do not fuse immediately. They must wait for the secondary oocyte to release the second polar body and finish maturing to an ootid and then an ovum. Finally, the two nuclei fuse, and a diploid (2n) zygote is formed.

- Is the secondary oocyte haploid?[23]
- When an oogonium undergoes meiosis, three cells result. How many of these are eggs, and why do only three cells result? When a spermatogonium undergoes meiosis, how many cells result?[24]

Before we move on to a discussion of the menstrual cycle, you will need more background information on oogenesis. The primary oocyte is not an isolated cell. It is found in a clump, surrounded by supporting cells called **granulosa cells**. The entire structure (oocyte plus granulosa cells) is known as a **follicle**. Granulosa cells assist in maturation. An immature primary oocyte is surrounded by a single layer of granulosa cells, forming a **primordial follicle**.

As a primordial follicle matures, granulosa cells proliferate to form several layers around the oocyte, and the oocyte itself forms a protective layer of mucopolysaccharides termed the **zona pellucida**. There may be several follicles in the ovary; they are surrounded and separated by cells termed **thecal cells**. Of the several maturing follicles, only one progresses to the point of ovulation each month; all others degenerate. The mature follicle is known as a **Graafian follicle**. During ovulation, the Graafian follicle bursts, releasing the secondary oocyte with its zona pellucida and protective granulosa cells into the fallopian tube. At this point the layer of granulosa cells surrounding the ovum is known as the **corona radiata**. The follicular cells remaining in the ovary after ovulation form a new structure called the **corpus luteum** (Figure 7).

---

[22] It only happens in *adult* males. Here, we're talking about events in the ovaries of a female while she's still in her mother's womb.

[23] Yes. After the first meiotic division, cell is haploid; the homologous chromosomes have been separated. They are, however, still replicated, hence the reason for meiosis II.

[24] Only one egg results. The three cells which result are two polar bodies plus one ovum. There are only three because the first polar body does not divide. In meiosis in the male, both cells derived from the first meiotic division go on to divide. Therefore, meiosis results in four cells in a male.

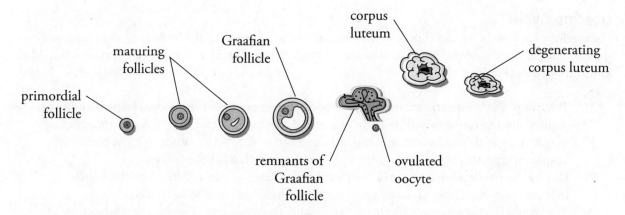

Figure 7 Fate of a Follicle

Estrogen is made and secreted by the granulosa cells (with help from the thecal cells) during the first half of the menstrual cycle. Both estrogen and progesterone are secreted by the corpus luteum during the second half of the cycle. Estrogen is a steroid hormone that plays an important role in the development of female secondary sexual characteristics, in the menstrual cycle, and during pregnancy. **Progesterone** is also a steroid hormone involved in the hormonal regulation of the menstrual cycle and pregnancy, but with different effects than estrogen.

The Menstrual Cycle

The **menstrual cycle** is (on average) a 28-day cycle that includes events occurring in the ovary (called the **ovarian cycle**), as well as events occurring in the uterus (referred to as the **uterine cycle**).

Ovarian Cycle

The ovarian cycle can be subdivided into three phases (see Figure 8 in a few pages):

1. During the **follicular phase**, a **primary follicle** matures and secretes estrogen. Rising estrogen levels have a positive feedback effect on granulosa cells, encouraging them to make even more estrogen. Maturation of the follicle is under the control of follicle stimulating hormone (FSH) from the anterior pituitary. The follicular phase lasts about 13 days.
2. In the **ovulatory phase**, a secondary oocyte is released from the ovary. This is triggered by a surge of luteinizing hormone (LH) from the anterior pituitary. The surge also causes the remnants of the follicle to become the corpus luteum. Ovulation typically occurs on day 14 of the cycle.
3. The **luteal phase** begins with full formation of the corpus luteum in the ovary. This structure secretes both estrogen and progesterone, and has a life span of about two weeks. The average length of the luteal phase is about 14 days.

The hormones secreted from the ovary during the ovarian cycle direct the uterine cycle.

Uterine Cycle

The uterine cycle covers the same 28 days that were discussed above, but the focus is on the preparation of the endometrium for potential **implantation** of a fertilized egg. The uterine cycle can also be subdivided into three phases (Figure 8):

1. The first phase is **menstruation**, triggered by the degeneration of the corpus luteum and subsequent drop in estrogen and progesterone levels. The sharp decrease in these hormones causes the previous cycle's endometrial lining to slough out of the uterus, producing the bleeding associated with this time period. Menstruation typically lasts about 5 days.
2. During the **proliferative phase** of the menstrual cycle, estrogen produced by the follicle induces the proliferation of a new endometrium. This phase lasts about 9 days.
3. After ovulation the **secretory phase** occurs, in which estrogen and progesterone produced by the corpus luteum further increase development of the endometrium, including secretion of glycogen, lipids, and other material. If pregnancy does not occur, death of the corpus luteum and decline in the secretion of estrogen and progesterone trigger menstruation once again. The secretory phase typically lasts about 14 days.

The menstrual cycle repeats every 28 days from puberty until **menopause** (at about age 50–60).

- At what stage of development is the endometrium when ovulation occurs?[25]
- Where is the secondary oocyte during the secretory phase?[26]

---

[25] The endometrium is at the proliferative phase, under the influence of ovarian estrogen.

[26] The secondary oocyte is traveling down the uterine tube toward the uterus. If it fails to implant in the uterus, the secretory phase ends and menstruation begins.

11.5

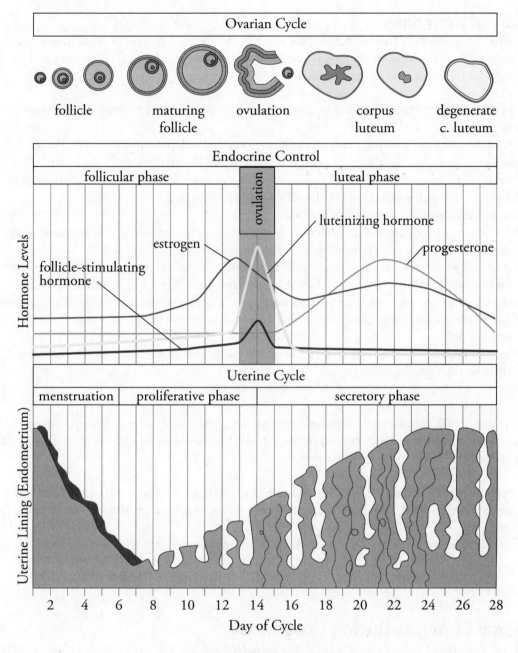

Figure 8 Menstrual Cycle

Summary of Hormones

The anterior pituitary and the hypothalamus play a role in the menstrual cycle by regulating the secretion of estrogen and progesterone from the ovary (see Figure 8 on the previous page). Estrogen and progesterone then regulate the events in the uterus. The following is a summary:

- GnRH from the hypothalamus stimulates the release of FSH and LH from the anterior pituitary.
- Under the influence of FSH, granulosa and thecal cells develop during the follicular phase and secrete estrogen. Secretion of GnRH, FSH, and LH is initially inhibited by estrogen; however, estrogen, which increases throughout the follicular stage, reaches a threshold near the end of this phase and has a positive effect on LH secretion.
- This sudden surge in LH causes ovulation.
- After ovulation, LH induces the follicle to become the corpus luteum and to secrete estrogen and progesterone (this marks the beginning of the secretory phase).
- If pregnancy does not occur, the combined high levels of estrogen and progesterone send feedback to strongly inhibit secretion of GnRH, FSH, and LH. When LH secretion drops, the corpus luteum regresses, no longer secretes estrogen or progesterone, and menstruation occurs.
- If LH levels remained high, how would this affect the secretion of estrogen and progesterone?[27]
- What would happen if the estrogen and progesterone levels in a woman's blood were kept artificially high for the entire month?[28]
- What would happen if the artificial hormones were suddenly taken away?[29]

Most birth control pills contain two hormones: estrogen and progestin (these are not necessarily the same as the hormones that are naturally secreted in the female, but have similar chemistry, so similar effects). The birth control pill works by doing three things:

1. Decreasing gonadotropin release, which inhibits ovulation since there will be no LH surge
2. Thickening the cervical mucus, making it harder for the sperm to get through to the fallopian tubes
3. Changing the composition of the endometrial wall, making it uninhabitable for a fertilized egg

Hormonal Changes During Pregnancy

There are still a couple of points we have not made completely clear: how can pregnancy occur if the uterine lining is lost each month, and why does the body discard the endometrium?

---

[27] If LH levels remained high, the corpus luteum would not regress, and estrogen and progesterone would also remain high, thus maintaining the endometrium so that menstruation would not occur. This is in effect what happens if an embryo is fertilized and implants, except the hormone in this case is not LH but hCG, human chorionic gonadotropin, an LH-like hormone (see the next section).

[28] The woman would not ovulate. That's what (most) birth control pills are: estrogen and progesterone.

[29] The endometrium would slough off, and the woman would menstruate. This is why there are 21 pills of one color and 7 pills of another color in most birth control pills. The 7 pills contain no hormones; they are either placebos or sometimes iron supplements. If a woman took the hormone pill every day and never took the 7 placebos, she would not menstruate. Also, the placebos are actually unnecessary; these 7 pills are only present in order to help establish the habit of taking a pill every day.

Recall the physiological reason for endometrial shedding is a decrease in estrogen and progesterone levels, which occurs as the corpus luteum degenerates. Why does the corpus luteum degenerate? Due to a decrease in luteinizing hormone. Why does LH decrease? Due to feedback inhibition from the high levels of estrogen and progesterone secreted by the corpus luteum.

Let's begin with why LH levels decrease. During pregnancy, ovulation should be prevented. This is achieved by constant high levels of estrogen and progesterone seen during pregnancy to inhibit secretion of LH by the pituitary; no LH surge, no ovulation. Constant high levels of estrogen inhibit LH release. The result is pregnancy without continued ovulation. The *secondary* result is the one we were trying to explain: when the corpus luteum secretes a lot of estrogen and progesterone during the menstrual cycle, LH levels drop, causing the corpus luteum to degenerate. The point is that the corpus luteum degenerates unless fertilization has occurred.

So how can pregnancy occur? If pregnancy is to occur, the endometrium must be maintained, because it is the site of gestation (i.e., where the embryo lives and is nourished). If fertilization takes place, within a few days a developing embryo becomes **implanted** in the endometrium, and a **placenta** begins to develop. The **chorion** is the portion of the placenta that is derived from the zygote. It secretes **human chorionic gonadotropin**, or **hCG,** which can take the place of LH in maintaining the corpus luteum. In the presence of hCG, the corpus luteum does not degenerate, estrogen and progesterone levels stay elevated, and menstruation does not occur. This answers the question of *how* pregnancy can occur. hCG is the hormone tested for in pregnancy tests because its presence confirms the presence of an embryo.

- Which of the following occur(s) during the menstrual cycle immediately prior to ovulation?[30]
  - I. A surge in luteinizing hormone release from the anterior pituitary
  - II. Completion of the second meiotic cell division by the oocyte
  - III. Shedding of the endometrium

- Which of the following statements concerning the menstrual cycle is/are true?[31]
  - I. The proliferative phase of the endometrium coincides with maturation of ovarian follicles.
  - II. The secretory phase of the endometrial cycle is dependent on secretion of estrogen from cells surrounding secondary oocytes.
  - III. Luteinizing hormone levels are highest during the menstrual phase of the endometrial cycle.

---

[30] **Statement I is true**. The LH surge *causes* ovulation. **Statement II is false**. Meiosis I is completed prior to ovulation. Meiosis II isn't completed until after fertilization. **Statement III is false**. Ovulation occurs around day 14 of the cycle. Menstruation begins at day 1.

[31] **Statement I is true**. Go back and review this section if you're unclear here. **Statement II is false**. It is secretion of estrogen and progesterone *by the corpus luteum* that drives the secretory phase. The corpus luteum is in the ovary, while the secondary oocyte is out in the uterine tube. **Statement III is false**. The luteinizing hormone level peaks during the proliferative phase, since this is when ovulation occurs.

11.6 DEVELOPMENT AND EMBRYOLOGY

Fertilization

Many animals perform sexual reproduction. Fertilization can occur internally or externally. In mammals, **internal fertilization** takes place inside the female after insemination through copulation. In other vertebrates (most reptiles, most birds, and some fish) fertilization occurs internally after **cloacal contact** (the **cloaca** is the posterior opening for intestinal, reproductive, and urinary tracts of some animal species).

In **external fertilization,** sperm and egg cells are joined outside the bodies of the reproducing individuals. Since sperm are more mobile in aqueous environments, many species use water to help with external fertilization. For example, many plants make use of external fertilization, especially ones without bright flowers or other means of attracting animals. In many aquatic animals (such as coral or hydra), eggs and sperm are simultaneously shed into the water, and sperm swim through water to fertilize the egg. In many fish species (including salmon) the female will deposit unfertilized eggs and the male will swim by and fertilize them.

In humans, a secondary oocyte is ovulated and enters the uterine tube. It is surrounded by the **corona radiata** (a protective layer of granulosa cells) and the **zona pellucida** (located just outside the egg cell membrane). The oocyte will remain fertile for about a day. If intercourse occurs, sperm are deposited near the cervix, and are activated, or **capacitated**. Sperm capacitation involves the dilution of inhibitory substances present in semen. Activated sperm will survive for two or three days. They swim through the uterus toward the secondary oocyte.

Fertilization is the fusion of a spermatozoan with the secondary oocyte (see Figure 9). It normally occurs in the uterine tube. In order for fertilization to occur, a sperm must penetrate the corona radiata and bind to and penetrate the zona pellucida. It accomplishes this using the **acrosome reaction**. The **acrosome** is a large vesicle in the sperm head containing hydrolytic enzymes which are released by exocytosis. After the corona radiata has been penetrated, an **acrosomal process** containing actin elongates toward the zona pellucida. The acrosomal process has **bindin**, a species-specific protein which binds to receptors in the zona pellucida. Finally, the sperm and egg plasma membranes fuse, and the sperm nucleus enters the secondary oocyte. In about 20 minutes, the secondary oocyte completes meiosis II, giving rise to an ootid and the second polar body. The ootid matures rapidly, becoming an **ovum**. Then the sperm and egg nuclei fuse, and the new diploid cell is known as a **zygote**.

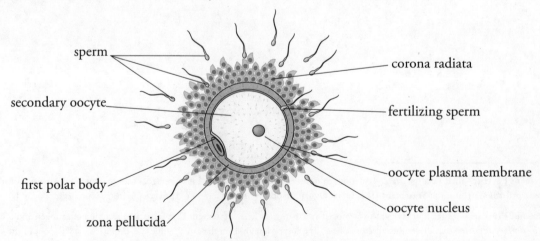

Figure 9 Fertilization

- Because of a particular disease, a man produces sperm without acrosomes. His spermatozoa are abnormal in that they:[32]
    - A. are immotile.
    - B. cannot undergo capacitation.
    - C. are incapable of fertilizing the egg.
    - D. can fertilize the eggs of many species.

Many changes occur after fertilization, to block penetration of an ovum by more than one sperm. In the **fast block** phase, the egg plasma membrane depolarizes. This prevents other spermatozoa from fusing with the egg cell membrane. The **slow block** (or **cortical reaction**) is due to Ca^{2+} release from the smooth ER. It causes the space between the zona pellucida and the plasma membrane to increase, the zona pellucida to harden, as well as egg activation (increased metabolism and protein synthesis). In other animals, post-fertilization events differ slightly. For example, in the sea urchin, vesicles migrate and fuse with the egg plasma membrane to increase the amount of plasma membrane in the egg, and a hard fertilization coat is formed.

Cleavage

The process of **embryogenesis** begins within hours of fertilization, but proceeds slowly in humans. The first stage is **cleavage**, in which the zygote undergoes many cell divisions to produce a ball of cells known as the **morula** (see Figure 10). The first cell division occurs about 36 hours after fertilization. The morula is the same size as the zygote, which indicates that the dividing cells spend most of their time in the S (synthesis) and M (mitotic phases), skipping the G_1 and G_2 (gap or growth phases).

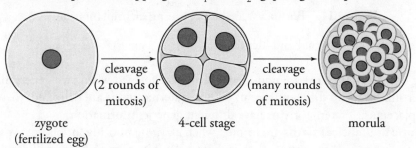

zygote
(fertilized egg)

cleavage
(2 rounds of
mitosis)

4-cell stage

cleavage
(many rounds
of mitosis)

morula

Figure 10   Cleavage

---

[32] Acrosomal enzymes are necessary for penetration of the corona radiata, and the acrosomal process is necessary for binding to and penetration of the zona pellucida. Sperm that lack an acrosome would be unable to complete these processes, which are necessary for fertilization (eliminate D, choice **C** is correct). The acrosome has nothing to do with motility (motility is the flagella's job; eliminate A), and capacitation is the activation of sperm in the female reproductive tract. It has nothing to do with the acrosome (eliminate choice B).

Blastulation

As cell divisions continue, the morula is transformed into a **blastocyst** (Figure 11). This process is known as **blastulation**. The blastocyst consists of a ring of cells called the **trophoblast** surrounding a cavity, and an **inner cell mass** adhering to the inside of the trophoblast at one end of the cavity. The **trophoblast** will give rise to the **chorion** (the zygote's contribution to the placenta). The inner cell mass will become the **embryo,** as well as some additional structures discussed below.

- If two inner cell masses form in the blastula, what will the result be?[33]

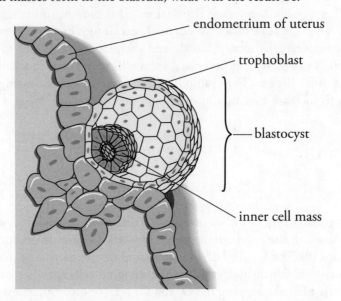

Figure 11   Blastocyst at the Beginning of Implantation

There are two kinds of twins: fraternal and identical.

- **Dizygotic** or **fraternal twins** are non-identical and are formed when two genetically different eggs are fertilized by two different sperm. When fraternal twins are delivered, there are typically two placentas. Fraternal twins have different genetic information.
- **Monozygotic** or **identical twins** are formed when a zygote, morula, or blastocyst splits into two separate embryos. If the cell mass splits before day five, two embryos will develop with separate placentas and separate amniotic sacs; this occurs about 2/3 of the time. After day five, splitting leads to two amniotic sacs but one placenta; this occurs about 1/3 of the time. Identical twins have identical genomic sequences.

Genetic mosaicism occurs when a genetic change (such as a mutation or genetic variation) occurs in one developing cell but not others. This change will be passed onto daughter cells. This leads to two or more populations of cells with different genotypes in one individual, who has developed from a single fertilized egg.

Genetic chimeras are formed when multiple fertilized eggs fuse. This leads to the development of a single organism composed of cells from different zygotes.

---

[33] The inner cell mass becomes the embryo. Two inner cell masses derived from a single zygote and enclosed by the same trophoblast will result in a pair of identical twins sharing the same placenta.

Implantation, Eggs, and the Placenta

The embryo is not the only important structure derived from the inner cell mass. There are three others: amnion, yolk sac, and allantois. The **amnion** surrounds a fluid-filled cavity which contains the developing embryo. **Amniotic fluid** is the "water" which "breaks" (is expelled) before humans give birth. The **yolk sac** is important in reptiles and birds because it contains the nourishing **yolk**. Mammals do not store yolk. Our yolk sac is important because it is the first site of red blood cell synthesis in the embryo. Finally, the **allantois** develops from the embryonic gut and forms the blood vessels of the **umbilical cord**, which transport blood between embryo and placenta in vertebrates that use a placenta.

- Each of the following has the same genome EXCEPT:[34]
  A. Chorion
  B. Amnion
  C. Yolk sac
  D. Endometrium

Some animals (birds, reptiles and mammals) evolved an amniotic egg, which allowed terrestrial vertebrates to sever ties with aquatic life. These organisms—called **amniotes**—can reproduce using a shell-encased amniotic egg, or the embryo and amniotic fluid can implant into the maternal uterus.

Animals can also be categorized by how they use eggs in reproduction. **Oviparous** animals lay eggs and there is little to no development of offspring in the mother. Animals that use internal fertilization lay shelled eggs, while animals that perform external fertilization lay eggs without shells. Most fish, most amphibians, most reptiles and all birds are oviparous. There are a few species of oviparous mammals, specifically **monotremes**, which include a few species of spiny anteaters as well as the platypus.

Ovoviviparous animals perform internal fertilization; the egg develops inside the mother to provide gas exchange, and then offspring are born alive. Some fish, some amphibians and some reptiles are ovoviviparous. **Marsupials** (mammals such as kangaroos and possums) are ovoviviparous.

Viviparous animals perform internal fertilization and do not use eggs. Instead, a placenta is used in development and offspring are born alive. All development occurs inside the mother and the placenta provides gas exchange. Very few fish, amphibians and reptiles, but most mammals (including us) are viviparous.

In humans, the developing blastocyst travels from the fallopian tube (the site of fertilization, cleavage and blastulation) to the uterus between 6 and 9 days after fertilization. It reaches the uterus and burrows into the endometrium, or implants, about a week after fertilization (Figure 11). The trophoblast secretes proteases that lyse endometrial cells. The blastocyst then sinks into the endometrium and is surrounded by it, absorbing nutrients through the trophoblast into the inner cell mass. The embryo receives a large part of its nutrition in this manner for the first few weeks of pregnancy. This is why the secretory phase of the **endometrial cycle** occurs: endometrial cells store glycogen, lipids, and other nutrients so that the early embryo may derive nourishment directly from the endometrium. Later, an organ develops which is specialized to facilitate exchange of nutrients, gases, and even antibodies between the maternal and embryonic bloodstreams: the placenta. Because it takes about three months for the placenta to develop, it is during the first trimester (three months) of pregnancy that hCG is essential for maintenance of the endometrium.

---

[34] The chorion, amnion, and yolk sac are all derived from the inner cell mass of the blastula, and therefore must have the same genome (eliminate A, B, and C). However, the endometrium is derived from the mother (it is the inner lining of the uterus), and would have a different genome than the embryo (choice **D** is correct).

- What happens if the corpus luteum is removed during the first trimester?[35]

During the last six months of pregnancy, the corpus luteum is no longer needed because the placenta itself secretes sufficient estrogen and progesterone for maintenance of the endometrium. Development of the placenta involves formation of placental villi. These are chorionic projections extending into the endometrium, into which fetal capillaries will grow. Surrounding the villi are sinuses (open spaces) filled with maternal blood.

- Does oxygen-containing blood pass from the mother into the developing fetus?[36]

Post-Implantation Development

We have examined embryogenesis from fertilization through blastulation. The next phase is **gastrulation** (Figure 12), when the **primary germ layers** (**ectoderm**, **mesoderm**, and **endoderm**) become distinct.

Animals with radial symmetry (animals in the phylum *Cnidaria*) undergo gastrulation differently from animals with bilateral symmetry. The radial animals develop only two germ layers, whereas bilateral animals develop three. Cnidarians are thus referred to as **diploblastic**, and all other animals are **triploblastic**. [Which two germ layers do jellyfish and hydra possess?[37]]

In primitive organisms, the **blastula** (equivalent to the blastocyst in humans) is a hollow ball of cells, and gastrulation involves the **invagination** (involution) of these cells to form layers. Imagine pushing your fist into a big soft round balloon to create an inner layer (contacting your fist) and an outer layer (contacting the air). The inner layer is the endoderm, and the outer layer is the ectoderm. The mesoderm (middle layer) develops from the endoderm. The cavity (where your fist is) is the primitive gut, or **archenteron**. The opening (where your wrist is) is the **blastopore**, and will give rise to the mouth or the anus. The whole structure is called the **gastrula**. Don't get confused: the gastrula has a blastopore; the blastula has no opening.

---

[35] The woman menstruates, and the embryo is lost. Remember, the role of hCG is to substitute for LH in stimulating the corpus luteum. The role of the corpus luteum is to make estrogen and progesterone, which maintain the endometrium.

[36] No. The placenta is like a lung in that it facilitates exchange of substances between the two bloodstreams without allowing actual mixing.

[37] Jellyfish and hydra possess ectoderm and endoderm. The ectoderm develops into structures such as the epidermis and nervous tissue; the endoderm develops into more internal structures (such as the gut and glands). Remember that in animals with three germ layers (triploblastic animals), the mesoderm develops from the endoderm.

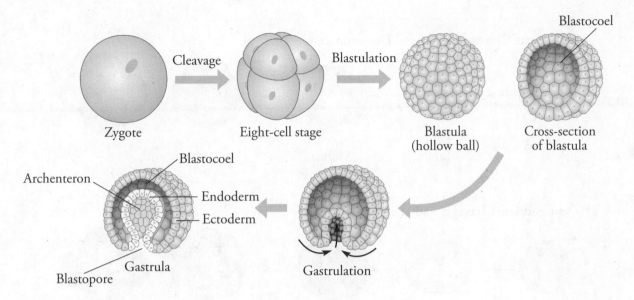

Figure 12   Gastrulation

Coelomates (animals with a body cavity) can be divided into two distinct lines of evolution: **protostomes** and **deuterostomes**, depending on how they perform gastrulation. When the blastocyst invaginates to produce the archenteron and blastopore, a second opening forms later to complete the digestive tube. One opening will become the mouth and the other will become the anus. "Stoma" refers to "mouth," and "proto" to "first," so protostomes develop a mouth from the first opening (blastopore) and an anus from the second opening. "Deutero" means "second," and in deuterostomes, the mouth develops from the second opening and the anus from the blastopore. Annelids, mollusks, and arthropods are protostomes, while echinoderms and chordates are deuterostomes. Roundworms are also protostomes, even though they are pseudocoelomates instead of coelomates.

Protostomes and deuterostomes also perform cleavage differently. Cleavage in protostomes is spiral and determinate. Spiral means that cell divisions become unequal early on in morula formation, resulting in some small and some large cells. In **spiral cleavage**, planes of cell division lie diagonal to the embryo's vertical axis, with the result being that smaller cells lie in grooves between larger cells. **Determinate** means that cell fate is decided upon early on. In contrast, deuterostomes perform radial and **indeterminate cleavage**. This means that cell divisions stay equal for a longer period of time. In **radial cleavage**, the planes of cell division align with the vertical axis either in parallel or perpendicularly, with the result that cells align on top of one another. Cells stay the same size as each other and retain totipotency (see section 11.7). [What might be the result if the cells of a deuterostome embryo were separated very early in their development?[38]]

---

[38] Each cell would go on to form a complete, normal animal. It is this property that makes it possible for identical twins to exist.

Protostome Cleavage: Spiral and Determinate

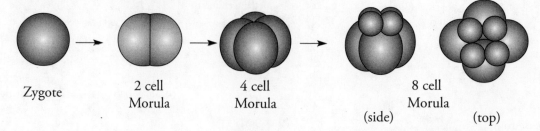

Zygote | 2 cell Morula | 4 cell Morula | 8 cell Morula (side) (top)

Deuterostome Cleavage: Radial and Indeterminate

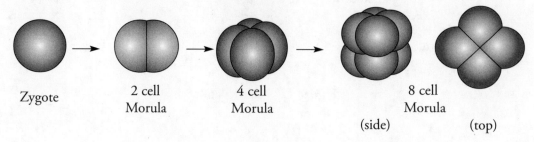

Zygote | 2 cell Morula | 4 cell Morula | 8 cell Morula (side) (top)

Figure 13 Cleavage in Protostomes and Deuterostomes

	Protostomes	**Deuterostomes**
Example animals	Annelids, mollusks, arthropods, roundworms	Echinoderms, chordates
Fate of first opening (blastopore)	Becomes mouth	Becomes anus
Fate of second opening	Becomes anus	Becomes mouth
Cleavage	Spiral and determinate	Radial and indeterminate

Table 4 Protostomes vs. Deuterostomes

In humans, things are a little different. The gastrula develops from a double layer of cells called the **embryonic disk**, instead of from a spherical blastula. But the end result is the same: three layers. You need to know what parts of the human body are derived from each layer:

Ectoderm	**Mesoderm**	**Endoderm**
• Entire nervous system • Pituitary gland (both lobes), adrenal medulla • Cornea and lens • Epidermis of skin and derivatives (hair, nails, sweat glands, sensory receptors) • Nasal, oral, anal epithelium	• All muscle, bone, and connective tissue • Entire cardiovascular and lymphatic system, including blood • Urogenital organs (kidneys, ureters, gonads, reproductive ducts) • Dermis of skin	• GI tract epithelium (except mouth and anus) • GI glands (liver, pancreas, etc.) • Respiratory epithelium • Epithelial lining of urogenital organs and ducts • Urinary bladder

Table 5 Fates of the Primary Germ Layers

Pay attention to what *types* of things are derived from each layer. One key thing to note is that **ectoderm** and *epithelium* are not synonymous. Epithelium outside the body (epidermis) is derived from ectoderm, but epithelium inside the body (gut lining) comes from endoderm.

In humans, the next step after gastrulation is **neurulation**, formation of the nervous system. It proceeds by invagination and pinching off of a layer of ectoderm along the dorsum (back) of the embryo to form the **dorsal neural groove**. This gives rise to the **neural tube**, which gives rise to the brain and spinal cord. Formation of the neural tube is induced by instructions from the underlying notochord, which is mesodermal in origin. It gives rise to the vertebral column. Other ectodermal cells migrate through the body to form peripheral nervous system ganglia.

Neurulation is one component of **organogenesis**, development of organ systems. By the eighth week of gestation, all major organ systems are present, and the **embryo** is now called a **fetus**. Even though the developmental process has attained staggering complexity, by the end of the first trimester the fetus is still only 5 cm long.

11.7

- During which trimester is the developing human most sensitive to toxins such as drugs and radiation?[39]
- A radioactive dye is detected only in the cells of placental villi. Weeks earlier, it must have been injected into the:[40]
  - A. inner cell mass.
  - B. trophoblast.
  - C. endometrium.
  - D. zygote.
- During gastrulation, do tissues derived from the trophoblast move inward to form the lining of the primitive gut?[41]

11.7 DIFFERENTIATION

The specialization of cell types during development is termed **differentiation** because as cells specialize, they become different from their parent cells and from each other. By specializing, a cell becomes better able to perform a particular task, while becoming less adept at other tasks. For example, a sensory neuron is the best vehicle for the transmission of a nerve impulse over great distances, but is quite incapable of obtaining nourishment on its own, or even of reproducing itself.

---

[39] During the first trimester, when the organs are being formed.

[40] The placenta is derived from the chorion, which is derived from the cells of the trophoblast, thus injecting a dye into the trophoblast would lead to its detection in the placental villi (choice **B** is correct). The inner cell mass ultimately becomes the embryo; thus dye injected into the inner cell mass would be detected in the embryo, not the placenta (eliminate A). The endometrium is derived from the mother and is only the site of implantation and placental development. It does not actually contribute to the placenta; thus dye injected into the endometrium would not be detected in the placenta (eliminate C). The zygote is the precursor to all embryonic and extraembryonic structures. Injecting a dye into the zygote would lead to its detection not only in the placenta, but also in the amnion, chorion, and embryo itself (eliminate D).

[41] No. Gastrulation involves only cells derived from the inner cell mass.

The zygote and morula have the potential to become any cell type in the blastocyst (inner cell mass or trophoblast). They are therefore known as **totipotent** cells. Cells in the inner cell mass of the blastocyst cannot become the trophoblast, but can differentiate into any of three primary germ layers, and can thus develop into any cell in an adult human (of which there are about 220 different types). These cells are called **pluripotent.** Cells of the primary germ layers are called **multipotent**. This means they can produce many (not all) cell types, and are more differentiated than pluripotent cells. Adult stem cells and umbilical cord blood stem cells are also multipotent.

There is a certain point in the development of a cell at which the cell fate becomes fixed; at this point the cell is said to be **determined**. **Determination** precedes differentiation. This means a cell is determined before it is visibly differentiated. Determination can be induced by a cell's environment, such as exposure to diffusible factors or neighboring cells, or it can be preprogrammed.

- During early embryonic development, cells near the developing notochord undergo an irreversible developmental choice to become skeletal muscle later in development, although they do not immediately change their appearance. This is an example of which of the following?[42]
  - A. Determination
  - B. Differentiation
  - C. Totipotency
  - D. Induction

11.8   BIRTH AND LACTATION

The technical term for birth is **parturition**. It is dependent on contraction of muscles in the uterine wall. The very high levels of progesterone secreted throughout pregnancy help repress contractions in uterine muscle, but near the end of pregnancy uterine excitability increases. This increased excitability is likely to be a result of several factors, including a change in the ratio of estrogen to progesterone, presence of the hormone **oxytocin** secreted by the posterior pituitary, and mechanical stretching of the uterus and cervix.

Weak contractions of the uterus occur throughout pregnancy. As pregnancy reaches full term, however, rhythmic **labor contractions** begin. It is thought that the onset of labor contractions is the result of a positive feedback reflex: Increased pressure on the cervix crosses a threshold that causes the posterior pituitary to increase the secretion of oxytocin. Oxytocin causes uterine contractions to increase in intensity, creating greater pressure on the cervix that stimulates still more oxytocin release and even stronger contractions.

The first stage of labor is dilation of the cervix. The second stage is the actual birth, involving movement of the baby through the cervix and birth canal, pushed by contraction of uterine (smooth) and abdominal (skeletal) muscle. The third stage is the expulsion of the placenta, after it separates from the wall of the uterus. Contractions of the uterus after birth help to minimize blood loss.

---

[42] A cell whose fate is fixed is said to be determined (choice **A** is correct) and is no longer totipotent (eliminate C). Since the cell's appearance hasn't changed, it is not yet differentiated (eliminate B). Although the question states that cells are located near the notochord, it does not say whether this location is the reason for their determination. They still might be cytoplasmically determined (eliminate D).

During pregnancy, milk production and secretion would be a waste of energy, but after parturition it is necessary. During puberty, estrogen stimulates development of breasts in women. Increased levels of estrogen and progesterone secreted by the placenta during pregnancy cause the further development of glandular and adipose breast tissue. But while these hormones stimulate breast development, they inhibit the release of **prolactin** and thus production of milk. After parturition, levels of estrogen and progesterone fall and milk production begins. Every time suckling occurs, the pituitary gland is stimulated by the hypothalamus to release a large surge of prolactin, prolonging the ability of the breasts to secrete milk. If the mother stops breast-feeding the infant, prolactin levels fall and milk secretion ceases. The converse is also true: Milk secretion can continue for years, as long as nursing continues. The breasts do not leak large amounts of milk when the infant is not nursing. This is because the posterior pituitary hormone **oxytocin** is necessary for **milk let-down** (release). Oxytocin is also released when suckling occurs.

11.8

Want More Practice?
Scan the QR code below to register your book for online chapter summaries, drills, practice tests, and more!

Hold Up!
How are you doing? We've covered a lot of ground, so before you jump into the General Chemistry section, how about a study break? Get a snack, take a walk, listen to a great song—give yourself a moment to relax before you do more studying. It's important not to burn yourself out when preparing for a big test!

General Chemistry

Periodic Table of the Elements

1 H 1.008																	2 He 4.0026
3 Li 6.94	4 Be 9.0122											5 B 10.81	6 C 12.011	7 N 14.007	8 O 15.999	9 F 18.998	10 Ne 20.180
11 Na 22.990	12 Mg 24.305											13 Al 26.982	14 Si 28.085	15 P 30.974	16 S 32.06	17 Cl 35.45	18 Ar 39.948
19 K 39.098	20 Ca 40.078	21 Sc 44.956	22 Ti 47.867	23 V 50.942	24 Cr 51.996	25 Mn 54.938	26 Fe 55.845	27 Co 58.933	28 Ni 58.693	29 Cu 63.546	30 Zn 65.38	31 Ga 69.723	32 Ge 72.630	33 As 74.922	34 Se 78.97	35 Br 79.904	36 Kr 83.798
37 Rb 85.468	38 Sr 87.62	39 Y 88.906	40 Zr 91.224	41 Nb 92.906	42 Mo 95.95	43 Tc (98)	44 Ru 101.07	45 Rh 102.91	46 Pd 106.42	47 Ag 107.87	48 Cd 112.41	49 In 114.82	50 Sn 118.71	51 Sb 121.76	52 Te 127.60	53 I 126.90	54 Xe 131.29
55 Cs 132.9	56 Ba 137.3	57–71 *	72 Hf 178.49	73 Ta 180.95	74 W 183.84	75 Re 186.21	76 Os 190.23	77 Ir 192.23	78 Pt 195.08	79 Au 196.97	80 Hg 200.59	81 Tl 204.38	82 Pb 207.2	83 Bi 208.98	84 Po [209]	85 At [210]	86 Rn [222]
87 Fr [223]	88 Ra 226.0	89–103 †	104 Rf [265]	105 Db [268]	106 Sg [271]	107 Bh [270]	108 Hs [277]	109 Mt [276]	110 Ds [281]	111 Rg [280]	112 Cn [285]	113 Nh [286]	114 Fl [289]	115 Mc [289]	116 Lv [293]	117 Ts [294]	118 Og [294]

*Lanthanide Series:

57 La 138.905	58 Ce 140.116	59 Pr 140.907	60 Nd 144.242	61 Pm [145]	62 Sm 150.36	63 Eu 151.964	64 Gd 157.25	65 Tb 158.925	66 Dy 162.500	67 Ho 164.930	68 Er 167.259	69 Tm 168.934	70 Yb 173.054	71 Lu 174.966

†Actinide Series:

89 Ac [227]	90 Th 232.038	91 Pa 231.035	92 U 238.028	93 Np [237]	94 Pu [244]	95 Am [243]	96 Cm [247]	97 Bk [247]	98 Cf [251]	99 Es [252]	100 Fm [257]	101 Md [258]	102 No [259]	103 Lr [262]

Chapter 12
Gchem Basics

Before starting your review of Gchem content, return to Section 2.1 for a general introduction to the SNS. There will be 30 Gchem questions on the DAT. They will occur after the 40 Biology questions and before the 30 Ochem questions.

The following chapters will review the Gchem content you should be familiar with for the DAT. The ADA publishes a list of topics tested on the DAT, usually called the "General Chemistry Specifications List." Go to the ADA website now and review the list; this will be the content you'll see in the next few chapters. As of 2023, you can expect to see a few questions on each of the following topics: stoichiometry and general concepts, gases, liquids and solids, solutions, acids and bases, chemical equilibria, thermodynamics, chemical kinetics, redox reactions, atomic and molecular structure, periodic properties, nuclear reactions, and Gchem laboratory techniques.

It is also worth checking to see if the content list has changed recently; sometimes last-minute changes are announced. For example, the Biology content list changed in January 2022 and was effective immediately! If some content changes are announced, don't worry. Go online via your Student Tools and check out the supplementary content posted for thisbook. We'll keep the Gchem content up to date there, so even if changes occur, we've got you covered.

You will not have access to a calculator in the SNS section, which means you'll need to do some calculations in your head and/or on your Noteboard. Before diving into Gchem, you may want to review Chapter 39 to brush up on some basic math.

In addition, there are some equations you'll need to memorize before the DAT. If an equation is in this book, you may need to use it on test day. Consider starting a summary list or a library of flash cards to help you memorize the Gchem equations sooner rather than later. Usually about half the Gchem questions require you to use an equation in some way; some questions will require you to plug in numbers and solve. Others will only require you to substitute numbers into an equation or two but won't require you to do the final calculation. Several of these questions will require you to combine equations together. You'll see lots of examples of each of these question types in the online drills you have access to by purchasing this book.

12.1 METRIC UNITS

Before we begin our study of chemistry, we will briefly go over metric units. Scientists use the *Système International d'Unitès* (the International System of Units), abbreviated SI, to express measurements of physical quantities. Six of the seven **base units** of SI are given below:

SI Base Unit	Abbreviation	Measures
meter	m	length
kilogram	kg	mass
second	s	time
mole	mol	amount of substance
kelvin	K	temperature
ampere	A	electric current

(The seventh SI base unit, the candela [cd], measures luminous intensity, but we will not need to worry about this one.) The units of any physical quantity can be written in terms of the SI base units. For example, the SI unit of speed is meters per second (m/s), the SI unit of energy (the joule) is kilograms times meters^2 per second^2 ($kg \cdot m^2/s^2$), and so forth.

Multiples of the base units that are powers of ten are often abbreviated and precede the symbol for the unit. For example, m is the symbol for milli-, which means 10^{-3} (one thousandth). So, one thousandth of a second, 1 millisecond, would be written as 1 ms. The letter M is the symbol for mega-, which means 10^6 (one million); a distance of one million meters, 1 megameter, would be abbreviated as 1 Mm. Some of the most common power-of-ten prefixes are given in the list below:

Prefix	Symbol	Multiple
nano-	n	10^{-9}
micro-	μ	10^{-6}
milli-	m	10^{-3}
centi	c	10^{-2}
kilo-	k	10^3
mega-	M	10^6

Two other units, ones that are common in chemistry, are the liter and the angstrom. The liter (abbreviated L) is a unit of volume equal to 1/1,000 of a cubic meter:

$$1,000 \text{ L} = 1 \text{ m}^3$$

$$1 \text{ L} = 1000 \text{ cm}^3$$

The standard SI unit of volume, the cubic meter, is inconveniently large for most laboratory work. The liter is a smaller unit. Furthermore, the most common way of expressing solution concentrations, **molarity** (*M*), uses the liter in its definition: *M* = moles of solute per liter of solution.

In addition, you will see the milliliter (mL) as often as you will see the liter. A simple consequence of the definition of a liter is the fact that one milliliter is the same volume as one cubic centimeter:

$$1 \text{ mL} = 1 \text{ cm}^3 = 1 \text{ cc}$$

While the volume of any substance can, strictly speaking, be expressed in liters, you rarely hear of a milliliter of gold, for example. Ordinarily, the liter is used to express the volumes of liquids and gases, but not solids.

The **angstrom**, abbreviated Å, is a unit of length equal to 10^{-10} m. The angstrom is convenient because atomic radii and bond lengths are typically around 1 to 3 Å.

Example 12-1: By how many orders of magnitude is a centimeter longer than an angstrom?

Solution: An **order of magnitude** is a factor of ten. Since 1 cm = 10^{-2} m and 1 Å = 10^{-10} m, a centimeter is 8 factors of ten, or 8 orders of magnitude, greater than an angstrom.

Remember that you do not have access to a calculator in the SNS section of the DAT, so you must do all calculations manually. To help prepare for this, you should read Chapter 39 in this book.

In addition, you should know the multiplication table up to 12 × 12, and should be comfortable multiplying most numbers by:

- Multiples of ten, such as 10, 100, 1000, etc.
- 20, 30, 40, 50, 60, 70, 80, and 90
- Decimals such as 0.1, 0.01, 0.001, etc.

It is worth remembering that any number to the exponent 0 is equal to 1. In other words, $x^0 = 1$, where x is any positive whole number. Finally, you should know how to square and cube the following numbers: 1–12, 20, 25, 30, 40, 50, 60, 70, 80, 90 and 100, or at least estimate these values. If you know these numbers, you will also be able to estimate square roots and cube roots for most numbers. For example, if you have to determine the cubed root of 450 (say, in a solubility and K_{sp} problem): if you know that 7^3 is 343 (or about 350 if you're estimating) and 8^3 is 512 (or close to 500 if you're estimating), then the cube root of 450 must be between 7 and 8. Estimations like this are necessary to answer general chemistry questions on the DAT, and will be sufficient for you to find the correct answer from multiple-choice options.

12.2   THE ELECTROMAGNETIC SPECTRUM

Electromagnetic radiation (EMR) refers to the waves (or their photons) of an electromagnetic field, propagating or radiating through space, carrying electromagnetic radiant energy. They do not require a medium to propagate, since they can travel through a vacuum of empty space. When an electromagnetic wave travels through a vacuum, its speed is constant at $c = 3 \times 10^8$ m/s.

The frequencies and wavelengths of electromagnetic waves span a huge range, and different ranges have been given specific names. This assignment is based on frequency, energy or wavelength and is known as the electromagnetic spectrum (EMS):

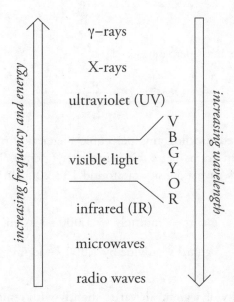

Figure 1   Electromagnetic Spectrum

EMR includes radio waves, microwaves, infrared, visible light, ultraviolet, X-rays, and gamma radiation. You should know these categories and their ranking from lowest frequency/energy (longest wavelength) to highest frequency/energy (shortest wavelength). Notice that visible light occupies only a small part of the EMS: ROYGBV ("Roy-Gee-Biv") stands for red, orange, yellow, green, blue, and violet. In terms of wavelengths, violet light has a wavelength (in vacuum) of about 400 nm and red light has a wavelength of about 700 nm; the other colors are in between.

Example 12-2: Which of the following statements is true regarding red photons and blue photons traveling through vacuum?

    A.   Red light travels faster than blue light and carries more energy.
    B.   Blue light travels faster than red light and carries more energy.
    C.   Red light travels at the same speed as blue light and carries more energy.
    D.   Blue light travels at the same speed as red light and carries more energy.

Solution: All electromagnetic waves, regardless of frequency, travel through vacuum at the same speed (at c or 3×10^8 m/s, eliminate A and B). Now, because blue light has a higher frequency than red light (remember ROYGBV, which lists the colors in order of increasing frequency), photons of blue light have higher energy than photons of red light. Therefore, D correct.

12.3 DENSITY

The **density** of a substance is its mass per volume:

$$\text{Density: } \rho = \frac{\text{mass}}{\text{volume}} = \frac{m}{V}$$

In SI units, density is expressed in kilograms per cubic meter (kg/m^3). However, in chemistry, densities are more often expressed in grams per cubic centimeter (g/cm^3). This unit of density is convenient because most liquids and solids have a density of around 1 to 20 g/cm^3. Here is the conversion between these two sets of density units:

$$g/cm^3 \rightarrow \text{multiply by } 1,000 \rightarrow kg/m^3$$

$$g/cm^3 \leftarrow \text{divide by } 1,000 \leftarrow kg/m^3$$

For example, water has a density of 1 g/cm^3 (it varies slightly with temperature, but this is the value the DAT will expect you to use). To write this density in kg/m^3, we would multiply by 1,000. The density of water is 1,000 kg/m^3. As another example, the density of copper is about 9,000 kg/m^3, so to express this density in g/cm^3, we would divide by 1,000: The density of copper is 9 g/cm^3.

Example 12-3: Diamond has a density of 3,500 kg/m^3. What is the volume, in cm^3, of a 1 3/4-carat diamond (where, by definition, 1 carat = 0.2 g)?

Solution: If we divide mass by density, we get volume, so, converting 3,500 kg/m^3 in 3.5 g/cm^3, we find that:

$$V = \frac{m}{\rho} = \frac{1.75 \, (0.2 \text{ g})}{3.5 \text{ g/cm}} = \frac{0.35 \text{ g}}{3.5 \text{ g/cm}} = 0.1 \text{ cm}^3$$

The density of a material varies with temperature and pressure. This variation is typically small for solids and liquids but much greater for gases. For most substances, increasing the pressure on an object decreases the volume and increases its density. Increasing the temperature of a substance decreases its density by increasing the volume. There are exceptions to these trends; water and ice are good examples of this. As you'll see in Chapter 15, solid ice is less dense than liquid water.

12.4 MOLECULAR FORMULAS

When two or more atoms form a covalent bond they create a **molecule**. For example, when two atoms of hydrogen (H) bond with one atom of oxygen (O), the resulting molecule is H_2O, water. A compound's **molecular formula** gives the identities and numbers of the atoms in the molecule. For example, the formula $C_4H_4N_2$ tells us that this molecule contains 4 carbon atoms, 4 hydrogen atoms, and 2 nitrogen atoms.

Example 12-4: What is the molecular formula of *para*-nitrotoluene?

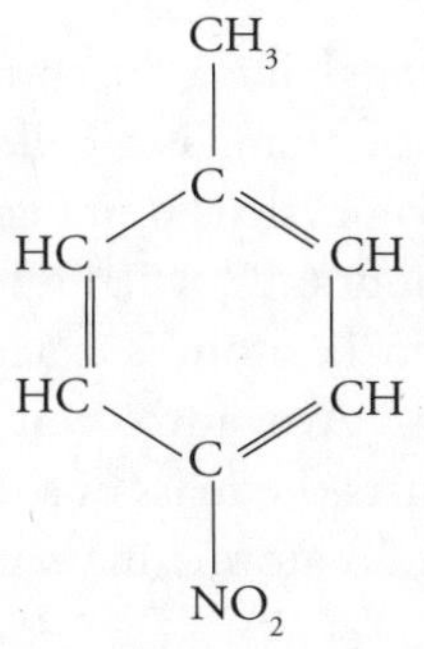

Solution: There are a total of seven C's, seven H's, one N, and two O's, so $C_7H_7NO_2$ is the molecular formula.

12.5 FORMULA AND MOLECULAR WEIGHT

If we know the chemical formula, we can figure out the **formula weight**, which is the sum of the atomic weights of all the atoms in the molecule. The unit for atomic weight is the **atomic mass unit**, abbreviated **amu**. (Note: Although *weight* is the popular term, it should really be *mass*.) One atomic mass unit is, by definition, equal to exactly 1/12 the mass of an atom of carbon-12 (^{12}C), the most abundant naturally occurring form of carbon. The periodic table lists the mass of each element; it is actually a weighted average of the atomic masses of all its naturally occurring forms (isotopes). For example, the atomic mass of hydrogen is listed as 1.0 (amu), and that of nitrogen as 14.0 (amu). Therefore, the formula weight for $C_4H_4N_2$ is:

$$4(12) + 4(1) + 2(14) = 80$$

(The unit *amu* is often not explicitly included.) When a compound exists as discrete molecules, the term **molecular weight** (**MW**) is usually used instead of formula weight. For example, the molecular weight of water, H_2O, is $2(1) + 16 = 18$. The term **formula weight** is usually used for *ionic* compounds, such as NaCl. The formula weight of NaCl is $23 + 35.5 = 58.5$.

Example 12-5: What is the formula weight of calcium phosphate, $Ca_3(PO_4)_2$?

Solution: The masses of the elements are Ca = 40 amu, P = 31 amu, and O = 16 amu. Therefore, the formula weight of calcium phosphate is:

$$3(40 \text{ amu}) + 2(31 \text{ amu}) + 8(16 \text{ amu}) = 310 \text{ amu}$$

12.6 THE MOLE

A **mole** is simply a particular number of things, like a dozen is any group of 12 things. One mole of anything contains 6.02×10^{23} entities. A mole of atoms is a collection of 6.02×10^{23} atoms; a mole of molecules contains 6.02×10^{23} molecules, and so on. This number, 6.02×10^{23}, is called **Avogadro's number**, denoted by N_A (or N_0). What is so special about 6.02×10^{23}? The answer is based on the atomic mass unit, which is defined so that the mass of a carbon-12 atom is exactly 12 amu. *The number of carbon-12 atoms in a sample of mass of 12 grams is 6.02×10^{23}.* Avogadro's number is the link between atomic mass units and grams. For example, the periodic table lists the mass of sodium (Na, atomic number 11) as 23.0. This means that 1 atom of sodium has a mass of 23 atomic mass units, or that 1 *mole* of sodium atoms has a mass of 23 *grams*.

Since 1 mole of a substance has a mass in grams equal to the mass in amus of 1 formula unit of the substance, we have the following formula:

$$\text{\# moles} = \frac{\text{mass in grams}}{\text{molecular weight (MW)}}$$

Example 12-6:

A. Which has the greater molecular weight: potassium dichromate ($K_2Cr_2O_7$) or lead azide (PbN_6)?
B. Which contains more molecules: a 1-mole sample of potassium dichromate or a 1-mole sample of lead azide?

Solution:

A. The molecular weight of potassium dichromate is:

$$2(39.1) + 2(52) + 7(16) = 294.2$$

and the molecular weight of lead azide is:

$$207.2 + 6(14) = 291.2$$

Therefore, potassium dichromate has the greater molecular weight.

B. Trick question. Both samples contain the same number of molecules, namely 1 mole of them. (Which weighs more: a pound of rocks or a pound of feathers?)

Example 12-7: How many molecules of hydrazine, N_2H_4, are in a sample whose mass is 96 grams?

Solution: The molecular weight of N_2H_4 is $2(14) + 4(1) = 32$. This means that 1 mole of N_2H_4 has a mass of 32 grams. Therefore, a sample that has a mass of 96 grams contains 3 moles of molecules, because the formula above tells us that:

$$n = \frac{96 \text{ g}}{32 \text{ g/mol}} = 3 \text{ moles}$$

Molecules of $N_2H_4 = (3 \text{ mol})(6.02 \times 10^{23} \text{ molecules/mol}) = 18.06 \times 10^{23} \text{ molecules} = 1.806 \times 10^{24} \text{ molecules}$.

12.7 EMPIRICAL FORMULAS

Let's look again at the molecule $C_4H_4N_2$. There are four atoms each of carbon and hydrogen, and half as many (two) nitrogen atoms. Therefore, the smallest whole numbers that give the same *ratio* of atoms (carbon to hydrogen to nitrogen) in this molecule are 2:2:1. If we use *these* numbers for the atoms, we get the molecule's **empirical formula**: C_2H_2N. In general, to reduce a molecular formula to the empirical formula, divide all the subscripts by their greatest common factor. Here are a few more examples:

Molecular Formula	Empirical Formula
$C_6H_{12}O_6$	CH_2O
$K_2S_2O_8$	KSO_4
$Fe_4Na_8O_{35}P_{10}$	$Fe_4Na_8O_{35}P_{10}$
$C_{30}H_{27}N_3O_{15}$	$C_{10}H_9NO_5$

Example 12-8: What is the empirical formula for ethylene glycol, $C_2H_6O_2$?

Solution: Dividing each of the subscripts of $C_2H_6O_2$ by 2, we get CH_3O.

12.8 PERCENTAGE COMPOSITION BY MASS

A molecule's molecular or empirical formula can be used to determine the molecule's percent mass composition. For example, let's find the mass composition of carbon, hydrogen, and nitrogen in $C_4H_4N_2$. Using the compound's empirical formula, C_2H_2N, will give us the same answer but the calculations will be easier because we'll have smaller numbers to work with. The empirical molecular weight is $2(12) + 2(1) + 14 = 40$, so each element's contribution to the total mass is:

$$\%C = \frac{2(12)}{40} = \frac{12}{20} = \frac{60}{100} = 60\%, \quad \%H = \frac{2(1)}{40} = \frac{1}{20} = \frac{5}{100} = 5\%, \quad \%N = \frac{14}{40} = \frac{7}{20} = \frac{35}{100} = 35\%$$

We can also use information about the percentage composition to determine a compound's empirical formula. Suppose a substance is analyzed and found to consist, by mass, of 70 percent iron and 30 percent oxygen. To find the empirical formula for this compound, the trick is to start with 100 grams of the substance. We choose 100 grams since percentages are based on parts in 100. One hundred grams of this substance would then contain 70 g of Fe and 30 g of O. Now, how many *moles* of Fe and O are present in this 100-gram substance? Since the atomic weight of Fe is 55.8 and that of O is 16, we can use the formula given above in Section 12.5 and find:

$$\# \text{ moles of Fe} = \frac{70 \text{ g}}{55.8 \text{ g/mol}} \approx \frac{70}{56} = \frac{5}{4} \quad \text{and} \quad \# \text{ moles of O} = \frac{30 \text{ g}}{16 \text{ g/mol}} = \frac{15}{8}$$

12.7

Because the empirical formula involves the ratio of the numbers of atoms, let's find the ratio of the amount of Fe to the amount of O:

$$\text{Ratio of Fe to O} = \frac{5/4 \text{ mol}}{15/8 \text{ mol}} = \frac{5}{4} \infty \frac{8}{15} = \frac{2}{3}$$

Since the ratio of Fe to O is 2:3, the empirical formula of the substance is Fe_2O_3.

Example 12-9: What is the percent composition by mass of each element in sodium azide, NaN_3?

    A.   Sodium 25%; nitrogen 75%
    B.   Sodium 35%; nitrogen 65%
    C.   Sodium 55%; nitrogen 45%
    D.   Sodium 65%; nitrogen 35%
    E.   Sodium 75%; nitrogen 26%

Solution: The molecular weight of this compound is $23 + 3(14) = 65$. Therefore, sodium's contribution to the total mass is:

$$\%Na = \frac{23}{65} \approx \frac{1}{3} \approx 33\%$$

Without even calculating nitrogen's contribution, we already see that B is best.

Example 12-10: What is the percent composition by mass of carbon in glucose, $C_6H_{12}O_6$?

Solution: The empirical formula for this compound is CH_2O, so the empirical molecular weight is $12 + 2(1) + 16 = 30$. Therefore, carbon's contribution to the total mass is:

$$\%C = \frac{12}{30} = 40\%$$

Example 12-11: What is the empirical formula of a compound that is, by mass, 90 percent carbon and 10 percent hydrogen?

Solution: A 100-gram sample of this compound would contain 90 g of C and 10 g of H. Since the atomic weight of C is 12 and that of H is 1, we have:

$$\text{\# moles of C} = \frac{90 \text{ g}}{12 \text{ g/mol}} = \frac{15}{2} \quad \text{and} \quad \text{\# moles of H} = \frac{10 \text{ g}}{1 \text{ g/mol}} = 10$$

Therefore, the ratio of the amount of C to the amount of H is:

$$\frac{15/2 \text{ mol}}{10 \text{ mol}} = \frac{3}{4}$$

12.8

Example 12-12: What is the percent, by mass of water, in the hydrate $MgCl_2 \cdot 5H_2O$?

Solution: The formula weight for this hydrate is $24.3 + 2(35.5) + 5[2(1) + 16] = 185.3$. Since water's total molecular weight in this compound is $5[2(1) + 16] = 90$, we see that water's contribution to the total mass is $\%H_2O = 90/185.3$, which is a little *less* than one-half (50 percent).

Example 12-13: In which of the following compounds is the mass percent of each of the constituent elements nearly identical?

    A.   NaCl
    B.   LiBr
    C.   HCl
    D. CaF_2
    E. BeF_2

Solution: The question is asking us to identify the compound made up of equal amounts, by mass, of two elements. Looking at the given compounds, we see that:

$$Na\ (23.0\ g/mol) \neq Cl\ (35.5\ g/mol)$$

$$Li\ (6.9\ g/mol) \neq Br\ (79.9\ g/mol)$$

$$H\ (1.0\ g/mol) \neq Cl\ (35.5\ g/mol)$$

$$Ca\ (40.1\ g/mol) \approx 2\ F\ (2 \times 19) = 38\ g/mol$$

$$Be\ (9.0\ g/mol) \neq 2\ F\ (2 \times 19) = 38\ g/mol$$

Therefore, D is best.

12.9   CHEMICAL EQUATIONS AND STOICHIOMETRIC COEFFICIENTS

The equation:

$$2\ Al + 6\ HCl \rightarrow 2\ AlCl_3 + 3\ H_2$$

describes the reaction of aluminum metal (Al) with hydrochloric acid (HCl) to produce aluminum chloride ($AlCl_3$) and hydrogen gas (H_2). The **reactants** are on the left side of the arrow, and the **products** are on the right side. A chemical equation is **balanced** if, for every element represented, the number of atoms on the left side is equal to the number of atoms on the right side. This illustrates the **Law of Conservation of Mass** (or of **Matter**), which says that the amount of matter (and thus mass) does not change in a chemical reaction. For a *balanced* reaction such as the one above, the coefficients (2, 6, 2, and 3) preceding each compound—which are known as **stoichiometric coefficients**—tell us in what proportion the reactants react and in what proportion the products are formed. For this reaction, 2 atoms of Al react

12.9

with 6 molecules of HCl to form 2 molecules of $AlCl_3$ and 3 molecules of H_2. The equation also means that 2 *moles* of Al react with 6 *moles* of HCl to form 2 *moles* of $AlCl_3$ and 3 *moles* of H_2.

The stoichiometric coefficients give the ratios of the number of molecules (or moles) that apply to the combination of reactants and the formation of products. They do *not* give the ratios by mass.

Balancing Equations

Balancing most chemical equations is simply a matter of trial and error. It's a good idea to start with the most complex species in the reaction. For example, let's look at the reaction below:

$$Al + HCl \rightarrow AlCl_3 + H_2 \text{ (unbalanced)}$$

Start with the most complex molecule, $AlCl_3$. To get 3 atoms of Cl on the product side, we need to have 3 atoms of Cl on the reactant side; therefore, we put a 3 in front of the HCl:

$$Al + 3\ HCl \rightarrow AlCl_3 + H_2 \text{ (unbalanced)}$$

We've now balanced the Cl's, but the H's are still unbalanced. Since we have 3 H's on the left, we need 3 H's on the right to accomplish this, so we put a coefficient of 3/2 in front of the H_2:

$$Al + 3\ HCl \rightarrow AlCl_3 + 3/2\ H_2$$

Notice that we put a 3/2 (*not* a 3) in front of the H_2, because a hydrogen molecule contains 2 hydrogen atoms. All the atoms are now balanced—we see 1 Al, 3 H's, and 3 Cl's on each side. Because it's customary to write stoichiometric coefficients as whole numbers, we simply multiply through by 2 to get rid of the fraction and write

$$2\ Al + 6\ HCl \rightarrow 2\ AlCl_3 + 3\ H_2$$

Example 12-14: Balance each of these equations:

A. $NH_3 + O_2 \rightarrow NO + H_2O$
B. $CuCl_2 + NH_3 + H_2O \rightarrow Cu(OH)_2 + NH_4Cl$
    $Cu(OH)_2 + 2\ NH_4Cl$
C. $C_3H_8 + O_2 \rightarrow CO_2 + H_2O$
D. $C_8H_{18} + O_2 \rightarrow CO_2 + H_2O$
    H_2O

Solution:

A. $4\ NH_3 + 5\ O_2 \rightarrow 4\ NO + 6\ H_2O$
B. $CuCl_2 + 2\ NH_3 + 2\ H_2O \rightarrow$
C. $C_3H_8 + 5\ O_2 \rightarrow 3\ CO_2 + 4\ H_2O$
D. $2\ C_8H_{18} + 25\ O_2 \rightarrow 16\ CO_2 + 18$

12.10 STOICHIOMETRIC RELATIONSHIPS IN BALANCED REACTIONS

Once the equation for a chemical reaction is balanced, the stoichiometric coefficients tell us the relative amounts of the reactant species that combine and the relative amounts of the product species that are formed. For example, recall that the reaction

$$2 \, Al + 6 \, HCl \rightarrow 2 \, AlCl_3 + 3 \, H_2$$

tells us that 2 moles of Al react with 6 moles of HCl to form 2 moles of $AlCl_3$ and 3 moles of H_2.

Example 12-15: If 108 grams of aluminum metal are consumed, how many grams of hydrogen gas will be produced?

Solution: Because the stoichiometric coefficients give the ratios of the number of moles that apply to the combination of reactants and the formation of products—not the ratios by mass—we first need to determine how many *moles* of Al react. Since the molecular weight of Al is 27, we know that 27 grams of Al is equivalent to 1 mole. Therefore, 108 grams of Al is 4 moles. Now we use the stoichiometry of the balanced equation: for every 2 moles of Al that react, 3 moles of H_2 are produced. So, if 4 moles of Al react, we'll get 6 moles of H_2. Finally, we convert the number of moles of H_2 produced to grams. The molecular weight of H_2 is 2(1) = 2. This means that 1 mole of H_2 has a mass of 2 grams. Therefore, 6 moles of H_2 will have a mass of 6(2 g) = 12 grams.

Example 12-16: How many grams of HCl are required to produce 534 grams of aluminum chloride?

Solution: First, we'll convert the desired mass of $AlCl_3$ into moles. The molecular weight of $AlCl_3$ is 27 + 3(35.5) = 133.5. This means that 1 mole of $AlCl_3$ has a mass of 133.5 grams. Therefore, 534 grams of $AlCl_3$ is equivalent to 534/133.5 = 4 moles. Next, we use the stoichiometry of the balanced equation. For every 2 moles of $AlCl_3$ that are produced, 6 moles of HCl are consumed. So, if we want to produce 4 moles of $AlCl_3$, we'll need 12 moles of HCl. Finally, we convert the number of moles of HCl consumed to grams. The molecular weight of HCl is 1 + 35.5 = 36.5. This means that 1 mole of HCl has a mass of 36.5 grams. Therefore, 12 moles of HCl will have a mass of 12(36.5 g) = 438 grams.

Example 12-17: Consider the following reaction:

$$CS_2 + 3 \, O_2 \rightarrow CO_2 + 2 \, SO_2$$

How much carbon disulfide must be used to produce 64 grams of SO_2?

Solution: Since the molecular weight of SO_2 is 32.1 + 2(16) = 64, we know that 64 grams of SO_2 is equivalent to 1 mole. From the stoichiometry of the balanced equation, we see that for every 1 mole of CS_2 that reacts, 2 moles of SO_2 are produced. Therefore, to produce just 1 mole of SO_2, we need 1/2 mole of CS_2. The molecular weight of CS_2 is 12 + 2(32.1) ≈ 76, so 1/2 mole of CS_2 has a mass of 38 grams.

12.10

12.11 THE LIMITING REAGENT

Let's look again at the reaction of aluminum with hydrochloric acid:

$$2\ Al + 6\ HCl \rightarrow 2\ AlCl_3 + 3\ H_2$$

Suppose that this reaction starts with 4 moles of Al and 18 moles of HCl. We have enough HCl to make 6 moles of $AlCl_3$ and 9 moles of H_2. *However,* there's only enough Al to make 4 moles of $AlCl_3$ and 6 moles of H_2. There isn't enough aluminum metal (Al) to make use of all the available HCl. As the reaction proceeds, we'll run out of aluminum. This means that aluminum is the **limiting reagent** here, because we run out of this reactive *first*, so it limits how much product the reaction can produce.

Now suppose that the reaction begins with 4 moles of Al and 9 moles of HCl. There's enough Al metal to produce 4 moles of $AlCl_3$ and 6 moles of H_2. But there's only enough HCl to make 3 moles of $AlCl_3$ and 4.5 moles of H_2. There isn't enough HCl to make use of all the available aluminum metal. As the reaction proceeds, we'll find that all the HCl is consumed before the Al is consumed. In this situation, HCl is the limiting reagent. Notice that we had more moles of HCl than we had of Al and the initial mass of the HCl was greater than the initial mass of Al. Nevertheless, the limiting reagent in this case was the HCl. The limiting reagent is the reactant that is consumed first, not necessarily the reactant that's initially present in the smallest amount.

Example 12-18: Consider the following reaction:

$$2\ ZnS + 3\ O_2 \rightarrow 2\ ZnO + 2\ SO_2$$

If 97.5 grams of zinc sulfide undergoes this reaction with 32 grams of oxygen gas, what will be the limiting reagent?

A. ZnS
B. O_2
C. ZnO
D. SO_2
E. There is no limiting reagent.

Solution: Since the molecular weight of ZnS is $65.4 + 32.1 = 97.5$ and the molecular weight of O_2 is $2(16) = 32$, this reaction begins with 1 mole of ZnS and 1 mole of O_2. From the stoichiometry of the balanced equation, we see that 1 mole of ZnS would react completely with $\dfrac{3}{2} = 1.5$ moles of O_2. Because we have only 1 mole of O_2, the O_2 will be consumed first; it is the limiting reagent, and the answer is B. Note that C and D can be eliminated immediately, because a limiting reagent is always a reactant.

12.11

12.12   SOME NOTATION USED IN CHEMICAL EQUATIONS

In addition to specifying what atoms or molecules are involved in a chemical reaction, an equation may contain additional information. One type of additional information that can be written right into the equation specifies the **phases** of the atoms or molecules in the reaction; that is, is the substance a solid, liquid, or gas? Another common condition is that a substance may be dissolved in water when the reaction proceeds. In this case, we'd say the substance is an aqueous solution. These four "states" are abbreviated and written in parentheses as follows:

Solid	(s)
Liquid	(l)
Gas	(g)
Aqueous	(aq)

These immediately follow the chemical symbol for the reactant or product in the equation. For example, the reaction of sodium metal with water, which produces sodium hydroxide and hydrogen gas, could be written like this:

$$2\ Na(s) + 2\ H_2O(l) \xrightarrow{\Delta} 2\ NaOH(aq) + H_2(g)$$

In some cases, the reactants are heated to produce the desired reaction. To indicate this, we write a "Δ"—or the word "heat"—above (or below) the reaction arrow. For example, heating potassium nitrate produces potassium nitrite and oxygen gas:

$$2\ KNO_3(s) \xrightarrow{\Delta} 2\ KNO_2(aq) + O_2(g)$$

Some reactions proceed more rapidly in the presence of a **catalyst**, which is a substance that increases the rate of a reaction without being consumed. For example, in the industrial production of sulfuric acid, an intermediate step is the reaction of sulfur dioxide and oxygen to produce sulfur trioxide. Not only are the reactants heated, but they are combined in the presence of vanadium pentoxide, V_2O_5. We indicate the presence of a catalyst by writing it below the arrow in the equation:

$$2\ SO_2 + O_2 \underset{V_2O_5}{\xrightarrow{\Delta}} 2\ SO_3$$

12.13   OXIDATION STATES

An atom's **oxidation state** (or **oxidation number**) is meant to indicate how the atom's "ownership" of its valence electrons changes when it forms a compound. For example, consider the formula unit NaCl. The sodium atom will transfer its valence electron to the chlorine atom, so the sodium's "ownership" of its valence electron has certainly changed. To indicate this, we'd say that the oxidation state of sodium is now +1 (or 1 *less* electron than it started with). On the other hand, chlorine accepts ownership of that 1 electron, so its oxidation state is –1 (that is, 1 *more* electron than it started with). Giving up ownership results in a more positive oxidation state; accepting ownership results in a more negative oxidation state.

This example of NaCl is rather special (and easy) since the compound is **ionic**, and we consider ionic compounds to involve the complete transfer of electrons. But what about a non-ionic (that is, a **covalent**) compound? *The oxidation state of an atom is the "charge" it would have if the compound were ionic.* Here's another way of saying this: the oxidation state of an atom in a molecule is the charge it would have if all the shared electrons were completely transferred to the more electronegative element. Note that for covalent compounds, this is not a real charge, just a bookkeeping trick.

The following list gives the rules for assigning oxidation states to the atoms in a molecule. If following one rule in the list causes the violation of another rule, the rule that is higher in the list takes precedence.

Rules for Assigning Oxidation States
1. The oxidation state of any element in its standard state is 0.
2. The sum of the oxidation states of the atoms in a neutral molecule must always be 0, and the sum of the oxidation states of the atoms in an ion must always equal the ion's charge.
3. Group 1 metals have a +1 oxidation state, and Group 2 metals have a +2 oxidation state.
4. Fluorine has a –1 oxidation state.
5. Hydrogen has a +1 oxidation state when bonded to something more electronegative than carbon, a –1 oxidation state when bonded to an atom less electronegative than carbon, and a 0 oxidation state when bonded to carbon.
6. Oxygen has a –2 oxidation state.
7. The rest of the halogens have a –1 oxidation state, and the atoms of the oxygen family have a –2 oxidation state.

12.13

It's worth noting a common exception to Rule 6: In peroxides (such as H_2O_2 or Na_2O_2), oxygen is in a –1 oxidation state.

As we will discuss later, the order of electronegativities of some elements can be remembered with the mnemonic FONClBrISCH (pronounced "fawn-cull-brish"). This lists the elements in order from the most electronegative (F) to the least electronegative (H). Hence, bonds from H to anything before C in FONClBrISCH will give hydrogen a +1 oxidation state, and bonds from H to anything *not* found in the list will give H a –1 oxidation state.

Let's find the oxidation number of manganese in $KMnO_4$. By Rule 3, K is +1, and by Rule 6, O is –2. Therefore, the oxidation state of Mn must be +7 in order for the sum of all the oxidation numbers in this electrically-neutral molecule to be zero (the unbreakable Rule 2).

Like many other elements, transition metals can assume different oxidation states, depending on the compound they're in. (Note, however, that a metal will never assume a negative oxidation state!) For example, iron has an oxidation number of +2 in $FeCl_2$ but an oxidation number of +3 in $FeCl_3$. The oxidation number of a transition metal is given as a Roman numeral in the name of the compound. Therefore, $FeCl_2$ is iron(II) chloride, and $FeCl_3$ is iron(III) chloride.

Example 12-19: Determine the oxidation state of the atoms in each of the following molecules:

A. NO_3^-
B. HNO_2
C. O_2
D. SF_4
E. Fe_3O_4

Solution:

A. By Rule 6, the oxidation state of O is –2; therefore, by Rule 2, the oxidation state of N must be +5.

B. By Rule 5, the oxidation state of H is +1, and by Rule 6, O has an oxidation state of –2. Therefore, by Rule 2, N must have an oxidation state of +3 in this molecule.

C. By Rule 1 (which is higher in the list than Rule 5 and thus takes precedence), each O atom in O_2 has an oxidation state of 0.

D. By Rule 4, F has an oxidation state of –1. So, by Rule 2, S has an oxidation state of +4.

E. By Rule 6, O has an oxidation state of –2. So, by Rule 2, Fe has an oxidation state of +8/3. (Notice that oxidation states do not have to be whole numbers.)

Want More Practice?
Scan the QR code below to register your book for online chapter summaries, drills, practice tests, and more!

12.13

Chapter 13
Atomic Structure

13.1 ELEMENTS AND THE PERIODIC TABLE

The elements are all displayed in the periodic table of the elements:

The horizontal rows are called **periods**. The vertical columns are called **groups** (or **families**).

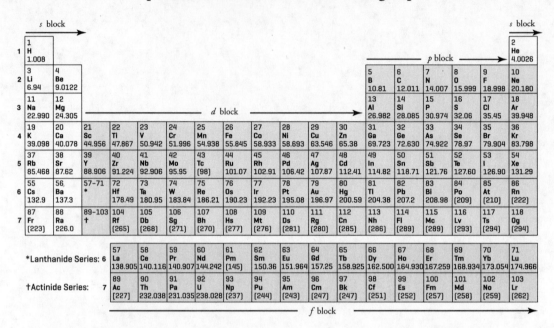

13.2 ATOMS

The smallest unit of any element is one **atom** of the element. All atoms have a central **nucleus**, which contains **protons** and **neutrons**, known collectively as **nucleons**. Each proton has an electric charge of +1 elementary unit; neutrons have no charge. Outside the nucleus, an atom contains electrons, and each **electron** has a charge of −1 elementary unit.

In every neutral atom, the number of electrons outside the nucleus is equal to the number of protons inside the nucleus. The electrons are held in the atom by the electrical attraction of the positively charged nucleus.

The number of protons in the nucleus of an atom is called its **atomic number**, **Z**. The atomic number of an atom uniquely determines what element the atom is, and Z may be shown explicitly by a subscript before the symbol of the element. For example, every beryllium atom contains exactly four protons, and we can write this as $_4$Be.

A proton and a neutron each have a mass slightly more than one atomic mass unit (1 amu = 1.66×10^{-27} kg), and an electron has a mass that's only about 0.05 percent the mass of either a proton or a neutron. So, virtually all the mass of an atom is due to the mass of the nucleus.

The number of protons plus the number of neutrons in the nucleus of an atom gives the atom's **mass number**, **A**. If we let N stand for the number of neutrons, then $A = Z + N$.

In designating a particular atom of an element, we refer to its mass number. One way to do this is to write A as a superscript. For example, if a beryllium atom contains 5 neutrons, then its mass number is $4 + 5 = 9$, and we would write this as ^9_4Be or simply as ^9Be. Another way is simply to write the mass number after the name of the elements, with a hyphen; ^9Be is beryllium-9.

13.3 ISOTOPES

If two atoms of the same element differ in their numbers of neutrons, then they are called **isotopes**. The atoms shown below are two different isotopes of the element beryllium. The atom on the left has 4 protons and 3 neutrons, so its mass number is 7; it's ^7Be (or beryllium-7). The atom on the right has 4 protons and 5 neutrons, so it's ^9Be (beryllium-9).

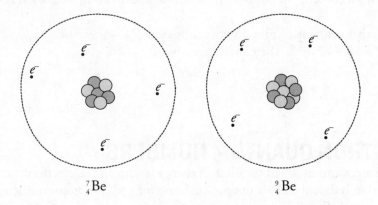

^7_4Be ^9_4Be

(These figures are definitely not to scale. If they were, each dashed circle showing the "outer edge" of the atom would literally be about 1,500 m—almost a mile across! The nucleus occupies only the *tiniest* fraction of an atom's volume, which is mostly empty space.) Notice that these atoms—like all isotopes of a given element—*have the same atomic number but different mass numbers.*

Example 13-1: An atom whose nucleus contains 7 neutrons and which has a mass number of 12 is an isotope of what element?

Solution: If $A = 12$ and $N = 7$, then $Z = A - N = 12 - 7 = 5$. The element whose atomic number is 5 is boron.

Atomic Weight

Elements exist naturally as a collection of their isotopes. The **atomic weight of an element** is a *weighted average* of the masses of its naturally occurring isotopes. For example, boron has two naturally occurring isotopes: boron-10, with an atomic mass of 10.013 amu, and boron-11, with an atomic mass of 11.009 amu. Since boron-10 accounts for 20 percent of all naturally occurring boron, and boron-11 accounts for the other 80 percent, the atomic weight of boron is

$$(20\%)(10.013 \text{ amu}) + (80\%)(11.009 \text{ amu}) = 10.810 \text{ amu}$$

and this is the value listed in the periodic table. (Recall that the atomic mass unit is defined so that the most abundant isotope of carbon, carbon-12, has a mass of precisely 12 amu.)

13.4 IONS

When a neutral atom gains or loses electrons, it becomes charged, and the resulting atom is called an **ion**. For each electron it gains, an atom acquires a charge of –1 unit, and for each electron it loses, an atom acquires a charge of +1 unit. A negatively charged ion is called an **anion**, while a positively charged ion is called a **cation**.

We designate how many electrons an atom has gained or lost by placing this number as a superscript after the chemical symbol for the element. For example, if a lithium atom loses 1 electron, it becomes the lithium cation Li^{1+}, or simply Li^+. If a phosphorus atom gains 3 electrons, it becomes the phosphorus anion P^{3-}.

Example 13-2: An atom contains 16 protons, 17 neutrons, and 18 electrons. What is this atom?

Solution: Any atom that contains 16 protons is a sulfur atom. Now, because $Z = 16$ and $N = 17$, the mass number, A, is $Z + N = 16 + 17 = 33$. Therefore, the answer is $^{33}S^{2-}$.

13.5 ELECTRON QUANTUM NUMBERS

Electrons held by an atom can exist only at discrete energy levels; that is, electron energy levels are **quantized**. This quantization is described by a unique "address" for each electron, consisting of four quantum numbers designating the shell, subshell, orbital, and spin.

The First Quantum Number

The first, or **principle**, quantum number is the **shell number**, n. It's related to the size and energy of an orbital. Loosely speaking, an **orbital** describes a three-dimensional region around the nucleus in which the electron is most likely to be found. The value of n can be any whole number starting with 1, and, generally, the greater the value of n, the greater the electron's energy and average distance from the nucleus. To determine the n of a specific electron, one should name the shell it occupies. For example, an electron in the $3s$ orbital has an $n = 3$.

The Second Quantum Number

An electron's second quantum number, the **subshell number**, is denoted by the letter l. It describes the *shape* (and energy) of an electron's orbital. The possible values for l depend on the value of n as follows: $l = 0, 1, 2,..., n - 1$. For example, if the principal quantum number is $n = 3$, then l could be 0, 1, or 2. Special letters are traditionally assigned to the values of l like this: the $l = 0$ subshell is called the **s subshell**, $l = 1$ is the **p subshell**, $l = 2$ is the **d subshell**, and the $l = 3$ subshell is the **f subshell**. The DAT primarily uses this spectroscopic notation—that is, *s, p, d,* and *f*—for the subshells.

The Third Quantum Number

An electron's third quantum number, the **orbital number**, is denoted by m_l. It describes the three-dimensional *orientation* of an orbital. The possible values of m_l depend on the value of l as follows: $m_l = -l, -(l-1),$ ..., $-1, 0,$ ..., $(l-1), l$. For example, if $l = 2$, then m_l could be $-2, -1, 0, 1,$ or 2. We use the possible values of the orbital quantum number to tell us how many orbitals are in each subshell.

13.5

- If $l = 0$, then m_l can only be equal to 0 (one possibility), so each s subshell has just 1 orbital.
- If $l = 1$, then m_l can equal $-1, 0, 1$ (three possibilities), so each p subshell has 3 orbitals.
- If $l = 2$, then $m_l = -2, -1, 0, 1,$ or 2 (five possibilities), so each d subshell has 5 orbitals.
- If $l = 3$, then there are seven possible values for m_l, so the f subshell contains 7 orbitals.

You should be able to recognize the shapes of the orbitals in the s and p subshells. Each s subshell has just one spherically symmetric orbital, and it's pictured as a sphere.

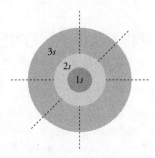

s orbitals
$(l = 0, m_l = 0)$

Each p subshell has three orbitals, each depicted as a dumbbell, with different spatial orientations.

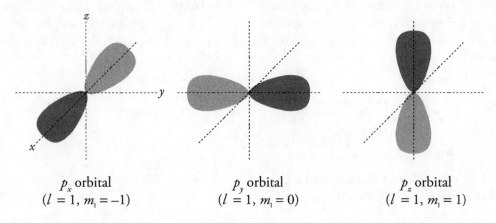

p_x orbital p_y orbital p_z orbital
$(l = 1, m_l = -1)$ $(l = 1, m_l = 0)$ $(l = 1, m_l = 1)$

The Fourth Quantum Number

An electron's fourth quantum number is the **spin number**, m_s, which designates the electron's intrinsic magnetism. Regardless of the values of the n, l, or m_l, the value of m_s can be either $+\frac{1}{2}$ (**spin up**) or $-\frac{1}{2}$ (**spin down**). Every orbital can accommodate 2 electrons, one spin up and one spin down. If an orbital is full, we say that the electrons it holds are "spin-paired."

Shell number, n	Subshell number, l	Orbital number, m_l	Spin number, m_s
size and energy of orbital	shape and energy of orbital	orientation of orbital	spin of electron in orbital
$n = 1, 2, 3, ...$	$l = 0, 1, 2, ... (n-1)$	$m_l = -l, -(l-1), ...$ $0 ... (l-1), l$	$m_s = \pm 1/2$

13.6   ELECTRON CONFIGURATIONS

Now that we've described the electron quantum numbers, let's see how we assign them to each electron in an atom. There are three basic rules:

1. *Electrons occupy the lowest energy orbitals available.* (This is the **Aufbau principle**.) Electron subshells are filled in order of increasing energy. The periodic table is logically constructed to reflect this fact, and therefore one can easily determine shell filling for specific atoms based on where they appear on the table. We will detail this in the next section on "Blocks."
2. *Electrons in the same subshell occupy available orbitals singly, before pairing up.* (This is known as **Hund's rule**.)
3. *No two electrons in the same atom can have the same set of four quantum numbers.* (This is the **Pauli exclusion principle**.)

For example, let's find the quantum numbers for all the electrons in an oxygen atom, which contains 8 electrons. Beginning with $n = 1$, the only allowed value of l is 0 (the s subshell), and the only allowed value of m_l is 0. There are, of course, two possible values for m_s, so the first two electrons have these quantum numbers:

	n	l	m_l	m_s
Electron #1:	1	0	0	$+\frac{1}{2}$
Electron #2:	1	0	0	$-\frac{1}{2}$

Therefore, these two electrons fill the only orbital in the $1s$ subshell. We write this as $1s^2$, to indicate that there are 2 electrons in the $1s$ subshell.

We still have six electrons left, so let's move on to $n = 2$. For $n = 2$, l can equal 0 (s subshell) or 1 (p subshell). When $l = 0$, m_l can only equal 0, and m_s can equal $+\frac{1}{2}$ or $-\frac{1}{2}$. So the next two electrons go in the $2s$ subshell:

	n	l	m_l	m_s
Electron #3:	2	0	0	$+\frac{1}{2}$
Electron #4:	2	0	0	$-\frac{1}{2}$

That is, we have 2 electrons in the 2s subshell: $2s^2$.

Now, for $l = 1$ (the p subshell), m_l can equal −1, 0, or 1. According to Hund's rule, we place one spin up electron in each of these three orbitals:

	n	l	m_l	m_s
Electron #5:	2	1	−1	+½
Electron #6:	2	1	0	+½
Electron #7:	2	1	1	+½

The eighth electron now pairs up with an electron in one of the 2p orbitals:

	n	l	m_l	m_s
Electron #8:	2	1	−1	−½

So, the last four electrons go in the 2p subshell: $2p^4$ (or more explicitly, $2p_x{}^2 2p_y{}^1 2p_z{}^1$).

The complete electron configuration for oxygen can now be written like this:

$$\text{Oxygen} = 1s^2 2s^2 2p^4$$

oxygen =   1s   2s   2p

↑ = spin-up electron
↓ = spin-down electron

Example 13-3: What's the maximum number of electrons that can go into any s subshell? Any p subshell? Any d? Any f?

Solution: An s subshell corresponds to $l = 0$. When $l = 0$, there's only 1 possible value for m_l (namely, 0). Since there are 2 possible values for m_s (+½ or −½), an s subshell can hold no more than $1 \times 2 = 2$ electrons.

A p subshell corresponds to $l = 1$. When $l = 1$, there are only 3 possible values for m_l (namely, −1, 0, or 1). Since there are again 2 possible values for m_s, a p subshell can hold no more than $3 \times 2 = 6$ electrons.

A d subshell corresponds to $l = 2$. When $l = 2$, there are only 5 possible values for m_l (namely, −2, −1, 0, 1, or 2). Since there are 2 possible values for m_s, a d subshell can hold no more than $5 \times 2 = 10$ electrons.

Finally, an f subshell corresponds to $l = 3$. When $l = 3$, there are only 7 possible values for m_l (namely, −3, −2, −1, 0, 1, 2, or 3). Since there are 2 possible values for m_s, an f subshell can hold no more than $7 \times 2 = 14$ electrons.

13.6

Example 13-4: Write down—and comment on—the electron configuration of argon (Ar, atomic number 18).

Solution: We have 18 electrons to successively place in the proper subshells, as follows:

$1s$:   2 electrons

$2s$:   2 electrons

$2p$:   6 electrons

$3s$:   2 electrons

$3p$:   6 electrons

13.6

Therefore,

$$[Ar] = 1s^22s^22p^63s^23p^6$$

Notice that $3s$ and $3p$ subshells have their full complement of electrons. In fact, the **noble gases** (those elements in the last column of the periodic table) all have their outer 8 electrons in filled subshells: 2 in the ns subshell plus 6 in the np. (The lone exception, of course, is helium; but its one and only subshell, the $1s$, is filled—with 2 electrons.) Because their 8 valence electrons are in filled subshells, we say that these atoms—Ne, Ar, Kr, Xe, and Rn—have a complete **octet**, which accounts for their remarkable chemical inactivity.

Blocks in the Periodic Table

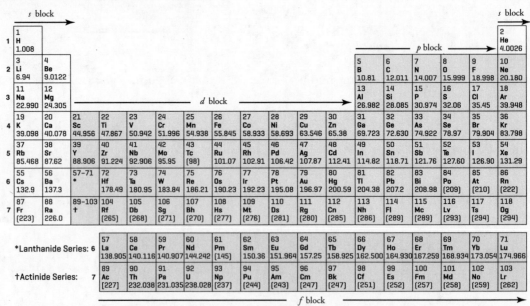

The periodic table can be divided into blocks, as shown on the previous page. The name of the block (*s, p, d,* or *f*) indicates the highest-energy subshell containing electrons in the ground-state of an atom within that block. For example, carbon is in the *p* block, and its electron configuration is $1s^2 2s^2 2p^2$; the highest-energy subshell that contains electrons (the $2p$) is a *p* subshell. The bold numbers next to the rows on the left indicate the period number; for example, potassium (K, atomic number 19) is in Period 4.

How do we use this block diagram to write electron configurations? To illustrate, let's say we want to write the configuration for chlorine ($Z = 17$). To get to $Z = 17$, imagine starting at $Z = 1$ (hydrogen) and filling up the subshells as we move along through the rows to $Z = 17$. (Notice that helium has been moved over next to hydrogen for purposes of this block diagram.) We'll first have $1s^2$ for the 2 atoms in Period 1, *s* block ($Z = 1$ and $Z = 2$); the $2s^2$ for the next 2 atoms, which are in Period 2, *s* block ($Z = 3$ and $Z = 4$); then $2p^6$ for the next 6 atoms, which are in Period 2, *p* block ($Z = 5$ through $Z = 10$); the $3s^2$ for the next 2 atoms, which are in Period 3, *s* block ($Z = 11$ and $Z = 12$); then, finally, $3p^5$ for the atoms starting with aluminum, Al, in Period 3, *p* block and counting through to chlorine, Cl. So, we've gone through the rows and blocks from the beginning and stopped once we hit the atom we wanted, and along the way we obtained $1s^2 2s^2 2p^6 3s^2 3p^5$. This is the electron configuration of chlorine.

The noble gases are often used as starting points, because they are at the end of the rows and represent a shell being completely filled; all that's left is to count over in the next row until the desired atom is reached. We find the closest noble gas whose atomic number is less than that of the atom whose configuration we want. In the case of chlorine ($Z = 17$), the closest noble gas with a smaller atomic number is neon ($Z = 10$). Starting with neon, we have 7 additional electrons to take care of. To get to $Z = 17$, we go through the 2 atoms in the *s* block of Period 3 ($3s^2$), then notice that Cl is the fifth element in the *p* block, giving us $3p^5$. Therefore, the electron configuration of chlorine is the same as that of neon plus $3s^2 3p^5$, which we can write like this: [Cl] = [Ne] $3s^2 3p^5$.

The simple counting through the rows and blocks works as long as you remember this simple rule: Whenever you're in the *d* block, *subtract 1 from the period number*. For example, the first row of the *d* block ($Z = 21$ through $Z = 30$) is in Period 4, but instead of saying that these elements have their outermost (or **valence**) electrons in the $4d$ subshell, we subtract 1 from the period number and say that these elements put their valence electrons in the $3d$ subshell.

In summary: The block in the table tells us in which subshell the outermost (valence) electrons of the atom will be. The period (row) gives the valence shell, n, as long as we remember the following fact about the atoms in the *d* block: electrons for an atom in the *d* block of Period n go into the subshell $(n-1)d$. For example, the electron configuration for scandium (Sc, atomic number 21) is [Ar]$4s^2 3d^1$. (Note: if you ever need to write the electron configuration for an element in the *f* block, the rule is: *In the f block, subtract 2 from the period number.*)

Example 13-5: What is the electron configuration of an aluminum atom?

Solution: Since aluminum (Al) has atomic number 13, a neutral aluminum atom must have 13 electrons, giving $1s^2 2s^2 2p^6 3s^2 3p^1$.

Example 13-6: What's the electron configuration of a zirconium atom ($Z = 40$)?

Solution: Zirconium (Zr) is in the *d* block of Period 5. After krypton (Kr, atomic number 36), we'll have $5s^2$ for the next 2 atoms in Period 5, *s* block ($Z = 37$ and $Z = 38$). Then, remembering the rule that electrons for an atom in the *d* block of Period n go into the subshell $(n - 1)d$, we know that the last two electrons will go in the $4d$ (not the $5d$) subshell. This gives us [Kr] $5s^2 4d^2$.

Electron Configurations of Ions

Recall that an ion is an atom that has acquired a nonzero electric charge. An atom with more electrons than protons is negatively charged and is called an anion; an atom with fewer electrons than protons is positively charged and is called a cation.

Atoms that gain electrons (anions) accommodate them in the first available orbital, the one with the lowest available energy. For example, fluorine (F, atomic number 9) has the electron configuration $1s^2 2s^2 2p^5$. When a fluorine atom gains an electron to become the fluoride ion, F^-, the additional electron goes into the $2p$ subshell, giving the electron configuration $1s^2 2s^2 2p^6$, which is the same as the configuration of neon. For this reason, F^- and Ne are said to be **isoelectronic**.

In order to write the electron configuration of an ion, we can use the blocks in the periodic table as follows. If an atom becomes an anion—that is, if it acquires one or more additional electrons—then we move to the *right* within the table by a number of squares equal to the number of electrons added in order to find the atom with the same configuration as the ion.

If an atom becomes a cation—that is, if it loses one or more electrons—then we move to the *left* within the table by a number of squares equal to the number of electrons lost in order to find the atom with the same configuration as the ion.

Example 13-7: What's the electron configuration of P^{3-}? Of Sr^+?

Solution: To find the configuration of P^{3-}, we locate phosphorus (P, atomic number 15) in the periodic table and move 3 places to the *right* (because we have an anion with a charge of 3^-); this lands us on argon (Ar, atomic number 18). Therefore, the electron configuration of the anion P^{3-} is the same as that of argon: $1s^2 2s^2 2p^6 3s^2 3p^6$.

To find the configuration of Sr^+, we locate strontium (Sr, atomic number 38) in the periodic table and move 1 place to the *left* (because we have a cation with charge 1+), thus landing on rubidium (Rb, atomic number 37). Therefore, the electron configuration of the anion Sr^+ is the same as that of rubidium: $[Kr] 5s^1$.

Electrons that are removed (*ionized*) from an atom always come from the valence level, which is usually the one with the highest energy, or the least stable orbital. For example, an atom of lithium, Li ($1s^2 2s^1$), becomes Li^+ ($1s^2$) when it absorbs enough energy for an electron to escape. However, recall from our discussion above that there are other factors that contribute to stability; namely, having a half-filled or filled d subshell. For **transition metals** (which are the elements in the d block), *the valence s electrons are always lost first; only after these are all gone do any d electrons get ionized.* For example, the electron configuration for the transition metal titanium (Ti, atomic number 22) is $[Ar] 4s^2 3d^2$. We might expect the electron configuration of the ion Ti^+ to be $[Ar] 4s^2 3d^1$ since the d electrons are slightly higher in energy. However, the *actual* configuration is $[Ar] 4s^1 3d^2$, and the valence electrons (the ones from the highest n level) are ALWAYS lost first. Similarly, the electron configuration of Ti^{2+} is not $[Ar] 4s^2$—it's actually $[Ar] 3d^2$.

Example 13-8: Which group I cation has the same electron configuration as the noble gas argon?

Solution: K^+ has the same electron configuration as argon.

Example 13-9: What's the electron configuration of Cu^+? Of Cu^{2+}? Of Fe^{3+}?

Solution: Copper (Cu, atomic number 29) is a transition metal, so it will lose its valence s electrons before losing any d electrons. Recall the anomalous electron configuration of Cu (to give it a filled $3d$ subshell): $[Ar]\, 4s^1 3d^{10}$. Therefore, the configuration of Cu^+ (the *cuprous* ion, Cu(I)) is $[Ar]\, 3d^{10}$, and that of Cu^{2+} (the *cupric* ion, Cu(II)) is $[Ar]\, 3d^9$. Since the electron configuration of iron (Fe, atomic number 26) is $[Ar]\, 4s^2 3d^6$, the configuration of Fe^{3+} (the *ferric* ion, Fe(III)) is $[Ar]\, 3d^5$, since the transition metal atom Fe first loses both of its valence s electrons, then once they're ionized, one of its d electrons.

13.7   ATOMIC STRUCTURE

Emission Spectra

Imagine a glass tube filled with a small sample of an element in gaseous form. When electric current is passed through the tube, the gas begins to glow with a color characteristic of that particular element. If this light emitted by the gas is then passed through a prism—which will separate the light into its component wavelengths—the result is the element's **emission spectrum**.

An atom's emission spectrum gives an energetic "fingerprint" of that element because it consists of a unique sequence of *bright* lines that correspond to specific wavelengths and energies. The energies of the photons, or particles of light that are emitted, are related to their frequencies, f, and wavelengths, λ, by the equation

$$E_{\text{photon}} = hf = h\frac{c}{\lambda}$$

where h is a universal constant called **Planck's constant** (6.63×10^{-34} J·s) and c is the speed of light.

The Bohr Model of the Atom

In 1913 the Danish physicist Niels Bohr realized that the model of atomic structure of his time was inconsistent with emission spectral data. In order to account for the limited numbers of lines that are observed in the emission spectra of elements, Bohr described a new model of the atom. In this model that would later take his name, he proposed that the electrons in an atom orbited the nucleus in circular paths, much as the planets orbit the Sun in the solar system. Distance from the nucleus was related to the energy of the electrons; electrons with greater amounts of energy orbited the nucleus at greater distances. However, the electrons in the atom cannot assume any arbitrary energy, but have *quantized* energy states, and thereby only orbit at certain allowed distances from the nucleus.

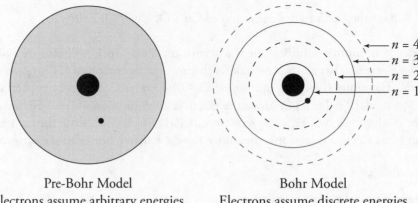

Pre-Bohr Model
Electrons assume arbitrary energies

Bohr Model
Electrons assume discrete energies

13.7

If an electron absorbs energy that's exactly equal to the difference in energy between its current level and that of an available higher lever, it "jumps" to that higher level. The electron can then "drop" to a lower energy level, emitting a photon whose energy is exactly equal to the difference between the levels. This model predicted that elements would have line spectra instead of continuous spectra, as would be the case if transitions between all possible energies could be expected. An electron could only gain or lose very specific amounts of energy due to the quantized nature of the energy levels. Therefore, only photons with certain energies are observed. These specific energies corresponded to very specific wavelengths, as seen in the emission line spectra.

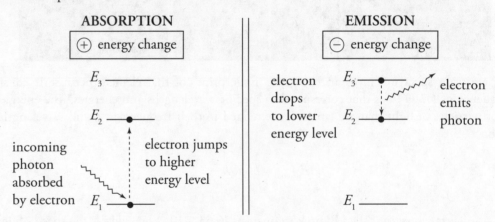

In the transition depicted below, an electron is initially in its **ground state** ($n = 1$), or its lowest possible energy level. When this electron absorbs a photon it jumps to a higher energy level, known as an **excited state** (in this case $n = 3$). Electrons excited to high energy don't always relax to the ground state in large jumps, rather they can relax in a series of smaller jumps, gradually coming back to the ground state. From this excited state the electron can relax in one of two ways, either dropping into the $n = 2$ level, or directly back to the $n = 1$ ground state. In the first scenario, we can expect to detect a photon with energy corresponding to the difference between $n = 3$ and $n = 2$. In the latter case we'd detect a more energetic photon of energy corresponding to the difference between $n = 3$ and $n = 1$.

Note: Distances between energy levels are not drawn to scale.

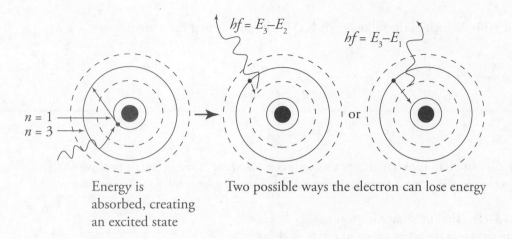

$hf = E_3 - E_2$

$hf = E_3 - E_1$

$n = 1$
$n = 3$

Energy is
absorbed, creating
an excited state

Two possible ways the electron can lose energy

or

The energies of these discrete energy levels were given by Bohr in the following equation, which only accurately predicted the behavior of atoms or ions containing one electron, now known as Bohr atoms. The value n in this case represents the energy level of the electron.

$$E_n = \frac{(-2.178 \times 10^{-18}\,\text{J})}{n^2}$$

Since we can calculate the energies of the levels of a Bohr atom, we can predict the wavelengths of photons emitted when excited electrons fall to the ground state. To do this, we calculate the energy differences between discrete levels by subtracting the initial energy of the electron from the final energy of the electron. We can find the energies of the two possible emitted photons shown above as follows:

$$\Delta E_{3 \to 2} = \frac{(-2.178 \times 10^{-18}\,\text{J})}{(2)^2} - \frac{(-2.178 \times 10^{-18}\,\text{J})}{(3)^2}$$

$$\Delta E_{3 \to 2} = -3.025 \times 10^{-19}\,\text{J}$$

$$\Delta E_{3 \to 1} = \frac{(-2.178 \times 10^{-18}\,\text{J})}{(1)^2} - \frac{(-2.178 \times 10^{-18}\,\text{J})}{(3)^2}$$

$$\Delta E_{3 \to 1} = -1.936 \times 10^{-18}\,\text{J}$$

Once the energy is calculated, the wavelength of the photon can be found by employing the relation $\Delta E = h\dfrac{c}{\lambda}$. Not all electron transitions produce photons we can see with the naked eye, but all transitions in an atom will produce photons either in the ultraviolet, visible, or infrared region of the electromagnetic spectrum.

Example 13-10: Which of the following is NOT an example of a Bohr atom?

A. H
B. He^+
C. Li^{2+}
D. H^+
E. Be^{3+}

Solution: A Bohr atom is one that contains only one electron. Since H^+ has a positive charge from losing the one electron in the neutral atom, thereby having no electrons at all, D is the answer.

Example 13-11: The first four electron energy levels of an atom are shown at the right, given in terms of electron volts. Which of the following gives the energy of a photon that could NOT be emitted by this atom?

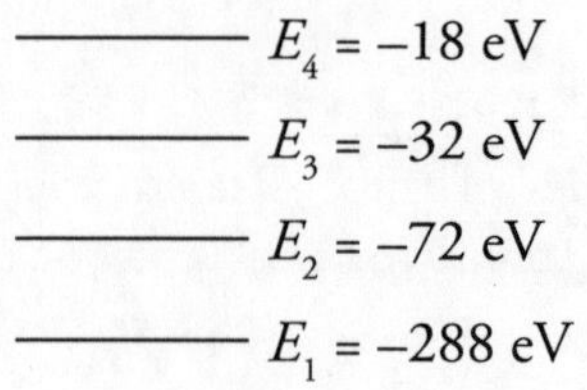

——————— $E_4 = -18$ eV

——————— $E_3 = -32$ eV

——————— $E_2 = -72$ eV

——————— $E_1 = -288$ eV

A. 14 eV
B. 40 eV
C. 44 eV
D. 54 eV
E. 216 eV

Solution: The difference between E_4 and E_3 is 14 eV, so a photon of 14 eV would be emitted if an electron were to drop from level 4 to level 3; this eliminates A. Similarly, the difference between E_3 and E_2 is 40 eV, so B is eliminated, and the difference between E_4 and E_2 is 54 eV, so D is eliminated. The difference between E_2 and E_1 is 216 eV so E is not the answer. The answer must be C; no two energy levels in this atom are separated by 44 eV.

13.8 NUCLEAR STRUCTURE

Nuclear Stability and Radioactivity

The protons and neutrons in a nucleus are held together by a force called the **strong nuclear force**. It's stronger than the electrical force between charged particles, since for all atoms besides hydrogen, the strong nuclear force must overcome the electrical repulsion between the protons. In fact, of the four fundamental forces of nature, the strong nuclear force is the most powerful.

radioactive
beryllium
nucleus

stable
beryllium
nucleus

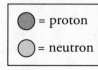

= proton

= neutron

Unstable nuclei are said to be **radioactive**, and they undergo a transformation to make them more stable, altering the number and ratio of protons and neutrons or just lowering their energy. Such a process is called **radioactive decay**, and we'll look at three types: **alpha**, **beta** and **gamma**. The nucleus that undergoes radioactive decay is known as the **parent**, and the resulting more stable nucleus is known as the **daughter**.

Alpha Decay

When a large nucleus wants to become more stable by reducing the number of protons and neutrons, it emits an alpha particle. An **alpha particle**, denoted by α, consists of 2 protons and 2 neutrons:

alpha particle

This is equivalent to a helium-4 nucleus, so an alpha particle is also denoted by He. Alpha decay reduces the parent's atomic number by 2 and the mass number by 4. For example, polonium-210 is an α-emitter. It undergoes alpha decay to form the stable nucleus lead-206:

$$\underbrace{^{210}_{84}\text{Po}}_{\text{parent}} \rightarrow \underbrace{^{206}_{82}\text{Pb}}_{\text{daughter}} + \underset{\text{ejected}}{^{4}_{2}\alpha}$$

Although alpha particles are emitted with high energy from the parent nucleus, this energy is quickly lost as the particle travels through matter or air. As a result, the particles do not typically travel far, and can be stopped by the outer layers of human skin or a piece of paper.

Beta Decay

There are actually three types of beta decay: β^-, β^+, and electron capture. Each type of beta decay involves the transmutation of a neutron into a proton, or vice versa, through the action of the **weak nuclear force**.

Beta particles are more dangerous than alpha particles since they are significantly less massive. They therefore have more energy and a greater penetrating ability. However, they can be stopped by aluminum foil or a centimeter of plastic or glass.

β^- **Decay**   When an unstable nucleus contains too many neutrons, it may convert a neutron into a proton and an electron (also known as a β^- **particle**), which is ejected. The atomic number of the resulting daughter nucleus is 1 greater than the radioactive parent nucleus, but the mass number remains the same. The isotope carbon-14, whose decay is the basis of radiocarbon dating of archaeological artifacts, is an example of a radioactive nucleus that undergoes β^- decay:

$$^{14}_{6}\text{C} \rightarrow {}^{14}_{7}\text{N} + \underset{\text{ejected}}{^{0}_{-1}\text{e}^-}$$

β^- decay is the most common type of beta decay, and when the DAT mentions "beta decay" without any further qualification, it means β^- decay.

β⁺ **Decay**   When an unstable nucleus contains too few neutrons, it converts a proton into a neutron and a positron, which is ejected. This is known as β⁺ **decay**. The positron is the electron's *antiparticle*; it's identical to an electron except its charge is positive. The atomic number of the resulting daughter nucleus is 1 less than the radioactive parent nucleus, but the mass number remains the same. The isotope fluorine-18, which can be used in medical diagnostic bone scans in the form $Na^{18}F$, is an example of a positron emitter:

$$\underset{9}{\overset{18}{}}F \quad \rightarrow \quad \underset{8}{\overset{18}{}}O \; + \; \underset{+1}{\overset{0}{}}e^{+} \quad \text{ejected}$$

Electron Capture   Another way for an unstable nucleus to increase the number of neutrons is to capture an electron from the closest electron shell (the $n = 1$ shell) and use it in the conversion of a proton into a neutron. Just like positron emission, **electron capture** causes the atomic number to be reduced by 1 while the mass number remains the same. The nucleus chromium-51 is an example of a radioactive nucleus that undergoes electron capture, becoming the stable nucleus vanadium-51:

$$\underset{24}{\overset{51}{}}Cr \; + \; \underset{-1}{\overset{0}{}}e^{-} \; \rightarrow \; \underset{23}{\overset{51}{}}V$$

Gamma Decay

A nucleus in an excited energy state—which is usually the case after a nucleus has undergone alpha or any type of beta decay—can "relax" to its ground state by emitting energy in the form of one or more photons of electromagnetic radiation. These photons are called **gamma photons** (symbolized by γ) and have a very high frequency and energy. Gamma photons (or gamma rays) have neither mass nor charge, and can therefore penetrate matter most effectively. A few inches of lead or about a meter of concrete will stop most gamma rays. Their ejection from a radioactive atom changes neither the atomic number nor the mass number of the nucleus. For example, after silicon-31 undergoes β⁻ decay, the resulting daughter nucleus then undergoes gamma decay:

$$\underset{14}{\overset{31}{}}Si \quad \xrightarrow{\beta^{-} \text{ decay}} \quad \underset{15}{\overset{31}{}}P^{*} \quad \xrightarrow{\gamma \text{ decay}} \quad \underset{15}{\overset{31}{}}P + \gamma \quad \text{emitted}$$

indicates nucleus
is in an excited
energy state

Notice that alpha and beta decay change the identity of the nucleus, but gamma decay does not. Gamma decay is simply an expulsion of energy.

Summary of Radioactive Decay

$$\boxed{N\downarrow \; Z\downarrow}$$ Alpha Decay

Decreases the number of neutrons *and* protons in large nucleus

Subtracts 4 from the mass number

Subtracts 2 from the atomic number

$$^{A}_{Z}X \xrightarrow{\;\alpha\;} \;^{A-4}_{Z-2}Y + \;^{4}_{2}\alpha$$

$$\boxed{N\downarrow \; Z\uparrow}$$ Beta$^-$ Decay

Decreases the number of neutrons, increases the number of protons

Adds 1 to the atomic number

$$^{A}_{Z}X \xrightarrow{\;\beta^-\;} \;^{A}_{Z+1}Y + \;^{0}_{-1}e^{-}$$

$$\boxed{N\uparrow \; Z\downarrow}$$ Beta$^+$ Decay

Increases the number of neutrons, decreases the number of protons

Subtracts 1 from the atomic number

$$^{A}_{Z}X \xrightarrow{\;\beta^+\;} \;^{A}_{Z-1}Y + \;^{0}_{+1}e^{+}$$

$$\boxed{N\uparrow \; Z\downarrow}$$ Electron Capture

Increases the number of neutrons, decreases the number of protons

Subtracts 1 from the atomic number

$$^{A}_{Z}X + \;^{0}_{-1}e^{-} \xrightarrow{\;EC\;} \;^{A}_{Z-1}Y$$

Gamma Decay

Brings an excited nucleus to a lower energy state

Doesn't change mass number or atomic number

$$^{A}_{Z}X^{*} \xrightarrow{\;\gamma\;} \;^{A}_{Z}X + \gamma$$

13.8

Example 13-12: Radioactive calcium-47, a known β^- emitter, is administered in the form of $^{47}CaCl_2$ by I.V. as a diagnostic tool to study calcium metabolism. What is the daughter nucleus of ^{47}Ca?

Solution: The β^- decay of ^{47}Ca is described by this nuclear reaction:

$$^{47}_{20}Ca \rightarrow \;^{47}_{21}Sc + \;^{0}_{-1}e^{-}$$

Therefore, the daughter nucleus is scandium-47.

Example 13-13: Americium-241 is used to provide intracavitary radiation for the treatment of malignancies. This radioisotope is known to undergo alpha decay. What is the daughter nucleus?

Solution: The α decay of ^{241}Am is described by this nuclear reaction:

$$^{241}_{95}\text{Am} \rightarrow\ ^{237}_{93}\text{Np} + ^{4}_{2}\alpha$$

Therefore, the daughter nucleus is neptunium-237.

Example 13-14: Vitamin B$_{12}$ can be prepared with *radioactive* cobalt (^{58}Co), a known β$^+$ emitter, and administered orally as a diagnostic tool to test for defects in intestinal vitamin B$_{12}$ absorption. What is the daughter nucleus of ^{58}Co?

Solution: The β$^+$ decay of ^{58}Co is described by this nuclear reaction:

$$^{58}_{27}\text{Co} \rightarrow\ ^{58}_{26}\text{Fe} + ^{0}_{+1}e^+$$

Therefore, the daughter nucleus is iron-58.

Example 13-15: A certain radioactive isotope is administered orally as a diagnostic tool to study pancreatic function and intestinal fat absorption. This radioisotope is known to undergo β$^-$ decay, and the daughter nucleus is xenon-131. What is the parent radioisotope?

Solution: The β$^-$ decay that results in ^{131}Xe is described by this nuclear reaction:

$$^{131}_{53}\text{I} \rightarrow\ ^{131}_{54}\text{Xe} + ^{0}_{-1}e^-$$

Therefore, the parent nucleus is iodine-131.

Example 13-16: Which of these modes of radioactive decay causes a change in the mass number of the parent nucleus?

    A. α
    B. β$^-$
    C. β$^+$
    D. γ
    E. Electron Capture

Solution: Gamma decay causes no changes in the number of protons or neutrons, so we can eliminate D. Beta decay (β$^-$, β$^+$, and EC) changes both N and Z by 1, but always such that the change in the sum $N + Z$ (which is the mass number, A) is zero. Therefore, we can eliminate B, C, and E. The answer is A.

Example 13-17: One of the naturally occurring radioactive series begins with radioactive ^{238}U. It undergoes a series of decays, one of which is: alpha, beta, beta, alpha, alpha, alpha, alpha, alpha, beta, beta, alpha, beta, alpha, beta. What is the final resulting nuclide of this series of decays?

13.8

Solution: Since there are so many individual decays, let's find the final daughter nucleus using a simple shortcut: For every alpha decay, we'll subtract 4 from the mass number (the superscript) and subtract 2 from the atomic number (the subscript); for every beta decay, we'll add 0 to the mass number and 1 to the atomic number. Since there are a total of 8 alpha-decays and 6 beta-decays, we get

$$\underset{92}{\overset{238}{}}U \xrightarrow{8\alpha} \underset{92 \ -8(2)}{\overset{238 \ -8(4)}{}} \xrightarrow{6\beta^- \ +6(0)}{+6(1)} = \underset{82}{\overset{206}{}} Pb$$

Therefore, the final daughter nucleus is lead-206.

Half Life

Different radioactive nuclei decay at different rates. The **half-life**, which is denoted by $t_{1/2}$, of a radioactive substance is the time it takes for one-half of some sample of the substance to decay, so the shorter the half-life, the faster the decay. The amount of a radioactive substance decreases exponentially with time, as illustrated in the following graph.

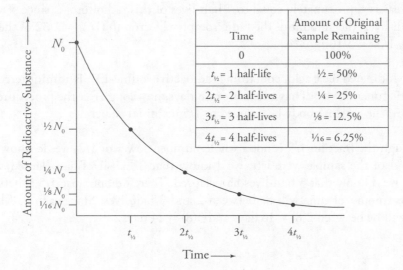

Time	Amount of Original Sample Remaining
0	100%
$t_{1/2}$ = 1 half-life	½ = 50%
$2t_{1/2}$ = 2 half-lives	¼ = 25%
$3t_{1/2}$ = 3 half-lives	⅛ = 12.5%
$4t_{1/2}$ = 4 half-lives	¹⁄₁₆ = 6.25%

For example, a radioactive sample with an initial mass of 80 grams and a half-life of 6 years will decay as follows:

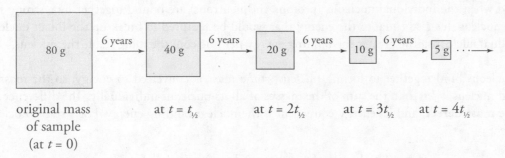

The equation for the exponential decay curve shown above is often written as $N = N_0 e^{-kt}$, but a simpler—and much more intuitive way—is

$$N = N_0 (1/2)^{t/t_{1/2}}$$

where $t_{1/2}$ is the half-life. For example, when $t = 3t_{1/2}$, the number of radioactive nuclei remaining, N, is $N_0(1/2)^3 = 1/8\, N_0$, just what we expect. If the form $N_0 e^{-kt}$ is used, the value of k (known as the **decay constant**) is inversely proportional to the half-life: $k = (\ln 2)/t_{1/2}$. The shorter the half-life, the greater the decay constant, and the more rapidly the sample decays.

Example 13-18: Cesium-137 has a half-life of 30 years. How long will it take for only 0.3 g to remain from a sample that had an original mass of 2.4 g?

Solution: Since 0.3 grams is 1/8 of 2.4 grams, the question is asking how long it will take for the radio-isotope to decrease to 1/8 its original amount. We know that this requires 3 half-lives, since $1/2 \times 1/2 \times 1/2 = 1/8$. So, if each half-life is 30 years, then 3 half-lives will be $3(30) = 90$ years.

Example 13-19: Radioisotope vitamin B_{12}, containing radioactive cobalt-58, is administered to diagnose a defect in a patient's vitamin-B_{12} absorption. If ^{58}Co has a half-life of 72 days, approximately what percentage of the radioisotope will still remain in the patient a year later?

Solution: One year is approximately equal to 5 half-lives of this radioisotope, since $5 \times 72 = 360$ days = 1 year. After 5 half-lives, the amount of the radioisotope will drop to $(1/2)^5 = 1/32$ of the original amount administered. So, $1/32 = 3/100 = 3\%$.

Example 13-20: Iodinated oleic acid, containing radioactive iodine-131, is administered orally to study a patient's pancreatic function. If ^{131}I has a half-life of 8 days, how long after the procedure will the amount of ^{131}I remaining in the patient's body be reduced to 1/5 its initial value?

Solution: Although the fraction 1/5 is not a whole-number power of 1/2, we do know that it's between 1/4 and 1/8. If 1/4 of the sample were left, we'd know that 2 half-lives had elapsed, and if 1/8 of the sample were left, we'd know that 3 half-lives had elapsed. Therefore, because 1/5 is between 1/4 and 1/8, we know that the amount of time will be between 2 and 3 half-lives. Since each half-life is 8 days, this amount of time will be between $2(8) = 16$ days and $3(8) = 24$ days.

Nuclear Binding Energy

Every nucleus that contains protons *and* neutrons has a **nuclear binding energy**. This is the energy that is released when the individual nucleons (protons and neutrons) are bound together by a strong force to form the nucleus. It's also equal to the energy that would be required to break up the intact nucleus into its individual nucleons. The greater the binding energy per nucleon, the more stable the nucleus.

When nucleons bind together to form a nucleus, some mass is converted to energy, so the mass of the combined nucleus is *less* than the sum of the masses of all its nucleons individually. The difference, Δm, is called the **mass defect**, and its energy equivalent *is* the nuclear binding energy. For a stable nucleus, the mass defect

$$\Delta m = \text{(total mass of separate nucleons)} - \text{(mass of nucleus)}$$

will always be positive.

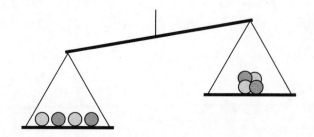

Nuclear binding energy, E_B, can be found from the mass defect using Einstein's equation for mass-energy equivalence: $E_B = (\Delta m)c^2$. In this equation, energy is measured in joules ($J = kg \cdot m^2 \cdot s^2$), mass is measured in kg, and the speed of light in vacuum, c, is a constant 3×10^8 m/s. If you plug 1 kg of mass into this equation, you will see that $E_B = (1 \text{ kg})(3 \times 10^8 \text{ m/s})^2 = 9 \times 10^{16}$ J. In other words, this equation implies that a mass of 1 kg is equal to a nuclear binding energy of 9×10^{16} J.

In the nuclear domain, masses are often expressed in atomic mass units (amu), where 1 amu $\approx 1.66 \times 10^{-27}$ kg, and energy is expressed in the unit electronvolts. In physics, an electronvolt (eV) is a measure of the amount of kinetic energy gained by a single electron accelerating from rest through an electric potential difference of one volt in vacuum. When used as a unit of energy, the numerical value of 1 eV $\approx 1.6 \times 10^{-19}$ J. In terms of these units, the equation for nuclear binding energy in joules, $E_B = (\Delta m)c^2$, can be written as E_B in eV:

For a mass of 1 amu, $E_B = (\Delta m)c^2 = (1 \text{ amu})c^2 = (1.66 \times 10^{-27} \text{ kg})(3 \times 10^8 \text{ m/s})^2 = 1.49 \times 10^{-10}$ J

Next, convert J to eV:

$$\frac{1 \text{ eV}}{1.6 \times 10^{-19} \text{J}} = \frac{x \text{ eV}}{1.49 \times 10^{-10} \text{J}}$$

$$x \text{ eV} = \frac{1.49 \times 10^{-10}}{1.6 \times 10^{-19} \text{J}} (1 \text{ eV}) \approx 931.5 \times 10^6 \text{ eV}$$

Because 10^6 eV = 1 MeV, 931.5×10^6 eV = 931.5 MeV. This means that a mass of 1 amu is equal to a nuclear binding energy of 931.5 MeV and generates the other equation for nuclear binding energy that you may need to use on the DAT: E_B (in MeV) = [Δm (in amu)] × 931.5 MeV/amu.

Example 13-21: The mass defect of a helium nucleus is 5×10^{-29} kg. What is its nuclear binding energy?

Solution: The equation $E_B = (\Delta m)c^2$ implies that 1 kg $\leftrightarrow 9 \times 10^{16}$ J, so a mass defect of 5×10^{-29} kg is equivalent to an energy of $(5 \times 10^{-29} \text{kg})(9 \times 10^{16} \text{J}) = 4.5 \times 10^{-12}$ J. (For practice, check that this binding energy is approximately equal to 30 MeV.)

Example 13-22: The mass defect of a triton (the nucleus of a tritium, $_1^3\text{H}$) is about 0.009 amu. What is its nuclear binding energy, in electronvolts?

Solution: In terms of amus and electronvolts, the equation for the nuclear binding energy is E_B(in eV) = [Δm(in amu)] × 931.5 MeV. Therefore, for the tritium nucleus, we have

$$E_B = (0.009) \times (931.5 \text{ MeV}) \approx 8.4 \text{ MeV}$$

Want More Practice?
Scan the QR code below to register your book for online chapter summaries, drills, practice tests, and more!

13.8

Chapter 14
Periodic Trends
and Bonding

14.1 GROUPS OF THE PERIODIC TABLE

We will use the electron configurations of the atoms to predict their chemical properties, including their reactivity and bonding patterns with other atoms.

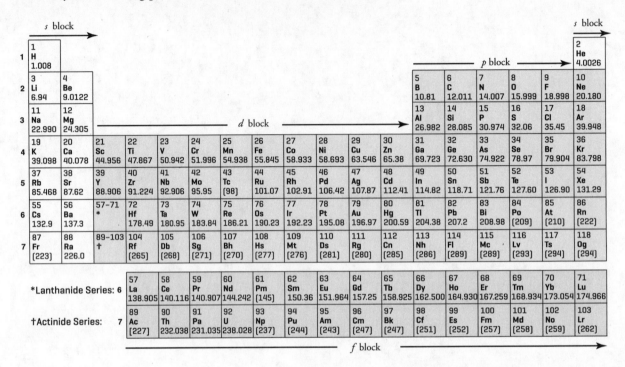

Recall that each horizontal row in the periodic table is called a **period**, and each vertical column is called a **group** (or **family**). Within any group in the periodic table, all of the elements have the same number of electrons in their outermost shell. For instance, the elements in Group II all have 2 electrons in their outermost shell. Electrons in an atom's outermost shell are called **valence** electrons, and it's the valence electrons that are primarily responsible for an atom's properties and chemical behavior.

Naming the Groups

Some groups (families) have special names.

Group	Name	Valence-Shell Configuration
Group I	*Alkali metals*	ns^1
Group II	*Alkaline earth metals*	ns^2
Group VII	*Halogens*	ns^2np^5
The *d* Block	*Transition metals*	
The *p* Block (except Group VIII)	*Representative elements*	
The *f* Block	*Rare earth metals*	
Group VIII	*Noble gases*	ns^2np^6

All noble gases (except helium) have 8 electrons in their outermost shells. Such a configuration is called an **octet**. The valence electron configuration of ns^2np^6 produces great stability, and most chemical behavior can be regarded as the quest of atoms to achieve such closed-shell stability.

Example 14-1: What is the only element with a closed valence shell, but not an octet?

Solution: He, along with H^- and Li^+, has a completed $n = 1$ shell with only 2 electrons, since the $n = 1$ shell can fit only 2 electrons.

Elements on the periodic table are classified as metal, nonmetal or metalloid. Here is a summary of how they differ:

	Metal	Nonmetal
Location on the periodic table	To the left of metalloids (see below)	Upper right
Examples	Alkali metals Alkaline earth metals Transition metals Rare earth metals (lanthanides and actinides)	H, C, N, O, P, S, Se Halogens Noble gases
CHEMICAL PROPERTIES:		
Ionization energy	Low	High
Electronegativity	Low	High
Valence electrons	Easily lost	Easily gained
Redox reactions	Good reducing agents	Good oxidizing agents
PHYSICAL PROPERTIES:		
Thermal conductance	High	Low
Electrical conductance	High	Low
Appearance	Metallic luster, shiny	Dull but can be colorful
At room temperature	Solid (except Hg) Malleable and ductile	Solid, liquid or gas Brittle

Most nonmetals gain electrons easily and have a wide range of chemical properties and reactivities. They typically have lower melting points and boiling point than metals.

Elements that possess qualities of both metals and nonmetals are called metalloids. These elements are:

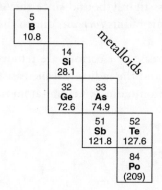

For the DAT, you should know which 7 elements are diatomic at standard state (H_2, N_2, O_2, F_2, Cl_2, Br_2, I_2). "Brinckle-hoff" is a good way to remember these (BrINCl HOF). You should also know the phases of the elements at standard state:

- 2 elements are liquid: mercury (Hg) and bromine (Br)
- 11 elements are gases: H, N, O, F, Cl and all noble gases (He, Ne, Ar, Kr, Xe, Rn)
- All other elements are solid in their standard state

Be careful with the halogens! At room temperature, they exist in all three states of matter: iodine and astatine are solids, bromine is a liquid, fluorine and chlorine are gases.

14.2   PERIODIC TRENDS

Shielding

Each filled shell between the nucleus and the valence electrons shields—or "protects"—the valence electrons from the full effect of the positively charged protons in the nucleus. This is called **nuclear shielding** or the **shielding effect**. As far as the valence electrons are concerned, the electrical pull by the protons in the nucleus is reduced by the negative charges of the electrons in the filled shells in between; the result is an effective reduction in the positive elementary charge, from Z to a smaller amount denoted by Z_{eff} (for *effective nuclear charge*).

Atomic and Ionic Radius

With progression across any period in the table, the number of protons increases, and hence their total pull on the outermost electrons increases, too. New shells are initiated only at the beginning of a period. So, as we go across a period, electrons are being added, but new shells are not; therefore, the valence electrons are more and more tightly bound to the atom because they feel a greater effective nuclear charge. Therefore, as we move from left to right across a period, **atomic radius** *decreases*.

However, with progression down a group, new shells are added and valence electrons experience increased shielding. The valence electrons are less tightly bound since they feel a smaller effective nuclear charge. Therefore, as we go down a group, atomic radius *increases* due to the increased shielding.

If we form an ion, the radius will decrease as electrons are removed (because the ones that are left are drawn in more closely to the nucleus), and the radius will increase as electrons are added. So, in terms of radius, we have $X^+ < X < X^-$; that is, cation radius < neutral-atom radius < anion radius.

Ionization Energy

Because the atom's positively charged nucleus holds the electrons in the atom, it takes energy to remove an electron. The amount of energy necessary to remove the least tightly bound electron from an isolated atom is called the atom's (**first**) **ionization energy** (often abbreviated **IE** or IE_1). As we move from left to right across a period, or up a group, the ionization energy *increases* since the valence electrons are more tightly bound. The ionization energy of any atom with a noble-gas configuration will always be very large. (For example, the ionization energy of neon is 4 times greater than that of lithium.) The **second ionization energy** (IE_2) of an atom, X, is the energy required to remove the least tightly bound electron from the cation X^+. Note that IE_2 will always be greater than IE_1.

Electron Affinity

The energy associated with the addition of an electron to an isolated atom is known as the atom's **electron affinity** (often abbreviated **EA**). If energy is *released* when the electron is added, the usual convention is to say that the electron affinity is negative; if energy is *required* in order to add the electron, the electron affinity is positive. The halogens have large negative electron affinity values, since the addition of an electron would give them the much-desired octet configuration. So they readily accept an electron to become an anion; the increase in stability causes energy to be released. On the other hand, the noble gases and alkaline earth metals have positive electron affinities; anions of these atoms are unstable. Electron affinities typically become more negative as we move to the right across a row or up a group (noble gases excepted), but there are anomalies in this trend.

Electronegativity

Electronegativity is a measure of an atom's ability to pull electrons to itself when it forms a covalent bond; the greater this tendency to attract electrons, the greater the atom's electronegativity. Electronegativity generally behaves as does ionization energy; that is, as we move from left to right across a period, electronegativity increases. As we go down a group, electronegativity decreases. You should know the order of electronegativity for these atoms:

$$F > O > N > Cl > Br > I > S > C > H$$

Summary of Periodic Trends

Atomic Radius	Ionization Energy	Electron Affinity	Electronegativity
← increases	*increases →*	*more negative →*	*increases →*

Example 14-2: Compared to calcium, beryllium is expected to have _____ electronegativity and _____ ionization energy.

Solution: Beryllium and calcium are in the same group, but beryllium is higher in the column. We therefore expect beryllium to have greater ionization energy and a greater electronegativity than calcium, since both of these periodic trends tend to increase as we go up within a group.

Example 14-3: Which of the following will have a greater value for phosphorus than for magnesium?

    A.   Atomic radius and ionization energy
    B.   Atomic radius and electronegativity
    C.   Ionization energy and electronegativity
    D.   Atomic radius, ionization energy, and electronegativity

Solution: Magnesium and phosphorus are in the same period (row), but phosphorus is farther to the right. We therefore expect phosphorus to have greater ionization energy and a greater electronegativity than magnesium, since both of these periodic trends tend to increase as we move to the right across a row. However, we expect the atomic radius of phosphorus to be smaller than that of magnesium, since atomic radii tend to *decrease* as we move to the right across a row. Therefore, the answer is C.

14.3   BONDING

How atoms interact with each other will depend largely on their placement in the periodic table and their electron configurations.

Lewis Dot Symbols

Each dot in the picture below represents one of fluorine's valence electrons. Fluorine is a halogen, whose general valence-shell configuration is ns^2np^5, so there are $2 + 5 = 7$ electrons in its valence shell. We simply place the dots around the symbol for the element, one on each side, and, if there are more than 4 valence electrons, we just start pairing them up. So, for fluorine, we'd have:

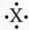

                                       unpaired electron

This is known as a **Lewis dot symbol**. Here are some others:

        K·   ·Mg·   ·Ḃ·   ·Ṡi·   :Ṗ·   :Ö: :C̤l: :N̈e:

(*Note*: Electrons in *d* subshells are not considered valence electrons.)

Example 14-4: Consider this Lewis dot symbol:

$$\cdot\overset{\displaystyle\cdot}{X}\cdot$$

X could represent what elements?

Solution: Since there are 4 dots in the Lewis symbol, X will be an element in Group 4 of the periodic table.

Covalent Bonds

A **covalent bond** is formed between atoms when each contributes one of its unpaired valence electrons. By sharing a pair of electrons to form a bond, each atom may acquire an octet configuration. For example, each of the fluorine atoms below can donate its unpaired valence electron to form a covalent bond and give the molecule F_2. The shared electrons are attracted by the nuclei of *both* atoms in the bond, which hold the atoms together.

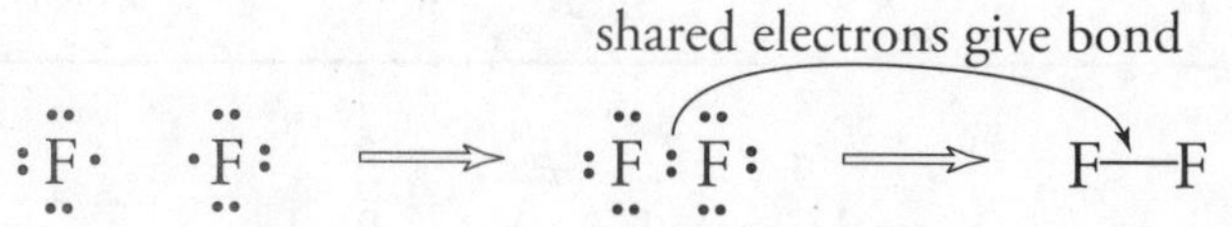

shared electrons give bond

$$:\ddot{F}\cdot \quad \cdot\ddot{F}: \implies :\ddot{F}:\ddot{F}: \implies F-F$$

When Lewis dot symbols for atoms are drawn together to show the bonding and non-bonding electrons in a molecule, the result is known as a **Lewis dot structure**.

Generally speaking, an atom can form one covalent bond for each unpaired valence electron. For example, consider an oxygen atom and two hydrogen atoms. The oxygen atom has 2 unpaired electrons. Each of the hydrogen atoms has 1 unpaired electron. So the oxygen atom can form 2 covalent bonds, and each of the hydrogen atoms can form 1 covalent bond to form the molecule H_2O.

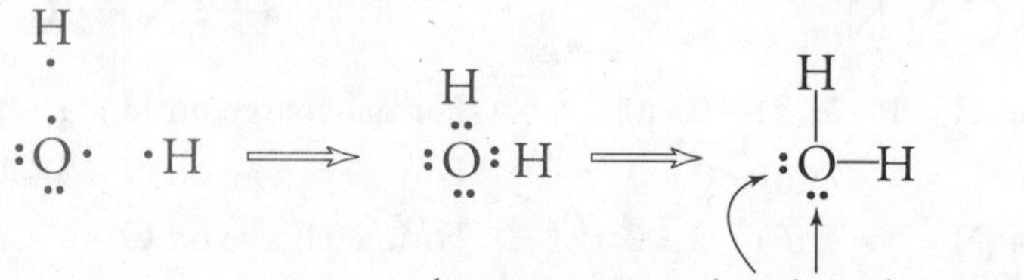

lone-pairs = nonbonding electrons
(unshared pairs of valence electrons)

We can also use Lewis dot structures to show atoms that form multiple covalent bonds; **double bonds** and **triple bonds**. Here are a couple of examples:

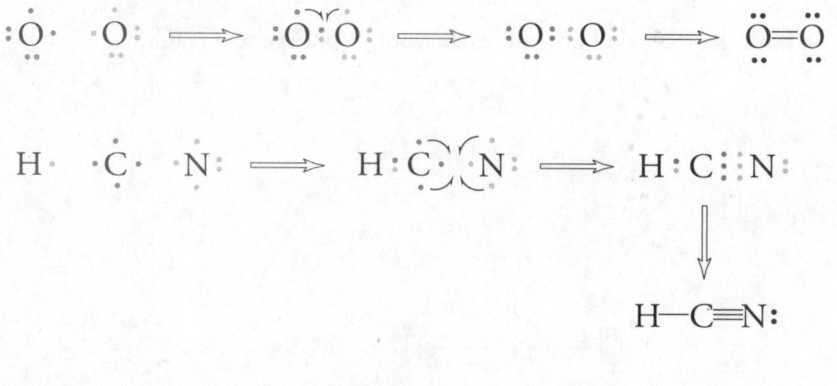

$$:\ddot{O}\cdot \quad \cdot\ddot{O} \implies :\ddot{O}:\ddot{O}: \implies :\ddot{O}::\ddot{O}: \implies \ddot{O}=\ddot{O}$$

$$H\cdot \quad \cdot\ddot{C}\cdot \quad \cdot N: \implies H:C:N: \implies H:C::N:$$

$$H-C\equiv N:$$

Formal Charge

The last Lewis dot structure shown above for the molecule consisting of 1 atom each of hydrogen, carbon, and nitrogen was drawn with C as the central atom. However, it could have been drawn with N as the central atom, and we could have still achieved closed-shell configurations for all the atoms:

$$H\cdot \quad \cdot\ddot{N}: \quad \cdot\ddot{C}\cdot \implies H:N::C: \implies H-N=C: \quad (?)$$

The problem is this doesn't give the correct structure for this molecule. The nitrogen atom is not actually bonded to the hydrogen. A helpful way to evaluate a proposed Lewis structure is to calculate the **formal charge** of each atom in the structure. These formal charges won't give the actual charges on the atoms; they'll simply tell us if the atoms are sharing their valence electrons in the "best" way possible, which will happen when the formal charges are all zero (or at least as small as possible). The formula for calculating the formal charge of an atom in a covalent compound is:

$$\text{Formal Charge (FC)} = V - \frac{1}{2}B - L$$

where V is the number of valence electrons, B is the number of bonding electrons, and L is the number of lone-paired (non-bonding) electrons. We'll show the calculations of the formal charges for each atom in both Lewis structures:

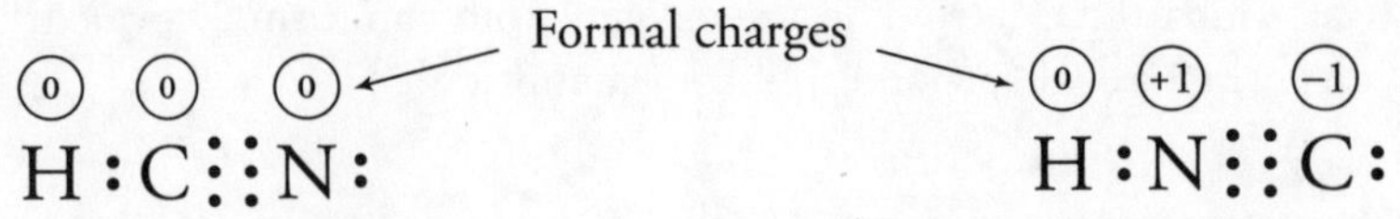

Formal charges

$\overset{\boxed{0} \quad \boxed{0} \quad \boxed{0}}{H:C::N:}$ $\overset{\boxed{0} \quad \boxed{+1} \quad \boxed{-1}}{H:N::C:}$

Formal charge on H = $1 - \frac{1}{2}(2) - 0 = 0$ Formal charge on H = $1 - \frac{1}{2}(2) - 0 = 0$

Formal charge on C = $4 - \frac{1}{2}(8) - 0 = 0$ Formal charge on N = $5 - \frac{1}{2}(8) - 0 = +1$

Formal charge on N = $5 - \frac{1}{2}(6) - 2 = 0$ Formal charge on C = $4 - \frac{1}{2}(6) - 2 = -1$

The best Lewis structures have a formal charge of zero on all the atoms. (Sometimes, this simply isn't possible, and then the best structure is the one that *minimizes* the magnitudes of the formal charges.) The fact that the HCN structure has formal charges of zero for all the atoms, but the HNC structure does not, tells us right away that the HCN structure is the better one.

Example 14-5: What's the formal charge on each atom in phosgene, $COCl_2$?

Solution:

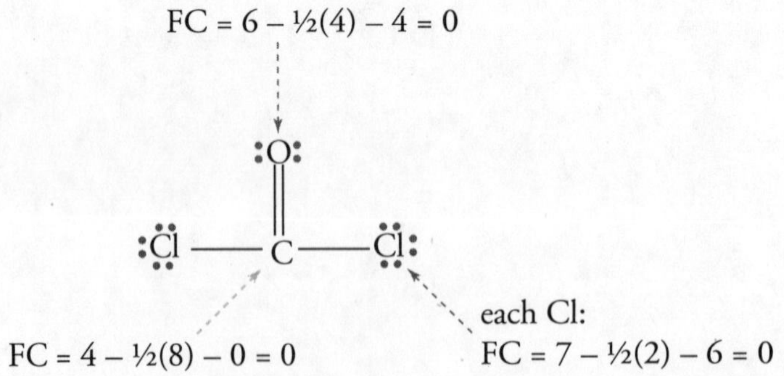

FC = $6 - \frac{1}{2}(4) - 4 = 0$

:O:
‖
:Cl — C — Cl:

each Cl:

FC = $4 - \frac{1}{2}(8) - 0 = 0$ FC = $7 - \frac{1}{2}(2) - 6 = 0$

Example 14-6: Which of the following is the best Lewis structure for CH_2O?

A. 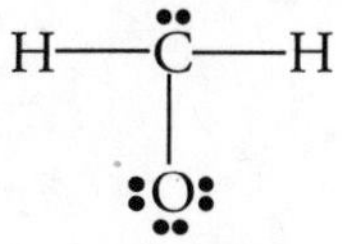 H—C̈—H   C. H—Ö—H   E. 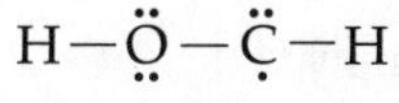   H—Ö̈—C̈—H
        | |
       :O: •C•

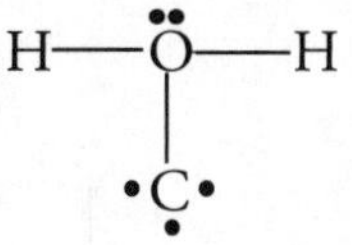

B. 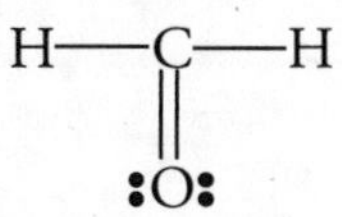 H—C—H   D. 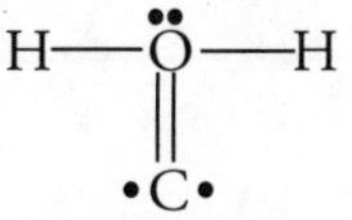 H—Ö—H
        ‖   ‖
       :O: •C•

Solution: When faced with a question like this on the DAT (and they're rather common), the first thing you should do is simply count the electrons. The correct structure for the molecule CH_2O must account for $4 + 2(1) + 6 = 12$ valence electrons. The structure in A has 14, the structure in C has 11, and the structure in E has 13. B and D both have 12 valence electrons. However, in D, oxygen is surrounded by 10 total electrons. This is not possible because oxygen, like all elements in the second row of the periodic table, cannot violate the octet rule and exceed 8 valence electrons. B, then, with 12 valence electrons and the least electronegative atom as the central atom, is the best choice.

Resonance

Let's draw the Lewis structure for sulfur dioxide.

:Ö—S̈=Ö

formal charges -----▶ (−1) (+1) (0)

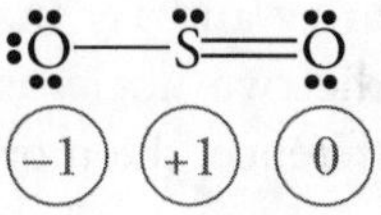

We could also draw the structure like this:

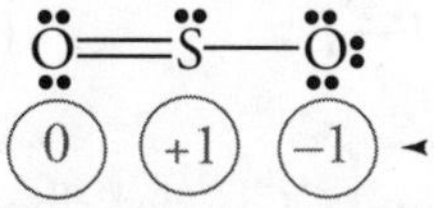

Ö=S̈—Ö:

(0) (+1) (−1) ◀----- formal charges

In either case, there's one S—O single bond and one S=O double bond. This would imply that the double-bonded O would be closer to the S atom than the single-bonded O. Experiment, however, reveals that the bond lengths are the same. Therefore, to describe this molecule, we say that it's an "average" (or, technically, a **resonance hybrid**) of the equivalent Lewis structures drawn above:

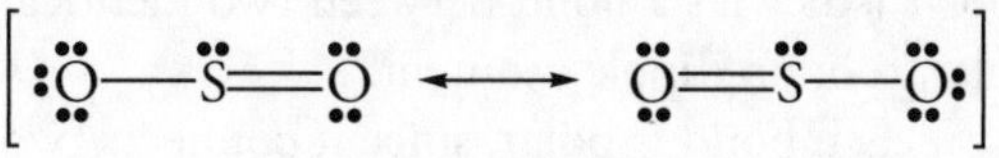

$$\left[:\ddot{O}—\ddot{S}=\ddot{O} \longleftrightarrow \ddot{O}=\ddot{S}—\ddot{O}: \right]$$

We can also symbolize the structure with a single picture, like this:

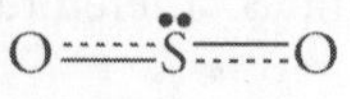

O-----S̈-----O

A molecule may be a resonance hybrid of more than two equivalent Lewis structures; for example, consider the carbonate ion, CO_3^{2-}:

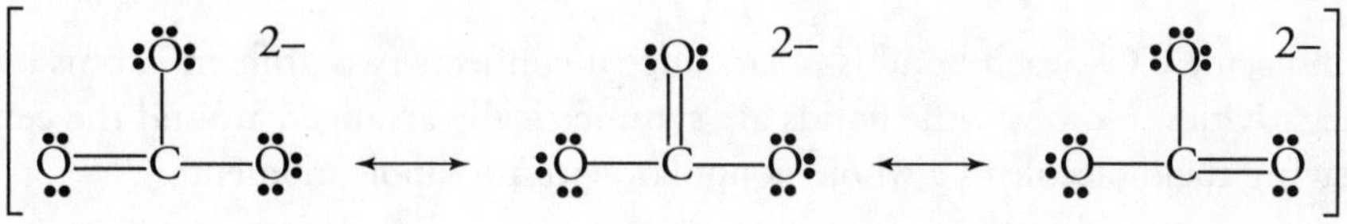

$$\left[\begin{array}{ccc} :\ddot{O}:\ ^{2-} & :O:\ ^{2-} & :\ddot{O}:\ ^{2-} \\ \ddot{O}=C—\ddot{O}: & :\ddot{O}—C—\ddot{O}: & :\ddot{O}—C=\ddot{O} \end{array} \right]$$

or, more simply,

$$
\begin{array}{c}
O \\
\| \\
O\text{-----}C\text{-----}O
\end{array} \quad ^{2-}
$$

Polar Covalent Bonds

Recall that electronegativity refers to an atom's ability to attract another atom's valence electrons when it forms a bond. Electronegativity, in other words, is a measure of how much an atom will "hog" the electrons that it's sharing with another atom.

Consider hydrogen fluoride:

$$H \colon \ddot{F} \colon$$

Fluorine is more electronegative that hydrogen (remember the order of electronegativity?), so the electron density will be greater near the fluorine than near the hydrogen. That means that the H—F molecule is partially negative (denoted by δ^-) on the fluorine side and partially positive (denoted by δ^+) on the hydrogen side. We refer to this as **polarity** and say that the molecule has a **dipole moment**. A bond is **polar** if the electron density between the two nuclei is uneven. This occurs if there is a difference in electronegativity, and the greater the difference, the more uneven the electron density and the greater the dipole moment.

electron density

$$H\text{—}\ddot{F}\colon \qquad \overset{\delta^+}{H}\text{—}\overset{\delta^-}{\ddot{F}}\colon \qquad \overset{\rightarrow}{H\text{—}F}$$

Example 14-7: For each of the molecules N_2, OCS, and CCl_4, describe the polarity of each bond and of the molecule as a whole.

Solution:

- The N≡N bond is nonpolar (since it's a bond between two identical atoms), and since this *is* the molecule, it's nonpolar, too; no dipole moment.
- For the molecule O=C=S, each bond is polar, since it connects two different atoms of unequal electronegativities. Furthermore, the O=C bond is more polar that then C=S bond, because the difference between the electronegativities of O and C is greater than the difference between the electronegativities of C and S. Therefore, the molecule as a whole is polar (that is, it has a dipole moment):

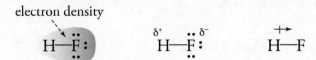

O=C=S ⟹ O=C=S

polar bonds   polar molecule

- For the molecule CCl_4, each bond is polar, since it connects two different atoms of unequal electronegativities. However, the bonds are symmetrically arranged around the central C atom, leaving the molecule as a whole nonpolar, with no dipole moment:

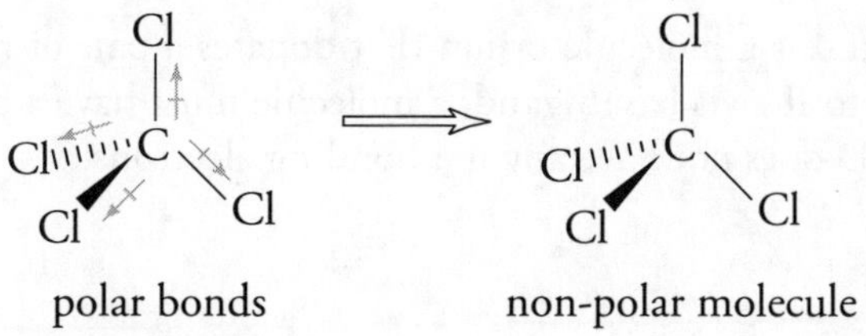

Cl
Cl⫸C⫸Cl ⟹ Cl⫸C⫸Cl
Cl   Cl   Cl   Cl

polar bonds   non-polar molecule

Coordinate Covalent Bonds

Sometimes, one atom will donate *both* of the shared electrons in a bond. That is called a **coordinate covalent bond**. For example, the nitrogen atom in NH_3 donates both electrons in its lone pair to form a bond to boron in the molecule BF_3 to give the coordinate covalent compound F_3BNH_3:

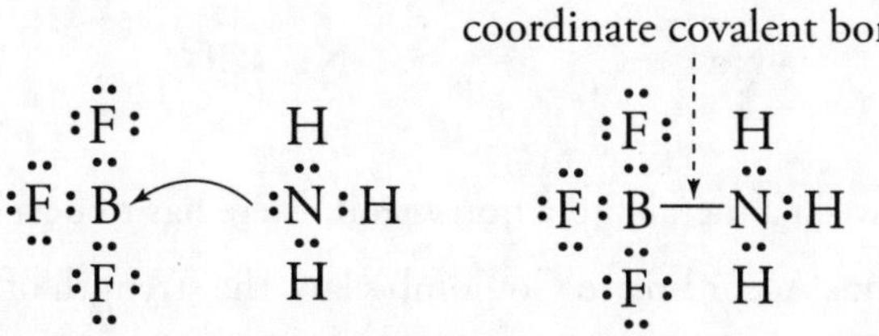

coordinate covalent bond

:F: H   :F: H
:F:B⤺ :N:H   :F:B—N:H
:F: H   :F: H

Since the NH_3 molecule donates a pair of electrons, it is known as a **Lewis base** or **ligand**. Since the BF_3 molecule accepts a pair of electrons, it's known as a **Lewis acid**. When a coordinate covalent bond breaks, the electrons that come from the ligand will leave *with* that ligand.

Example 14-8: Identify the Lewis acid and the Lewis base in the following reaction, which forms a coordination complex:

$$4\ NH_3 + Zn^{2+} \rightarrow Zn(NH_3)_4^{2+}$$

Solution: Each of the NH_3 molecules donates its lone pair to the zinc atom, thus forming four coordinate covalent bonds. Since the zinc ion accepts these electron pairs, it's the Lewis acid; since each ammonia molecule donates an electron pair, they are Lewis bases (or ligands):

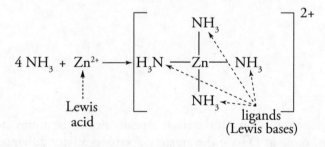

Example 14-9: Which one of the following anions *cannot* behave as a Lewis base/ligand?

   A. F^-
   B. OH^-
   C. NH_2^-
   D. BH_4^-
   E. NO_3^-

Solution: A Lewis base/ligand is a molecule or ion that donates a pair of nonbonding electrons. So, in order to even be a candidate for Lewis base/ligand, a molecule must have a pair of nonbonding electrons in the first place. The ion in D does not have any nonbonding electrons.

Ionic Bonds

While sharing valence electrons is one way atoms can achieve the stable octet configuration, the octet may also be obtained by gaining or losing electrons. For example, a sodium atom will give its valence electron to an atom of chlorine. This results in a sodium cation (Na^+) and a chloride anion (Cl^-), which form sodium chloride. They're held together by the electrostatic attraction between a cation and anion; this is an **ionic bond**.

$$Na \quad \cdot \overset{\cdot\cdot}{\underset{\cdot\cdot}{Cl}} : \quad \Longrightarrow \quad Na^{\oplus} \quad : \overset{\cdot\cdot}{\underset{\cdot\cdot}{Cl}} :^{\ominus}$$

For an ionic bond to form between a metal and a non-metal, there has to be a big difference in electronegativity between the two elements. According to Coulomb's law, the strength of the bond is proportional to the charges on the ions, and it decreases as the ions get farther apart. The potential energy of two charges, q_1 and q_2, is proportional to $q_1 q_2 / r$, where r is the distance between them. (*Note*: The *force* is proportional to $q_1 q_2 / r^2$.) We can use this to estimate the relative strength of ionic systems. For example, consider MgO and NaCl. For MgO, we have $PE_{MgO} \propto (+2)(-2)/r$, while for NaCl, we have $PE_{NaCl} \propto (+1)(-1)/r$. First, note that these potential energies are *negative*; this tells us that each ionic system is more stable than the ions separated from each other. Second, the ratio of these potential energies is equal to $-4/-1 = 4$ (assuming that the values of r are very nearly the same). Therefore, the MgO "bond" is expected to be about 4 times stronger than the NaCl "bond."

Example 14-10: Which of the following is most likely an ionic compound?

   A. NO
   B. HI
   C. ClF
   D. KBr
   E. CO

Solution: A diatomic compound is ionic if the electronegativities of the atoms are very different. Of the atoms listed in the choice, those in D have the greatest electronegativity difference (K is an alkali metal, and Br is a halogen); K will give up its lone valence electron to Br, forming an ionic bond.

14.4 VSEPR THEORY

The shapes of simple molecules are predicted by **valence shell electron-pair repulsion (VSEPR) theory**. There's one rule: Since electrons repel one another, electron pairs, whether bonding or nonbonding, attempt to move as far apart as possible.

For example, the bonding electrons in magnesium hydride, MgH_2, repel one another and attempt to move as far apart as possible. In this molecule, two pairs of electrons point in opposite directions:

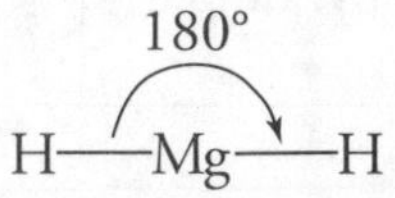

$$H{\longrightarrow}Mg{\longrightarrow}H \quad 180°$$

The angle between the bonds is 180°. A molecule with this shape is said to be linear.

Molecular shape depends on the **geometric family** to which the molecule belongs, and a molecule's geometric identity is based solely on its number of electron groups. While both bonding and nonbonding pairs of electrons are counted as individual electron groups, double and triple bonds count only as *one* electron group (even though they involve two and three pairs of electrons, respectively). To illustrate, here are the number of electron groups of the *central atom* in each of these molecules:

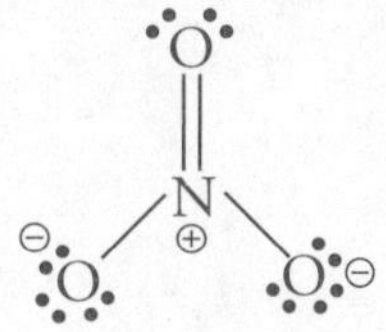

3 electron groups	4 electron groups	5 electron groups

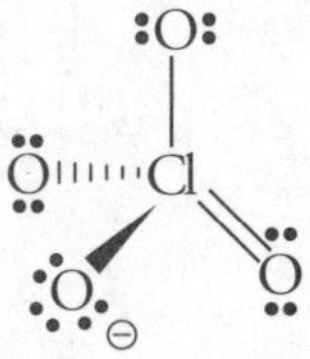

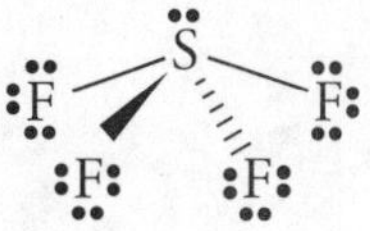

Once you've determined the molecule's geometric family, you can then determine the molecule's overall shape by counting the number of nonbonding pairs of electrons on the central atom. Notice that when there are no lone electron pairs, the shape of the molecule is the same as the geometry.

Geometric Family	# Electron Pairs on Central Atom	Shape		Bond Angles
Linear	0	Linear		180°
Trigonal Planar	0	Trigonal Planar	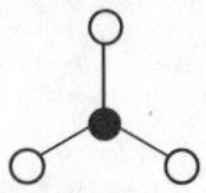	120°
	1	Bent	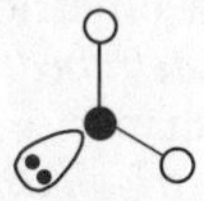	116°
Tetrahedral	0	Tetrahedral	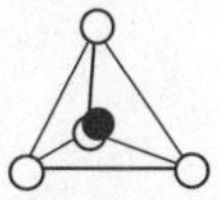	109.5°
	1	Trigonal Pyramidal	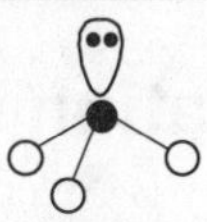	107°
	2	Bent	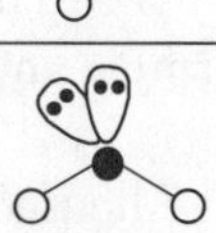	104.5°

14.4

| Trigonal Bipyramidal | 0 | Trigonal Bipyramidal | 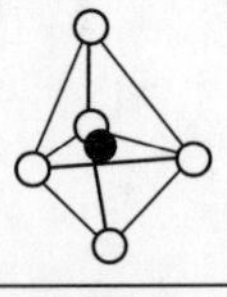 | 90° 120° 180° |
| Octahedral | 0 | Octahedral | 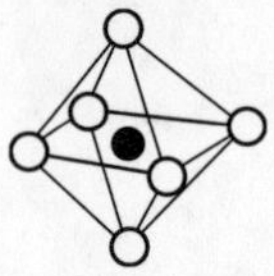 | 90° 180° |

Example 14-11: Determine the geometric family and predict the shape of each of the following molecules:

A. H_2O
B. BrF_3
C. $XeOF_4$
D. NH_3
E. NH_4^+

Solution:

A. geometric family: *tetrahedral* shape: *bent*

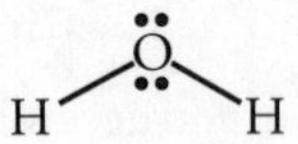

B. geometric family: *trigonal bipyramidal* shape: *T-shaped*

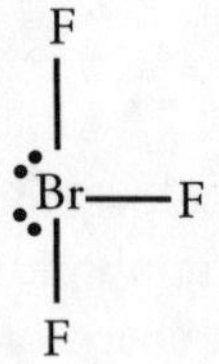

C. geometric family: *octahedral* shape: *square pyramid*

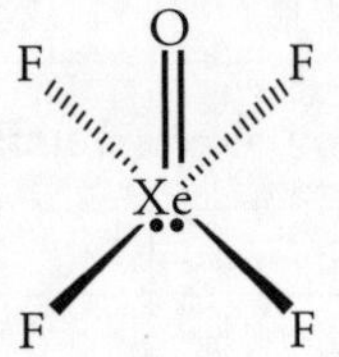

D. geometric family: *tetrahedral* shape: *trigonal pyramid*

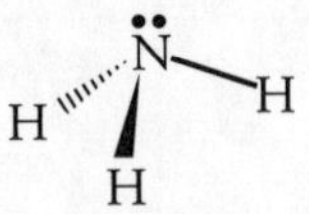

E. geometric family: *tetrahedral* shape: *tetrahedral*

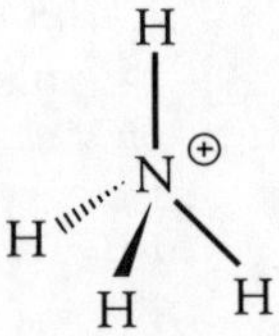

A Note on Hybridization

Although hybridization theory is covered in more detail in the Organic Chemistry section, it's useful here to briefly outline how to determine an atom's hybridization.

Every pair of electrons must be housed in an electronic orbital (either an *s, p, d,* or *f*). For example, the carbon atom in methane, CH_4, has *four* pairs of electrons surrounding it (four single covalent bonds plus no lone pairs) so it must provide *four* electronic orbitals to house these electrons. Orbitals always get "used" in the following order:

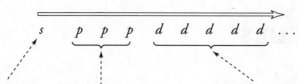

The single *s* orbital always gets used first.

The *p* orbitals get used up next. There are three *p* orbitals that may be used.

The *d* orbitals get used only after the *s* and *p* orbitals are full. There are five available *d* orbitals.

So, since the carbon atom in methane must provide *four* orbitals, we just count: 1...2...3...4:

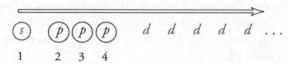

Therefore, the hybridization of the carbon atom in methane is $s + p + p + p$, which is written as sp^3. The sum of the exponents in the hybridization nomenclature tells us how many orbitals of this type are used. So, in methane, there are $1 + 3 = 4$ hybrid orbitals. The following table gives the hybridization of the central atom for each of the geometric families:

Number of Electron Groups	Geometric Family	Hybridization of Central Atom
2	Linear	sp
3	Trigonal Planar	sp^2
4	Tetrahedral	sp^3
5	Trigonal bipyramidal	sp^3d
6	Octahedral	sp^3d^2

Example 14-12: Determine the hybridization of the central atom in each of the following molecules from the previous example:

A. H_2O
B. BrF_3
C. $XeOF_4$
D. NH_3
E. NH_4^+

Solution:

A. Hybridization of O is sp^3.
B. Hybridization of Br is sp^3d.
C. Hybridization of Xe is sp^3d^2.
D. Hybridization of N is sp^3.
E. Hybridization of N is sp^3.

14.5 TYPES OF SOLIDS

Ionic Solids

An **ionic solid** is held together by the electrostatic attraction between cations and anions in a lattice structure. The bonds that hold all the ions together in the crystal lattice are the same as the bonds that hold each pair of ions together. Ionic bonds are strong, and most ionic substances (like NaCl and other salts) are solid at room temperature. As discussed previously, the strength of the bonds is primarily dependent on the magnitudes of the ion charges, and to a lesser extent, the size of the ions according to Coulomb's Law. The greater the charge, the stronger the force of attraction between the ions. The smaller the ions, the more they are attracted to each other.

Network Solids

In a **network solid**, atoms are connected in a **lattice** of covalent bonds, meaning that all interactions between atoms are covalent bonds. Like in an ionic solid, in a network solid the *inter*molecular forces are identical to the *intra*molecular forces. You can think of a network solid as one big molecule. Network solids are very strong, and tend to be very hard solids at room temperature. Diamond (one of the allotropes of carbon) and quartz (a form of silica, SiO_2) are examples of network solids.

Metallic Solids

A sample of metal can be thought of as a covalently bound lattice of nuclei and their inner shell electrons, surrounded by a "sea" or "cloud" of electrons. At least one valence electron per atom is not bound to any one particular atom and is free to move throughout the lattice. These freely roaming valence electrons are called **conduction electrons**. As a result, metals are excellent conductors of electricity and heat, and are malleable and ductile. Metallic bonds vary widely in strength, but almost all metals are solids at room temperature.

Molecular Solids

The particles at the lattice points of a crystal of a molecular solid are molecules. These molecules are held together by one of three types of *inter*molecular interactions—hydrogen bonds, dipole-dipole forces, or London dispersion forces. These attractive forces are discussed in detail in the next section. Since these forces are *significantly* weaker than ionic, network, or metallic bonds, molecular compounds typically have much lower melting and boiling points than the other types of solids above. Molecular solids are often liquids or gases at room temperature, and are more likely to be solids as the strength of their intermolecular forces increase.

14.6 INTERMOLECULAR FORCES

Liquids and solids are sometimes held together by intermolecular forces such as dipole-dipole forces and London dispersion forces. **Intermolecular forces** are the relatively weak interactions that take place between neutral molecules.

Polar molecules are attracted to ions, producing **ion-dipole** forces. **Dipole-dipole forces** are the attractions between the positive end of one polar molecule and the negative end of another polar molecule. (Hydrogen bonding [which we will look at more closely below] is the strongest dipole-dipole force.) A permanent dipole in one molecule may induce a dipole in a neighboring nonpolar molecule, producing a momentary **dipole-induced dipole force**. Finally, an instantaneous dipole in a nonpolar molecule may induce a dipole in a neighboring nonpolar molecule. The resulting attraction is known as a **London dispersion force**. London dispersion forces are very weak and transient interactions between the instantaneous dipoles in nonpolar molecules. They are the weakest of all intermolecular interactions, and they're the "default" force; all a molecule needs to experience it is electrons, and the more electrons it has, the greater the dispersion force. For nonpolar molecules, it's the only intermolecular force present. Many substances whose molecules experience only dispersion forces are gases at room temperature.

A final note: Dipole forces, hydrogen bonding, and London forces are *all* collectively known as **van der Waals forces**. However, you may sometimes see the term "van der Waals forces" used to mean only London dispersion forces.

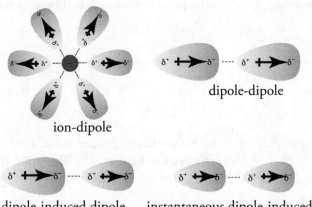

ion-dipole

dipole-dipole

dipole-induced dipole

instantaneous dipole-induced dipole
(London dispersion force)

Despite being weak, intermolecular forces can have a profound impact on the physical properties of a particular molecule. Specifically, substances with stronger intermolecular forces will exhibit greater melting points, greater boiling points, greater viscosities, and lower vapor pressures than similar compounds with weaker intermolecular forces. This is particularly true for hydrogen bonding.

14.6

Hydrogen Bonding

Hydrogen bonding is the strongest type of intermolecular force between neutral molecules. Two molecules form a hydrogen bond when the partially positive hydrogen of one molecule attracts the lone pair on a partially negative atom of another molecule. Specifically, *hydrogen bonds occur only between the H attached to an N, O, or F atom* and a lone pair on another N, O, or F atom. The most famous example of a substance that experiences hydrogen bonding is water:

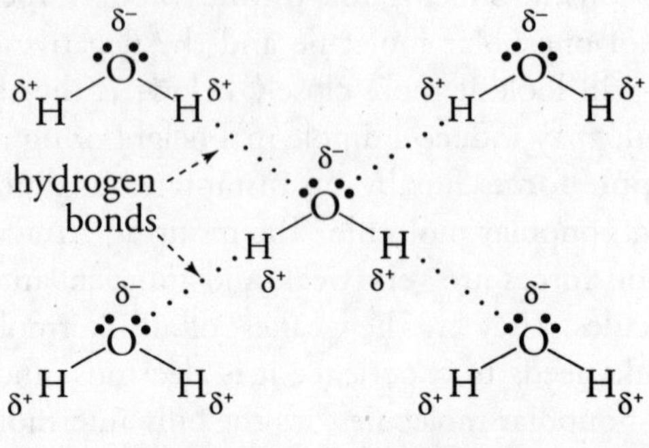

One of the consequences of hydrogen bonding is the high boiling points of compounds such as NH_3, H_2O, and HF. The boiling points of these hydrides are higher than those of hydrides of other elements from Groups V, VI, and VII (the groups where N, O, and F reside). For example, the boiling point of the Group V hydride H_2S is approximately –50°C, while that of H_2O is (of course) 100°C.

Example 14-13: Identify the binary mixture that *cannot* experience hydrogen bonding with each other:

- A. NH_3 / H_2O
- B. H_2O / HF
- C. HF / CO_2
- D. H_2S / HCl
- E. NH_2CH_3/CO

Solution: Hydrogen bonding occurs when an H covalently bonded to an F, O, or N electrostatically interacts with another F, O, or N (which doesn't need to have an H). Therefore, A, B, C, and E can all experience hydrogen bonding. D, however, cannot, and this is the answer.

Want More Practice?
Scan the QR code below to register your book for online chapter summaries, drills, practice tests, and more!

Chapter 15
Phases

15.1 PHYSICAL CHANGES

Matter can undergo physical changes as well as chemical changes. Melting, freezing, and boiling are all examples of physical changes. A key property of a physical change is that no *intra*molecular bonds are made or broken; a physical change affects only the *inter*molecular forces between molecules or atoms. For example, ice melting to become liquid water does not change the molecules of H_2O into something else. Melting reflects the disruption of the attractive interactions between the molecules.

Every type of matter experiences intermolecular forces such as dispersion forces, dipole interactions, and hydrogen bonding. All molecules have some degree of attraction towards each other (dispersion forces at least), and it's the intermolecular interactions that hold matter together as solids or liquids. The strength and the type of intermolecular forces depend on the identity of the atoms and molecules of a substance and vary greatly. For example, $NaCl(s)$, $H_2O(l)$ and $N_2(g)$ all have different kinds and strengths of intermolecular forces, and these differences give rise to their widely varying melting and boiling points.

Phase Transitions

Physical changes are closely related to temperature. What does temperature tell us about matter? Temperature is a measure of the amount of internal kinetic energy (the energy of motion) that molecules have. The average kinetic energy of the molecules of a substance directly affects its **state** or **phase**: whether it's a **solid, liquid,** or **gas.** Kinetic energy is also related to the degree of disorder, or **entropy**: In general, the higher the average kinetic energy of the molecules of a substance, the greater its entropy.

solid liquid gas

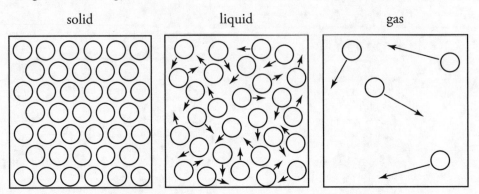

If we increase the temperature at a given pressure, a solid typically transforms into liquid and then into gas. What causes the phase transitions as the temperature increases? Phase changes are simply the result of breaking (or forming) intermolecular interactions. At low temperatures, matter tends to exist as a solid and is held together by intermolecular interactions. The molecules in a solid may jiggle a bit, but they're restricted to relatively fixed positions and form an orderly array, because the molecules don't have enough kinetic energy to overcome the intermolecular forces. Solids are the most ordered and least energetic of the phases. As a solid absorbs heat its temperature increases, meaning the average kinetic energy of the molecules increases. This causes the molecules to move around more, loosening the intermolecular interactions and increasing the entropy. When enough energy is absorbed for the molecules to move freely around one another, the solid melts and becomes liquid. At the molecular level, the molecules in a liquid are still in contact and interact with each other, but they have enough kinetic energy to escape fixed positions. Liquids have more internal kinetic energy and greater entropy than solids. If enough heat is absorbed by the liquid, the kinetic energy increases until the molecules have enough speed to escape intermolecular forces and vaporize into the gas phase. Molecules in the gas phase move freely of one another and experience very little, if any, intermolecular forces. Gases are the most energetic and least ordered of the phases.

To illustrate these phase transitions, let's follow ice through the transitions from solid to liquid to gas. Ice is composed of highly organized H_2O molecules held rigidly by hydrogen bonds. The molecules have limited motion. If we increase the temperature of the ice, the molecules will eventually absorb enough heat to move around, and the organized structure of the molecules will break down as fixed hydrogen bonds are replaced with hydrogen bonds in which the molecules are *not* in fixed positions. We observe the transition as ice melting into liquid water. If we continue to increase the temperature, the kinetic energy of the molecules eventually becomes great enough for the individual molecules to overcome all hydrogen bonding and move freely. This appears to us as vaporization, or boiling of the liquid into gas. At this point the H_2O molecules zip around randomly, forming a high-entropy, chaotic swarm. All the phase transitions are summarized here.

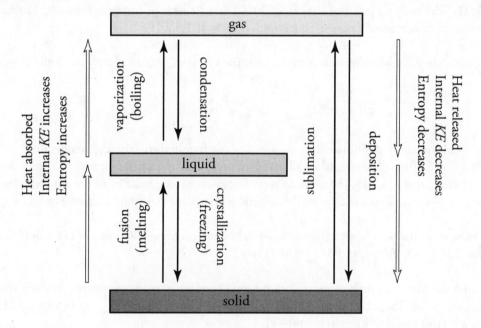

15.2 HEATS OF PHASE CHANGES

When matter undergoes a phase transition, energy is either absorbed or released. The amount of energy required to complete a transition is called the **heat of transition,** symbolized ΔH. For example, the amount of heat that must be absorbed to change a solid into liquid is called the **heat of fusion**, and the energy absorbed when a liquid changes to gas is the **heat of vaporization**. Each substance has a specific heat of transition for each phase change, and the magnitude is directly related to the strength and number of the intermolecular forces that substance experiences.

The amount of heat required to cause a change of phase depends on two things: the type of substance and the amount of substance. For example, the heat of fusion for H_2O is 6.0 kJ/mol. So, if we wanted to melt a 2 mol sample of ice (at 0°C), 12 kJ of heat would need to be supplied. The heat of vaporization for H_2O is about 41 kJ/mol, so vaporizing a 2 mol sample of liquid water (at 100°C) would require 82 kJ of heat. If that 2 mol sample of steam (at 100°C) condensed back to liquid, 82 kJ of heat would be released. In general, the amount of heat, q, accompanying a phase transition is given by:

$$q = n \times \Delta H_{\text{phase change}}$$

where n is the number of moles of the substance. If ΔH and q are positive, heat is absorbed; if ΔH and q are negative, heat is released.

Example 15-1: The melting point of iron is 1,530°C, and its heat of fusion is 64 cal/g. How much heat would be required to completely melt a 50 g chunk of iron at 1,530°C?

Solution: Since the heat of transition is given in units of cal/g, we can simply multiply it by the given mass

$$q = m \times \Delta H_{\text{fusion}} = (50g) \times 64 \text{ cal/g} = 3200 \text{ cal}$$

By the way, a **calorie** is, by definition, the amount of heat required to raise the temperature of 1 gram of water by 1°C. The SI unit of heat (and of all forms of energy) is the **joule**. Here's the conversion between joules and calories: 1 cal ≈ 4.2 J. (The popular term *calorie*—the one most of us are concerned with day to day when we eat—is actually a kilocalorie [10^3 cal] and is sometimes written as Calorie [with a capital C]).

Example 15-2: What happens when a container of liquid water (holding 100 moles of H_2O) at 0°C completely freezes? (*Note:* $\Delta H_{\text{fusion}} = 6$ kJ/mol, and $\Delta H_{\text{vap}} = 41$ kJ/mol.)

Solution: In order for ice to melt, it must absorb heat; therefore, the reverse process—water freezing into ice—must *release* heat. The heat of transition from liquid to solid is $-\Delta H_{\text{fusion}}$, so in this case the heat of transition is $q = (100 \text{ mol})(-6 \text{ kJ/mol}) = -600$ kJ.

15.3 CALORIMETRY

In between phase changes, matter can absorb or release energy without undergoing transition. We observe this as an increase or a decrease in the temperature of a substance. When a sample is undergoing a phase change, it absorbs or releases heat *without* a change in temperature, so when we talk about a temperature change, we are considering only cases where the phase doesn't change. One of the most important facts about physical changes of matter is this (and it will bear repeating):

When a substance absorbs or releases heat, one of two things can happen: either its temperature changes *or* it will undergo a phase change *but not both at the same time.*

The amount of heat absorbed or released by a sample is proportional to its change in temperature. The constant of proportionality is called the substance's **heat capacity, C**, which is the product of its **specific heat, c**, and its mass, m; that is, $C = mc$. We can write the equation $q = C\Delta T$ in this more explicit form:

$$q = mc\Delta T$$

where

> q = heat added to (or released by) a sample
> m = mass of the sample
> c = specific heat of the substance
> ΔT = temperature change

A substance's specific heat is an *intrinsic* property of that substance and tells us how resistant it is to changing its temperature. For example, the specific heat of liquid water is 1 calorie per gram-°C. (This is actually the definition of a **calorie**: the amount of heat required to raise the temperature of 1 gram of water by 1°C.) The specific heat of copper, however, is much less; only 0.09 cal/g-°C. So, if we had a 1 g sample of water and 1 g sample of copper and each absorbed 10 calories of heat, the resulting changes in the temperatures would be

$$\Delta T_{water} = \frac{q}{mc_{water}} \qquad\qquad \Delta T_{copper} = \frac{q}{mc_{copper}}$$

$$= \frac{10 \text{ cal}}{(1 \text{ g})(1\frac{\text{cal}}{\text{g-°C}})} \qquad\qquad = \frac{10 \text{ cal}}{(1 \text{ g})(0.09\frac{\text{cal}}{\text{g-°C}})}$$

$$= 10°C \qquad\qquad\qquad = 111°C$$

That's a big difference! So, while it's true that the temperature change is proportional to the heat absorbed, it's *inversely* proportional to the substance's heat capacity. A substance like water, with a relatively high specific heat, will undergo a smaller change in temperature than a substance (like copper) with a lower specific heat.

A few notes:

1. The specific heat of a substance also depends upon phase. For example, the specific heat of ice is different from that of liquid water.
2. The SI unit for energy is the joule, not the calorie. You may see specific heats (and heat capacities) given in terms of joules rather than calories. Remember, the conversion between joules and calories is 1 cal ≈ 4.2 J.
3. Specific heats may also be given in terms of Kelvins rather than degrees Celsius; that is, you may see the specific heat of water, say, given as 4.2 J/g K rather than 4.2 J/g°C. However, since the size of a Celsius degree is the same as a Kelvin (that is, if two temperatures differ by 1°C, they also differ by 1K), the numerical value of the specific heat won't be any different if Kelvins are used.

Example 15-3: The specific heat of tungsten is 0.03 cal/g-°C. If a 50-gram sample of tungsten absorbs 100 calories of heat, what will be the change in temperature of the sample?

Solution: From the equation $q = mc\Delta T$, we find that

$$\Delta T = \frac{q}{mc} = \frac{100 \text{ cal}}{(50 \text{ g})(0.03 \text{ cal/g°C})} = \frac{2}{3/100} \text{°C} = 67 \text{°C}$$

15.4   PHASE TRANSITION DIAGRAM

Let's consider the complete range of phase changes from solid to liquid to gas. The process in this direction requires the input of heat. As heat is added to the solid, its temperature increases until it reaches its melting point. At that point, absorbed heat is used to change the phase to liquid, not to increase the temperature. Once the sample has been completely melted, additional heat again causes its temperature to rise, until the boiling point is reached. At that point, absorbed heat is used to change the phase to gas, not to increase the temperature. Once the sample has been completely vaporized, additional heat again causes its temperature to rise. We can summarize all this with a **phase transition diagram**, which plots the temperature of the sample versus the amount of heat absorbed. The figure below is a typical phase transition diagram.

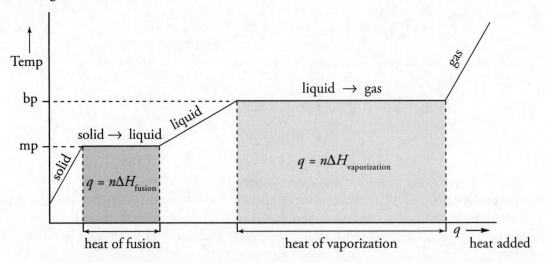

The horizontal axis represents the amount of heat added, and the vertical axis is the corresponding temperature of the substance. Notice the flat lines when the substance reaches its melting point (mp) and boiling point (bp). *During a phase transition, the temperature of the substance does not change.* Also, the greater the value for the heat of transition, the longer the flat line. A substance's heat of vaporization is always greater than its heat of fusion. The sloped lines show how the temperature changes (within a phase) as heat is added. Since $\Delta T = q/C$, the slopes of the non-flat lines are equal to $1/C$, the reciprocal of the substance's heat capacity in that phase.

Example 15-4: How much heat (in calories) is necessary to raise the temperature of 2 g of solid H_2O from 0°C to 85°C? (*Note:* Heat of fusion for water = 80 cal/g and the specific heat of water is 1 cal/g °C.)

Solution: There are two steps here: (1) melt the ice at 0°C to liquid water at 0°C, and (2) heat the water from 0°C to 85°C.

$$
\begin{aligned}
q_{total} &= q_1 + q_2 \\
&= m\Delta H_{fusion} + mc_{water}\Delta T \\
&= (2 \text{ g})(80 \text{ cal/g}) + (2 \text{ g})(1 \text{ cal/g}°C)(85°C) \\
&= (160 \text{ cal}) + (170 \text{ cal}) \\
&= 330 \text{ cal}
\end{aligned}
$$

15.4

Phase Diagrams

The phase of a substance doesn't depend just on the temperature; it also depends on the pressure. For example, even at high temperatures, a substance can be squeezed into the liquid phase if the pressure is high enough, and at low temperature, a substance can enter the gas phase if that pressure is low enough. A substance's **phase diagram** shows how its phases are determined by temperature and pressure. The figure below is a generic example of a phase diagram.

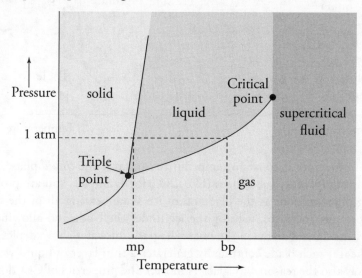

The boundary lines between phases represent points at which the two phases are in equilibrium. For example, a glass of liquid water at 0°C containing ice cubes is a two-phase system, and if its temperature and pressure were plotted in a phase diagram, it would be on the solid-liquid boundary line. Crossing a boundary line implies a phase transition. Notice that the solid phase is favored at low temperatures and high pressures, while the gas phase is favored at high temperatures and low pressures.

If we draw a horizontal line at the "1 atm" pressure level, the temperature at the point where this line crosses the solid-liquid boundary is the substance's **normal melting point**, and the temperature at the point where the line crosses the liquid-gas boundary is the **normal boiling point**.

15.4

The **triple point** is the temperature and pressure at which all three phases exist simultaneously in equilibrium.

The **critical point** marks the end of the liquid-gas boundary. Beyond this point, the substance displays properties of both a liquid (such as high density) and a gas (such as low viscosity). If a substance is in this state—where the liquid and gas phases are no longer distinct—it's called a **supercritical fluid**, and no amount of increased pressure can force the substance back into its liquid phase.

The Phase Diagram for Water

Water is the most common of a handful of substances that are denser in the liquid phase than in the solid phase. As a result, the solid-liquid boundary line in the phase diagram for water has a slightly *negative* slope, as opposed to the usual positive slope for most other substances. Compare these diagrams:

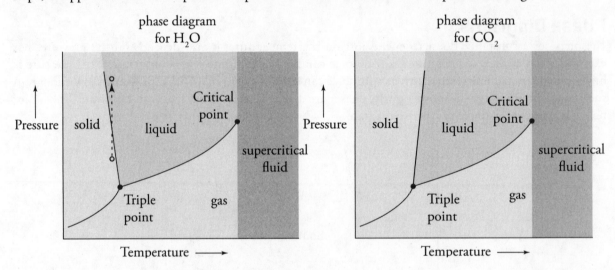

For H_2O, an increase in pressure at constant temperature can favor the *liquid* phase, not the solid phase, as would be the case for most other substances (like CO_2, for example). You are probably already familiar with the following phenomenon: as the blade of an ice skate bearing all of the weight of the skater contacts the ice, the pressure increases, melting the ice under the blade and allowing the skate to glide over the liquid water. (The dashed arrow in the phase diagram for water above depicts this effect.) As the skater moves across the ice, each blade continually generates a thin layer of liquid water that refreezes as the blade passes. (This is also the reason why glaciers move.) The properties of CO_2 don't allow for skating because solid CO_2 will never turn to liquid when the pressure is increased. (And now you know why solid CO_2 is called *dry ice*!)

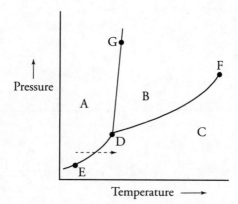

Example 15-5: In which region of the diagram above is the substance in the gas phase?

Solution: The gas phase is favored at high temperatures and low pressure, so we know that region C represents the gas phase.

Example 15-6: In which part of the diagram is gas in equilibrium with liquid?

Solution: The liquid phase is represented by region B and the gas phase by region C. Therefore, an equilibrium between liquid and gas phases is represented by a point on the boundary between regions B and C. This boundary is the "line" DF.

Example 15-7: The dashed arrow in the diagram indicates what type of phase transition?

Solution: The arrow shows a substance in the solid phase (region A) moving directly to the gaseous phase (region C) without melting first. The phase transition from solid to gas is called sublimation.

Want More Practice?
Scan the QR code below to register your book for online chapter summaries, drills, practice tests, and more!

Chapter 16
Gases

16.1 GASES AND THE KINETIC-MOLECULAR THEORY

Unlike the condensed phases of matter (solids and liquids), **gases** have no fixed volume. A gas will fill all the available space in a container. Gases are *far* more compressible than solids or liquids, and their densities are very low (roughly 1 kg/m³), about three to four orders of magnitude less than solids and liquids. But the most striking difference between a gas and a solid or liquid is that the molecules of a gas are free to move over large distances.

The most important properties of a gas are its **pressure, volume,** and **temperature.** How these macroscopic properties are related to each other can be derived from some basic assumptions concerning the *microscopic* behavior of gas molecules. These assumptions are the foundation of the **kinetic-molecular theory.**

Kinetic-molecular theory, a model for describing the behavior of gases, is based on the following assumptions:

1. The molecules of a gas are so small compared to the average spacing between them that the molecules themselves take up essentially no volume.
2. The molecules of a gas are in constant motion, moving in straight lines at constant speeds and in random directions between collisions. The collisions of the molecules with the walls of the container define the **pressure** of the gas (the average force exerted per unit area), and all collisions—molecules striking the walls and each other—are *elastic* (that is, the total kinetic energy is the same after the collision as it was before). Since each molecule moves at a constant speed between collisions and the collisions are elastic, the molecules of a gas experience no intermolecular forces.
3. The molecules of a gas span a distribution of speeds, and the average kinetic energy of the molecules is directly proportional to the absolute temperature (the temperature in kelvins) of the sample: $KE_{avg} \propto T$.

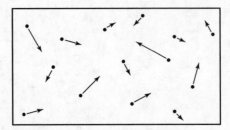

A gas that satisfies all these requirements is said to be an **ideal gas.** Most real gases behave like ideal gases under ordinary conditions, so the results that follow from the kinetic-molecular theory can be applied to real gases.

Units of Volume, Temperature, and Pressure

Volume

The SI unit for volume is the cubic meter (m³), but in chemistry, the **cubic centimeter** (**cm³** or **cc**) and **liter** (**L**) are commonly used. One cubic meter is equal to one thousand liters.

$$1 \text{ cm}^3 = 1 \text{ cc} = 1 \text{ mL} \quad \text{and} \quad 1 \text{ m}^3 = 1000 \text{ L}$$

Temperature

Temperature may be expressed in degrees Fahrenheit, degrees Celsius, or in kelvins (not degrees Kelvin). In scientific work, the Celsius scale is popular, where water freezes at 0°C and boils at 100°C (at standard atmospheric pressure). However, the "proper" unit for expressing temperatures is the kelvin (K), and this is the one we use when talking about gases (because of assumption #3 stated above for the kinetic-molecular theory). The relationship between kelvins and degrees Celsius is simple:

$$T \text{ (in K)} = T \text{ (in °C)} + 273.15$$

When dealing with gases, the best unit for expressing temperature is the kelvin (K). This scale, also known as the absolute temperature scale, is used because all gases would theoretically attain a zero value as pressure is lowered to a perfect vacuum. From a practical perspective, all of the gas laws equations on the DAT require the use of absolute temperatures.

Pressure

Since pressure is defined as force per unit area, the SI unit for pressure is the **pascal** (abbreviated **Pa**), where $1 \text{ Pa} = 1 \text{ N/m}^2$. The unit is inconveniently small for normal calculations involving gases (for example, a nickel sitting on a table exerts about 140 Pa of pressure), so several alternative units for pressure are usually used.

At sea level, atmospheric pressure is about 101,300 pascals (or 101.3 kPa); this is 1 **atmosphere** (1 **atm**). Related to the atmosphere is the **torr**, where 1 atm = 760 torr. (Therefore, 1 torr is about the same as the pressure exerted by a nickel sitting on a table.) At 0°C, 1 torr is equal to 1 **mm Hg** (**millimeter of mercury**), so we generally just take 1 atm to equal 760 mm Hg:

$$1 \text{ atm} = 760 \text{ torr} = 760 \text{ mm Hg}$$

Standard Temperature and Pressure

Standard Temperature and Pressure (STP) means a temperature of 0°C (273.15 K) and a pressure of 1 atm.

Example 16-1: A temperature of 273°C is equivalent to what temperature in kelvins?

Solution: Temperature (in K) = 273°C + 273 = 546 K

16.2 THE IDEAL GAS LAW

The volume, temperature, and pressure of an ideal gas are related by a simple equation called the **ideal gas law**. Most real gases under ordinary conditions act very much like ideal gases, so the ideal gas law applies to most gas behavior:

> **Ideal Gas Law**
> $$PV = nRT$$

where

P = the pressure of the gas in atmospheres
V = the volume of the container in liters
n = the number of moles of the gas
R = the universal gas constant, 0.0821 L atm/K mol
T = the absolute temperature of the gas (that is, T in kelvins)

Questions on gas behavior typically take one of two forms. The first type of question simply gives you some facts, and you use $PV = nRT$ to determine a missing variable. In the second type, "before" and "after" scenarios are presented for which you determine the effect of changing the volume, temperature, or pressure. In this case, you apply the ideal gas law twice, once for each scenario. We'll solve a typical example of each type of question.

1. If two moles of helium at 27°C fill a 3 L balloon, what is the pressure?

Take the ideal gas law, solve it for P, then plug in the numbers (and don't forget to convert the temperature in °C to kelvins!):

$$PV = nRT$$

$$P = \frac{nRT}{V}$$

$$P = \frac{(2 \text{ mol})(0.082 \text{ L atm/K mol})(300 \text{ K})}{3 \text{ L}}$$

$$P = 16 \text{ atm}$$

2. Argon, at a pressure of 2 atm, fills a 100 mL vial at a temperature of 0°C. What would the pressure of the argon be if we increase the volume to 500 mL, and the temperature is 100°C?

We're not told how much argon (the number of moles, n) is in the vial, but it doesn't matter since it doesn't change. Since R is also a constant, the ratio of PV/T, which is equal to nR, remains constant. Therefore,

$$\frac{P_1 V_1}{T_1} = \frac{P_2 V_2}{T_2} \quad \Rightarrow \quad P_2 = P_1 \frac{V_1}{V_2} \frac{T_2}{T_1}$$

$$P_2 = (2 \text{ atm})\left(\frac{0.1 \text{ L}}{0.5 \text{ L}}\right)\left(\frac{373 \text{ K}}{273 \text{ K}}\right)$$

$$P_2 = 0.55 \text{ atm}$$

P-V-T **Gas Laws in Systems Where** *n* **Is Constant**

As we saw in answering Question 2 above, the amount of gas often remains the same, and the *n* drops out. Our work can be simplified even further if the pressure, temperature, or volume is also held constant. (And remember: When working with the gas laws, *temperature* always means *absolute temperature* [that is, *T* in kelvins].)

- If the pressure is constant, the volume is proportional to the temperature: $V \propto T$

This is known as **Charles's law**. If the pressure is to remain constant, then a gas will expand when heated and contract when cooled. If the temperature of the gas is increased, the molecules will move faster, hitting the walls of the container with more force; in order to keep the pressure the same, the frequency of the collisions would need to be reduced. This is accomplished by expanding the volume. With more available space, the molecules strike the walls less often in order to compensate for hitting them harder.

- If the temperature is constant, the pressure is inversely proportional to the volume: $P \propto 1/V$

This is known as **Boyle's law**. If the volume decreases, the molecules have less space to move around in. As a result, they'll collide with the walls of the container more often, and the pressure increases. On the other hand, if the volume of the container increases, the gas molecules have more available space and collide with the wall less often, resulting in a lower pressure.

- If the volume is constant, the pressure is proportional to the temperature: $P \propto T$

If the temperature goes up, so does the pressure. This should make sense when you consider the origin of pressure. As the temperature increases, the molecules move faster. As a result, they strike the walls of the container surface more often and with greater speed.

We can summarize the statements like this:

In a system with constant *n*:

At constant P : $\dfrac{V_1}{T_1} = \dfrac{V_2}{T_2}$

At constant T : $P_1 V_1 = P_2 V_2$

At constant V : $\dfrac{P_1}{T_1} = \dfrac{P_2}{T_2}$

If only *n* (which tells us the amount of gas) stays constant, we have the **combined gas law** (which we used to answer Question 2 above):

Combined Gas Law (constant *n*)

$$\frac{P_1 V_1}{T_1} = \frac{P_2 V_2}{T_2}$$

Example 16-2: Helium, at a pressure of 3 atm, occupies a 16 L container at a temperature of 30°C. What would be the volume of the gas if the pressure were increased to 5 atm and the temperature lowered to –20°C?

Solution: We use the combined gas law after remembering to convert the given temperatures to kelvin:

$$\frac{P_1 V_1}{T_1} = \frac{P_2 V_2}{T_2} \quad \Rightarrow \quad V_2 = V_1 \frac{P_1}{P_2} \frac{T_2}{T_1} = (16\ \text{L})\left(\frac{3\ \text{atm}}{5\ \text{atm}}\right)\left(\frac{253\ \text{K}}{303\ \text{K}}\right) \approx (16\ \text{L})\left(\frac{3}{5}\right)\left(\frac{250\ \text{K}}{300\ \text{K}}\right) = 8\ \text{L}$$

All of these laws follow from the ideal gas law and can be derived easily from it. They tell us what happens when n and P are constant, when n and T are constant, when n and V are constant, and in the case of the combined gas law, when n alone is constant. But what about n when P, V, and T are constant? That law of gases was proposed by Avogadro:

- If two equal-volume containers hold gas at the same pressure and temperature, then they contain the same number of particles (regardless of the identity of the gas).
  Avogadro's law can be used to determine the **standard molar volume** of an ideal gas at STP, which is the volume that one mole of a gas—any *ideal* gas—would occupy at 0°C and 1 atm of pressure:

$$V = \frac{nRT}{P} = \frac{(1\ \text{mol})(0.0821\ \tfrac{\text{L atm}}{\text{K mol}})(273\ \text{K})}{1\ \text{atm}} = 22.4\ \text{L}$$

To give you an idea of how much this is, 22.4 L is equal to the total volume of three basketballs.

Avogadro's law and the **standard molar volume** of a gas can be used to simplify some gas law problems. Consider the following question:

3. Given the Haber process, $3\ H_2(g) + N_2(g) \rightarrow 2\ NH_3(g)$, if you start with 5 L of $H_2(g)$ and 4 L of $N_2(g)$ at STP, what will the volume of the three gases be when the reaction is complete?

We can answer this question by using the ideal gas law, or we can recognize that the only thing changing is n (the number of moles of each gas) and use the standard molar volume. If we further recognize that the standard molar volume is the same for all three gases, and it is this value that we'd use to convert each given volume into moles (and then vice versa), we can use the balanced equation to quickly determine the answer.

Since we need 3 L of H_2 for every 1 L of N_2, and we have 4 L of N_2 but only 5 L of H_2, H_2 will be the limiting reagent, and its volume will be zero at the end of the reaction. Since 1 L of N_2 is needed for every 3 L of H_2, we get

$$5\ \text{L of}\ H_2 \times \frac{1\ \text{L of}\ N_2}{3\ \text{L of}\ H_2} = 1.7\ \text{L of}\ N_2$$

So the amount of N_2 remaining will be $4 - 1.7 = 2.3$ L. The volume of NH_3 produced is

$$5 \text{ L of H}_2 \times \frac{2 \text{ L of NH}_3}{3 \text{ L of H}_2} = 3.3 \text{ L of NH}_3$$

Therefore, the final volume will be 2.3L of N_2 + 3.3L of NH_3 = 5.6L of gases total.

Example 16-3: Three moles of oxygen gas are present in a 10 L chamber at a temperature of 25°C. What is the pressure of the gas (in atm)?

Solution: Since 25°C = 298 K, the ideal gas law gives

$$P = \frac{nRT}{V} = \frac{(3)(0.08)(298)}{10} \text{ atm} \approx \frac{(3)(0.1)(300)}{10} \text{ atm} \approx 9 \text{atm}$$

Example 16-4: An ideal gas at 2 atm occupies a 5-liter tank. It is then transferred to a new tank with a volume of 12 liters. If temperature is held constant throughout, what is the new pressure?

Solution: Since n and T are constants, we can use Boyle's law to find

$$P_1 V_1 = P_2 V_2 \quad \Rightarrow \quad P_2 = P_1 \frac{V_1}{V_2} = (2 \text{ atm}) \frac{5 \text{ L}}{12 \text{ L}} = \frac{5}{6} \text{ atm}$$

Example 16-5: A 6-liter container holds $H_2(g)$ at a temperature of 400 K and a pressure of 3 atm. If the temperature is increased to 600 K, what will be the pressure?

Solution: Since n and V are constants, we can write

$$\frac{P_1}{T_1} = \frac{P_2}{T_2} \quad \Rightarrow \quad P_2 = P_1 \frac{T_2}{T_1} = (3 \text{ atm}) \frac{600 \text{ K}}{400 \text{ K}} = 4.5 \text{ atm}$$

Example 16-6: How many atoms of helium are present in 11.2 liters of the gas at $P = 1$ atm and $T = 273$ K?

Solution: $P = 1$ atm and $T = 273$ K define STP, so 1 mole of an ideal gas would occupy 22.4 L. A volume of 11.2 L is exactly half this so it must correspond to a 0.5 mole sample. Since 1 mole of helium contains 6.02×10^{23} atoms, 0.5 mole contains half this many: 3.01×10^{23}.

Remember from Chapter 12 that density = $\frac{m}{V}$ and $n = \frac{m}{M}$. The ideal gas law can also be used to be calculate the density of a gas (in g/L):

$$PV = nRT$$

$$PV = \frac{m}{M} RT$$

$$\frac{PM}{RT} = \frac{m}{V} = \rho$$

16.3 DALTON'S LAW OF PARTIAL PRESSURES

Consider a mixture of, say, three gases in a single container.

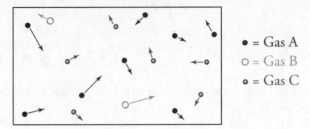

- ● = Gas A
- ○ = Gas B
- ◉ = Gas C

The total pressure is due to the collisions of all three types of molecules with the container walls. The pressure that the molecules of Gas A alone exert is called the **partial pressure** of Gas A, denoted by p_A. Similarly, the pressure exerted by the molecules of Gas B alone and the pressure exerted by the molecules of Gas C alone are p_B and p_C.

Dalton's law of partial pressures says that the total pressure is simply the sum of the partial pressures of all the constituent gases. In this case, then, we'd have:

Dalton's Law

$$P = p_A + p_B + p_C$$

So, if we know the partial pressures, we can determine the total pressure. We can also work backward. Knowing the total pressure, we can figure out the individual partial pressures. All that is required is the mole fraction. For example, in the diagram above, there are a total of 16 molecules: 8 of Gas A, 2 of Gas B, and 6 of Gas C. Therefore, the mole fraction of Gas A is $X_A = 8/16 = 1/2$, the mole fraction of Gas B is $X_B = 2/16 = 1/8$, and the mole fraction of Gas C is $X_C = 6/16 = 3/8$. *The partial pressure of a gas is equal to its mole fraction times the total pressure.* For example, if the total pressure in the container above is 8 atm, then

$$p_A = X_A P = \frac{1}{2} P = \frac{1}{2}(8 \text{ atm}) = 4 \text{ atm}$$

$$p_B = X_B P = \frac{1}{8} P = \frac{1}{8}(8 \text{ atm}) = 1 \text{ atm}$$

$$p_C = X_C P = \frac{3}{8} P = \frac{3}{8}(8 \text{ atm}) = 3 \text{ atm}$$

Example 16-7: A mixture of neon and nitrogen contains 0.5 mol Ne(*g*) and 2 mol N_2(*g*). If the total pressure is 20 atm, what is the partial pressure of the neon?

Solution: The mole fraction of Ne is

$$X_{Ne} = \frac{n_{Ne}}{n_{Ne} + n_{N_2}} = \frac{0.5}{(0.5 + 2)} = \frac{0.5}{2.5} = \frac{1}{5}$$

Therefore,

$$p_{Ne} = X_{Ne}P = \frac{1}{5}P = \frac{1}{5}(20 \text{ atm}) = 4 \text{ atm}$$

Example 16-8: A vessel contains a mixture of three gases: A, B, and C. There is twice as much A as B and half as much C as A. If the total pressure is 300 torr, what is the partial pressure of Gas C?

    A.   60 torr
    B.   75 torr
    C.   100 torr
    D.   120 torr

Solution: The question states that there is twice as much A as B, and it also says (backward) there is twice as much A as C. So the amounts of B and C are the same, and each is half the amount of A. Since this is a multiple-choice question, instead of doing algebra we'll just plug in the choices and find the one that works. The only one that works is B, so that $p_A = 150$ torr, $p_B = 75$ torr, and $p_C = 75$ torr, for a total of 300 torr.

Example 16-9: If the ratio of the partial pressures of a pair of gases mixed together in a sealed vessel is 3:1 at 300 K, what would be the ratio of their partial pressures at 400 K?

Solution: Remember that the partial pressure of a gas is the way that we talk about the amount of gas in a mixture. The question states that the ratio of partial pressures of two gases is 3:1. That just means there's three times more of one than the other. Regardless of the temperature, if the vessel is sealed, then there will always be three times more of one than the other.

16.4   GRAHAM'S LAW OF EFFUSION

The escape of a gas molecule through a very tiny hole (comparable in size to the molecules themselves) into an evacuated region is called **effusion**:

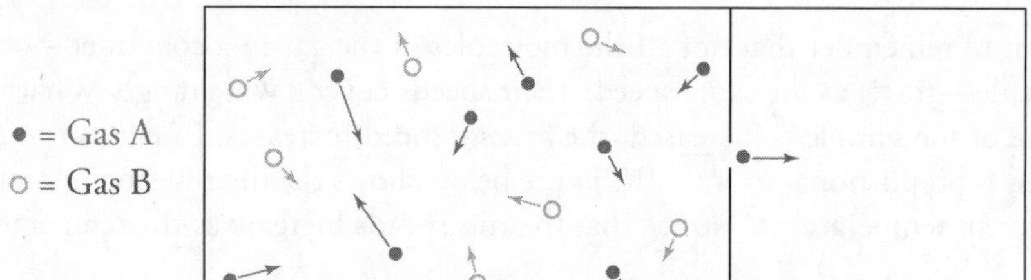

The gases in the left-hand container are at the same temperature, so their average kinetic energies are the same. If Gas A and Gas B have different molar masses, the heavier molecules will move, on average, slower than the lighter ones will. We can be even more precise. The average kinetic energy of a molecule of Gas A is $\frac{1}{2}m_A(v_A^2)_{avg}$, and the average kinetic energy of a molecule of Gas B is $\frac{1}{2}m_B(v_B^2)_{avg}$. Setting these equal to each other, we get

$$\frac{1}{2}m_A(v_A^2)_{avg} = \frac{1}{2}m_B(v_B^2)_{avg} \implies \frac{(v_A^2)_{avg}}{(v_B^2)_{avg}} = \frac{m_B}{m_A} \implies \frac{\text{rms } v_A}{\text{rms } v_B} = \sqrt{\frac{m_B}{m_A}}$$

(The abbreviation **rms** stands for *root-mean-square*; it's the square root of the mean [average] of the square of speed. Therefore, rms *v* is a convenient measure of the average speed of the molecules.) For example, if Gas A is hydrogen gas (H_2, molecular weight = 2) and Gas B is oxygen gas (O_2, molecular weight = 32), the hydrogen molecules will move, on average,

$$\sqrt{\frac{m_B}{m_A}} = \sqrt{\frac{32}{2}} = \sqrt{16} = 4$$

times faster than the oxygen molecules.

This result—which follows from one of the assumptions of the kinetic-molecular theory (namely that the average kinetic energy of the molecules of a gas is proportional to the temperature)—can be confirmed experimentally by performing an effusion experiment. Which gas should escape faster? The rate at which a gas effuses should depend directly on how fast its molecules move; the faster they travel, the more often they'd "collide" with the hole and escape. So we'd expect that if we compared the effusion rates for Gases A and B, we'd get a ratio equal to the ratio of their average speeds (if the molecules of Gas A travel 4 times faster than those of Gas B, then Gas A should effuse 4 times faster). Since we just figured out that the ratio of their average speeds is equal to the reciprocal of the square root of the ratio of their masses, we'd expect the ratio of their effusion rates to be the same. This result is known as **Graham's law of effusion**:

Graham's Law of Effusion

$$\frac{\text{rate of effusion of Gas A}}{\text{rate of effusion of Gas B}} = \sqrt{\frac{\text{molar mass of Gas B}}{\text{molar mass of Gas A}}}$$

Let's emphasize the distinction between the relationships of temperature to the kinetic energy and to the speed of the gas. The molecules of two different gases at the same temperature have the same average kinetic energy. But the molecules of two different gases at the same temperature don't have the same average *speed*. Lighter molecules travel faster, because the kinetic energy depends on both the mass and the speed of the molecules.

Also, it's important to remember that not all the molecules of the gas in a container—even if there's only one type of molecule—travel at the same speed. Their speeds cover a wide range. What we *can* say is that as the temperature of the sample is increased, the *average* speed increases. In fact, since $KE \propto T$, the root-mean-square speed is proportional to $\sqrt{T}$. The figure below shows the distribution of molecular speeds for a gas at three different temperatures. Notice that the rms speeds increase as the temperature is increased.

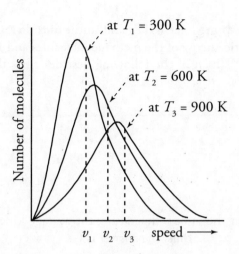

at $T_1 = 300$ K

at $T_2 = 600$ K

at $T_3 = 900$ K

v_1 v_2 v_3 speed ⟶

Example 16-10: A container holds methane (CH_4) and sulfur dioxide (SO_2) at a temperature of 227°C. Let v_M denote the rms speed of the methane molecules and v_S the rms speed of the sulfur dioxide molecules. Which of the following best describes the relationship between these speeds?

A. $v_S = 16\, v_M$
B. $v_S = 2\, v_M$
C. $v_S = v_M$
D. $v_M = 2\, v_S$
E. $v_M = 16\, v_S$

Solution: The molecular weight of methane is $12 + 4(1) = 16$, and the molecular weight of sulfur dioxide is $32 + 2(16) = 64$. Therefore

$$\frac{v_M}{v_S} = \sqrt{\frac{m_S}{m_M}} = \sqrt{\frac{64}{16}} = \sqrt{4} = 2 \quad \Rightarrow \quad v_M = 2v_S$$

So, D is the answer.

Example 16-11: In a laboratory experiment, Chamber A holds a mixture of four gases: 1 mole each of chlorine, fluorine, nitrogen, and carbon dioxide. A tiny hole is made in the side of the chamber, and the gases are allowed to effuse from Chamber A into an empty container. When 2 moles of gas have escaped, which gas will have the greatest mole fraction in Chamber A?

Solution: The gas with the greatest mole fraction remaining in Chamber A will be the gas with the *slowest* rate of effusion. This is the gas with the highest molecular weight. Of the gases in the chamber, Cl_2 has the greatest molecular weight.

Example 16-12: A balloon holds a mixture of fluorine, $F_2(g)$, and helium, $He(g)$. If the rms speed of helium atoms is 540 m/s, what is the rms speed of the fluorine molecules?

Solution: The molecular weight of F_2 is $2(19) = 38$, and the molecular weight of He is 4. Therefore,

$$\frac{v_{F_2}}{v_{He}} = \sqrt{\frac{m_{He}}{m_{F_2}}} = \sqrt{\frac{4}{38}} \approx \sqrt{\frac{1}{9}} = \frac{1}{3} \quad \Rightarrow \quad v_{F_2} \approx \frac{1}{3}v_{He} = \frac{1}{3}(540 \tfrac{m}{s}) = 180 \tfrac{m}{s}$$

Example 16-13: A container holds methane (CH_4) and sulfur dioxide (SO_2) at a temperature of 227°C. Let KE_M denote the average kinetic energy of the methane molecules and KE_S the average kinetic energy of the sulfur dioxide molecules. Which of the following best describes the relationship between these energies?

    A. $KE_S = 4\ KE_M$
    B. $KE_S = 3\ KE_M$
    C. $KE_M = KE_S$
    D. $KE_M = 3KE_S$
    E. $KE_M = 4\ KE_S$

Solution: Since both gases are at the same temperature, the average kinetic energies of their molecules will be the *same* (remember: $KE_{avg} \propto T$). Thus, the answer is C.

16.5   APPROACHING IDEAL-GAS BEHAVIOR

Let's review two of the assumptions that were listed for the kinetic-molecular theory:

1. The molecules of an ideal gas are so small compared to the average spacing between them that the molecules themselves take up essentially no volume.
2. The molecules of an ideal gas experience no intermolecular forces.

Under some conditions, these assumptions don't hold up very well, and the laws for ideal gases don't apply to real gases. In particular, *high pressures and low temperatures cause real gases to deviate most from ideal-gas behavior.* (Incidentally, these are the conditions under which a gas can liquefy.) Therefore, in reality, the actual volume and pressure for a real gas are less than those values obtained from applying the ideal gas law to that gas. That is, $P_{real} < P_{ideal}$ because the real gases *do* experience intermolecular forces, reducing collision with the walls of the container. And $V_{real} < V_{ideal}$ because molecules of real gases *do* have volume that reduces the effective volume of the container (since the molecules take up space, there is less space in the container for all the other particles to occupy).

So, when are gases at their "most ideal"? For most gases, low pressure and high temperature lead to ideality. Also, the lower the molecular weight or the smaller the size of its molecules, the more "ideal" its behavior. Additionally, monatomic gases display ideal behavior more readily than do diatomic (or higher-atomic) gases. Finally, the weaker the intermolecular forces present, the more likely the gas will behave ideally.

Example 16-14: Of the following, which gas would behave most like an ideal gas if all were at the same temperature and pressure?

   A. $H_2O(g)$
   B. $CH_3OH(g)$
   C. $HF(g)$
   D. $NH_3(g)$
   E. $CH_4(g)$

16.5

Solution: The molecules of a perfect (ideal) gas experience no intermolecular forces, so the gas in this list that will behave most like an ideal gas will be the one that has the weakest intermolecular forces. H_2O, CH_3OH (methanol), HF, and NH_3 experience hydrogen-bonding, while CH_4 experiences only weak dispersion forces. Therefore, E is the answer.

Want More Practice?
Scan the QR code below to register your book for online chapter summaries, drills, practice tests, and more!

Chapter 17
Solutions

17.1   DISSOLUTION AND SOLUBILITY

A **solution** forms when one substance **dissolves** into another, forming a *homogeneous* mixture. The process of dissolving is known as **dissolution**. For example, sugar dissolved into iced tea is a solution. A substance present in a relatively smaller proportion is called a **solute**, and a substance present in a relatively greater proportion is called a **solvent**. The process that occurs when the solvent molecules surround the solute molecules is known as **solvation**; if the solvent is water, the process is called **hydration**.

Solutions can involve any of the three phases of matter. For example, you can have a solution of two gases, of a gas in a liquid, of a solid in a liquid, or of a solid in a solid (an *alloy*). However, most of the solutions with which you're familiar have a liquid as the solvent. Salt water has solid salt (NaCl) dissolved into water, seltzer water has carbon dioxide gas dissolved in water, and vinegar has liquid acetic acid dissolved in water. In fact, most of the solutions that you commonly see have water as the solvent: lemonade, tea, soda pop, and corn syrup are examples. When a solution has water as the solvent, it is called an **aqueous** solution.

The **concentration** of a solution tells you how much solute is dissolved in the solvent. A **concentrated solution** has a greater amount of solute per unit volume than a solution that is **dilute**. A **saturated** solution is one in which no more solute will dissolve. At this point, we have reached the **molar solubility** of the solute for that particular solvent, and the reverse process of dissolution, called **precipitation**, occurs at the same rate as dissolving. Both the solid form and the dissolved form of the solute are said to be in **dynamic equilibrium**.

Solubility refers to the amount of solute that will saturate a particular solvent. Solubility is specific for the type of solute and solvent. For example, 100 mL of water at 25°C becomes saturated with 40 g of dissolved NaCl, but it would take 150 g of KI to saturate the same volume of water at this temperature. And both of these salts behave differently in methanol than in water. Solubility also varies with temperature, increasing or decreasing with temperature depending upon the solute and solvent. The solubility of most (but not all) solids in liquids increases with increasing temperature, and the solubility of gases in liquids decreases with increasing temperature.

Concentration Measurements

Molarity (*M*) expresses the concentration of a solution in terms of moles of solute per volume (in liters) of solution:

$$\text{Molarity } (M) = \frac{\text{\# moles of solute}}{\text{\# liters of solution}}$$

Concentration is denoted by enclosing the solute in brackets. For instance, "$[Na^+] = 1.0\ M$" indicates a solution whose concentration is equivalent to 1 mole of sodium ions per liter of solution.

Molality (*m*) expresses concentration in terms of moles of solute per *mass* (in kilograms) of solvent:

$$\text{Molality } (m) = \frac{\text{\# moles of solute}}{\text{\# kg of solvent}}$$

Molality is particularly useful when measuring properties that involve temperature because, unlike molarity, molality does not change with temperature. And, since a liter of water has a mass of one kilogram, the molar and molal concentrations of dilute aqueous solutions are nearly the same.

Mole fraction simply expresses the fraction of moles of a given substance (which we'll denote here by S) relative to the total moles in a solution:

$$\text{mole fraction of S} = X_S = \frac{\text{\# moles of substance S}}{\text{total \# moles in solution}}$$

Mole fraction is a useful way to express concentration when more than one solute is present.

Diluting a solution involves combining a solution of higher concentration (or molarity, *M*) with water, in order to make a solution with a lower concentration. You can calculate how to do this, starting with a certain volume (*V*) of the initial (i) solution and ending with a final (f) solution:

$$M_i V_i = M_f V_f$$

You may also have learned this equation as $C_1 V_2 = C_2 V_2$, where *C* stands for concentration.

How do we know which solutes are soluble in which solvents? Well, that's easy:

Like dissolves like.

Solutes will dissolve best in solvents where the intermolecular forces being broken in the solute are being replaced by equal (or stronger) intermolecular forces between the solvent and the solute.

Electrolytes

When ionic substances dissolve, they **dissociate** into ions. Free ions in a solution are called **electrolytes** because the solution can conduct electricity. Some salts dissociate completely into individual ions, while others only partially dissociate (that is, a certain percentage of the ions will remain paired, sticking close to each other rather than being independent and fully surrounded by solvent). Solutes that dissociate completely (like ionic substances) are called **strong electrolytes**, and those that remain ion-paired to some extent are called **weak electrolytes**. (Covalent compounds that don't dissociate into ions are **non-electrolytes**.) Solutions of strong electrolytes are better conductors of electricity than those of weak electrolytes.

Different ionic compounds will dissociate into different numbers of particles. Some won't dissociate at all, and others will break up into several ions. The **van't Hoff** (or **ionizability**) **factor** (**i**) tells us how many ions one unit of a substance will produce in a solution. Ionic bonds dissociate in solution, increasing the number of particles and thus i. Strong bases and strong acids will also have an $i > 1$ because they also fully dissociate in water. Covalent bonds do not dissociate in water, so a molecule with all covalent bonds will have $i = 1$. For the sake of the DAT, weak acids and weak bases also have $i = 1$. There are no molecules with $i < 1$. For example:

- Glucose ($C_6H_{12}O_6$) is non-ionic and contains all covalent bonds, so it does not dissociate. Therefore, $i = 1$. Indeed, the van't Hoff factor for almost all biomolecules (hormones, proteins, steroids, etc.) is 1.
- NaCl dissociates into Na^+ and Cl^-. Therefore, $i = 2$.
- HNO_3 dissociates into H^+ and NO_3^-. Therefore, $i = 2$.
- $CaCl_2$ dissociates into Ca^{2+} and 2 Cl^-. Therefore, $i = 3$.

Example 17-1: Of the following, which is the *weakest* electrolyte?

    A. NH_4I
    B.   LiF
    C.   AgBr
    D. H_2O_2
    E.   NaCl

Solution: All ionic compounds, whether soluble or not, are defined as strong electrolytes, so A, B, C, and E are eliminated. D, hydrogen peroxide, is a covalent compound that does not produce an appreciable number of ions upon dissolution and thus is a weak electrolyte. D is the best answer.

Example 17-2: A researcher adds 0.4 kg of $CaBr_2$ (MW = 200 g/mol) to 10 L (= 10 kg) of water, in which it dissolves completely.

    A.   What is the molality of the calcium bromide in the solution?
    B.   What is the concentration of bromide ion in the solution?
    C.   How much water would the researcher need to add to the solution in order to decrease the concentration by a factor of 4?
    D.   How does the molarity of the calcium bromide in the solution compare to the molality? Is it slightly lower, slightly higher, or exactly equal?

Solution:

A. Since the molecular weight of $CaBr_2$ is 0.2 kg/mol, a 0.4 kg sample represents 2 moles. Then by definition we have

$$\text{Molality } (m) = \frac{\#\text{ moles of solute}}{\#\text{ kg of solvent}} = \frac{2\text{ mol}}{10\text{ kg}} = 0.2m$$

B. Since $CaBr_2$ dissociates into one Ca^{2+} ion and 2 Br^- ions, the concentration of bromide ion in the solution is $2(0.2\ M) = 0.4\ M$.

C. Let x be the number of liters of additional water added to the solution. If the concentration is to be decreased by a factor of 4 (that is, to 0.05 M), then

$$\frac{2\text{ mol}}{10\text{ L} + x\text{ L}} = 0.05M \quad \Rightarrow \quad \frac{2}{10 + x} = \frac{5}{100} \quad \Rightarrow \quad x = 30$$

D. Since the solution contains both the solvent and the solute, the number of liters of solution is slightly *greater* than 10 L. Therefore, the molarity will be slightly *lower* than the molality.

Solubility Rules

There are two sets of solubility rules that show up time and time again on the DAT. The first set governs the solubility of salts in water. Memorize them.

Salt Solubility Rules

1. All Group I (Li^+, Na^+, K^+, Rb^+, Cs^+) and ammonium (NH_4^+) salts are *soluble*.
2. All nitrate (NO_3^-), perchlorate (ClO_4^-), and acetate ($C_2H_3O_2^-$) salts are *soluble*.
3. All silver (Ag^+), lead (Pb^{2+}/ Pb^{4+}), and mercury (Hg_2^{2+}/ Hg^{2+}) salts are *insoluble, except* for their nitrates, perchlorates, and acetates.

The second set governs the general solubility of solids and gases in liquids, as a function of the temperature and pressure. Unlike the solubility rules for salts in water, which are 99.9 percent reliable, the rules below should be taken as just rules of thumb because they are only 95 percent reliable (still not bad). Memorize these, too:

Phase Solubility Rules

1. The solubility of solids in liquids tends to increase with increasing temperature.
2. The solubility of gases in liquids tends to decrease with increasing temperature.
3. The solubility of gases in liquids tends to increase with increasing pressure.

Example 17-3: Which of the following salts is expected to be *insoluble* in water?

A. CsOH
B. NH_4NO_3
C. $CaCO_3$
D. $AgClO_4$
E. Na_2CO_3

Solution: According to the solubility rules for salts in water, A, B, D, and E are expected to be soluble. C is therefore the best answer.

Example 17-4: Which of the following acids could be added to an unknown salt solution and NOT cause precipitation?

A. HCl
B. HI
C. H_2SO_4
D. HNO_3
E. HBr

Solution: According to the solubility rules for salts, all nitrate (NO_3^-) salts are soluble. Therefore, only the addition of nitric acid guarantees that any new ion combination would be soluble. D is the correct answer.

17.2 COLLIGATIVE PROPERTIES

Colligative properties depend on the *number* of solute particles in the solution rather than the *type* of particle. For example, when any solute is dissolved into a solvent, the boiling point, freezing point, and vapor pressure of the solution will be different from those of the pure solvent. For colligative properties, *the identity of the particle is not important.* That is, for a 1 *M* solution of *any* solute, the change in a colligative property will be the same no matter what the size, type, or charge of the solute particles. Remember to consider the van't Hoff factor when accounting for particles: One mole of sucrose ($i = 1$) will have the same number of particles *in solution* as 0.5 mol of NaCl ($i = 2$), and therefore will have the same effect on a colligative property. Thus, we can consider the effective concentration to be the product *iM* (or *im*); this is the concentration of particles present.

The four colligative properties we'll study for the DAT are vapor-pressure depression, boiling-point elevation, freezing-point depression, and osmotic pressure.

Vapor-Pressure Depression

Think about being at the ocean or a lake in the summer. The air is always more humid (moist) than in the middle of a parking lot. Why? Because some of the water molecules gain enough energy to get into the gas phase, so we see a dynamic equilibrium setup between the molecules in the liquid phase and the molecules in the gas (vapor) phase.

Vapor pressure is the pressure exerted by the gaseous phase of a liquid that evaporated from the exposed surface of the liquid. The weaker a substance's intermolecular forces, the higher its vapor pressure and the more easily it evaporates. For example, if we compare diethyl ether, $H_5C_2OC_2H_5$, and water, we notice that while water undergoes hydrogen bonding, diethyl ether does not, so despite its greater molecular mass, diethyl ether will vaporize more easily and have a higher vapor pressure than water. Easily vaporized liquids—liquids with *high* vapor pressure—like diethyl ether are said to be **volatile.**

Now let's think about what happens to vapor pressure when the liquid contains a dissolved solute. The solute molecules are attached to solvent molecules and act as "anchors." As a result, more energy is required to enter the gas phase since the solvent molecules need to break away from their interactions with the solute before they can enter the gas phase. In fact, the boiling point of a liquid is defined as the temperature at which the vapor pressure of the solution is equal to the atmospheric pressure over the solution. Thus, at sea level, where the atmospheric pressure is 760 torr, the solution must have a vapor pressure of 760 torr in order to boil. Adding more solute to the same solution will decrease its vapor pressure. Boiling will still take place when vapor pressure is 760 torr, but more heat will have to be supplied to reach this vapor pressure, and thus the solution will boil at a higher temperature. For example, salted water (say, for cooking spaghetti) boils at a higher temperature than unsalted water.

If we have a solution of two liquids, A and B, then the total vapor pressure is equal to the partial vapor pressure of A plus the partial vapor pressure of B. That is, $P = p_A + p_B$, which is known as **Dalton's law.** To calculate the partial pressures, we use **Raoult's law** (also known as the **ideal solution law**), which says that the partial vapor pressure of A (or B) is proportional to its mole fraction in the solution:

Raoult's Law
$$p_A = X_A P^\circ_A$$

In this equation, P°_A stands for the vapor pressure of *pure* A. Therefore, $P = X_A P^\circ_A + X_B P^\circ_B$. Notice that the presence of B causes X_A to be less than 1, so p_A is lower than P°_A; this is **vapor-pressure depression**. In fact, because $X_A = 1 - X_B$, we can write the formula for vapor-pressure depression in terms of B like this:

Vapor-Pressure Depression
$$\Delta P_A = -X_B P^\circ_A$$

Most solutions deviate from Raoult's law. For example, consider once again a solution containing a mixture of two liquids, A and B. If the intermolecular attractions between A and B are weaker than those between A and A or between B and B, then the molecules will escape from the liquid solution into the gas phase more easily than they would from pure A or pure B. Therefore, their partial vapor pressures will be higher than predicted by Raoult's law. Overall, Raoult's law works well when describing the effects of adding a non-volatile solute, and when describing dilute solutions.

Example 17-5: A solution is formed by mixing 0.6 mol of benzene with 0.2 mol of toluene. At the temperature of the solution, the vapor pressure of pure benzene is 96 torr, and the vapor pressure of pure toluene is 28 torr.

    A.   What is the mole fraction of toluene in the solution?

    B.   By how much is the vapor pressure of benzene lowered due to the presence of toluene in this solution?

    C.   What is the total vapor pressure of the solution?

Solution:

    A.   The mole faction of toluene in the solution is

$$X_T = \frac{n_T}{n_B + n_T} = \frac{0.2}{0.6 + 0.2} = \frac{0.2}{0.8} = \frac{1}{4}$$

    B.   Using the equation for vapor-pressure depression, we find that

$$\Delta P_B = -X_T P^{\circ}{}_B = -\frac{1}{4}(96 \text{ torr}) = -24 \text{ torr}$$

    C.   Combining Dalton's law with Raoult's law, we find that

$$P = p_B + p_T = X_B P^{\circ}{}_B + X_T P^{\circ}{}_T = \frac{3}{4}(96 \text{ torr}) + \frac{1}{4}(28 \text{ torr}) = 72 + 7 = 79 \text{ torr}$$

Boiling-Point Elevation

When a liquid boils, the molecules in the liquid acquire enough energy to overcome the intermolecular forces and break free into the gas phase. The liquid molecules escape as a vapor at the surface between the liquid and air. But what happens when a non-volatile solute is added to the liquid? The solute particles are attached to solvent molecules and act as "anchors." As a result, more energy is required since you not only have to convert the solvent into the gas phase, but you first have to break the interaction with the solute. What happens to the boiling point? In order for the molecules to escape, they need more energy than they did without the solute. This translates into an elevation of the boiling point. The increase in boiling point is directly related to the number of particles in solution and the type of solvent. For a given solvent, the more solute particles, the greater the boiling-point elevation. For problems involving boiling-point elevation, the concentration of particles is measured in *molality* because it remains constant with temperature. Also, you have to consider that some compounds dissociate when they dissolve, so the equation for boiling-point elevation includes the van't Hoff factor, i:

Boiling-Point Elevation
$$\Delta T_b = k_b i m$$

In this equation, k_b is the solvent's boiling-point elevation constant, i is the solute's van't Hoff factor, and m is the molal concentration of the solution. For water, $k_b \approx 0.5°C \, / \, m$.

Freezing-Point Depression

What happens when we add a solute to a liquid, then try to freeze the solution? Solids are held together by attractive intermolecular forces. During freezing, the molecules in a liquid will assemble into an orderly, tightly packed array. However, the presence of solute particles will interfere with efficient arrangement of the solvent molecules into a solid lattice. As a result, a liquid will be less able to achieve a solid state when a solute is present, and the freezing point of the solution will decrease. (Or, equivalently, the melting point of a solid containing a solute is decreased.) The good news is that the formula for freezing-point depression has exactly the same form as the formula for boiling-point elevation, except that the temperature is going down instead of up (that is, the equation for freezing-point *depression* has a *minus* sign whereas the equation for boiling-point *elevation* has a *plus* sign).

Freezing-Point Depression
$$\Delta T_f = -k_f i m$$

In this equation, k_f is the solvent's freezing-point depression constant, i is the solute's van't Hoff factor, and m is the molal concentration of the solution. For water, $k_f \approx 1.9°C/m$.

Example 17-6: What is the boiling point of a 2 m aqueous solution of sodium chloride?

Solution: The value of i for NaCl is $1 + 1 = 2$, so the change in the boiling point of the water is given by

$$\Delta T_b = k_b i m = (0.5°C/m)(2)(2 \, m) = 2°C$$

Therefore, the boiling point is $100°C + 2°C = 102°C$.

Example 17-7: What is the freezing point of a 1 m solution of barium fluoride in water?

Solution: The value of i for BaF_2 is $1 + 2 = 3$, so the change in the freezing point of the water is given by

$$\Delta T_f = -k_f i m = -(1.9°C/m)(3)(1 \, m) = -5.7°C$$

Therefore, the freezing point is $0°C + (-5.7°C) = -5.7°C$

Osmotic Pressure

Osmosis describes the net movement of water across a semipermeable membrane from a region of low solute concentration to a region of higher solute concentration in an effort to dilute the higher concentration solution. The semipermeable membrane prohibits the transfer of solutes, but allows water to traverse through it. In the following figure, the net movement of water will be to the right:

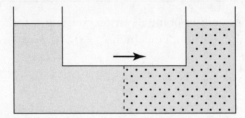

Osmotic pressure (Π) can be defined as the pressure it would take to *stop* osmosis from occurring. If a pressure gauge were added to the same system, osmotic pressure could be measured.

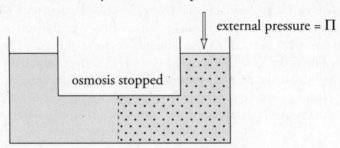

external pressure = Π

osmosis stopped

The osmotic pressure of a solution is given by the **van't Hoff equation**:

$$\Pi = MiRT$$

where Π is osmotic pressure in atm, M is the molarity of the solution, i is the van't Hoff factor, R is the universal gas constant (0.0821 L atm/K mol), and T is the temperature in kelvins.

Again, changes in osmotic pressure are affected only by the number of particles in solution (taking into account the van't Hoff factor), not by the identity of those particles.

Want More Practice?
Scan the QR code below to register your book for online chapter summaries, drills, practice tests, and more!

Chapter 18
Kinetics

18.1   REACTION MECHANISM: AN ANALOGY

Chemical **kinetics** is the study of how reactions take place and how fast they occur. (Kinetics tells us nothing about the *spontaneity* of a reaction, however! We'll study that a little later.)

Consider this scenario: A group of people are washing a pile of dirty dishes and stacking them up as clean, dry dishes. Our "reaction" has dirty dishes as starting material, and clean, dry dishes as the product:

$$\text{dirty dish} \rightarrow \text{clean-and-dry dish}$$

But what about a *soapy* dish? We know it's part of the process, but the equation doesn't include it. When we break down the pathway of a dirty dish to a clean-and-dry dish, we realize that the reaction happens in several steps, a sequence of **elementary** steps that show us the reaction **mechanism:**

1. dirty dish $\rightarrow$ soapy dish
2. soapy dish $\rightarrow$ rinsed dish
3. rinsed dish $\rightarrow$ clean-and-dry dish

The soapy and rinsed dishes are reaction **intermediates**. They are necessary for the conversion of dirty dishes to clean-and-dry dishes, but don't appear either in the starting material or products. If you add up all the reactants and products, the intermediates cancel out, and you'll have the overall equation.

In the same way, we write chemical reactions as if they occur in a single step:

$$2\,NO + O_2 \rightarrow 2\,NO_2$$

But in reality, things are a little more complicated, and reactions often proceed through intermediates that we don't show in the chemical equation. The truth for the reaction above is that it occurs in two steps:

1. $2\,NO \rightarrow N_2O_2$
2. $N_2O_2 + O_2 \rightarrow 2\,NO_2$

The N_2O_2 comes and goes during the reaction, but isn't part of the starting material or products. N_2O_2 is a reaction intermediate.

There's an important difference, however, between our dirty dishes example and a chemical reaction that has to do with intermediates. While we can actually *see* the intermediate stages as we wash the dishes (the soapy and rinsed dishes), we *cannot* see nor isolate intermediates in a chemical reaction. In kinetics, these are known as **reactive intermediates** and are generally used up as fast as they are formed (this is sometimes known as the **steady-state approximation**).

Rate-Determining Step

What determines the rate of a reaction? Consider our friends doing the dishes.

1. dirty dish $\rightarrow$ soapy dish   Bingo washes at 5 dishes per minute.
2. soapy dish $\rightarrow$ rinsed dish   Ringo rinses at 8 dishes per minute.
3. rinsed dish $\rightarrow$ clean-and-dry dish   Dingo dries at 3 dishes per minute.

What will be the rate of the overall reaction? Thanks to Dingo, the dishes move from dirty to clean-and-dry at only 3 dishes a minute. It doesn't matter how fast Bingo and Ringo wash and rinse; the dishes will pile up behind Dingo. The **rate-determining step** is Dingo's drying step, and true to its name, it determines the overall rate of reaction.

The slowest step in a process determines the overall reaction rate.

This applies to chemical reactions as well. For our chemical reaction given above, we have

$$2\,NO \rightarrow N_2O_2 \quad \text{(fast)}$$

$$N_2O_2 + O_2 \rightarrow 2\,NO_2 \quad \text{(slow)}$$

The second step is the slowest, and it will determine the overall rate of reaction. No matter how fast the first step moves along, the intermediates will pile up in front of the second step as it plods along. The slow step dictates the rate of the overall reaction.

Once again, there's an important difference between our dishes analogy and a chemical reaction: While the dishes pile up behind Dingo, in a chemical reaction the intermediates will not pile up. Rather they will shuttle back and forth between reactants and products until the slow step takes it forward. This would be like taking a rinsed dish and getting it soapy again, until Dingo is ready for it!

18.2   REACTION RATE

The **rate** of a reaction indicates how fast reactants are being consumed or how fast products are being formed. The reaction rate depends on several factors. Since the reactant molecules must collide and interact in order for old bonds to be broken and new ones to be formed to generate the product molecules, anything that affects these collisions and interactions will affect the reaction rate. The reaction rate is determined by:

1. how frequently the reactant molecules collide,
2. the orientation of the colliding molecules, and
3. their energy.

Activation Energy

Every chemical reaction has an **activation energy** (E_a), or the minimum energy required of reactant molecules during a molecular collision in order for the reaction to proceed to products. If the reactant molecules don't possess this much energy, their collisions won't be able to produce the products and the reaction will not occur. If the reactants possess the necessary activation energy, they can reach a high-energy (and short-lived!) **transition state**, also known as the **activated complex**. For example, if the reaction is $A_2 + B_2 \rightarrow 2\,AB$, the activated complex might look something like this:

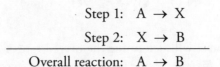

Now that we have introduced all species that might appear throughout the course of a chemical reaction, we can illustrate the energy changes that occur as a reaction occurs in a **reaction coordinate diagram**. Consider the following two-step process and its reaction coordinate graph below:

$$\text{Step 1:} \quad A \rightarrow X$$
$$\text{Step 2:} \quad X \rightarrow B$$
$$\overline{\text{Overall reaction:} \quad A \rightarrow B}$$

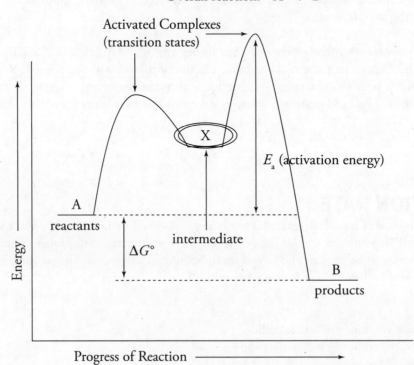

Notice that the transition state is always an energy maximum, and is therefore distinct from an intermediate. Remember that reaction intermediates (shown as X in this case) are produced in an early step of the mechanism, and are later used up so they do not appear as products of the overall reaction. The intermediate is shown here as a local minimum in terms of its energy, but has more energy than either the reactants or products. The high energy intermediate is therefore highly reactive, making it difficult to isolate.

Since the progress of the reaction depends on the reactant molecules colliding with enough energy to generate the activated complex, we can make the following statements concerning the reaction rate:

1. *The lower the activation energy, the faster the reaction rate.* The reaction coordinate above suggests that the second step of the mechanism will therefore be the slow step, or the rate-determining step, since the second "hill" of the diagram is higher.
2. *The greater the concentrations of the reactants, the faster the reaction rate.* Favorable collisions are more likely as the concentrations of reactant molecules increase.
3. *The higher the temperature of the reaction mixture, the faster the reaction rate.* At higher temperatures, more reactant molecules have a sufficient energy to overcome the activation-energy barrier, and molecules collide at a higher frequency, so the reaction can proceed at a faster rate.

Notice in the reaction coordinate diagram above that the $\Delta G°$ of the reaction has no bearing on the rate of the reaction, and vice versa. Thermodynamic factors and kinetic factors *do not affect each other* (a concept the DAT loves to ask about).

18.3   CATALYSTS

Catalysts provide reactants with a different route, usually a shortcut, to get to products. A **catalyst** will almost always make a reaction go faster by either speeding up the rate-determining step or providing an optimized route to products. A catalyst that accelerates a reaction does so *by lowering the activation energy* of the rate-determining step, and therefore the energy of the highest-energy transition state:

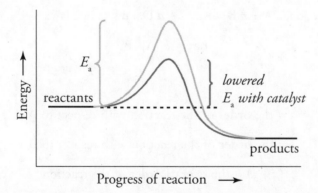

The key difference between a reactant and a catalyst is that the reactants are converted to products, but *a catalyst remains unchanged at the end of a reaction.* A catalyst can undergo a temporary change during a reaction, but it is always converted back to its original state. Like reaction intermediates, catalysts aren't included in the overall reaction equation.

Our dish crew could use a catalyst. Picture Dingo walking to pick up each wet dish, drying it on both sides, and walking back to place it in the clean dish stack. Now imagine a helper, Daisy, who takes the wet dish from Ringo, then walks it over to Dingo, and while he dries and stacks, she returns with another wet dish. This way, Dingo can dry 5 dishes a minute instead of 3, and the overall dish-cleaning rate increases to 5 dishes a minute. Daisy is the catalyst, but the chain of events in the overall reaction remains the same.

In the same way, chemical reactions can be catalyzed. Consider the decomposition of ozone:

$$O_3(g) + O(g) \rightarrow 2\,O_2(g)$$

This reaction actually takes place in two steps and is catalyzed by nitric oxide (NO):

1. **NO(g)** + $O_3(g) \rightarrow NO_2(g) + O_2(g)$
2. $NO_2(g) + O(g) \rightarrow$ **NO(g)** + $O_2(g)$

NO(g) is necessary for this reaction to proceed at a noticeable rate, and even undergoes changes itself during the process. But NO(g) remains unchanged at the end of the reaction and makes the reaction occur much faster than it would in its absence. NO(g), a product of automobile exhaust, is a catalyst in ozone destruction.

18.4   RATE LAWS

The **rate law** for a chemical reaction is an equation that links the reaction rate with the concentrations or pressures of the reactants, using a rate constant (k). The data for rate laws are determined by the *initial rates* of reaction and typically are given as the **rate at which the reactant disappears**. You'll rarely see products in a rate law expression, usually only reactants. What does a rate law tell us? Although a reaction needs all the reactants to proceed, *only those that are involved in the rate-determining step (the slow step) are part of the rate law expression*. Some reactants may not affect the reaction rate at all, and so they won't be a part of the rate law expression.

Let's look at a generic reaction, $a\,A + b\,B \rightarrow c\,C + d\,D$, and its rate law:

$$\text{rate} = k\,[A]^x[B]^y$$

where

x = the **order** of the reaction with respect to A

y = the **order** of the reaction with respect to B

$(x + y)$ = the **overall order** of the reaction

k = the rate constant

The rate law can only be determined *experimentally*. You *can't* get the orders of the reactants, not to mention the rate constant k, just by looking at the balanced equation. The exception to this rule is for an *elementary step* in a reaction mechanism. The rate law is first order for a unimolecular elementary step and second order for a bimolecular elementary step. The individual order of the reactants in a rate law will follow from their stoichiometry in the rate-determining step (similar to the way they're included in an equilibrium constant).

In the following example, we will work through how to determine the rate law from a set of reaction rate data. These are challenging questions and rarely on the DAT, but read through this example once to make sure you understand how to do this, just in case. We will use the reaction

$$A + B + C \rightarrow D + E$$

Experiment	[A]	[B]	[C]	Initial reaction rate [M/s]
1	0.2 M	0.1 M	0.05 M	1×10^{-3}
2	0.4 M	0.1 M	0.05 M	2×10^{-3}
3	0.2 M	0.2 M	0.05 M	4×10^{-3}
4	0.2 M	0.1 M	0.10 M	1×10^{-3}

From the experimental data, we can determine the orders with respect to the reactants—that is, the exponents x, y, and z in the equation

$$\text{rate} = k[A]^x[B]^y[C]^z$$

and the overall order of the reaction, $x + y + z$.

Let's first find the order of the reaction with respect to Reactant A. As we go from Experiment 1 to Experiment 2, only [A] changes, so we can use the data to figure out the order of the reaction with respect to Reactant [A]. We notice that the value of [A] doubled, and the reaction rate doubled. Therefore, the reaction rate is proportional to [A], and $x = 1$.

Next, let's look at [B]. As we go from Experiment 1 to Experiment 3, only [B] changes. When [B] is doubled, the rate is quadrupled. Therefore, the rate is proportional to $[B]^2$, and $y = 2$.

Finally, let's look at [C]. As we go from Experiment 1 to Experiment 4, only [C] changes. When [C] is doubled, the rate is unaffected. This tells us that the reaction rate does not depend on [C], so $z = 0$.

Therefore, the rate law has the form

$$\text{rate} = k[A][B]^2$$

The reaction is first order with respect to [A], second order with respect to [B], zero order with respect to [C], and third order overall. In general, if a reaction rate increases by a factor f when the concentration of a reactant increases by a factor c, and $f = c^x$, then we can say that x is the order with respect to that reactant.

The Rate Constant

From the experimental data, you can also calculate the rate constant, k. For the reaction we looked at above, we found that the rate law is given by: rate $= k[A][B]^2$. Solving this for k, we get

$$k = \frac{\text{rate}}{[A][B]^2}$$

Now, just pick any experiment in the table, and using the results of Experiment 1, you'd find that

$$k = \frac{\text{rate}}{[A][B]^2} = \frac{1 \times 10^{-3}}{(0.2)(0.1)^2} = 0.5$$

Any of the experiments will give you the same value for k because it's a constant for any given reaction. That is, each reaction has its own rate constant, which takes into account such factors as the frequency of collisions, the fraction of the collisions with the proper orientation to initiate the desired bond changes, and the activation energy. It is worth noting that if you add a catalyst (thus decreasing E_a) or increase the temperature, both the rate and the rate constant (k) will increase.

The units of the rate constant are not necessarily uniform from one reaction to the next. Reactions of different orders will have rate constants bearing different units. In order to obtain the units of the rate constant one must keep in mind that the rate, on the left side of the equation, must always have units of M/s as it measures the change in concentration of a species in the reaction over time. The units given to the rate constant must, when combined with the units of the concentrations in the rate equation, provide M/s.

Below is a generic second order rate equation.

$$\text{Rate} = k[A][B]$$

Assuming that the concentrations of both A and B are in molarity (M), then in order to give the left side of the equation units of M/s, the units of the rate constant must be $M^{-1}s^{-1}$. If the rate were third order, the units would be $M^{-2}s^{-1}$, or if first order then simply s^{-1}.

Example 18-1: A reaction is run without a catalyst and is found to have an activation energy of 140 kJ/mol and a heat of reaction, ΔH, of 30 kJ/mol. In the presence of a catalyst, however, the activation energy is reduced to 120 kJ/mol. What will be the heat of reaction in the presence of the catalyst?

A. −10 kJ/mol
B. 10 kJ/mol
C. 30 kJ/mol
D. 50 kJ/mol
E. 110 kJ/mol

18.4

Solution: Catalysts affect only the kinetics of a reaction, not the thermodynamics. The heat of the reaction will be the same with or without a catalyst. The answer is C.

Experiment	[A]	[B]	Initial reaction rate (M/s)
1	0.01 M	0.01 M	4.0×10^{-3}
2	0.01 M	0.02 M	8.0×10^{-3}
3	0.02 M	0.02 M	1.6×10^{-2}
4	0.04 M	0.02 M	3.2×10^{-2}

Example 18-2: Based on the data given above, determine the rate law for the reaction A + B → C.

A. Rate = $k[B]$
B. Rate = $k[A][B]$
C. Rate = $k[A]^2[B]$
D. Rate = $k[A][B]^2$
E. Rate = $k[A]^2[B]^2$

Solution: Comparing Experiments 1 and 2, we notice that when [B] doubled (and [A] remained unchanged), the reaction rate doubled. Therefore, the reaction is first order with respect to [B]; this eliminates D and E. Now, comparing Experiments 3 and 4, we notice that when [A] doubled (and [B] remained unchanged), the reaction rate also doubled. This means that the reaction is first order with respect to [A] as well. Therefore, the answer is B.

Example 18-3: Which of the following gives the form of the rate law for the balanced reaction?

$$4A + 2B \rightarrow C + 3D$$

A. Rate = $k[A]^4[B]^2$
B. Rate = $k[A]^2[B]$
C. Rate = $k[C][D]^3/[A]^4[B]^2$
D. Rate = $k[C][D]$
E. Cannot be determined from the information given

Solution: Unless the given reaction is the rate-determining, elementary step, we have no way of knowing what the rate law is. The answer is E.

Want More Practice?
Scan the QR code below to register your book for online chapter summaries, drills, practice tests, and more!

Chapter 19
Equilibrium

19.1 EQUILIBRIUM

Many reactions are reversible, and situations can occur in which the forward and reverse reactions come into a balance called **equilibrium**. How does equilibrium come about? The process is *dynamic*; once equilibrium is established, both forward and reverse reactions are still taking place, but the composition of the reaction does not change. However, let's begin at the starting line. Before any bonds are broken or made, the reaction flask contains only reactants and no products. As the reaction proceeds, products begin to form and eventually build up, and some of them begin to revert to reactants. That is, once products are formed, both the forward and reverse reactions are occurring. Ultimately, the reaction will come to equilibrium, a state at which both the forward and reverse reactions occur at the same constant rate. At equilibrium, the overall concentration of reactants and products remains the same, but at the molecular level, they are continually interconverting. Because the forward and reverse processes balance one another perfectly, we don't observe any change in concentrations.

> *When a reaction is at equilibrium (and only at equilibrium), the rate of the forward reaction is equal to the rate of the reverse reaction.*

Equilibria occur for *closed reactions* (which means no new reactants, products, or other changes are imposed).

The Equilibrium Constant

Each reaction will tend towards its own equilibrium and, for a given temperature, will have an **equilibrium constant, K_{eq}**. For the generic, balanced reaction

$$a\,A + b\,B \rightleftharpoons c\,C + d\,D$$

the equilibrium expression is given by:

$$K_{eq} = \frac{[C]^c[D]^d}{[A]^a[B]^b}$$

This is known as the **mass-action ratio**, where the square brackets represent the molar concentrations at equilibrium.

The constant K is often given a subscript to indicate the type of reaction it represents. For example, K_a (for acids), K_b (for bases), and K_{sp} (for solubility product) are all equilibrium constants. The equilibrium expression is derived from the ratio of the concentration of products to reactants at equilibrium, as follows:

1. Products are in the numerator, and reactants are in the denominator. They are in brackets because the equilibrium expression comes from the *concentrations* (at equilibrium) of the species in the reaction.
2. The coefficient of each species in the reaction becomes an exponent on its concentration in the equilibrium expression.
3. Solids and pure liquids are *not* included, because their concentrations don't change. (A substance that's a solid or pure liquid in the reaction is often indicated by an "[s]" or "[l]" subscript, respectively. We're also allowed to omit solvents in dilute solutions because the solvents are in vast excess and their concentrations do not change.)
4. Aqueous dissolved particles are included.
5. If the reaction is gaseous, we can use the partial pressure of each gas as its concentration. The equilibrium constant determined with pressures will be different than with concentrations because of their different units. The constant using partial pressures is often termed K_p.

The value of K_{eq} is constant at a given temperature for a particular reaction, no matter what ratio of reactants and products are given at the beginning of the reaction. That is, any closed system will proceed towards its equilibrium ratios of products and reactants even if you start with all products, or a mixture of some reactants and some products. You can even open the flask and add more of any reactant or product, and the system will change until it has reached the K_{eq} ratio. We'll discuss this idea in detail in just a moment, but right now focus on this:

The value of K_{eq} for a given reaction is a constant at a given temperature.

If the temperature changes, then a reaction's K_{eq} value will change.

The value of K_{eq} tells you the direction the reaction favors:

$K_{eq} < 1 \rightarrow$ reaction favors the reactants
$K_{eq} = 1 \rightarrow$ reaction balances reactants and products
$K_{eq} > 1 \rightarrow$ reaction favors the products

We will see in later how K_{eq} and $\Delta G°$ are related, and essentially tell us the same things about whether a reaction favors the reactants or the products.

Example 19-1: What is the equilibrium constant for this reaction:

$$2\,NO \rightleftharpoons N_2 + O_2?$$

Solution: The mass-action ratio is products over reactants. Stoichiometric coefficients become exponents on the concentrations, not coefficients inside the square brackets. Therefore, the coefficient of 2 for the reactant NO means the denominator will be $[NO]^2$.

$$\frac{[N_2][O_2]}{[NO]^2}$$

Example 19-2: When the reaction $2A + B \rightleftharpoons 2C$ reaches equilibrium, $[A] = 0.1\ M$ and $[C] = 0.2\ M$. If the value of K_{eq} for this reaction is 8, what is $[B]$ at equilibrium?

Solution: The expression for K_{eq} is $\dfrac{[C]^2}{[A]^2[B]}$. We now solve for $[B]$ and substitute in the given values:

$$K_{eq} = \frac{[C]^2}{[A]^2[B]} \rightarrow [B] = \frac{[C]^2}{[A]^2 K_{eq}} = \frac{(0.2)^2}{(0.1)^2(8)} = \frac{2^2}{8} = 0.5$$

19.2 THE REACTION QUOTIENT

The equilibrium constant expression is a ratio: the concentration of the products divided by those of the reactants, each raised to the power equal to its stoichiometric coefficient in the balanced equation. If the reaction is not at equilibrium, the same expression is known simply as the **reaction quotient, Q**. For the generic, balanced reaction

$$a\,A + b\,B \rightleftharpoons c\,C + d\,D$$

the reaction quotient is given by:

$$Q = \frac{[C]^c\,[D]^d}{[A]^a\,[B]^b}$$

where the square brackets represent the molar concentrations of the species. The point now is that the concentrations in the expression Q do *not* have to be the concentrations at equilibrium. (If the concentrations are the equilibrium concentrations, the Q will equal K_{eq}.)

Comparing the value of Q to K_{eq} tells us in what direction the reaction will proceed. The reaction will strive to reach a state in which $Q = K_{eq}$. So, if Q is less than K_{eq}, then the reaction will proceed in the forward direction (in order to increase the concentration of the products and decrease the concentration of the reactants) to increase Q to the K_{eq} value. On the other hand, if Q is greater than K_{eq}, then the reaction will proceed in the reverse direction (in order to increase the concentrations of the reactants and decrease the concentrations of the products) to reduce Q to K_{eq}.

K_{eq} is the condition the reaction will try to achieve.

If $Q = K_{eq}$, the reaction is at equilibrium.

$$Q \Longrightarrow K_{eq} \Longleftarrow Q$$

If $Q < K_{eq}$,
reaction proceeds in
the **forward** direction
so Q gets closer to K_{eq}.

If $Q > K_{eq}$,
reaction proceeds in
the **reverse** direction
so Q gets closer to K_{eq}.

Example 19-3: The value of the equilibrium constant for the reaction

$$2\ COF_2(g) \rightleftharpoons CO_2(g) + CF_4(g)$$

is $K_{eq} = 2$. If a 1 L reaction container currently holds 1 mole each of CO_2 and CF_4 and 0.5 mole of COF_2, then which direction is favored?

Solution: The expression for Q is $\dfrac{[CO_2][CF_4]}{[COF_2]^2}$. Therefore, the value of Q is:

$$\frac{(1)(1)}{(0.5)^2} = 4$$

Since $Q > K_{eq}$, the reverse reaction will be favored.

19.3 LE CHÂTELIER'S PRINCIPLE

A system at equilibrium will try to neutralize any imposed change (or stress) in order to reestablish equilibrium. This is called **Le Châtelier's principle.** For example, if you add more reactant to a system that is at equilibrium, the system will react by favoring the forward reaction to consume that reactant and reestablish equilibrium.

To illustrate, let's look at the Haber process for making ammonia:

$$N_2(g) + 3\ H_2(g) \rightleftharpoons 2\ NH_3(g) + \text{heat}$$

Let's assume the reaction is at equilibrium, and see how it reacts to disturbances to the equilibrium by changing the concentration of the species, the pressure, or the temperature.

Adding Ammonia

If we add ammonia, the system is no longer at equilibrium, and there is an excess of product. How can the reaction reestablish equilibrium? By consuming some of the added ammonia, the ratio of products to reactant would decrease towards the equilibrium ratio, so the reverse reaction will be favored (we say the system "shifts to the left"), converting ammonia into nitrogen and hydrogen, until equilibrium is restored.

You can see how this follows from comparing the reaction quotient of the disturbed system to the equilibrium constant. If we add ammonia to the reaction mixture, then $[NH_3]$ increases, and the reaction quotient, Q, becomes greater than K_{eq}. As a result, the reaction will proceed in the reverse direction to reduce Q to K_{eq}.

Removing Ammonia

If we remove the product, ammonia, then the forward reaction will be favored—the reaction "shifts to the right"—in order to reach equilibrium again. Again, you can see how this follows from comparing the reaction quotient of the disturbed system to the equilibrium constant. If we remove ammonia from the reaction mixture, then $[NH_3]$ decreases, and the reaction quotient, Q, becomes smaller than K_{eq}. As a result, the reaction will proceed in the forward direction to increase Q to K_{eq}.

Adding Hydrogen

If we add some reactant, say $H_2(g)$, then the forward reaction will be favored—the reaction "shifts to the right"—to reach equilibrium again. This follows from comparing the reaction quotient of the disturbed system to the equilibrium constant. If we add hydrogen to the reaction mixture, the $[H_2]$ increases, and the reaction quotient, Q, becomes smaller than K_{eq}. As a result, the reaction will proceed in the forward direction to increase Q to K_{eq}.

Removing Nitrogen

If we remove some reactant, say $N_2(g)$, then the reverse reaction will be favored—the reaction "shifts to the left"—to reach equilibrium again. Again, this follows from comparing the reaction quotient of the disturbed system to the equilibrium constant. If we remove nitrogen from the reaction mixture, then $[N_2]$ decreases, and the reaction quotient, Q, becomes larger than K_{eq}. As a result, the reaction will proceed in the reverse direction in order to decrease Q to K_{eq}.

Changing the Volume of the Reaction Container

The Haber process is a gaseous reaction, so a change in volume will cause the partial pressures of the gases to change. Specifically, a decrease in volume of the reaction container will cause the partial pressures of the gases to increase; an increase in volume reduces the partial pressures of the gases in the mixture. If the number of moles of gas on the left side of the reaction does not equal the number of moles of gas on the right, then a change in pressure will disrupt the equilibrium ratio, and the system will react to reestablish equilibrium.

How does the system react? Let's first assume the volume is reduced so that the pressure increases. Look back at the equation for the Haber process: There are 4 moles of gas on the reactant side (3 of H_2 plus 1 of N_2) for every 2 moles of NH_3 gas formed. If the reaction shifts to the right, four moles of gas can be condensed into 2 moles, reducing the pressure to reestablish equilibrium. On the other hand, if the volume is increased so that the pressure decreases, the reaction will shift to the left, increasing the pressure to reestablish equilibrium.

To summarize: Consider a gaseous reaction (at equilibrium) with unequal numbers of moles of gas of reactants and products. If the volume is reduced, increasing the pressure, a net reaction occurs favoring the side with the smaller total number of moles of gas. If the volume is expanded, decreasing the pressure, a net reaction occurs favoring the side with the greater total number of moles of gas. (This is only true for reactions involving gases.)

Changing the Temperature of the Reaction Mixture

Heat can be treated as a reactant or a product just like all the chemical reactants and products. Adding or removing heat (by increasing or decreasing the temperature) is like adding or removing any other reagent. Exothermic reactions release heat (which we note on the right side of the equation like a product), and the ΔH will be negative. Endothermic reactions consume heat (which we note on the left side of the equation like a reactant), and the ΔH will be positive.

The Haber process is an exothermic reaction. So, if you increase the temperature at which the reaction takes place once it's reached equilibrium, the reaction will shift to the left to consume the extra heat, thereby producing more reactants. If you decrease the temperature at which the reaction takes place once it's reached equilibrium, the reaction will shift to the right to produce extra heat, thereby producing more product.

Since the reverse of an exothermic reaction is an endothermic one (and vice versa), every equilibrium reaction involves an exothermic reaction and an endothermic reaction. We can then say this: *Lowering* the temperature favors the *exothermic* reaction, while *raising* the temperature favors the *endothermic* one. Keep in mind that, unlike changes in concentration or pressure, changes in temperature *will* affect the reaction's K_{eq} value, depending on the direction the reaction shifts to reestablish equilibrium.

Note that the above changes are specific to the system *once it is at equilibrium*. The kinetics of the reaction are a different matter. Remember, all reactions proceed faster when the temperature is increased, and this is true for the Haber process. Indeed, in industry this reaction is typically run at around 500°C, despite the fact that the reaction is exothermic. The reason is that a fast reaction with a 10 percent yield of ammonia may end up being better overall than a painfully slow reaction with a 90 percent yield of ammonia. Heating a reaction gets it to equilibrium faster. Once it's there, adding or taking away heat will affect the equilibrium as predicted by Le Châtelier's principle.

Adding a Catalyst

Adding a catalyst to a reaction that's already at equilibrium has no effect. Because it increases the rate of both the forward and reverse reactions equally, the equilibrium amounts of the species are unchanged. So, the introduction of a catalyst would cause no disturbance. Remember that a catalyst increases the reaction rate but does *not* affect the equilibrium.

Example 19-4: Nitrogen dioxide gas can be formed by the endothermic reaction shown below. Which of the following changes to the equilibrium would *not* increase the formation of NO_2?

$$N_2O_4(g) \rightleftharpoons 2NO_2(g) \qquad \Delta H = +58 \text{ kJ}$$

A. An increase in the temperature
B. A decrease in the volume of the container
C. Adding additional N_2O_4
D. Removing NO_2 as it is formed
E. All of the above would increase the formation of NO_2.

Solution: Since ΔH is positive, this reaction is endothermic, and we can think of heat as a reactant. So if we increase the temperature (thereby "adding a reactant," namely heat), the equilibrium would shift to the right, thus increasing the formation of NO_2. This eliminates A. Adding reactant (C) or removing product (D) would also shift the equilibrium to the right. The answer must be B. A decrease in the volume of the container would increase the pressure of the gases, causing the equilibrium to shift in favor of the side with the fewer number of moles of gases; in this case, that would be to the left.

19.4 SOLUBILITY PRODUCT CONSTANT

All salts have characteristic solubilities in water. Some, like NaCl, are very soluble, while others, like AgCl, barely dissolve at all. The extent to which a salt will dissolve in water can be determined from its **solubility product constant**, K_{sp}. The solubility product is simply another equilibrium constant, one in which the reactants and products are just the undissolved and dissolved salts.

For example, let's look at the dissolution of magnesium hydroxide in water:

$$Mg(OH)_2(s) \rightleftharpoons Mg^{2+}(aq) + 2\ OH^-(aq)$$

At equilibrium, the solution is *saturated*; the rate at which ions go into solution is equal to the rate at which they precipitate out. The equilibrium expression is

$$K_{sp} = [Mg^{2+}][OH^-]^2$$

Notice that we leave the $Mg(OH)_2$ out of the equilibrium expression because it's a pure solid. (The "concentration of a solid" is meaningless when discussing the equilibrium between a solid and its ions in a saturated aqueous solution.)

Solubility Computations

Let's say you know the K_{sp} for a solid, and you're asked to find out just how much of it can dissolve into water; that is, you're asked to determine the salt's **molar solubility**, the number of moles of that salt that will saturate a liter of water.

To find the solubility of $Mg(OH)_2$, we begin by figuring out how much of each type of ion we'll have once we have x moles of the salt. Since each molecule dissociates into 1 magnesium ion and 2 hydroxide ions, if x moles of this salt have dissolved, the solution contains x moles of Mg^{2+} ions and $2x$ moles of OH^- ions:

$$Mg(OH)_2(s) \rightleftharpoons Mg^{2+}(aq) + 2OH^-(aq)$$

$$x \rightleftharpoons x + 2x$$

So, if x stands for the number of moles of $Mg(OH)_2$ that have dissolved per liter of saturated solution (which is what we're trying to find), then $[Mg^{2+}] = x$ and $[OH^-] = 2x$. Substituting these into the solubility product expression gives us

$$K_{sp} = [Mg^{2+}][OH^-]^2$$

$$= x\,(2x)^2 = x\,(4x^2) = 4x^3$$

It is known that K_{sp} for $Mg(OH)_2$ at 25°C is about 1.6×10^{-11}. So, if we set this equal to $4x^3$, we can solve for x. We get $x \approx 1.6 \times 10^{-4}$. This means that a solution of $Mg(OH)_2$ at 25°C will be saturated at a $Mg(OH)_2$ concentration of $1.6 \times 10^{-4}\,M$.

Example 19-5: The solubility product for lithium phosphate, Li_3PO_4, is $K_{sp} = 2.7 \times 10^{-9}$. How many moles of this salt would be required to form a saturated, 1 L aqueous solution?

Solution: The equilibrium is $Li_3PO_4(s) \rightleftharpoons 3Li^+(aq) + PO_4^{3-}(aq)$. If we let x denote $[PO_4^{3-}]$, then we have $[Li^+] = 3x$. Therefore, $K_{sp} = (3x)^3 \times x = 27x^4$; setting this equal to $2.7 \times 10^{-9} = 27 \times 10^{-10}$ we find that

$$27x^4 = 27 \times 10^{-10} \quad \rightarrow \quad x = (10^{-10})^{1/4} = 10^{-2.5} = 10^{0.5} \times 10^{-3} \approx 3.2 \times 10^{-3}$$

Therefore, 3.2×10^{-3} mol will be required.

19.5   ION PRODUCT

The **ion product** is the reaction quotient for a solubility reaction. That is, while K_{sp} is equal to the product of the concentrations of the ions in a solution when the solution is saturated (that is, *at equilibrium*), the ion product—which we'll denote by Q_{sp}—has exactly the same form as the K_{sp} expression, but the concentrations don't have to be those at equilibrium. The reaction quotient allows us to make predictions about what the reaction will do:

$Q_{sp} < K_{sp} \rightarrow$ more salt can be dissolved
$Q_{sp} = K_{sp} \rightarrow$ solution is saturated
$Q_{sp} > K_{sp} \rightarrow$ excess salt will precipitate

For example, let's say we had a liter of solution containing 10^{-4} mol of barium chloride and 10^{-3} mol of sodium sulfate, both of which are soluble salts:

$$BaCl_2(s) \rightarrow Ba^{2+}(aq) + 2Cl^-(aq)$$

$$Na_2SO_4(s) \rightarrow 2Na^+(aq) + SO_4^{2-}(aq)$$

When you mix two salts in a solution, ions can recombine to form new salts, and you have to consider the new salt's K_{sp}. Barium sulfate, $BaSO_4$, is a slightly soluble salt, and at 25°C, its K_{sp} is 1.1×10^{-10}. Its dissolution equilibrium is

$$BaSO_4(s) \rightleftharpoons Ba^{2+}(aq) + SO_4^{2-}(aq)$$

19.5

Its ion product is $Q_{sp} = [Ba^{2+}][SO_4^{2-}]$, so in this solution, we have $Q_{sp} = (10^{-4})(10^{-3}) = 10^{-7}$, which is much greater than its K_{sp}. Since $Q_{sp} > K_{sp}$, the reverse reaction would be favored, and $BaSO_4$ would precipitate out of solution.

19.6   THE COMMON-ION EFFECT

Let's consider again a saturated solution of magnesium hydroxide:

$$Mg(OH)_2(s) \rightleftharpoons Mg^{2+}(aq) + 2OH^-(aq)$$

What would happen if we now added some sodium hydroxide, NaOH, to this solution? Since NaOH is very soluble in water, it will dissociate completely:

$$NaOH(s) \rightarrow Na^+(aq) + OH^-(aq)$$

The addition of NaOH has caused the amount of hydroxide ion—the **common ion**—in the solution to increase. This disturbs the equilibrium of magnesium hydroxide; since the concentration of a product of that equilibrium is increased, Le Châtelier's principle tells us that the system will react by favoring the reverse reaction, producing solid $Mg(OH)_2$, which will precipitate. Therefore, the molar solubility of the slightly soluble salt [in this case, $Mg(OH)_2$] is decreased by the presence of another solute (in this case, NaOH) that supplies a common ion. This is the **common-ion effect**.

Want More Practice?
Scan the QR code below to register your book for online chapter summaries, drills, practice tests, and more!

Chapter 20
Acids and Bases

20.1 DEFINITIONS

There are three different definitions of acids and bases.

Arrhenius Acids and Bases

Arrhenius gave us the most straightforward definitions of acids and bases:

Acids ionize in water to produce hydrogen (H^+) ions.
Bases ionize in water to produce hydroxide (OH^-) ions.

For example, HCl is an acid,

$$HCl \rightarrow H^+ + Cl^-$$

and NaOH is a base:

$$NaOH \rightarrow Na^+ + OH^-$$

It's important to remember that H^+ does not exist by itself. Rather, it will combine with a molecule of water to give H_3O^+. However, for purposes of the DAT, it doesn't matter which of the two you use: H^+ or H_3O^+.

Brønsted-Lowry Acids and Bases

Brønsted and Lowry offered the following definitions:

Acids are proton (H^+) donors.
Bases are proton (H^+) acceptors.

This definition of an acid is essentially the same idea as put forth by Arrhenius. The subtlety is apparent in their definition of a base. A Brønsted-Lowry base is a substance that is capable of accepting a proton. While hydroxide ions qualify as Brønsted-Lowry bases, many other compounds fit this definition as well.

If we consider the reversible reaction below:

$$H_2CO_3 + H_2O \rightleftharpoons H_3O^+ + HCO_3^-$$

then according to the Brønsted-Lowry definition, H_2CO_3 and H_3O^+ are acids; HCO_3^- and H_2O are bases. The Arrhenius and Brønsted-Lowry definitions of acid and bases are the most important ones for DAT General Chemistry.

Lewis Acids and Bases

Lewis's definitions of acids and bases are the broadest of all:

> *Lewis acids are electron-pair acceptors.*
> *Lewis bases are electron-pair donors.*

If we consider the reversible reaction below:

$$AlCl_3 + H_2O \rightleftharpoons (AlCl_3OH)^- + H^+$$

then according to the Lewis definition, $AlCl_3$ and H^+ are acids because they accept electron pairs; H_2O and $(AlCl_3OH)^-$ are bases because they donate electron pairs. Lewis acid/base reactions frequently result in the formation of coordinate covalent bonds, as discussed earlier. For example, in the reaction above, water acts as a Lewis base since it donates both of the electrons involved in the coordinate covalent bond between OH^- and $AlCl_3$. $AlCl_3$ acts as a Lewis acid, since it accepts the electrons involved in this bond.

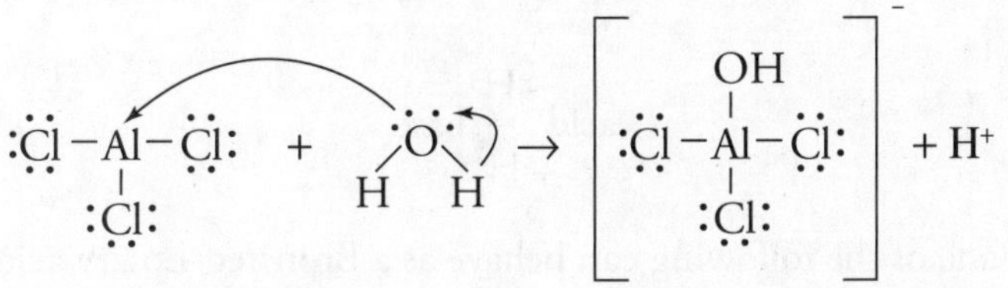

20.2 CONJUGATE ACIDS AND BASES

When a Brønsted-Lowry acid donates an H^+, the remaining structure is called the **conjugate base** of the acid. Likewise, when a Brønsted-Lowry base bonds with an H^+ in solution, this new species is called the **conjugate acid** of the base. To illustrate these definitions, consider this reaction:

acid–base conjugates

$$NH_3 + H_2O \rightleftharpoons NH_4^+ + OH^-$$

acid–base conjugates

Considering only the forward direction, NH_3 is the base and H_2O is the acid. The products are the conjugate acid and base of the reactants: NH_4^+ is the conjugate acid of NH_3, and OH^- is the conjugate base of H_2O:

acid ------------> conjugate base

$$NH_3 + H_2O \rightleftharpoons NH_4^+ + OH^-$$

base ------------> conjugate acid

Now consider the reverse reaction in which NH_4^+ is the acid and OH^- is the base. The conjugates are the same as for the forward reaction: NH_3 is the conjugate base of NH_4^+, and H_2O is the conjugate acid of OH^-:

$$
\begin{array}{c}
\text{conjugate} \\
\text{base} \longleftarrow \text{acid} \\
NH_3 + H_2O \rightleftharpoons NH_4^+ + OH^- \\
\text{conjugate} \\
\text{acid} \longleftarrow \text{base}
\end{array}
$$

The difference between a Brønsted-Lowry acid and its conjugate base is that the base is missing an H^+. The difference between a Brønsted-Lowry base and its conjugate acid is that the acid has an extra H^+.

Forming conjugates:

$$\text{acid} \underset{+ H^+}{\overset{- H^+}{\rightleftharpoons}} \text{base}$$

Example 20-1: Which one of the following can behave as a Brønsted-Lowry acid but not a Lewis acid?

A. CF_4
B. $NaAlCl_4$
C. HF
D. Br_2
E. NaCl

Solution: A Brønsted-Lowry acid donates an H^+, while a Lewis acid accepts a pair of electrons. Since a Brønsted-Lowry acid must have an H in the first place, only C can be the answer.

Example 20-2: What is the conjugate base of HBrO (hypobromous acid)?

Solution: To form the conjugate base of an acid, simply remove an H^+. Therefore, the conjugate base of HBrO is BrO^-.

20.3   THE STRENGTHS OF ACIDS AND BASES

Brønsted-Lowry acids can be placed into two big categories: *strong* and *weak*. Whether an acid is strong or weak depends on how completely it ionizes in water. A **strong** acid is one that dissociates completely (or very nearly so) in water; hydrochloric acid, HCl, is an example:

$$HCl(aq) + H_2O(l) \rightarrow H_3O^+(aq) + Cl^-(aq)$$

This reaction goes essentially to completion.

On the other hand, hydrofluoric acid, HF, is an example of a **weak** acid, since its dissociation in water,

$$HF(aq) + H_2O(l) \rightleftharpoons H_3O^+(aq) + F^-(aq)$$

does not go to completion; most of the HF remains undissociated.

If we use HA to denote a generic acid, its dissociation in water has the form:

$$HA(aq) + H_2O(l) \rightleftharpoons H_3O^+(aq) + A^-(aq)$$

The strength of the acid is directly related to how much the products are favored over the reactants. The equilibrium expression for this reaction is:

$$K_a = \frac{[H_3O^+][A^-]}{[HA]}$$

This is written as K_a, rather than K_{eq}, to emphasize that this is the equilibrium expression for an acid-dissociation reaction. In fact, K_a is known as the **acid-ionization** (or **acid-dissociation**) **constant** of the acid (HA). If $K_a > 1$, then the products are favored, and we say the acid is strong; if $K_a < 1$ then the reactants are favored, and the acid is weak. We can also rank the relative strengths of acids by comparing their K_a values: The larger the K_a value, the stronger the acid; the smaller the K_a value, the weaker the acid.

The acids for which $K_a > 1$—the strong acids—are so few that you should memorize them:

Common Strong Acids	
Hydroiodic acid	HI
Hydrobromic acid	HBr
Hydrochloric acid	HCl
Perchloric acid	$HClO_4$
Sulfuric acid	H_2SO_4
Nitric acid	HNO_3

The values of K_a for these acids are so large that most tables of acid ionization constants don't even list them. On the DAT, you may assume that any acid that's not in this list is a weak acid. (Other acids that fit the definition of *strong* are so uncommon that it's very unlikely they would appear on the test. For example, $HClO_3$ has a pK_a of –1, and could be considered strong, but it is definitely one of the weaker strong acids and is not likely to appear on the DAT.)

Example 20-3: In a 1 M aqueous solution of boric acid (H_3BO_3, $K_a = 5.8 \times 10^{-10}$), which of the following species will be present in solution in the greatest quantity?

    A. H_3BO_3
    B. $H_2BO_3^-$
    C. HBO_3^{2-}
    D. H_3O^+
    E. BO_3^{3-}

Solution: The equilibrium here is $H_3BO_3(aq) + H_2O(l) \rightleftharpoons H_3O^+(aq) + H_2BO_3^-(aq)$. Boric acid is a weak acid (it's not on the list of strong acids), so the equilibrium lies to the left (also, notice how small its K_a value is). So, there'll be very few H_3O^+ or $H_2BO_3^-$ ions in a solution but plenty of undissociated H_3BO_3. The answer is A.

Example 20-4: Why is HF a weak acid, while HCl, HBr, and HI are strong acids?

Solution: F is smaller than Cl, Br, or I. The more stable an acid's conjugate base is, the stronger the acid. Larger anions are better able to spread out their negative charge, making them more stable. HF is the weakest of the H-X acids because it has the least stable conjugate base due to its size.

Example 20-5: Of the following acids, which one would dissociate to the greatest extent (in water)?

    A. HCN (hydrocyanic acid), $K_a = 6.2 \times 10^{-10}$
    B. HNCO (cyanic acid), $K_a = 3.3 \times 10^{-4}$
    C. HClO (hypochlorous acid), $K_a = 2.9 \times 10^{-8}$
    D. HBrO (hypobromous acid), $K_a = 2.2 \times 10^{-9}$
    E. H_2S (hydrosulfuric acid), $K_a = 1.1 \times 10^{-7}$

Solution: The acid that would dissociate to the greatest extent would have the greatest K_a value. Of the choices given, HNCO (B) has the greatest K_a value.

We can apply the same ideas as above to identify strong and weak *bases*. If we use B to denote a generic base, its dissolution in water has the form:

$$B(aq) + H_2O(l) \rightleftharpoons HB^+(aq) + OH^-(aq)$$

The strength of the base is directly related to how much the products are favored over the reactants. If we write the equilibrium constant for this reaction, we get:

$$K_b = \frac{[HB^+][OH^-]}{[B]}$$

This is written as K_b, rather than K_{eq}, to emphasize that this is the equilibrium expression for a base-dissociation reaction. In fact, K_b is known as the **base-ionization** (or **base-dissociation**) **constant**. We can rank the relative strengths of bases by comparing their K_b values: The larger the K_b value, the stronger the base; the smaller the K_b value, the weaker the base.

For the DAT and general chemistry, you should know about the following strong bases that may be used in aqueous solutions:

Common Strong Bases
Group 1 hydroxides (Ex: NaOH)
Group 1 oxides (Ex: Li_2O)
Some group 2 hydroxides ($Ba(OH)_2$, $Sr(OH)_2$, $Ca(OH)_2$)
Metal amides (Ex: $NaNH_2$)

Weak bases include ammonia (NH_3) and amines, as well as the conjugate bases of many weak acids, as we'll discuss in the following.

The Relative Strengths of Conjugate Acid-Base Pairs

Let's once again look at the dissociation of HCl in water:

$$HCl(aq) + H_2O(l) \rightarrow H_3O^+(aq) + Cl^-(aq)$$

no basic properties

The chloride ion (Cl^-) is the conjugate base of HCl. Since this reaction goes to completion, there must be no reverse reaction. Therefore, Cl^- has no tendency to accept a proton and thus does not act as a base. The conjugate base of a strong acid has no basic properties in water.

On the other hand, hydrofluoric acid, HF, is a weak acid since its dissociation is not complete:

$$HF(aq) + H_2O(l) \rightleftharpoons H_3O^+(aq) + F^-(aq)$$

Since the reverse reaction does take place to a significant extent, the conjugate base of HF, the fluoride ion, F^-, *does* have some tendency to accept a proton, and so behaves as a weak base. The conjugate base of a weak acid is a weak base.

In fact, the weaker the acid, the more the reverse reaction is favored, and the stronger its conjugate base. For example, hydrocyanic acid (HCN) has a K_a value of about 5×10^{-10}, which is much smaller than that of hydrofluoric acid ($K_a \approx 7 \times 10^{-4}$). Therefore, the conjugate base of HCN, the cyanide ion, CN^-, is a stronger base than F^-.

The same ideas can be applied to bases:

1. The conjugate acid of a strong base has no acidic properties in water. For example, the conjugate acid of LiOH is Li^+, which does not act as an acid in water.
2. The conjugate acid of a weak base is a weak acid (and the weaker the base, the stronger the conjugate acid). For example, the conjugate acid of NH_3 is NH_4^+, which is a weak acid.

Example 20-6: Of the following anions, which is the strongest base?

A. I⁻
B. CN⁻
C. NO_3^-
D. Br⁻
E. HSO_4^-

Solution: Here's another way to ask the same question: Which of the following anions has the weakest conjugate acid? Since HI, HNO_3, H_2SO_4 and HBr are all strong acids, while HCN is a weak acid, CN⁻ (B) has the weakest conjugate acid, and is thus the strongest base.

Amphoteric Substances

Take a look at the dissociation of carbonic acid (H_2CO_3), a weak acid:

$$H_2CO_3(aq) + H_2O(l) \rightleftharpoons H_3O^+(aq) + HCO_3^-(aq) \quad (K_a = 4.5 \times 10^{-7})$$

The conjugate base of carbonic acid is HCO_3^-, which also has an ionizable proton. Carbonic acid is said to be **polyprotic**, because it has more than one proton to donate.

Let's look at how the conjugate base of carbonic acid dissociates:

$$HCO_3^-(aq) + H_2O(l) \rightleftharpoons H_3O^+(aq) + CO_3^{2-}(aq) \quad (K_a = 4.8 \times 10^{-11})$$

In the first reaction, HCO_3^- acts as a base, but in the second reaction it acts as an acid. Whenever a substance can act as either an acid or a base, we say that it is **amphoteric**. The conjugate base of a weak polyprotic acid is always amphoteric, because it can either donate or accept another proton. Also notice that HCO_3^- is a weaker acid than H_2CO_3; in general, every time a polyprotic acid donates a proton, the resulting species will be a weaker acid than its predecessor.

20.4   THE ION-PRODUCT CONSTANT OF WATER

Water is amphoteric. It reacts with itself in a Brønsted-Lowry acid-base reaction, one molecule acting as the acid, the other as the base:

$$H_2O(l) + H_2O(l) \rightleftharpoons H_3O^+(aq) + OH^-(aq)$$

This is called the autoionization (or self-ionization) of water. The equilibrium expression is:

$$K_w = [H_3O^+][OH^-]$$

This is written as K_w, rather than K_{eq}, to emphasize that this is the equilibrium expression for the autoionization of water; K_w is known as the ion-product constant of water. Only a very small fraction of the water molecules will undergo this reaction, and it's known that at 25°C,

$$K_w = 1.0 \times 10^{-14}$$

(Like all other equilibrium constants, K_w varies with temperature; it increases as the temperature increases. However, because 25°C is so common, this is the value you should memorize.) Since the number of H_3O^+ ions in pure water will be equal to the number of OH^- ions, if we call each of their concentrations x, then $x^2 = K_w$, which gives $x = 1 \times 10^{-7}$. That is, the concentration of both types of ions in pure water is $1 \times 10^{-7}\ M$. (In addition, K_w is constant at a given temperature, regardless of the H_3O^+ concentration.)

If the introduction of an acid increases the concentration of H_3O^+ ions, then the equilibrium is disturbed, and the reverse reaction is favored, decreasing the concentration of OH^- ions. Similarly, if the introduction of a base increases the concentration of OH^- ions, then the equilibrium is again disturbed; the reverse reaction is favored, decreasing the concentration of H_3O^+ ions. However, in either case, the product of $[H_3O^+]$ and $[OH^-]$ will remain equal to K_w.

For example, suppose we add 0.002 moles of HCl to water to create a 1-liter solution. Since the dissociation of HCl goes to completion (it's a strong acid), it will create 0.002 moles of H_3O^+ ions, so $[H_3O^+]$ = 0.002 M. Since H_3O^+ concentration has been increased, we expect the OH^- concentration to decrease, which it does:

$$[OH^-] = \frac{K_w}{[H_3O^+]} = \frac{1 \times 10^{-14}}{2 \times 10^{-3}} = 5 \times 10^{-12}\ M$$

20.5 pH

The pH scale measures the concentration of H^+ (or H_3O^+) ions in a solution. Because the molarity of H^+ tends to be quite small and can vary over many orders of magnitude, the pH scale is logarithmic:

$$pH = -\log[H^+]$$

This formula implies that $[H^+] = 10^{-pH}$. Since $[H^+] = 10^{-7}\ M$ in pure water, the pH of water is 7. At 25°C, this defines a pH neutral solution. If $[H^+]$ is greater than $10^{-7}\ M$, then the pH will be less than 7, and the solution is said to be acidic. If $[H^+]$ is less than $10^{-7}\ M$, the pH will be greater than 7, and the solution is basic (or alkaline). Notice that a *low* pH means a *high* $[H^+]$ and the solution is *acidic*; a *high* pH means a *low* $[H^+]$ and the solution is basic.

pH > 7   basic solution

pH = 7   neutral solution

pH < 7   acidic solution

The range of the pH scale for most solutions falls between 0 and 14, but some strong acids and bases extend the scale past this range. For example, a 10 M solution of HCl will fully dissociate into H^+ and Cl^-. Therefore, the $[H^+] = 10\ M$, and the pH = –1.

20.5

An alternate measurement expresses the acidity or basicity in terms of the hydroxide ion concentration, $[OH^-]$, by using pOH. The same formula applies for hydroxide ions as for hydrogen ions:

$$pOH = -\log[OH^-]$$

This formula implies that $[OH^-] = 10^{-pOH}$.

Acids and bases are inversely related: the greater the concentration of H^+ ions, the lower the concentration of OH^- ions, and vice versa. Since $[H^+][OH^-] = 10^{-14}$ at 25°C, the values of pH and pOH satisfy a special relationship at 25°C:

$$pH + pOH = 14$$

So, if you know the pOH of a solution, you can find the pH, and vice versa. For example, if the pH of a solution is 5, then the pOH must be 9. If the pOH of a solution is 2, then the pH must be 12.

On the DAT, it will be helpful to be able to figure out the pH even in cases where the H^+ concentration isn't exactly equal to the whole-number power of 10. In general, if y is a number between 1 and 10, and you're told that $[H^+] = y \times 10^{-n}$ (where n is a whole number) then the pH will be between $(n-1)$ and n. For example, if $[H^+] = 6.2 \times 10^{-5}$, then the pH is between 4 and 5.

Relationships Between Conjugates

pK_a and pK_b

The definitions of pH and pOH both involve the opposite of a logarithm. In general, "p" of something is equal to the $-\log$ of that something. Therefore, the following definitions won't be surprising:

$$pK_a = -\log K_a$$

$$pK_b = -\log K_b$$

Because H^+ concentrations are generally very small and can vary over such a wide range, the pH scale gives us more convenient numbers to work with. The same is true for pK_a and pK_b. Remember that the larger the K_a value, the stronger the acid. Since "p" means "take the negative log of...," the *lower* the pK_a value, the stronger the acid. For example, acetic acid (CH_3COOH) has a K_a of 1.75×10^{-5}, and hypochlorous acid (HClO) has a K_a of 2.9×10^{-8}. Since the K_a of acetic acid is larger than that of hypochlorous acid, we know this means that more molecules of acetic acid than hypochlorous acid will dissociate into ions in aqueous solution. In other words, acetic acid is stronger than hypochlorous acid. The pK_a of acetic acid is 4.8, and the pK_a of hypochlorous acid is 7.5. The acid with the lower pK_a value is the stronger acid. The same logic applies to pK_b: the lower the pK_b value, the stronger the base.

K_a and K_b

Let's now look at the relationship between the K_a and the K_b for an acid-base conjugate pair by working through an example question. Let K_a be the acid-dissociation constant for formic acid (HCOOH) and let K_b stand for the base-dissociation constant of its conjugate base (the formate ion, HCOO⁻). If K_a is equal to 5.6×10^{-11}, what is $K_a \times K_b$?

The equilibrium for the dissociation of HCOOH is:

$$HCOOH(aq) + H_2O(l) \rightleftharpoons H_3O^+(aq) + HCOO^-(aq)$$

so:

$$K_a = \frac{[H_3O^+][HCOO^-]}{[HCOOH]}$$

The equilibrium for the dissociation of HCOO⁻ is:

$$HCOO^-(aq) + H_2O(l) \rightleftharpoons HCOOH(aq) + OH^-(aq)$$

so:

$$K_b = \frac{[HCOOH][OH^-]}{[HCOO^-]}$$

Therefore,

$$K_a K_b = \frac{[H_3O^+][HCOO^-]}{[HCOOH]} \times \frac{[HCOOH][OH^-]}{[HCOO^-]} = [H_3O^+][OH^-]$$

We now immediately recognize this product as K_w, the ion-product constant of water, whose value (at 25°C) is 1×10^{-14}.

This calculation wasn't special for HCOOH; we can see that the same thing will happen for any acid and its conjugate base. So, for any acid-base conjugate pair, we'll have:

$$K_a K_b = K_w = 1 \times 10^{-14}$$

This gives us a way to quantitatively relate the strength of an acid and its conjugate base. For example, the value of K_a for HF is about 7×10^{-4}; therefore, the value of K_b for its conjugate base, F⁻, is about 1.4×10^{-11}. For HCN, $K_a \approx 5 \times 10^{-10}$, so K_b for CN⁻ is 2×10^{-5}.

It also follows from our definitions and logarithm algebra that for an acid-base conjugate pair at 25°C, we'll have:

$$pK_a + pK_b = 14$$

Example 20-7: What is the pH of a solution at 25°C whose hydroxide ion concentration is $1 \times 10^{-4}\ M$?

Solution: Since pOH = −log[OH⁻], we know that pOH = 4. Therefore, the pH is 10.

Example 20-8: Orange juice has a pH of 3.5. What is its [H⁺]?

Solution: Because pH = −log[H⁺], we know that $[H^+] = 10^{-pH}$. For orange juice, then, we have $[H^+] = 10^{-3.5} = 10^{0.5-4} = 10^{0.5} \times 10^{-4} = \sqrt{10} \times 10^{-4} \approx 3.2 \times 10^{-4}\ M$.

Example 20-9: If 99% of the H_3O^+ ions are removed from a solution whose pH was originally 3, what will be its new pH?

Solution: If 99% of the H_3O^+ ions are removed, then only 1% remain. This means that the number of H_3O^+ ions is now only 1/100 of the original. If $[H_3O^+]$ is decreased by a factor of 100, then the pH is *increased* by 2—to pH 5 in this case—since log 100 = 2.

pH Calculations

For Strong Acids

Strong acids dissociate completely, so the hydrogen ion concentration will be the same as the concentration of the acid. That means that you can calculate the pH directly from the molarity of the solution. For example, a 0.01 M solution of HCl will have $[H^+] = 0.01\ M$ and pH = 2.

For Weak Acids

Weak acids come to equilibrium with their dissociated ions. In fact, for a weak acid at equilibrium, the concentration of undissociated acid will be much greater than the concentration of hydrogen ion. To get the pH of a weak acid solution, you need to use the equilibrium expression.

Let's say you add 0.2 mol of HCN (hydrocyanic acid, a weak acid) to water to create a 1-liter solution, and you want to find the pH. Initially, [HCN] = 0.2 M, and none of it has dissociated. If x moles of HCN are dissociated at equilibrium, then the equilibrium concentration of HCN is 0.2 − x. Now, since each molecule of HCN dissociates into one H⁺ ion and one CN⁻ ion, if x moles of HCN have dissociated, there'll be x moles of H⁺ and x moles of CN⁻:

	HCN	$\rightleftharpoons$	H⁺	+	CN⁻
initial:	0.2 M		0 M		0 M
at equilibrium:	(0.2 − x) M		x M		x M

(Actually, the initial concentration of H^+ is 10^{-7} M, but it's so small that it can be neglected for this calculation.) Our goal is to find x, because once we know $[H^+]$, we'll know the pH. So, we set up the equilibrium expression:

$$K_a = \frac{[H^+][CN^-]}{[HCN]} = \frac{x^2}{0.2 - x}$$

It's known that the value of K_a for HCN is 4.9×10^{-10}. Because the K_a is so small, not that much of the HCN is going to dissociate. (This assumption, that x added to or subtracted from a number is negligible, is always a good one when $K < 10^{-4}$ [the usual case found on the DAT].) That is, we can assume that x is going to be a very small number, insignificant compared to 0.2; therefore, the value $(0.2 - x)$ is almost exactly the same as 0.2. By substituting 0.2 for $(0.2 - x)$, we can solve the equation above for x:

$$\frac{x^2}{0.2} \approx 4.9 \times 10^{-10}$$
$$x^2 \approx 1 \times 10^{-10}$$
$$\therefore x \approx 1 \times 10^{-5}$$

Since $[H^+]$ is approximately 1×10^{-5} M, the pH is about 5.

We simplified the computation by assuming that the concentration of hydrogen ion $[H^+]$ was insignificant compared to the concentration of undissociated acid $[HCN]$. Since it turned out that $[H^+] \approx 10^{-5}$ M, which is much less than $[HCN] = 0.2$ M, our assumption was valid. On the DAT, you should always simplify the math wherever possible.

Example 20-10: If 0.7 mol of benzoic acid (C_6H_5COOH, $K_a = 6.6 \times 10^{-5}$) is added to water to create a 1-liter solution, what will be the pH?

Solution: Initially $[C_6H_5COOH] = 0.7$ M, and none of it has dissociated. If x moles of C_6H_5COOH are dissociated at equilibrium, then the equilibrium concentration of C_6H_5COOH is $0.7 - x$. Now, since each molecule of C_6H_5COOH dissociates into one H^+ ion and one $C_6H_5COO^-$ ion, if x moles of C_6H_5COOH have dissociated, there'll be x moles of H^+ and x moles of $C_6H_5COO^-$:

	C_6H_5COOH	$\rightleftharpoons$	H^+	$+$	$C_6H_5COO^-$
initial:	0.7 M		0 M		0 M
at equilibrium:	$(0.7 - x)$ M		x M		x M

(Again, the initial concentration of H^+ is 10^{-7} M, but it's so small that it can be neglected.) Our goal is to find x, because once we know $[H^+]$, we'll know the pH. So, we set up the equilibrium expression:

$$K_a = \frac{[H^+][C_6H_5COO^-]}{[C_6H_5COOH]} = \frac{x^2}{0.7 - x} \approx \frac{x^2}{0.7}$$

20.5

and then solve the equation for x:

$$\frac{x^2}{0.7} \approx 6.6 \times 10^{-5}$$

$$x^2 \approx 4.6 \times 10^{-5} = 46 \times 10^{-6}$$

$$\therefore x \approx 7 \times 10^{-3}$$

Since $[H^+]$ is approximately $7 \times 10^{-3}\ M \approx 10^{-2}\ M$, the pH is a little more than 2, say 2.2.

20.6 NEUTRALIZATION REACTIONS

When an acid and a base are combined, they will react in what is called a **neutralization reaction**. Oftentimes this reaction will produce a salt and water. Here's an example:

$$HCl\ +\ NaOH\ \rightarrow\ NaCl\ +\ H_2O$$

| acid | base | salt | water |

This type of reaction takes place when, for example, you take an antacid to relieve excess stomach acid. The antacid is a weak base, usually carbonate, that reacts in the stomach to neutralize acid.

If a strong acid and strong base react (as in the example above), the resulting solution will be pH neutral (which is why we call it a neutralization reaction). However, if the reaction involves a weak acid or weak base, the resulting solution will generally not be pH neutral.

No matter how weak an acid or base is, when mixed with an equimolar amount of a strong base or acid, we can expect complete neutralization. It has been found experimentally that all neutralizations have the same exothermic "heat of neutralization," the energy released from the reaction that is the same for all neutralizations: $H^+ + OH^- \rightarrow H_2O$.

As you can see from the reaction above, equal molar amounts of HCl and NaOH are needed to complete the neutralization. To determine just how much base (B) to add to an acidic solution (or how much acid (A) to add to a basic solution) in order to cause complete neutralization, we just use the following formula:

$$a \times [A] \times V_A = b \times [B] \times V_B$$

where a is the number of acidic hydrogens per formula unit and b is a constant that tells us how many H_3O^+ ions the base can accept.

For example, let's calculate how much $0.1\ M$ NaOH solution is needed to neutralize 40 mL of a $0.3\ M$ HCl solution:

$$V_B = \frac{a \times [A] \times V_A}{b \times [B]} = \frac{1 \times (0.3\ M) \times (40\ mL)}{1 \times (0.1\ M)} = 120\ mL$$

Example 20-11: Binary mixtures of equal moles of which of the following acid-base combinations will lead to a complete (99⁺%) neutralization reaction?

  I.   HCl and NaOH
 II.   HF and NH$_3$
III.   HNO$_3$ and NaHCO$_3$

Solution: Remember, regardless of the strengths of the acids and bases, all neutralization reactions (including these three) go to completion.

20.7   HYDROLYSIS OF SALTS

A **salt** is an ionic compound, consisting of a cation and an anion. In water, the salt dissociates into ions, and depending on how these ions react with water, the resulting solution will be either acidic, basic, or pH neutral. To make the prediction, we notice that there are essentially two possibilities for both the cation and the anion in a salt:

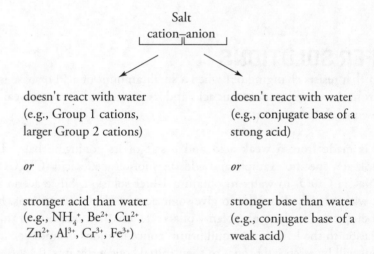

Salt
cation–anion

doesn't react with water
(e.g., Group 1 cations,
larger Group 2 cations)

or

stronger acid than water
(e.g., NH$_4^+$, Be^{2+}, Cu^{2+},
Zn^{2+}, Al^{3+}, Cr^{3+}, Fe^{3+})

doesn't react with water
(e.g., conjugate base of a
strong acid)

or

stronger base than water
(e.g., conjugate base of a
weak acid)

Whether the salt solution will be acidic, basic, or pH neutral depends on which combination of possibilities (four total) from the diagram above applies. The reaction of a substance—such as a salt or an ion—with water is called a hydrolysis reaction, a more general use of the term since the water molecule may not be split. Let's look at some examples.

If we dissolve NaCl in water, Na$^+$ and Cl$^-$ ions go into solution. Na$^+$ ions are Group 1 ions and do not react with water. Since Cl$^-$ is the conjugate base of a strong acid (HCl), it also doesn't react with water. These ions just become hydrated (surrounded by water molecules). Therefore, the solution will be pH neutral.

How about NH$_4$Cl? In a solution it will break into NH$_4^+$ and Cl$^-$. The ammonium ion is a stronger acid than water (it's the conjugate acid of NH$_3$, a weak base), and Cl$^-$ will not react with water. As a result, a solution of this salt will be acidic and have a pH less than 7, and NH$_4$Cl is called an acidic salt.

20.7

Now let's consider sodium acetate, $Na(CH_3COO)$. In a solution it will break into Na^+ and CH_3COO^-. Na^+ is a Group 1 cation and does not react with water. However, CH_3COO^- is a stronger base than water since it's the conjugate base of acetic acid (CH_3COOH), a weak acid. Therefore, a solution of the salt will be basic and have a pH greater than 7, and $NaCH_3COO$ is a basic salt.

Finally, let's consider NH_4CN. In a solution it will break into NH_4^+ and CN^-. NH_4^+ is a stronger acid than water, and CN^- is a stronger base than water (it's the conjugate base of HCN, a weak acid). So, which one wins? In a case like this, we need to know the K_a value for the reaction of the cation with water with the K_b value for the reaction of the anion with water and compare these values. Since:

$$NH_4^+(aq) \ + \ H_2O(l) \rightleftharpoons NH_3(aq) \ + \ H_3O^+(aq) \quad (K_a = 6.3 \times 10^{-10})$$

$$CN^-(aq) \ + \ H_2O(l) \rightleftharpoons HCN(aq) \ + \ OH^-(aq) \quad (K_b = 1.6 \times 10^{-5})$$

we see that in this case K_b of $CN^- > K_a$ of NH_4^+, so the forward reaction of the second reaction will dominate the forward reaction of the first reaction, and the solution will be basic.

20.8 BUFFER SOLUTIONS

A **buffer** is a solution that resists changing pH when a small amount of acid or base is added. The buffering capacity comes from the presence of a weak acid and its conjugate base (or a weak base and its conjugate acid) in roughly equal concentrations.

One type of buffer is made from a weak acid and a salt of its conjugate base. To illustrate how a buffer works, let's look at a specific example and add 0.1 mol of acetic acid (CH_3COOH) and 0.1 mol of sodium acetate ($NaCH_3COO$) to water to obtain a 1-liter solution. Since acetic acid is a weak acid ($K_a = 1.75 \times 10^{-5}$), it will partially dissociate to give some acetate (CH_3COO^-) ions. However, the salt is soluble and will dissociate completely to give plenty of acetate ions. The addition of this common ion will shift the acid dissociation to the left, so the equilibrium concentrations of undissociated acetic acid molecules and acetate ions will be essentially equal to their initial concentrations, 0.1 M.

$$CH_3COOH \ + \ H_2O \rightleftharpoons H_3O^+ \ + \ CH_3COO^-$$

Since buffer solutions are designed to resist changes in pH, let's first figure out the pH of this solution. Writing the expression for the equilibrium constant gives:

$$K_a = \frac{[H_3O^+][CH_3COO^-]}{[CH_3COOH]}$$

which we can solve for $[H_3O^+]$:

$$[H_3O^+] = \frac{K_a[CH_3COOH]}{[CH_3COO^-]} \qquad \text{(Equation 1)}$$

Since the equilibrium concentrations of both CH_3COOH and CH_3COO^- are 0.1 M, this equation tells us that:

$$[H_3O^+] = \frac{K_a[CH_3COOH]}{[CH_3COO^-]} = \frac{K_a(0.1\ M)}{0.1\ M} = 1.75 \times 10^{-5}$$

and pH $= -\log[H_3O^+]$, so:

$$pH = -\log(1.75 \times 10^{-5})$$
$$pH = 4.76$$

Okay, now let's see what happens if we add a little bit of strong acid, 0.005 mol HCl, for example. HCl will dissociate completely in a solution into 0.005 mol of H^+ ions and 0.005 mol of Cl^- ions. The chloride ions will have no effect on the equilibrium or the pH. The additional protons will shift the buffer equilibrium to the left, and the acetate ions react with additional H_3O^+ ions to produce additional acetic acid molecules. As a result, the concentration of acetate ions will drop by 0.005, from 0.1 M to 0.095 M; the concentration of acetic acid will increase by 0.005, from 0.1 M to 0.105 M. This will cause the pH to drop from 4.76 to 4.71, a decrease of just 0.05. If we had added this HCl to a liter of pure water, the pH would have dropped from 7 to 2.3! The buffer solution we created was effective at resisting a large drop in pH because it had enough base (acetate ions) to neutralize the additional acid.

Now let's see what happens if we add a little bit of strong base, 0.005 mol KOH, for example. KOH will dissociate completely in a solution into 0.005 mol of K^+ ions and 0.005 mol of OH^- ions. The potassium ions will have no effect, but the OH^- ions will shift the buffer equilibrium to the right; they'll react with acetic acid molecules to produce more acetate ions ($CH_3COOH + OH^- \rightarrow CH_3COO^- + H_2O$). As a result, the concentration of acetic acid will drop by 0.005, from 0.1 M to 0.095 M; the concentration of acetate ions will increase by 0.005, from 0.1 M to 0.105 M. The pH will thus increase from 4.76 to 4.80, an increase of just 0.04. If we had added this KOH to a liter of pure water, the pH would have increased from 7 to 11.7! Again the buffer solution we created was effective at resisting a large rise in pH because it had enough acid to neutralize the additional base.

The Henderson–Hasselbalch equation describes the derivation of pH as a measure of acidity and is useful for estimating the pH of a buffer solution and finding the equilibrium pH in acid-base reactions.

$$pH = pK_a + \log\left(\frac{[\text{conjugate base}]}{[\text{weak acid}]}\right)$$

You should understand what this equation is used for and what it means, but you will not have to use it for advanced calculations on test day. For example, if you are exactly half way through a deprotonation reaction, the concentration of the weak acid you started with will be equal to the concentration of the conjugate base (or [acid] = [conjugate base]). This means the Henderson–Hasselbalch equation reduces down to pH $= pK_a + \log(1)$ and since $\log(1) = 0$, pH $= pK_a$. In fact, this equation is used to give a good definition of pK_a: the pH where you are exactly halfway through deprotonating an acid.

20.8

Example 20-12: What could be added to a solution of HCN to create a buffer?

Solution: HCN is a weak acid, so we would look for a salt of its conjugate base, CN⁻. NaCN is such a salt.

Example 20-13: As hydrogen ions are added to an acidic buffer solution, what happens to the concentrations of undissociated acid and conjugate base?

Solution: The conjugate base, A⁻, reacts with the added H⁺ to form HA, so the conjugate base decreases and the undissociated acid increases.

Example 20-14: As hydrogen ions are added to an alkaline buffer solution, what happens to the concentrations of base and conjugate acid?

Solution: The base, B, reacts with the added H⁺ to form HB⁺, so the base decreases and the conjugate acid increases.

20.9 ACID-BASE TITRATIONS

An **acid-base titration** is an experimental technique used to determine the identity of an unknown weak acid (or weak base) by determining its pK_a (or pK_b). Titrations can also be used to determine the concentration of *any* acid or base solution (whether it be known or unknown). The procedure consists of adding a strong acid (or a strong base) of *known* identity and concentration—the **titrant**—to a solution containing the unknown base (or acid). (One never titrates an acid with an acid or a base with a base.) While the titrant is added in small, discrete amounts, the pH of the solution is recorded (with a pH meter).

If we plot the data points (the pH value vs. the volume of titrant added), we obtain a graph called a titration curve. Let's consider a specific example: the titration of HF (a weak acid) with NaOH (a strong base).

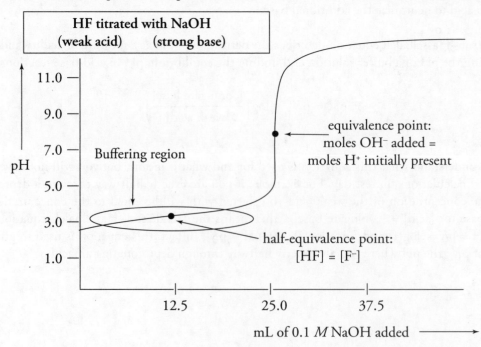

When the amount of titrant added is 0, the pH is of course just the pH of the original, pure solution of HF. Then, as NaOH is added, an equivalent amount of HF will be neutralized according to the reaction:

$$NaOH + HF \rightarrow Na^+ + F^- + H_2O$$

As HF is neutralized, the pH will increase. But from the titration curve, we can see that the pH is certainly not increasing very rapidly as we add the first 20 or so mL of NaOH. This should tell you that at the beginning of this titration the solution is behaving as a buffer. As HF is being converted into F^-, we are forming a solution that contains a weak acid and its conjugate base. This section of the titration curve, where the pH changes very gradually, is called the **buffering domain** (or **buffering region**).

Now, as the experiment continues, the solution suddenly loses its buffering capability, and the pH increases dramatically. At some point during this drastic increase, all HF is neutralized, and no acid remains in the solution. Every new molecule of OH^- that is added remains in solution. Therefore, the pH continues to increase rapidly until the OH^- concentration in the solution is not that much different from the NaOH concentration in the titrant. From here on, the pH doesn't change very much and the curve levels off.

There is a point during the drastic pH increase at which just enough NaOH has been added to completely neutralize all the HF. This is called the **acid-base equivalence point**. At this point, we simply have Na^+ ions and F^- ions in the solution. Note that the solution should be *basic* here. In fact, from what we know about the behavior of conjugates, we can state the following facts about the equivalence point of different titrations:

- For a weak acid (titrated with a strong base), the equivalence point will occur at a pH > 7.
- For a weak base (titrated with a strong acid), the equivalence point will occur at a pH < 7.
- For a strong acid (titrated with a strong base) or for a strong base (titrated with a strong acid), the equivalence point will occur at pH = 7.

Therefore, by just looking at the pH at the equivalence point of our titration, we can tell whether the acid (or base) we were titrating was weak or strong.

Recall the purpose of this titration experiment: to determine the pK_a (or pK_b) of the unknown weak acid (or weak base). From the titration curve, determine the volume of titrant added at the equivalence point; call it $V_{at\ equiv}$. A key question is this: What's in a solution when the volume of added titrant is $1/2\ V_{at\ equiv}$? Let's return to our titration of HF by NaOH. We can read from its titration curve that $V_{at\ equiv} = 25$ mL. When the amount of NaOH added was $1/2\ V_{at\ equiv} = 12.5$ mL, the solution consisted of equal concentrations of HF and F^-, i.e., enough NaOH was added to convert 1/2 of the HF to F^-. (After all, when the amount of titrant added was twice as much, $V_{at\ equiv} = 25$ mL, *all* of the HF had been converted to F^-. So naturally, when 1/2 as much was added, only 1/2 was converted.) Therefore, at this point—called the **half-equivalence point**—we have:

$$[HF]_{at\ half-equiv} = [F^-]_{at\ half-equiv} = 1/2\ [HF]_{original}$$

The Henderson–Hasselbalch equation then tells us that:

$$pH_{at\ half-equiv} = pK_a + \log\left(\frac{[F^-]_{at\ half-equiv}}{[HF]_{at\ half-equiv}}\right) = pK_a + \log 1 = pK_a$$

The pK_a of HF equals the pH at the half-equivalence point. For our curve, we see that this occurs around pH 3.2, so we conclude that the pK_a of HF is about 3.2.

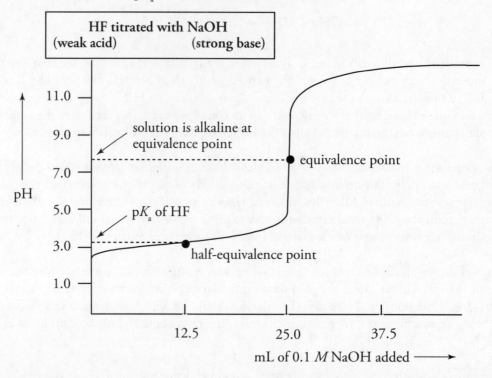

Compare the sample titration curves for a weak base titrated with a strong acid to the one for a weak acid titrated with a strong base (like the one we just looked at). Note the pH at the equivalence point (relative to pH 7) for each curve.

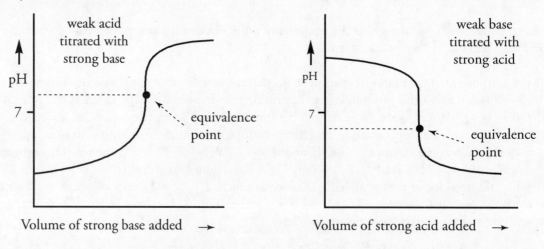

As mentioned, the titration curve for a strong acid-strong base titration would have the equivalence point at a neutral pH of 7, as shown on the next page.

20.9

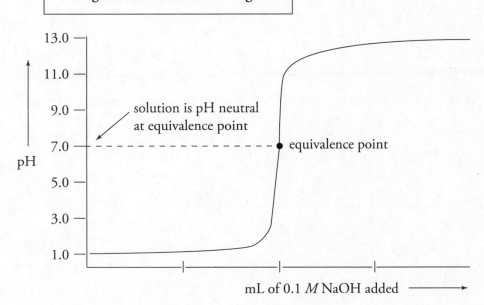

strong acid titrated with a strong base

solution is pH neutral
at equivalence point

equivalence point

pH

mL of 0.1 M NaOH added ⟶

20.9

The titration curve for the titration of a polyprotic acid (like H_2SO_4 or H_3PO_4) will have more than one equivalence point. The number of equivalence points is equal to the number of ionizable hydrogens the acid can donate.

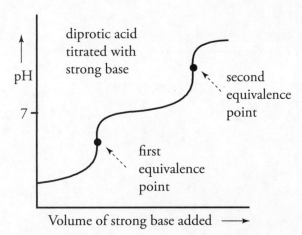

diprotic acid
titrated with
strong base

pH

7

second
equivalence
point

first
equivalence
point

Volume of strong base added ⟶

Example 20-15: A 50 mL solution of HCOOH (formic acid) is titrated with 0.2 M NaOH. The equivalence point is reached when 40 mL of the NaOH solution has been added. What was the original concentration of the formic acid solution?

Solution: Using our formula $a \times [A] \times V_A = b \times [B] \times V_B$, we find that

$$[A] = \frac{b \times [B] \times V_B}{a \times V_A} = \frac{1 \times (0.2\ M) \times (40\ \text{mL})}{1 \times (50\ \text{mL})} = 0.16\ M$$

Want More Practice?
Scan the QR code below to register your book for online chapter summaries, drills, practice tests, and more!

Chapter 21
Thermodynamics

21.1 SYSTEM AND SURROUNDINGS

Why does anything happen? Why does a creek flow downhill, a volcano erupt, a chemical reaction proceed? It's all **thermodynamics**: the transformation of energy from one form to another. The laws of thermodynamics underlie any event in which energy is transformed.

In thermodynamics we have to designate a "starting line" and a "finish line" to be able to describe how energy flows in chemical reactions and physical changes. To do this we use three distinct designations to describe energy flow: the system, the surroundings, and the thermodynamic universe (or just universe).

The system is the thing we're looking at: a melting ice cube, a solid dissolving into water, a beating heart, anything we want to study. Everything else: the table the ice cube sits on and the surrounding air, the beaker that holds the solid and the water, the chest cavity holding the heart, is known collectively as the surroundings. The system and the surroundings taken together form the thermodynamic universe.

We need to define these terms so that we can assign a direction—and therefore a sign, either (+) or (–)—to energy flow. For chemistry (and for physics), we define everything in terms of what's happening to the *system*.

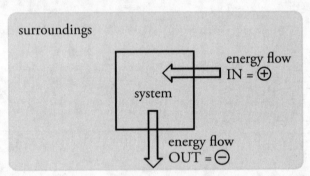

Consider energy flowing from the surroundings into the system, like the heat flowing from the table to the ice cube that's sitting on it. What is happening in the system? As energy flows in (here it's heat), the molecules in the system absorb it and start to jiggle faster. Eventually enough energy is absorbed to cause the ice to melt. Overall, the energy of the system *increased*, and we therefore give it a (+) sign. What about water when it freezes? Here, energy (once again, heat) leaves the water (our system), and the water molecules' jiggling slows down. The energy of the system has *decreased*, and we therefore assign a (–) sign to energy flow. Finally, energy that flows into the system flows out of the surroundings, and energy that flows out of the system flows into the surroundings. Therefore, we can make these statements:

1. When energy flows into a system from the surroundings, the energy of the system increases and the energy of the surroundings decreases.
2. When energy flows out of a system into the surroundings, the energy of the system decreases and the energy of the surroundings increases.

Keep this duality in mind when dealing with energy.

21.2 THE FIRST LAW OF THERMODYNAMICS

The **First Law of Thermodynamics** says that the total energy of the universe is constant. Energy may be transformed from one form to another, but it cannot be created or destroyed. Because of this, it must be transferred into some other form such as heat (q) or work (w). Thus, we have the following mathematical statement of the first law:

$$\Delta E = q + w$$

This law is usually analyzed using gases in metal containers, holding some parameters constant and changing others. For example:

- **Isobaric** process: pressure of the system stays constant; volume and temperature change relative to each other.
- **Isochoric** process: volume of the system stays constant; temperature and pressure change relative to each other.
- **Isothermal**: temperature of the system stays constant; pressure and volume change relative to each other.
- **Adiabatic** process: no heat flows in or out of the system (so $q = 0$); pressure, volume and temperature all change relative to each other.

You should be familiar with definitions for these four terms, as they describe the four types of thermodynamic processes.

21.3 THE SECOND LAW OF THERMODYNAMICS

Entropy

There are several different ways to state the **Second Law of Thermodynamics**, each appropriate to the particular system under study, but they're all equivalent. One way to state this law is that the disorder of the universe increases in a spontaneous process. For this to make sense, let's examine what we mean by the term *spontaneous*. For example, water will spontaneously splash and flow down a waterfall, but it will not spontaneously collect itself at the bottom and flow up the cliff. A bouncing ball will come to rest, but a ball at rest will not suddenly start bouncing. If the ball is warm enough, it's got the energy to start moving, but heat—the disorganized, random kinetic energy of the constituent atoms—will not spontaneously organize itself and give the ball an overall kinetic energy to start it moving. From another perspective, heat will spontaneously flow from a plate of hot food to its cooler surroundings, but thermal energy in the cool surroundings will not spontaneously concentrate itself and flow into the food. None of these processes would violate the first law, but they do violate the second law.

Nature has a tendency to become increasingly disorganized, and another way to state the second law is that *all processes tend to run in a direction that leads to maximum disorder.* Think about spilling milk from a glass. Does the milk ever collect itself together and refill the glass? No, it spreads out randomly over the table and floor. In fact, it needed the glass in the first place just to have any shape at all. Likewise, think about the helium in a balloon: It expands to fill its container, and if we empty the balloon, the helium diffuses randomly throughout the room. The reverse doesn't happen. Helium atoms don't collect themselves from the atmosphere and move into a closed container. The natural tendency of *all* things is to increase their disorder.

We measure disorder or randomness as **entropy**. The greater the disorder of a system, the greater is its entropy. Entropy is represented by the symbol S, and the change in entropy during a reaction is represented by the symbol ΔS. The change in entropy is determined by the equation:

$$\Delta S = S_{products} - S_{reactants}$$

If randomness increases—or order decreases—during the reaction, then ΔS is positive for the reaction. If randomness decreases—or order increases—then ΔS is negative. For example, let's look at the decomposition reaction for carbonic acid:

$$H_2CO_3 \rightleftharpoons H_2O + CO_2$$

In this case, one molecule breaks into two molecules, and disorder is increased. That is, the atoms are less organized in the water and in carbon dioxide molecules than they are in the carbonic acid molecule. The entropy is increasing for the forward reaction. Let's look at the reverse process: If CO_2 and H_2O come together to form H_2CO_3, we've decreased entropy because the atoms in two molecules have become more organized by forming one molecule.

In general, entropy is predictable in many cases:

- Liquids have more entropy than solids.
- Gases have more entropy than solids or liquids.
- Particles in a solution have more entropy than undissolved solids.
- Two moles of a substance have more entropy than one mole.
- The value of ΔS for a reverse reaction has the same magnitude as that of the forward reaction, but with opposite sign: $\Delta S_{reverse} = -\Delta S_{forward}$.

While the overall drive of nature is to increase entropy, reactions can occur in which entropy decreases, but we must either put in energy or gain energy from making more stable bonds. (We'll explore this further when we discuss Gibbs free energy.)

Example 21-1: Of the following reactions, which would have the greatest positive entropy change?

A. $2\ NO(g) + O_2(g) \rightarrow 2\ NO_2(g)$
B. $2\ HCl(aq) + Mg(s) \rightarrow MgCl_2(aq) + H_2(g)$
C. $2\ H_2O(g) + Br_2(g) + SO_2(g) \rightarrow 2\ HBr(g) + H_2SO_4(aq)$
D. $2\ I^-(aq) + Cl_2(g) \rightarrow I_2(s) + 2\ Cl^-(aq)$
E. $N_2(g) + 3H_2(g) \rightarrow 2NH_3(g)$

Solution: The reactions in A, C, and D all describe processes involving a decrease in randomness, that is, an increase in order. However, the process in B has a highly ordered solid on the left, but a highly disordered gas on the right, so we'd expect this reaction to have a positive entropy change.

21.4 ENTHALPY

Enthalpy is a measure of the heat energy that is released or absorbed when bonds are broken and formed during a reaction that's run at constant pressure. The symbol for enthalpy is H. Some general principles about enthalpy prevail over all reactions:

- When a bond is formed, energy is released: $\Delta H < 0$.
- Energy must be put into a bond in order to break it: $\Delta H > 0$.

In a chemical reaction, energy must be put into the reactants to break their bonds. Once the reactant bonds are broken, the atoms rearrange to form products. As the product bonds form, energy is released. The enthalpy of a reaction is given by the difference between the enthalpy of the products and the enthalpy of the reactants.

$$\Delta H = H_{products} - H_{reactants}$$

The enthalpy change, ΔH, is also known as the **heat of reaction**.

If the products of a chemical reaction have stronger bonds than the reactants, then more energy is released in the making of product bonds than was put in to break the reactant bonds. In this case, energy is released overall from the system, and the reaction is **exothermic**. The products are in a lower energy state than the reactants, and the change in enthalpy, ΔH, is negative, since heat flows out of the system. If the products of a chemical reaction have weaker bonds than the reactants, then more energy is put in during the breaking of reactant bonds than is released in the making of product bonds. In this case, energy is absorbed overall, and the reaction is **endothermic**. The products are in a higher energy state than the reactants, and the change in enthalpy, ΔH, is positive, since heat had to be added to the system from the surroundings.

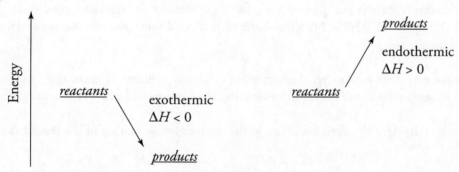

Enthalpy is a **state function**, which means that changes are independent of the pathway of the reaction.

Example 21-2: For the endothermic reaction

$$2\ CO_2(g) \rightarrow 2\ CO(g) + O_2(g)$$

will $\Delta H + \Delta S$ be positive or negative?

Solution: Since we're told that the reaction is endothermic, we know that ΔH is positive. Now, what about ΔS? Has the disorder increased or decreased? On the reactant side, we have one type of gas molecule, while on the right we have two. The reaction increases the numbers of gas molecules, so this describes an increase in disorder. ΔS is positive.

21.5 CALCULATION OF ΔH_{rxn}

The heat of reaction (ΔH_{rxn}) can be calculated in a number of ways. Each of these will lead to the same answer given accurate starting values. The three most important methods to be familiar with are the use of heats of formation (ΔH_f), Hess's law of heat summation, and the summation of individual bond enthalpies.

Standard State Conditions

Essentially every process is affected by temperature and pressure, so scientists have a convention called **standard state conditions** for which most constants, heats of formation, enthalpies, and so on are determined. In the standard state, the temperature is 298 K (25°C) and 1 atm pressure. All solids and liquids are assumed to be pure, and solutions are considered to be at a concentration of 1 M. Values that have been determined at standard state are designated by a ° superscript: $\Delta H°$, for example. Be careful not to confuse *standard state* with *standard temperature and pressure* (STP). STP is at 0°C, while standard state is at 25°C.

Heat of Formation

The **heat of formation**, $\Delta H°_f$, is the amount of energy required to make one mole of a compound *from its constituent elements in their natural or standard state*. The convention is to assign elements in their standard state forms a $\Delta H°_f$ of zero. For example, the $\Delta H°_f$ of C(s) (as graphite) is zero. Diatomic molecules, such as O_2, H_2, Cl_2 and so on are also defined as zero, rather than their atomic forms (such as O, Cl, etc.), because the diatomic state is the *natural* state for these elements at standard conditions. For example, $\Delta H°_f = 0$ for O_2, but for O, $\Delta H°_f = 249$ kJ/mol at standard conditions, because it takes energy to break the O=O double bond.

When a compound's $\Delta H°_f$ is positive, then an input of heat is required to make that compound from its constituent elements. When $\Delta H°_f$ is negative, making the compound from its elements gives off heat.

You can calculate the $\Delta H°$ of a reaction if you know the heats of formation of the reactants and products:

$$\Delta H°_{rxn} = (\Sigma n \times \Delta H°_{f,\ products}) - (\Sigma n \times \Delta H°_{f,\ reactants})$$

In the above equation, "n" denotes the stoichiometric coefficient applied to each species in a chemical reaction as written. $\Delta H°_f$ of a given compound is the heat needed to form one mole, and as such if two moles of a molecule are needed to balance a reaction, one must double the corresponding $\Delta H°_f$ in the heat equation. If only half a mole is required, one must divide the $\Delta H°_f$ by 2.

Hess's Law of Heat Summation

Hess's law states that if a reaction occurs in several steps, then the sum of the energies absorbed or given off in all the steps will be the same as that for the overall reaction. This is due to the fact that enthalpy is a state function, so ΔH is independent of the pathway of the reaction.

For example, the combustion of carbon to form carbon monoxide proceeds by a two-step mechanism:

1. $C(s) + O_2(g) \rightarrow CO_2(g)$ $\quad\quad \Delta H_1 = -394$ kJ
2. $CO_2(g) \rightarrow CO(g) + 1/2\ O_2(g)$ $\quad \Delta H_2 = +283$ kJ

To get the overall reaction, we add the two steps:

$$C(s) + 1/2\ O_2(g) \rightarrow CO(g)$$

So, to find ΔH for the overall reaction, we just add the enthalpies of the steps:

$$\Delta H_{rxn} = \Delta H_1 + \Delta H_2 = -394 \text{ kJ} + 283 \text{ kJ} = -111 \text{ kJ}$$

It's important to remember the following two rules when using Hess's law:

1. *If a reaction is reversed, the sign of ΔH is reversed too.*
   For example, for the reaction $CO_2(g) \rightarrow C(s) + O_2(g)$, we'd have $\Delta H = +394$ kJ.

2. *If an equation is multiplied by a constant, then ΔH must be multiplied by that same constant.*
   For example, for $1/2\ C(s) + 1/2\ O_2(g) \rightarrow 1/2\ CO_2(g)$, we'd have $\Delta H = -197$ kJ.

Example 21-3: The combustion of methanol is given by this reaction:

$$2CH_3OH(g) + 3O_2(g) \rightarrow 2CO_2(g) + 4H_2O(g),\ \Delta H = -1352 \text{ kJ}$$

A. How much heat is produced when 16 g of oxygen gas reacts with excess methanol?
B. Is the reaction exothermic or endothermic? Does it result in an increase or in a decrease in entropy?
C. How many moles of carbon dioxide are produced when 676 kJ of heat is produced?

Solution:

A. The molecular weight of O_2 is 2(16) = 32 g/mol, so 16 g represents one-half mole. If 1352 kJ of heat is released when 3 moles of O_2 react, then just (1/6)(1352 kJ) = 225 kJ of heat will be released when one-half mole of O_2 reacts.
B. Because ΔH is negative, the reaction is exothermic. And since 6 moles of gaseous products are being formed from just 5 moles of gaseous reactants, the disorder (entropy) has increased.
C. The stoichiometry of the given balanced reaction tells us that 2 moles of CO_2 are produced when 1352 kJ of heat is produced. So, half as much CO_2 (that is, 1 mole) is produced when half as much heat, 676 kJ, is produced.

Example 21-4: What is $\Delta H°$ for the following reaction under standard conditions if the $\Delta H°_f$ of $CH_4(g)$ = –75 kJ/mol, $\Delta H°_f$ of $CO_2(g)$ = –393 kJ/mol, and $\Delta H°_f$ of $H_2O(l)$ = –286 kJ/mol?

$$CH_4(g) + 2O_2(g) \rightarrow CO_2(g) + 2H_2O(l)$$

Solution: Using the equation for $\Delta H°_{rxn}$, we find that

$$\Delta H°_{rxn} = (\Delta H°_f CO_2 + 2\,\Delta H°_f H_2O) - (\Delta H°_f CH_4 + 2\,\Delta H°_f O_2)$$

$$= (-393 \text{ kJ/mol} + 2(-286) \text{ kJ/mol}) - (-75 \text{ kJ/mol} + 0 \text{ kJ/mol})$$

$$= -890 \text{ kJ/mol}$$

Summation of Bond Enthalpies

Enthalpy itself can be viewed as the energy stored in the chemical bonds of a compound. Bonds have characteristic enthalpies that denote how much energy is required to break them homolytically (often called the bond dissociation energy, or BDE).

An important distinction can be made here in the difference in sign of ΔH for making a bond versus breaking a bond. One must, necessarily, infuse energy into a system to break a chemical bond. As such, the ΔH for this process is positive; it is endothermic. On the other hand, creating a bond between two atoms must have a negative value of ΔH. It therefore gives off heat and is exothermic. If this weren't the case it would indicate that the bonded atoms were higher in energy than they were when unbound; such a bond would be unstable and immediately dissociate.

Therefore, we have a very important relation that can help you on the DAT:

> Energy is needed to break a bond.
>
> Energy is released in making a bond.

From this we come to the third method of determining ΔH_{rxn}. If a question provides a list of bond enthalpies, ΔH_{rxn} can be determined through the following equation:

$$\Delta H_{rxn} = \Sigma \text{ (BDE bonds broken)} - \Sigma \text{ (BDE bonds formed)}$$

One can see that if stronger bonds are being formed than those being broken, then ΔH_{rxn} will be negative. More energy is released than supplied and the reaction is exothermic. If the opposite is true and breaking strong bonds takes more energy than is regained through the making of weaker product bonds, then the reaction is endothermic.

21.5

Example 21-5: Given the table of average bond dissociation energies below, calculate ΔH_{rxn} for the combustion of methane.

Bond	Average Bond Dissociation Energy (kJ/mol)
C—H	413
O—H	467
C=O	799
C=N	615
H—Cl	427
O=O	495

Solution: First determine how many of each type of bond are broken in the reactants and formed in the products based on the stoichiometry of the balanced equation. Then using the bond dissociation energies we can calculate the enthalpy change:

$$\Delta H_{rxn} = \Sigma \text{ (BDE bonds broken)} - \Sigma \text{ (BDE bonds formed)}$$

$$\Delta H_{rxn} = (4(\text{C—H}) + 2(\text{O=O})) - (2(\text{C=O}) + 4(\text{O—H}))$$

$$= (4(413) + 2(495)) - (2(799) + 4(467))$$

$$= -824 \text{ kJ/mol}$$

You may notice that the two methods did not produce exactly the same answer. This is due to the fact that bond energies are reported as the average of many examples of that type of bond, whereas heats of formation are determined for each individual chemical compound. The exact energy of a bond will be dependent not only on the two atoms bonded together but also the chemical environment in which they reside. The average bond energy gives an approximation of the strength of an individual bond, and as such, the summation of bond energies give an approximation of ΔH_{rxn}.

Example 21-6: Which of the following substances does NOT have a heat of formation equal to zero at standard conditions?

A. $F_2(g)$
B. $Cl_2(g)$
C. $Br_2(g)$
D. $I_2(s)$
E. $H_2(g)$

Solution: Heat of formation, $\Delta H°_f$, is zero for a pure element in its natural phase at standard conditions. All of the choices are in their standard state, except for bromine, which is a liquid, not a gas, at standard conditions. The correct answer is C.

21.6   GIBBS FREE ENERGY

The magnitude of the change in **Gibbs free energy**, ΔG, is the energy that's available (free) to do useful work from a chemical reaction. The spontaneity of a reaction is determined by changes in enthalpy and in entropy, and G includes both of these quantities. Now we have a way to determine whether a given reaction will be spontaneous. In some cases—namely, when ΔH and ΔS have different signs—it's easy. For example, if ΔH is negative and ΔS is positive, then the reaction will certainly be spontaneous (because the products have less energy and more disorder than the reactants; there are two tendencies for a spontaneous reaction: to decrease enthalpy and/or to increase entropy). If ΔH is positive and ΔS is negative, then the reaction will certainly be nonspontaneous (because the products would have more energy and less disorder than the reactants).

But what happens when ΔH and ΔS have the *same* sign? Which factor—enthalpy or entropy—will dominate and determine the spontaneity of the reaction? The sign of the single quantity ΔG will dictate whether or not a process is spontaneous, and we calculate ΔG from this equation:

> **Change in Gibbs Free Energy**
> $$\Delta G = \Delta H - T\Delta S$$

where T is the absolute temperature (in kelvins). And now, we can say this:

- $\Delta G < 0$ $\rightarrow$ spontaneous in the forward direction
- $\Delta G = 0$ $\rightarrow$ reaction is at equilibrium
- $\Delta G > 0$ $\rightarrow$ nonspontaneous in the forward direction

If ΔG for a reaction is positive, then the value of ΔG for the *reverse* reaction has the same magnitude but is negative. Therefore, the reverse reaction is spontaneous.

ΔG and Temperature

The equation for ΔG shows us that the entropy ($T\Delta S$) term depends directly on temperature. At low temperatures, the entropy doesn't have much influence on the free energy, and ΔH is the dominant factor in determining spontaneity. But as the temperature increases, the entropy term becomes more significant relative to ΔH and can dominate the value for ΔG. In general, the universe tends towards increasing disorder (positive ΔS) and stable bonds (negative ΔH), and a favorable combination of these will make a process spontaneous. The following chart summarizes the combinations of ΔH and ΔS that determine ΔG and spontaneity.

ΔH	ΔS	ΔG	Reaction is...?
–	+	–	spontaneous
+	+	– at sufficiently high T + at low T	spontaneous nonspontaneous
–	–	+ at high T – at sufficiently low T	nonspontaneous spontaneous
+	–	+	nonspontaneous

Important note: While values of ΔH are usually reported in terms of kJ, values of ΔS are usually given in terms of J. When using the equation $\Delta G = \Delta H - T\Delta S$, make sure that your ΔH and ΔS are expressed *both* in kJ or *both* in J.

Example 21-7: What must be true about a spontaneous, endothermic reaction with regard to ΔG, ΔH, or ΔS?

Solution: Since the reaction is spontaneous, we know that ΔG is negative, and since we know the reaction is endothermic, we also know that ΔH is positive. The equation $\Delta G = \Delta H - T\Delta S$ then tells us that ΔS must be positive.

21.7 REACTION ENERGY DIAGRAMS

A chemical reaction can be graphed as it progresses in a reaction energy diagram. True to its name, a reaction energy diagram plots the free energy of the total reactions versus the conversion of reactants to products.

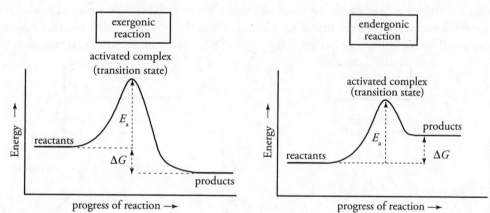

The ΔG of the overall reaction is the difference between the energy of the products and the energy of the reactants: $\Delta G_{rxn} = G_{products} - G_{reactants}$. When the value of $T\Delta S$ is very small, then ΔG can approximate ΔH, with the difference between the energy of products and reactants being very close to the heat of reaction, ΔH.

Recall that the activation energy, E_a, is the extra energy the reactants required to overcome the activation barrier, and it determines the kinetics of the reaction. The higher the barrier, the slower the reaction proceeds towards equilibrium; the lower the barrier, the faster the reaction proceeds towards equilibrium. However, E_a does *not* determine the equilibrium, and an eternally slow reaction (very big E_a) can have a very favorable (large) K_{eq}.

Kinetics vs. Thermodynamics

Just because a reaction is thermodynamically favorable (i.e., spontaneous) does not automatically mean that it will be taking place rapidly. **Do not confuse kinetics with thermodynamics** (this is something the DAT will try to get you to do many times!). They are separate realms. *Thermodynamics predicts the spontaneity (and the equilibrium) of reactions, not their rates.* If you had a starting line and a finish line, thermodynamics tells you how far you will go, while kinetics tells you how quickly you will get there. A classic example to illustrate this is the formation of graphite from diamond. Graphite and diamond are two of the several different forms (**allotropes**) of carbon, and the value of ΔG° for the reaction $C_{(diamond)} \rightarrow C_{(graphite)}$ is about –2900 J. Because ΔG° is negative, this reaction is spontaneous under standard conditions. But it's *extremely* slow. Even diamond heirlooms passed down through many generations are still in diamond form.

Reversibility

Reactions follow the principle of microscopic reversibility: The reverse reaction has the same magnitude for all thermodynamic values (ΔG, ΔH, and ΔS) but of the opposite sign, and the same reaction pathway, but in reverse. This means that the reaction energy diagram for the reverse reaction can be drawn by simply using the mirror image of the forward reaction. The incongruity you should notice is that E_a is different for the forward and reverse reactions. Coming from the products side towards the reactants, the energy barrier will be the difference between $G_{products}$ and the energy of the activated complex.

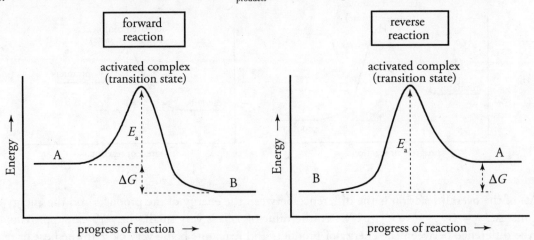

The Thermodynamics of Catalysts

The addition of a catalyst will affect the rate of a reaction, but not the equilibrium. A catalyst provides a different pathway for the reactants to get to the products, and lowers the activation energy, E_a. But a catalyst does not change any of the thermodynamic quantities such as ΔG, ΔH, and ΔS of a reaction.

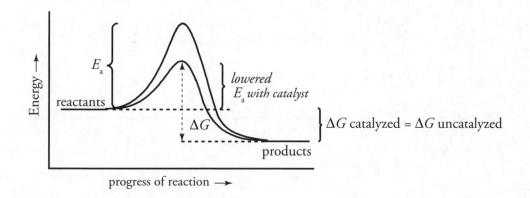

21.8   THERMODYNAMICS AND EQUILIBRIUM

In the previous section, we stated that if ΔG was negative we could expect a reaction to proceed spontaneously in the forward direction, with the opposite being true when ΔG is positive. When a system proceeds in one direction or another there will be a change in the relative values of products and reactants, and the reaction will proceed until equilibrium is achieved and $\Delta G = 0$. Therefore, there must be a relationship between ΔG and the reaction quotient Q, as well as the equilibrium constant K_{eq}. This relationship is given in the following equation:

$$\Delta G = \Delta G° + RT \ln Q$$

You will not have to use this equation in calculations on test day, but should understand what it means. Remember that Q is used when a reaction is not at equilibrium (Section 19.2). ΔG is a statement of spontaneity of a reaction in one direction or another and ΔG always equals zero at equilibrium. In other words, when $Q = K_{eq}$ (equilibrium), $\Delta G = 0$. This leads to an alternate version of this equation:

$$0 = \Delta G° + RT \ln K_{eq} \quad \text{or} \quad \Delta G° = -RT \ln K_{eq}$$

ΔG changes with changing reaction composition until it reaches zero at equilibrium. As the superscript denotes, $\Delta G°$ is the Gibbs free energy for a reaction under standard conditions. It is a constant at constant temperature.

These equations tell us three important things:

1.   When $\Delta G° < 0$, $K_{eq} > 1$ and the products are favored at equilibrium.
2.   When $\Delta G° = 0$, $K_{eq} = 1$; products and reactants are present in equal amounts at equilibrium.
3.   When $\Delta G° > 0$, $K_{eq} < 1$ and reactants are favored at equilibrium.

The difference between the heights of the reactants and products on any reaction coordinate diagram is $\Delta G°$. As we know from analyzing these plots, if the reactants are higher than the products, we expect the products to be favored. This would give us the expected negative value of $\Delta G°$, and likewise a value of K_{eq} greater than 1.

Want More Practice?
Remember to register your book online for chapter summaries, drills, practice tests, and more!

Chapter 22
Electrochemistry

22.1 OXIDATION-REDUCTION REACTIONS

Recall that the **oxidation number** (or **oxidation state**) of each atom in a molecule describes how many electrons it is donating or accepting in the overall bonding of the molecule. Many elements can assume different oxidation states depending on the bonds they make. A reaction in which the oxidation numbers of any of the reactants change is called an **oxidation-reduction** (or **redox**) reaction.

In a redox reaction, atoms gain or lose electrons as new bonds are formed. The total number of electrons does not change, of course; they're just redistributed among the atoms. When an atom loses electrons, its oxidation number increases; this is **oxidation**. When an atom gains electrons, the oxidation number decreases; this is **reduction**. A mnemonic device is helpful:

LEO the lion says GER

LEO: Lose Electrons = Oxidation

GER: Gain Electrons = Reduction

Another popular mnemonic is

OIL RIG

OIL: Oxidation Is electron Loss

RIG: Reduction Is electron Gain

An atom that is oxidized in a reaction loses electrons to another atom. We call the oxidized atom a **reducing agent** or **reductant**, because by giving up electrons, it reduces another atom that gains the electrons. On the other hand, the atom that gains the electrons has been **reduced**. We call the reduced atom an **oxidizing agent** or **oxidant**, because it oxidizes another atom that loses the electrons.

Take a look at this redox reaction:

$$Fe + 2HCl \rightarrow FeCl_2 + H_2$$

The oxidation state of iron changes from 0 to +2. The oxidation state of hydrogen changes from +1 to 0. (The oxidation state of chlorine remains at −1.) So, iron has lost two electrons, and two protons (H^+) have gained one electron each. Therefore, the iron has been oxidized, and the hydrogens have been reduced. In order to better see the exchange of electrons, a redox reaction can be broken down into a pair of **half-reactions** that show the oxidation and reduction separately. These **ion-electron** equations show only the actual oxidized or reduced species—and the electrons involved—in an electron-balanced reaction. For the redox reaction shown above, the ion-electron half-reactions are:

$$\text{oxidation:} \quad Fe \rightarrow Fe^{2+} + 2e^-$$
$$\text{reduction:} \quad 2H^+ + 2e^- \rightarrow H_2$$

22.2 GALVANIC CELLS

Because a redox reaction involves the transfer of electrons, and the flow of electrons constitutes an electric current that can do work, we can use a spontaneous redox reaction to generate an electric current. A device for doing this is called a **galvanic** (or **voltaic**) **cell**, the main features of which are shown in the figure below.

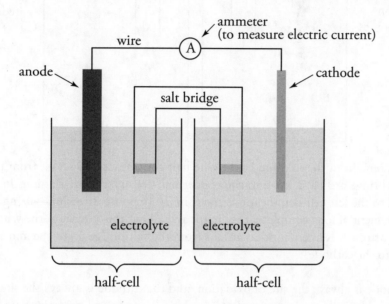

One **electrode**, generally comprised of a metal (labeled the **anode**) gets oxidized, and the electrons its atoms lose travel along the wire to a second metal electrode (labeled the **cathode**). It is at the cathode that reduction takes place. In this way, the anode acts as an electron source, while the cathode acts as an electron sink. Electrons always flow through the conducting wire from the anode to the cathode. This electron flow is the electric current that is produced by the spontaneous redox reaction between the electrodes.

Let's look at a specific galvanic cell, with the anode made of zinc, and the cathode made of copper. The anode is immersed in a $ZnSO_4$ solution, the cathode is immersed in a $CuSO_4$ solution, and the half cells are connected by a **salt bridge** containing an aqueous solution of KNO_3. When the electrodes are connected by a wire, zinc atoms in the anode are oxidized ($Zn \rightarrow Zn^{2+} + 2e^-$), and the electrons travel through the wire to the cathode. There, the Cu^{2+} ions in the solution pick up these electrons and get reduced to copper metal ($Cu^{2+} + 2e^- \rightarrow Cu$), which accumulates on the copper cathode. The sulfate anions balance the charge on the Zn^{2+}, but do not participate in any redox reaction, and are therefore known as spectator ions.

22.3

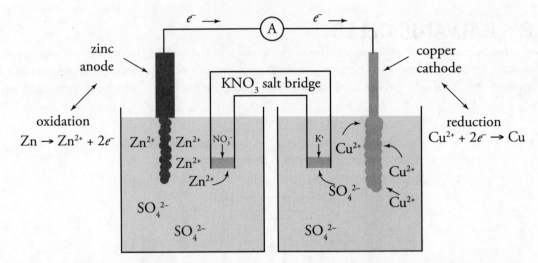

The Zn^{2+} ions that remain in the solution in the zinc half-cell attract NO_3^- ions from the salt bridge, and K^+ ions in the salt bridge are attracted into the copper half-cell. Notice that anions in the solution travel from the right cell to the left cell—and cations travel in the opposite direction—using the salt bridge as a conduit. This movement of ions completes the circuit and allows the current in the wire to continue, until the zinc strip is consumed. Remember that anions from the salt bridge go to the anode and cations from the salt bridge go to the cathode.

Notice that the anode is always the site of oxidation, and the cathode is always the site of reduction. One way to help remember this is just to notice that "a" and "o" (anode and oxidation) are both vowels, while "c" and "r" (cathode and reduction) are both consonants. Another popular mnemonic is "an ox, red cat" for "anode = oxidation, reduction = cathode."

We often use a shorthand notation, called a **cell diagram**, to identify the species present in a galvanic cell. Cell diagrams are read as follows:

Anode | Anodic solution (concentration) | | Cathodic solution (concentration) | Cathode

If the concentrations are not specified in the cell diagram, you should assume they are 1 M.

22.3   STANDARD REDUCTION POTENTIALS

To determine whether the redox reaction of a cell is spontaneous and can produce an electric current, we need to figure out the cell voltage. Each half-reaction has a potential (E), which is the cell voltage it would have if the other electrode were the standard reference electrode. (*Note*: We usually consider cells at standard conditions: 25°C, 1 atm pressure, aqueous solutions at 1 M concentrations, and with substances in their standard states. To indicate standard conditions, we use a ° superscript on quantities such as E and ΔG.) By definition, the standard reference electrode is the site of the redox reaction $2\,H^+ + 2e^- \rightarrow H_2$, which is assigned a potential of 0.00 volts.

Half Reaction	Standard Potential, $E°$ (volts)
$Au^{3+}(aq) + 3e^- \rightarrow Au(s)$	1.50
$Pt^{2+}(aq) + 2e^- \rightarrow Pt(s)$	1.20
$Pd^{2+}(aq) + 2e^- \rightarrow Pd(s)$	0.99
$Ag^{2+}(aq) + 2e^- \rightarrow Ag(s)$	0.80
$Cu^{2+}(aq) + 2e^- \rightarrow Cu(s)$	0.34
$2H^+(aq) + 2e^- \rightarrow H_2(g)$	0.00
$Pb^{2+}(aq) + 2e^- \rightarrow Pb(s)$	−0.13
$Fe^{2+}(aq) + 2e^- \rightarrow Fe(s)$	−0.44
$Zn^{2+}(aq) + 2e^- \rightarrow Zn(s)$	−0.76
$Al^{3+}(aq) + 3e^- \rightarrow Al(s)$	−1.67
$Mg^{2+}(aq) + 2e^- \rightarrow Mg(s)$	−2.36
$Li^+(aq) + 1e^- \rightarrow Li(s)$	−3.05

By adding the half-reaction potential for a given pair of electrodes, we get the cell's overall voltage. Tables of half-reaction potentials are usually given for reductions only. Since each cell has a reduction half-reaction and an oxidation half-reaction, we get the potential of the oxidation by simply reversing the sign of the corresponding reduction potential.

For example, the standard reduction potential for the half-reaction $Cu^{2+} + 2e^- \rightarrow Cu$ is +0.34 V. The standard reduction potential for the half-reaction $Zn^{2+} + 2e^- \rightarrow Zn$ is −0.76 V. Reversing the zinc reduction to an oxidation, we get $Zn \rightarrow Zn^{2+} + 2e^-$, with a potential of +0.76 V. Therefore, the overall cell voltage for the zinc-copper cell is (+0.76 V) + (+0.34 V) = +1.10 V:

$$
\begin{array}{lll}
\text{oxidation:} & Zn \rightarrow Zn^{2+} + 2e^- & E° = +0.76 \text{ V} \\
\text{reduction:} & Cu^{2+} + 2e^- \rightarrow Cu & E° = +0.34 \text{ V} \\
\hline
& Zn + Cu^{2+} \rightarrow Zn^{2+} + Cu & E° = +1.10 \text{ V}
\end{array}
$$

The free-energy change, $\Delta G°$, for a redox reaction whose cell voltage is $E°$ is given by the equation

$$\Delta G° = -nFE°$$

where n is the number of moles of electrons transferred and F stands for a **faraday** (the magnitude of the charge of one mole of electrons, approximately 96,500 coulombs). Since a reaction is spontaneous if $\Delta G°$ is negative, this equation tells us that the redox reaction in a cell will be spontaneous if the cell voltage is positive. Since the cell voltage for our zinc-copper cell was +1.10 V, we know the reaction will be spontaneous and produce an electric current that can do work.

> If the cell voltage is positive, then the reaction is spontaneous.
>
> If the cell voltage is negative, then the reaction is nonspontaneous.

Let's do another example and consider what would happen if the zinc electrode in our cell above were replaced by a gold electrode, given that the **standard reduction potential** for the reaction $Au^{3+} + 3e^- \rightarrow$ Au is $E° = +1.50$ V. The redox reaction that we're investigating is

$$Au + Cu^{2+} \rightarrow Au^{3+} + Cu$$

Let's first break this down into half-reactions:

$$Au \rightarrow Au^{3+} + 3e^- \qquad\qquad E° = -1.50 \text{ V}$$

$$Cu^{2+} + 2ee^- \rightarrow Cu \qquad\qquad E° = +0.34 \text{ V}$$

The overall reaction is not electron balanced; but by multiplying the first half-reaction by 2 and the second half-reaction by 3, we get

$$
\begin{aligned}
2Au &\rightarrow 2Au^{3+} + 6e^- & E° &= -1.50 \text{ V} \\
3Cu^{2+} + 6e^- &\rightarrow 3Cu & E° &= +0.34 \text{ V} \\
\hline
2Au + 3Cu^{2+} &\rightarrow 2Au^{3+} + 3Cu & E° &= -1.16 \text{ V}
\end{aligned}
$$

The final equation is now electron balanced. Notice that although we multiplied the half-reactions by stoichiometric coefficients, we did *not* multiply the potentials by those coefficients. You never multiply the potential by a coefficient, even if you multiply a half-reaction by a coefficient to get the balanced equation for the reaction. This is because the potentials are *intrinsic* to the identities of the species involved and do not depend on the number of moles of the species.

Because the cell voltage is negative, this reaction would not be spontaneous. However, it would be spontaneous in the other direction; that is, if copper were the *anode* and gold the *cathode*, then the potential of the cell would be +1.16 V, which implies a spontaneous reaction.

Oxidizing and Reducing Agents

We can also use reduction potentials to determine whether reactants are good or poor oxidizing or reducing agents. For example, let's look again at the half-reactions in our original zinc-copper cell. The half-reaction $Zn^{2+} + 2e^- \rightarrow Zn$ has a standard potential of -0.76 V, and the half-reaction $Cu^{2+} + 2e^- \rightarrow Cu$ has a standard potential of $+0.34$ V. The fact that the reduction of Zn^{2+} is nonspontaneous means that the oxidation of Zn is spontaneous, so Zn would rather give up electrons. If it does, this means that Zn acts as a reducing agent because in giving up electrons it reduces something else. The fact that the reduction of Cu^{2+} has a positive potential tells us that this reaction would be spontaneous at standard conditions. In other words, Cu^{2+} is a good oxidizing agent because it's looking to accept electrons, thereby oxidizing something else. So, in general, if a reduction half-reaction has a large negative potential, then the product is a good reducing agent. On the other hand, if a reduction half-reaction has a large positive potential, then the reactant is a good oxidizing agent. Now, whether something is a "good" oxidizing or reducing agent depends on what it's being compared to. So, to be more precise, we should say this:

> The more negative the reduction potential, the weaker the reactant is as an oxidizing agent, and the stronger the product is as a reducing agent.
>
> The more positive the reduction potential, the stronger the reactant is as an oxidizing agent, and the weaker the product is as a reducing agent.

For example, given that $Pb^{2+} + 2e^- \rightarrow Pb$ has a standard potential of -0.13 V, and $Al^{3+} + 3e^- \rightarrow Al$ has a standard potential of -1.67 V, what could we conclude? Well, since Al^{3+} has a large negative reduction potential, the product, aluminum metal, is a good reducing agent. In fact, because the reduction potential of Al^{3+} is more negative than that of Pb^{2+}, we'd say that aluminum is a stronger reducing agent than lead.

Example 22-1: What is the standard cell voltage for the reduction of Ag^+ by Al?

Solution: The half-reactions are

$$Ag^+ + e^- \rightarrow Ag \qquad E° = 0.80 \text{ V}$$
$$Al \rightarrow Al^{3+} + 3e^- \qquad E° = +1.67 \text{ V}$$

Although we would multiply both sides of the first half-reaction by the stoichiometric coefficient 3 before adding it to the second one to give the overall, electron-balanced redox reaction, we don't bother to do that here. The question is asking only for $E°$, and the potentials of the half-reactions are not affected by stoichiometric coefficients. Adding the potentials of these half-reactions gives us the overall cell voltage: $E° = 2.47$ V.

Example: 22-2 Is the reaction below spontaneous?

$$2Au + 3Fe^{2+} \rightarrow 2Au^{3+} + 3Fe$$

Solution: If the cell voltage $E°$ is negative, then the reaction is nonspontaneous, and if $E°$ is positive, then the reaction is spontaneous. The half-reactions are

$$2 (Au \rightarrow Au^{3+} + 3e^-) \qquad E° = -1.50 \text{ V}$$
$$3 (Fe^{2+} + 2e^- \rightarrow Fe) \qquad E° = -0.44 \text{ V}$$

The question is really asking only about $E°$, and the potentials of the half-reactions are *not* affected by stoichiometric coefficients (2 and 3, in this case). Since each of these half-reactions has a negative value for $E°$, the cell voltage (obtained by adding them) will also be negative, so the reaction is not spontaneous.

Example 22-3: Of the following, which is the strongest reducing agent?

  A. Zn
  B. Fe
  C. Pd
  D. Pd^{2+}
  E. Au^{3+}

Solution: Remember the rule: The more negative the reduction potential, the stronger the product is as a reducing agent. Zn (A) is the product of a redox half-reaction whose potential is -0.76 V. Fe (B) is the product of a redox half-reaction whose potential is -0.44 V. So, we know we can eliminate B. Pd (C) is the product of a redox half-reaction whose potential is $+0.99$ V, so C is eliminated. Finally, in order for Pd^{2+} or Au^{3+} to be a reducing agent, they would have to be oxidized—that is, lose more electrons. A cation getting further oxidized? Not likely, especially when there's a neutral metal (A) that is happier to do so.

Example 22-4: Which of the following best approximates the value of $\Delta G°$ for this reaction:

$$2Al + 3Cu^{2+} \rightarrow 2Al^{3+} + 3Cu?$$

A. $-(12)(96,500)$ J
B. $-(6)(96,500)$ J
C. $+(6)(96,500)$ J
D. $+(12)(96,500)$ J
E. It cannot be determined from the information given.

Solution: The half-reactions are

$$2\ (Al \rightarrow Al^{3+} + 3e^-) \qquad E° = +1.67 \text{ V}$$
$$3\ (Cu^{2+} + 2e^- \rightarrow Cu) \qquad E° = 0.34 \text{ V}$$

so the overall cell voltage is $E° = 2.01$ V ≈ 2 V. Because the number of electrons transferred is $n = 2 \times 3 = 6$, the equation $\Delta G° = -nFE°$ tells us that A is the answer:

$$\Delta G° = -(6)(95,500)(2) \text{ J} = -(12)(96,500) \text{ J}$$

22.4 ELECTROLYTIC CELLS

Unlike a galvanic cell, an **electrolytic cell** *uses* an external voltage source (such as a battery) to *create an electric current* that forces a nonspontaneous redox reaction to occur. This is known as **electrolysis**. A typical example of an electrolytic cell is one used to form sodium metal and chlorine gas from molten NaCl.

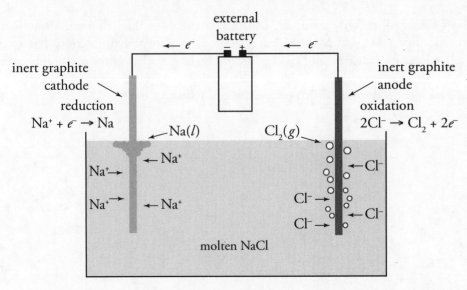

The half-reactions for converting molten NaCl into sodium and chlorine are:

$$Na^+ + e^- \rightarrow Na(l) \qquad E° = -2.71 \text{ V}$$
$$2Cl^- \rightarrow Cl_2(g) + 2e^- \qquad E° = -1.36 \text{ V}$$

The standard voltage for the overall reaction is –4.07 V, which means the reaction is *not* spontaneous. The electrolytic cell shown above uses an external battery to remove electrons from chloride ions and forces sodium ions to accept them. In so doing, the sodium ions are reduced to sodium metal, and the chloride ions are oxidized to produce chlorine gas, which bubbles out of the electrolyte.

Electrolytic cells are also used for plating a thin layer of metal on top of another material, a process known as **electroplating**. If a fork is used as the cathode in an electrolytic cell whose electrolyte contains silver ions, silver will precipitate onto the fork, producing a silver-plated fork. Other examples of metal plating include gold-plated jewelry, and plating tin or chromium onto steel (for tin cans and car bumpers).

Galvanic vs. Electrolytic Cells

Notice that in both galvanic cells and electrolytic cells, the anode is the site of oxidation, and the cathode is the site of reduction. Furthermore, electrons in the external circuit always move from the anode to the cathode. The difference, of course, is that a galvanic cell uses a spontaneous redox reaction to create an electric current, whereas an electrolytic cell uses an electric current to force a nonspontaneous redox reaction to occur.

It follows that in a galvanic cell, the anode is negative and the cathode is positive, since electrons are spontaneously moving from a negative to a positive charge. However, in an electrolytic cell the anode is positive and the cathode is negative, since electrons are being forced to move where they don't want to go.

Galvanic	Electrolytic
Reduction at cathode Oxidation at anode Electrons flow from anode to cathode Anions migrate to anode Cations migrate to cathode	
Spontaneously generates electrical power $(-\Delta G)$	Nonspontaneous, requires an external electric power source $(+\Delta G)$
Total $E°$ of reaction is positive	Total $E°$ of reaction is negative
Anode is negative	Anode is positive
Cathode is positive	Cathode is negative

Want More Practice?
Remember to register your book
online for chapter summaries,
drills, practice tests, and more!

Chapter 23
Gchem Lab Techniques

23.1   BASIC TECHNIQUES

Calorimetry

This is the science of measuring the amount of heat that can be generated (in an exothermic process), consumed (in an endothermic process) or dissipated by a sample. A calorimeter is a device that can be used to measure the heat of a reaction. A Styrofoam cup can be used as a calorimeter because it has well-insulated walls to prevent heat exchange with the environment. In order to measure heats of reactions, reactants are often enclosed in a calorimeter, the reaction is initiated, and the temperature difference before and after the reaction is measured and then used to evaluate the enthalpy change of the reaction. A calorimeter may be operated under constant pressure, or constant volume. Before using a calorimeter, it is important to know its heat capacity. This is the amount of heat required to raise the temperature of the entire calorimeter by 1 K, and it is usually determined experimentally before or after actual measurements of the heat of reaction. This is done by transferring a known amount of heat into the calorimeter and measuring its temperature increase. Because the temperature differences are very small, sensitive thermometers are required for these measurements.

Electrolysis

In chemistry and manufacturing, electrolysis is a method of using a direct electric current to drive an otherwise non-spontaneous chemical reaction. Electrolysis is commercially important for separating elements from naturally occurring sources, such as ores, using an electrolytic cell. The electrolysis of water can be used to produce hydrogen and oxygen.

Burning and Glowing Splint Tests

A splint is a strip of thin wood, which can be used in a test for a combustible gas. A sample of the gas is trapped in a tube with a stopper. A splint is lit and held near the opening of the tube, then the stopper is removed. In larger samples, the end of the splint may be placed into the tube. If the gas is combustible, the mixture ignites. This may give either a visible flame or an audible sound. This test is often used to test for the presence of hydrogen (which ignites with a distinctive "squeaky pop" sound) and for O_2. If the gas is not combustible, the burning splint will be extinguished; carbon dioxide, nitrogen, and argon are all inert gases.

The glowing splint test is similar. Here, a splint is lit, allowed to burn for a few seconds, then blown out by mouth or by shaking. While the tip is still glowing, the splint is introduced to the gas sample. In the presence of oxygen (or other oxidizing gases such as nitrous oxide), the splint reignites and burns back to life.

Water Displacement as a Method to Determine Density of an Object

Here, a submerged object displaces a volume of liquid equal to the volume of the object. Since 1 mL of water has a volume of 1 cm^3, the amount of water displaced can measure the volume of the solid. Density is then calculated via ρ = m/V. It's important to remember that objects with the same mass but different volume have different densities.

Other Techniques

Sometimes the technique questions test concepts you've learned about in earlier chapters, such as *colligative properties* (Section 17.2) or ***titration*** (Section 20.9). Also, some techniques are used in both general and chemistry lab settings, so you could also see questions on extraction, crystallization, precipitation, chromatography, or distillation. These techniques are covered in Chapter 29.

23.2   EQUIPMENT

You should be familiar with the function of certain laboratory equipment, or what equipment could be used to do certain things.

A **buret** (Figure 1) is a device used in analytical chemistry for the dispensing of variable, measured amounts of a chemical solution. A **pipette** (Figure 2) is similar, and can dispense precise volumes of a liquid, but of only one volume at a time. A certain pipette can be calibrated to deliver varying volumes, but only one volume can be dispensed at a time. In other words, a buret is distinguished from a pipette by the fact that for the buret, the quantity delivered is variable. For example, in a titration, one solution is dispensed with a pipette, and another solution is added to it from a buret in aliquots of varying size.

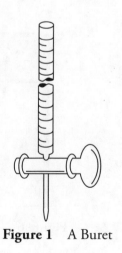

Figure 1   A Buret

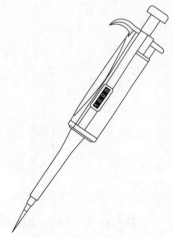

Figure 2   A Pipette

Laboratory or Erlenmeyer flasks (Figure 3) are commonly used glassware vessels. They can be used for making or storing solutions. Erlenmeyer flasks are not usually used to measure liquids since their markings are relatively imprecise and the walls of the container are sloped. **Volumetric flasks** (Figure 4) are calibrated to contain a precise volume at a particular temperature, but only *one* volume. For example, a 50 mL volumetric flask will measure 50.00 mL very precisely, and this will be the only volume you can measure from it.

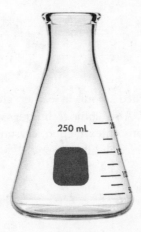

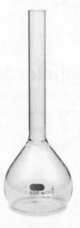

Figure 3   An Erlenmeyer Flask

Figure 4   A Volumetric Flask

A **graduated cylinder** (Figure 5) is the most common and versatile piece of laboratory equipment used to measure the volume of a liquid. Graduated cylinders are generally more accurate and precise than laboratory flasks and beakers. However, they are less accurate and precise than a volumetric pipette or volumetric flask for the *one* volume they are calibrated to measure.

A **beaker** (Figure 6) is a simple container for stirring, mixing, and heating liquids commonly used in many laboratories. Beakers are generally cylindrical in shape, with a flat bottom and a small spout (or "beak") to help with pouring. Beakers are available in a wide range of sizes and are not typically used to measure volumes.

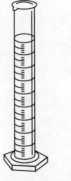

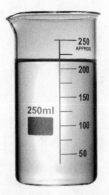

Figure 5   A Graduated Cylinder

Figure 6   A Beaker

23.3 SAFETY

These questions usually test common sense, safety equipment or acids and bases.

23.3

Equipment	Purpose	Alternatives
Safety Goggles	• Can be worn over regular glasses • Tighten the strap at the back • Do not wear contact lenses in the lab • Wear at all times when managing compounds and fragile glass materials	• Safety glasses offer less protection • A face shield offers more protection • Special safety glasses must be worn to block UV rays and lasers
Laboratory Coat	• Worn over regular clothing • Protects skin and clothes from compounds • Should only be worn within the laboratory	• Many styles available • Can also wear a rubber apron for additional protection
Gloves	• Protects hands from chemicals	• Many different types available (thin, thick, different materials)
Fumehood	• When using poisonous gas	• Can wear a gas mask to handle poisonous gas outside the fumehood

When diluting acidic solutions, remember to always add acid to water to make a more dilute solution. Heat is released when strong acids are mixed with water, so if you add water to acid, the solution can boil and splash.

To clean up a strong acid or strong base spill: neutralize a strong acid (or base) spill with a complementary weak base (or acid), then clean up with a paper towel or sponge.

23.4 DATA ANALYSIS

Data is often evaluated on precision and accuracy. **Precision** can be defined as reproducibility in measurement, or how little multiple measured values vary from each other. **Accuracy** is defined as how close a measured value is to a true or accepted value.

Give Yourself A Break
Avoid burnout and give yourself a little study break before you continue on to the next chapter. Go for a walk, get some fresh air, or get a snack and give yourself a moment to breathe and let all of this soak in.

Organic Chemistry

Before starting your review of Ochem content, return to Section 2.1 for a general introduction to the SNS. There will be 30 Ochem questions on the DAT. They will occur at the end of the SNS, after 40 Biology and 30 Gchem questions.

The following chapters will review the Ochem content you should be familiar with for the DAT. The ADA publishes a list of topics tested on the DAT, usually called the "Organic Chemistry Specifications List." Go to the ADA website now and review the list; this will be the content you'll see in the next few chapters. As of 2023, you can expect to see 2-4 questions each on stereochemistry, nomenclature, acid-base chemistry, and aromatics and bonding. Most versions of the DAT have 4-6 questions on mechanisms (energetics and structure) and another 4-6 questions on chemical and physical properties of molecules. Finally, about 1/3 of the Ochem questions are usually on individual reactions of the major functional groups and combinations of reactions to synthesize compounds.

It is also worth checking to see if the content list has changed recently; sometimes last-minute changes are announced. For example, the Biology content list changed in January 2022 and was effective immediately! If some content changes are announced, don't worry. Go online and check out the supplementary content posted for this book. We'll keep the Ochem content up to date there, so even if changes occur, we've got you covered.

There are a decent number of reactions you'll need to memorize before the DAT. If a reaction is in this book, you may need to use it on test day. Consider starting a summary list or a library of flash cards to help you memorize the Ochem reactions sooner rather than later. Recognizing reagents can be an efficient way to answer mechanism questions. You'll see lots of examples of Ochem question types in the online drills you have access to by purchasing this book.

Chapter 24
Ochem Nomenclature

This section covers the fundamentals of nomenclature in organic chemistry. Although this section will require memorization as your primary study technique, it is in your best interest to be comfortable reading, hearing, and using this terminology. Although most of the terminology that appears on the DAT is IUPAC, some common nomenclature is also used.

24.1 CARBON CHAINS

Let's start with some common carbon chain prefixes and alkane names:

Number of carbon atoms in a row	Prefix	Alkane	Name
1	meth-	CH_4	methane
2	eth-	CH_3CH_3	ethane
3	prop-	$CH_3CH_2CH_3$	propane
4	but-	$CH_3CH_2CH_2CH_3$	butane
5	pent-	$CH_3(CH_2)_3CH_3$	pentane
6	hex-	$CH_3(CH_2)_4CH_3$	hexane
7	hept-	$CH_3(CH_2)_5CH_3$	heptane
8	oct-	$CH_3(CH_2)_6CH_3$	octane
9	non-	$CH_3(CH_2)_7CH_3$	nonane
10	dec-	$CH_3(CH_2)_8CH_3$	decane

In the case of an all-carbon containing ring, these are preceded by the prefix **cyclo-**. Hence, a six-membered ring containing all $-CH_2-$ units is called *cyclohexane*.

Nomenclature For Substituents	
Substituent	**Name**
$-CH_3$	methyl
$-CH_2CH_3$	ethyl
$-CH_2CH_2CH_3$	propyl
$H_3C-\overset{\displaystyle H}{\underset{\displaystyle \vert}{C}}-CH_3$	isopropyl
$-CH_2CH_2CH_2CH_3$	butyl (or *n*-butyl)
$-CH_2-CH\diagup\begin{smallmatrix}CH_3\\CH_3\end{smallmatrix}$	isobutyl
$CH_3\underset{\vert}{CH}CH_2CH_3$	*sec*-butyl
$-\overset{\displaystyle CH_3}{\underset{\displaystyle CH_3}{\overset{\vert}{\underset{\vert}{C}}}}-CH_3$	*tert*-butyl (or *t*-butyl)

Common Functional Groups

Recognizing common functional groups is important for the DAT. Here are the groups you need to know:

R = alkyl group = hydrogen substituents group (or H), X = halogen (F, Cl, Br, I)

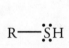

| alkane | alkene or olefin | alkyne | alkyl halide | alcohol |

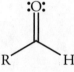 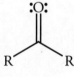 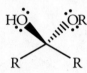

| thiol | ether | epoxide or oxirane | phenol |

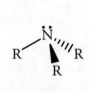

| aldehyde | ketone | hemiacetal | acetal |

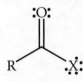

| amine | imine | carboxylic acid |

| acid halide | acid anhydride | ester | amide |

24.2   ABBREVIATED LINE STRUCTURES

The prevalence of carbon-hydrogen (C–H) bonds in organic chemistry has led chemists to use an abbreviated drawing system, merely for convenience. Just imagine having to draw every C–H bond for a large molecule like a steroid or polymer! Abbreviated line structures use only a few simple rules:

1. Carbons are represented simply as vertices.
2. C–H bonds are not drawn.
3. Hydrogens bonded to any atom other than carbon must be shown.

To illustrate rules 1 and 2, pentane can be represented using the full Lewis structure,

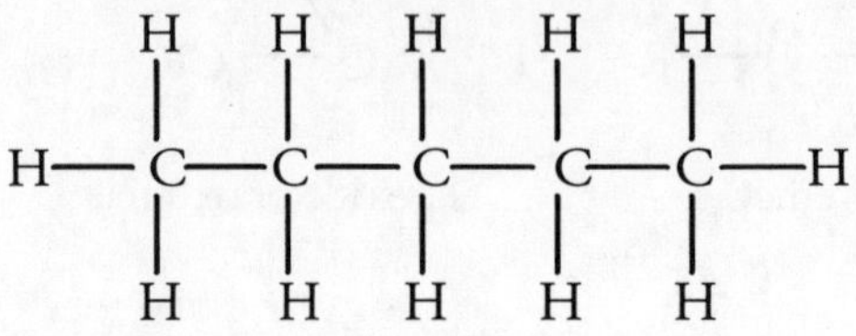

or using the abbreviated line structure.

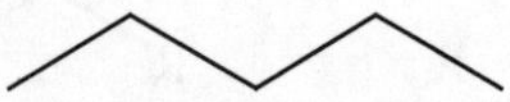

Although C–H bonds are not drawn, the number of hydrogens required to complete carbon's valency are assumed. To clarify this, let's look more closely at the abbreviated line structure of pentane:

These three carbon atoms are each bonded to two other carbon atoms. In order to complete carbon's valency, we assume there are two hydrogens bonded to each of these carbons.

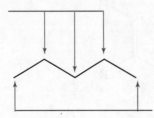

These two carbon atoms are each bonded to one other carbon atom. In order to complete carbon's valency, we assume there are three hydrogens bonded to each of these carbons.

This must be correct, because if we draw out all of the hydrogens in pentane, we get the full Lewis structure shown above.

To illustrate rule 3 above, consider dimethyl amine:

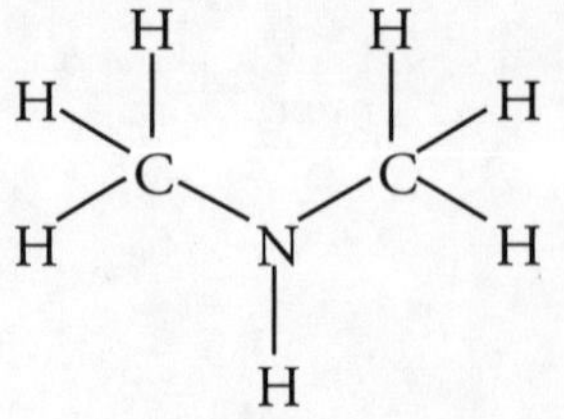

full Lewis structure 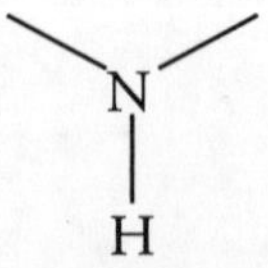   abbreviated line
                                        structure

Remember that hydrogens bonded to carbon can be assumed (the methyl groups in dimethyl amine, for example), but hydrogens bonded to any other atom must be shown. Lone pairs of electrons are often omitted.

Example 24-1: Translate each of the following Lewis structures into an abbreviated line structure:

A.

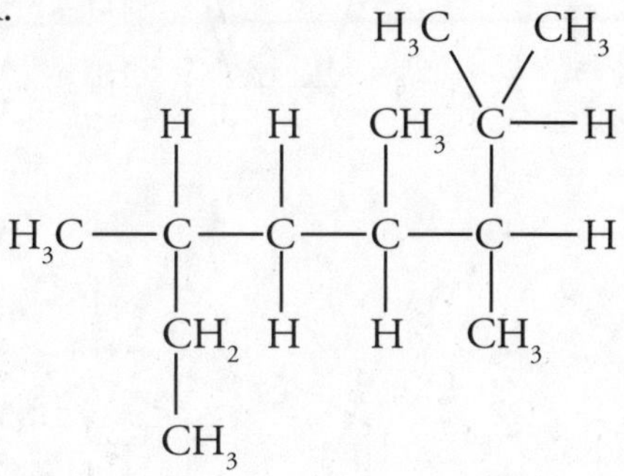

B.

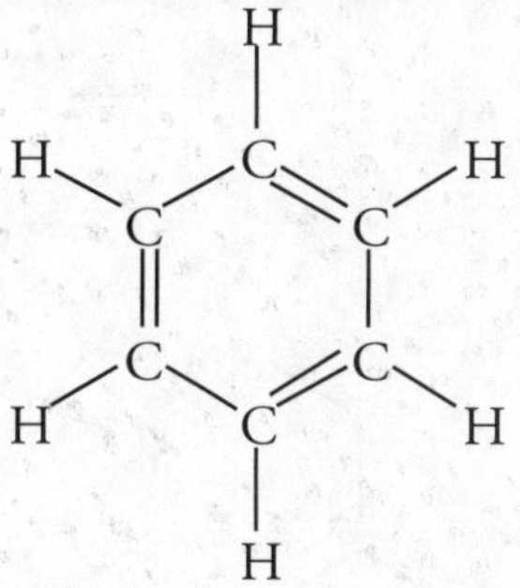

C.

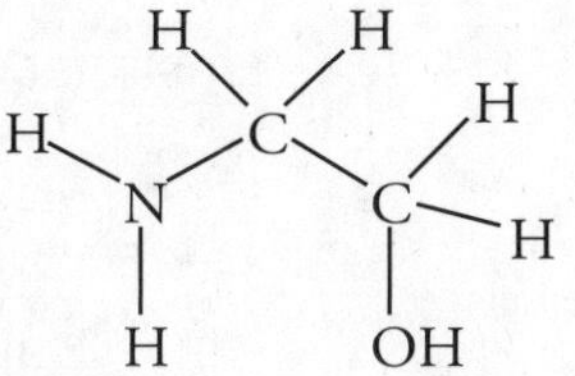

D.

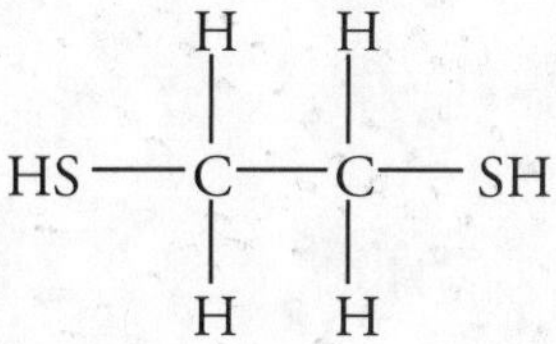

Solution:

A.

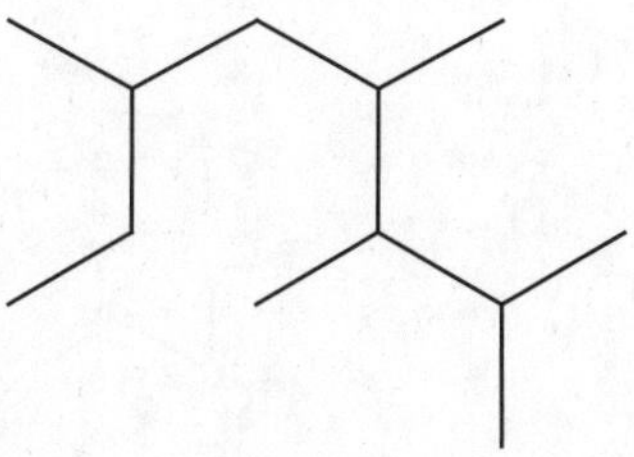

B.

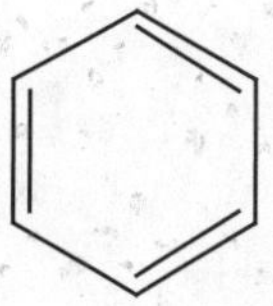

C.

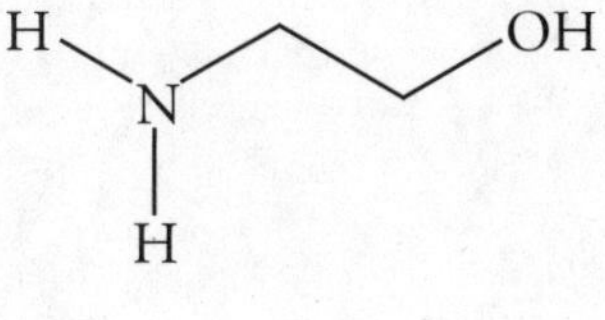

D.

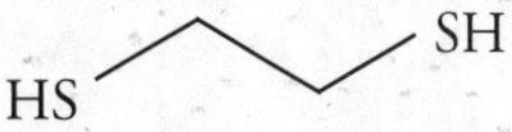

Example 24-2: Translate each of the following abbreviated line structures into a Lewis structure:

A.

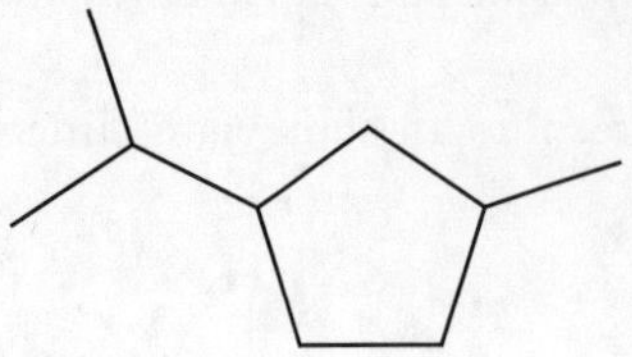

B.

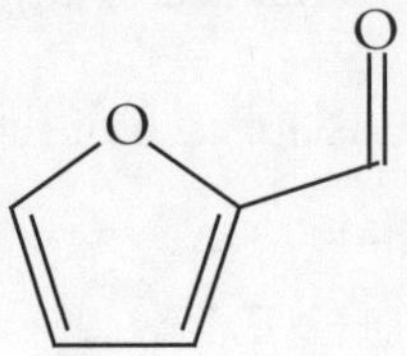

C.

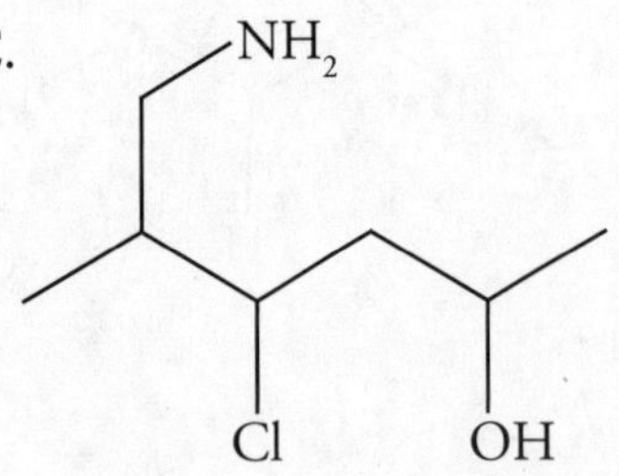

D.

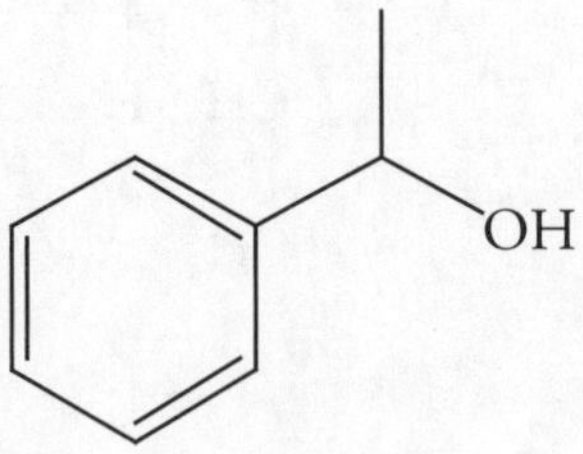

Solution:

A.

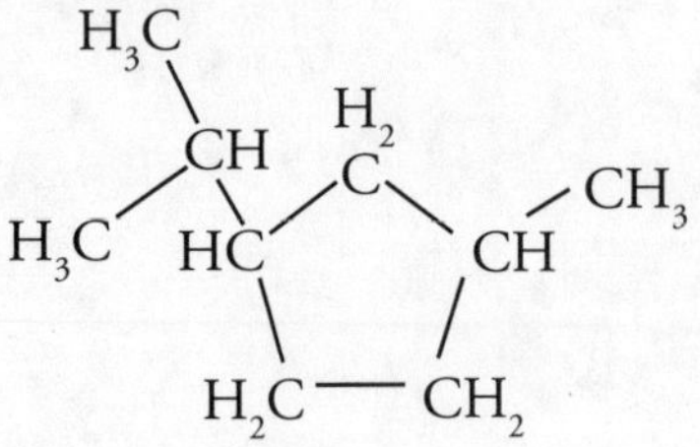

B.

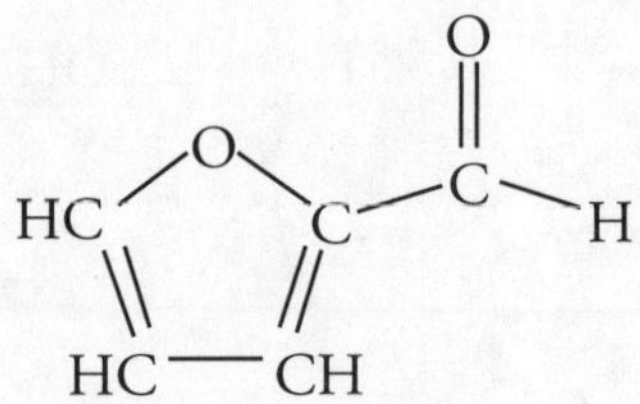

C.

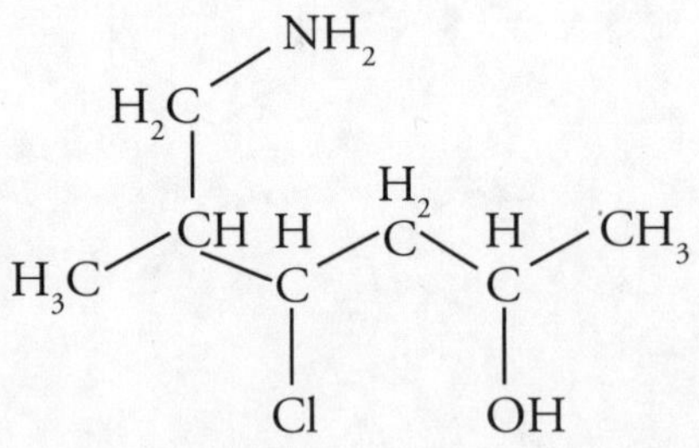

D.

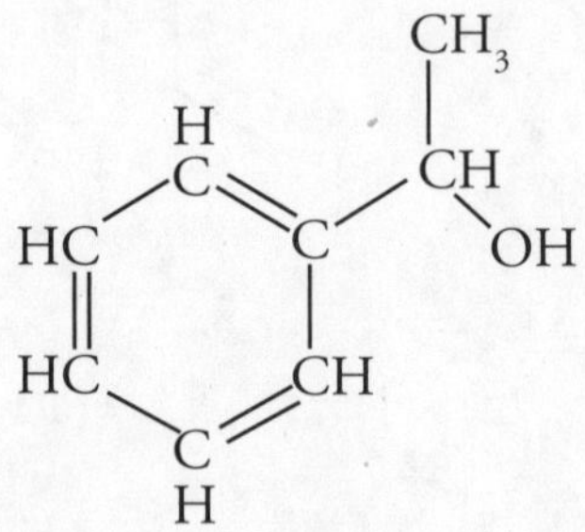

24.3 NOMENCLATURE OF ALKANES

Alkanes are named by a set of simple rules. One particular alkane (shown below) will be used to illustrate this process:

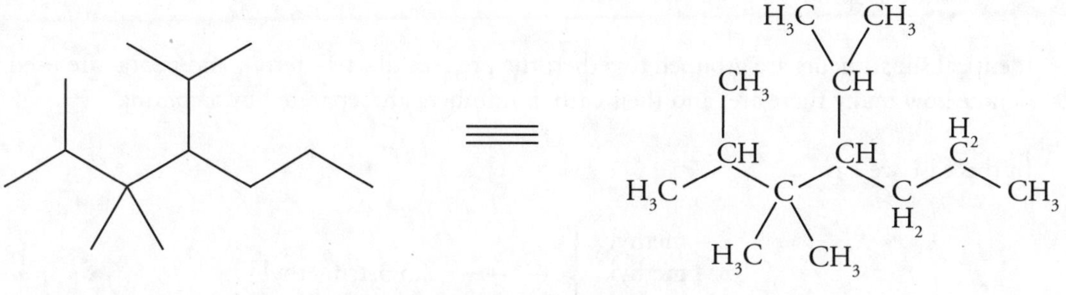

1. Identify the longest continuous carbon chain. The names of these chains are given in the first table in this chapter; go back there now if you need a refresher. If there are two possible chains of equal length, pick the one with more substituents.

   The longest chain in the compound above is a 7-carbon chain, which is called heptane. This chain is shown below, outlined by dashed lines.

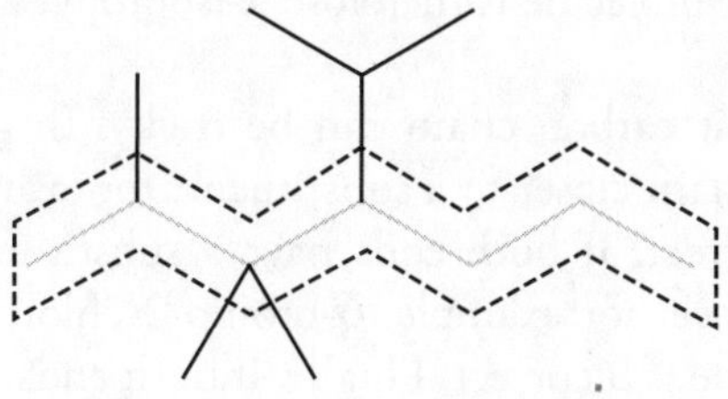

2. Identify any substituents on this chain. The names of some common hydrocarbon substituents are given in the second table in this chapter.

   There are four substituents in this example: three methyl groups and one isopropyl group.

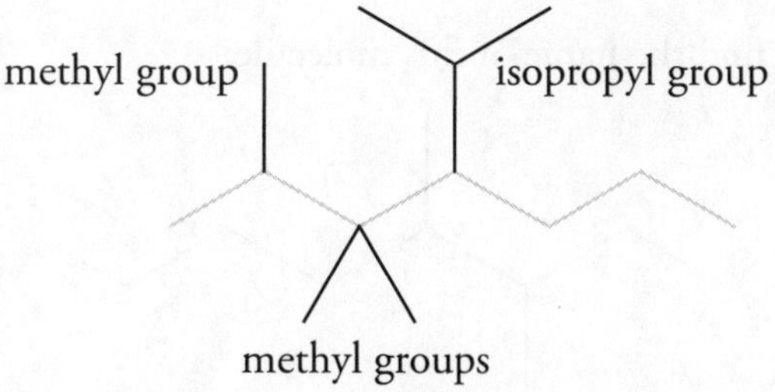

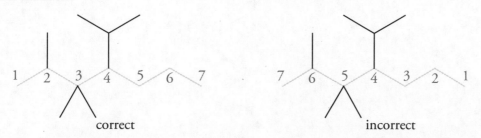

3. Number the carbons of the main chain such that the substituents are on the carbons with lower numbers.

Now each substituent can be associated with the carbon atom to which it's attached:

2 – methyl
3 – methyl
3 – methyl
4 – isopropyl

4.   Identical substituents are grouped together; the prefixes di-, tri-, tetra-, and penta- are used to denote how many there are, and their carbon numbers are separated by a comma.

In this case we have

2 – methyl
3 – methyl   ⟶   2,3,3-trimethyl
3 – methyl

5.   Alphabetize the substituents, ignoring the prefixes di-, tri-, etc. and *n*-, *sec*-, *tert*-, and separate numbers from words by a hyphen and numbers from numbers by a comma. Note that "iso" is not a prefix but is part of the substituent name, so it is NOT ignored when alphabetizing.

The complete name for our molecule is therefore 4-isopropyl-2,3,3-trimethylheptane.

Sometimes, numbering the longest carbon chain can be tricky. In general you should number carbon atoms starting at the end of the chain closer to a substituent; for example, 2,5-dimethyloctane is correct, while 4,7-dimethyloctane is incorrect. If both ends have a substituent of equal distance from the end, look for the next point of difference; for example, 6-bromo-2-chloro-3-methylheptane is correct, while 2-bromo-6-chloro-5-methylheptane is incorrect. Finally, if both ends have a different substituent of equal distance from the end and no other points of difference, use alphabetical order to determine priority; for example, 2-bromo-6-chloroheptane is correct because alphabetically, bromine comes before chlorine. Therefore, bromine is assigned the second carbon position, and chlorine is assigned the sixth carbon position. 6-bromo-2-chloroheptane is incorrect. Draw out each of the examples above to work through what each rule means and how you can use it on the DAT.

Let's do another example and find the name of this molecule:

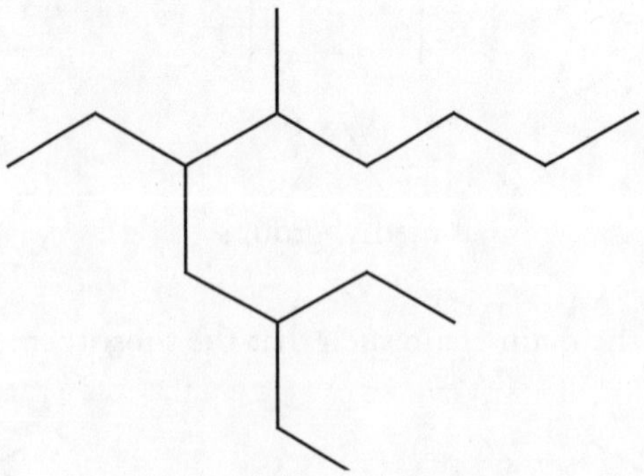

1. The longest continuous carbon chain is a 10-carbon chain, called decane.

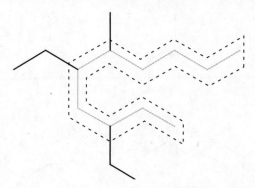

2. There are three substituents on this chain: two ethyl groups and a methyl group.

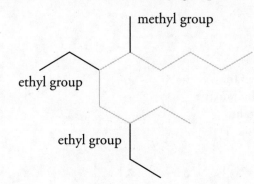

3. The correct numbering of the carbons in the main chain is as follows:

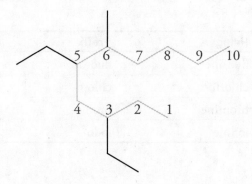

4. The substituents are now identified as:
    3,5-diethyl
    6-methyl

5. The complete name of the molecule is therefore 3,5-diethyl-6-methyldecane.

Example 24-3: Name each of the following alkanes:

(a)

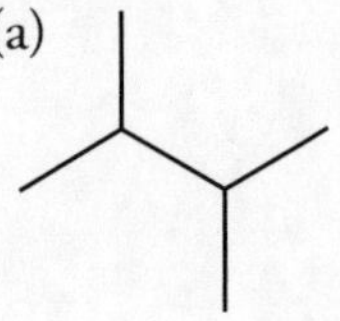

(b)

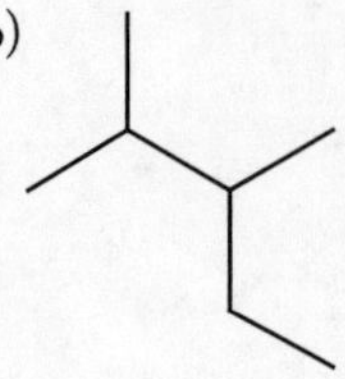

(c)

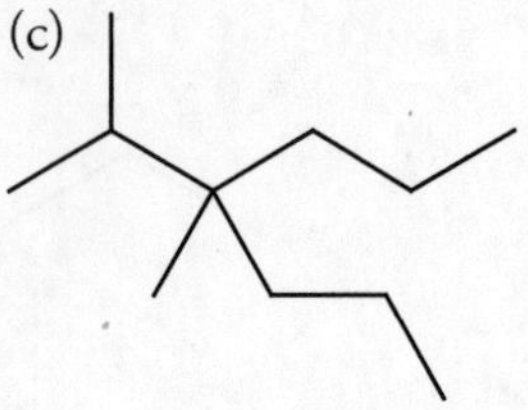

(d)

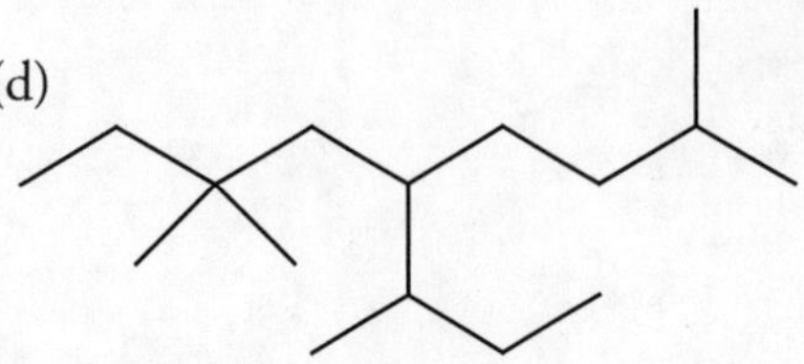

(e)

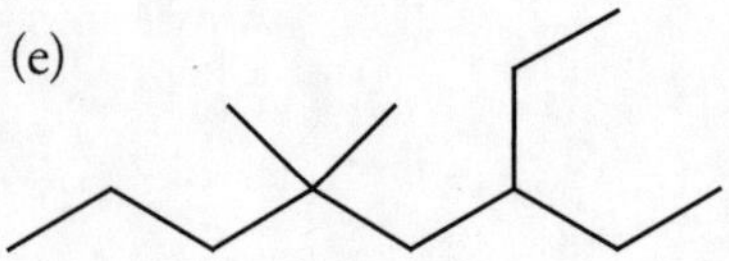

Solution:

A. 2,3-dimethylbutane
B. 2,3-dimethylpentane
C. 4-isopropyl-4-methylheptane
D. 5-*sec*-butyl-2,7,7-trimethylnonane
E. 3-ethyl-5,5-dimethyloctane

24.4 NOMENCLATURE OF HALOALKANES

Alkanes with halogen (F, Cl, Br, I) substituents follow the same set of rules as simple alkanes. Halogens are named using these prefixes:

Halogen	Prefix
fluorine	fluoro-
chlorine	chloro-
bromine	bromo-
iodine	iodo-

By applying the same rules as for naming simple alkanes, verify the following names:

Structure   Name

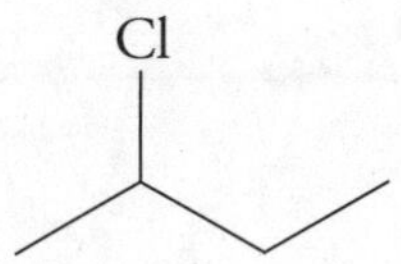

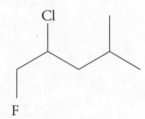

2-chlorobutane

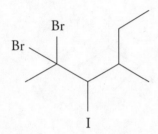

2-chloro-1-fluoro-4-methylpentane

2, 2-dibromo-3-iodo-4-methylhexane

Example 24-4: Name each of the following haloalkanes:

A.   B.

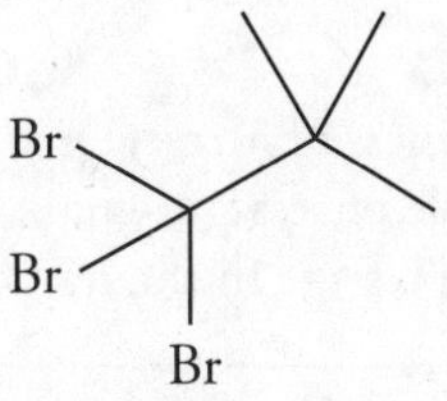

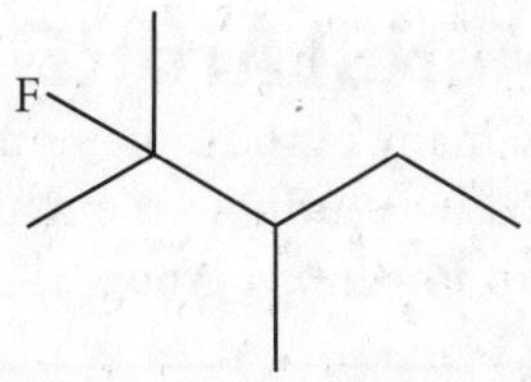

C. 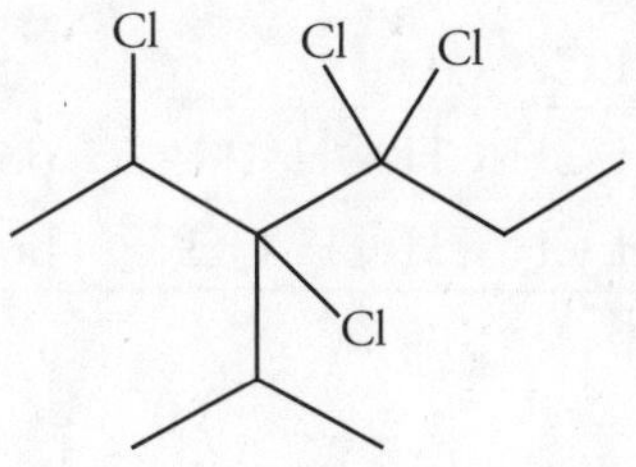   D.

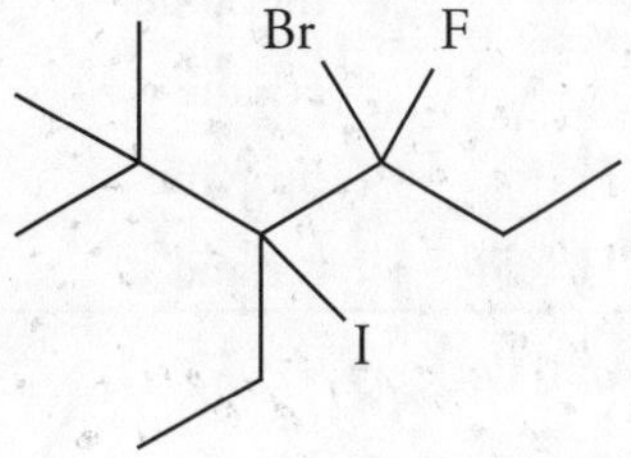

Solution:

A.   1,1,1-tribromo-2,2-dimethylpropane
B.   2-fluoro-2,3-dimethylpentane
C.   2,3,4,4-tetrachloro-3-isopropylhexane
D.   4-bromo-3-ethyl-4-fluoro-3-iodo-2,2-dimethylhexane

24.4

Example 24-5: For each name, draw the structure:

A.   3-chloro-2,2-dimethylbutane
B.   3-bromo-4-chloro-5,5-diethylnonane
C.   2,3-dibromo-1,1-diiodopropane
D.   3,4-difluoro-2,2,3-trimethylpentane

Solution:

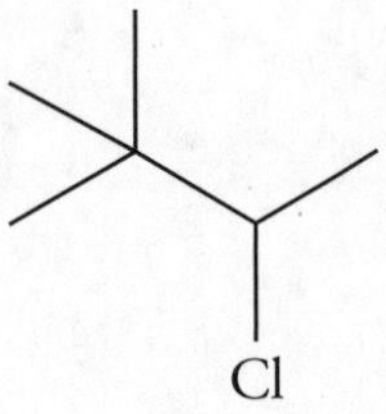

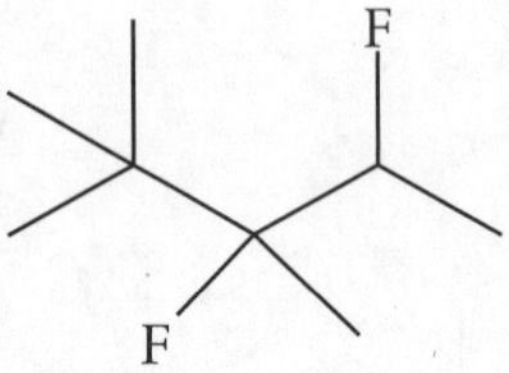

24.5   NOMENCLATURE OF ALCOHOLS

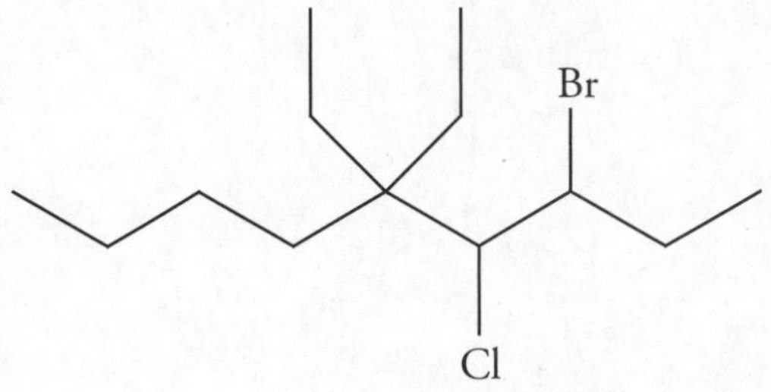

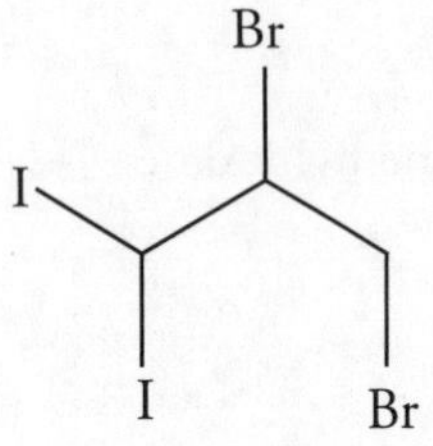

Alcohols also follow many of the same nomenclature rules as alkanes. **Hydroxyl groups** (–OH), however, are typically denoted by a suffix to the main alkyl chain. The table of straight-chain alcohols given below shows that to denote a hydroxyl group, the suffix –ol replaces the last –e in the name of the alkane.

Alkanes		Alcohols	
Structure	**Name**	**Structure**	**Name**
CH_4	methane	CH_3OH	methanol
CH_3CH_3	ethane	CH_3CH_2OH	ethanol
$CH_3CH_2CH_3$	propane	$CH_3CH_2CH_2OH$	propanol
$CH_3CH_2CH_2CH_3$	butane	$CH_3CH_2CH_2CH_2OH$	butanol

When the position of the hydroxyl group needs to be specified, the number is placed after the name of the longest carbon chain and before the –*ol* suffix, separated by hyphens. For example:

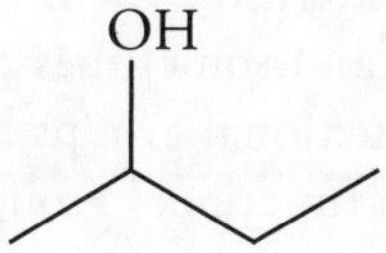

butan-2-ol
(or 2 butanol)
or *sec*-butanol

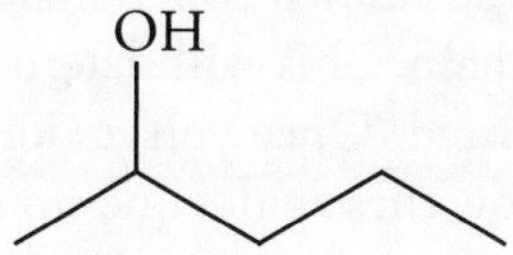

pentan-2-ol
(or 2-pentanol)

Priorities are assigned (the way the main carbon chain is numbered) to give the lowest number to the hydroxyl group. For example:

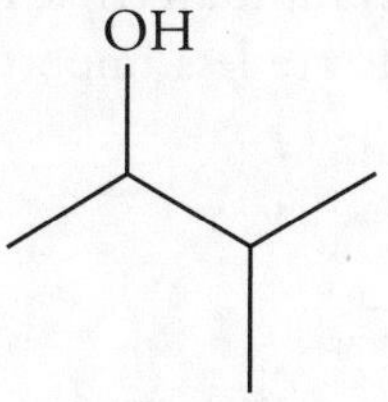

3-methylbutan-2-ol
not
2-methylbutan-3-ol

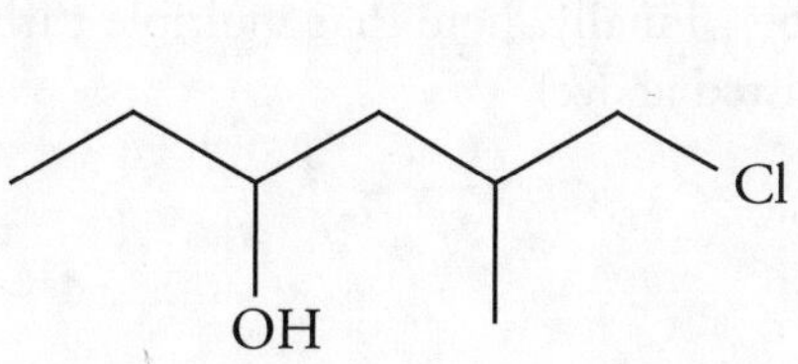

6-chloro-5-methylhexan-3-ol

Example 24-6: Name each of the following molecules:

A.

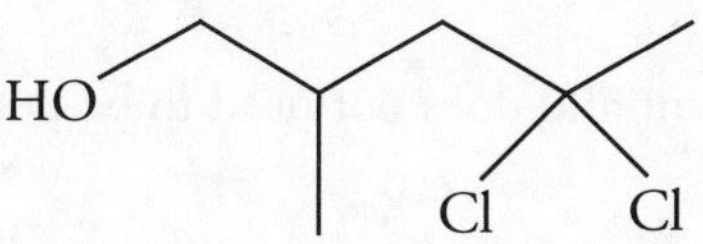

B.

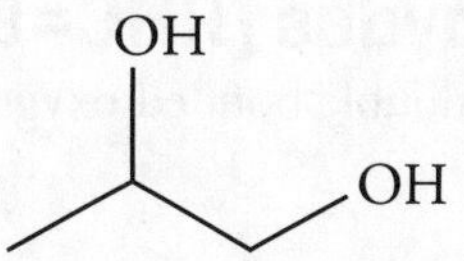

C.

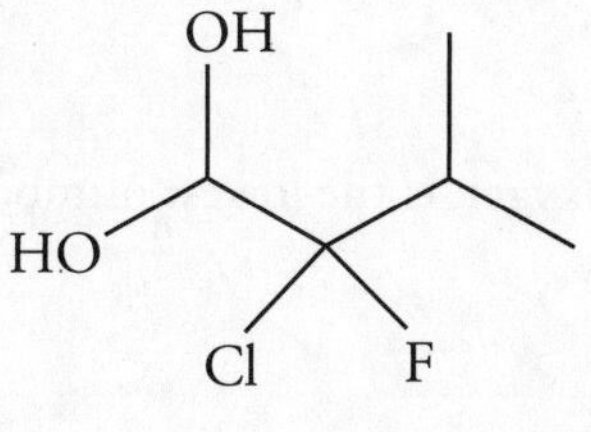

D.

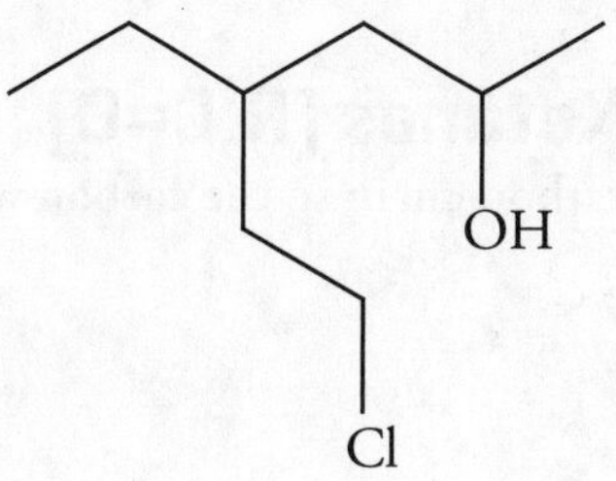

Solution:

A. 4,4-dichloro-2-methylpentanol (the "-1-" is assumed if no number is given)
B. propan-1,2-diol (or 1,2-propandiol)
C. 2-chloro-2-fluoro-3-methylbutan-1,1-diol
D. 6-chloro-4-ethylhexan-2-ol

24.6   ADDITIONAL FUNCTIONAL GROUPS

If a molecule contains additional functional groups, you must determine the most important functional group in the carbon chain. This will determine the base name and sometimes dictates how the carbon skeleton will be numbered. Once you've done this, all other functional groups and halogens are considered substituents. Follow these guidelines to determine the main functional group:

Carboxylic acid > Ester > Acid halide > Amide > Aldehyde > Ketone > Alcohol > Amine > C=C > C≡C

Naming Alkenes ($R_2C=CR_2$) and Alkynes ($RC≡CR$)

Number the carbon chain so the double/triple bond gets the lowest number. This numbering system must go through the double or triple bond. Double bonds are more important than triple bonds and should get the lower number. Finally, note that multiple carbon-carbon bonds are less important than other functional groups (listed above).

Naming Ethers (R–O–R')

There are two options on how to name these. First, you can name the two alkyl groups in alphabetical order and add the word "ether." The other option is to choose the longest R-group as the principal chain, number the other R-group, and name an "alkoxy."

Naming Aldehydes (RHC=O)

The carbon with the double bonded oxygen is C1 by default and does not need to be numbered. Add the suffix "al."

Naming Ketones ($R_2C=O$)

Number the carbon chain so the carbon with double-bonded oxygen is the lowest number. Add the suffix "one."

Naming Carboxylic Acids (RCOOH)

The carbon with the double-bonded oxygen is C1 by default and does not need to be numbered. Add the suffix "oic acid."

Naming Esters (RCOOR')

Esters are alkyl derivatives of carboxylic acids. A complete ester name is a version of alkyl alkanoate. The easiest way to deal with naming esters is to recognize the carboxylic acid and the alcohol they can be prepared from. For example, the general ester RCO_2R' can be derived from the carboxylic acid RCO_2H and the alcohol HOR'. The first component of an ester name (the alkyl) is derived from the alcohol, R'OH. The second component of an ester name (the "oate") is derived from the carboxylic acid, RCO_2H. As above, since the carboxylic acid group is at the end of the chain, it must be C1.

Example 24-7: Name each of the following molecules. You may want to start by drawing each structure out in longer form.

24.6

A. $CH_3CH(Cl)CH(Cl)C(CH_3)_2CH_2CH(C_2H_5)CH_2CH_3$
B. $C_6H_{11}Br$
C. $CH_3C(CH_3)CBrCCCH_2CH_3$
D. $CH_3CH_2C(C_2H_5)_2CH(OH)CH_3$
E. $C(CH_3)_3OC_2H_5$
F. $CH_3CHC(CH_3)ClCHO$
G. $CH_3COCHCHCH_2F$
H. CH_3COOH
I. $CH_3CH(OCH_3)CH(CH[CH_3]_2)CCCOOH$
J. $CH_3CH_2COOCH_3$
K. $CH_3CH_2CH_2COOCH(CH_3)_2$

Solution:

A. 2,3-dichloro-6-ethyl-4,4-dimethyloctane
B. Bromocyclohexane
C. 3-bromo-2-methylhept-2-ene-4-yne
D. 3,3-diethylpent-2-ol
E. *tert*-butyl ethyl ether or 1-ethoxy-1,1-dimethyl ethane
F. 2-chloro-2-methylbutanal
G. 5-fluoro-pent-3-ene-2-one
H. Ethanoic acid
I. 5-methoxy-4-isopropyl-hex-2-ynoic acid
J. Methyl propanoate
K. Isopropyl butanoate

Chapter 25
Structure and Bonding

25.1 BONDING IN ORGANIC MOLECULES

The chemistry of organic molecules is dominated by the reactivity of covalent bonds. An understanding of the fundamentals of covalent bonding can provide the intuitive grasp necessary to answer a wide range of questions in organic chemistry. This chapter will briefly outline the basic principles that must be mastered in order to successfully complete organic chemistry passages on the DAT. These include hybridization, sigma (σ) bonding, pi (π) bonding, structural formulas, electron delocalization, resonance stabilization, bond length, bond energy, isomerism, chirality, and optical activity.

Hybridization

In order to rationalize observed chemical and structural trends, chemists developed the concept of orbital hybridization. In this model, one imagines a mathematical combination of atomic orbitals centered on the same atom to produce a set of composite, **hybrid** orbitals. For example, consider an s and a p orbital on an atom.

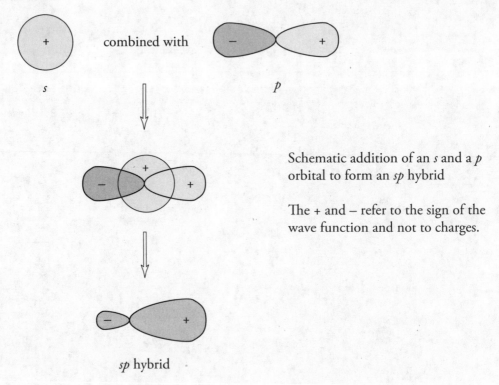

Schematic addition of an s and a p orbital to form an sp hybrid

The + and − refer to the sign of the wave function and not to charges.

Notice that the new orbital is highly directional; this allows for better overlap when bonding.

There will be two such sp hybrid orbitals formed because two orbitals (the s and the p) were originally combined; that is, the total number of orbitals is conserved in the formation of hybrid orbitals. For this reason, the number of hybrid orbitals on a given atom of hybridization sp^x is $1 + x$ (1 for the s, x for the p's), where x may be either 1, 2, or 3.

The percentages of the *s* character and *p* character in a given sp^x hybrid orbital are listed below:

sp^x hybrid orbital	s character	p character
sp	50%	50%
sp^2	33%	67%
sp^3	25%	75%

To determine the hybridization for most atoms in simple organic molecules, add the number of attached atoms to the number of non-bonding electron pairs (non-delocalized) and use the brief table below (which also gives the ideal bond angles and molecular geometry). The number of attached atoms plus the number of lone pairs is equal to the number of orbitals combined to make the new hybridized orbitals.

# of attached atoms + # of lone pairs	Hybridization	Bond Angles (ideal)	Molecular Geometry
2	sp	180°	linear
3	sp^2	120°	trigonal planar
4	sp^3	109.5°	tetrahedral

sp hybridization:

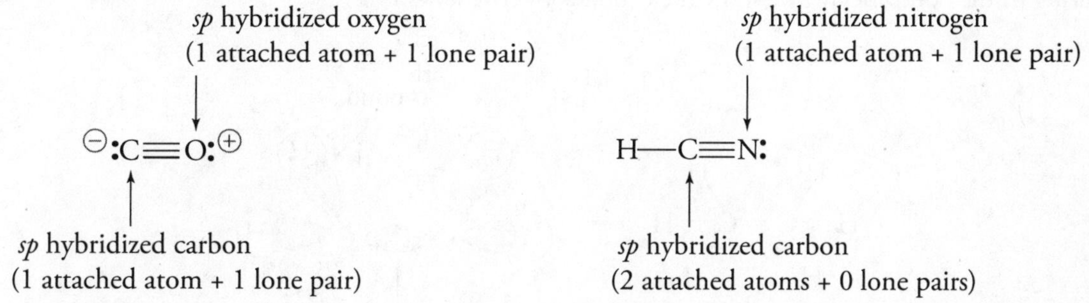

sp hybridized oxygen
(1 attached atom + 1 lone pair)

sp hybridized nitrogen
(1 attached atom + 1 lone pair)

$$^{\ominus}:C \equiv O:^{\oplus}$$

$$H - C \equiv N:$$

sp hybridized carbon
(1 attached atom + 1 lone pair)

sp hybridized carbon
(2 attached atoms + 0 lone pairs)

sp² hybridization:

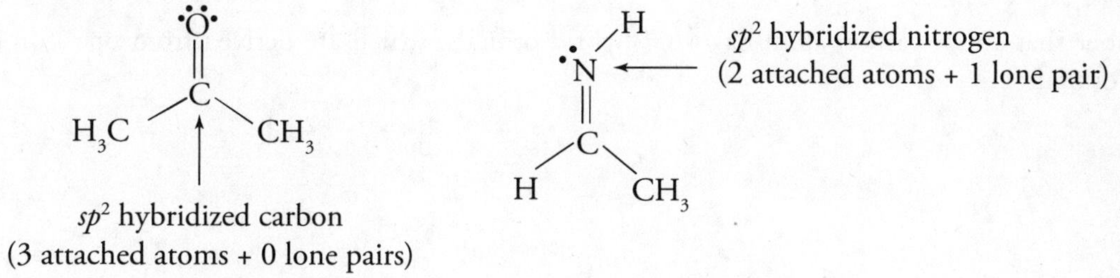

sp² hybridized nitrogen
(2 attached atoms + 1 lone pair)

sp² hybridized carbon
(3 attached atoms + 0 lone pairs)

sp^3 hybridization:

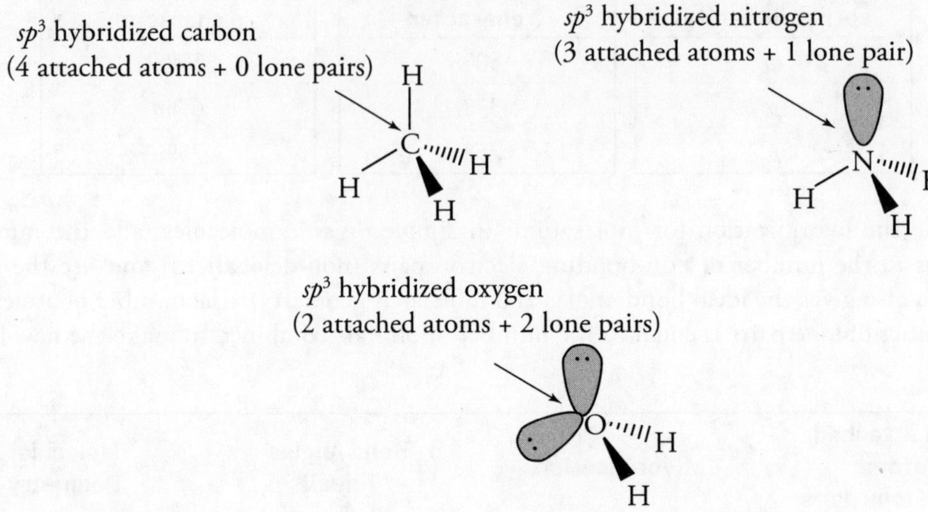

sp^3 hybridized carbon
(4 attached atoms + 0 lone pairs)

sp^3 hybridized nitrogen
(3 attached atoms + 1 lone pair)

sp^3 hybridized oxygen
(2 attached atoms + 2 lone pairs)

Sigma (σ) Bonds

A σ **bond** consists of two electrons that are localized between two nuclei. It is formed by the end-to-end overlap of one hybridized orbital (or an *s* orbital in the case of hydrogen) from each of the two atoms participating in the bond. Below, we show the σ bonds in ethane, C_2H_6:

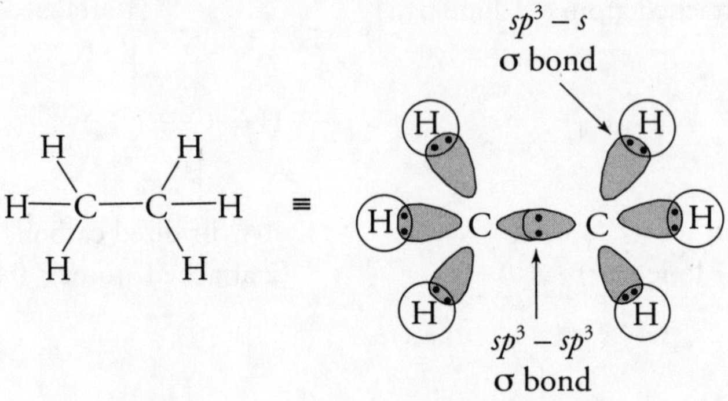

$sp^3 - s$
σ bond

$sp^3 - sp^3$
σ bond

Remember that an sp^3 carbon atom has 4 sp^3 hybrid orbitals, which are derived from one *s* orbital and three *p* orbitals.

Example 25-1: Label the hybridization of the orbitals comprising the σ bonds in the molecules shown below:

A.

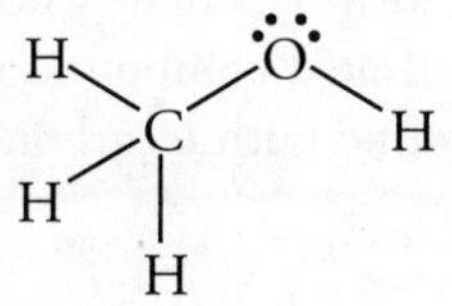

B.

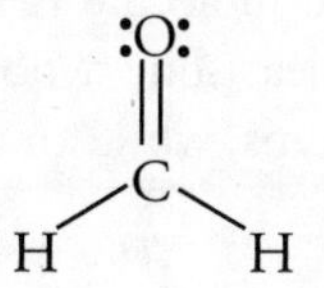

C.

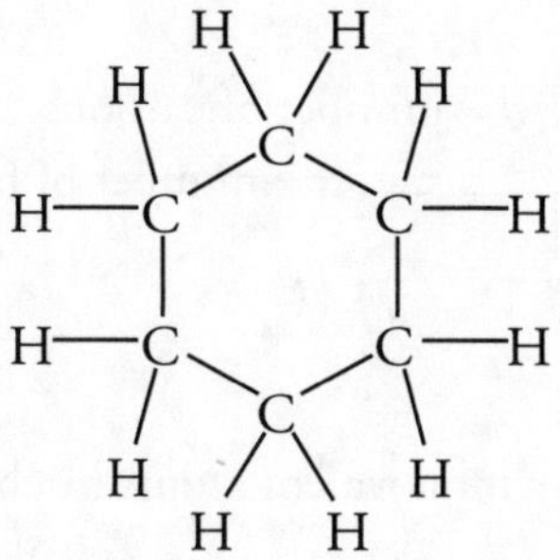

D.

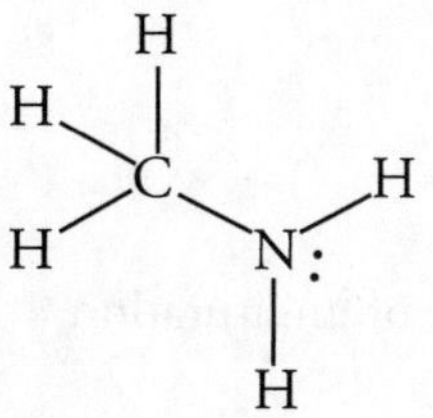

Solution:

A. Bonds to H are sp^3-s σ bonds. The C–O bond is an sp^3-sp^3 σ bond.
B. The bonds to H are sp^2-s σ bonds. The C=O bond contains an sp^2-sp^2 σ bond. (It's also composed of a π bond, which we'll discuss in the next section.)
C. All C–C bonds are sp^3-sp^3 σ bonds, while all C–H bonds are sp^3-s σ bonds.
D. All bonds to H are sp^3-s σ bonds. The C–N bond is an sp^3-sp^3 σ bond.

Pi (π) Bonds

A π **bond** is composed of two electrons that are localized to the region that lies on opposite sides of the plane formed by the two bonded nuclei and immediately adjacent atoms, not directly between the two nuclei as with a σ bond. A π bond is formed by the proper, parallel, side-to-side alignment of two unhybridized p orbitals on adjacent atoms. (An sp^2 hybridized atom has three sp^2 orbitals—which come from one s and two p orbitals—plus one p orbital that remains unhybridized.) Below, we show the π bonds in ethene, C_2H_4:

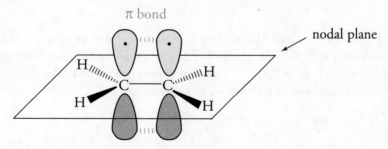

In any multiple bond, there is only one σ bond; the remainder are π bonds. Therefore:

a single bond: composed of 1 σ bond
a double bond: composed of 1 σ bond and 1 π bond
a triple bond: composed of 1 σ bond and 2 π bonds

25.2 STRUCTURAL FORMULAS

By definition, an organic molecule is said to be **saturated** if it contains no π bonds and no rings; it is **unsaturated** if it has at least one π bond or a ring. A saturated compound with n carbon atoms has exactly $2n + 2$ hydrogen atoms, while an unsaturated compound with n carbon atoms has fewer than $2n + 2$ hydrogens.

The formula below is used to determine the **degree of unsaturation** (d) of simple organic molecules:

$$\text{degree of unsaturation} = \frac{(2n + 2) - x}{2}$$

n = number of carbons
x = number of hydrogens

- x represents the number of hydrogens and any monovalent atoms (such as the halogens: F, Cl, Br, or I).
- Since the number of oxygens has no effect, it is generally ignored.
- For nitrogen-containing compounds, replace each N by 1 C and 1 H when using this formula.

One degree of unsaturation indicates the presence of one π bond or one ring; two degrees of unsaturation means there are two π bonds (two separate double bonds or one triple bond), or one π bond and one ring, or two rings, and so on. The presence of heteroatoms can also affect the degree of unsaturation in a molecule. This is best illustrated through a series of related molecules that all have one degree of unsaturation.

Butene (C_4H_8) has one degree of unsaturation, since $d = [(2 \cdot 4 + 2) - 8]/2 = 1$, in the form of a double bond:

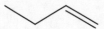

4-Chlorobutene (C_4H_7Cl) also has one degree of unsaturation, but the number of hydrogens is different. Each halogen atom (fluorine, chlorine, bromine, iodine) or other monovalent atom "replaces" one hydrogen atom, so $d = [(2 \cdot 4 + 2) - (7 + 1)]/2 = 1$:

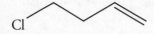

Methoxyethene (C_3H_6O) also has one degree of unsaturation. Each oxygen (or other divalent atom) "replaces" one carbon and two hydrogen atoms (CH_2 groups are sometimes referred to as methylene groups), so $d = [(2(3 + 1) + 2) - (6 + 2)]/2 = 1$. Since a divalent atom can take the place of a methylene group, it doesn't affect the degree of unsaturation, and can be ignored.

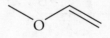

Methyl vinyl amine (C_3H_7N) has one degree of unsaturation as well. Each nitrogen (or other trivalent atom) "replaces" one carbon and one hydrogen atom. The formula thus gives $d = [(2(3 + 1) + 2)-(7 + 1)]/2 = 1$:

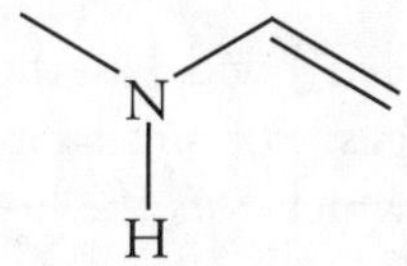

Example 25-2: Determine the degree of unsaturation of each of these molecules. Which, if any, are saturated?

A. C_6H_8
B. C_4H_6O
C. $C_{20}H_{30}O$
D. C_3H_8O
E. C_3H_5Br

Solution:

A. $d = [(2{\cdot}6 + 2)-8]/2 = 3$.
B. Ignore the oxygen atom; $d = [(2{\cdot}4 + 2)-6]/2 = 2$.
C. Ignore the oxygen atom; $d = [(2{\cdot}20 + 2)-30]/2 = 6$.
D. Ignore the oxygen atom; $d = [(2{\cdot}3 + 2)-8]/2 = 0$. This molecule is saturated.
E. Since Br is a halogen, we treat it like a hydrogen, so $d = [(2{\cdot}3 + 2)-(5 + 1)]/2 = 1$.

25.3 BOND LENGTH AND BOND DISSOCIATION ENERGY

While the term **bond length** makes good intuitive sense (the distance between two nuclei that are bonded to one another), **bond dissociation energy (BDE)** is not quite as intuitive. Bond dissociation energy is the energy required to break a bond homolytically. In **homolytic bond cleavage**, one electron of the bond being broken goes to each fragment of the molecule. In this process two radicals form. This is *not* the same thing as **heterolytic bond cleavage** (also known as **dissociation**). In heterolytic bond cleavage, both electrons of the electron pair that make up the bond end up on the same atom; this forms both a cation and an anion.

$$(H_3C)_3C — H \longrightarrow C(CH_3)_3^{\bullet} + H^{\bullet}$$

homolytic bond cleavage

$$(H_3C)_3C — Cl \longrightarrow C(CH_3)_3^{\oplus} + Cl^{\ominus}$$

heterolytic bond cleavage

These two processes are very different and hence have very different energies associated with them. Here, we will only consider homolytic bond dissociation energies.

When one examines the relationship between bond length and bond dissociation energy for a series of similar bonds, an important trend emerges: For similar bonds, *the higher the bond order, the shorter and stronger the bond.* The following table, which lists the bond dissociation energies (BDE, in kcal/mol) and the bond lengths (r, in angstroms, where 1 Å = 10^{-10} m) for carbon-carbon and carbon-oxygen bonds, illustrates this trend:

	C–C	C=C	C≡C	C–O	C=O	C≡O
BDE	83	144	200	86	191	256
r (in Å)	1.54	1.34	1.20	1.43	1.20	1.13

An important caveat arises because of the varying atomic radii: *bond length/BDE comparisons should only be made for <u>similar</u> bonds.* Thus, carbon-carbon bonds should be compared only to other carbon-carbon bonds; carbon-oxygen bonds should be compared only to other carbon-oxygen bonds, and so on.

Recall the shapes of unhybridized atomic orbitals: *s* orbitals are spherical about the atomic nucleus, while *p* orbitals are elongated "dumbbell"-shaped about the atomic nucleus.

s orbital ⬤   𝟾 p orbital

When comparing the same type of bonds, the greater the *s* character in the component orbitals, the shorter the bond (because *s* orbitals are closer to the nucleus than *p* orbitals). A greater percentage of *p* character also leads to a more directional hybrid orbital that is farther from the nucleus and thus a longer bond. In addition, when comparing the same types of bonds, *the longer the bond, the weaker it is; the shorter the bond, the stronger it is.* In the following diagram, compare all the C–C bonds and all the C–H bonds:

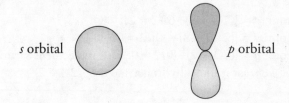

Bond	Bond length	Bond	Bond length
C–C (*sp – sp*)	1.21 Å	C–H (*sp – s*)	1.06 Å
C–C (*sp – sp³*)	1.46 Å	C–H (*sp³ – s*)	1.10 Å

25.4   ISOMERISM

Constitutional Isomerism

Constitutional (or, less precisely, *structural*) **isomers** are compounds that have the same molecular formula but whose atoms are connected together differently. Take pentane (C_5H_{12}), for example. *n*-pentane is a fully-saturated hydrocarbon that has two additional constitutional isomers:

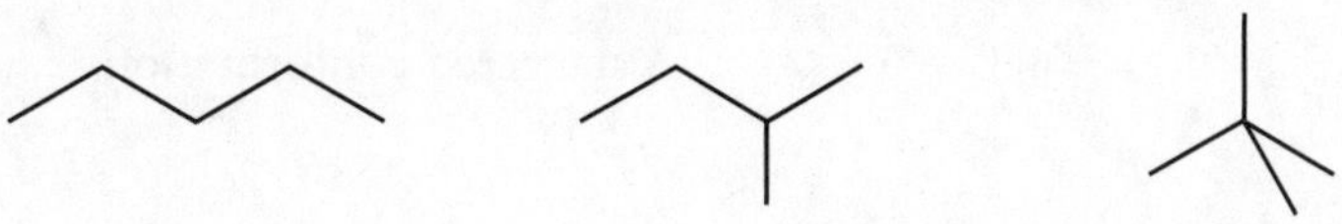

n-pentane   Isopentane   Neopentane

Example 25-3: Draw (and name) all the constitutional isomers of hexane, C_6H_{14}. (*Hint*: There are five of them altogether.)

Solution:

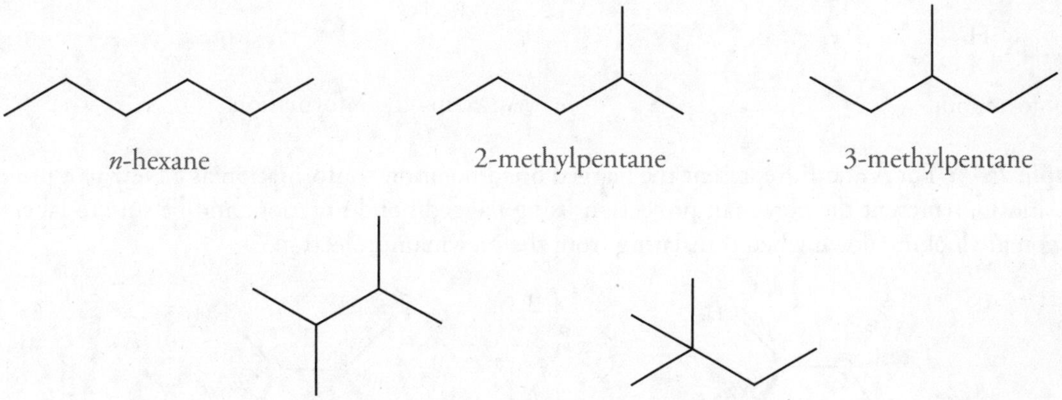

n-hexane   2-methylpentane   3-methylpentane

2, 3-dimethylbutane   2, 2-dimethylbutane

Conformational Isomerism

Conformational isomers are compounds that have the same molecular formula and the same atomic connectivity, but which differ from one another by rotation about a (single) σ bond. In truth, they are the exact same molecule. For saturated hydrocarbons there are two orientations of σ bonds attached to adjacent sp^3 hybridized carbons on which we will concentrate. These are the **staggered** conformation and the **eclipsed** conformation. In staggered conformations a σ bond on one carbon bisects the angle formed by two σ bonds on the adjacent carbon. In an eclipsed conformation a σ bond on one carbon directly lines up with a σ bond on an adjacent carbon. Both conformations can be visualized using either the flagged bond notation, or the Newman projection, as shown with ethane (C_2H_6) below.

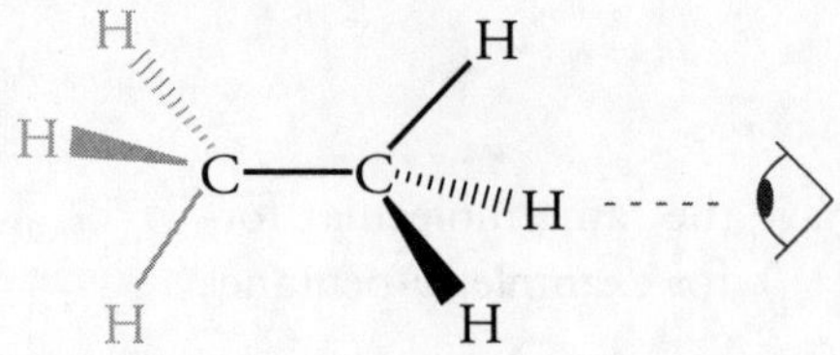

25.4

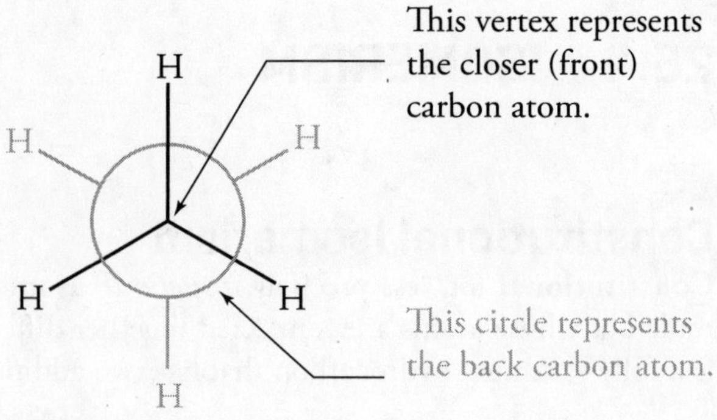

This vertex represents the closer (front) carbon atom.

If we were to look down the C–C bond from the left, we would see:

This circle represents the back carbon atom.

A staggered conformation

A staggered conformation

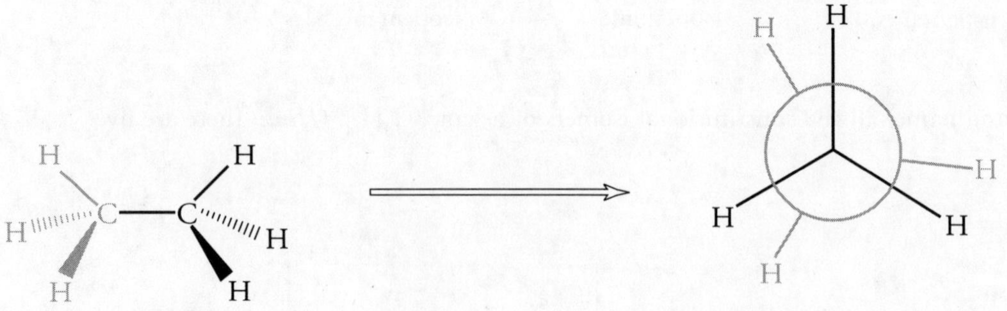

An eclipsed conformation

An eclipsed conformation

Example 25-4: For A and B, represent the flagged bond notation conformation as a Newman projection. For C and D, represent the Newman projection using flagged bond notation, and be sure to label which bond you are looking down when translating from the Newman projection.

A.

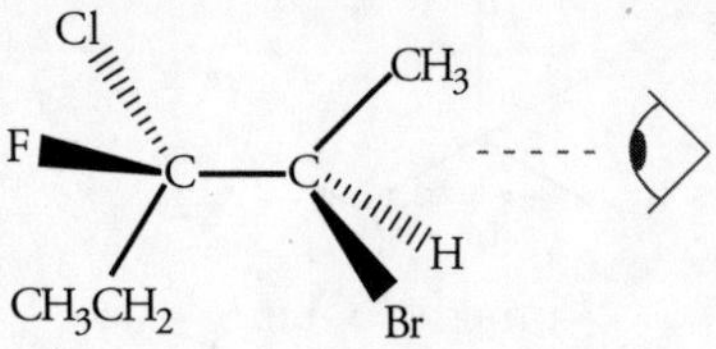

B.

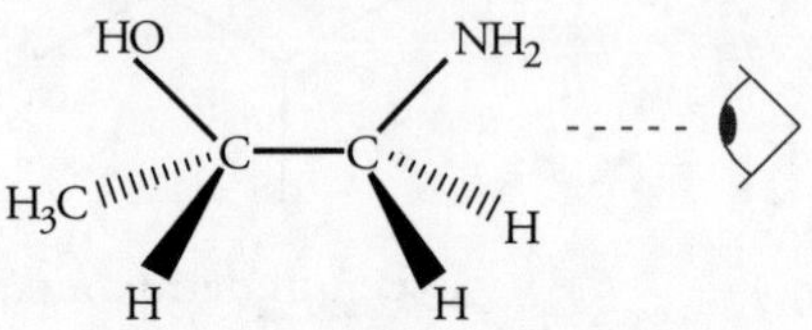

C.

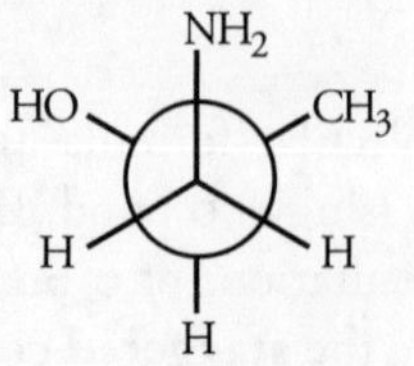

D.

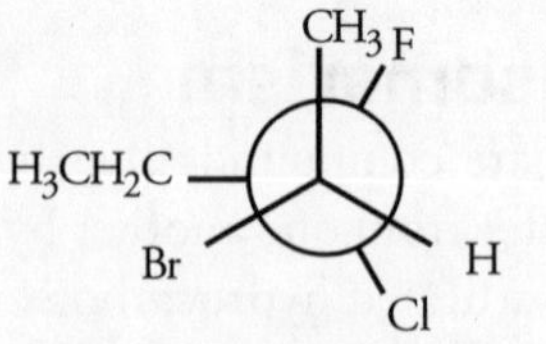

Solution:

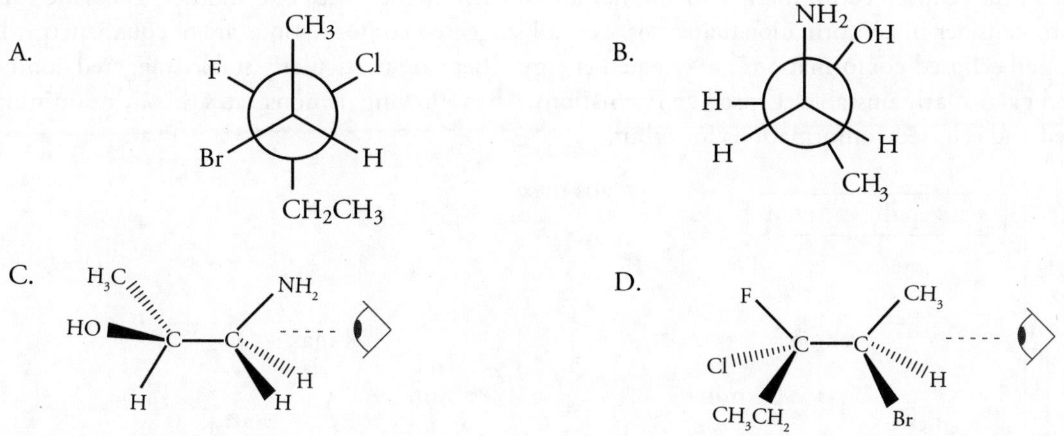

A.

B.

C.

D.

Using these notations, we turn our attention to the conformational analysis of hydrocarbons as demonstrated for *n*-butane.

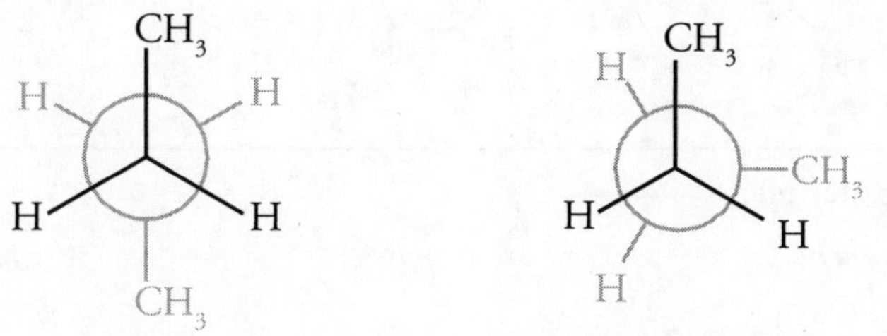

staggered conformation

less crowded
more stable

eclipsed conformation

more crowded
electronic repulsion
less stable

The σ bonds should
actually directly
line up with each other.
For clarity here,
they are not
directly aligned.

It's important to note, however, that there are an infinite number of conformations for a molecule that has free rotation around a C–C bond, and that all of these other conformations are energetically related to the staggered and eclipsed conformations on which we will concentrate. For example, relative to the carbon atom in the rear of a Newman projection, the front carbon atom could be rotated any number of degrees. Any change in the rotation of one carbon, relative to its adjacent neighbor, is a change in molecular conformation.

What are the relative stabilities of the staggered conformations, the eclipsed conformations, and the infinite number of conformations that are in between them? A staggered conformation is more stable than an eclipsed conformation for two reasons. First, the staggered conformation is more stable than the eclipsed conformation because of electronic repulsion. Covalent bonds repel one another simply because they are composed of (negatively charged) electrons. That being the case, the staggered conformation is more stable than the eclipsed, since in the staggered conformation, the σ bonds are as far apart as possible, while in the eclipsed conformation they are directly aligned with one another. The other major reason the staggered conformation is more stable than the eclipsed conformation is steric hindrance. It is more favorable to have atoms attached to the σ bonds in the roomier staggered conformation where they are 60° apart, rather than the eclipsed conformation where they are directly aligned with one another. There are further aspects to consider in conformational analysis. Not all staggered conformations are of equal energy. Likewise, not all eclipsed conformations are of equal energy. There are particularly stable staggered conformations and particularly unstable eclipsed conformations. The following demonstrates this by examining all staggered and eclipsed conformations for *n*-butane.

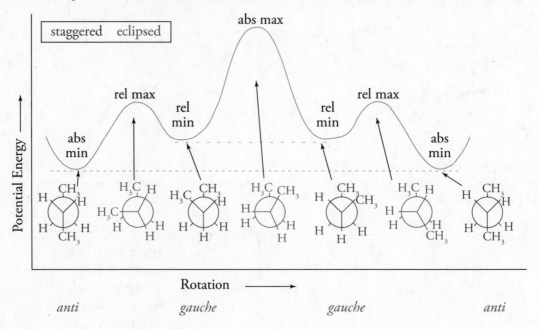

We begin our discussion with the most stable conformation of *n*-butane. This staggered conformation is referred to as the ***anti* conformation** and arises when the two largest groups attached to adjacent carbons are 180° apart. This produces the most sterically favorable, and hence the most energetically favorable (lowest energy) conformation. Now we proceed through a series of 60° rotations around the C2–C3 σ bond until we return to the initial conformation (360°). In our first rotation, we go from the *anti* staggered to an eclipsed conformation and observe the relative energy maximum that results from the alignment of the methyls and hydrogens. Next, as we rotate another 60°, we fall again into a staggered conformation that resides in a relative energy minimum. Notice that this energy minimum is not as low as the *anti* conformation. In this structure the methyl substituents are closer together than in the *anti* conformation. They are now 60° apart; this is referred to as a ***gauche* conformation**. A *gauche* conformation arises when the two largest groups on adjacent carbon atoms are in a staggered conformation 60° apart. In our next 60° rotation we travel to the absolute maximum on our potential energy diagram. In this eclipsed conformation, the two methyl groups are directly aligned behind one another and are therefore in the most crowded and unfavorable environment. As we continue our rotation, we fall from the absolute energy maximum and go through the corresponding staggered and eclipsed conformations encountered before.

Example 25-5: Draw a Newman projection for the most stable conformation of each of these compounds:

A. 2,2,5,5-tetramethylhexane (about the C3–C4 bond)
B. 2,2-dimethylpentane (about the C2–C3 bond)
C. 1,2-ethandiol

Solution:

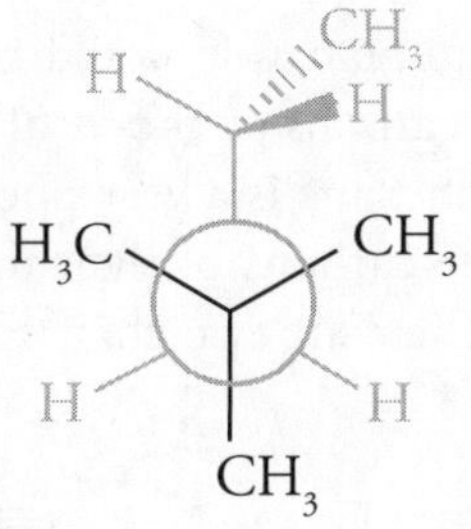

C. In this molecule, the *gauche* conformation is more stable than the *anti* conformation, because an intramolecular hydrogen bond can be formed in the *gauche* but not in the *anti* conformation.

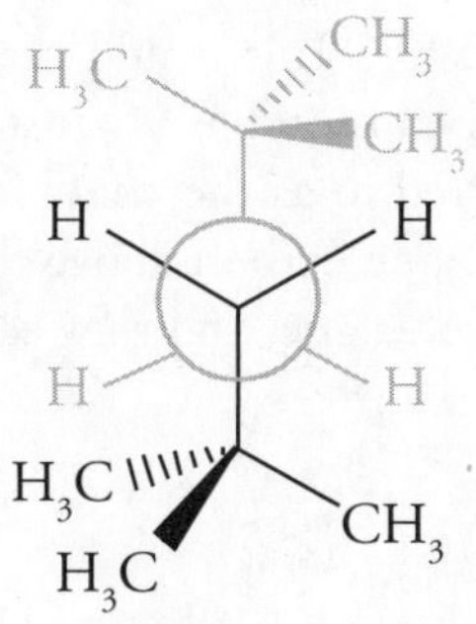

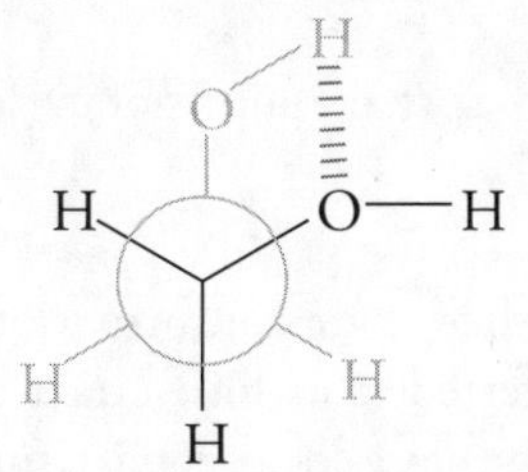

Remember that it's usually the case that the *anti* conformation is the more stable. In general, the two largest groups on adjacent carbon atoms would like to be *anti* to one another since this will minimize steric interactions. However, if the two groups are not too large and can form intramolecular hydrogen bonds with one another, then the *gauche* conformation can be more stable.

Thus far we've limited our discussion of conformational isomers to molecules with unrestricted rotation around σ bonds. Let's now consider the conformational analysis of two very common cycloalkanes, cyclopentane (C_5H_{10}) and cyclohexane (C_6H_{12}).

In cyclopentane, the pentagonal bond angle is 108° (close to normal tetrahedral of 109°), so we might expect cyclopentane to be a planar structure. If all of the carbons of cyclopentane were in a plane, however, all of the carbon-hydrogen σ bonds on adjacent carbons would eclipse each other. In order to compensate for the eclipsed C–H σ bonds, cyclopentane has one carbon out of the plane of the other carbons and so adopts a puckered conformation. This puckering allows the carbon-hydrogen σ bonds on adjacent carbons to be somewhat staggered, and thus reduces the energy of the compound. This puckered form of cyclopentane is referred to as the "envelope" form.

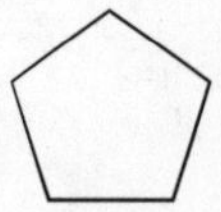

Cyclopentane

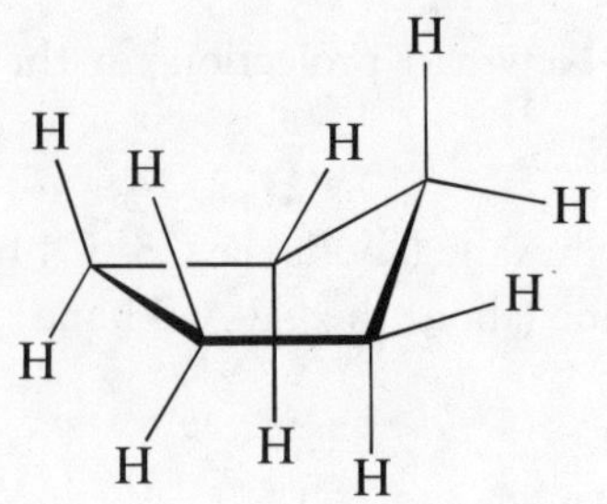

If cyclohexane were planar, it would have bond angles of 120°. This would produce considerable strain on *sp³* hybridized carbons as the ideal bond angle should be around 109°. Instead, the most stable conformation of cyclohexane is a very puckered molecule referred to as the **chair form**. In the chair conformation, four of the carbons of the ring are in a plane with one carbon above the plane and one carbon below the plane. There are two chair conformations for cyclohexane, and they easily interconvert at room temperature:

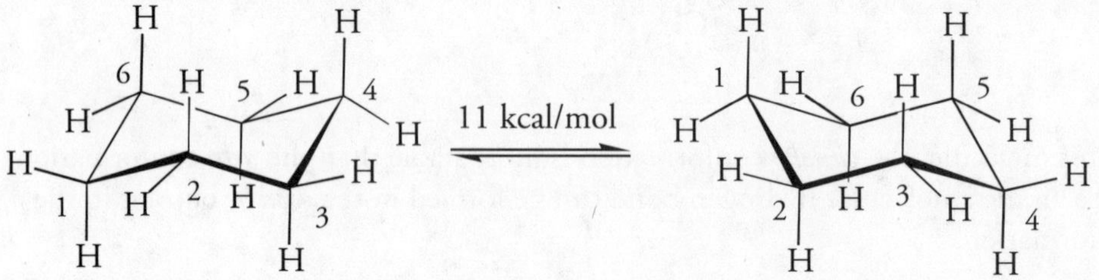

Chair representations of cyclohexane

As one chair conformation flips to the other chair conformation, it must pass through several other less stable conformations including some (referred to as **half-chair** conformations) that reside at energy maxima and one (the **twist boat** conformation) at a local energy minimum (but still of much higher energy than the chair conformations). The **boat** conformation represents a transition state between twist boat conformations. It is important to remember, however, that all of these conformations are much more unstable than the chair conformations and thus do not play an important role in cyclohexane chemistry.

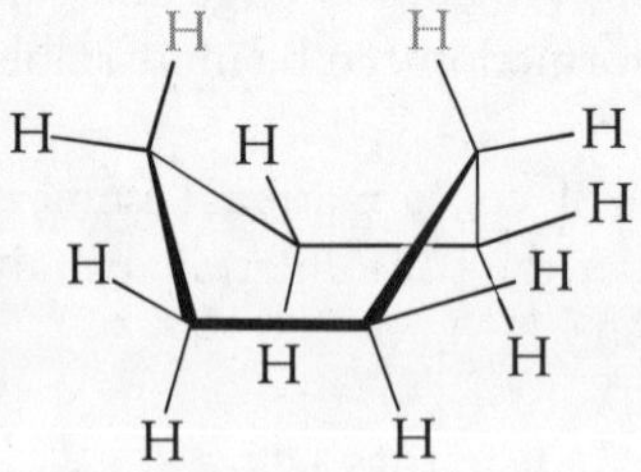

Boat conformation

Notice that there are two distinct types of hydrogens in the chair forms of cyclohexane. Six of the hydrogens lie on the equator of the ring of carbons. These hydrogens are referred to as **equatorial** hydrogens. The other six hydrogens lie above or below the ring of carbons, three above and three below; these are called **axial** hydrogens.

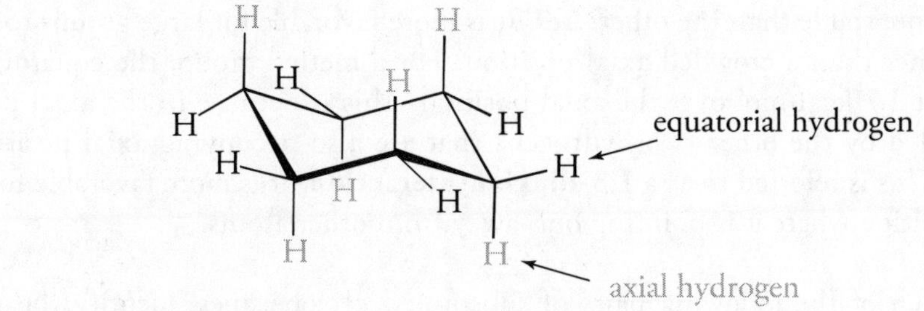

There is an energy barrier of about 11 kcal/mol between the two equivalent chair conformations of cyclo-hexane. At room temperature there is sufficient thermal energy to inter-convert the two chair conforma-tions about 10,000 times per second. Note that when a hydrogen (or any substituent group) is axial in one chair conformation, it becomes equatorial when cyclohexane flips to the other chair conformation. The same is also true for an equatorial hydrogen which flips to an axial position when the chair forms inter-convert. This property is demonstrated for deuterocyclohexane:

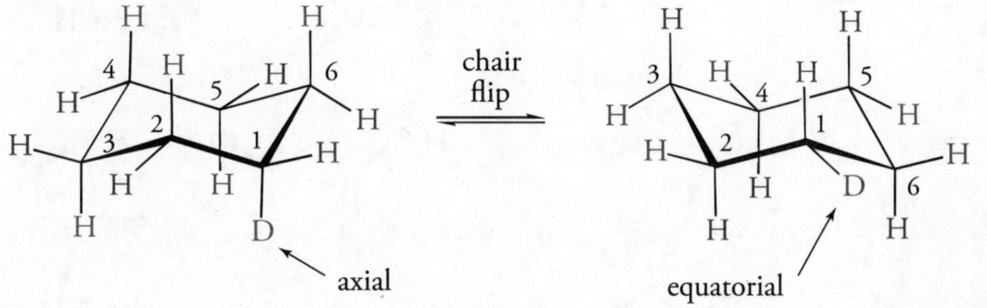

Also notice that each carbon has a bond on the top or above the other bond. For example, C1 on the left (above) has a hydrogen in the top/up position and a deuterium in the bottom/down position. Just like the axial position alternates up and down around a cyclohexane ring, so does which bond is on the top and which is on the bottom. In other words, for the molecule on the left above, the axial bond is on the top for carbons 2, 4, and 6. The axial bond is on the bottom for carbons 1, 3, and 5. When drawn in wedge/dash form, wedge bonds are pointing up and go in the top position. Dashed bonds are pointing down and go in the bottom position. These factors become important when examining substituted cyclohexanes. Let's first consider methylcyclohexane. The methyl group can occupy either an equatorial or axial position:

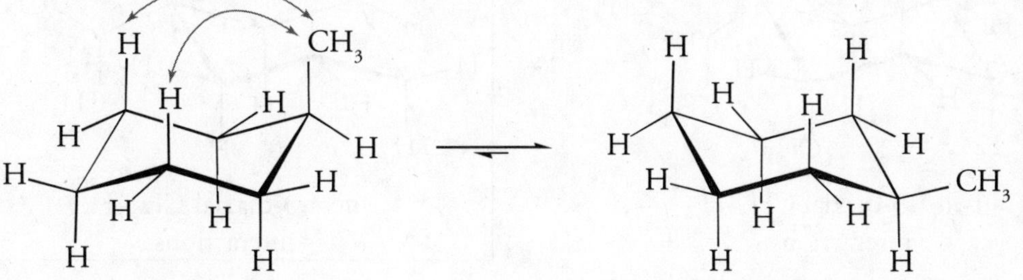

two 1,3-diaxial CH_3–H
interactions

no 1,3-diaxial CH_3–H
interactions

25.4

Is one conformation more stable than the other? Yes. It is more favorable for large groups to occupy the equatorial position rather than a crowded axial position. For a methyl group, the equatorial position is more stable by about 1.7 kcal/mol over the axial position. This is because in the axial position, the methyl group is crowded by the other two hydrogens that are also occupying axial positions on the same side of the ring. This is referred to as a **1,3-diaxial interaction**. It is more favorable for methyl to be in an equatorial position where it is pointing out, away from other atoms.

Example 25-6: In each of the following pairs of substituted cyclohexanes, identify the more stable isomer:

A.

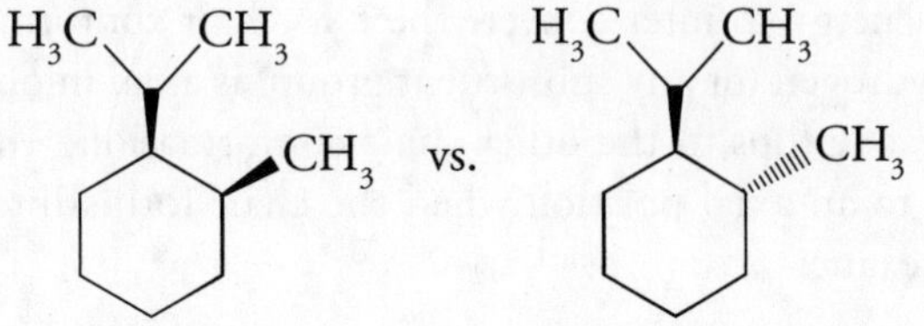

C.

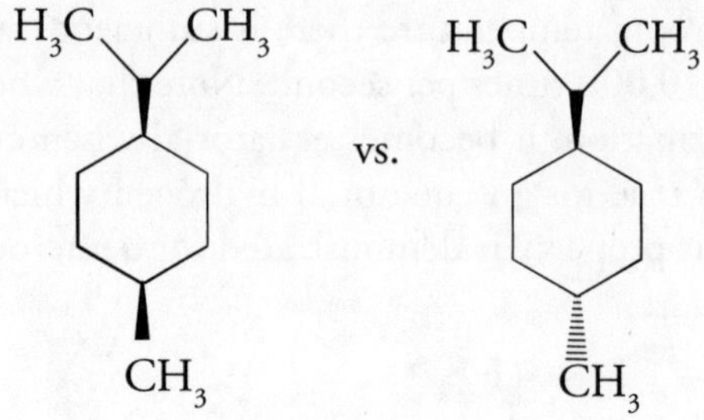

B.

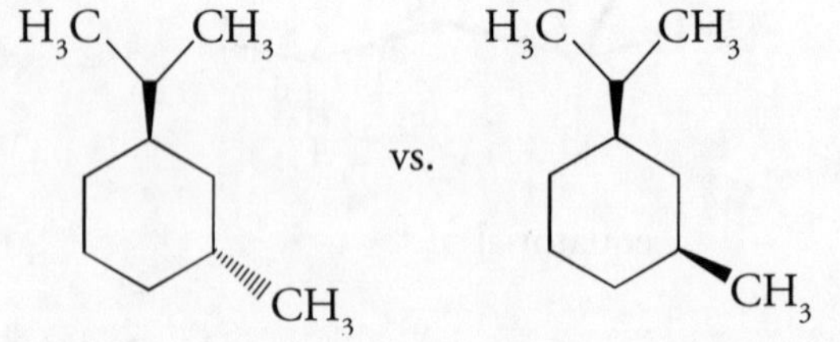

D.

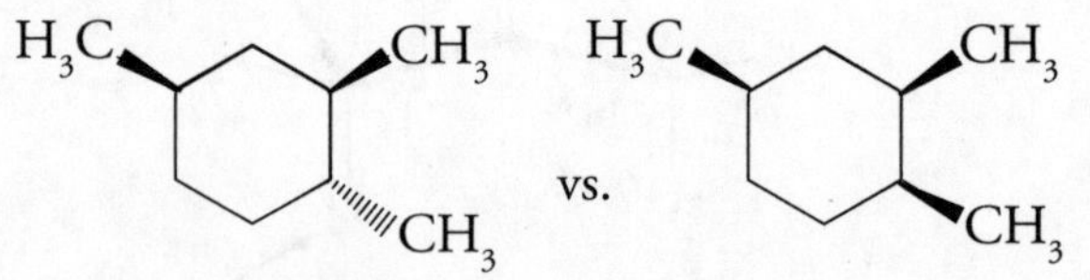

Solution: Draw chair conformations of each isomer and compare them to see which is more stable. As a good rule of thumb, it's best to first put the bulkier (i.e., larger) substituent in a roomier equatorial position and decide if it's the more stable of the two chair conformations; it usually is. Also remember that wedge bonds are pointing up and go in the top position. Dashed bonds are pointing down and go in the bottom position. This will help you draw the structures below.

A.

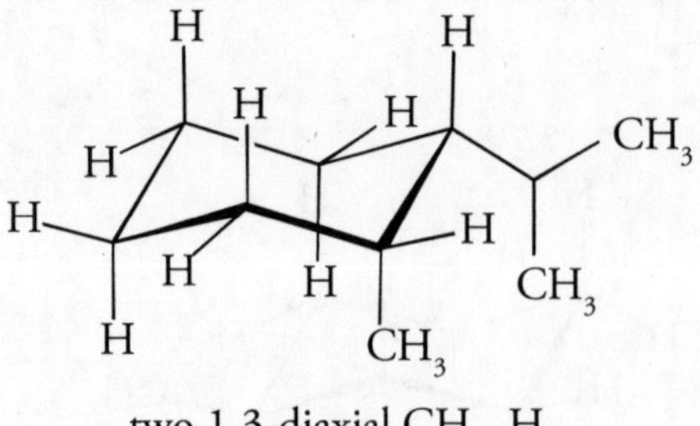

This is the more stable isomer.

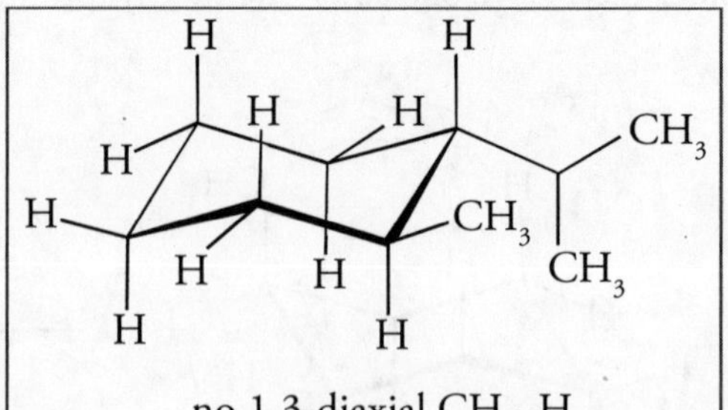

two 1,3-diaxial CH_3–H interactions

vs.

no 1,3-diaxial CH_3–H interactions

B.

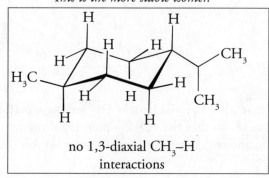

This is the more stable isomer.

vs.

two 1,3-diaxial CH₃–H
interactions

no 1,3-diaxial CH₃–H
interactions

25.4

C.

This is the more stable isomer.

vs.

two 1,3-diaxial CH₃–H
interactions

no 1,3-diaxial CH₃–H
interactions

D.

This is the more stable isomer.

vs.

no 1,3-diaxial CH₃–H
interactions

two 1,3-diaxial CH₃–H
interactions

Stereoisomerism

Stereoisomerism is of major importance in DAT Ochem. **Stereoisomers** are molecules that have the same molecular formula and connectivity but which differ from one another only in the spatial arrangement of the atoms. They cannot be interconverted by rotation of σ bonds. For example, consider the following two molecules:

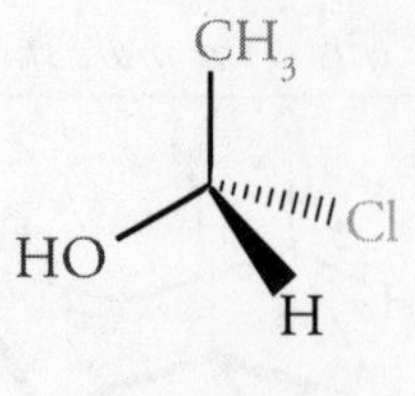

Molecule I 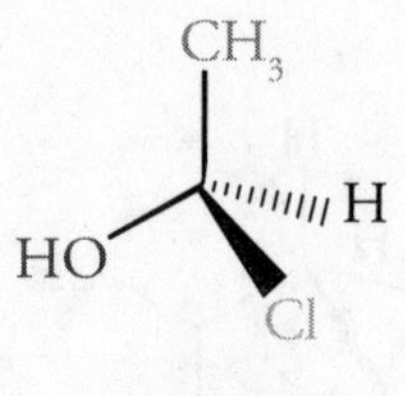   Molecule II

Both molecules have the same molecular formula, C_2H_5ClO, with the same atoms bonded to each other. However, if one superimposes II onto I without any rotation, the result is:

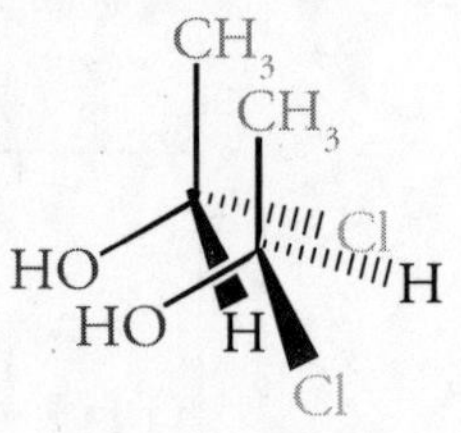

Note that while the –CH$_3$ and –OH groups superimpose, the –Cl and –H do not. Likewise, if we rotate Molecule II so that the –OH is pointing directly up (12 o'clock) and the –CH$_3$ is pointing at about 7 o'clock, and then attempt to superimpose II on I, the result is:

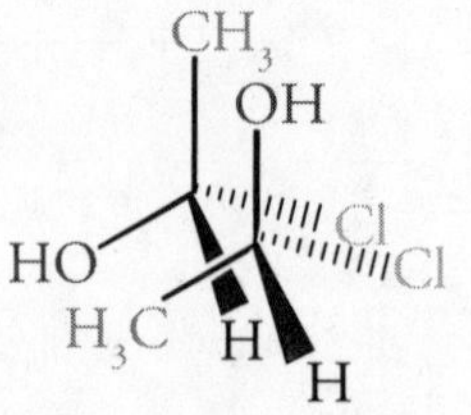

While the –Cl and the –H groups are now superimposed, the –CH$_3$ and the –OH are not. No matter how one rotates Molecules I and II, two of the substituent groups will be superimposed, while the other two will not. Hence they are indeed different molecules: They are stereoisomers.

Chirality

Any molecule that cannot be superimposed on its mirror image is said to be **chiral**, while a molecule that *can* be superimposed on its mirror image has a plane of symmetry and is said to be **achiral**. It's important that you be able to identify **chiral centers**. For carbon or nitrogen, a chiral center will have four different groups bonded to it. Note that since a carbon atom has four different groups attached to it, it must be sp^3 hybridized with (approximately) 109° bond angles and tetrahedral geometry. Such a carbon atom is also sometimes referred to as a **stereocenter**, a **stereogenic center**, or an **asymmetric center**.

Example 25-7: Identify all the chiral centers in the following molecules and determine how many possible stereoisomers each compound has by placing a star next to each chiral center. (Note: the number of possible stereoisomers equals 2^n, where n is the number of chiral centers.)

A.

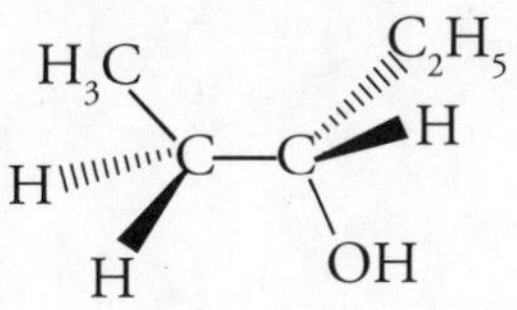

B.

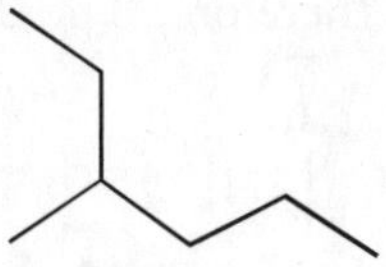

C.

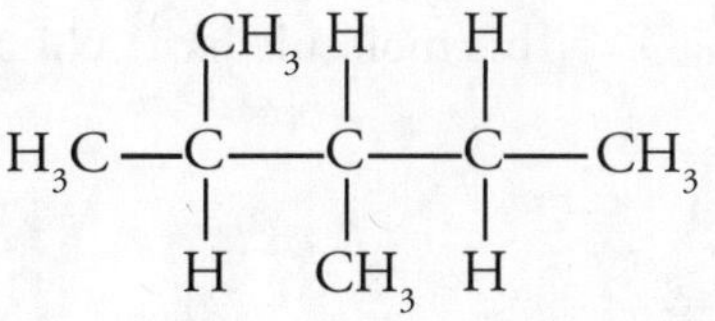

D.

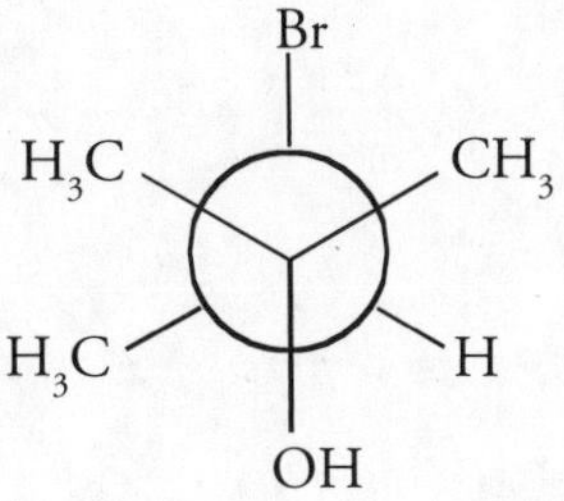

E.

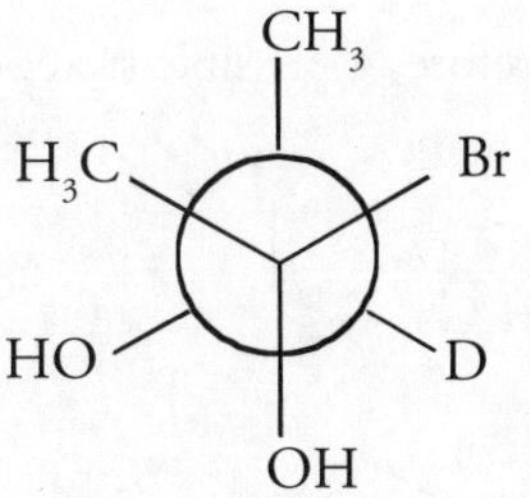

F.

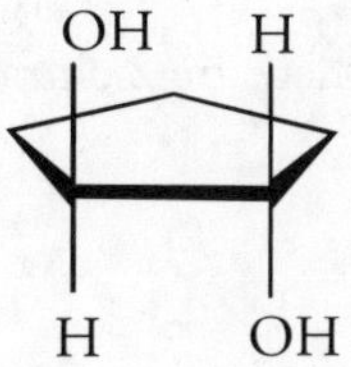

G.

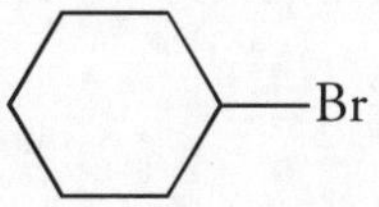

H.

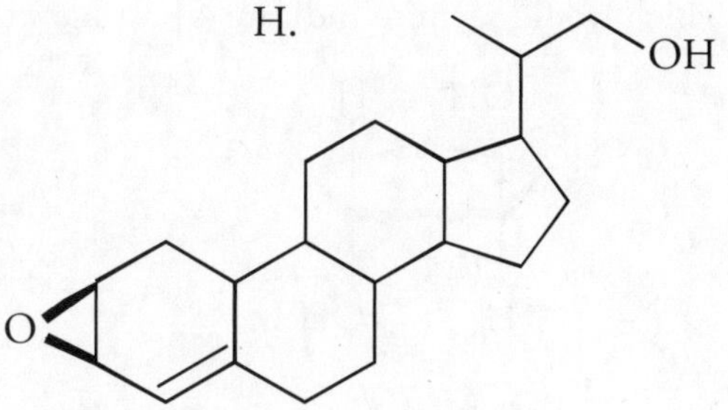

I.

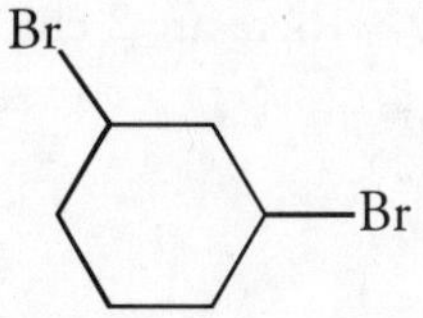

Solution:

A. This molecule has no chiral centers.

B. This molecule has 1 chiral center and, therefore, 2 possible stereoisomers:

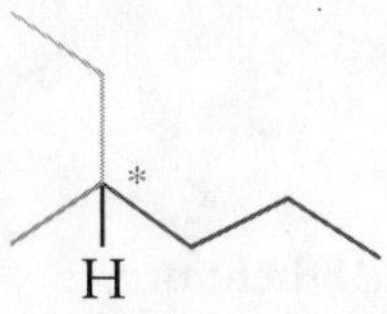

C. There is 1 chiral center and, therefore, 2 possible stereoisomers:

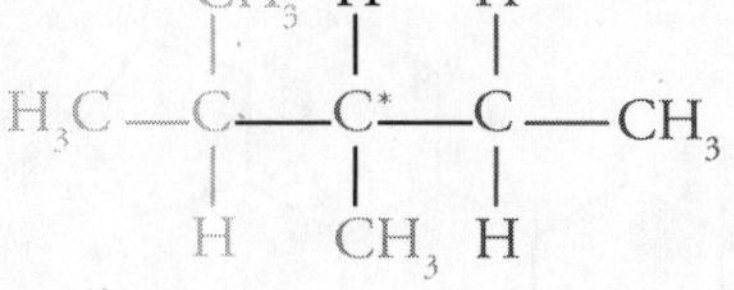

D. This molecule has 1 chiral center and, therefore, 2 possible stereoisomers:

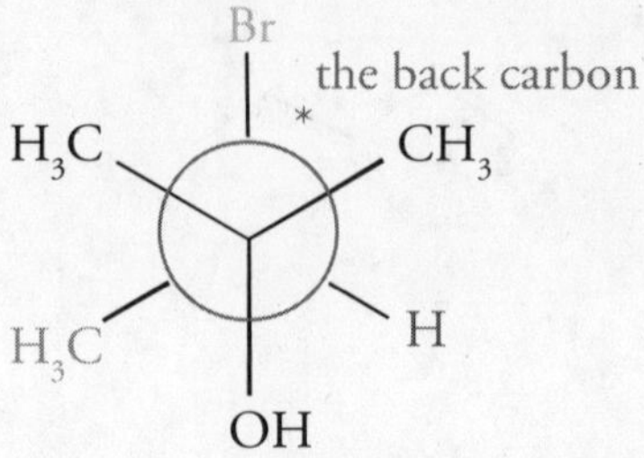

E. There are 2 chiral centers and, therefore, 4 possible stereoisomers:

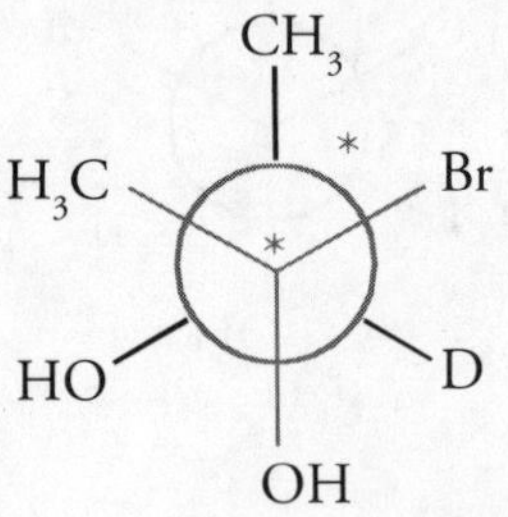

F. There are 2 chiral centers, which would seem to indicate 4 possible stereoisomers:

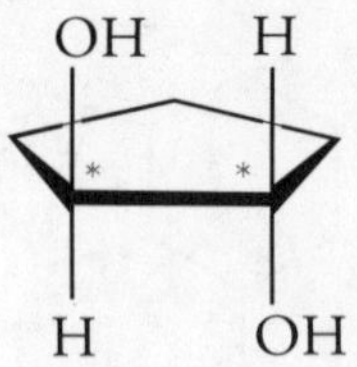

However, there are only 3, because the following "2" molecules are actually the same:

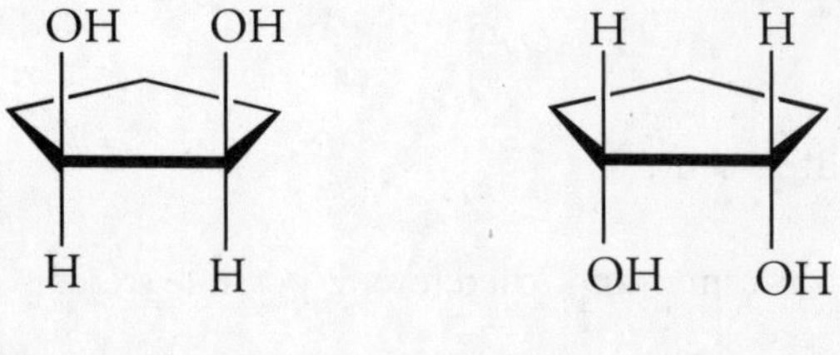

G. This molecule has no chiral centers.

H. This molecule has 9 chiral centers and, therefore, $2^9 = 512$ possible stereoisomers:

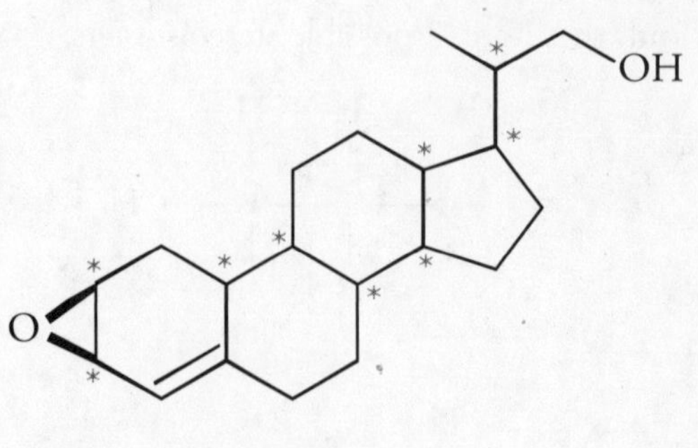

I.   Although there are two chiral centers,

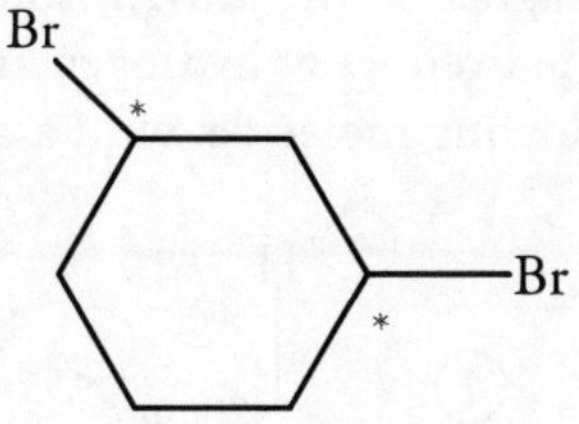

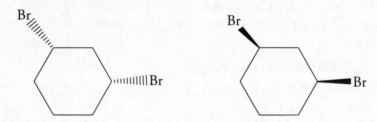

there are 3, not 4 stereoisomers, because—see (f) on the previous page—the following "two" molecules are actually the same:

Absolute Stereocenter Configuration

Chiral centers (carbon or nitrogen atoms bearing four different substituents) can be assigned an **absolute configuration**. There is an arbitrary set of rules for assigning absolute configuration to a stereocenter (known as the **Cahn-Ingold-Prelog rules**), which can be illustrated using Molecule A:

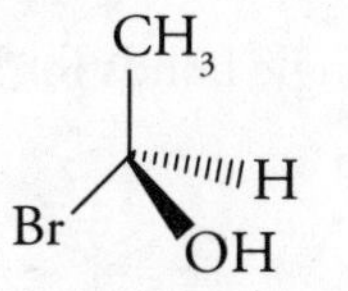

Molecule A

1.   Priority is assigned to the four different substituents on the chiral center according to increasing atomic number of the atoms directly attached to the chiral center. Going one atom out from the chiral center, bromine has the highest atomic number and is given highest priority, #1; oxygen is next and is therefore #2; carbon is #3, and the hydrogen is the lowest priority group, #4:

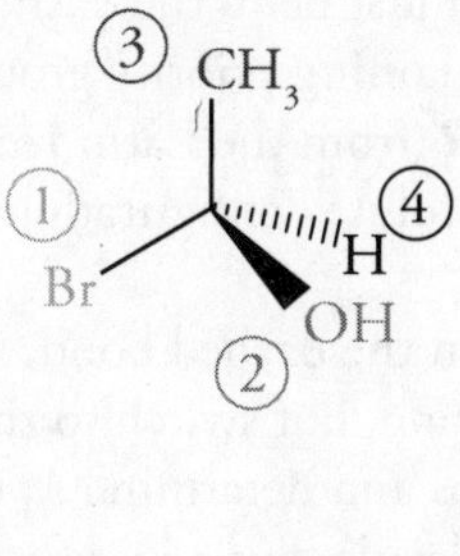

If isotopes are present, then priority among these are assigned on the basis of atomic weight with the higher priority being assigned to the heavier isotope (since they are all of the same atomic number). For example, the isotopes of hydrogen are ^1H, ^2H = D (deuterium), and ^3H = T (tritium), and for the following molecule, we'd assign priorities as shown:

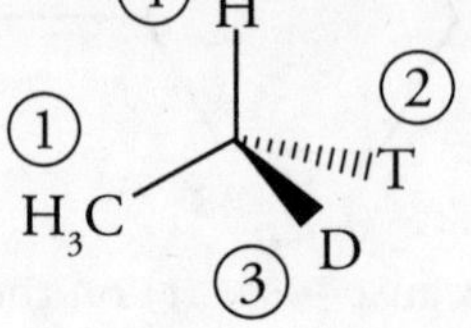

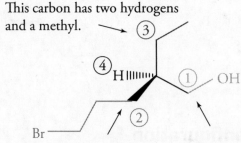

If two identical atoms are attached to a stereocenter, then the next atoms in both chains are examined until a difference is found. Once again, this is done by atomic number. Note the following example:

This carbon has two hydrogens and a methyl. ⟶ ③

④ H‖‖‖‖‖ ① OH

②

This carbon has two hydrogens followed by a –CH₂CH₂Br.

This carbon has two hydrogens and an –OH.

2. A multiple bond is counted as two single bonds for both of the atoms involved. For example:

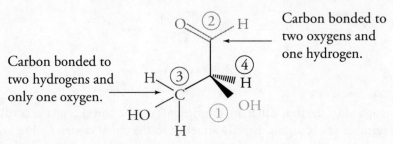

Carbon bonded to two oxygens and one hydrogen.

Carbon bonded to two hydrogens and only one oxygen.

3. Once priorities have been assigned, the lowest priority group needs to point directly away from the viewer; in other words, it must be in the dashed position. Then trace a path from highest priority group to lowest remaining priority group. If the path traveled is *clockwise*, then the absolute configuration is **R** (from the Latin *rectus*, right). Conversely, if the path traveled is *counterclockwise*, then the absolute configuration is **S** (from the Latin *sinister*, left).

4. If the lowest-priority group is not on the dashed bond, swap it with whatever group is there. Then determine absolute configuration, but switch to the opposite as your final answer. In other words, if you swap two groups and determine *R*, the final answer is actually *S*. Another option is to mentally rotate the molecule, but a lot of students struggle to do this quickly and accurately. We'll see some instances of both options in the following examples.

The two-dimensional representation (on the left) of the following hypothetical molecule is known as the "Fischer projection," named after famous organic chemist Emil Fischer.

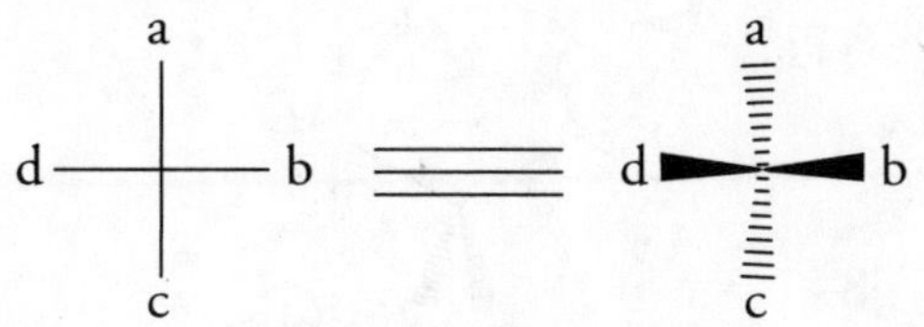

The Fischer projection is a simplification of the actual three-dimensional structure. In the Fischer projection, as shown on the right, vertical lines are assumed to go back into the page, and horizontal lines are assumed to come out of the page. The lowest-priority group needs to be on the top or bottom position of a Fischer projection. If this is not the case, hold one group in place and rotate the other three either clockwise or counter clockwise. This essentially rotates around a C–C single bond. When you use this strategy, you do NOT need to switch the *R/S* absolute configuration.

Example 25-8: Assign absolute configurations to the following molecules.

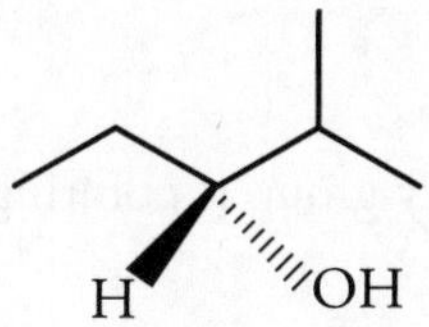

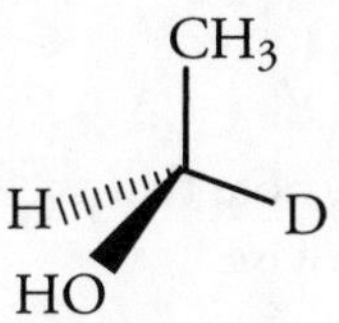

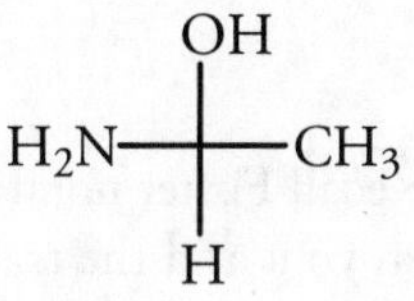

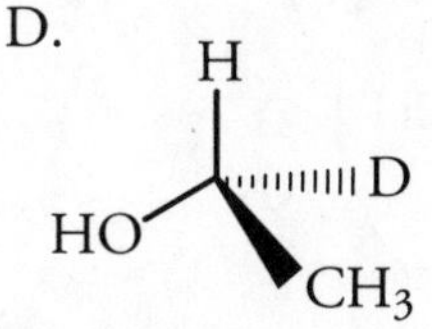

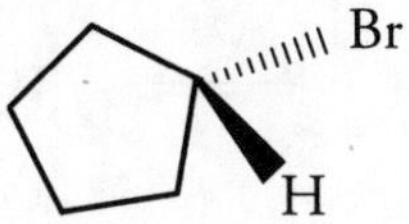

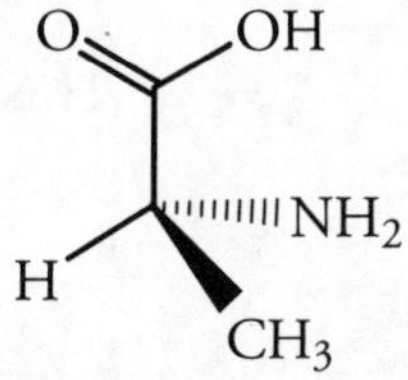

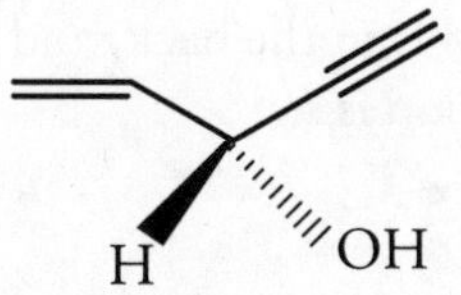

Solution:

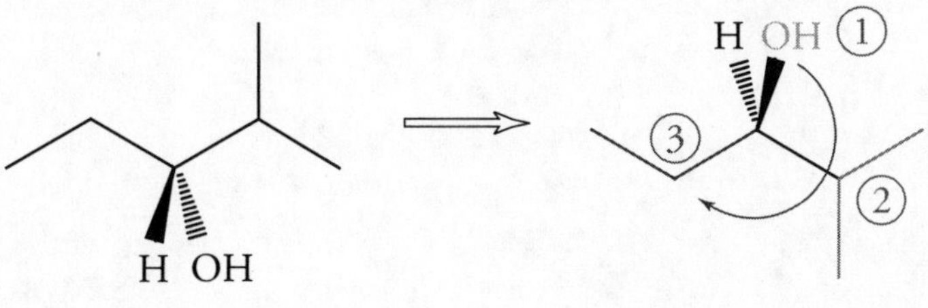

A. *R.* Either rotate the molecule so the lowest priority group is in the back, or simply trace it as it stands and invert the configuration (since the lowest priority group is coming toward you):

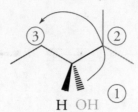

B.   *R.* The lowest priority group is already pointing away from you and the trace is clockwise.

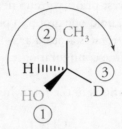

C.   *S.* Recall Fisher notation for molecules, note that the lowest priority group is pointing away from you, and the trace is counterclockwise.

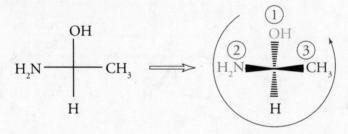

D.   *R.* The lowest priority group is neither going into nor coming out of the plane of the page. One method is to rotate the molecule so the lowest priority group is in the back, and redraw the molecule. Since the path is traveled clockwise, the configuration is *R.*

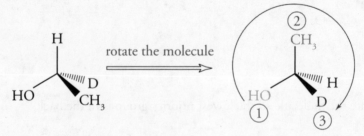

Here's a trick to help in the rotation of molecules. Exchanging two groups on a chiral center necessarily changes the absolute configuration. So in this case, it is perhaps most convenient to exchange any two groups such that the lowest priority group is going into the page:

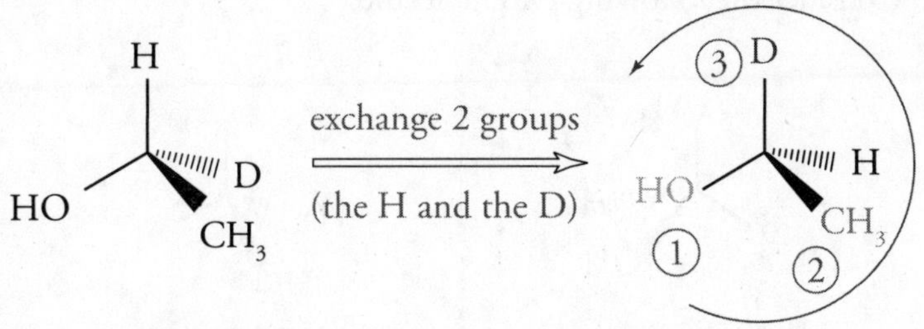

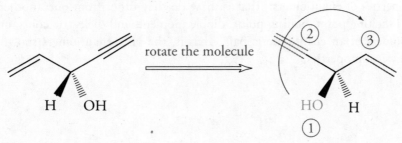

Note that this trace is going counterclockwise. Remember, however, that we exchanged two groups (the hydrogen and the deuterium), which necessarily changes the absolute configuration. Since the counterclockwise trace in the altered molecule means an *S* configuration, the true configuration is *R*.

E.   Because this molecule is not chiral, we cannot assign it an absolute configuration.

F.   *S*. Rotate so the lowest priority group is in back,

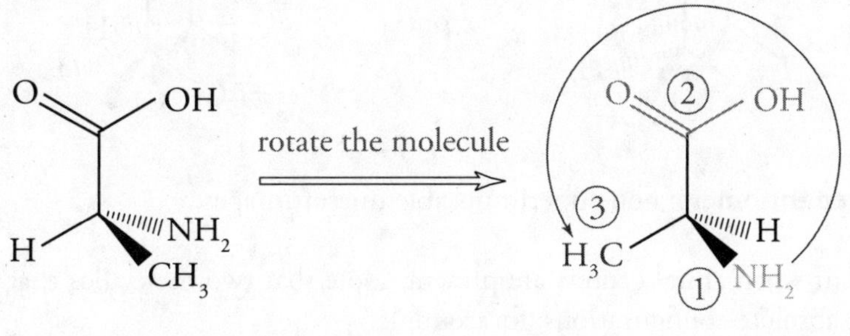

or exchange two groups, –H and –NH₂:

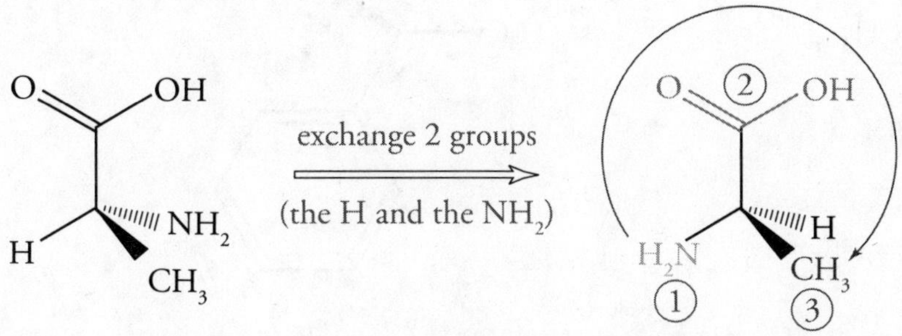

Clockwise trace.
But remember that two groups on the chiral center were exchanged, so the absolute configuration of the given molecule is the opposite; therefore, *S*.

G.   *R*. Rotate so the lowest priority group is in the back:

Enantiomers

It is important to be able to identify chiral centers because, as we have seen, when there are four different groups attached to a centralized carbon, there are two distinct arrangements or configurations possible for these groups in space. Consider the following two molecules:

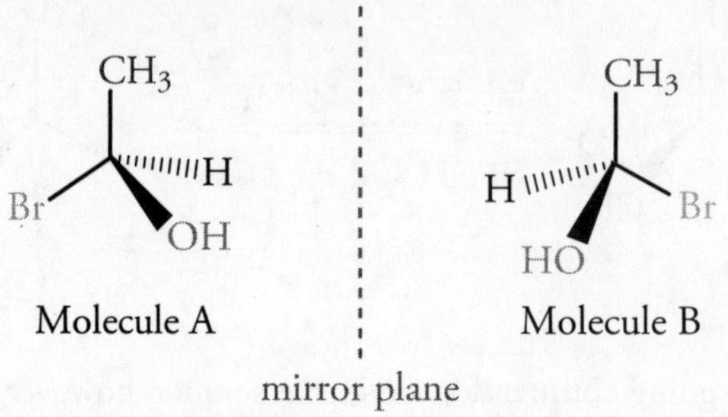

Molecule A   Molecule B

mirror plane

Molecule A has one chiral center with four different groups attached. Notice that Molecule B also has a chiral center and that the four groups attached to it are the same as those in Molecule A. Observe the mirror plane that has been drawn between Molecules A and B. Molecules A and B are mirror images of each other, but they are not superimposable; therefore, they are chiral.

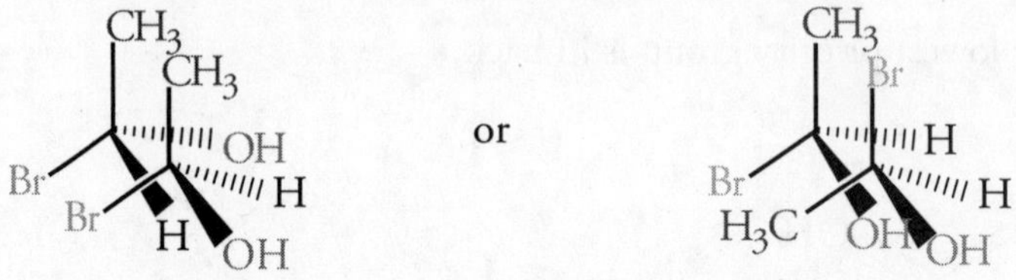

or

These molecules are **enantiomers**: non-superimposable mirror images.

Enantiomers can occur when chiral centers are present. Note that two molecules that are enantiomers will always have opposite absolute configurations; for example:

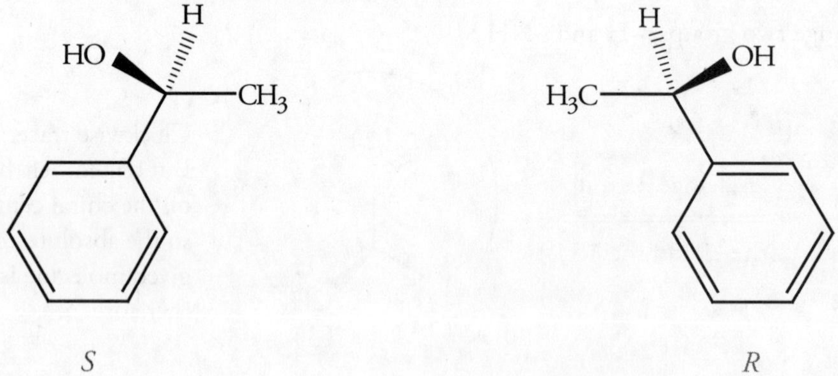

S   R

What are the properties of enantiomers? That is, how do they differ from one another? Most chemical properties such as melting point, boiling point, dipole moment, and dielectric constant are the same for both pure enantiomers of an enantiomeric pair. That is, the pure enantiomers shown above will have many identical physical properties.

Optical Activity

One important property that differs between enantiomers is the manner in which they interact with plane-polarized light. A compound that rotates the plane of polarized light is said to be **optically active**. A compound that rotates plane-polarized light clockwise is said to be **dextrorotatory** (*d*), also denoted by (+), while a compound that rotates plane-polarized light in the counterclockwise direction is said to be **levorotatory** (*l*), also denoted by (−). The magnitude of rotation of plane-polarized light for any compound is called its **specific rotation**. This property is dependent on the structure of the molecule, the concentration of the sample, and the path length through which the light must travel.

A pair of enantiomers will rotate plane-polarized light with equal magnitude, but in opposite directions. For example, pure (+)-2-bromobutanoic acid has a specific rotation of +39.5°, while (−)-2-bromobutanoic acid has a specific rotation of −39.5°.

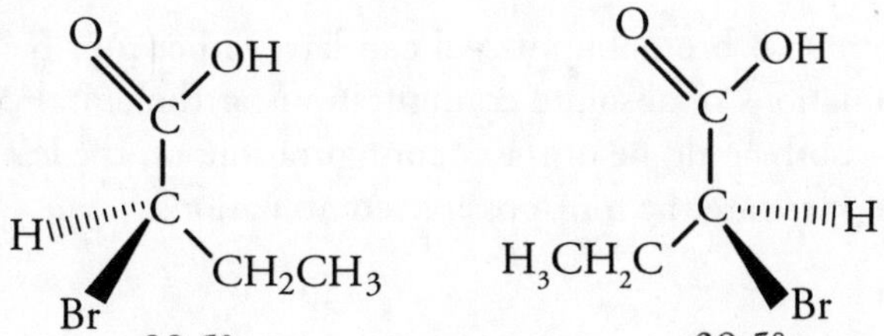

(+) and (−)-2-bromobutanoic acid

What do you think the specific rotation of an equimolar mixture of the two enantiomers above will be? Since one enantiomer will rotate plane-polarized light in one direction, while the other enantiomer will rotate light by the same magnitude in the opposite direction, the specific rotation of a 50/50 mixture of enantiomers—a **racemic mixture**—is 0°. Therefore, a racemic mixture of enantiomers, also known as a *racemate*, is not optically active.

Example 25-9: What is the specific rotation of the *R* enantiomer of 2-bromobutanoic acid? Of the *S* enantiomer?

Solution:

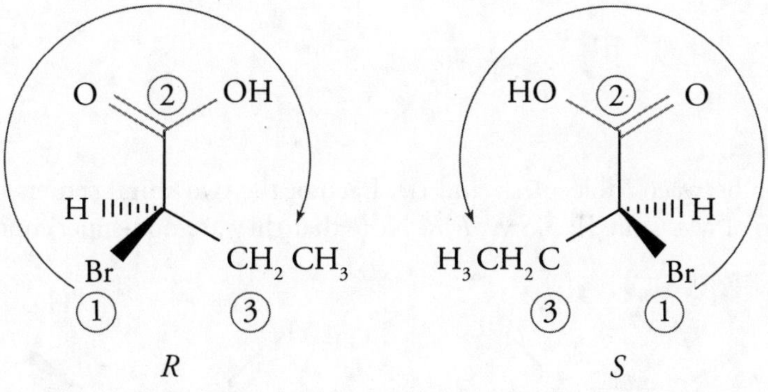

The magnitude of rotation cannot be predicted; it must be experimentally determined. It just so happens in this case that the *R* enantiomer has the (+) rotation [while the *S* enantiomer has the (−) rotation]. But be careful: *This is only coincidental. (+) and (−) say nothing about whether the absolute configuration is R or S.* There is no correlation between the sign of rotation and the absolute configuration.

Diastereomers

In the preceding discussions on stereoisomerism we have focused on molecules that have only one chiral center. What about molecules with multiple stereocenters? Remember that the number of possible stereoisomers is 2^n, where n is the number of chiral centers. If there is one chiral center, then there are two possible stereoisomers: the enantiomeric pair R and S. Two chiral centers means there are four possible stereoisomers. Consider the following molecule (3-bromobutan-2-ol), for example:

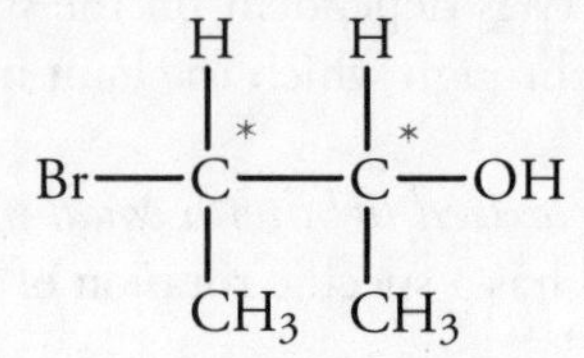

Each of the two chiral centers in 3-bromobutan-2-ol can have either R or S absolute configuration. This leads to four possible combinations of absolute configurations at the chiral centers. Both carbons could be of the S configuration, or both could be of the R configuration; or, the left carbon could be R and the right carbon S, or vice versa. Here are the four possible combinations:

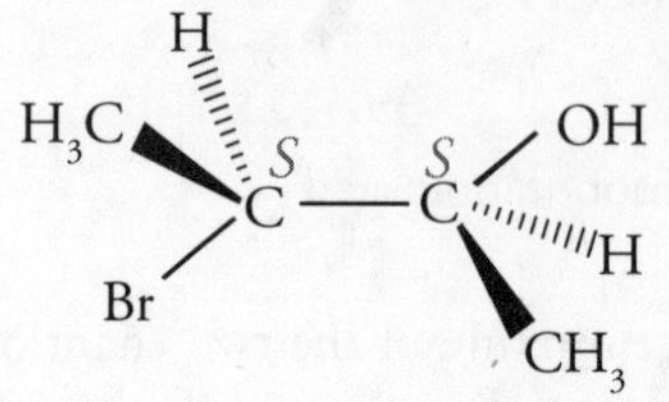

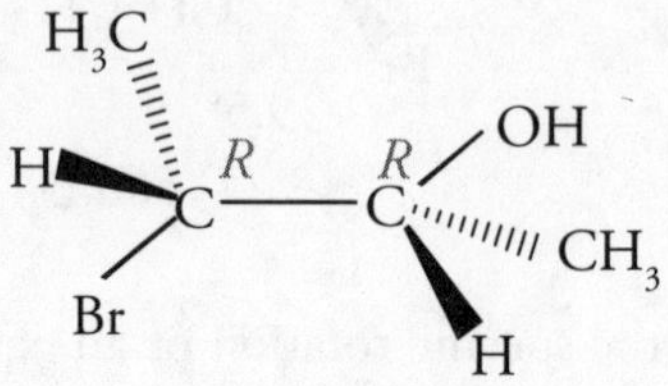

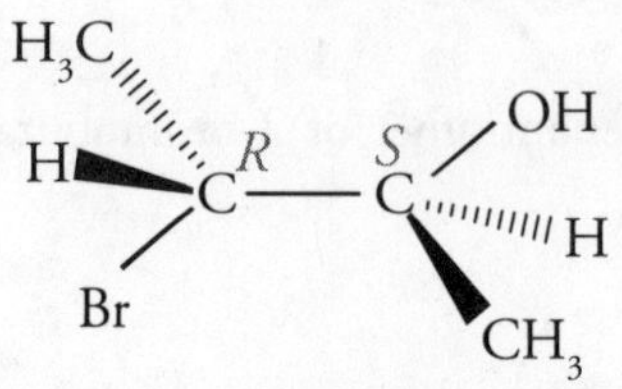

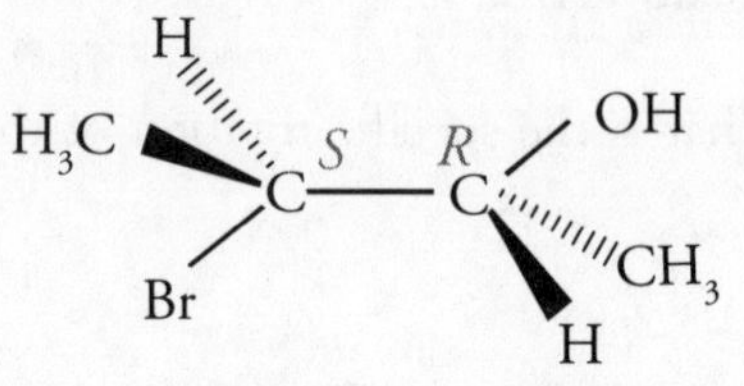

What's the relationship between Molecules I and II? Each of the two chiral centers in Molecule I is of the opposite configuration of Molecule II: S,S vs. R,R. Note that they are non-superimposable mirror images:

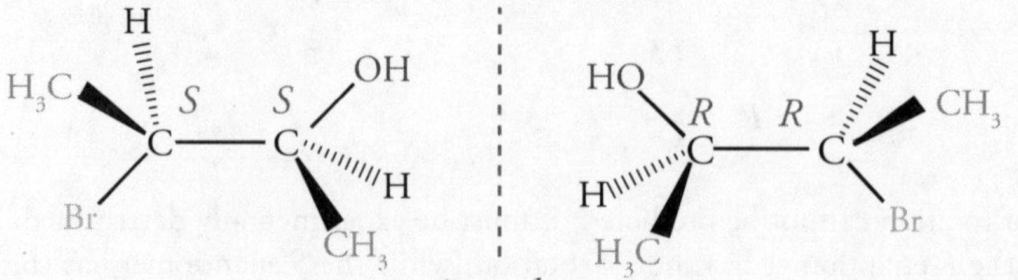

Therefore, these molecules are enantiomers. What about Molecules III and IV? Once again, each of the two chiral centers in Molecule III is of the opposite configuration of those in Molecule IV. This makes Molecules III and IV an enantiomer pair, just as we noted for Molecules I and II above. Is there a relationship between Molecules I and III?

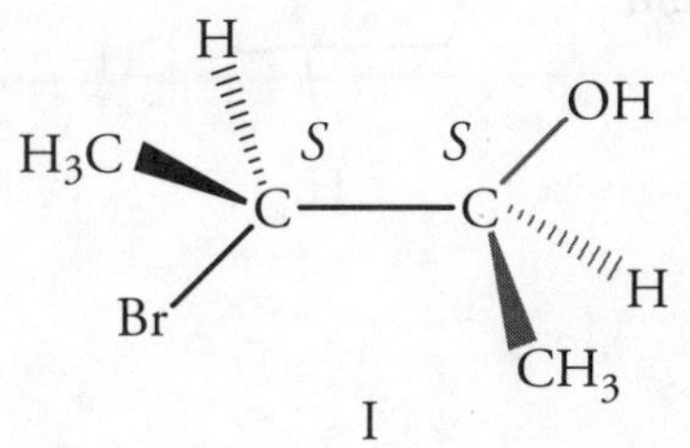

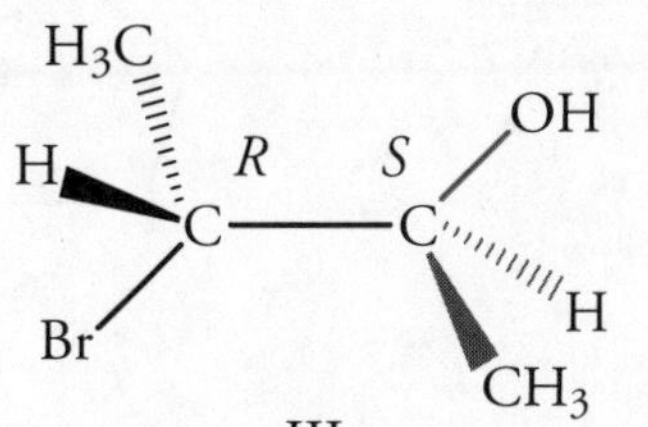

By mentally moving Molecule III to the left and aligning it over Molecule I, we see that the right chiral centers of both molecules are directly superimposable (*S* superimposes onto *S*). Also note that no matter what we do, we cannot get the left chiral centers of Molecules I and III to superimpose (*S* does not superimpose onto *R*).

Molecules I and III are diastereomers. **Diastereomers** are stereoisomers that are not enantiomers. That is, diastereomers are stereoisomers that are non-superimposable, non-mirror images. The same is true for Molecules I and IV. One of the chiral centers is of the same absolute configuration, while the other chiral center is of the opposite configuration:

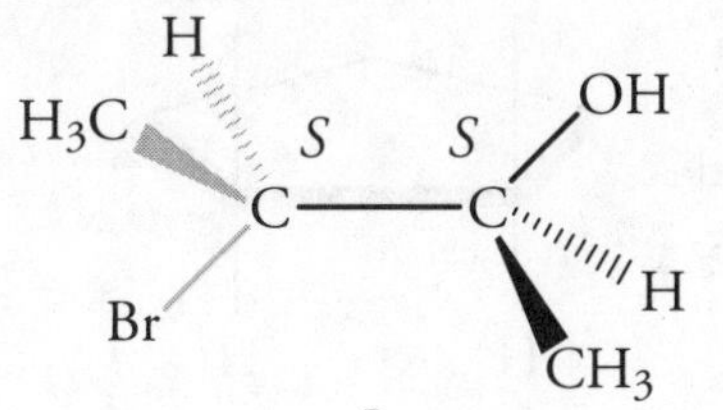

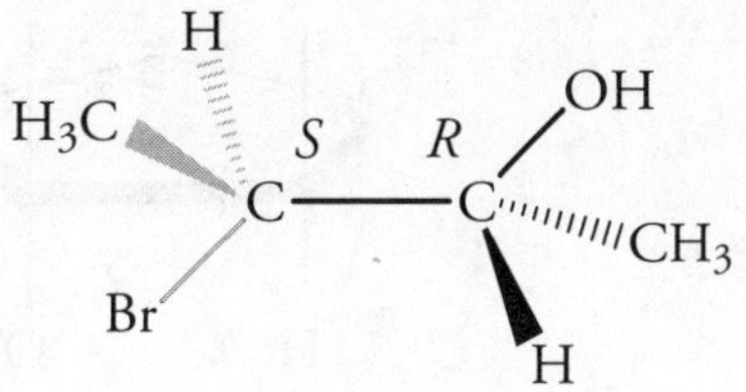

The figure below summarizes all possible stereochemical relationships between isomers containing two stereocenters. Inverting at least one, but not all, of the chiral centers within a molecule will form a diastereomer of that molecule. Enantiomers can be formed by inverting every stereocenter within the molecule.

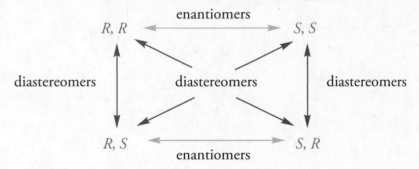

Example 25-10: For each pair of molecules below, state the relationship between them.

A.

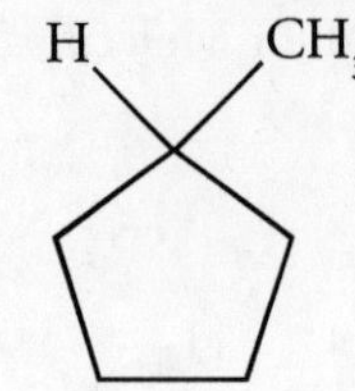

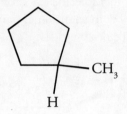

and

B.

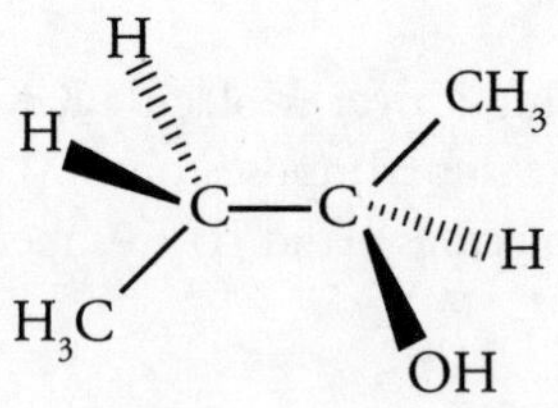

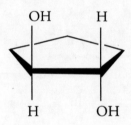

and

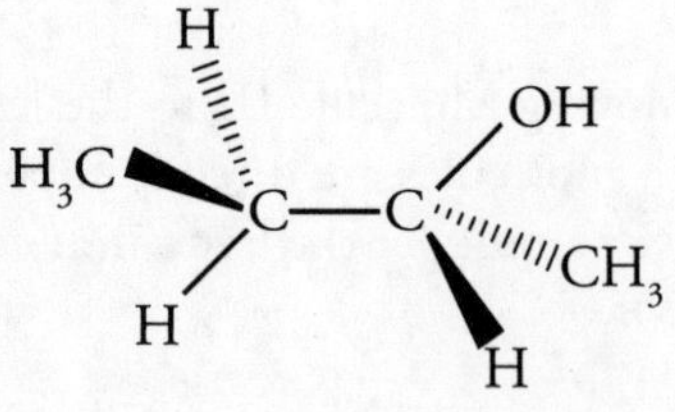

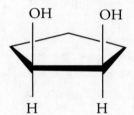

C.

OH   H

and

OH   OH

H   OH

H   H

D.

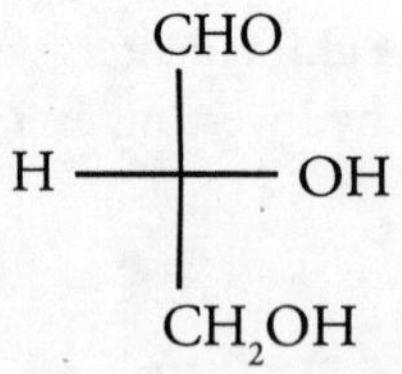

CHO

H —— OH

CH₂OH

and

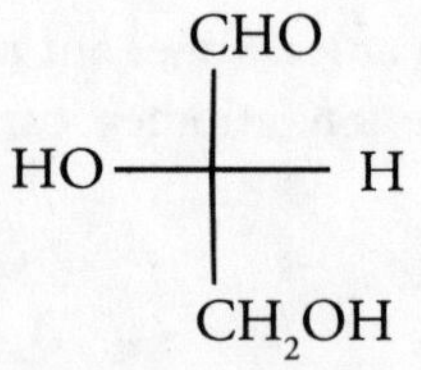

CHO

HO —— H

CH₂OH

E.

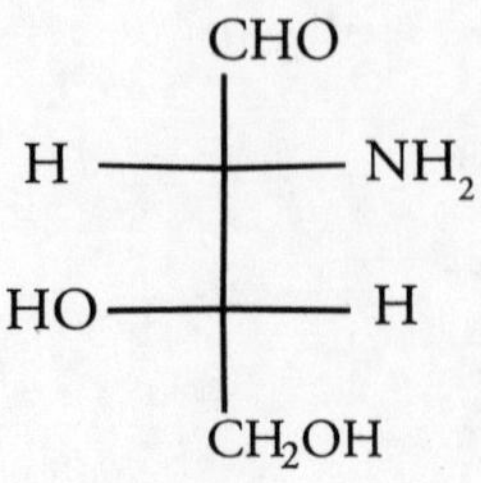

CHO

H —— NH₂

HO —— H

CH₂OH

and

CH₂OH

H —— OH

H —— NH₂

CHO

25.4

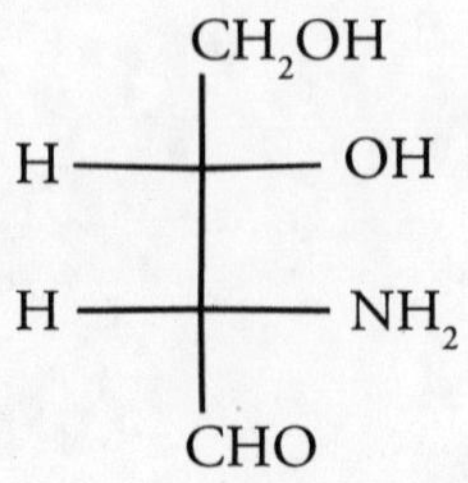

Solution:

A. The molecules are superimposable and therefore identical.

B. The molecules are identical. (The left carbon is not a chiral center.)

C. Diastereomers.

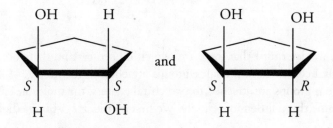

D. Enantiomers.

E. Diastereomers.

While the structures of diastereomers are similar, their physical and chemical properties can vary dramatically. They can have different melting points, boiling points, solubilities, dipole moments, specific rotations, etc. Most importantly for the DAT, the specific rotation of diastereomers is also different, but *there is no relationship between the specific rotations of diastereomers as there is for enantiomers.* There is no way to predict the specific rotation of one diastereomer if you know the degree of rotation of another.

*Note that C and E in the above problem are a special type of diastereomer called an **epimer**, meaning that they differ at only one chiral center. There is also a special type of epimer called an **anomer**, which is an epimer due to ring closure. These types of diastereomers are important in carbohydrate chemistry, but it is very unlikely that the DAT will ask you about them.

Meso Compounds

Let's look at another molecule with more than one stereocenter. Consider 2,3-butanediol:

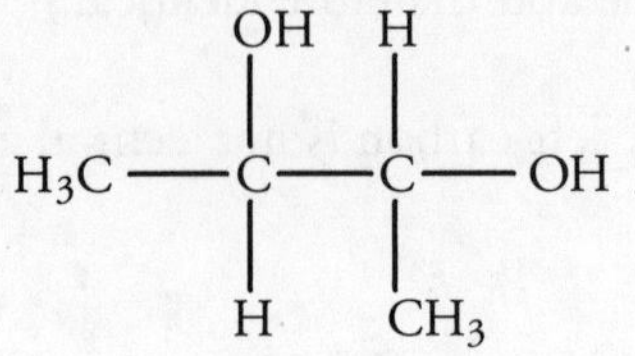

Upon inspection, we determine that there are two chiral centers and therefore four possible stereoisomers. Notice that both chiral centers have the same groups attached to them: –H, –CH$_3$, –OH, and –CH(OH)CH$_3$. When the same four groups are attached to two chiral centers, the molecule can have an internal plane of symmetry. Let's examine this a little more closely. We first consider 2,3-butanediol's R,R stereoisomer and the S,S stereoisomer:

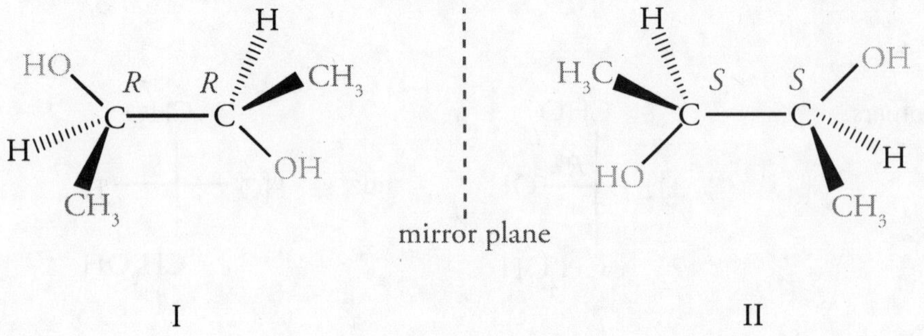

mirror plane

I   II

There are two things to notice here. First, I and II are non-superimposable mirror images and therefore enantiomers. Second, in both I and II there is no internal plane of symmetry. This is demonstrated for Molecule II:

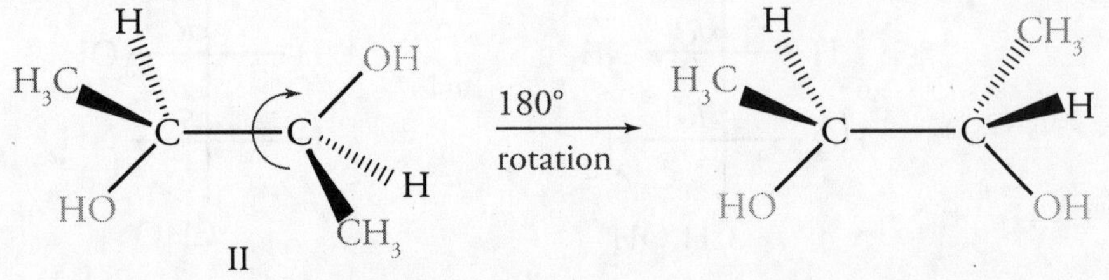

The –OH's line up on the two chiral centers, but the –CH$_3$'s and –H's do not. The optical rotation of a 50/50 mixture of Molecules I and II would measure zero because this is a racemic mixture.

Now look at the *R,S* stereoisomer and its mirror image:

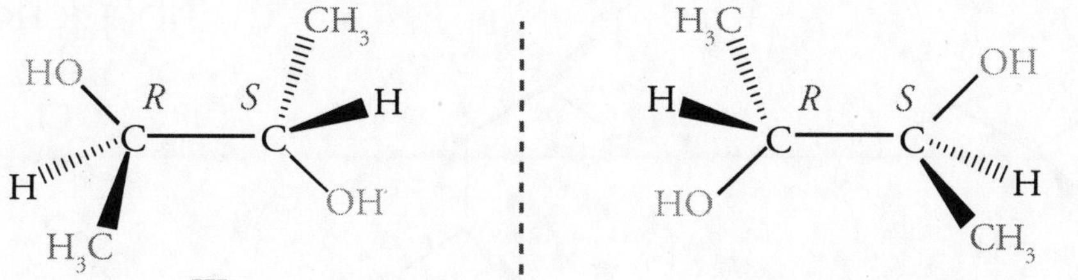

III

III and IV are actually
the same molecule.

Rotate the entire molecule
so that the two –OH groups
are as in III.

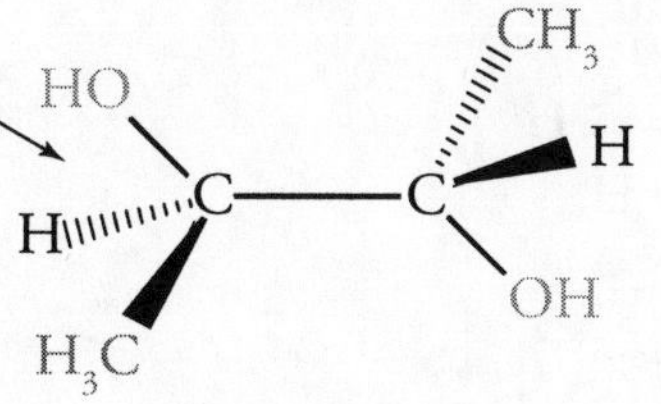

IV

It turns out that Molecules III and IV are directly superimposable and therefore identical. This is because
there is an internal plane of symmetry within the molecule.

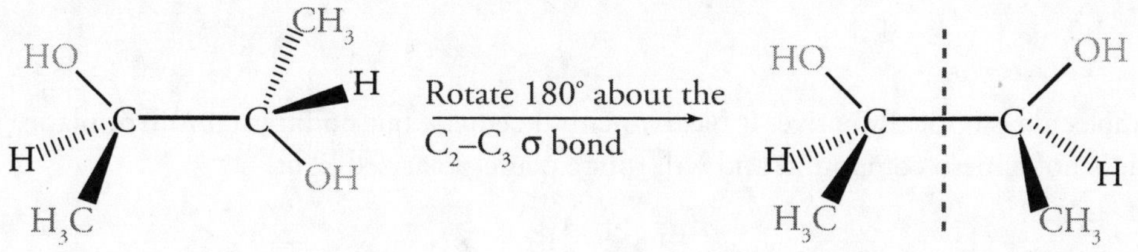

III

Rotate 180° about the
C_2–C_3 σ bond

One side of the molecule is the
mirror image of the other side.
This is a *meso* compound.

When there's an internal plane of symmetry in a molecule that contains chiral centers, the compound is
called a **meso** compound. Then, 2,3-butanediol has only *three* stereoisomers, not four. Molecules I and
II are enantiomers, while III and IV are the same molecule. Molecule III (or IV) is an example of a meso
compound. Meso compounds have chiral centers but are not optically active because one side of the molecule is a mirror image of the other. In a sense, the optical activity imparted by one side of the molecule
is canceled by its other side.

Example 25-11: Which of the following molecules are optically active?

A.

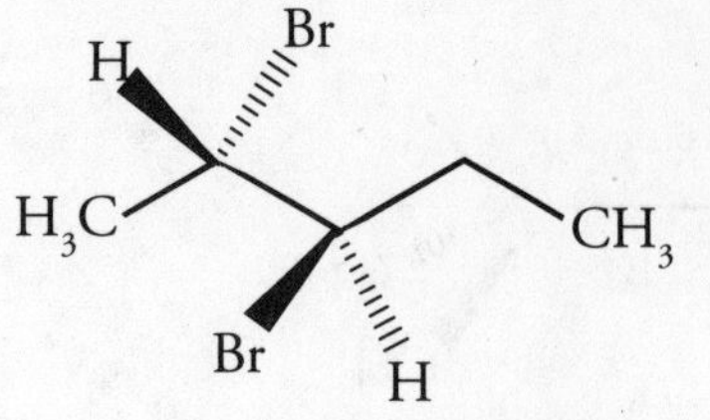

B.

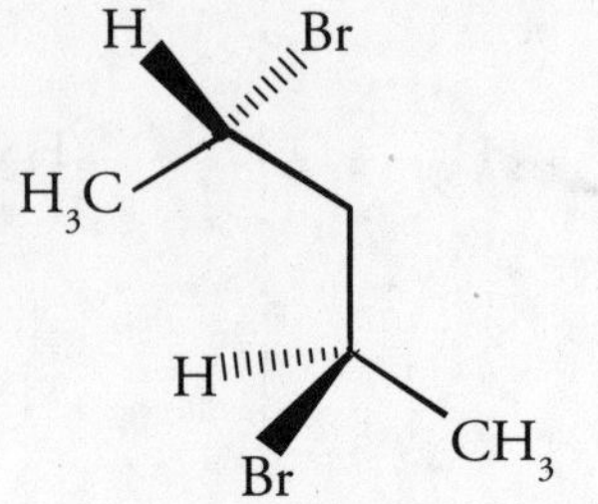

C. $HOCH_2CHCH_2OH$
   |
   Cl

D.

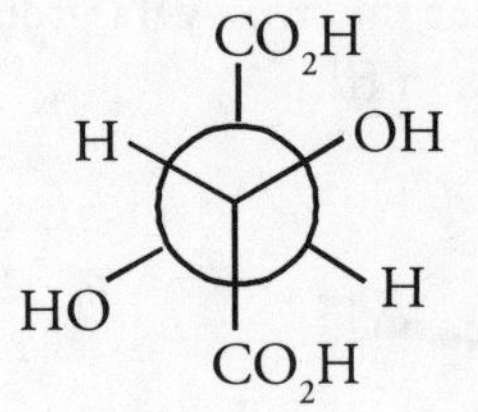

E.

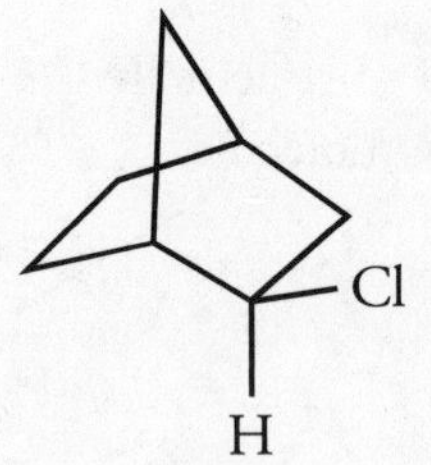

F.

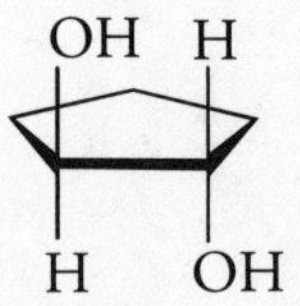

G.

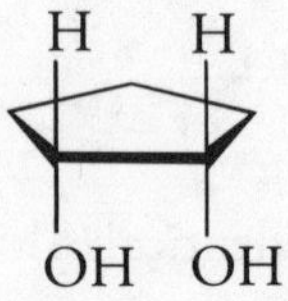

Solution:

A. This molecule is optically active. It has two chiral centers, but no internal mirror plane. There-fore, it is not a meso compound and will rotate plane-polarized light.

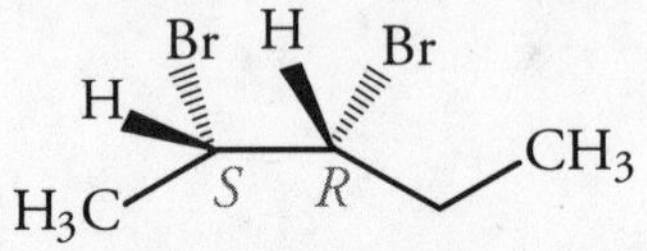

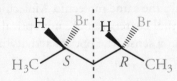

B. This molecule is a meso compound due to its two chiral centers and internal mirror plane. It will be optically inactive. Be sure to look for rotations around σ bonds in order to find the mirror planes of some molecules.

C. This molecule has no chiral centers, so will have no optical activity.

25.4

D. By rotating around the C–2 to C–3 bond to put the molecule into an eclipsed conformation, you can see that there is an internal mirror plane in the molecule. Since C–2 and C–3 are also chiral centers with four different substituents, this is a meso compound, and will be optically inactive.

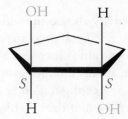

E. This molecule has three chiral centers (the two bridgehead carbons are chiral), but no plane of symmetry. It is therefore chiral and optically active.

F. There is no mirror image in this molecule even though it has two chiral centers (they have the same absolute configuration). It will therefore be optically active.

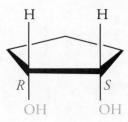

G. This molecule does have an internal mirror plane, and its two chiral centers have opposite absolute configurations. It is therefore meso, and not optically active.

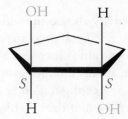

Geometric Isomers

Geometric isomers are diastereomers that differ in orientation of substituents around a ring or a double bond. Cyclic hydrocarbons and double bonds (alkenes) are constrained by their geometry, meaning they do not rotate freely about all bonds. So, there's a difference between having substituents on the same side of the ring (or double bond) and having substituents on opposite sides. For example, the following are geometric isomers of 1,2-dimethylcyclohexane:

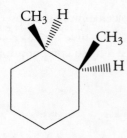

cis-1,2-Dimethylcyclohexane 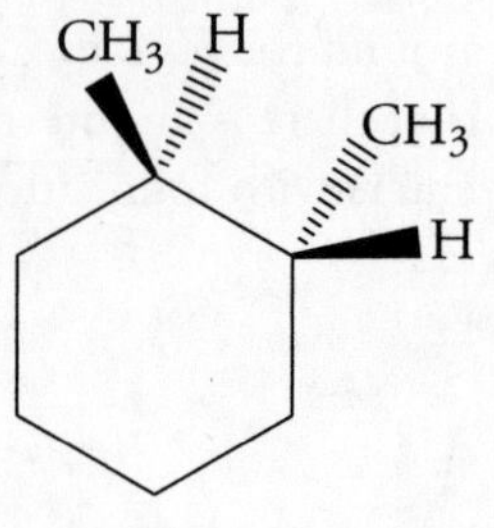   trans-1,2-Dimethylcyclohexane

Priority of substituent groups is assigned the same way as for absolute configuration. On carbon 1 (at the top of the cyclohexane), the methyl group is given higher priority than H, and the same is true on carbon 2 (on the right). The molecule in which the two higher-priority groups are on the same side is termed *cis*, and the molecule in which the two higher-priority groups are on opposite sides of the ring is termed *trans*. *Cis* and *trans* nomenclature is used when hydrogen and hydrocarbon groups are being compared or when at least one hydrogen atom is present on each carbon. If more complicated groups or substituents are present, *E/Z* is used instead.

The same-side/opposite-side substituent relativity also occurs with double bonds, but in this case the stereochemistry is officially designated by *Z* or *E*. *E/Z* notation is a completely unambiguous way to specify the appropriate stereochemistry at the double bond. In this system, a high and low priority group are assigned at each carbon of the double bond based on atomic number, just as with absolute configuration. If the two high priority groups are on the *same* side, the configuration at the double bond is *Z* (from the German *zusammen*, meaning *together*). On the other hand, if the two high priority groups are on opposite sides of the double bond, the configuration is referred to as *E* (from the German *entgegen*, meaning *opposite*). The geometric isomers of 2-bromo-1-chloropropene and of 1,2-dibromoethene are shown below:

Highest priority groups (Br and Cl) on same side, so *Z*.

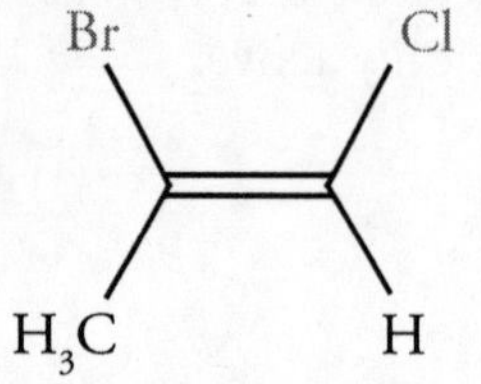

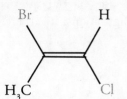

Highest priority groups (Br and Cl) on opposite side, so *E*.

(*Z*)-2-bromo-1-chloropropene   (*E*)-2-bromo-1-chloropropene

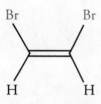   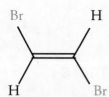

cis-1,2-dibromoethene   trans-1,2-dibromoethene

SUMMARY OF ISOMERS

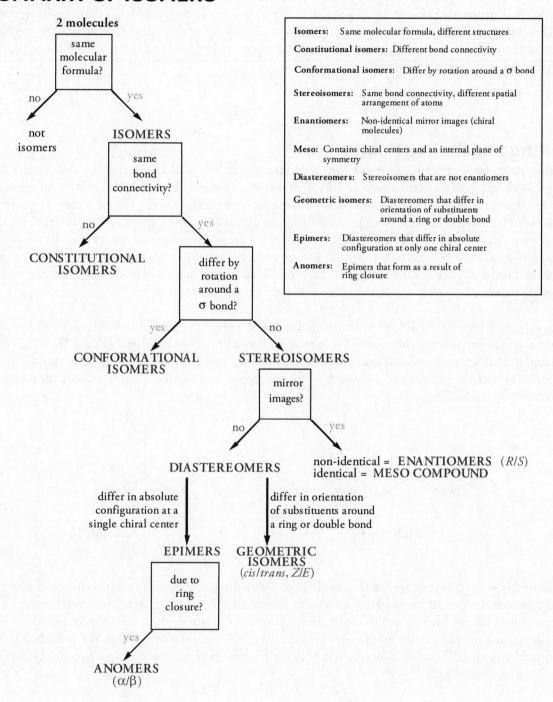

2 molecules

same molecular formula?

no → **not isomers**

yes → **ISOMERS**

same bond connectivity?

no → **CONSTITUTIONAL ISOMERS**

yes → differ by rotation around a σ bond?

yes → **CONFORMATIONAL ISOMERS**

no → **STEREOISOMERS**

mirror images?

no → **DIASTEREOMERS**

yes → non-identical = **ENANTIOMERS** (*R/S*)
identical = **MESO COMPOUND**

DIASTEREOMERS

differ in absolute configuration at a single chiral center → **EPIMERS**

differ in orientation of substituents around a ring or double bond → **GEOMETRIC ISOMERS** (*cis/trans*, *Z/E*)

EPIMERS

due to ring closure?

yes → **ANOMERS** (α/β)

Isomers: Same molecular formula, different structures

Constitutional isomers: Different bond connectivity

Conformational isomers: Differ by rotation around a σ bond

Stereoisomers: Same bond connectivity, different spatial arrangement of atoms

Enantiomers: Non-identical mirror images (chiral molecules)

Meso: Contains chiral centers and an internal plane of symmetry

Diastereomers: Stereoisomers that are not enantiomers

Geometric isomers: Diastereomers that differ in orientation of substituents around a ring or double bond

Epimers: Diastereomers that differ in absolute configuration at only one chiral center

Anomers: Epimers that form as a result of ring closure

25.5 PHYSICAL PROPERTIES OF HYDROCARBONS

The **physical properties** of organic molecules that you need to know for the DAT are **melting point**, **boiling point**, and **solubility**. For melting point and boiling point, consider interactions between identical molecules. For solubility, we'll consider interactions between the solute (dissolved substance) and the solvent (dissolving liquid).

Melting and Boiling Points

Melting point (**mp**) and **boiling point** (**bp**) are indicators of how well identical molecules interact with (attract) each other. Nonpolar molecules, like hydrocarbons, interact principally because of an attractive force known as the London dispersion force, one of the intermolecular (van der Waals) forces. This force exists between temporary dipoles formed in nonpolar molecules as a result of a temporary asymmetric electron distribution. Such intermolecular forces must be overcome to melt a nonpolar compound (solid → liquid) or to boil a nonpolar compound (liquid → gas). The greater the attractive forces between molecules, the more energy will be required to get the compound to melt or boil. The weaker these forces, the lower the melting or boiling point.

Many factors determine the degree to which molecules of a given compound will interact. For hydrocarbons, the most significant of these factors is *branching*. Branching tends to inhibit van der Waals forces by reducing the surface area available for intermolecular interaction. Thus, branching tends to reduce attractive forces between molecules and to lower both melting point and boiling point. Consider the following two constitutional isomers:

Molecule I	Molecule II
n-octane	2,4-dimethylhexane

Molecule I, *n*-octane, is unbranched. Molecule II, 2,4-dimethylhexane, is a branched isomer of *n*-octane. Although each compound has the same molecular formula, C_8H_{18}, these two constitutional isomers have dramatically different melting points and boiling points. *n*-Octane requires much more energy to melt or boil, because unbranched, it experiences greater van der Waals forces than does the branched isomer 2,4-dimethylhexane. Therefore, *n*-octane has both a higher melting point and a higher boiling point than does 2,4-dimethylhexane.

The second factor influencing melting point and boiling point for hydrocarbons is molecular weight. The greater the molecular weight of a compound, the more surface area there is to interact, the greater the number of van der Waals interactions, and the higher the melting point and boiling point. Therefore, hexane—a six-carbon alkane—has a higher mp and bp than propane, a three-carbon alkane.

The influence of molecular weight on melting point and boiling point is readily seen when considering the following trends for hydrocarbons:

- Small hydrocarbons (1 to 3 carbons) tend to be gases at room temperature.
- Intermediate hydrocarbons (4 to 16 carbons) tend to be liquids at room temperature.
- Large hydrocarbons (more than 16 carbons) tend to be (waxy) solids at room temperature.

25.5

Melting Point / Boiling Point Rules:

1. Increasing branching decreases mp and bp
2. Increasing molecular weight increases mp and bp

Example 25-12: Rank the following six hydrocarbons in order of increasing boiling point:

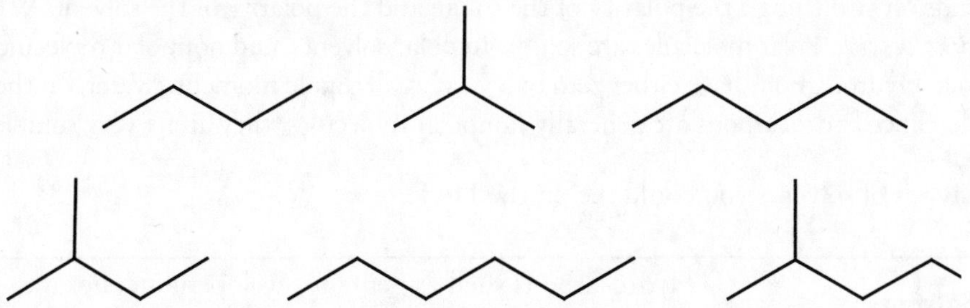

Solution: Since branching lowers the boiling point, each of the branched hydrocarbons has a lower boiling point than the unbranched hydrocarbon of the same molecular formula. Also, the larger the molecule, the greater the surface area over which van der Waals forces can act, so heavier molecules have higher boiling points. We can now put the whole sequence in order of increasing bp:

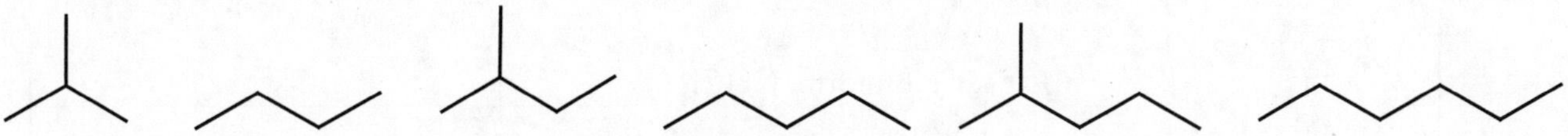

Increasing Boiling Point

Example 25-13: Rank the following three compounds in order of increasing boiling point:

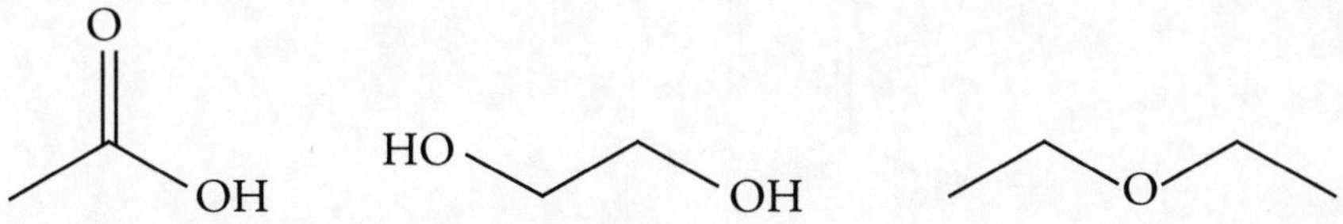

Solution: Hydrogen bonding is another intermolecular force that can affect melting and boiling points. (Remember that hydrogen bonding occurs between a **hydrogen-bond donor**—a hydrogen attached to a nitrogen, oxygen, or fluorine atom, and a **hydrogen-bond acceptor**—a lone pair of electrons on a nitrogen, oxygen, or fluorine in another molecule.) The more hydrogen-bond donors and hydrogen-bond acceptors there are in a molecule, the higher the boiling and melting points will be. This is because the hydrogen bonds, like dispersion forces, act to hold the molecules together, resisting the change to becoming either a liquid or a gas. The first molecule, acetic acid ($C_2H_4O_2$), has one hydrogen-bond donor and four hydrogen-bond acceptors (each lone electron pair on the oxygen atoms). The second molecule,

1,2-ethanediol ($C_2H_6O_2$), has two hydrogen-bond donors and four hydrogen-bond acceptors. The third molecule, diethyl ether ($C_4H_{10}O$), has two hydrogen-bond acceptors, but no hydrogen-bond donors. From this we can now correctly assign the order of their boiling points:

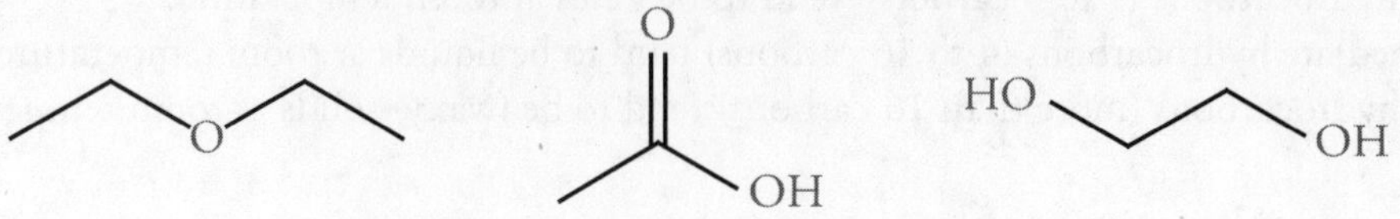

25.5

Increasing Boiling Point

Solubility

Solubility depends on two things: the polarity of the solute and the polarity of the solvent. When it comes to solubility, *like dissolves like*. Polar molecules are soluble in polar solvents, and nonpolar molecules are soluble in nonpolar solvents. Hydrocarbons have either zero or a very small dipole moment. Water, on the other hand, is a polar molecule. Since hydrocarbons are generally nonpolar molecules, they aren't very soluble in water.

Here are some types of solvents you could see on the DAT:

Nonpolar Solvents	• Hydrocarbons such as pentane, cyclopentane, hexane, cyclohexane, benzene, toluene
Versatile **Aprotic Solvents**	• These solvents can dissolve a range of polar and nonpolar solutes • Diethyl ether, Et$_2$O • Tetrahydrofuran, THF 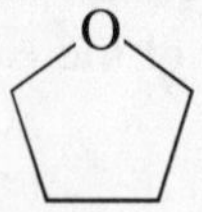 • Chloroform, CHCl$_3$
Polar Protic Solvents	• Water • Alcohols, especially MeOH, EtOH • Carboxylic acids such as formic acid, acetic acid
Polar Aprotic Solvents	• Dimethylformamide, DMF 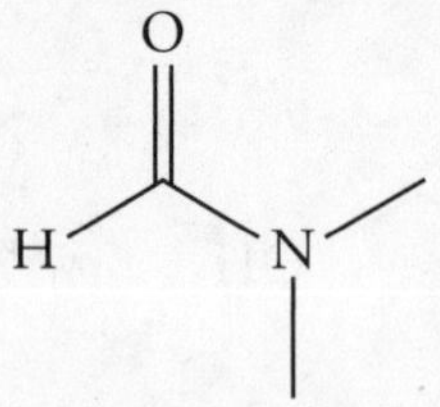 • Dimethyl sulfoxide, DMSO 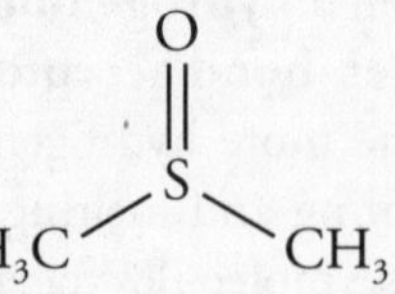 • Acetone 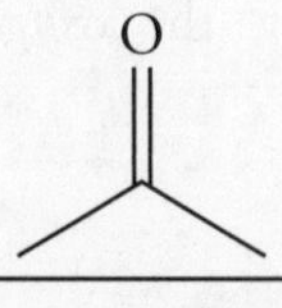

25.6   THE ORGANIC CHEMIST'S TOOLBOX

In the following chapters, we will frequently discuss several fundamental principles necessary to understand the reactivity of organic molecules. These "tools" are collected here.

Reaction Intermediates

Most organic reactions proceed through one of the following three types of intermediate species:

1. carbocations (carbonium ions),
2. alkyl radicals,
3. carbanions.

There is a fourth type of intermediate you could see on the DAT, the halonium ion (or usually the bromonium ion more specifically). However, these only occur in a small number of reactions. We'll discuss these more in Chapter 27.

Carbocations, or **carbonium ions**, are positively charged species with a full positive charge on carbon. The reactivity of these species is determined by what type of carbon bears the positive charge. On the DAT, carbocations will always be sp^2 hybridized with an empty p orbital.

Alkyl radicals are reaction intermediates that contain one unpaired electron. The reactivity of these species is determined by what type of carbon bears the lone radical electron. Even though these species are not positively charged, they are electron deficient, like carbocations. Consequently, the reactivity trends for alkyl radicals are the same as those for carbocations. Alkyl radicals on the DAT will be sp^2 hybridized with the unpaired electron in an unhybridized p orbital.

Carbanions are negatively charged species with a full negative charge localized on carbon. The reactivity of these species is determined by what type of carbon bears the negative charge. On the DAT, carbanions are usually sp^3 hybridized with the lone pair in an sp^3-hybridized orbital.

It's essential to understand the stabilities of reaction intermediates, because generally the major product of a reaction is derived from the most stable intermediate. Organic intermediates are stabilized in two major ways: **Inductive effects** stabilize charge through σ bonds, while **resonance effects** stabilize charge by delocalization through π bonds. We discuss each of these in the sections that follow. One final thing to remember here: secondary carbocations can undergo rearrangements to become a more stable tertiary carbocation. This can occur by either a 1,2-hydride (H^-) shift or a 1,2-methide ($CH3^-$) shift, which you'll see in the next chapter. If both are possible, the hydride shift will occur. Neither radical nor carbanion intermediates can rearrange.

Stability Continuum			
Carbocations	3°	2°	1°	methyl
Alkyl Radicals	3°	2°	1°	methyl
Carbanions	methyl	1°	2°	3°
	more stable	→	less stable
	less reactive	→	more reactive
	lower energy	→	higher energy

Inductive Effects

All substituent groups surrounding a reaction intermediate can be thought of as electron-withdrawing groups or electron-donating groups. **Electron-withdrawing** groups pull electrons toward themselves through σ bonds. **Electron-donating** groups donate (push) electron density away from themselves through σ bonds. Groups *more* electronegative than carbon tend to withdraw, while groups *less* electronegative than carbon tend to donate. On the DAT, alkyl substituents are always electron-donating groups.

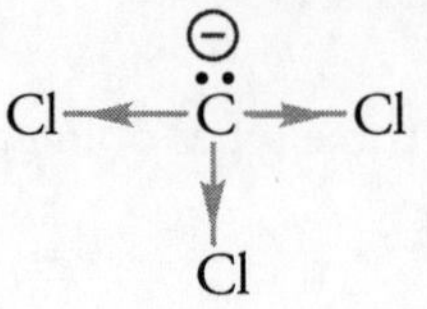

Electron
Withdrawal

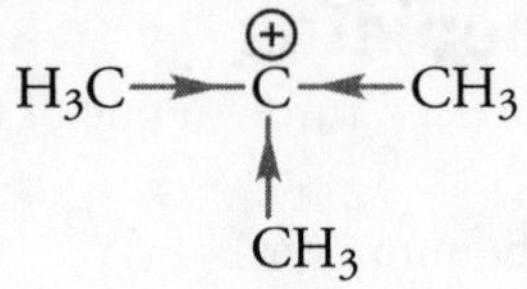

Electron
Donation

Electron-donating groups tend to stabilize electron-deficient intermediates (carbocations and radicals), while electron-withdrawing groups tend to stabilize electron-rich intermediates (carbanions). The stabilization of reaction intermediates by the sharing of electrons through σ bonds is called the **inductive effect**.

Example 25-14: Inductive effects frequently alter the reactivity of molecules. Justify the fact that trichloroacetic acid ($pK_a = 0.6$) is a stronger acid than acetic acid ($pK_a = 4.8$).

Solution: The chlorine atoms in trichloroacetic acid are electron withdrawing. This decreases the amount of electron density elsewhere in the molecule, especially in the O–H bond. With less electron density, the O–H bond is weaker, making it more acidic than the O–H bond in acetic acid.

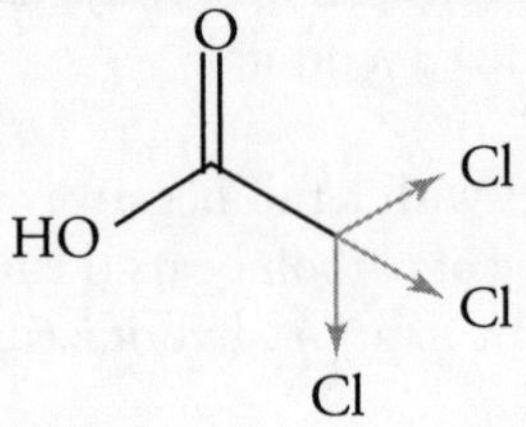

An alternative explanation would be to consider the stability of the conjugate bases of these acids.

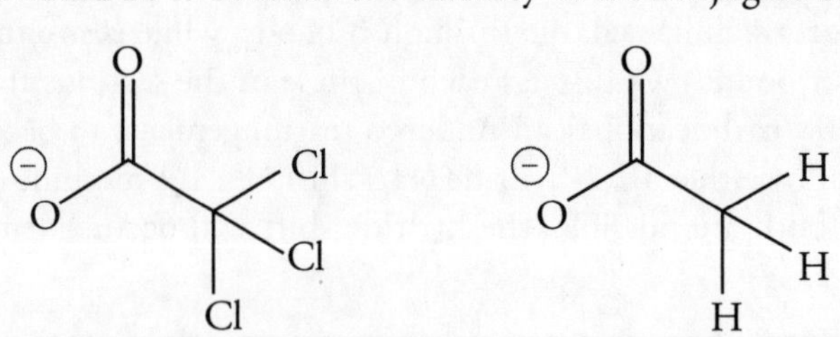

The chlorine atoms in trichloroacetate anion distribute the negative charge better, making it more stable than the acetate anion. Remember from general chemistry that the stronger the acid, the weaker (the more stable) the conjugate base. Therefore, because trichloroacetate anion is a weaker base (is more stable) than acetate anion, trichloroacetic acid is a stronger acid than acetic acid.

Resonance Stabilization

While induction works through σ bonds, resonance stabilization occurs in conjugated π systems. A **conjugated system** is one containing three or more atoms that each bear a *p* orbital. These orbitals are aligned so they are all parallel, creating the possibility of delocalized electrons.

Electrons that are confined to one orbital, either a bonding orbital between two atoms or a lone-pair orbital, are said to be **localized**. When electrons are allowed to interact with orbitals on adjacent atoms, they are no longer confined to their original "space," and so are termed **delocalized**. Consider the allyl cation:

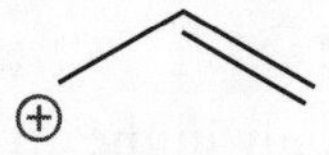

The electrons in the π bond can interact with the empty *p* orbital on the carbon bearing the positive charge. This is illustrated by the following resonance structures:

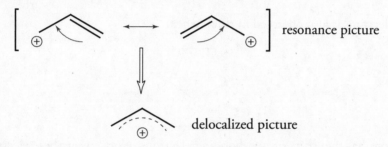

resonance picture

delocalized picture

The electron density is spread out—delocalized—over the entire 3-carbon framework in order to stabilize the carbocation. So, we might say of the allyl cation that both the electrons and the positive charge are delocalized.

As the allyl cation demonstrates, it often happens that a single Lewis structure for a molecule is not sufficient to most accurately represent the molecule's true structure. It is important to remember that resonance structures are just multiple representations of the actual structure. The molecule does not become one resonance structure or another; it exists as a combination of all resonance structures, although all may not contribute equally. All resonance structures must be drawn to give an accurate picture of the real nature of the molecule. In the case of the allyl cation, the two structures are identical and will have equivalent energy. They will also contribute equally to the delocalized picture of what the molecule really looks like. This average of all resonance contributors is called the **resonance hybrid**.

Benzene (C_6H_6) is another common molecule that exhibits resonance. Looking at a Lewis representation of benzene might lead one to believe that there are two distinct types of carbon-carbon bonds: single σ bonds (this structure of benzene has three such bonds) and double bonds (of which there are also three):

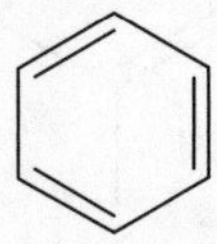

benzene

Thus one might expect two distinct carbon-carbon bond lengths: one for the single bonds, and one for the double bonds. Yet experimental data clearly demonstrate that all the C–C bond lengths are identical in benzene. All the carbons of benzene are sp^2 hybridized, so they each have an unhybridized p orbital. Two structures can be drawn for benzene, which differ only in the location of the π bonds. The true structure of benzene is best pictured as a resonance hybrid of these structures. Perhaps a better representation of benzene shows both resonance contributors, like this:

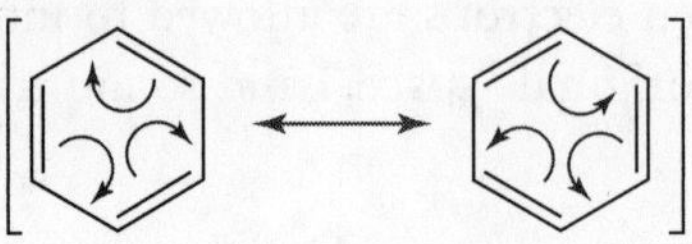

25.6

Notice that these resonance structures differ only in the arrangement of their π electrons, not in the locations of the atoms. All six unhybridized p orbitals are aligned parallel with one another. This alignment of adjacent unhybridized p orbitals allows for delocalization of π electrons over the entire ring. Whenever we have a delocalized π system (aligned p orbitals), resonance structures can be drawn.

Delocalization of electrons is also observed in thiophene:

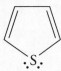

Here, the sulfur atom has two pairs of non-bonding electrons. Notice that these electrons are one atom away from two π bonds. One pair of these electrons is actually in an unhybridized p orbital, such that it can be delocalized into the cyclic π system. Here are the representative resonance structures:

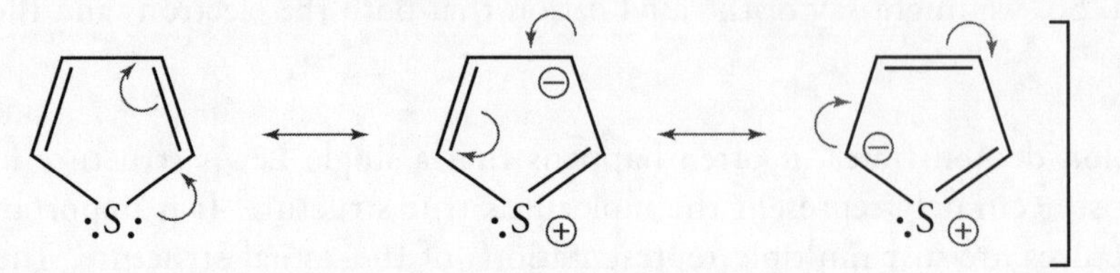

The other pair of electrons, however, is in a hybrid orbital and cannot delocalize into the π system. Here, the delocalization of sulfur's electrons imparts aromatic stability to the molecule (see Section 26.2). The hybridization of the sulfur is therefore most correctly represented as sp^2.

Let's consider one more example:

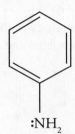

:NH$_2$

The nitrogen in aniline has an unshared electron pair that is one atom removed from a cyclic π system. Again, these electrons can be delocalized by overlap of the lone pair-containing orbital with the p orbitals of the benzene ring. This can be demonstrated by the following resonance structures:

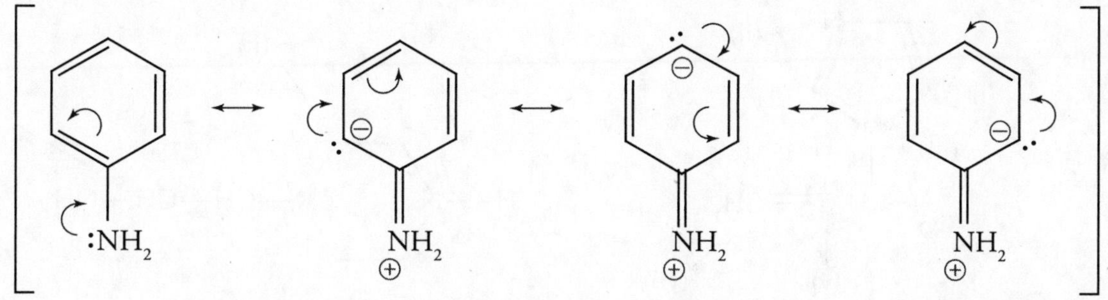

In this case, the delocalization of the nitrogen's electrons disrupts the aromaticity of the benzene ring and is therefore less favorable. Experimental determination of the nitrogen's bond angles reveals that they are actually intermediate between 120° and 109°, so the hybridization of the nitrogen can best be described not as sp^2 or sp^3, but as something intermediate between them. The important point, however, is that the electrons are at least somewhat delocalized into the π system. Therefore, the nitrogen's hybridization is not strictly sp^3.

25.6

Example 25-15: For the following molecules, indicate the hybridization and idealized bond angles for the indicated atoms.

A.

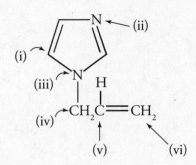

B.

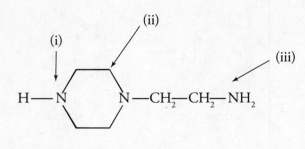

C.

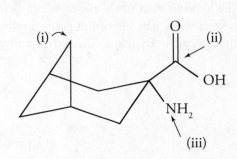

D.

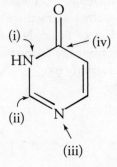

E.

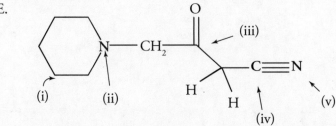

F.

Solution: Remember to always draw the electrons on nitrogen if they are not drawn in the structure.

A. (i) sp^2, 120° (ii) sp^2, 120° (iii) sp^2, 120° (The lone pair is delocalized, so it's not counted.)
    (iv) sp^3, 109° (v) sp^2, 120° (vi) sp^2, 120°
B. (i) sp^3, 109° (ii) sp^3, 109° (iii) sp^3, 109°
C. (i) sp^3, 109° (ii) sp^2, 120° (iii) sp^3, 109°
D. (i) sp^2, 120° (ii) sp^2, 120° (iii) sp^2, 120° (iv) sp^2, 120°
E. (i) sp^3, 109° (ii) sp^3, 109° (iii) sp^2, 120° (iv) sp, 180° (v) sp, 180°
F. (i) sp^3, 109° (ii) sp, 180° (iii) sp^3, 109° (iv) sp^3, 109°

So why all this focus on resonance? In general, π electrons—in alkenes and alkynes, for example—are (relatively) chemically reactive; just think of all the reactions you have studied involving π electrons (for instance, the protonation of a π bond).

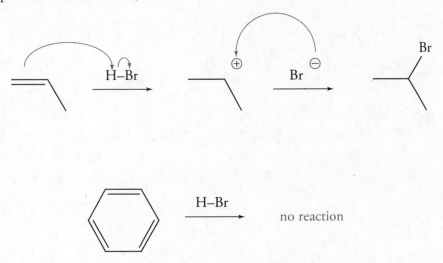

However, the π electrons of benzene do not react with the strong acid HBr. (Due to its aromaticity, benzene has a particularly stable delocalized system. For more on this see Chapter 27.) The localized π electrons of the alkene do react with HBr producing the addition product shown. Since it's important to recognize molecules that are stabilized by resonance delocalization, we'll next review the three basic principles of resonance delocalization.

25.6

1. Resonance structures usually involve electrons that are adjacent to (one atom away from) a π bond or an unhybridized p orbital. Here are some examples of molecules that are stabilized by resonance delocalization:

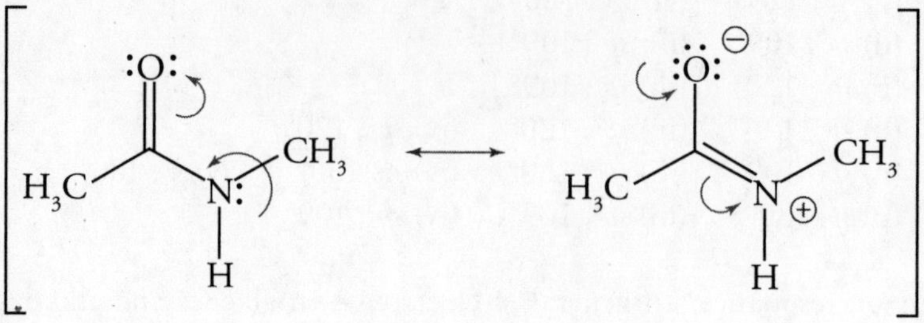

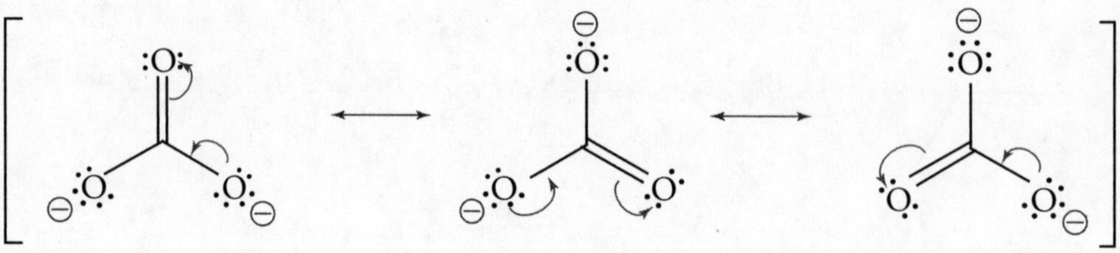

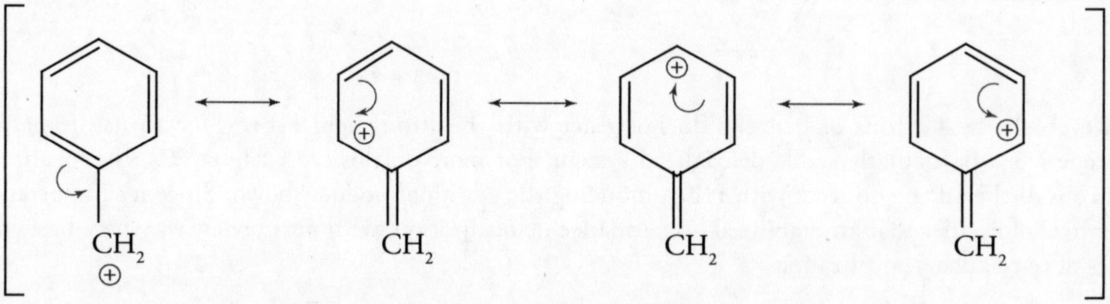

2. Resonance structures of lowest energy are the most important. Remember that the evaluation of resonance structures involves primarily three criteria:
   (i) Resonance contributors in which the octet rule is satisfied (for all the atoms it should be) are more important than ones in which it is not.
   (ii) Resonance contributors that minimize separation of charge are better than those with a large separation of charge.
   (iii) In structures that have separation of charge, the more important resonance contributor has negative charge on the more electronegative atom, and positive charge on the less electronegative atom.

3. Resonance structures can never be drawn through atoms that are truly sp^3 hybridized. Remember that an sp^3 hybridized atom is one with a total of four σ bonds and non-bonding electron pairs.

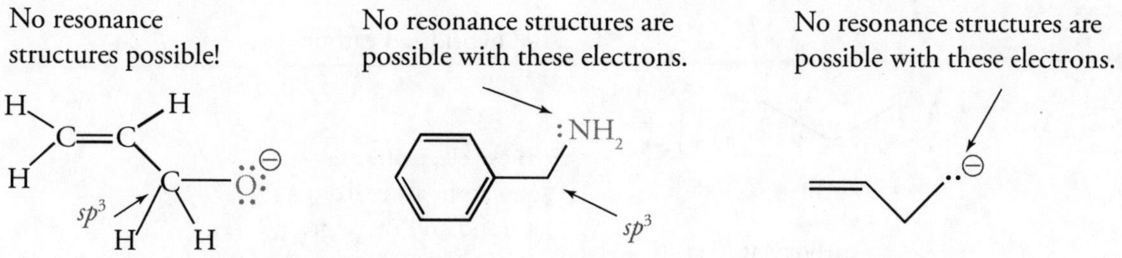

No resonance
structures possible!

No resonance structures are
possible with these electrons.

No resonance structures are
possible with these electrons.

Ochem Acidity

To demonstrate some applications of resonance theory, here are some examples that examine acidity of functional groups. Subsequent chapters will examine the application of resonance theory to the properties of nucleophilicity and basicity.

What happens when a molecule acts as an acid? A Brønsted-Lowry acid is a molecule that donates a proton (H^+). Since H^+ is donated, it is usually the case that the atom which donates the proton takes on a negative charge. The extent to which that negative charge is stabilized determines the relative acidity of the compound. Consider these examples:

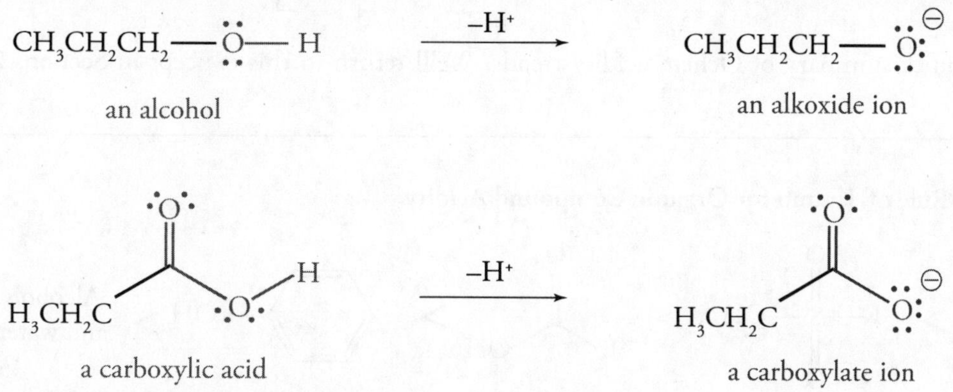

$$CH_3CH_2CH_2 - \overset{..}{\underset{..}{O}} - H \xrightarrow{-H^+} CH_3CH_2CH_2 - \overset{..}{\underset{..}{O}}{}^{\ominus}$$

an alcohol   an alkoxide ion

a carboxylic acid   a carboxylate ion

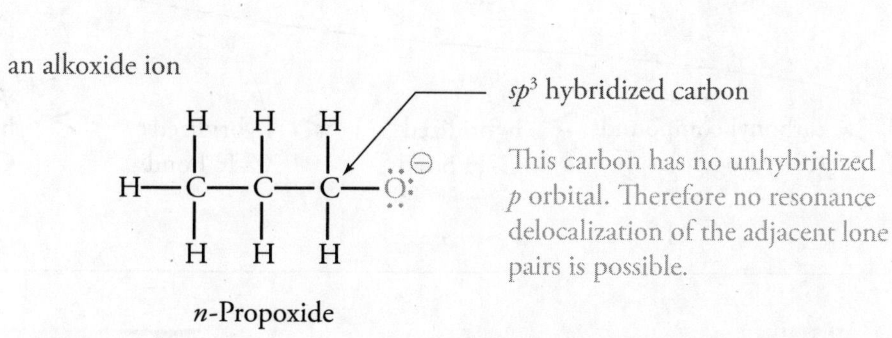

an alkoxide ion

sp³ hybridized carbon

This carbon has no unhybridized p orbital. Therefore no resonance delocalization of the adjacent lone pairs is possible.

n-Propoxide

The electrons on the oxygen in the alkoxide ion above have no adjacent empty p orbital or π system. Therefore, they are localized and highly reactive. This makes the alkoxide ion a very strong base (much like OH⁻).

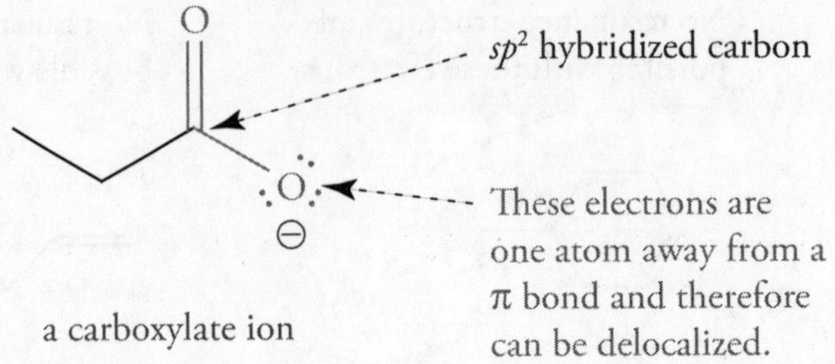

a carboxylate ion

sp^2 hybridized carbon

These electrons are one atom away from a π bond and therefore can be delocalized.

In the carboxylate ion, the electrons on the negatively charged oxygen are adjacent to a π bond and can therefore be delocalized. This leads to greater stability of the carboxylate anion and thus to higher acidity of the conjugate acid. The following demonstrates resonance stabilization for the carboxylate ion. (Note: These two resonance structures are identical and therefore of equal energy.)

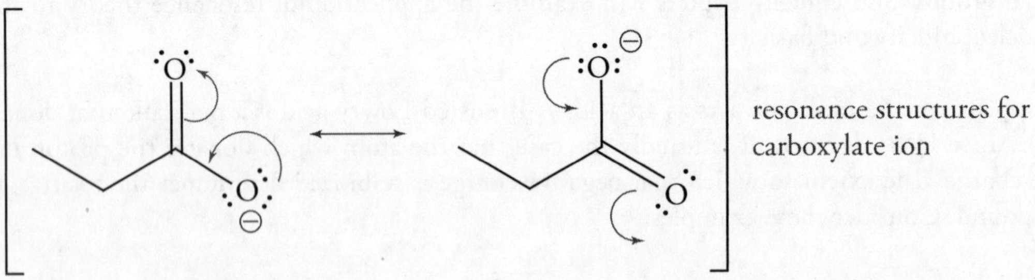

resonance structures for carboxylate ion

Here is a quick summary of Ochem acidity trends. We'll return to this concept in Sections 26.5, 28.1, and 28.2.

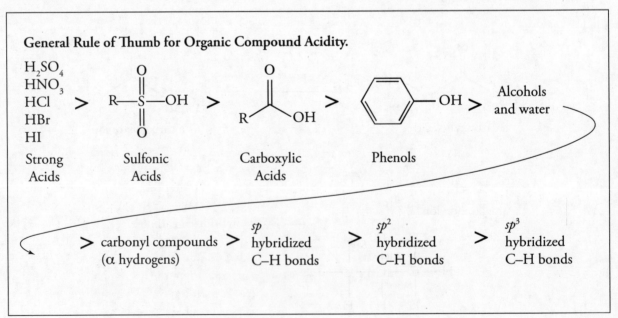

General Rule of Thumb for Organic Compound Acidity.

H_2SO_4
HNO_3
HCl
HBr
HI

Strong Acids

Sulfonic Acids

Carboxylic Acids

Phenols

Alcohols and water

> carbonyl compounds (α hydrogens) > sp hybridized C–H bonds > sp^2 hybridized C–H bonds > sp^3 hybridized C–H bonds

Example 25-16: Of the following two molecules, which one would you expect to be the stronger acid?

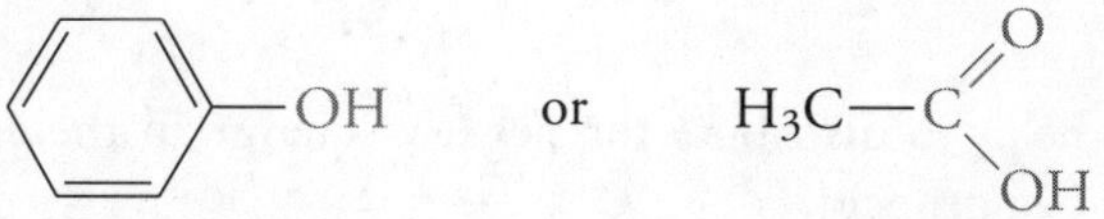

Phenol   or   Acetic acid

Solution: We examine the conjugate base of each acid in order to determine which one will have the more stabilized anion. Since both conjugate bases have electrons that can be delocalized, the question is: Which conjugate base is more stabilized by resonance delocalization?

Let's examine the resonance structures for the phenoxide and the acetate ions:

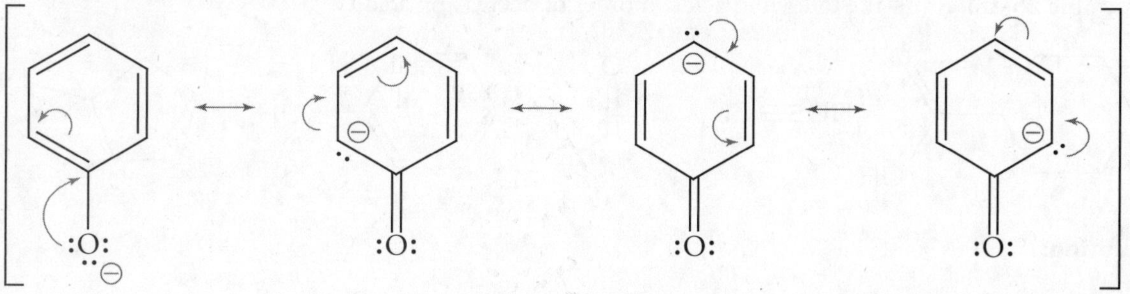

resonance structures for
the phenoxide ion

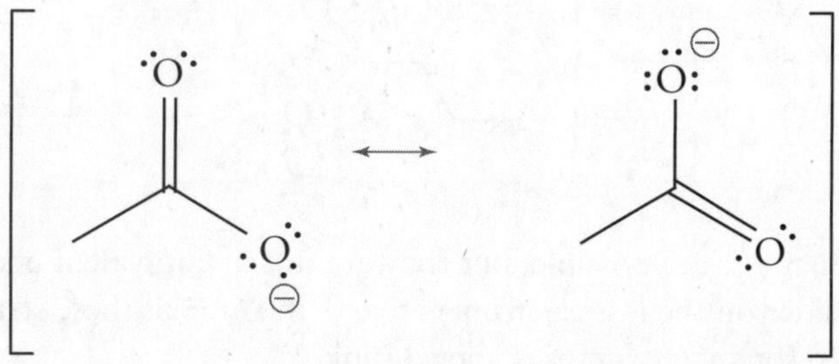

resonance structures for
the acetate ion

The resonance structures for the acetate ion are of equivalent energy with the negative charge on electronegative oxygen in both structures. In examining the resonance structures for the phenoxide ion, notice that although there are four resonance structures, three of them have the negative charge on carbon rather than on the electronegative oxygen. Also note that the three phenoxide resonance structures that have negative charge on carbon disrupt the aromaticity of the benzene ring. So, acetate ion is more resonance stabilized than phenoxide ion and hence acetic acid is a stronger acid.

Example 25-17: Use resonance structures to explain why *para*-nitrophenol (pK_a = 7.2) is a stronger acid than phenol (pK_a = 10).

Solution: The nitro group helps to distribute the negative charge in the corresponding conjugate base, making *para*-nitrophenol a stronger acid.

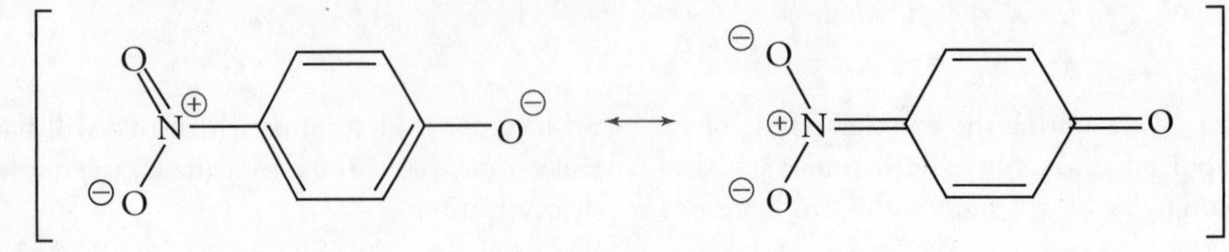

Example 25-18: Rank the following acids in order of decreasing acidity.

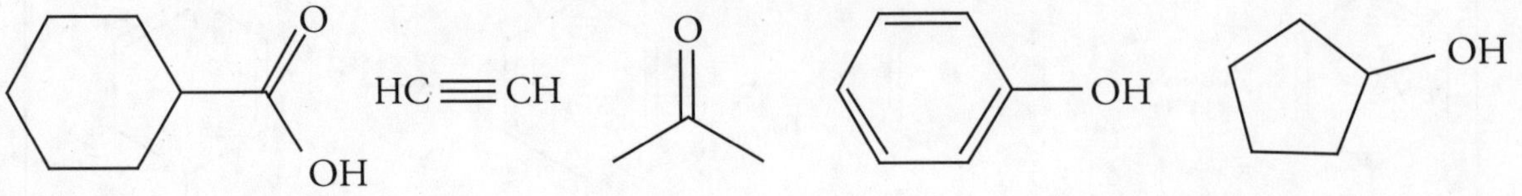

Solution:

1.   For this molecule, there are two good resonance structures of equivalent energy with negative charge on the electronegative oxygen, so rank 1st.

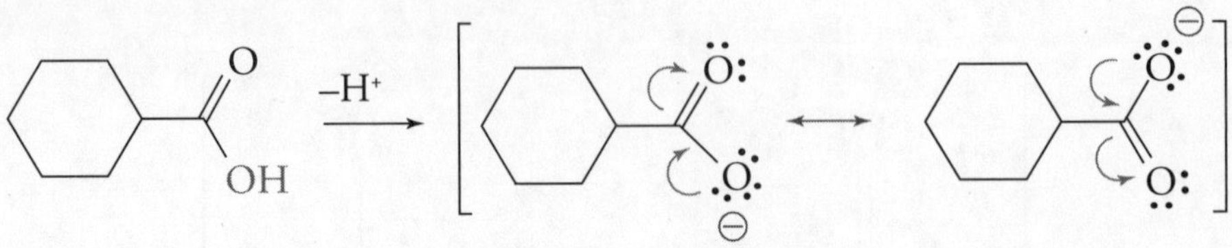

2.   Four resonance structures are possible, but they are not of equivalent energy. In addition, the negative charge resides on the less electronegative C in three of these structures. Therefore, it's not as good as the resonance structures above; rank 2nd.

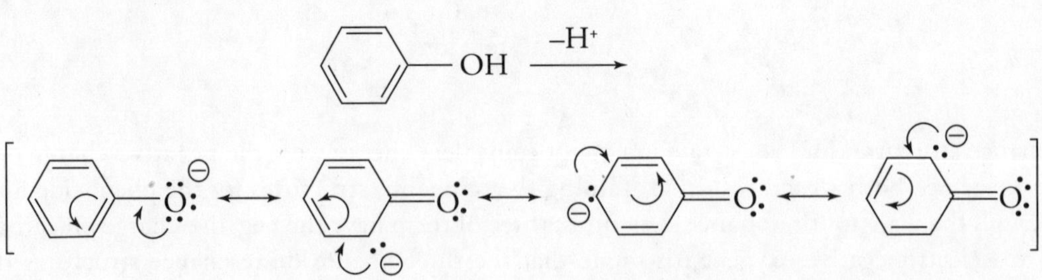

3.   There are no possible resonance structures for this molecule, but the negative charge resides on an electronegative oxygen; rank 3rd.

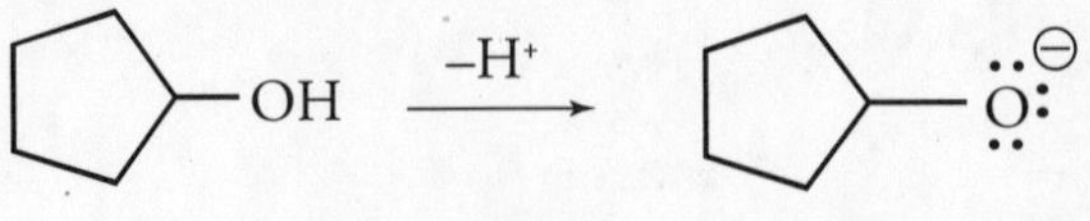

4. The hydrogens next to the carbonyl carbon are acidic because there are two resonance structures for the conjugate base of a ketone. One is stable with the negative charge on oxygen, and one is higher in energy with the negative charge on carbon. Even though it has resonance, it is less acidic than cyclopentanol because some of the charge resides on the carbon; rank 4th.

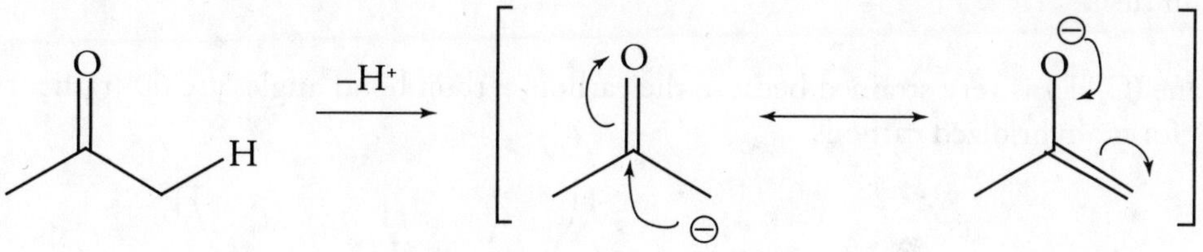

5. There are no possible resonance structures for this molecule, and the negative charge is on carbon, an atom with low electronegativity; rank 5th.

Ochem Bases

In addition to common acids, you should also recognize some bases. The strong bases you may see on the DAT include:

- Group I hydroxides (e.g., NaOH)
- Group I oxides (e.g., Li_2O)
- Some group II hydroxides: $Ba(OH)_2$, $Ca(OH)_2$, $Sr(OH)_2$
- Metal amides ($^-NR_2$), e.g., $NaNH_2$
- Alkoxides (^-OMe, ^-OEt, etc.)
- Metal alkoxides (NaOMe, NaOEt, etc.)

There are two bulky (or sterically hindered) bases you should recognize for the DAT:

Potassium *tert*-butoxide or KOtBu:

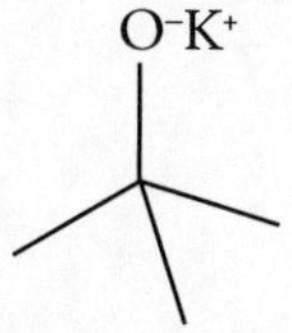

Lithium diisopropylamide or LDA:

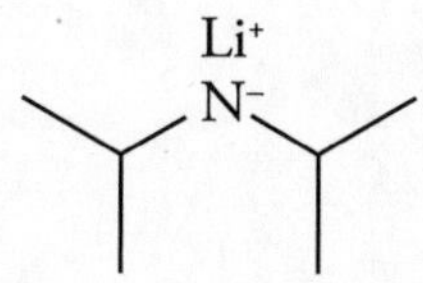

Ring Strain

The last item in our toolbox is a feature of organic molecules that, unlike inductive and resonance effects, contributes to instability in a molecule: **ring strain**. Ring strain arises when bond angles between ring atoms deviate from the ideal angle predicted by the hybridization of the atoms. Let's examine several cycloalkanes in turn.

Cyclopropane (C_3H_6) is very strained because the carbon-carbon bond angles are 60° rather than the idealized 109° for sp^3 hybridized carbons.

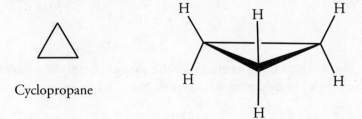

Cyclopropane

Cyclobutane (C_4H_8) might be expected to have 90° carbon-carbon bond angles. However, one of the carbons is bent out of the plane of the ring by about 20°, such that all of the carbon-carbon bond angles are 88°. The distortion of the cyclobutane ring minimizes the eclipsing of carbon-hydrogen σ bonds on adjacent carbon atoms.

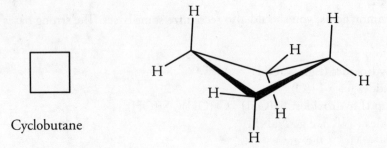

Cyclobutane

The deviation of the bond angles from the normal tetrahedral 109° causes cyclopropane and cyclobutane to be unstable. The strain weakens the carbon-carbon bonds and increases reactivity of these cycloalkanes in comparison to other alkanes. For example, while it is essentially impossible to cleave the average alkane C–C single bond via hydrogenation, C–C bonds in these highly strained cyclic molecules are significantly more reactive. However, they are still much less reactive than C=C double (π) bonds.

Here are the hydrogenation reactions of cyclopropane and cyclobutane:

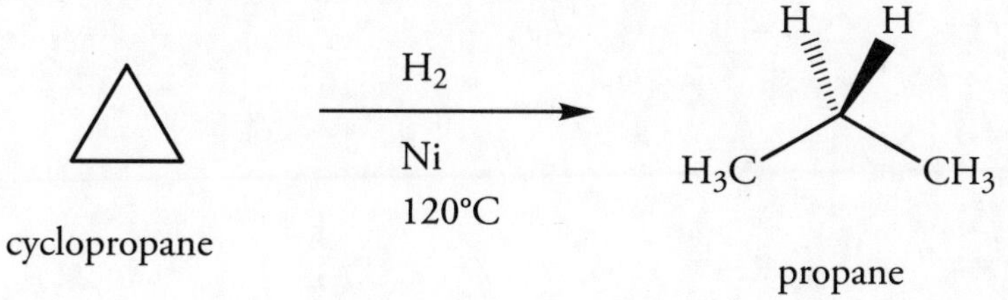

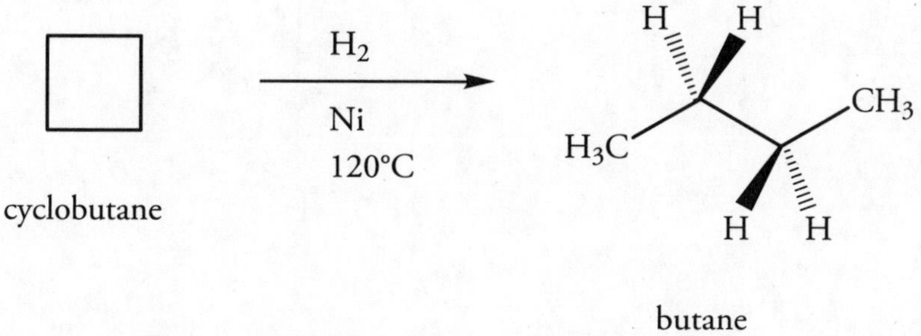

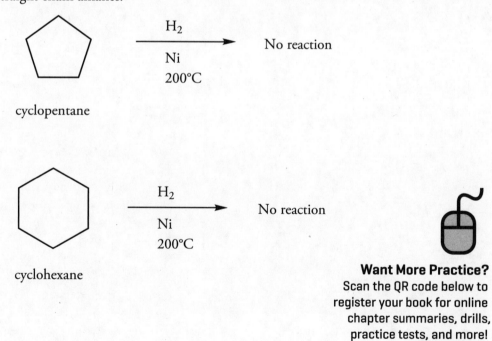

Unlike cyclopropane and cyclobutane, cyclopentane has a low degree of ring strain, and cyclohexane is strain free. Both molecules have near-tetrahedral bond angles (109°) due to the conformations they adopt. Consequently, these cycloalkanes do not undergo hydrogenation reactions under normal conditions, and react similarly to straight chain alkanes:

Want More Practice?
Scan the QR code below to register your book for online chapter summaries, drills, practice tests, and more!

Chapter 26
Substitution and Elimination Reactions

In Chapter 25 we explored the fundamentals of structure and stereochemistry. In this chapter we will discuss three major reaction types: free radical halogenations (FRHs), nucleophilic substitutions, and elimination reactions. We will examine these reactions in the context of five functional groups: alkanes, haloalkanes, alcohols, ethers, and amines.

These reactions are defined by bonding changes that occur over the course of the reaction. In both FRHs and substitution reactions, one σ bond in the starting material is converted into a new σ bond in the product. Let's take a closer look at the two most common types of substitution reactions. In elimination reactions, two single bonds are removed and a double bond is formed.

For both nucleophilic substitution reactions and elimination reactions, there are two options for how the mechanism could proceed. Let's jump into Chapter 26 and look at how these reactions happen and what you need to know for the DAT.

26.1   FREE RADICAL HALOGENATION

We will now examine the basic principles of **free-radical halogenation**, an important reaction of alkanes on the DAT, by focusing on the mechanism of this reaction. Free-radical halogenation is a reaction that proceeds by a multi-step mechanism that includes **initiation**, **propagation**, and **termination** (and is often subject to **inhibition** by molecular oxygen).

Initiation

A free radical reaction can be initiated by light or heat. In a light-initiated reaction, a photon ($E = h\nu$) collides with (usually) a molecular halogen such as Cl_2 or Br_2, causing homolytic cleavage of a bond (see Section 24.3). This results in the formation of two halogen radicals.

Homolytic Cleavage: One electron goes with each atom of the bond being broken. This produces two radicals.

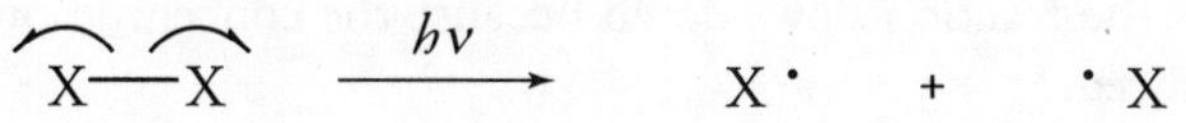

$$X-X \xrightarrow{h\nu} X\cdot \; + \; \cdot X$$

Propagation

For every halogen radical formed in the initiation step, about 10,000 alkyl halide molecules are formed in the propagation steps of this chain reaction. In the first step of the propagation reactions, a halogen radical collides with an alkane molecule (R–H), causing homolytic cleavage of a C–H bond with formation of a molecule of hydrogen halide (H–X) and an alkyl radical (R·).

In the next step of the propagation, the alkyl halide product is formed. This is accomplished by the collision of an alkyl radical (R·) with molecular halogen (X–X). This collision results in the homolytic cleavage of the molecular halogen so that a molecule of alkyl halide (R–X) product is formed and a halogen radical (X·) is regenerated.

$$R-H \; + \; \cdot X \longrightarrow R\cdot \; + \; H-X$$

$$R\cdot \; + \; X-X \longrightarrow R-X \; + \; \cdot X$$

The halogen radical then proceeds to collide with another alkane molecule, continuing the propagation of the chain reaction. Therefore, one halogen radical is able to lead to the production of many, many alkyl halide products since the halogen radical is always regenerated in the process.

Termination

The propagation of the chain reaction continues until one of the reactive radicals of the propagation steps combines with another radical. This can be accomplished by the combination of two halogen radicals (X·) to form a molecule of molecular halogen (X–X), or the combination of two alkyl radicals (R·) to form a molecule of alkane (R–R), or finally, by the combination of an alkyl radical (R·) with a halogen radical (X·) to form an alkyl halide (R–X). The consumption of reactive radicals stops the propagation of the chain reaction.

$$X\cdot + \cdot X \rightarrow X\text{–}X$$

$$R\cdot + \cdot R \rightarrow R\text{–}R$$

$$R\cdot + \cdot X \rightarrow R\text{–}X$$

Inhibition

Finally, as previously stated, the free-radical halogenation reaction is inhibited by molecular oxygen. This occurs when an alkyl radical reacts with a molecule of molecular oxygen to form a less reactive alkyl peroxy radical (R—O—O·). The reaction slows down because the concentration of the more reactive alkyl radical intermediate is reduced.

$$R\cdot + O{=}O \rightleftharpoons R\text{—}O\text{—}O\cdot$$

Summary of Free-Radical Halogenation of Alkanes Mechanism

Initiation: A step that yields a net increase in the number of radicals.

$$(1) \quad X\text{—}X \xrightarrow[\text{or heat}]{h\nu} 2\,X\cdot$$

Propagation: A step that yields no net change in the number of radicals.

$$(2) \quad R\text{—}H + \cdot X \longrightarrow R\cdot + H\text{—}X$$

$$(3) \quad R\cdot + X\text{—}X \longrightarrow R\text{—}X + X\cdot$$

Then (2), (3), (2), (3), . . .

Termination: A step that yields a net decrease in the number of radicals.

$$(4) \quad X\cdot + X\cdot \longrightarrow X\text{—}X$$

$$(5) \quad R\cdot + R\cdot \longrightarrow R\text{—}R$$

$$(6) \quad R\cdot + X\cdot \longrightarrow R\text{—}X$$

Inhibition: Inhibition by molecular oxygen slows down the reaction by reducing the amount of reactive radical intermediate. This is reversible.

$$(7) \quad R\cdot + O_2 \rightleftharpoons R\text{—}O\text{—}O\cdot$$

Stereochemistry of Free-Radical Halogenation

When the halogen radical collides with the alkane, it abstracts a hydrogen from an sp^3 hybridized tetrahedral carbon atom in a homolytic cleavage that results in the formation of a molecule of H–X and a carbon radical intermediate. The next important point to consider is the hybridization of the intermediate alkyl carbon radical. As the hydrogen radical is abstracted, the resulting carbon radical rehybridizes to place the single electron in an unhybridized p orbital. The geometry is planar with 120° bond angles, and the lone electron resides above and below the plane of the molecule in an unhybridized p orbital.

sp³ hybridized   *sp² hybridized*

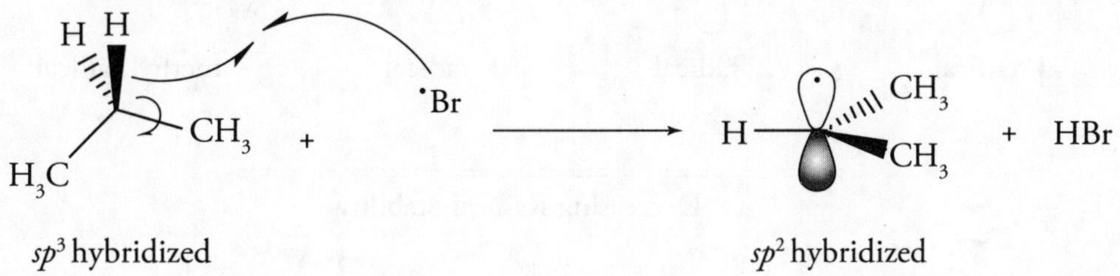

When the alkyl radical then reacts with a molecule of molecular halogen in the next step of the reaction, the carbon-halogen bond can form on either side of the plane defined by the sp^2 hybridized atom. This leads to racemization at carbon if its substitution is unsymmetrical, since bond formation can occur to an equal extent from either side of the unhybridized p orbital.

Racemization of an Unsymmetrical Alkyl Radical

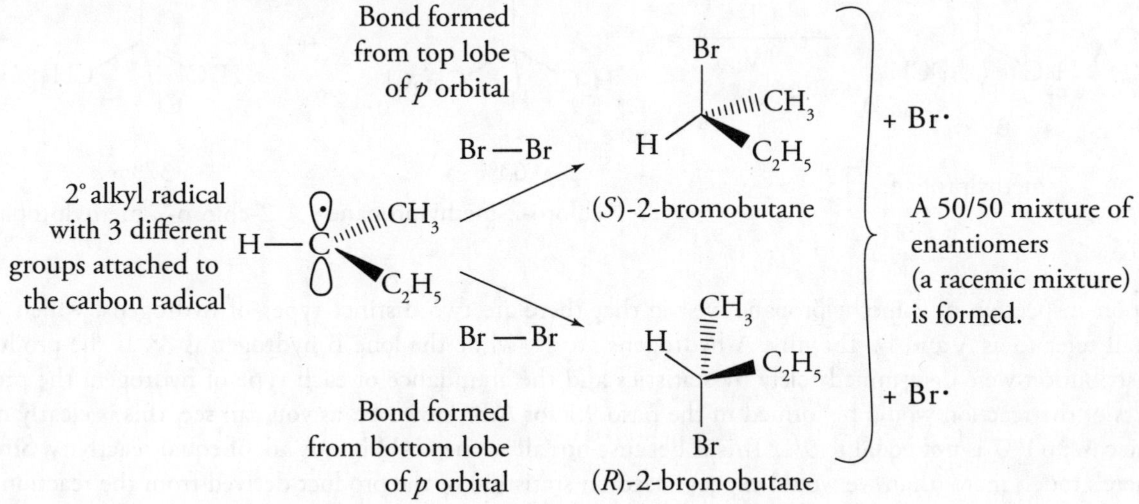

Stability of Alkyl Radicals

Next we examine the relative stability of carbon alkyl radicals. Free radicals are like carbocations in the sense that they have an unfilled p orbital (one electron for a radical vs. zero electrons for a carbocation). Also, like carbocations (see Section 24.6) alkyl substituents on carbon increase the relative stability of the radical.

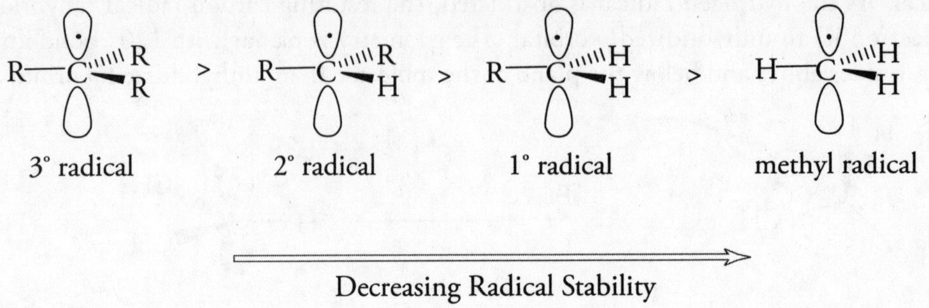

3° radical > 2° radical > 1° radical > methyl radical

Decreasing Radical Stability

Selectivity

The varying stabilities of alkyl radicals have a profound effect on the selectivity of these reactions. First, we will look at the free-radical chlorination of 2-methylpropane.

2-methylpropane

63%
1-chloro-2-methylpropane

37%
2-chloro-2-methylpropane

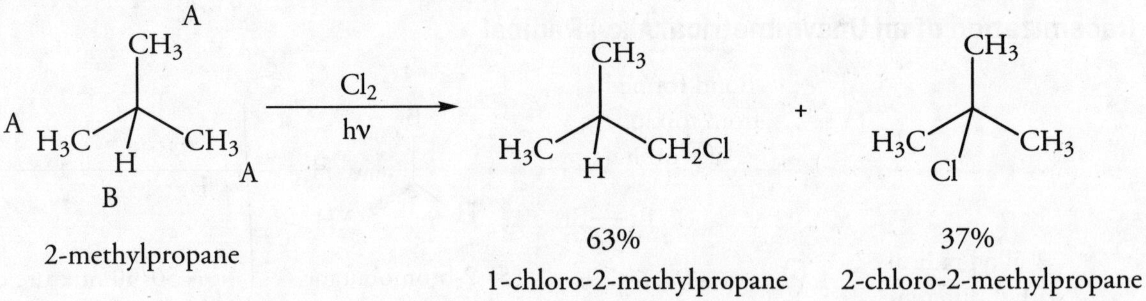

Upon inspection of 2-methylpropane we see that there are two distinct types of hydrogens, which we shall refer to as A and B. The nine A hydrogens are 1°, while the lone B hydrogen is 3°. If the product distribution were determined solely by statistics and the abundance of each type of hydrogen, the products of the reaction would be formed in the ratio 9:1 for A:B. However, as you can see, this is clearly not the case; 63/37 is not equal to 9/1. This is because not all of the C–H bonds are of equal reactivity. Since there's much more (than we would expect based on statistics) of the product derived from the reaction at position B, we can infer that position B is more reactive than position A. In order to calculate the selectivity of the different positions, one needs to factor out the number of reactive sites:

$$\text{Selectivity} = \frac{\text{reactivity}}{\text{\# of sites available}}$$

Therefore, in this case we have:

$$\frac{\text{selectivity of 3°}}{\text{selectivity of 1°}} = \frac{(\text{reactivity at 3°}) / (\text{\# of 3° sites})}{(\text{reactivity at 1°}) / (\text{\# of 1° sites})} = \frac{37/1}{63/9} = \frac{37}{7} = 5.3$$

We now consider the corresponding free radical bromination of 2-methylpropane. The bromine radical is less reactive than the corresponding chlorine radical. The lower reactivity of the bromine radical results in a much higher selectivity (3° > 2° > 1°) in the bromination reaction compared to the corresponding chlorination reaction. The reason for this is beyond the scope of the DAT, but you should have a sense of the degree of selectivity, which has been quantified and is on the order of 1640:82:1 (see the calculations below).

Bromination of Alkanes is Much More Selective than Chlorination

Reaction Rate

	R_3CH (3°)	>	R_2CH_2 (2°)	>	RCH_3 (1°)
Bromination:	1640.0		82.0		1
Chlorination:	5.3		3.9		1

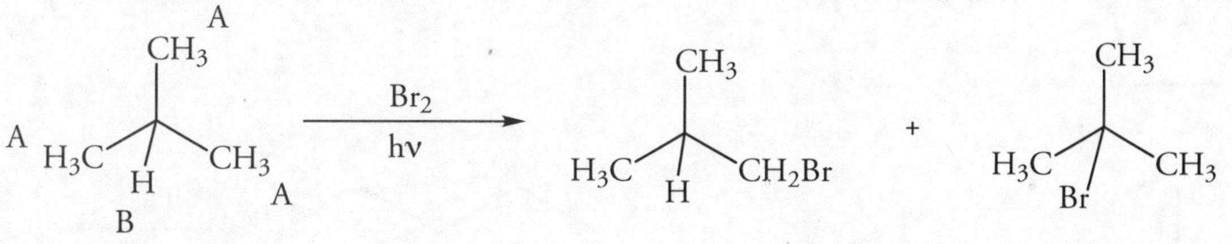

2-methylpropane 1-bromo-2-methylpropane 2-bromo-2-methylpropane

$$\text{species ratio} = \frac{\text{1-bromo-2-methylpropane}}{\text{2-bromo-2-methylpropane}} = \frac{\#\,1°\,H}{\#\,3°\,H} \times \frac{\text{reactivity of 1°\,H}}{\text{reactivity of 3°\,H}} = \frac{9}{1} \times \frac{1}{1640} = \frac{9}{1640}$$

Therefore,

$$\%\,\textit{1-bromo-2-methylpropane} = \frac{9}{9+1640} \times 100\% = 0.5\% \qquad \%\,\textit{2-bromo-2-methylpropane} = \frac{1640}{9+1640} \times 100\% = 99.5\%$$

The reason for the lower selectivity in the chlorination of an alkane is that it is more exothermic than the corresponding bromination reaction. In the bromine case, only one of the two propagation steps is exothermic (the other is endothermic). For this reason, bromination is slower and more selective than chlorination.

Enthalpies for Radical Halogenation of Methane

$$CH_4 + X_2 \rightarrow CH_3X + HX$$

X	$\Delta H°$ (kcal/mol)
F	−102.8
Cl	−24.7
Br	−7.3
I	+12.7

Propagation Steps of Radical Bromination of Methane

Step	$\Delta H°$ (kcal/mol)
$CH_4 + Br^{\bullet} \rightarrow CH_3^{\bullet} + HBr$	+18
$CH_3^{\bullet} + Br_2 \rightarrow CH_3Br + Br^{\bullet}$	−25

It is predicted from the enthalpy values in the table above that fluorine should be a very unselective reagent. This is, in fact, experimentally observed.

Example 26-1: Predict the organic product(s) from the following free-radical halogenation reactions. For the brominations, determine the major and minor products.

A.

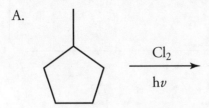

D.

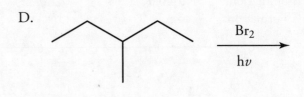

B.

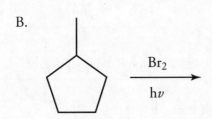

E.

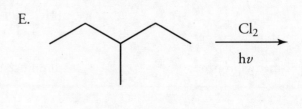

C.

Solution:

A.

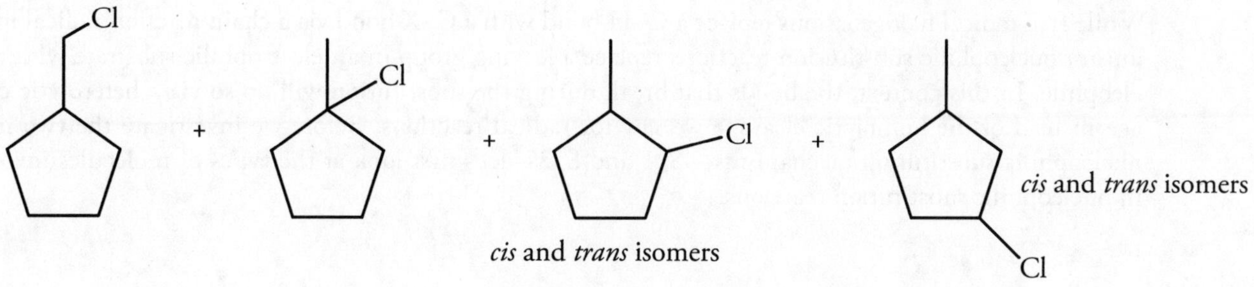

Cl
+
Cl
+
Cl
+
cis and trans isomers
cis and trans isomers
Cl

B.

Br
Br
+
+
Br
+
major
minor
cis and trans
cis and trans
Br

C.

Cl
+
Cl

D.

Br
+
+
Br
Br
+
Br
major
minor
minor
minor

E.

Cl
+
Cl
+
Cl
+
Cl

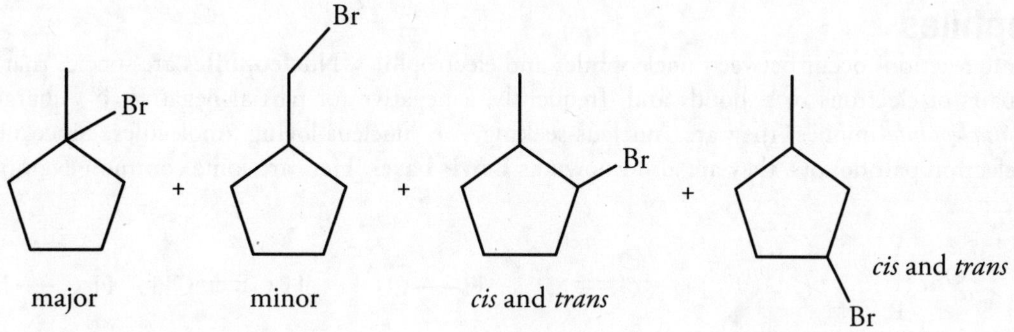

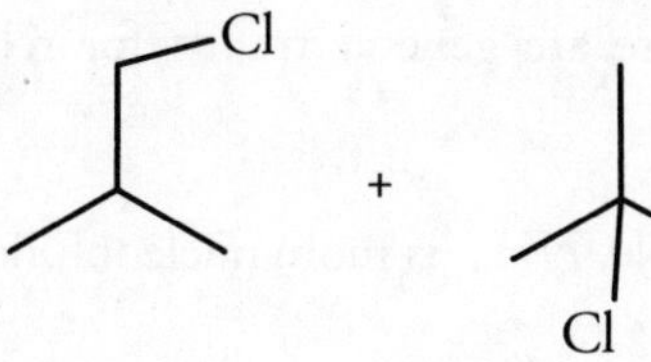

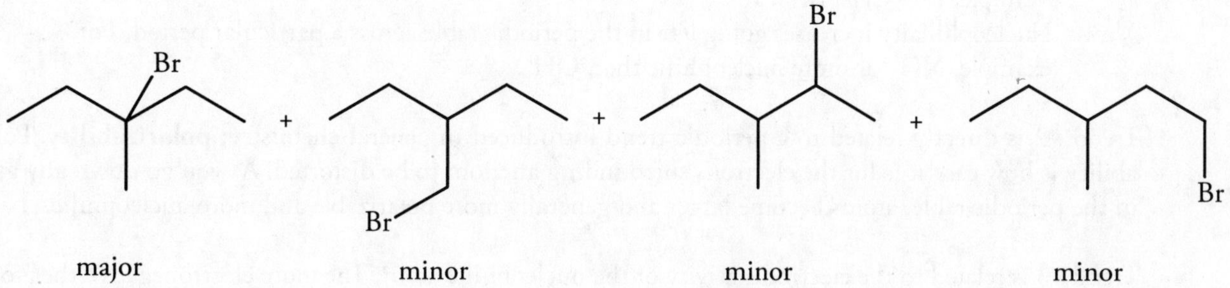

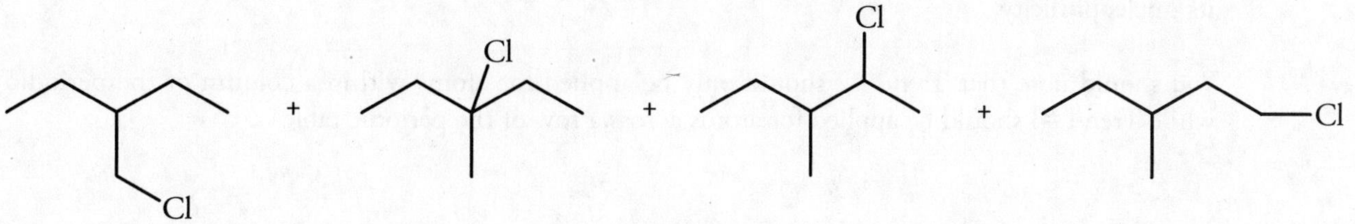

26.2 NUCLEOPHILIC SUBSTITUTIONS

While free-radical halogenations replace a C–H bond with a C–X bond via a chain reaction radical mechanism, nucleophilic substitution reactions replace a leaving group in an electrophilic substrate with a nucleophile. In this context, the bonds that break during the substitution will do so via a heterolytic cleavage instead of the homolytic cleavage we saw for radical reactions. Before we investigate the two main nucleophilic substitution mechanisms—S_N1 and S_N2—let's first look at the types of molecules involved in nucleophilic substitution reactions.

Nucleophiles

Most organic reactions occur between nucleophiles and electrophiles. **Nucleophiles** are species that have unshared pairs of electrons or π bonds and, frequently, a negative (or partial negative, δ^-) charge. As the name *nucleophile* implies, they are "nucleus-seeking" or "nucleus-loving" molecules. Since nucleophiles are electron pair donors, they are also known as **Lewis bases**. Here are some common examples of nucleophiles:

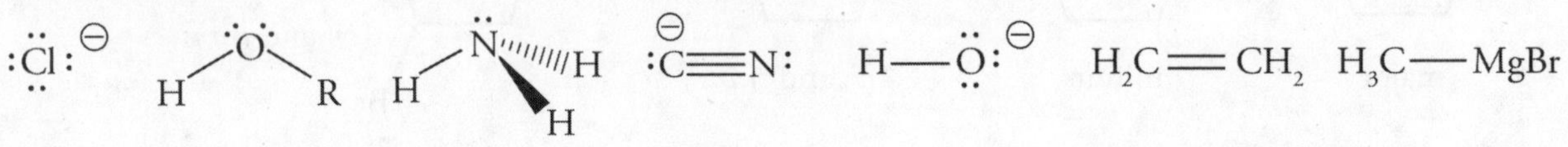

Nucleophilicity is a measure of how "strong" a nucleophile is. There are general trends for relative nucleophilicities:

1. Nucleophilicity increases as negative charge increases. For example, NH_2^- is more nucleophilic than NH_3.
2. Nucleophilicity increases going down the periodic table within a particular group. For example, $F^- < Cl^- < Br^- < I^-$.
3. Nucleophilicity increases going left in the periodic table across a particular period. For example, NH_2^- is more nucleophilic than OH^-.

Trend #2 is directly related to a periodic trend introduced in general chemistry: **polarizability**. Polarizability is how easy it is for the electrons surrounding an atom to be distorted. As you go down any group in the periodic table, atoms become larger and generally more polarizable and more nucleophilic.

Trend #3 is related to the electronegativity of the nucleophilic atom. The more electronegative the atom is, the better it is able to support its negative charge. Therefore, the less electronegative an atom is, the higher its nucleophilicity.

You should note that Trend #2 should only be applied for atoms within a column of the periodic table, while Trend #3 should be applied for atoms across a row of the periodic table.

Example 26-2: In each of the following pairs of molecules, identify the one that is more nucleophilic.

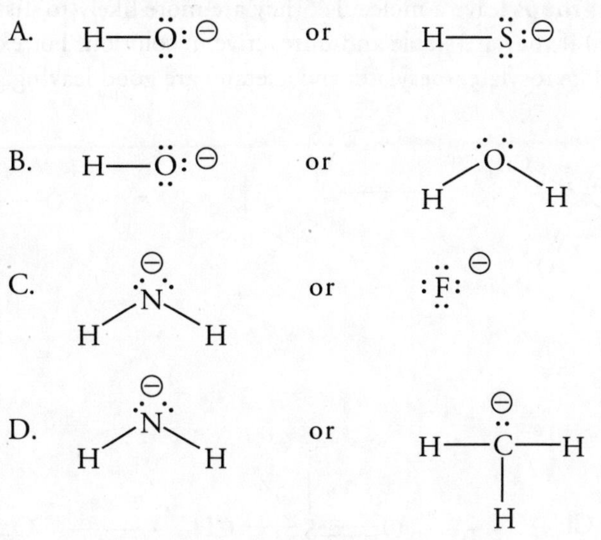

A. H—Ö:⊖   or   H—S̈:⊖

B. H—Ö:⊖   or   H—O—H (bent, :O: with H and H)

C. H—N̈—H (with ⊖)   or   :F̈:⊖

D. H—N̈—H (with ⊖)   or   H—C̈—H with H below (⊖)

Solution:

A. SH⁻, since by Trend #2 above, S is more nucleophilic than O.
B. OH⁻, because OH⁻ carries a negative charge, while H_2O does not (Trend #1, previous page).
C. NH_2^-, since F is more electronegative than N.
D. CH_3^-, because N is more electronegative than C.

Electrophiles

Electrophiles are electron-deficient species. They have a full or partial positive (δ^+) charge and "love electrons." Frequently, they have an incomplete octet. **Electrophilicity** is a measure of how strong an electrophile is. Since electrophiles are electron pair acceptors, they are also known as **Lewis acids**. Here are some common examples of electrophiles:

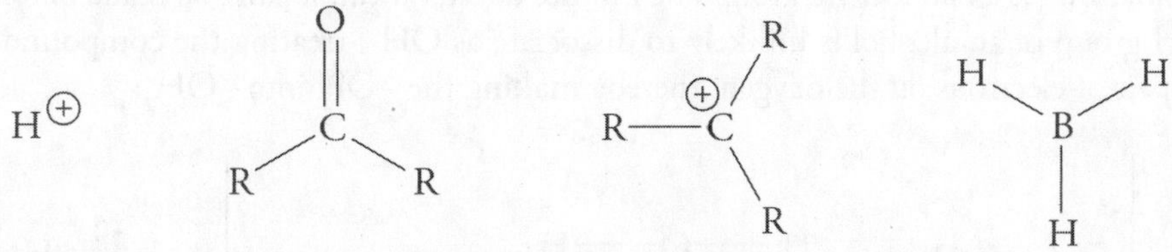

H⊕   R—C(=O)—R   R—C⁺(R)(R)   H—B(H)—H

In all organic reactions (except free-radical and pericyclic reactions), nucleophiles are attracted—and donate a pair of electrons—to electrophiles. When the electrophile accepts the electron pair (a Lewis acid/Lewis base reaction), a new covalent bond forms between the two species, which we can represent symbolically like this:

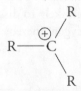

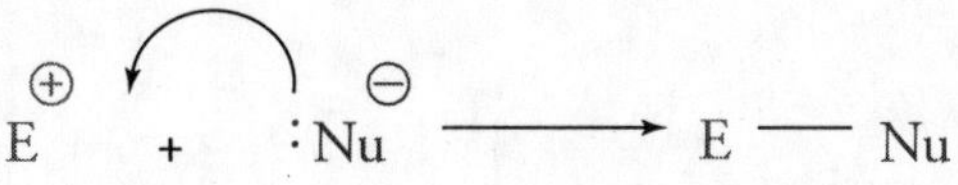

E⊕   +   :Nu⊖   ⟶   E—Nu

Leaving Groups

Not surprisingly, **leaving groups** leave a molecule. They are more likely to dissociate from their substrate (that is, do their "leaving") if they are stable and unreactive in solution. For example, leaving groups that are resonance-stabilized (like tosylate, mesylate, and acetate) are good leaving groups:

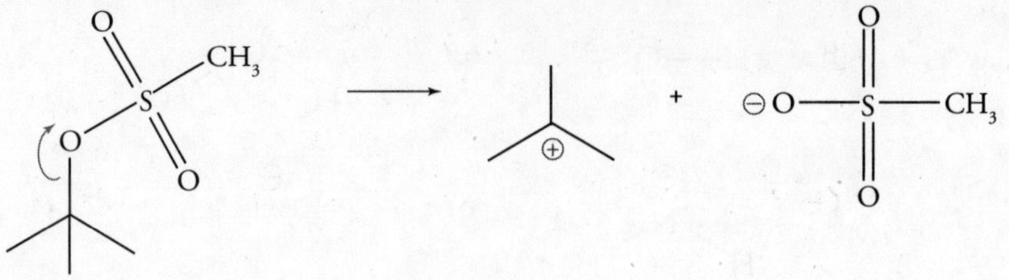

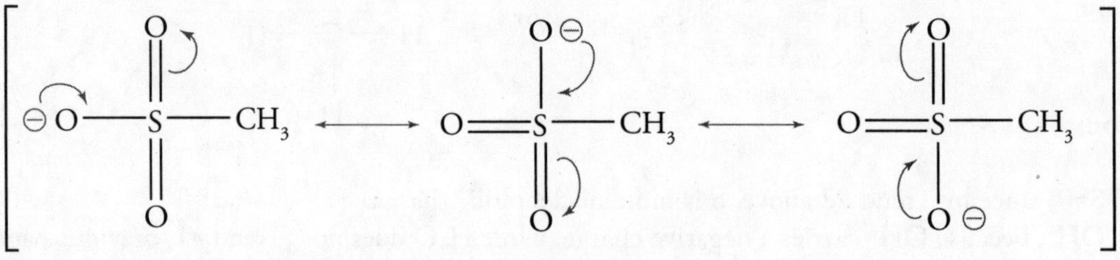

Resonance Structures of the Mesylate Leaving Group

I⁻, Br⁻, and Cl⁻ are conjugate bases of strong acids and so are essentially neutral (in acid/base properties, not in charge). They are good leaving groups because their negative charge is stabilized due to their large size. F⁻ is small and the conjugate base of a weak acid; it is therefore a weak base, somewhat reactive, and not a good leaving group. Strong bases (HO⁻, RO⁻, NH₂⁻, etc.) are great electron donors because they cannot stabilize their negative charge very well, making them very reactive. As a result, these groups are more likely to stay bound to their substrate rather than dissociate in solution. As you might expect, strong bases are therefore bad leaving groups.

Just because something is a bad leaving group one minute doesn't mean it can't be made better. For example, while the −OH group of an alcohol is unlikely to dissociate as OH⁻, treating the compound with acid protonates a lone pair of electrons on the oxygen, thereby making the −OH into −OH₂⁺:

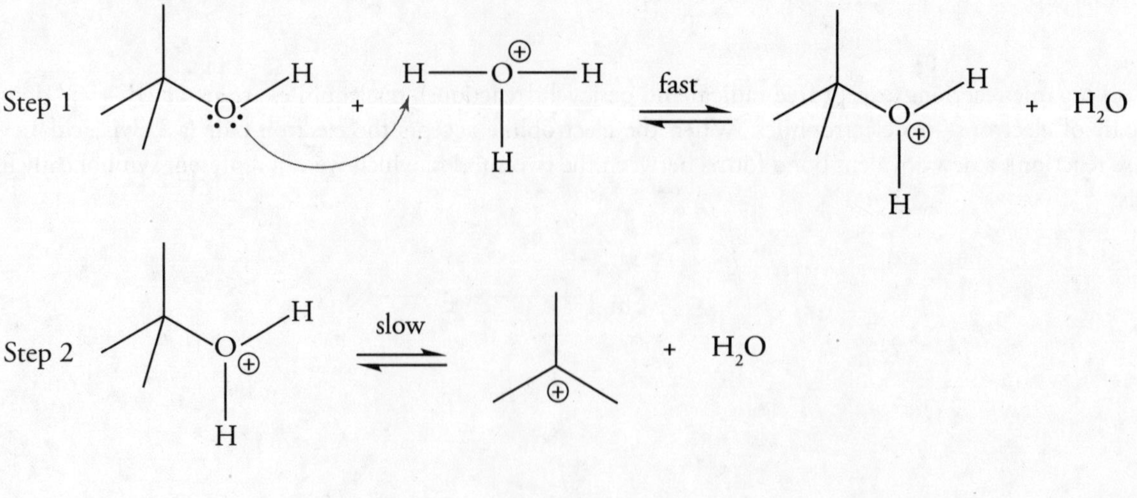

The altered group can dissociate as a neutral water molecule, and voila—no negative charge to stabilize. Water is a great leaving group because it is stable and unreactive. This trick will work for any of the strong bases listed above and is the reason why many organic reactions are acid catalyzed.

There are other options for the –OH group of an alcohol; it can be **mesylated**, **tosylated**, or converted into a halide:

Toyslation:
OH → OTs

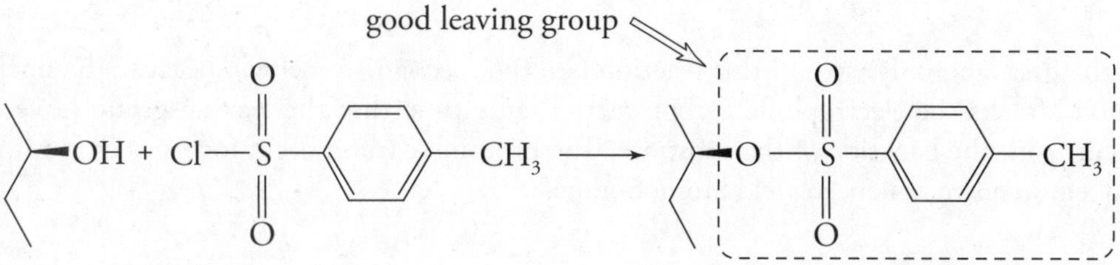

an organic tosylate (R–OTs)

Mesylation
OH → OMs

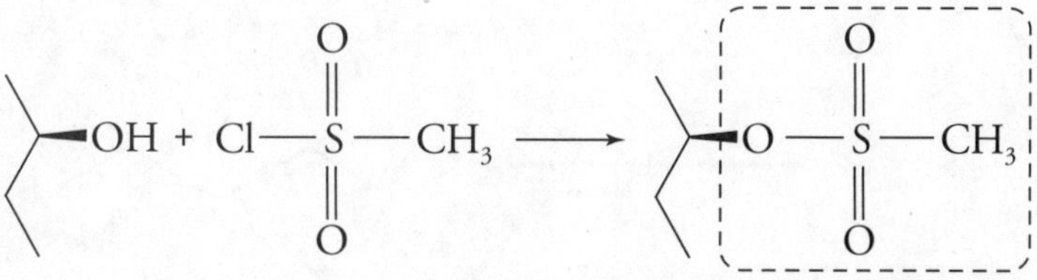

an organic mesylate (R–OMs)

Switch OH
to a halide:
OH → X

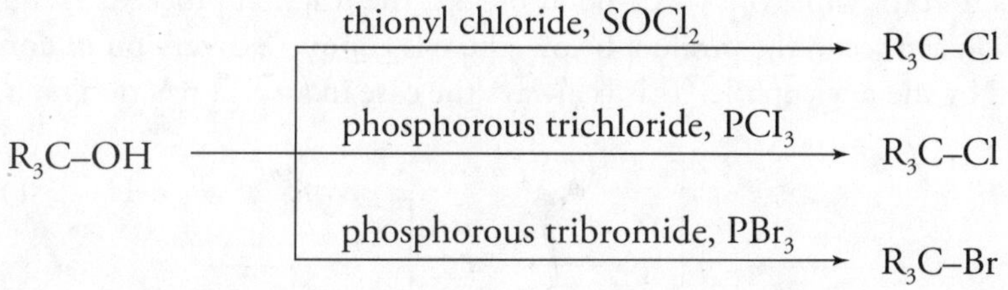

These are all ways to turn a poor leaving group (unstable and reactive OH^-) into a good leaving group. We'll see specific examples of alcohol-to-halide reactions in Section 26.5.

S_N2 Reactions

The first nucleophilic mechanism we'll examine is the S_N2 mechanism. Typical electrophiles (also known as substrates) for this type of reaction are alkyl halides. Alkyl halides are alkanes that contain at least one halogen (fluorine, chlorine, bromine or iodine). Since halogen atoms are very electronegative, most halides (Cl^-, Br^-, I^-) make good leaving groups. Hence, the chemistry of alkyl halides involves substitution and elimination reactions.

Let us first consider an example of an S_N2 substitution reaction of an alkyl halide. When 1-iodobutane is treated with a Br^- nucleophile, an S_N2 reaction occurs in which bromide replaces the I^- group (known as the leaving group) to yield 1-bromobutane.

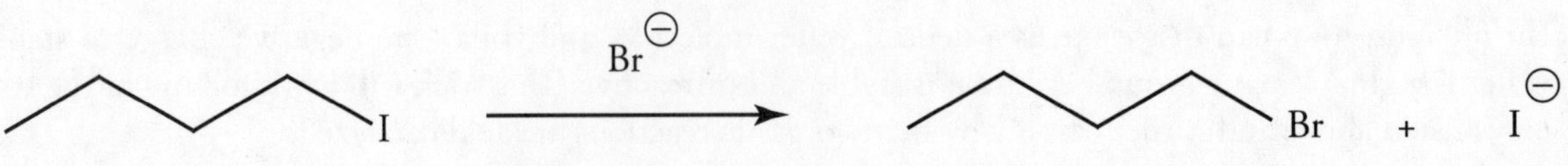

1-iodobutane   1-bromobutane

In the first (and only) step of this reaction (see the mechanism below), because the nucleophilic bromide anion attacks the electrophilic carbon at the same time that the leaving group leaves, the attack must occur from the backside of the substrate. The bromine-carbon bond forms as the iodine-carbon bond is broken, in a single step, to yield bromobutane.

S$_N$2 Mechanism

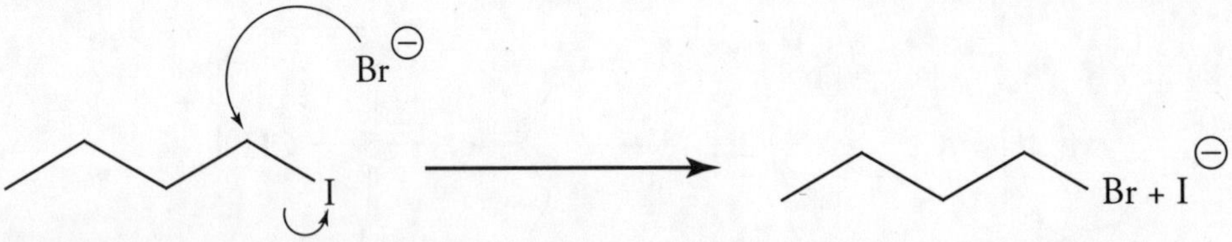

Let's look at a chiral substrate in order to see the stereochemical implications of this concerted mechanism. When (R)-1-deutero-1-chloroethane is treated with iodide, the typical backside attack occurs. As the new C–I bond begins to form while the C–Cl bond breaks, the reaction proceeds through a **pentavalent transition state**. As you can see in the product below, there is complete **inversion of configuration** at the carbon being attacked by the nucleophile. This is always the case in an S$_N$2 reaction on a chiral substrate.

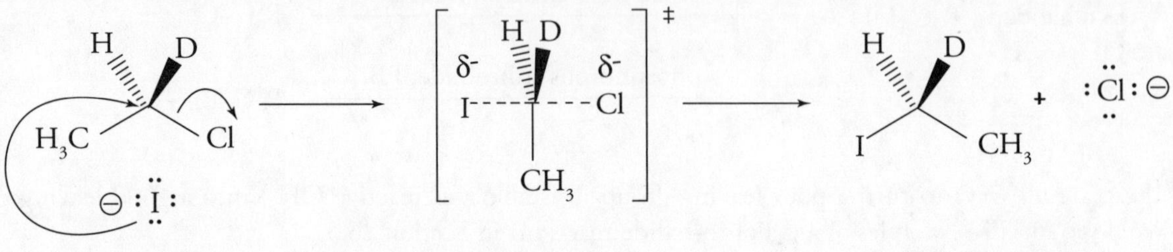

backside attack   pentavalent   inverted product

transition state

Furthermore, the rate of the reaction is a function of two variables—that is, **bimolecular**. The rate of the reaction depends on the concentrations of both the nucleophile and the electrophile, and is equal to the product of the rate constant (k), the concentration of the nucleophile ([I$^-$]), and the concentration of the electrophile ([R–Cl]).

$$\text{reaction rate} = k[\text{nucleophile}][\text{electrophile}]$$

We can now explain what we mean when we say that this reaction proceeds by an "S$_N$2" mechanism. The "S" indicates that it is a <u>s</u>ubstitution reaction mechanism, the subscript "N" indicates that it is <u>n</u>ucleophilic, and the "2" indicates that it is <u>b</u>imolecular. The rate of the reaction depends not only on the concentration of the electrophile, but also on the degree of substitution of the electrophilic carbon. Since the transition state is sterically crowded with five groups attached, the more bulky those groups are, the harder it is for the nucleophile to gain access to the reactive site. Therefore, less substituted substrates react faster than more substituted ones.

The last factor to consider in substitution reactions is the solvent. To favor an S_N2 mechanism, protic solvents such as water and alcohols should be avoided. Since these hydrogen bonding solvents are able to strongly solvate the nucleophile, they hinder the backside attack necessary for the concerted reaction. To prevent this interference, polar, aprotic solvents such as acetone, DMF (dimethylformamide), or DMSO (dimethylsulfoxide) should be used. Their polar nature allows the charged nucleophiles and leaving groups to remain dissolved, but they are not as efficient at completely solvating the nucleophile.

S_N1 Reactions

Over the course of S_N1 substitution reactions, a carbocation (carbonium ion) forms. So let's take a moment to review the relative stability of carbocations. Remember that the formation of charged species from neutral ones is generally an energetically disfavorable process; that is, it is energetically *uphill*. But some ions are more stable than others. For alkyl cations, the relative stabilities are given below.

3° carbocation   2° carbocation   1° carbocation   methyl carbocation

Decreasing carbocation stability

The order of stabilities for carbocations is thought to be the result of the electron-donating ability of alkyl groups. (The mechanism of this interaction is beyond the scope of the DAT.)

Now that we have reviewed the basics of carbocation stability, let's consider an example where a chiral halide undergoes an S_N1 substitution reaction. When (R)-3-bromo-3-methylhexane is treated with H_2O, a racemic mixture of 3-methylhexan-3-ol is formed:

(R)-3-bromo-3-methylhexane   (R)-3-methylhexan-3-ol   (S)-3-methylhexan-3-ol

S_N1 substitution occurs in two distinct steps, unlike S_N2 reactions that occur in one step. In the first step of the S_N1 reaction, a planar carbocation with 120° bond angles forms (see mechanism below). This occurs when the leaving group falls off (dissociates). This is the slow step of the mechanism, or the rate limiting step. In the final step of this reaction, **racemization** occurs as the nucleophile attacks equally *on either side* of the carbocation. The result is a racemic mixture.

S$_N$1 Mechanism

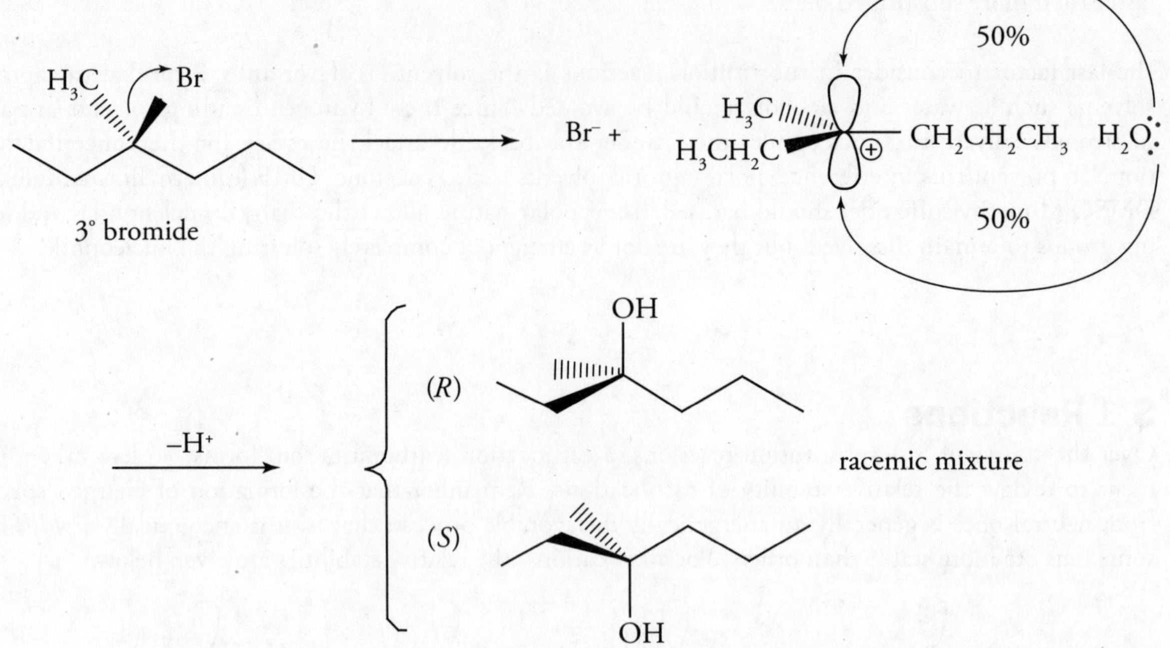

Unlike the S$_N$2 reaction explained above where the rate of the reaction was a function of two variables, the S$_N$1 reaction rate is a function of only one variable, that is, **unimolecular**. The rate of the S$_N$1 reaction depends only upon the concentration of the electrophile (the species that loses the leaving group over the course of the reaction). The rate of the reaction is equal to the product of the rate constant (k), and the electrophile concentration ([R–Br]):

$$\text{reaction rate} = k[\text{electrophile}]$$

As before, we can now explain what we mean when we say that this reaction proceeds by an "S$_N$1" mechanism. The "S" indicates that it is a substitution reaction mechanism, the subscript "N" indicates that it is nucleophilic, and the "1" indicates that it is unimolecular.

The rate of the reaction depends not only on the concentration of the electrophile, but also on the degree of substitution of the electrophilic carbon. Since the dissociation of the leaving group is the slow step of the mechanism, anything that makes that step more favorable will speed up the reaction. As was just discussed, the more substituted the carbocation intermediate, the more stable it is. Therefore, more substituted substrates will dissociate to make more stable intermediates faster, speeding up the rate of the entire reaction.

To favor an S$_N$1 mechanism, protic solvents such as water and alcohols should be used. The role of the solvent is twofold. The protic solvent helps to stabilize the forming carbocation and solvate the leaving group, thereby facilitating the first, or slow, step of the mechanism. Secondly, the solvent then behaves as the nucleophile in a **solvolysis** reaction, attacking the carbocation intermediate. This produces an alcohol product if water is used as the solvent and an ether if the reaction is run in an alcoholic solvent.

Alcohols undergo substitution reactions just as alkyl halides do. They can undergo either S_N1 or S_N2 substitution reactions depending upon the degree of substitution of the alcohol. Alcohols are treated with strong mineral acids to make their bad –OH leaving group into a good one (H_2O). In S_N2 reactions, the conjugate base of the mineral acid will attack while the leaving group leaves. In S_N1 reactions, the water will first dissociate, followed by a nucleophilic attack of the halide ion on the carbocation intermediate.

While this chapter focuses on substitution and elimination reactions, since alcohols are an important class of compounds for the DAT because of their distinctive properties, we will discuss them in more detail later.

Example 26-3: Predict whether the following substitution reactions will proceed via an S_N1 or an S_N2 mechanism.

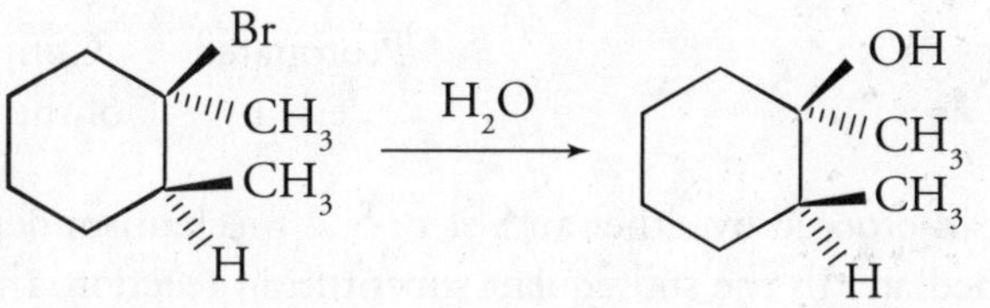

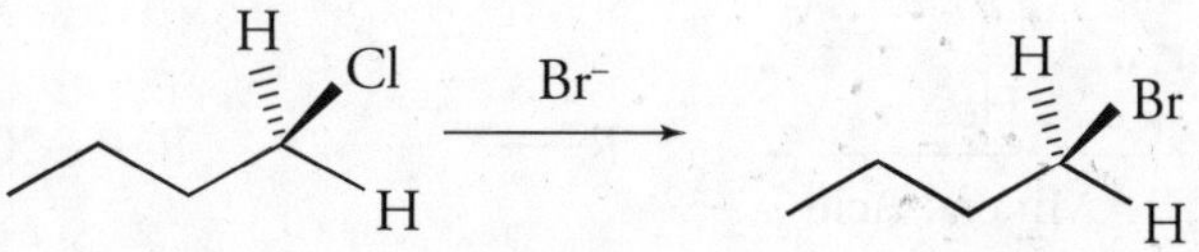

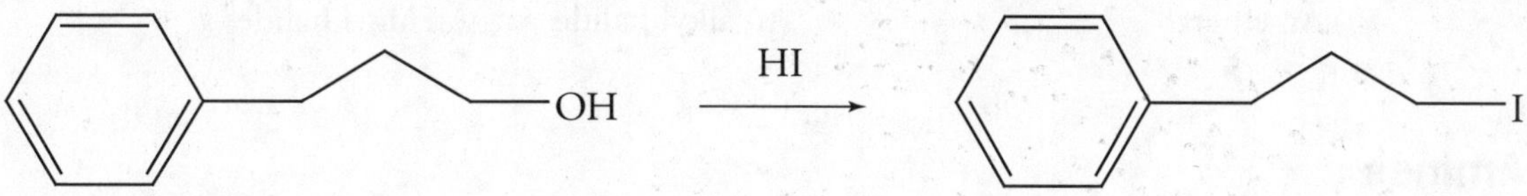

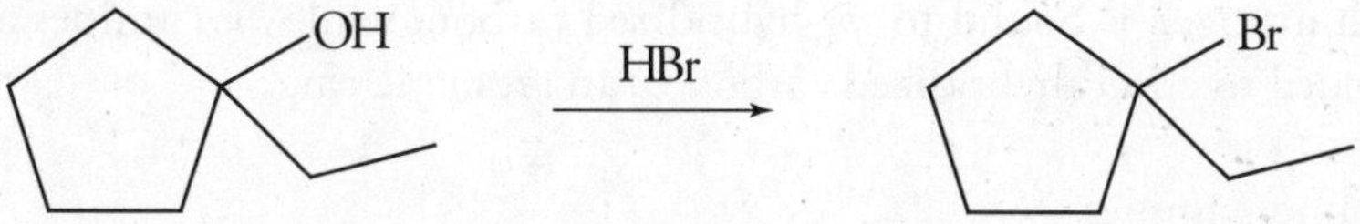

Solution:

A. 3° bromide, S_N1
B. 1° chloride, S_N2
C. 1° alcohol, S_N2
D. 3° alcohol, S_N1

Substitution Reactions with Other Functional Groups

Ethers

Ethers are weak bases that are generally quite chemically unreactive in the absence of strong acids. The chemical reactions that ethers participate in are due to the weak basicity of the ether oxygen. Let's consider a reaction in which an ether is cleaved in the presence of strong acid. The acid protonates the oxygen of the ether, converting a poor leaving group into a good leaving group.

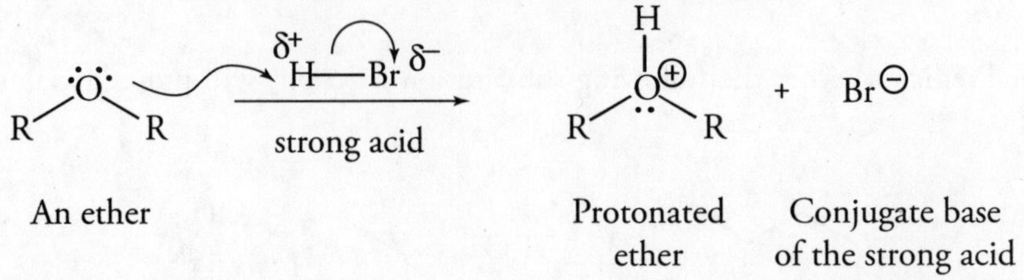

An ether   strong acid   Protonated ether   Conjugate base of the strong acid

At this point, the reaction can proceed by either an S_N1 or S_N2 mechanism depending on the structure of the protonated ether intermediate. In the subsequent substitution reaction, the halide (X^-) from the acid acts as the nucleophile. The ether cleavage reaction ultimately yields two molecules of haloalkane. Here is the general reaction:

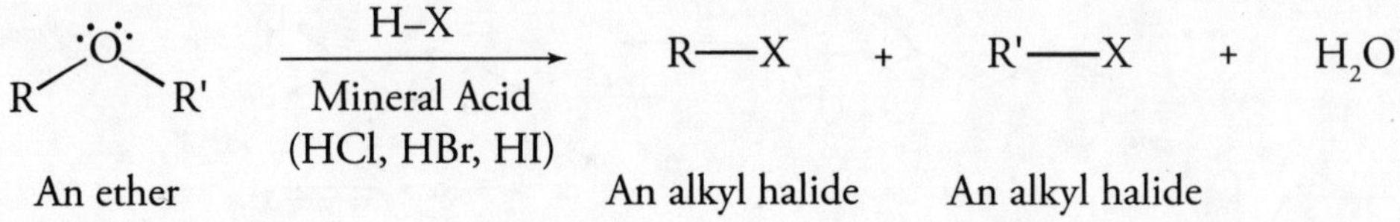

An ether   Mineral Acid (HCl, HBr, HI)   An alkyl halide   An alkyl halide

Amines

Organic compounds that contain nitrogen are of fundamental importance in biological systems. The most common class of nitrogen-containing compounds are referred to as **amines** and have the general structure of $R–NH_2$. Amines can be further classified as either **alkyl amines** or **aryl amines**. *Alkyl* amines are compounds in which nitrogen is bound to sp^3-hybridized carbon, while *aryl* amines are compounds in which nitrogen is bonded to an sp^2-hybridized carbon of an aromatic ring.

Below are a few examples of common amines.

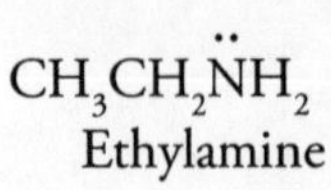

$CH_3CH_2NH_2$
Ethylamine

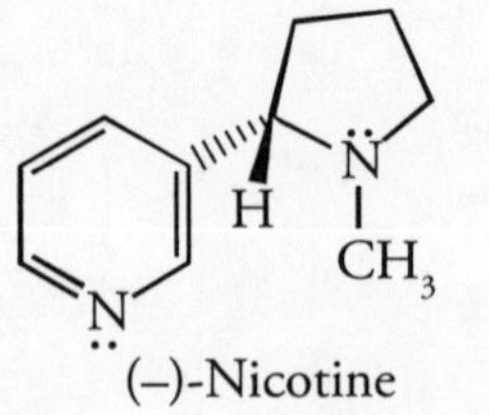

(–)-Nicotine

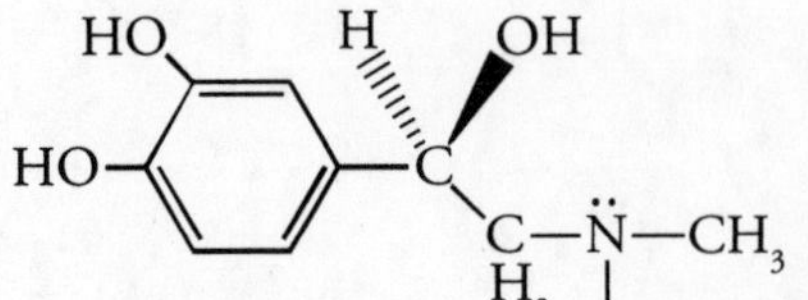

Epinephrine

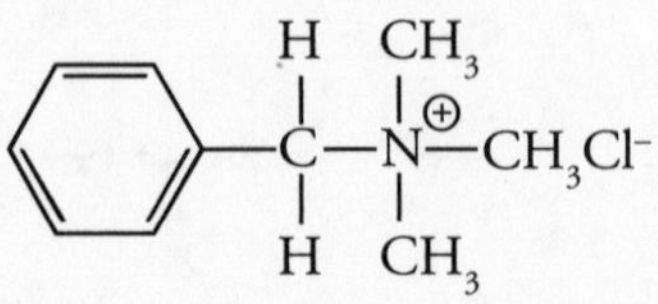

Benzyltrimethyl-ammonium chloride

Amines can be further categorized as primary amines, secondary amines, tertiary amines, and quaternary ammonium ions.

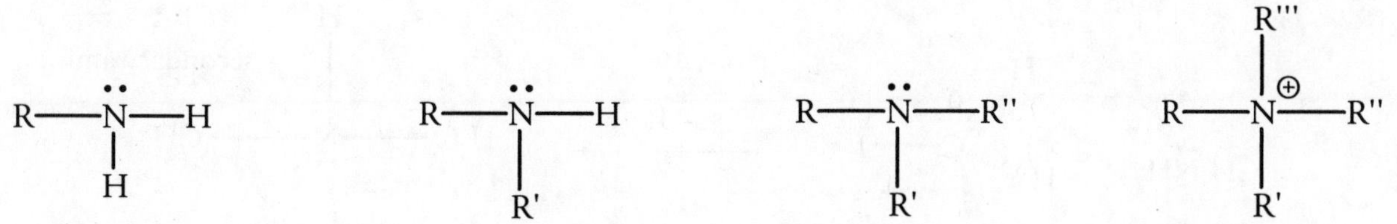

| A primary amine | A secondary amine | A tertiary amine | A quaternary ammonium ion |

Next, we'll examine the structure and bonding of alkyl amines. As an example we will look at the simple alkyl amine, methyl amine, CH_3NH_2. Notice that the nitrogen has three σ bonds and one lone electron pair. Its hybridization is therefore sp^3 with approximately 109° bond angles. The molecular geometry of an alkyl amine is pyramidal.

An interesting phenomenon of alkyl amines is that they undergo rapid pyramidal inversion at the sp^3-hybridized nitrogen. This rapid process has a low energy barrier (energy of activation) of only 6 to 7 kcal/mol, so that at room temperature the two pyramidal forms of the alkyl amine readily interconvert between one another. Because of this rapid interconversion, amines are not chiral.

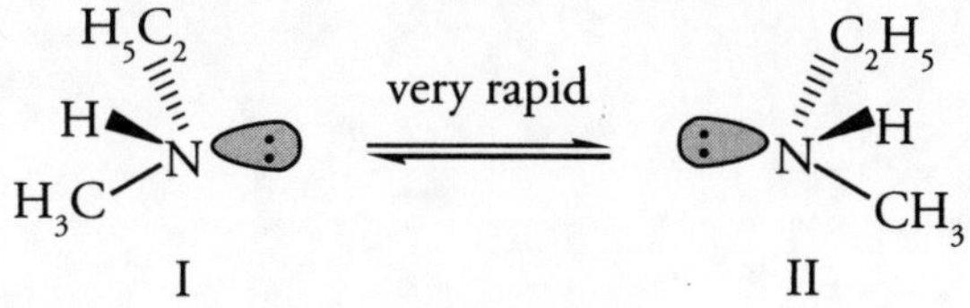

Methylethylamine
(Energy of activation for inversion only about 6–7 kcal/mol)

Alkylation of Amines

We now examine an important reaction of amines: alkylation. Alkyl amines can participate in S_N2 type substitution reactions because of their lone electron pairs. We now consider an example of an exhaustive alkylation of methylamine with methyl iodide.

In this S_N2 substitution reaction, the lone pair of electrons on the nitrogen of the alkyl amine serves as the nucleophile by attacking the electrophilic, sterically-unhindered carbon atom of methyl iodide. The primary amine, methylamine, first reacts with methyl iodide, to form a 2° amine. The 2° amine then reacts with another molecule of methyl iodide to form a 3° amine. Finally, the 3° amine reacts with yet another molecule of methyl iodide to yield a quaternary ammonium ion.

26.3

Notice that the quaternary ammonium ion no longer has a lone electron pair and can no longer act as a nucleophile.

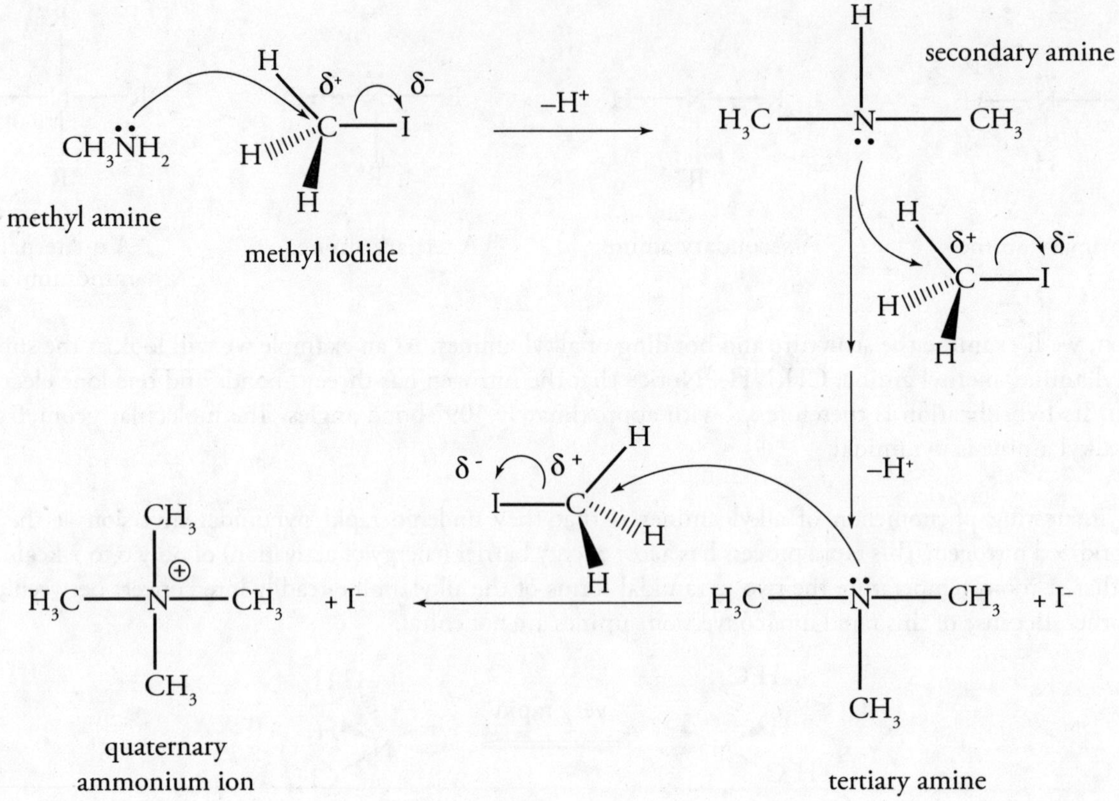

26.3 ELIMINATION REACTIONS

Elimination reactions are defined by the bonding changes that occur over the course of a reaction. In an elimination reaction, two σ bonds in the starting material are converted into a π bond in the product. You should note that this is the reverse pathway of an addition reaction (which we'll review in the next chapter).

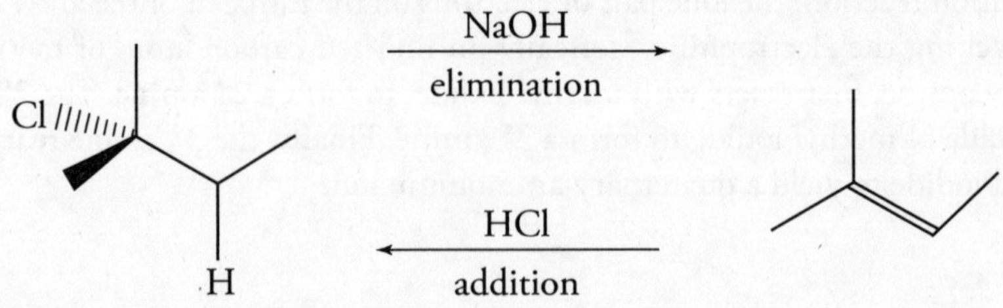

In the example above, the two σ bonds in the starting material that are broken are the C–Cl and the adjacent C–H bond. The π bond that forms in the product is the C=C double bond.

E1 Reactions

Like substitution, elimination can be either a unimolecular (E1) or a bimolecular (E2) process. E1 elimination, like S_N1 substitution, occurs via a 2-step mechanism.

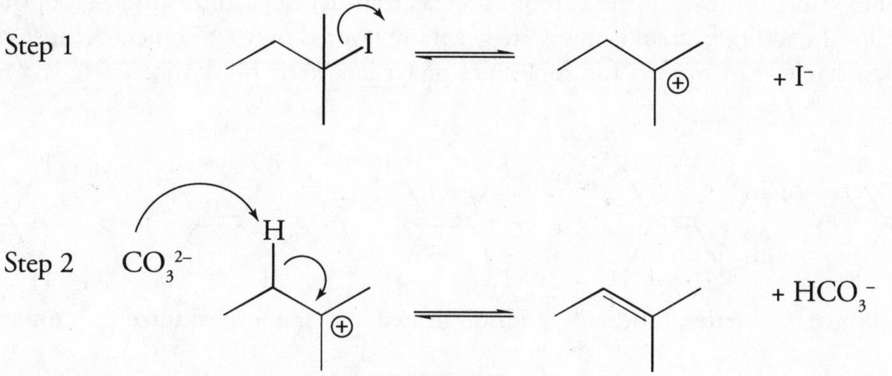

Step 1

Step 2

The iodide anion ionizes by falling off the carbon to which it was attached (Step 1), leaving behind a carbocation. A weak base then removes a proton on the carbon next to the carbon formerly attached to iodine (Step 2), leaving behind its electrons to form a C=C double bond.

E1 works best with 3° substrates, because they best support the positive charge after the leaving group leaves (remember, 3° > 2° > 1° for carbocation stability). Furthermore, in the E1 mechanism, the overall rate of the reaction is proportional only to the concentration of the substrate: rate = k[R–LG]. It's important to note that the base must remove a proton that is adjacent to the leaving group for elimination to proceed.

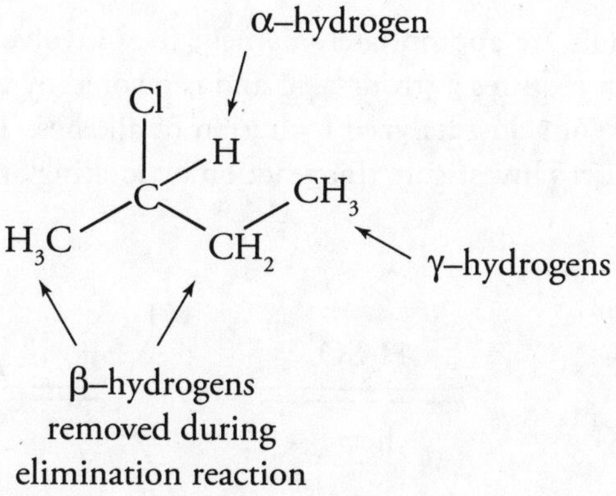

α–hydrogen

CH₃

γ–hydrogens

β–hydrogens
removed during
elimination reaction

If no adjacent protons exist, elimination cannot occur directly.

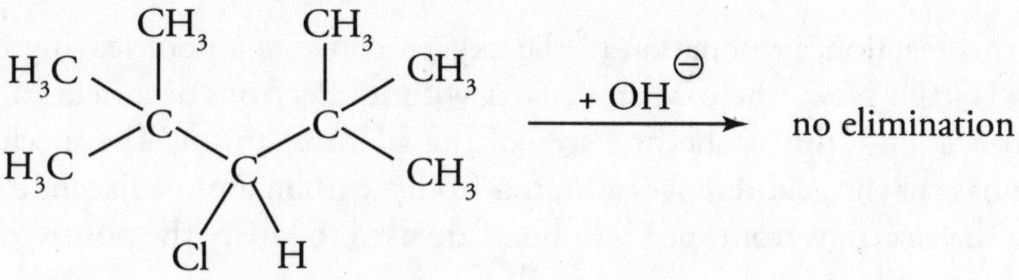

+ OH⁻   no elimination

Here we have only
α and γ-protons

If there is more than one type of adjacent proton that can be removed from the carbocation intermediate by the base to give different alkenes as products, the more highly substituted alkene is usually formed in the greatest amount because it is thermodynamically favored. In other words, more substituted double bonds are more stable because alkene carbons are electron deficient and carbon groups act as electron-donating groups. In addition, *trans* isomers are generally favored over *cis* isomers because *cis/Z* geometric isomers are less stable than *trans/E* and molecules prefer less steric hindrance. Here is a summary of alkene stability:

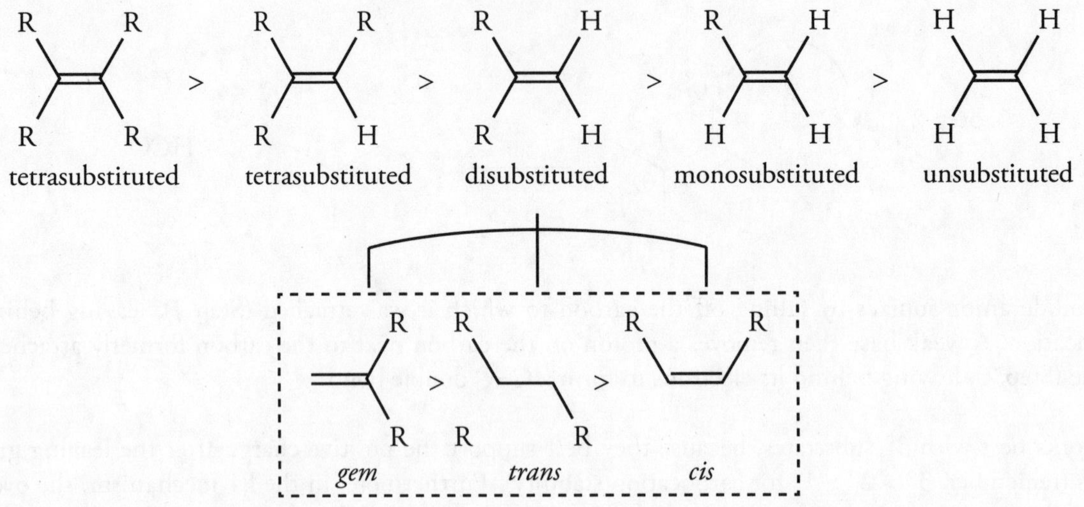

Overall, regioselectivity and stereoselectivity of E1 reactions are thus determined by the relative stabilities of the products.

Dehydration reactions of alcohols are appropriately named; they involve the loss of a molecule of water to form an alkene. This reaction requires a strong acid and is favored by high temperatures. Dehydration of alcohols is simply the reverse of acid-catalyzed hydration of alkenes. This reaction is also an excellent example of an E1 mechanism. Let's investigate this reaction by looking at the dehydration of *tert*-butanol under anhydrous conditions.

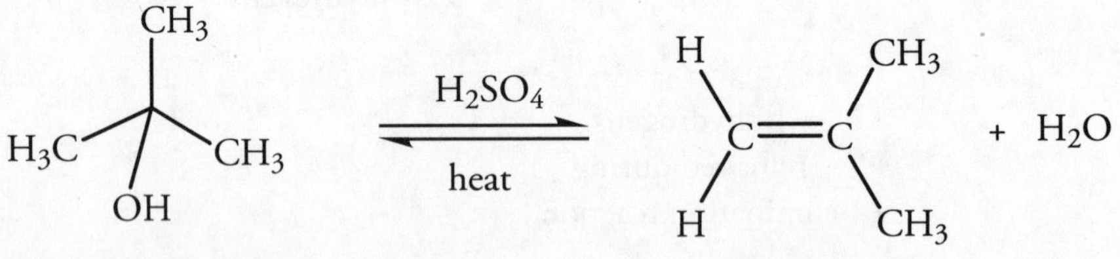

In the first step of this reaction, protonation of the oxygen converts a poor leaving group (–OH) into a good leaving group (H_2O). Next, the oxygen departs with its electrons as a neutral water molecule and leaves behind a carbocation—this is the first step of the E1 mechanism. The mechanism is completed when the conjugate base of the acid removes a proton from a carbon atom adjacent to the carbon bearing the positive charge. The electrons from the C–H bond are used to satisfy the positively-charged carbon by forming a carbon-carbon π bond.

E1 Mechanism

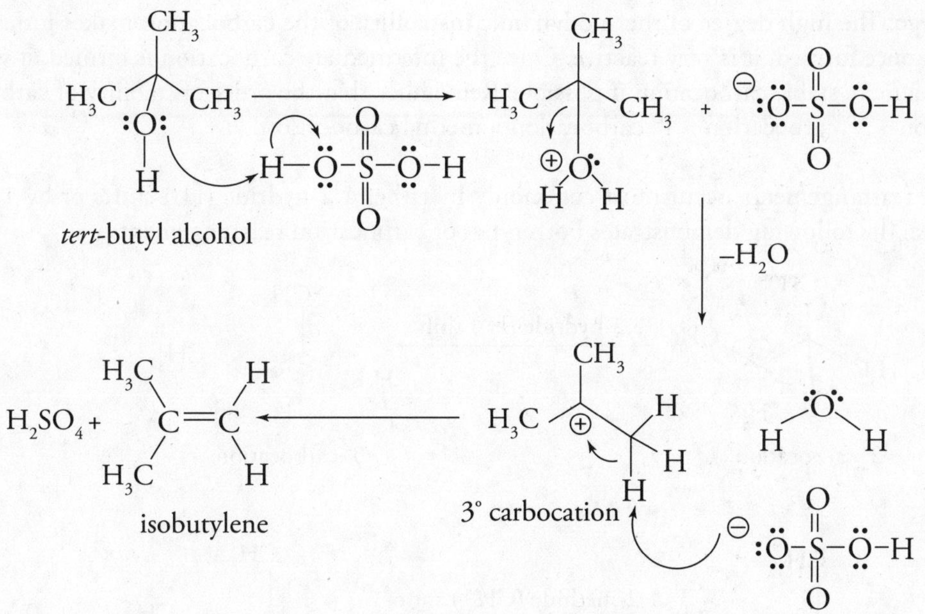

tert-butyl alcohol

isobutylene

3° carbocation

Remember that any proton on a carbon adjacent to a carbocation may be removed to form an alkene, but the major organic product will be the most substituted alkene since it is thermodynamically most stable. The following example, the dehydration of 3-methylpentan-2-ol, will clarify this point.

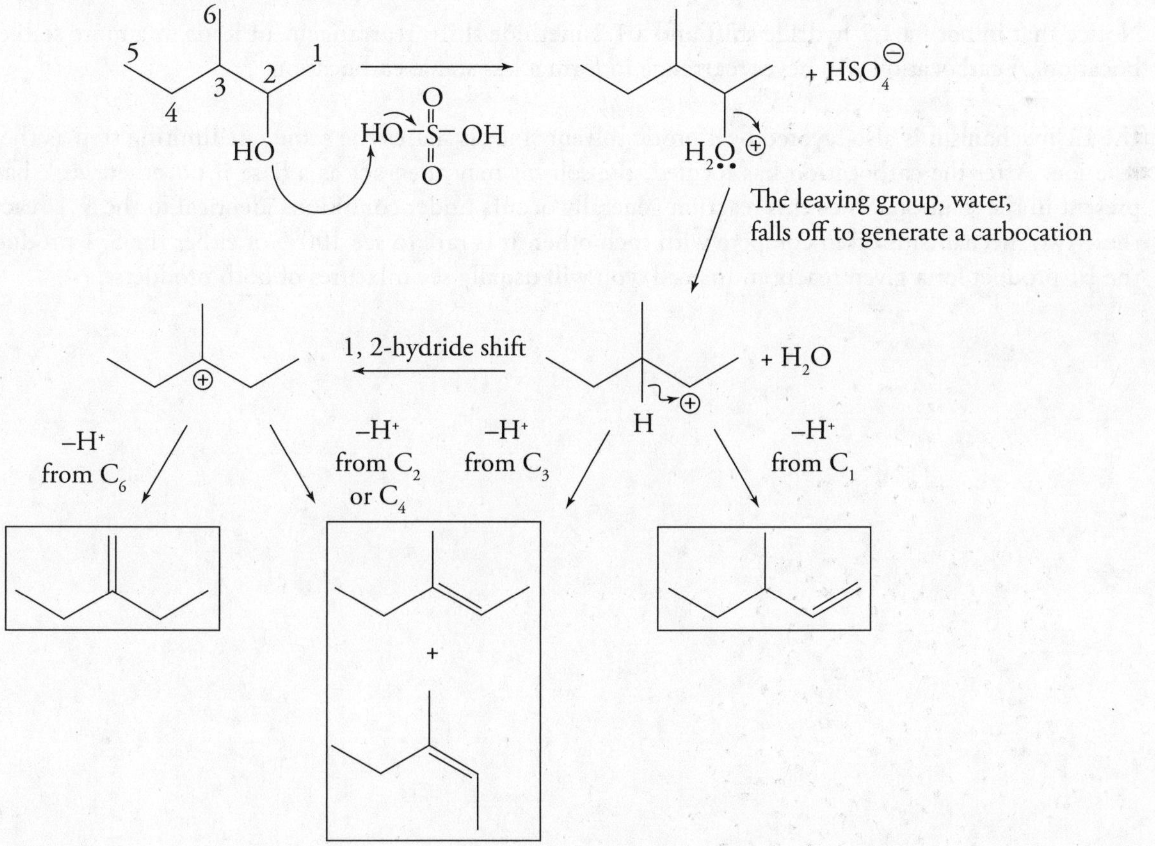

The leaving group, water, falls off to generate a carbocation

1, 2-hydride shift

+ H₂O

−H⁺ from C₆

−H⁺ from C₂ or C₄

−H⁺ from C₃

−H⁺ from C₁

The alcohol dehydration reaction above is an example of **carbocation rearrangement**. Carbocations are thermodynamically unstable due to the electron deficiency (no octet of electrons) on the carbon with the positive charge. The high degree of thermodynamic instability of the carbocation makes it quite difficult to form, and once formed, it is very reactive. Once the intermediate carbocation is formed, it will quickly rearrange to a more stable carbocation if possible. Remember that the order of stability of carbocations is: 3° carbocation > 2° carbocation > 1° carbocation > methyl carbocation.

Carbocation rearrangements occur most commonly by either 1,2-hydride (H⁻) shifts or by 1,2-methide (CH₃⁻) shifts. The following demonstrates both types of carbocation rearrangements.

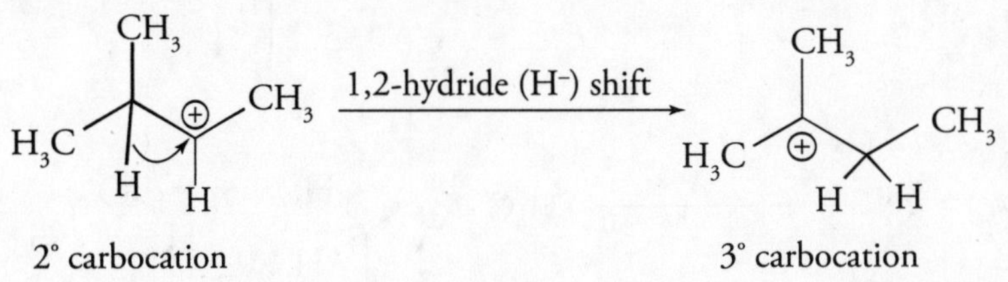

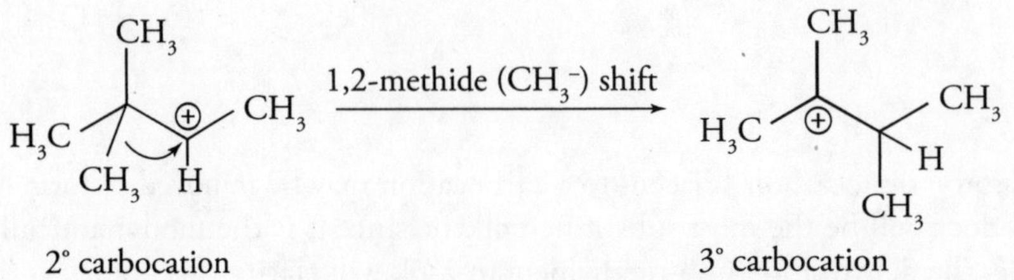

Notice that in both a 1,2-hydride shift and a 1,2-methide shift, rearrangement leads to a more stable carbocation. A carbocation will never rearrange to form a less stable carbocation.

The E1 mechanism is also favored by a protic solvent since it shares the same rate limiting step as the S_N1 reaction. After the carbocation has formed, the solvent may then act as a base if no other weak base is present in the solution. Since this reaction generally occurs under conditions identical to the S_N1 reaction, these two mechanisms often compete with each other. It is rare to see 100% of either the S_N1 product or the E1 product for a given reaction. Instead, you will usually see mixtures of both products.

Example 26-4: Determine the major organic product (A, B, C, or D) from each of the following dehydration reactions:

(i)

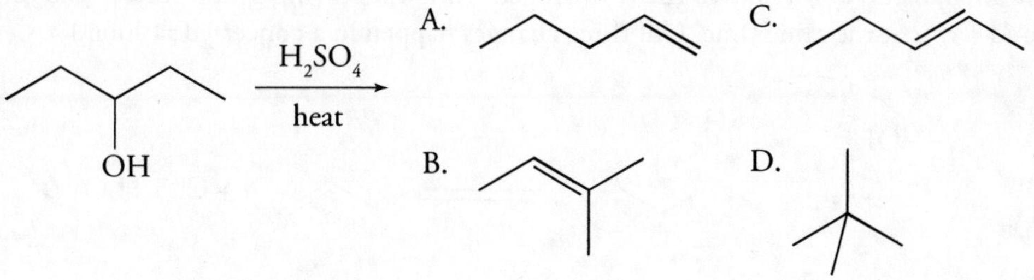

H_2SO_4 / heat

A.

B.

C.

D.

(ii)

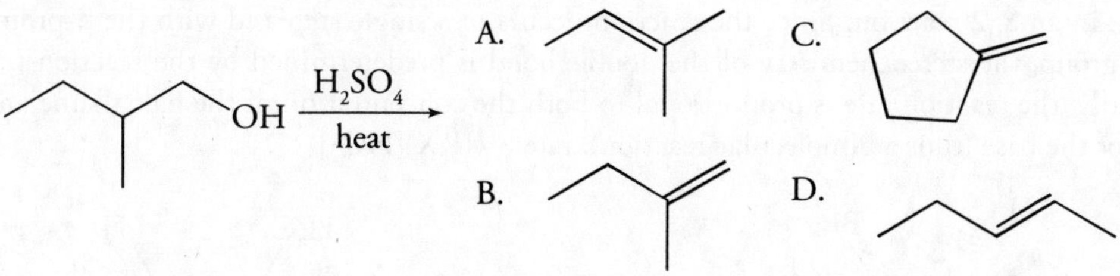

H_2SO_4 / heat

A.

B.

C.

D.

(iii)

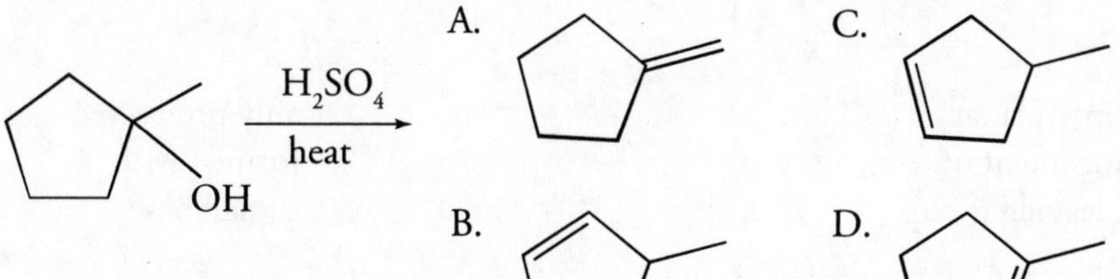

H_2SO_4 / heat

A.

B.

C.

D.

(iv)

H_2SO_4 / heat

A.

B.

C.

D.

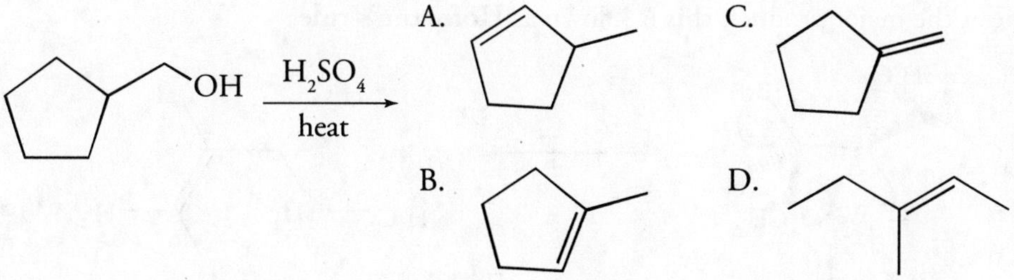

Solution:

(i)   C
(ii)   A (Note that carbocation rearrangement would occur.)
(iii) D
(iv)   B, carbocation rearrangement

26.3

E2 Reactions

E2 elimination, just as S_N2 substitution, proceeds via a 1-step mechanism. A strong base (generally hydroxide or an alkoxide ion) removes the β-hydrogen while the leaving group leaves. The carbon-carbon double bond forms at the same time. (All three changes happen in a concerted fashion.)

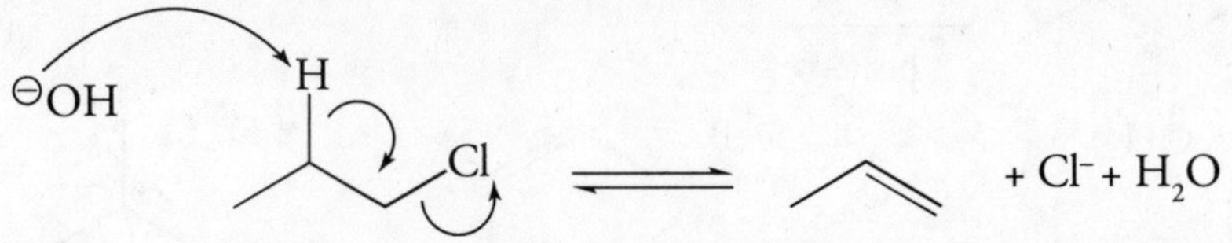

While all other reactions we've examined thus far work with both alkyl halides and alcohols as substrates, only alkyl halides may act as the substrate for E2 reactions. The E2 mechanism works best if the proton to be removed is *anti* to the leaving group, similar to the way the nucleophile must approach from the backside in an S_N2 reaction. Since the reaction occurs in a single step and with the β-proton *anti* to the leaving group, the stereochemistry of the double bond is predetermined by the reaction transition state. Expectedly, the reaction rate is proportional to both the concentration of the haloalkane and the concentration of the base (thus a bimolecular reaction): rate = k[RX][HO⁻].

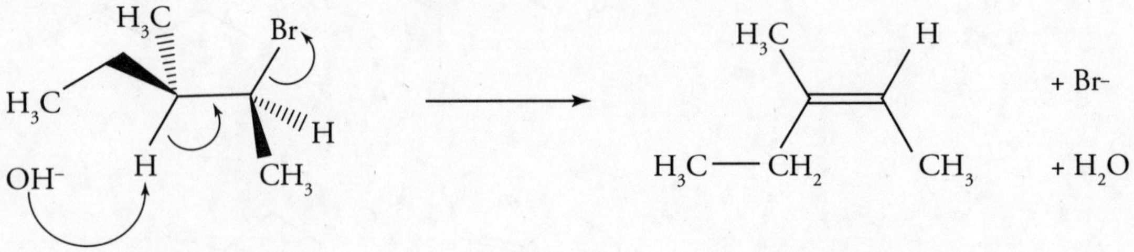

antiperiplanar
arrangement of
H and leaving group

only product
formed with
small base

The choice of base in an E2 mechanism has a large impact on the regiochemistry of the reaction. As shown above, small bases will remove the proton from the most substituted carbon, thereby yielding the most substituted, most stable alkene as the major product; this is known as **Zaitsev's rule**. However, if a bulky base is used (usually *tert*-butoxide or LDA), steric hindrance prevents the thermodynamic product from being formed. Instead, the base will remove the most accessible β-proton, yielding the least substituted alkene as the major product; this is known as **Hofmann's rule**.

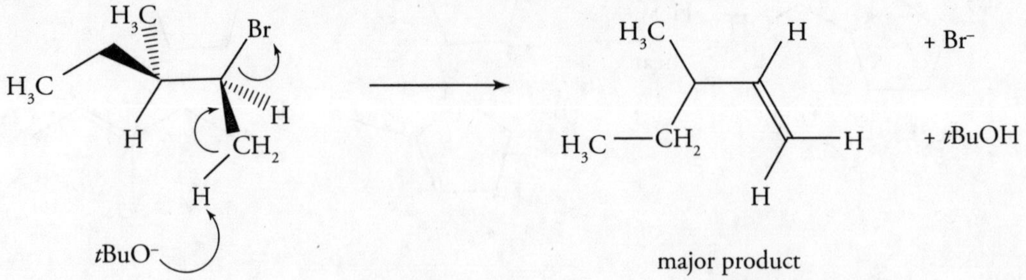

major product
formed with
bulky base

The elimination pathway in many instances may compete with the substitution pathway. This is because a base can also act as a nucleophile. Generally speaking, strong bases such as OH⁻ or OR⁻ yield exclusively the elimination product(s) unless the substrate is primary. We'll discuss this more shortly.

Example 26-5: A chemist has a compound, C_4H_9Cl, which she believes to be either *n*-butyl chloride or *t*-butyl chloride.

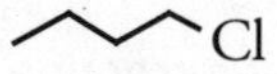

n-butyl chloride

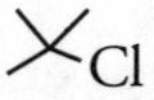

$\times$Cl

t-butyl chloride

She reacts the compound with a base and gets an alkene, C_4H_8. She determines that the rate of reaction is independent of the concentration of base used. Therefore, her original compound was which form of C_4H_9Cl?

Solution: Because the rate of the reaction is independent of the hydroxide concentration, it is only dependent on the concentration of the alkyl chloride, and hence, E1. E1 works best with 3° halides, so C_4H_9Cl must be *t*-butyl chloride.

26.4 S$_N$ VERSUS E REACTIONS

Now that we have reviewed both S$_N$ and E reactions, let's compare them:

Reaction dominance with increasing electrophile substitution

$\longrightarrow$

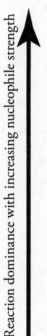

Reaction dominance with increasing nucleophile strength

S$_N$2
- rate = $k[E^+][Nu^-]$
- one step
- backside attack
- requires strong Nu$^-$
- inversion of configuration
- methyl > 1° > 2° >> 3°

S$_N$1
- rate = $k[E^+]$
- two steps
- carbocation intermediate
- requires good Nu$^-$
- results in racemization
- 3° > 2° >> 1° > methyl

E2
- rate = $k[E^+][B^-]$
- one step
- antiperiplanar geometry
- requires strong base (B$^-$)
- small base gives most substituted alkene; bulky base gives least substituted
- 3° > 2° > 1°

E1
- rate = $k[E^+]$
- two steps
- carbocation intermediate
- requires weak base (B$^-$)
- major product is most substituted alkene; *trans* > *cis*
- 3° > 2° >> 1°

On the DAT, you will likely have to determine which reaction mechanism will occur for a given set of reagents. Here is how you can pick your reaction mechanism:

1. If you are given rate law or kinetic data, use this to determine if a reaction is occurring via a unimolecular or bimolecular mechanism.
2. Compare base, nucleophile (Nu), and electrophile (EP) characteristics:

Base Strength	Nu Strength	Methyl EP	1° EP	2° EP	3° EP
Strong	Strong	S_N2	$E2 < S_N2$	$E2 > S_N2$	E2
Strong	Weak	No reaction	E2	E2	E2
Weak	Strong	S_N2	S_N2	S_N2	$S_N1 > E1$
Weak	Weak	No reaction	No reaction	S_N1 and E1	S_N1 and E1

3. Consider solvent effects. Polar aprotic solvents are used for SN2 and E2 reactions, while polar protic solvents are used for SN1 and E1 reactions.
4. Watch for changes in temperature. Higher temperatures favor elimination reactions over substitution reactions (E > SN).

Comparing nucleophile and base strength can be tricky. Here is an example of some common reagents you could see on the DAT:

	Strong Nucleophile	Weak Nucleophile
Strong Base	^-OH, ^-OMe, ^-OEt, $^-CH_3$, $^-NH_2$	^-OtBu, LDA
Weak Base	Cl^-, Br^-, I^-, ^-CN, ^-SH, $^-SCH_3$, azide (N_3^-), phthalimide, alkene	H_2O, F^-, CH_3COO^-, HCO_3^-, CO_3^{2-}, H_2SO_4, HSO_4^-, SO_4^{2-}, MeOH, EtOH, iPrOH, tBuOH, Me_2O, Et_2O, NH_3, $MeNH_2$, $EtNH_2$, Me_2NH, Me_3N

26.5 PROPERTIES AND REACTIONS OF ALCOHOLS

We've seen that alcohols are a very useful class of chemicals because of their diverse reactivity. Let's review a few other properties of this important functional group, such as their intermolecular interactions and acidity.

Hydrogen Bonding

In order to examine the effect of hydrogen bonding in alcohols, let's examine two molecules that are isomers of one another, *n*-butanol and diethyl ether. Both have the same molecular formula ($C_4H_{10}O$), yet there is a dramatic difference in their boiling points (117°C for *n*-butanol vs. 34.6°C for diethyl ether). This difference arises from the ability of *n*-butanol to form intermolecular hydrogen bonds, while diethyl ether cannot. Alcohols form intermolecular hydrogen bonds because they have hydroxyl (–OH) groups. This results from a strong dipole in which the hydroxyl group's proton acquires a substantial partial positive charge (δ^+) and the oxygen acquires a substantial partial negative charge (δ^-). The partial positive hydrogen can interact electrostatically with a non-bonding pair of electrons on a nearby oxygen, resulting in a hydrogen bond. On the other hand, diethyl ether has an oxygen atom with non-bonding electrons, but all hydrogen atoms are bound to carbons. Since carbon and hydrogen have similar electronegativity values, the bond is not very polarized, and these hydrogens cannot participate in hydrogen bonding. It's important to remember that a hydrogen bond is not a covalent bond; in this case it's an intermolecular interaction.

Intermolecular hydrogen bonding between molecules of *n*-butanol

molecular weight = 74
b.p. = 117°C

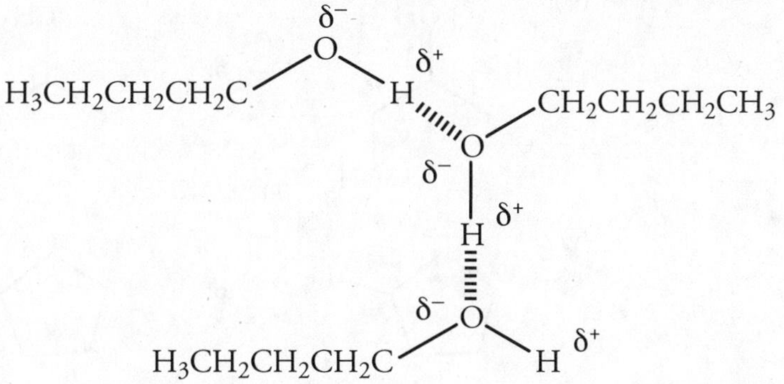

Intermolecular hydrogen bonding is not possible between molecules of diethyl ether

molecular weight = 74
b.p. = 34.6°C

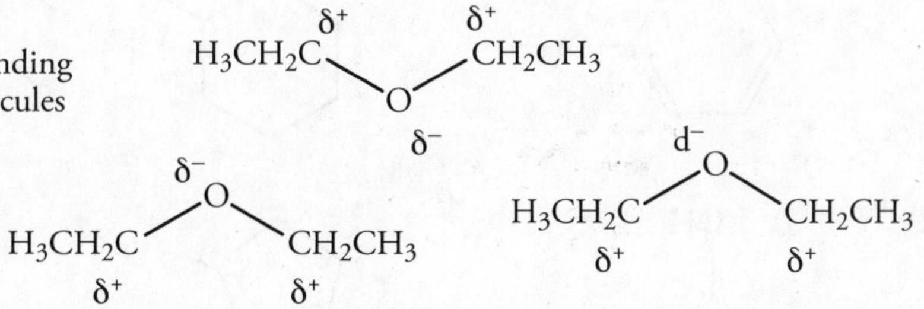

Example 26-6: For each of the following pairs of compounds, predict which molecule will have the higher boiling point.

(i)

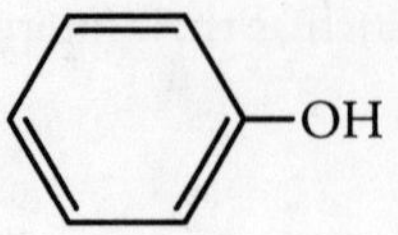

OH or Br

(ii)

or OH

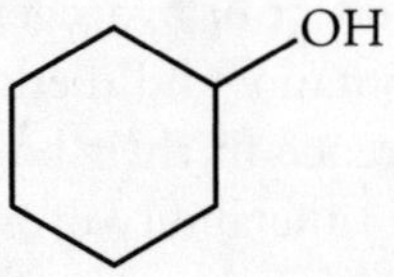

(iii)

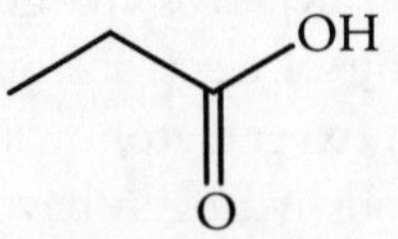

OH or CH₃

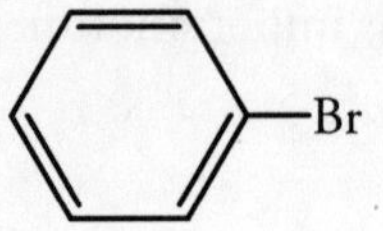

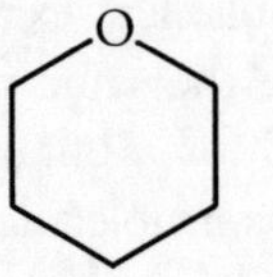

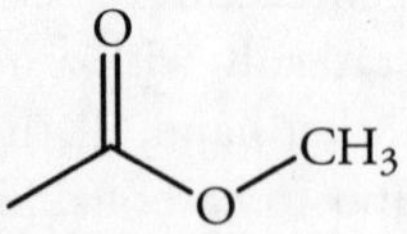

(iv)

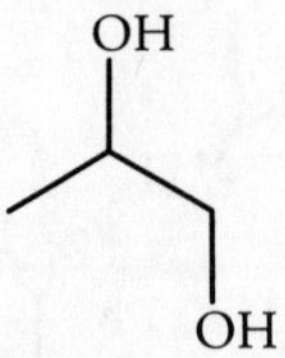

or

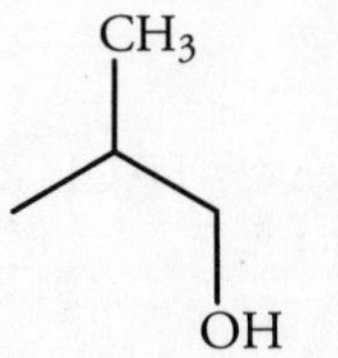

(v)

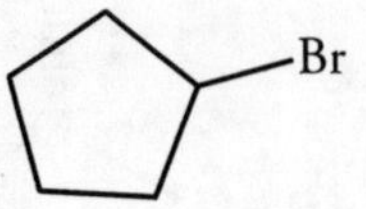

Br or CH₃

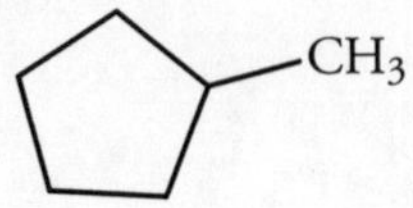

Solution:

(i)

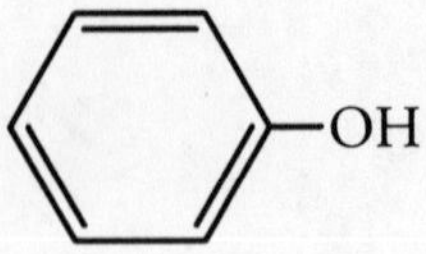

OH

(ii)

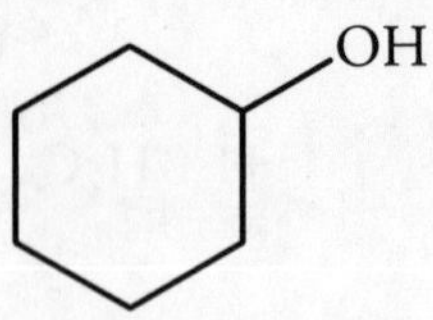

OH

(iii)

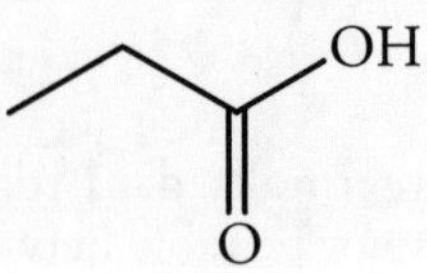

OH

(iv)

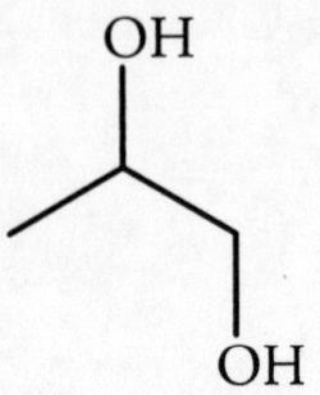

(v)

Br

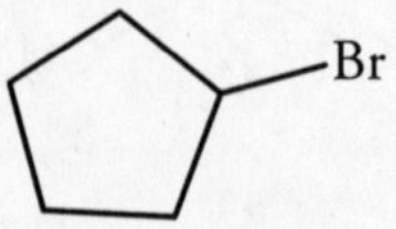

(primarily because of its greater mass)

The hydrogen bonding pattern in phenols provides insight into *inter*molecular vs. *intra*molecular hydrogen bonding. Let's consider the two isomers, *para*-nitrophenol (also called 4-nitrophenol) and *ortho*-nitrophenol (also called 2-nitrophenol). First, examine the hydrogen bonding pattern in *para*-nitrophenol. Notice that hydrogen bonding can occur with both the nitro and the hydroxyl groups in this molecule and that the bonding is exclusively intermolecular. That is, all hydrogen bonding takes place between individual molecules of *para*-nitrophenol. These hydrogen bonding interactions hold molecules of *para*-nitrophenol together and increase their boiling and melting points. Now, examine the hydrogen bonding pattern in *ortho*-nitrophenol. Notice that for this molecule, the nitro group and the hydroxyl group are in close proximity so that intramolecular hydrogen bonding can occur between the hydrogen of the hydroxyl group and a lone pair of electrons on the nitro group on the same molecule. These intramolecular hydrogen bonding interactions decrease the amount of intermolecular hydrogen bonding interactions that can occur between molecules, thereby decreasing the melting and boiling points of *ortho*-nitrophenol relative to *para*-nitrophenol.

para-nitrophenol
Intermolecular hydrogen bonding

ortho-nitrophenol
Intramolecular hydrogen bonding

Acidity

In this section, we're building on the Ochem acidity content you first saw in Section 25.6. You'll get a little more practice with Ochem acidity content in Sections 28.1 and 28.2. The acidity of a compound is determined by the ease with which it can lose a proton (H^+). Alcohols are a relatively acidic functional group for the same reason that they engage in hydrogen bonding: the large difference in electronegativity between oxygen and hydrogen. If an alcohol like methanol is deprotonated, an alkoxide ion is formed. The alkoxide is a relatively stable species, compared to a carbanion, for example, since the negative charge that results from this reaction is located on the very electronegative oxygen atom.

Methanol   Methoxide   Proton
ion

Phenols are considerably more acidic than alcohols, but are not as acidic as carboxylic acids. The increased acidity of phenols relative to alcohols is due to the fact that the phenoxide ion can be stabilized by resonance, while alkoxide ions cannot. This is demonstrated by the following:

Resonance Structures for the Phenoxide Ion

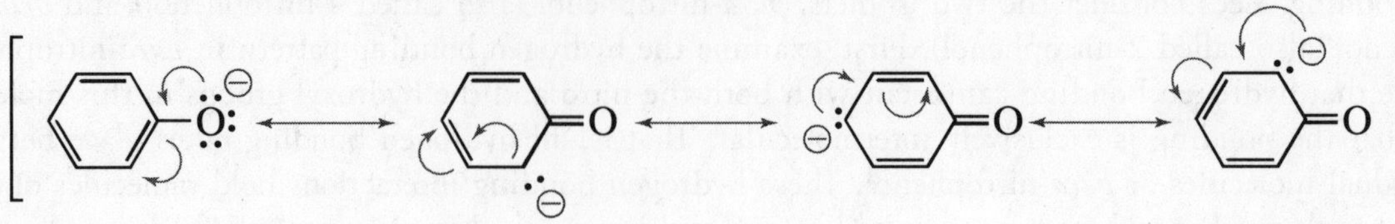

Electron-withdrawing substituents on phenols increase their acidity. As an example, consider *para*-nitrophenol. The nitro group is strongly electron withdrawing and greatly stabilizes the phenoxide ion through resonance stabilization. Once the *para*-nitrophenol is deprotonated, it's easy to see how the nitro group can withdraw electrons through the delocalized π system such that the negative charge on the phenoxide oxygen can be delocalized all the way to an oxygen atom of the nitro group. This electron-withdrawing resonance stabilization of the nitro group increases the acidity of *para*-nitrophenol as compared to a phenol that does not have electron-withdrawing substituents.

Effects of Substituents on Acidity

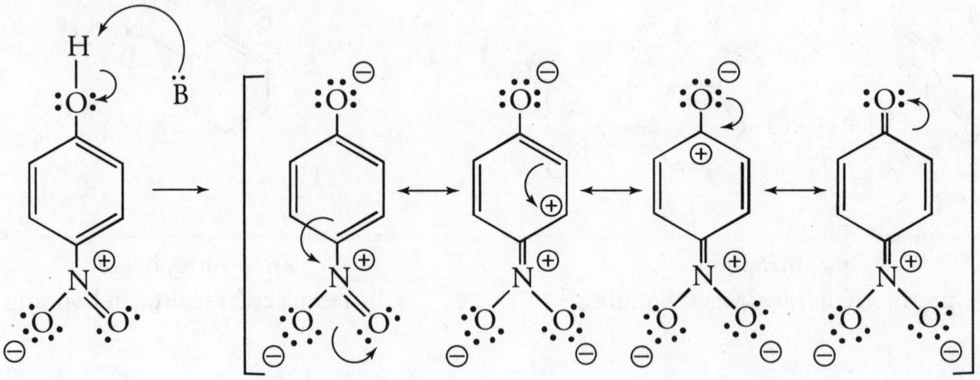

On the other hand, consider a substituted phenol that has an electron-*donating* group rather than an electron-*withdrawing* group. A good example of this is *para*-methoxyphenol. Here, it is easy to see how once *para*-methoxyphenol is deprotonated, the negative charge on the oxygen can be destabilized by the donation of a lone pair of electrons from the methoxy oxygen so a negative charge is placed on a carbon that's adjacent to the negatively charged phenoxide oxygen. Electron-donating groups tend to destabilize a phenoxide ion and decrease the acidity of substituted phenols.

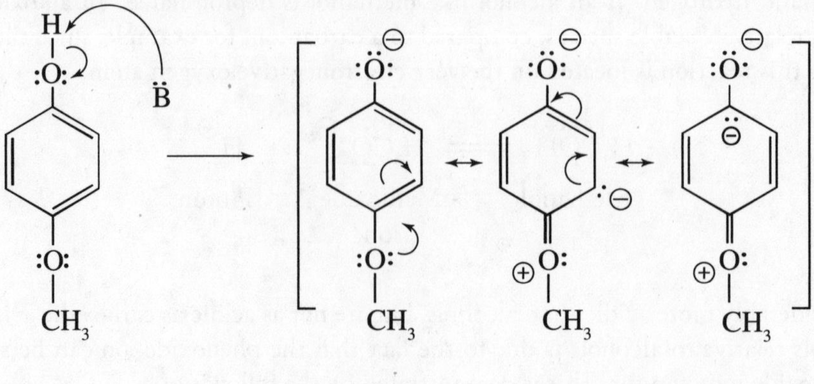

Example 26-7: For each of the following groups of four phenols, rank them in order of decreasing acidity.

(i)

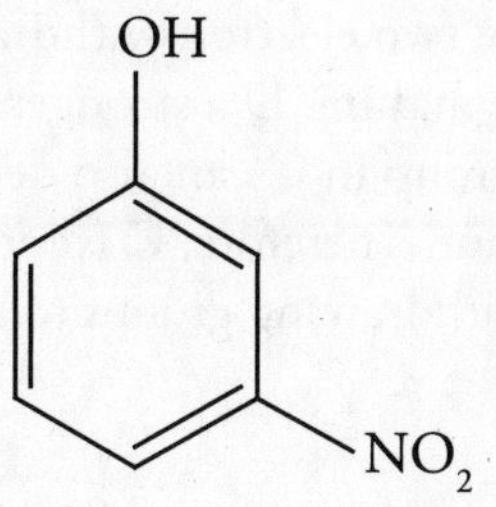

A 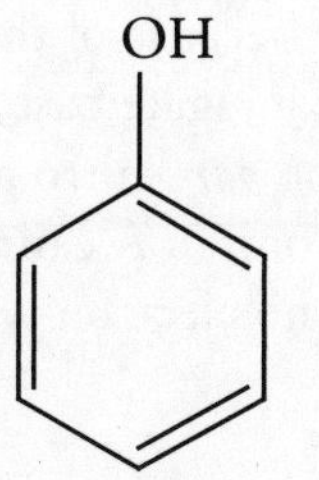   B 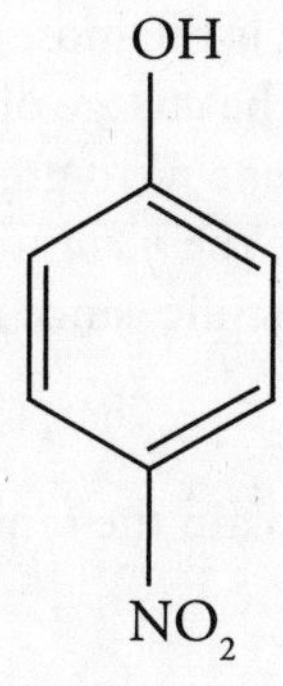   C 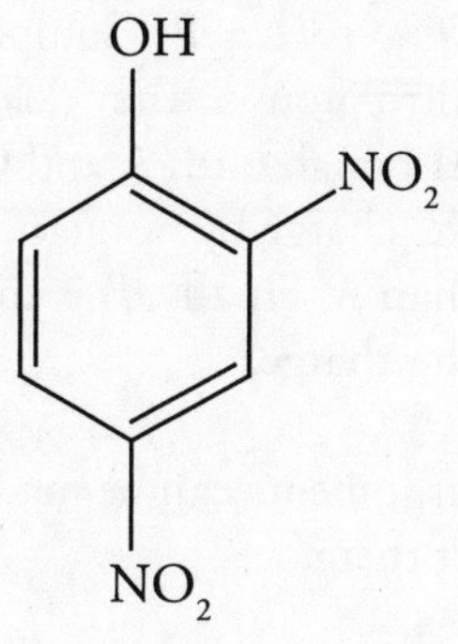   D

(ii)

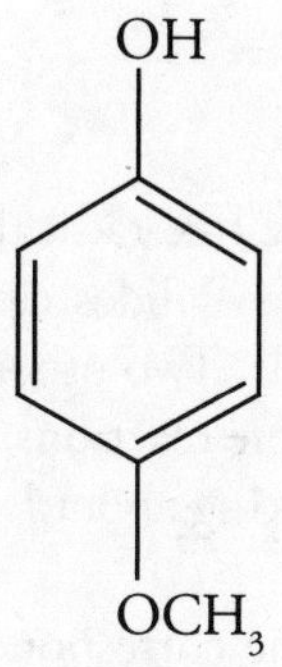

A 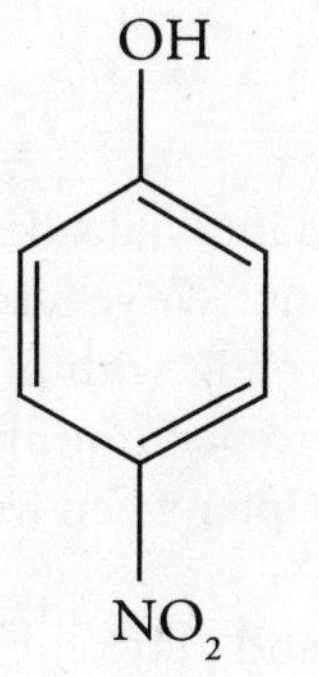   B 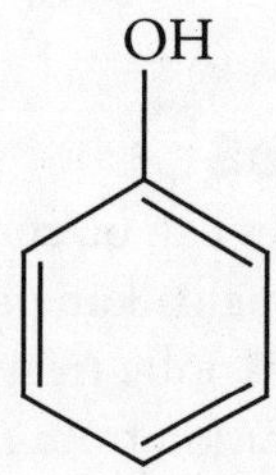   C 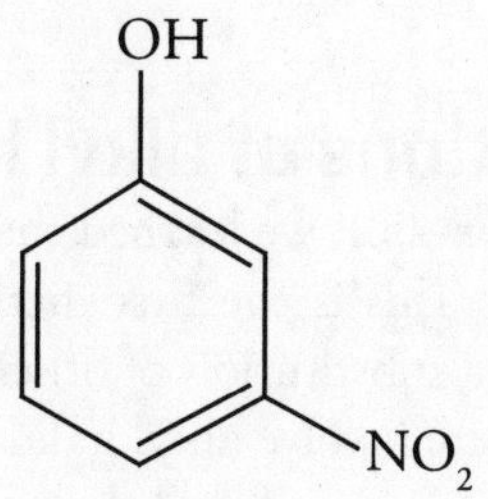   D

(iii)

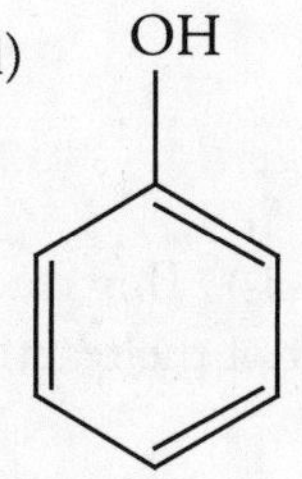

A 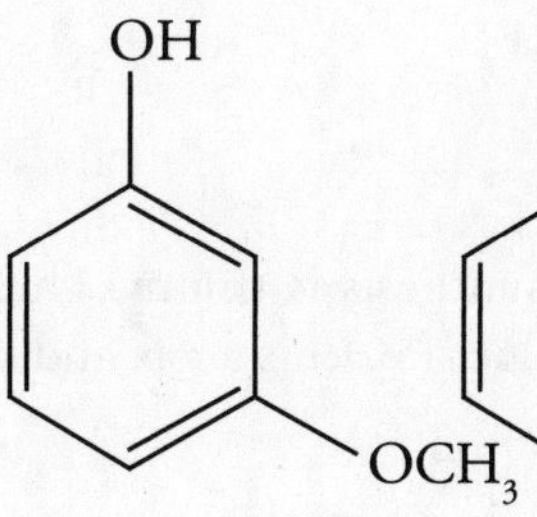   B 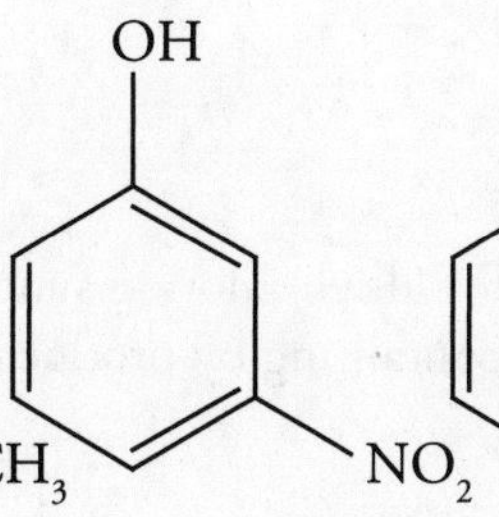   C 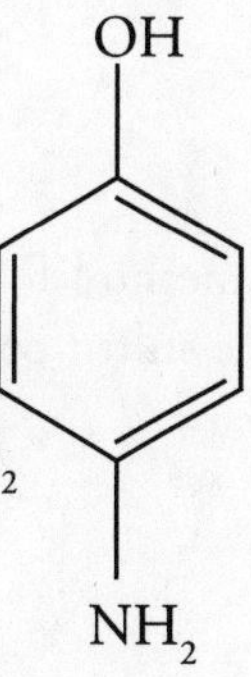   D

26.5

Solution:

(i) D > C > A > B. Compound D is the most acidic because of the two electron-withdrawing nitro groups. They delocalize the charge of the conjugate base, making D a stronger acid. Although both A and C have one nitro group, the *para*-nitro group in C can also delocalize the charge by resonance, while the *meta*-nitro group in A cannot. Therefore, C is more acidic than A. Finally, B is the least acidic, since it has no electron-withdrawing groups to stabilize the charge.

Similar arguments can be made to explain the rankings for the four phenols in (ii) and (iii). See if you can construct them.

(ii) B > D > C > A

(iii) C > A > B > D

Reactions of alkyl halides

In Section 25.1, we learned that alkanes can be converted into haloalkanes by the free-radical halogenation reaction. This is the first method of haloalkane synthesis. We've also seen how halides can be interconverted via substitution of other halides, or by treating alcohols with mineral acids. Two other methods presented here involve alkyl halide preparation from the corresponding alcohol. These reactions shouldn't be a surprise; we introduced them at the beginning of this chapter when we were talking about leaving groups!

One common reagent used to produce alkyl bromides and alkyl chlorides is the corresponding phosphorus trihalide compound (PBr_3 or PCl_3). For example, they can be used to convert isobutyl alcohol into isobutyl bromide or isobutyl chloride. Here is an example:

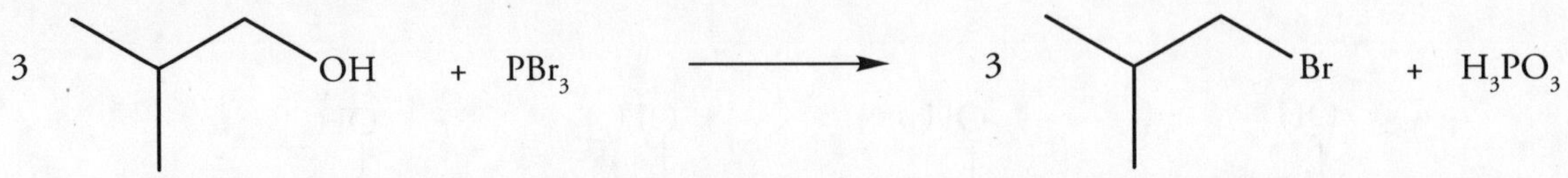

$$3 \quad \text{(isobutyl alcohol)} \quad OH \quad + \quad PBr_3 \quad \longrightarrow \quad 3 \quad \text{(isobutyl bromide)} \quad Br \quad + \quad H_3PO_3$$

Another common method for alkyl chloride synthesis is thionyl chloride ($SOCl_2$). This reaction is very convenient since the sulfur containing by-product (SO_2) is a gas and bubbles out of the reaction flask.

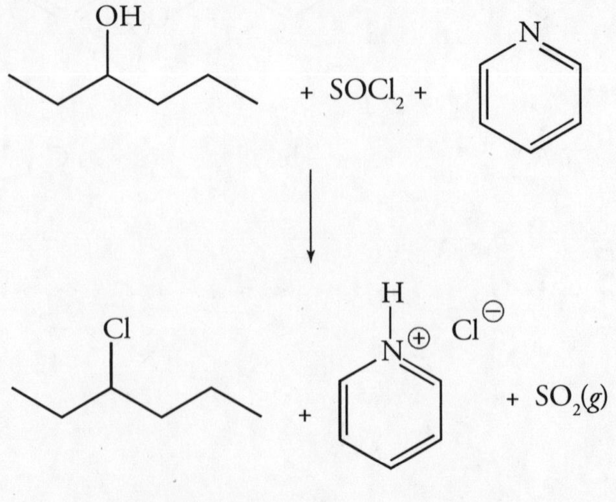

Want More Practice?
Remember to register your book online for chapter summaries, drills, practice tests, and more!

Chapter 27
Electrophilic Addition Reactions

27.1 REACTIONS OF ALKENES AND ALKYNES

Electrophilic Addition Reactions

Addition reactions are defined by the bonding changes that occur over the course of a reaction. In an addition reaction, a π bond in the starting material is broken, and two σ bonds in the product result. You should note that this is the reverse pathway of elimination reactions (see Section 26.3).

Recall that a carbon-carbon π bond is formed by the proper alignment of two adjacent unhybridized *p* orbitals. The electrons are localized in a region that lies above and below the plane defined by the central carbons and immediately adjacent atoms.

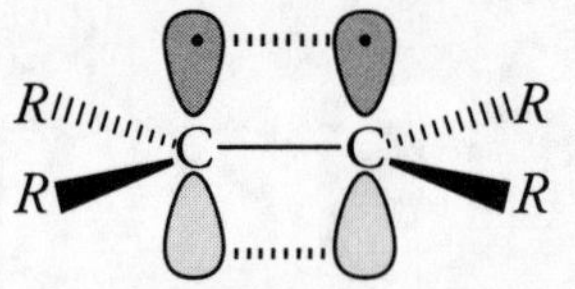

R = any alkyl group or hydrogen

These π electrons are more loosely held than σ electrons and can be nucleophilic. It is this property of π bonds that allows electrophilic additions to occur.

Before we turn to the specific electrophilic addition reactions that are important to be familiar with for the DAT, be aware that trying to memorize the nitty-gritty details of each reaction is not the best use of your time. For many of the reactions below, mechanisms are shown to highlight the similarities or differences between reactions. You do not need to memorize details of all mechanisms. You should, however, pay particular attention to the general addition mechanism and the regio- and stereochemistry of all reactions. In this chapter, we will review 13 electrophilic addition reactions. For each, keep track of reagents, whether the reaction happens via a Markovnikov mechanism, whether carbocation rearrangements can occur, and whether the reaction forms *syn*, *anti*, or both types of products. We will start by looking at the common Markovnikov reactions (monohalogenation via HX, acid catalyzed hydration, and oxymercuration/demercuration). Next we'll look at two anti-Markovnikov reactions (hydroboration/oxidation and monohalogenation with ROOR). Finally, we'll look at all the other electrophilic addition reactions (dihalogenation, halohydrin formation, epoxidation, two options for diol formation, and three common reagents that can hydrogenate alkenes and alkynes).

Markovnikov Additions

H—X Addition

The first reaction we will examine is addition of a strong mineral acid (H—Cl, H—Br, or H—I) to a carbon-carbon π bond. Consider the reaction between 3-methyl-1-butene and H—Br.

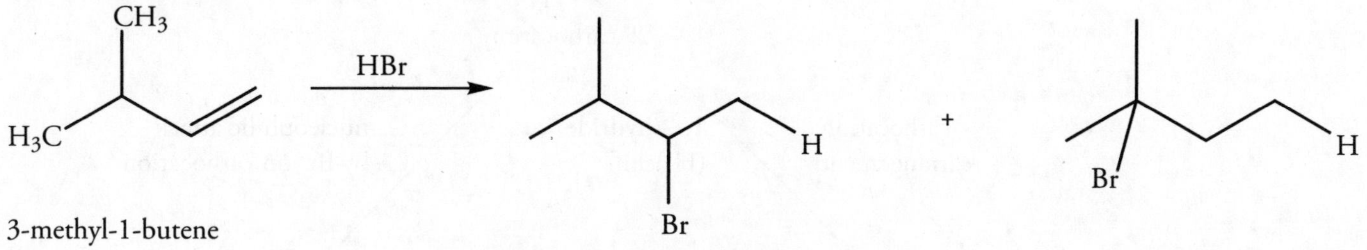

3-methyl-1-butene

(R),(S)-2-bromo-3-methylbutane
(Both enantiomers of 2-bromo-3-methylbutane
formed in equal amounts.)

2-bromo-2-methylbutane

In the first step of this reaction (shown below), the π electrons are protonated to form a new C–H σ bond, a carbocation, and a bromide ion. Notice that the more substituted carbon receives the positive charge, and the less substituted carbon (more hydrogens) receives the new C–H σ bond. The formation of the most stable carbocation intermediate corresponds to **Markovnikov's rule**. That is, given a choice, the most stable carbocation intermediate is always formed. Once the carbocation intermediate is formed, it can have two fates. The carbocation may undergo nucleophilic attack by the bromide ion, in a fashion similar to the fast step in an S_N1 reaction. As in the S_N1 reaction, the planarity of the carbocation intermediate results in a racemic mixture of products, in this case both (R) and (S)-2-bromo-3-methylbutane. Alternatively, this carbocation can rearrange to a more stable 3° carbocation by means of a 1,2-hydride (H⁻) shift, which is subsequently attacked by bromide yielding the achiral molecule 2-bromo-2-methylbutane.

Let's look at the mechanism:

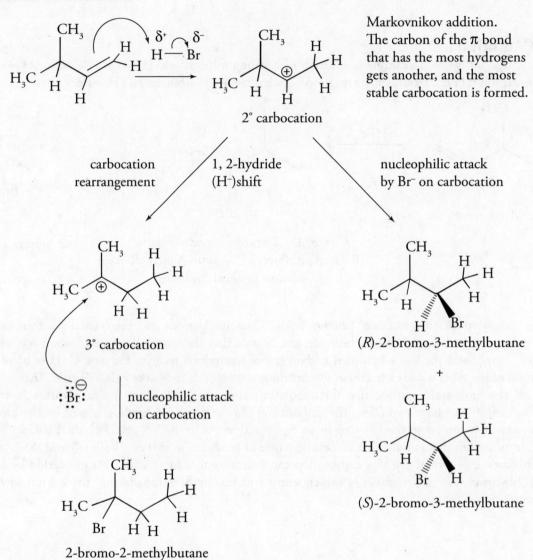

Markovnikov addition. The carbon of the π bond that has the most hydrogens gets another, and the most stable carbocation is formed.

Acid-Catalyzed Hydration of Alkenes

In acid-catalyzed hydration of alkenes, the alkene is added to an acid-water solution (a 50/50 mixture of sulfuric acid and water is typical) and allowed to react until the alcohol product is formed. Sulfuric acid is the ideal strong acid in this reaction, because unlike Cl^- or Br^-, its conjugate base, HSO_4^-, is non-nucleophilic. As such, there should be no nucleophile to compete with water for the carbocation. Note that this is a reversible reaction. (For a description of alcohol dehydration [an elimination reaction], see Section 26.3.) The following represents some typical examples of acid catalyzed alkene hydration reactions.

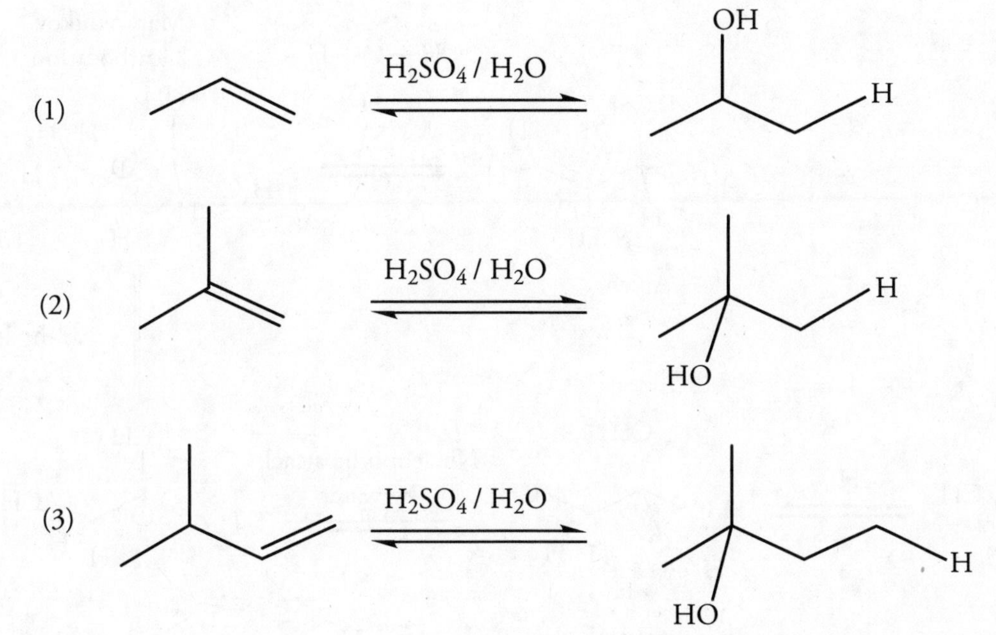

There are a few important points to note about the above hydration reactions. First, notice that all of the alcohols that are formed correspond to the Markovnikov addition product; this is because of the reaction mechanism. Shown below is the mechanism for Reaction 1 above.

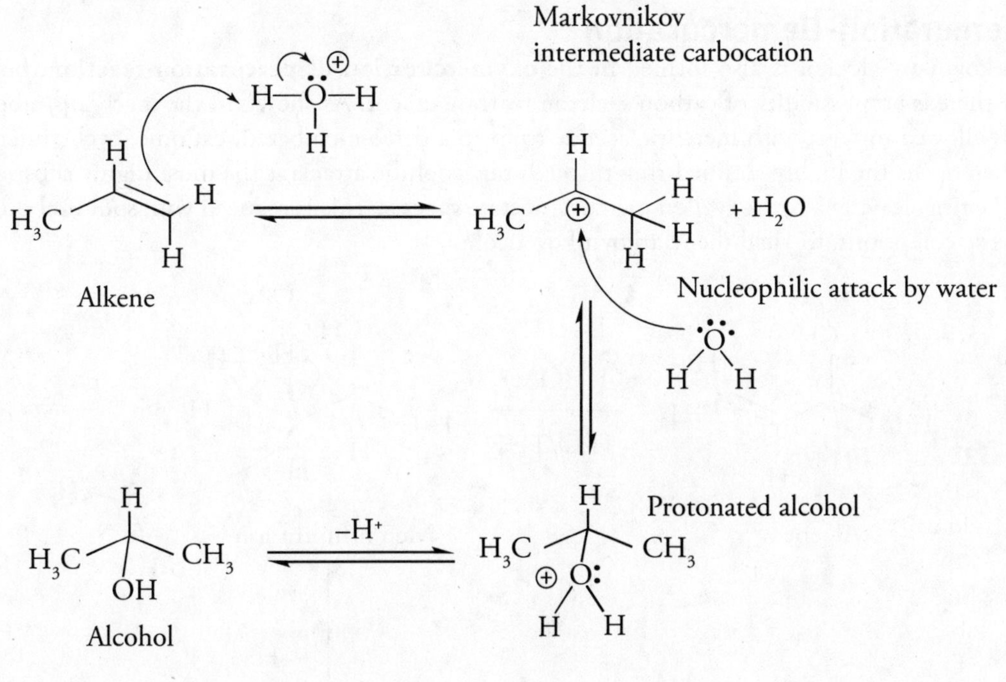

In the first step of this reaction, the π bond of the alkene is protonated to form the Markovnikov carbocation intermediate—the carbon of the π bond that has the most hydrogens to begin with receives the C–H σ bond, and the most substituted carbon is the recipient of the positive charge. Next, the carbocation is attacked by a nucleophilic water molecule to form the protonated alcohol. The protonated alcohol then quickly loses a proton to form the product. The following mechanism for reaction 3 above depicts how acid-catalyzed hydration reactions are prone to carbon skeleton rearrangements.

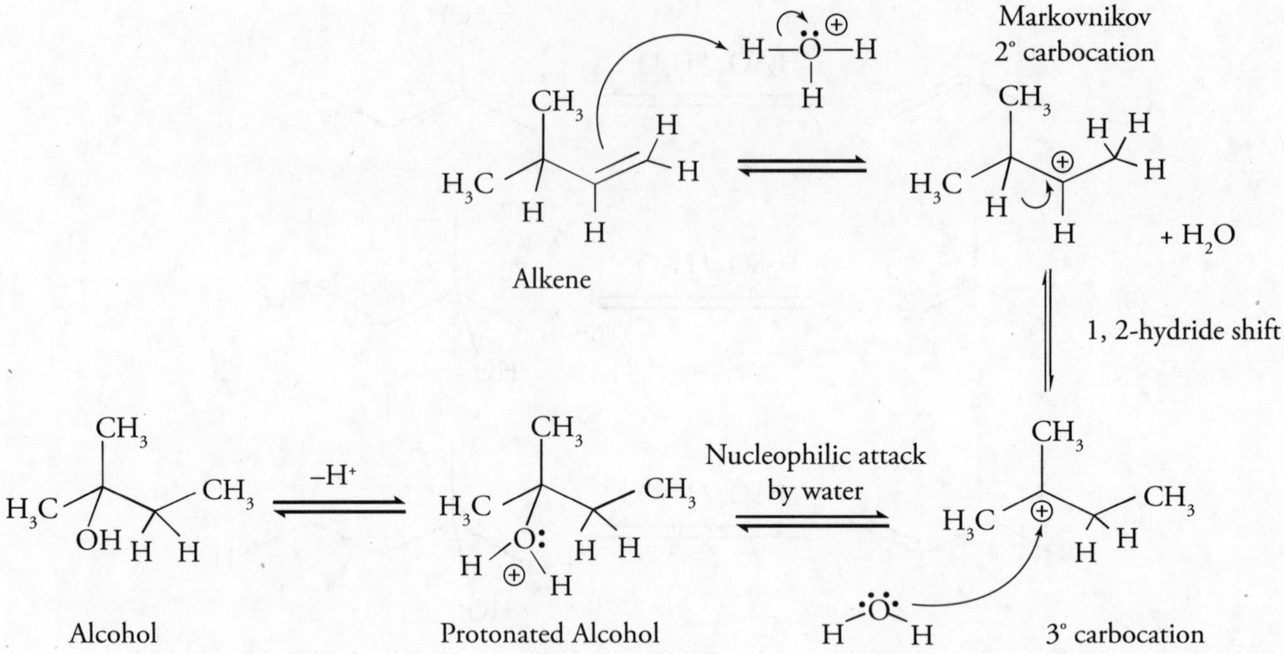

As you can see, if the original Markovnikov carbocation can rearrange to a more stable carbocation, it will.

Oxymercuration-Demercuration

The Markovnikov alcohol is also formed in the **oxymercuration-demercuration reaction**, but in this reaction there is no possibility of carbon skeleton rearrangement. As shown in the mechanism below, the alkene is allowed to react with mercuric acetate to form a three-membered, cationic, cyclic intermediate. Water then opens the highly strained ring through nucleophilic attack at the most highly substituted carbon in the ring, leaving a hydroxyalkyl mercuric acetate species. This is reduced with sodium borohydride, under basic conditions, to yield the Markovnikov alcohol.

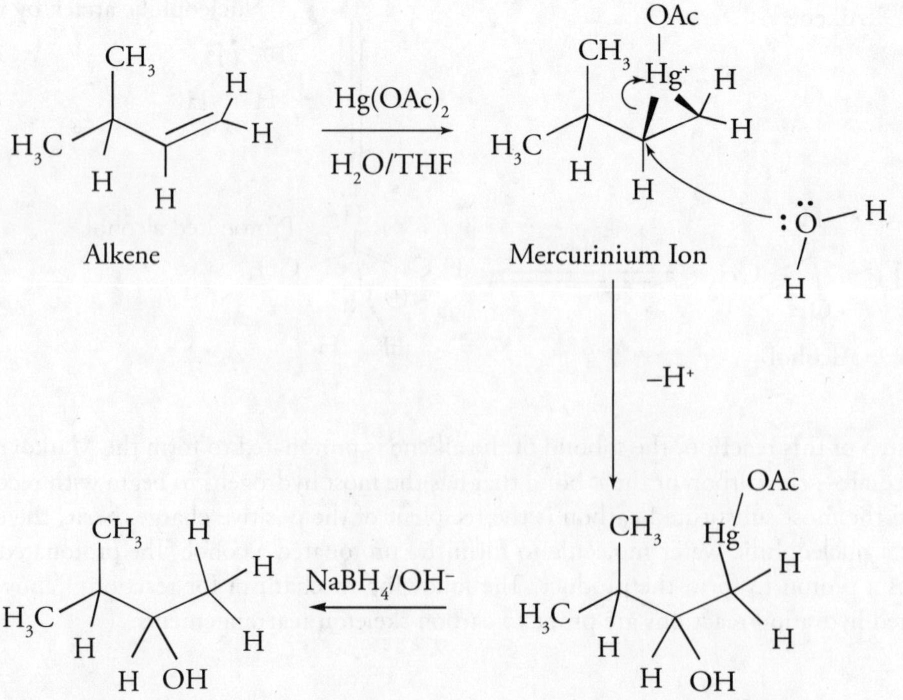

The cyclic, cationic intermediate is key in the selective formation of the Markovnikov alcohol. It may seem counterintuitive to think that water, a nucleophile, would attack the more substituted carbon of the ring, since this site is more sterically challenging than the less substituted side. The reason behind this choice of regiochemistry lies in the examination of possible resonance structures of the cation.

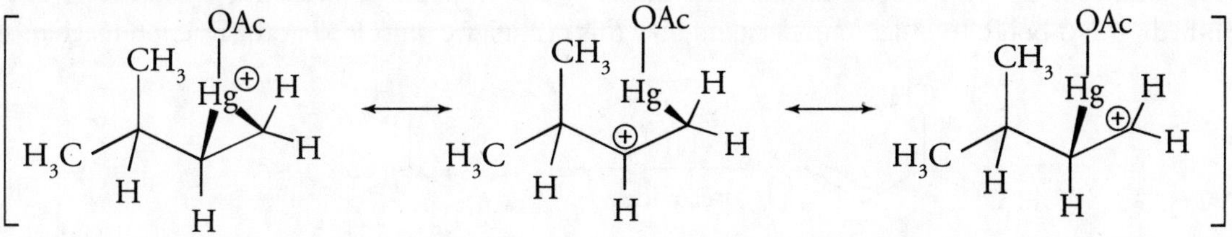

As in any molecule with multiple possible resonance structures, the resulting electronic structure of the above molecule will be a mix of the three, weighted with respect to the stability of each. The carbocation in the middle structure is more highly substituted, and thus energetically favorable to the one on the right. As such this carbon will bear a greater portion of the cationic charge, and be more attractive to nucleophiles.

This type of 3-membered cyclic intermediate plays a role in many reactions, a few of which will be mentioned shortly. In each case, so long at the species is cationic, the attack which opens the ring, and subsequent substitution, takes place at the more highly substituted of the ring carbons.

Anti-Markovnikov Addition

Hydroboration-Oxidation

Alcohols can be synthesized in an anti-Markovnikov fashion, with the hydroxyl occupying the least substituted of the two carbons of the double bond, through a process known as **hydroboration**. In this reaction the alkene is treated with BH_3 (either in solution as in BH_3–THF, or neat in the dimeric form, B_2H_6) to form an intermediate organoborane compound. The organoborane intermediate is then oxidized with hydrogen peroxide (H_2O_2) under basic conditions to form the anti-Markovnikov alcohol. These properties are demonstrated by the following two reactions.

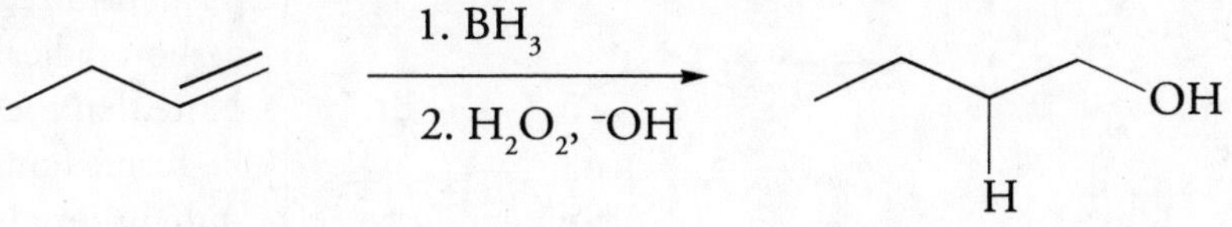

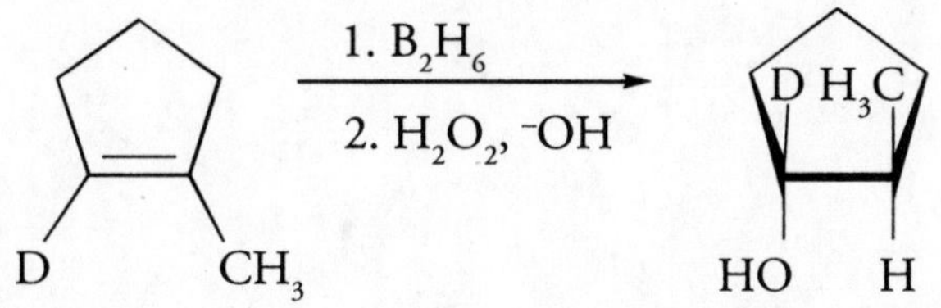

Notice that the –OH ends up on the less substituted carbon instead of the more substituted carbon. Furthermore, the stereochemistry of the addition to the π bond is *syn*. Both the hydrogen that is added and the –OH end up on the same side of the former C=C double bond.

HBr Addition in the Presence of Peroxides

Chemists have also developed tools to produce halogenated alkanes in anti-Markovnikov fashion. When an alkene is treated with H–Br in the presence of peroxides (R–O–O–R), H and Br are added to the π bond with the opposite regiochemistry than is seen in the addition of HX without peroxides. The less substituted carbon of the π bond ends up with a bond to bromine; the more substituted carbon of the π bond receives a new carbon-hydrogen σ bond. In order to understand how this occurs, we must look at the reaction mechanism.

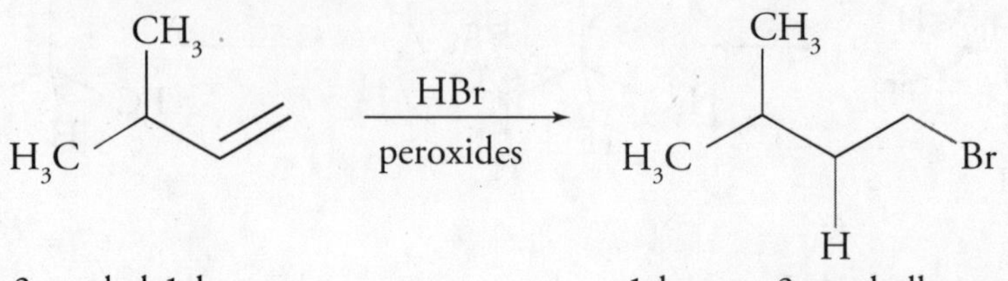

3-methyl-1-butene   1-bromo-3-methylbutane

Homolytic bond cleavage of the O–O bond of the peroxide molecule occurs in the first step of this reaction, generating two R–O• radicals. One R–O• radical then abstracts a hydrogen atom from HBr in another homolytic bond cleavage, to form a molecule of alcohol and a bromine radical. The lone electron of the bromine radical forms a σ bond with the less substituted carbon of the π bond such that the other electron of the π bond resides on the more substituted carbon. The order of stability for radicals is 3° > 2° > 1°, just as it is for carbocations. The alkyl radical then collides with a molecule of H–Br and abstracts a hydrogen atom in a homolytic bond cleavage resulting in the formation of the alkyl halide product and another bromine radical. Note that this peroxide effect only works for H–Br; it is not observed with H–Cl or H–I.

Initiation Steps

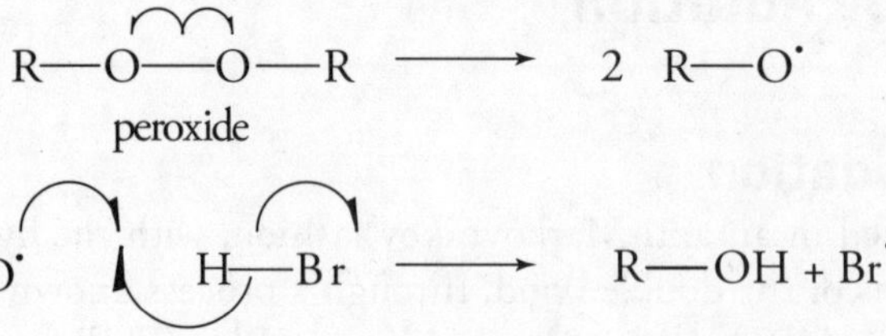

peroxide

Propagation Steps

3-methyl-1-butene

sp²-hybridized, carbon radical intermediate. Note that the C–H σ bond can be formed on either side of the unhybridized *p* orbital.

1-bromo-3-methylbutane

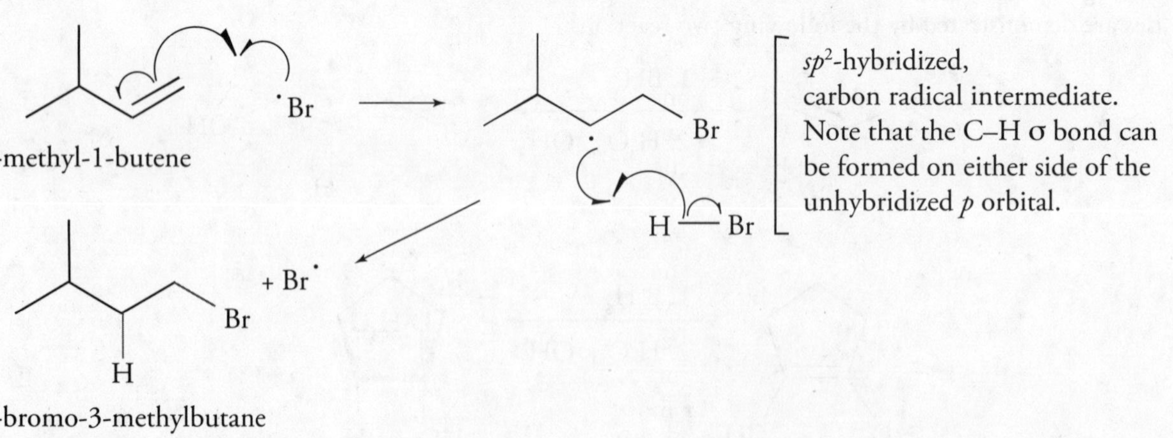

Remember, the most important features to focus on for the DAT for all of the reactions described above are the regiochemistry differences. Therefore, be sure you know which reactions follow Markovnikov addition rules, and which follow anti-Markovnikov addition.

Additional Electrophilic Addition Reactions

X$_2$ Addition

Whereas the addition of HX is an effective technique to monohalogenate double bonds, dihalogenation is known to occur through treatment of alkenes with diatomic halogens.

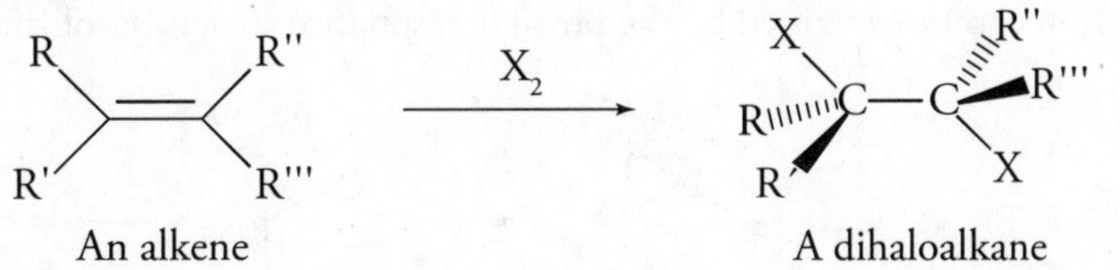

An alkene   A dihaloalkane

Consider the reaction that occurs when cyclopentene is treated with bromine (Br$_2$). In the first step of this reaction, the nucleophilic π electrons attack molecular bromine to yield a bromonium ion and a bromide anion in an S$_N$2 reaction. At first glance it would not appear that molecular bromine would be very electrophilic. However, when an electron-rich π bond comes close to a molecule of Br$_2$, it induces a dipole in the Br$_2$ molecule so that one side of the molecule becomes slightly negatively charged while the other side becomes slightly positively charged. This provides the initial driving force for the reaction. Let's look at a mechanism:

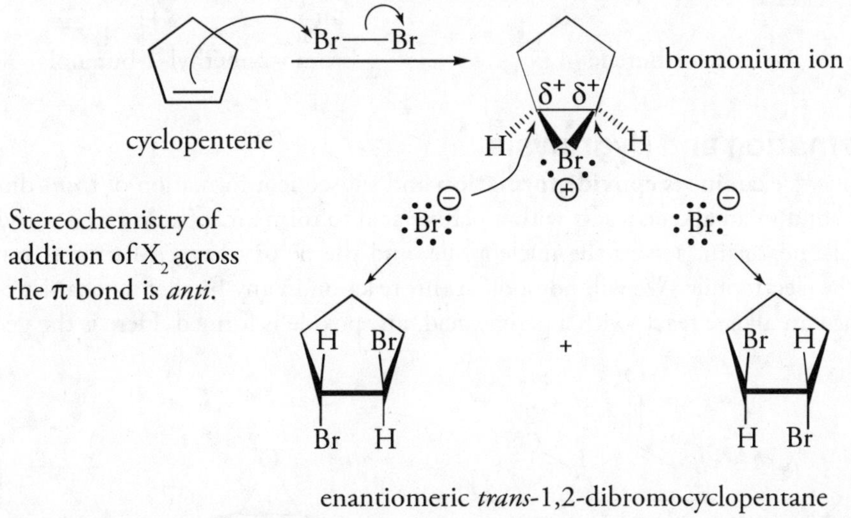

enantiomeric *trans*-1,2-dibromocyclopentane

As is the case with the previously mentioned mercurinium ion, the positive charge on this bridged bromine pulls electrons away from the two carbons to which it is attached, causing them to become slightly positive and electrophilic. These electrophilic carbon atoms are susceptible to nucleophilic attack by bromide ions from the opposite side of the bridged structure. As the nucleophilic bromide ion attacks the bridged structure, it forms a bromine-carbon σ bond. Simultaneously, one of the carbon-bromine bonds of the bridged structure breaks; this reaction is essentially an S$_N$2 substitution. It is important to be aware of the stereochemistry of addition of the two bromines to the π bond. Notice that two chiral centers are formed in this particular reaction, and the two products that are formed (depending upon whether the bromide ion attacks the right or left carbon of the bridged bromonium ion) are nonsuperimposable mirror images of each other—that is, enantiomers. Since attack at either carbon of the bridged intermediate is equally likely, equal amounts of enantiomers are formed giving a racemic mixture. Also, it is important to note that the two bromine atoms are added across the double bond in anti-fashion. This is a result of the S$_N$2-like backside attack by the second bromine atom on the carbon of the bromonium ion.

Halohydrin Formation

If an alkene is treated with Br_2 in water, an intermediate bromonium ion is formed, which subsequently undergoes nucleophilic attack by water. This yields a halohydrin, a molecule in which a bromine atom and an $-OH$ from water have been added across the carbon-carbon π bond. If the bromonium ion is unsymmetrical, the nucleophile will prefer to attack the more substituted carbon atom of the bridged structure for the same reason we saw water attack the more substituted carbon in the oxymercuration reaction. Again, this phenomenon can be explained by the possible resonance structures of the cation.

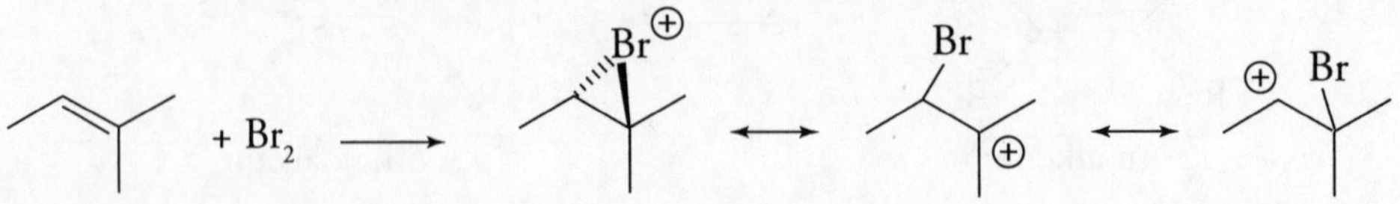

The more substituted carbon bears the greater partial positive charge, thanks to its greater inductive stabilization of this charge. As such, the ring opening attack by water occurs at the more substituted carbon, in *anti*-fashion. This reaction also technically occurs via a Markovnikov mechanism.

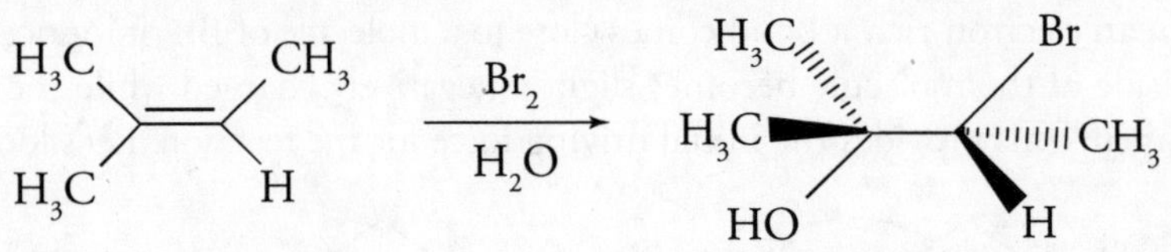

2-methyl-2-butene   3-bromo-2-methyl-2-butanol

Epoxide Formation and Hydrolysis

The next reaction we examine is **epoxide formation** and subsequent formation of *trans*-diols. In this type of reaction, a π bond in an alkene reacts with a peroxy acid to form an epoxide and a carboxylic acid. The π bond of the alkene, again, acts as the nucleophile, and the peroxy oxygen furthest from the carbonyl oxygen acts as the electrophile. We will not look at this reaction in any further mechanistic detail. The key point is that when an alkene reacts with a peroxy acid, an epoxide is formed. Here is the general reaction:

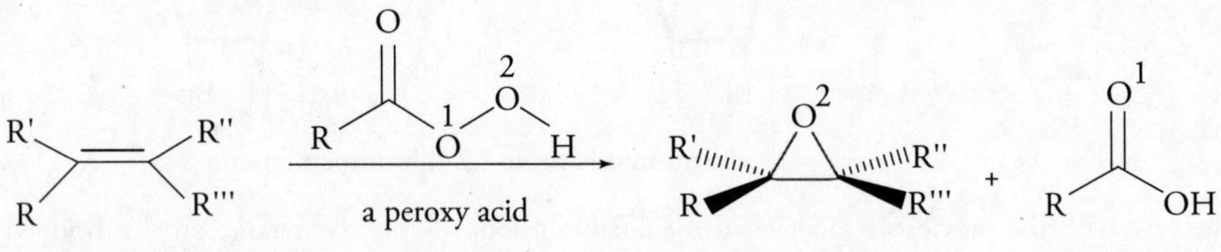

an alkene   a peroxy acid   an epoxide   a carboxylic acid

Here is a specific example of epoxidation followed by acidic or basic hydrolysis. This reaction forms a *trans*-diol:

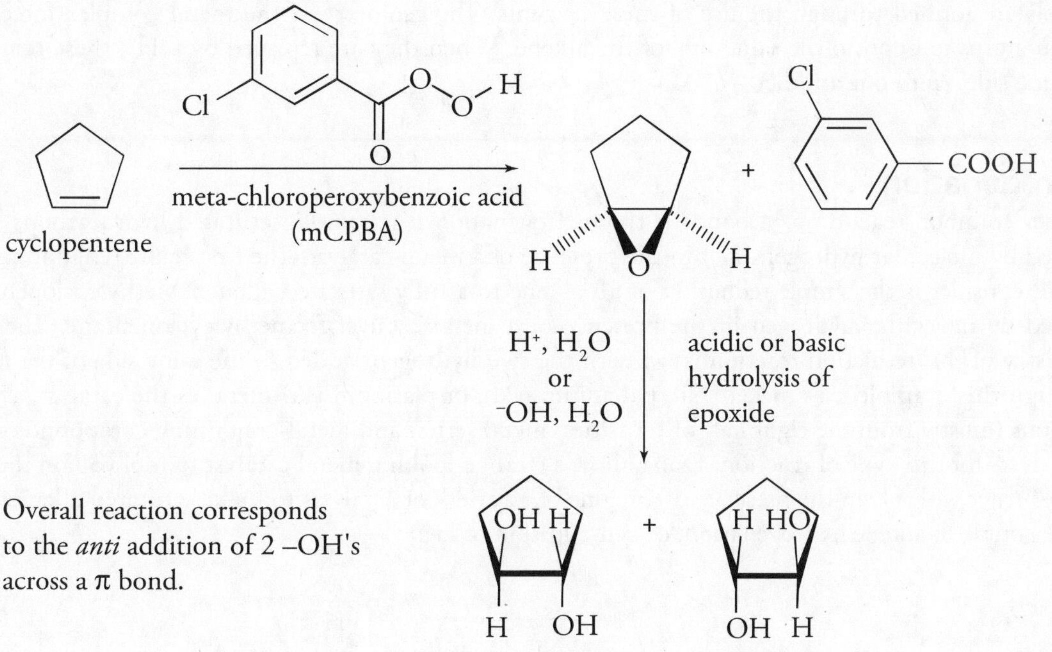
Cl
O
O
H
O
Cl
COOH
+
meta-chloroperoxybenzoic acid
(mCPBA)
cyclopentene
H
O
H
H⁺, H₂O
or
⁻OH, H₂O
acidic or basic
hydrolysis of
epoxide
Overall reaction corresponds
to the *anti* addition of 2 –OH's
across a π bond.
OH H
+
H HO
H OH
OH H

Enantiomeric *trans* diols

It is also important to note that when an epoxide is hydrolyzed under acidic or basic conditions, a *trans*-1,2-diol is formed.

Oxidation with Dilute $KMnO_4$

When alkenes are treated with dilute $KMnO_4$ (potassium permanganate) or OsO_4 (osmium tetraoxide), *cis*-diols are formed. The stereochemistry of this reaction requires *syn*-addition of two –OH's across the π bond. Here is an example:

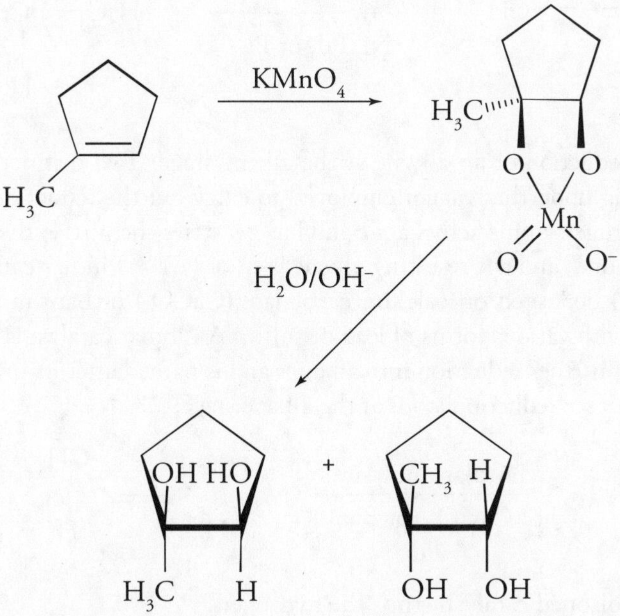
KMnO₄
H₃C
H₃C
O
O
Mn
O
O⁻
H₂O/OH⁻
OH HO
+
CH₃ H
H₃C H
OH OH

The organometallic intermediate in the above mechanism (similarly valid for OsO_4) is the reason only *cis*-diols are formed through the use of these reagents. The geometry of the metal complex forces both oxygen atoms to bond to the same side of the alkene. When they are replaced by OH^-, these remain on the same side, *cis* to one another.

Hydrogenation

Another common reaction of π bonds is the hydrogenation reaction. Unsaturated hydrocarbons can be reduced by molecular hydrogen (H_2) in the presence of a metal catalyst. The first hydrogenation reaction we will consider is the simple reduction of an alkene to a fully saturated alkane. Methylcyclopentene is reduced by molecular hydrogen in the presence of a metal catalyst to methylcyclopentane. The stereo-chemistry of this reduction reaction is *syn* with the two hydrogens added to the same side of the π bond. Although this example uses nickel (Ni), palladium (Pd), or platinum (Pt) metal as the catalyst, a variety of metals (mostly from the right half of transition metal series) and metal-containing compounds can act as catalysts for this type of reaction. Don't allow a strange-looking metal catalyst to fool you on the DAT; alkenes react with H_2 in the presence of any one of a variety of catalysts to make saturated alkanes. Here is an example of alkene hydrogenation, or syn-addition of H_2:

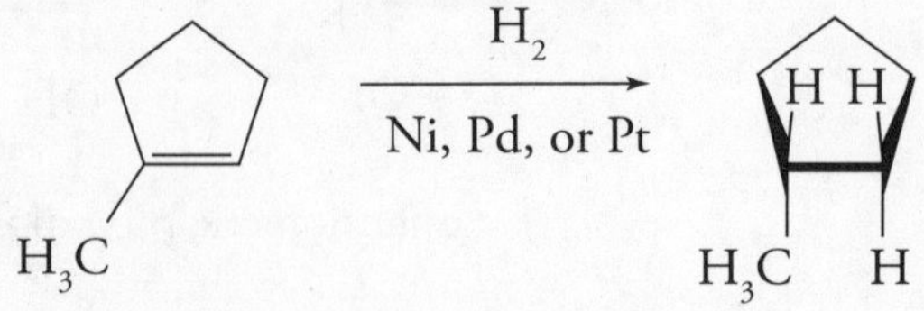

Next, we will explore hydrogenations of alkynes, compounds that have carbon-carbon triple bonds. If an alkyne is reduced by molecular hydrogen (H_2) in the presence of a metal catalyst, it will be reduced all the way to the alkane. This is demonstrated by the reduction of 2-pentyne all the way to the fully satu-rated pentane. Here is one example of π bond hydrogenation in alkynes:

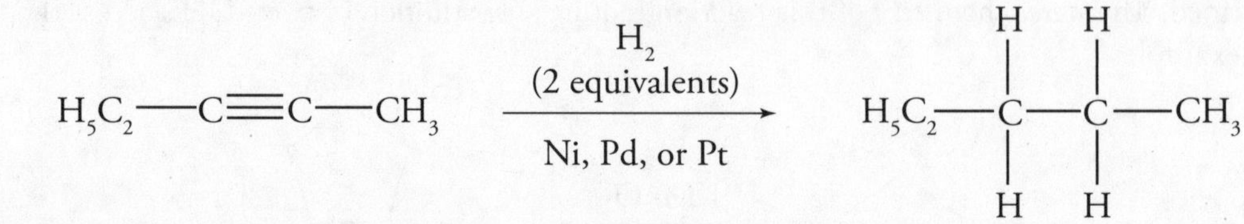

It is possible to stop the reduction of an alkyne at the alkene stage. Two distinct stereochemistries of addi-tion are possible depending upon the reagent employed to carry out the reduction. If a **Lindlar catalyst** is used, addition of two hydrogen atoms across a π bond has *syn* stereochemistry; the two hydrogens are added to the same side of the π bond, and the resulting alkene is *cis* or (Z). A Lindlar catalyst is heterogeneous and consists of palladium (Pd) deposited on calcium carbonate ($CaCO_3$) or barium sulfate ($BaSO_4$). These re-agents are then poisoned with various forms of lead or sulfur. A Lindlar catalyst is used for hydrogenation of alkynes to alkenes without further reduction into alkanes and is named after its inventor Herbert Lindlar. In the example below, you can see reduction stops at the alkene stage:

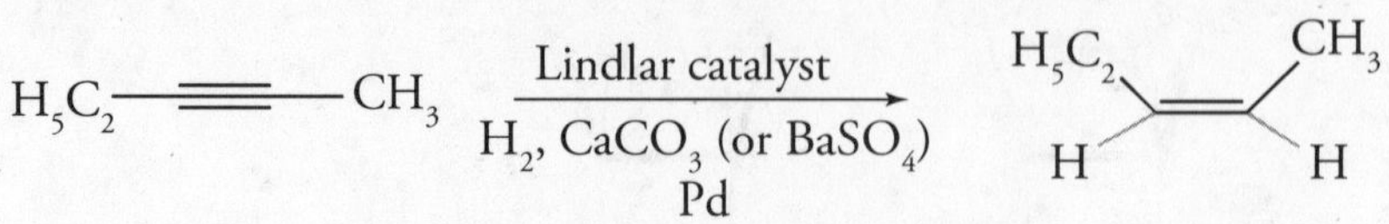

Poisoned catalyst–stops the hydrogen
reduction of alkyne at the alkene stage

On the other hand, it is also possible to stop the reduction of an alkyne at the alkene stage with the resulting alkene being of the *trans* or (*E*) stereochemistry. This is accomplished with a reagent that consists of sodium metal in the presence of liquid ammonia. In this reaction, two hydrogens are added across a π bond of the alkyne with an *anti*-stereochemistry such that the two hydrogens are added on opposite sides of the π bond. As with the Lindlar catalyst, reduction stops at the alkene stage.

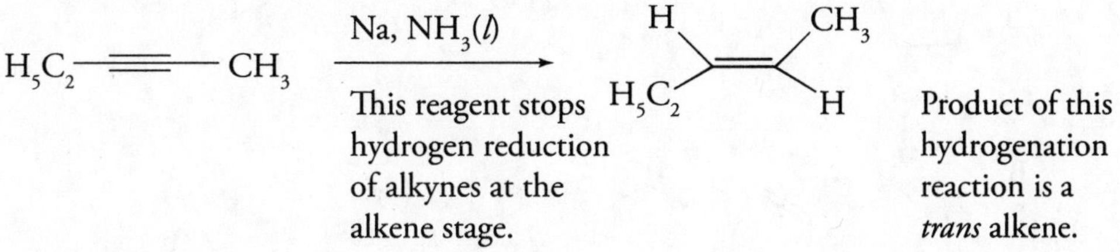

$$H_5C_2 \overset{}{=\!=\!=} CH_3 \xrightarrow{\text{Na, NH}_3(l)}$$

This reagent stops hydrogen reduction of alkynes at the alkene stage.

Product of this hydrogenation reaction is a *trans* alkene.

Ozonolysis

In the first step of this reaction, ozone (O$_3$) reacts with a π bond to form a cyclic intermediate called an ozonide. This intermediate is then hydrolyzed in a reductive workup step, resulting in cleavage of the double bond to yield aldehyde and/or ketone products. Here is how you can predict the products of an ozonolysis reaction: whatever is attached to a π bond of the alkene (an alkyl group or a hydrogen) remains attached in the aldehyde or ketone product, and there is an additional carbonyl group.

Here is a general example:

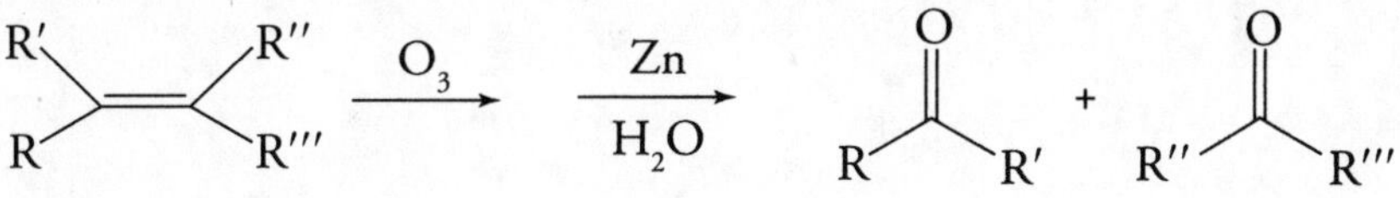

$$\underset{R}{\overset{R'}{\diagdown}}C=C\underset{R'''}{\overset{R''}{\diagup}} \xrightarrow{O_3} \xrightarrow{\underset{H_2O}{Zn}} \quad \underset{R}{\overset{O}{\diagdown}}\underset{R'}{\diagup} + \underset{R''}{\overset{O}{\diagdown}}\underset{R'''}{\diagup}$$

Here are two specific examples:

Here are two specific examples illustrated with chemical structures.

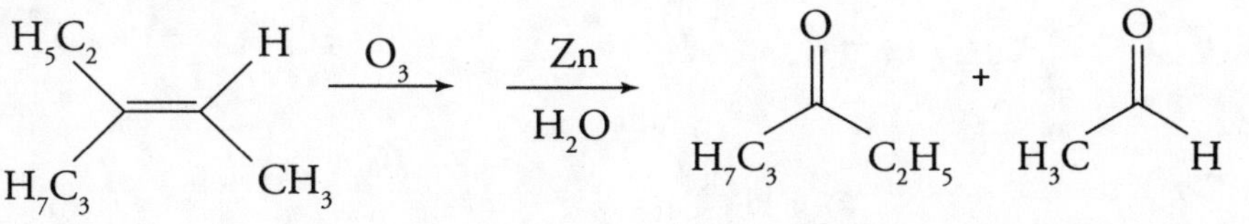

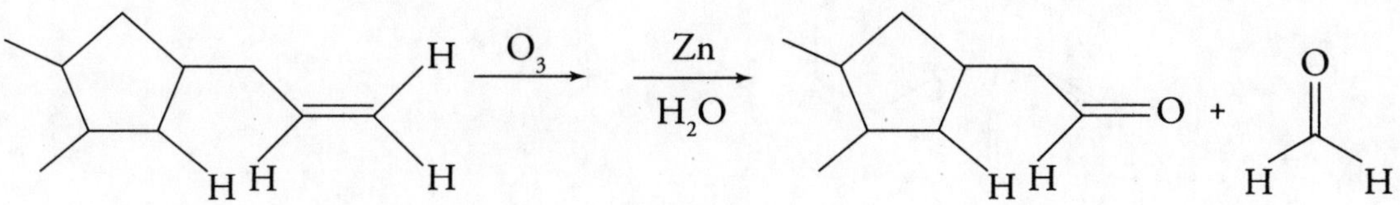

Example: 27-1 Predict the products of ozonolysis for the following reactions:

A.

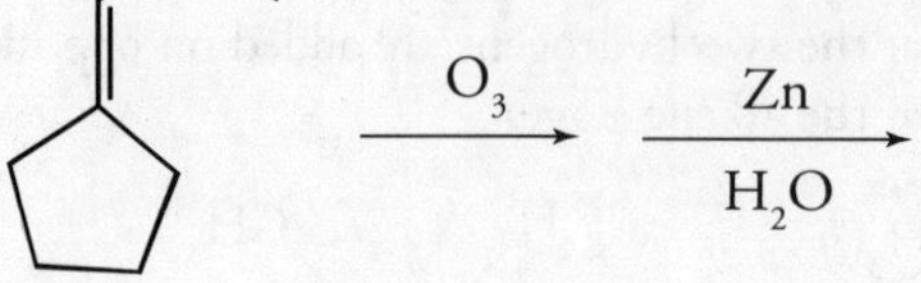

B.

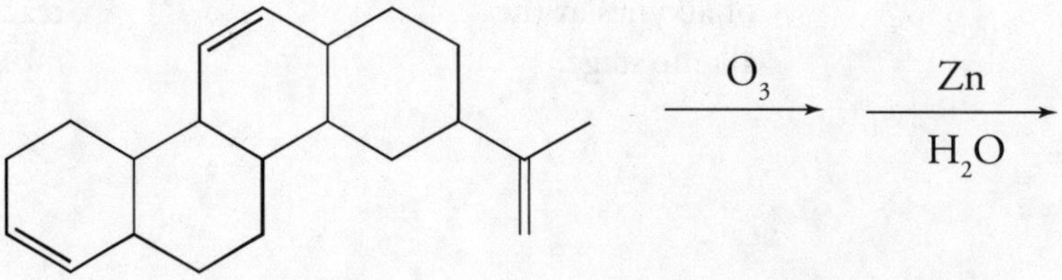

C.

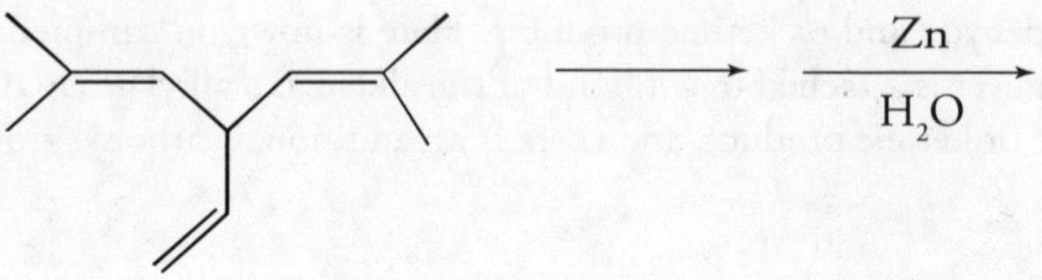

Solution:

A.

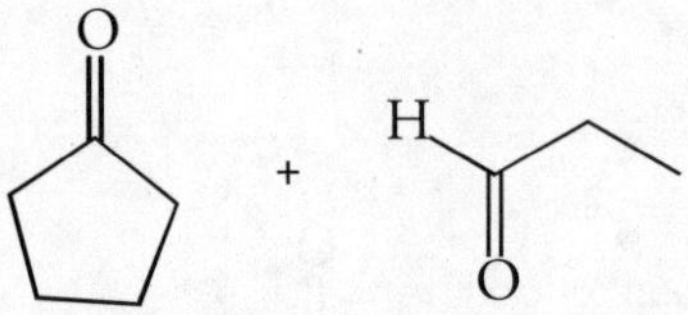

B.

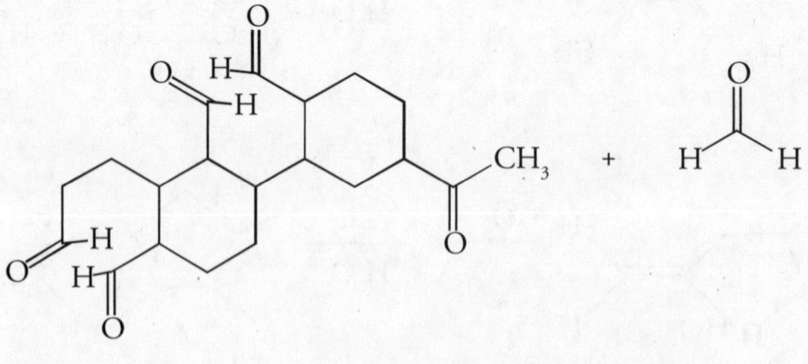

C.

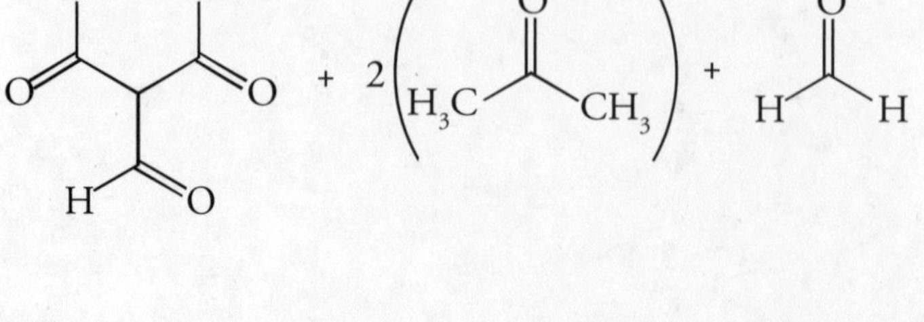

Example 27-2: Predict the principal organic product for each of the following reactions:

A.

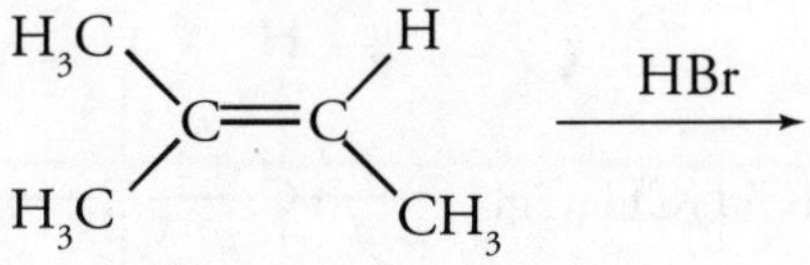

$$\xrightarrow{\text{HBr}}$$

B.

$$(H_3C)_2HCH_2CH_2CH_2CHC=CH_2 \xrightarrow[\text{peroxides}]{\text{HBr}}$$

C.

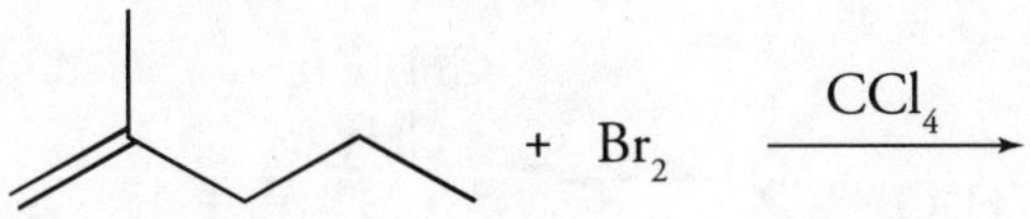

$$+ \ Br_2 \xrightarrow{\text{CCl}_4}$$

D.

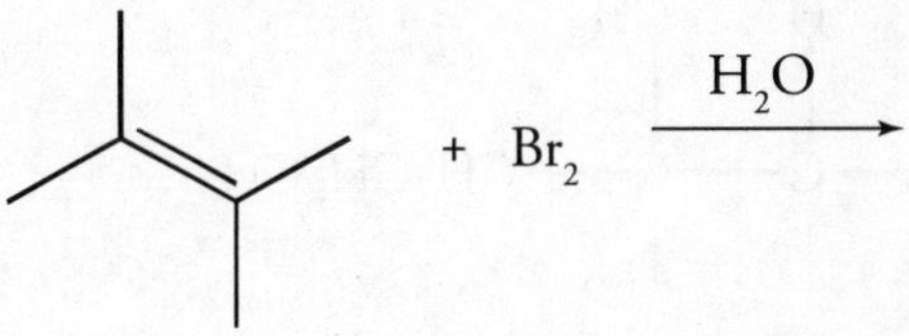

$$+ \ Br_2 \xrightarrow{\text{H}_2\text{O}}$$

E.

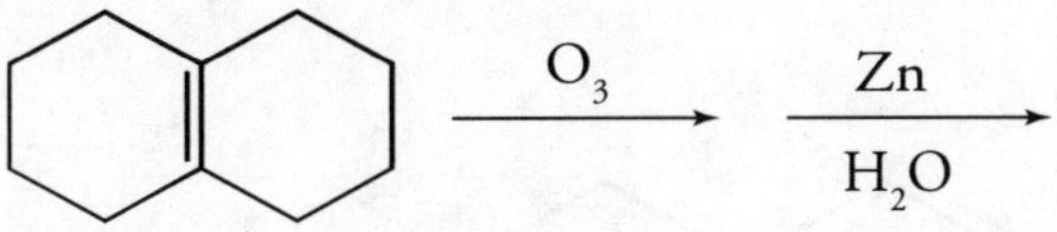

$$\xrightarrow{O_3} \xrightarrow[\text{H}_2\text{O}]{\text{Zn}}$$

F.

$$\text{1-hexyne} \xrightarrow[\text{Pt}]{2 \ H_2}$$

G.

$$\xrightarrow[\text{NH}_3(l)]{\text{Na}}$$

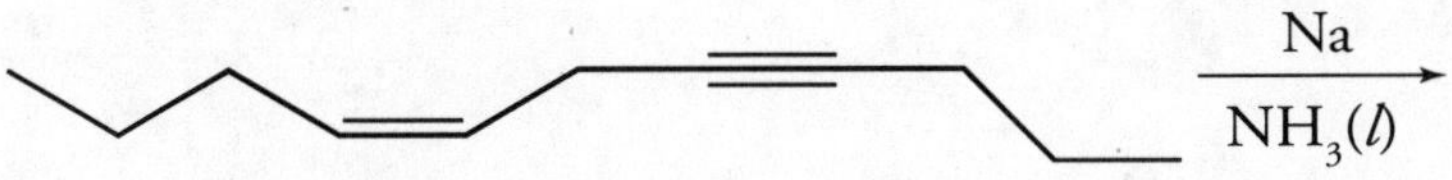

H.

$$\text{2-hexyne} \xrightarrow[\substack{\text{Pd} \\ \text{H}_2, \text{CaCO}_3 \\ \text{quinoline}}]{\substack{\text{Lindlar} \\ \text{catalyst}}}$$

I.

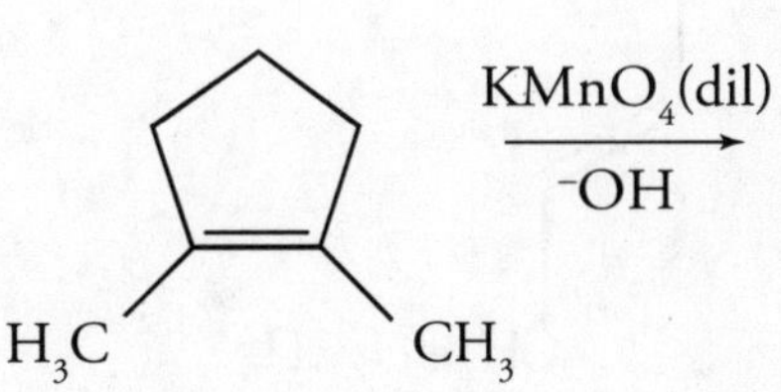

$$\xrightarrow[\text{-OH}]{\text{KMnO}_4(\text{dil})}$$

J.

$$\xrightarrow{\text{peroxy acid}} \xrightarrow[\text{H}_2\text{O}]{\text{H}^+}$$

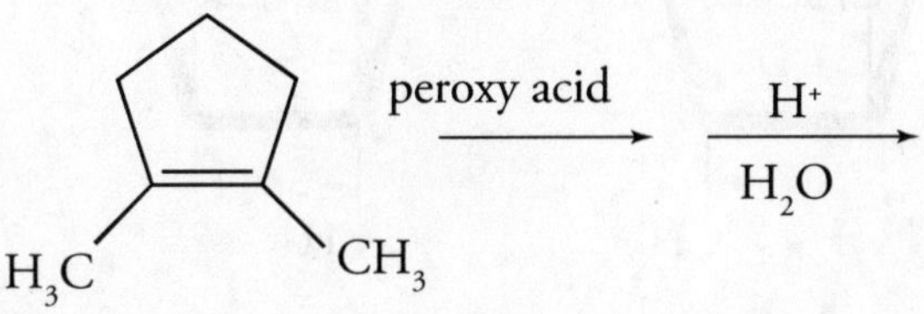

Solution:

A.

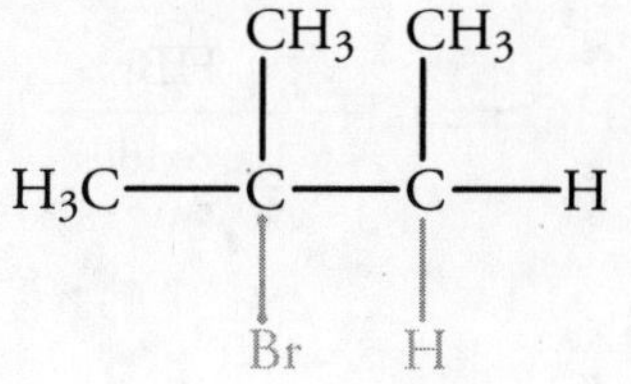

$$H_3C-\overset{\overset{\displaystyle CH_3}{|}}{\underset{\underset{\displaystyle Br}{|}}{C}}-\overset{\overset{\displaystyle CH_3}{|}}{\underset{\underset{\displaystyle H}{|}}{C}}-H$$

B.

$$(CH_3)_2CHCH_2CH_2CH_2-\overset{\overset{\displaystyle H}{|}}{\underset{\underset{\displaystyle H}{|}}{C}}-\overset{\overset{\displaystyle H}{|}}{\underset{\underset{\displaystyle H}{|}}{C}}-Br$$

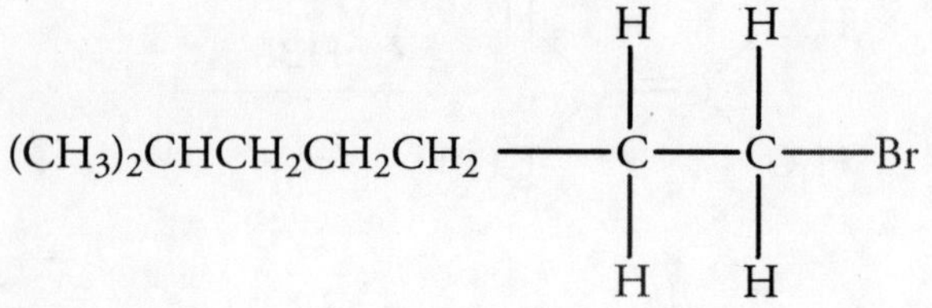

C.

$$H-\overset{\overset{\displaystyle H}{|}}{\underset{\underset{\displaystyle Br}{|}}{C}}-\overset{\overset{\displaystyle CH_3}{|}}{\underset{\underset{\displaystyle Br}{|}}{C}}-CH_2CH_2CH_3$$

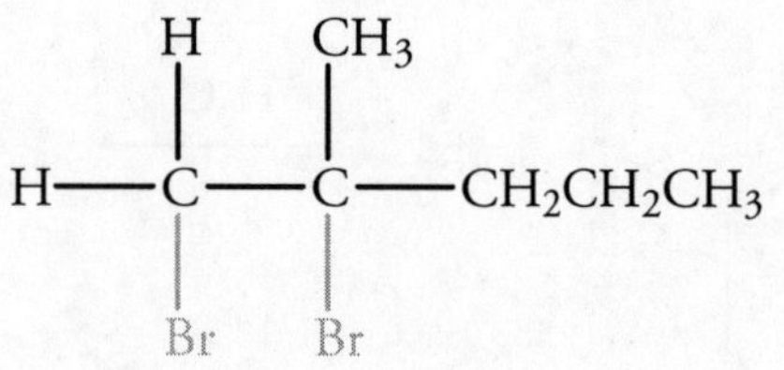

D.

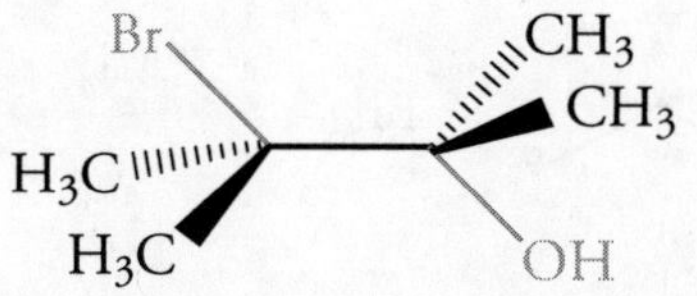

E.

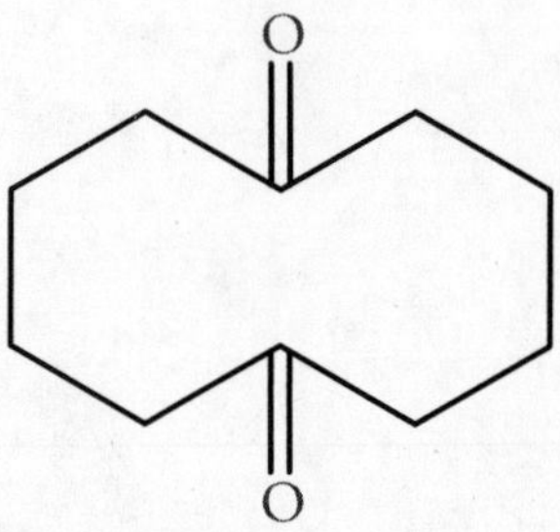

F.

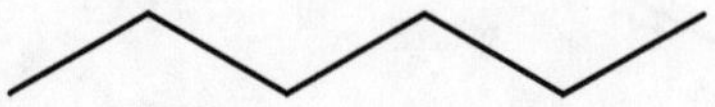

G.

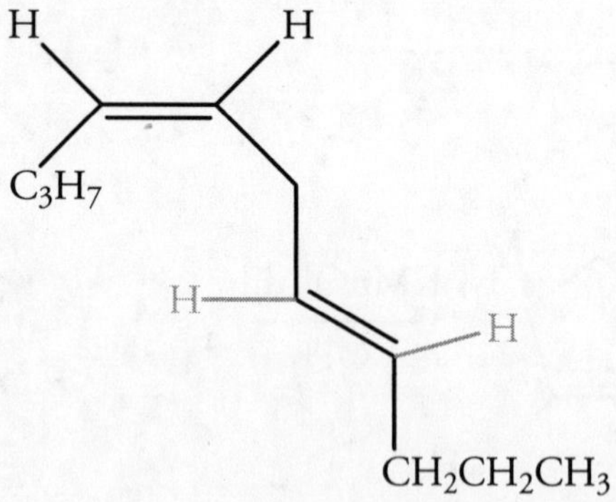

H.

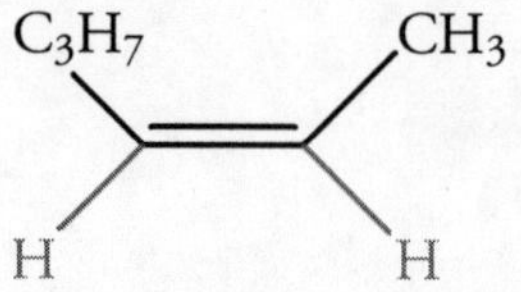

I.

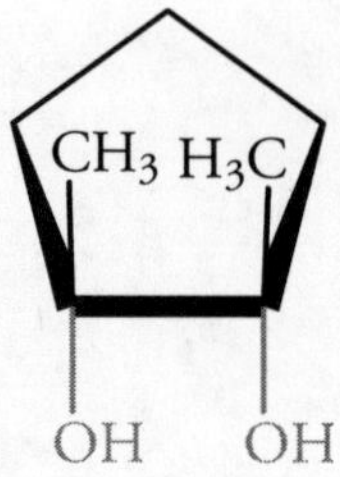

J.

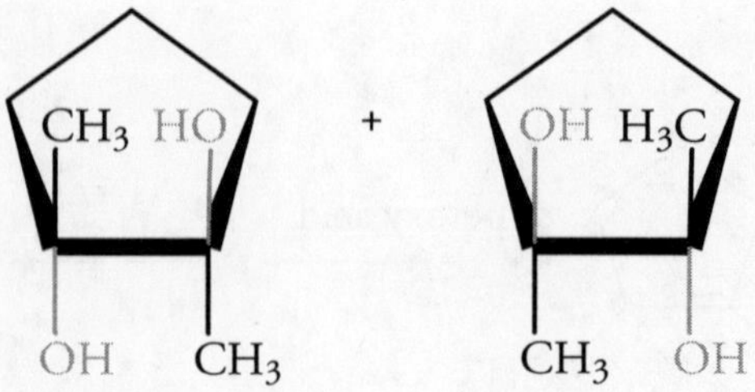

27.2 AROMATIC COMPOUNDS

Here are the criteria that must be satisfied in order for a compound to be considered **aromatic**:

1. The compound must possess a **cyclic system** in which every atom of the ring has an unhybridized p orbital such that the π electrons of the ring can delocalize through them.
2. The cyclic delocalized p orbital system must be flat and planar.
3. The delocalized p orbital system must possess a **Hückel number** of π electrons.

Hückel numbers are of the form $4n + 2$, where $n = 0, 1, 2, 3, \ldots$ When $n = 0$, we have 2 π electrons; when $n = 1$, we have 6 π electrons; when $n = 2$, we have 10 π electrons; and so on. This Hückel number of π electrons imparts an aromatic stability to delocalized, flat, planar systems of p orbitals because it corresponds to a closed-shell configuration with all bonding orbitals filled.

Some Aromatic Compounds

  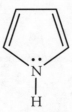

| all carbons sp^2 flat and planar 6 p electrons | all carbons sp^2 flat and planar 2 p electrons | all carbons sp^2 flat and planar 6 p electrons | all carbons sp^2 flat and planar 6 p electrons |

Some Non-aromatic Compounds

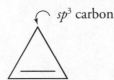  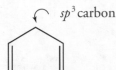

| 2 π electrons but an sp^3 carbon through which the π electrons cannot delocalize | all carbons sp^2 but only 4 π electrons | all carbons sp^2 but 8 π electrons | only 4 π electrons and a sp^3 carbon through which the π electrons cannot delocalize |

Example 27-3: Which of the following molecules are aromatic?

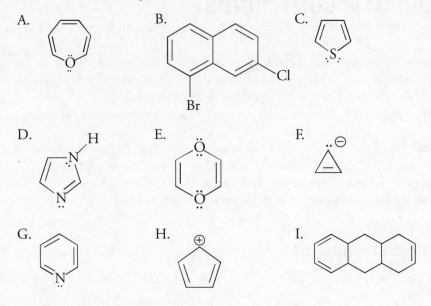

A.   B.   C.

D.   E.   F.

G.   H.   I.

Solution: Only B, C, D, and G are aromatic; the rest are not.

Nomenclature of Substituted Benzenes

There are several benzene-based molecules you should recognize for the DAT:

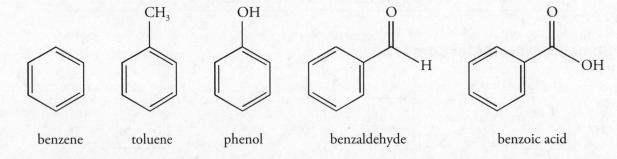

benzene   toluene   phenol   benzaldehyde   benzoic acid

A second substituent can be in one of three different positions relative to the first. These three positions are called the *ortho* (abbreviated *o-*), *meta* (abbreviated *m-*), and *para* (abbreviated *p-*) positions. Let's add a second substituent to benzoic acid as an example:

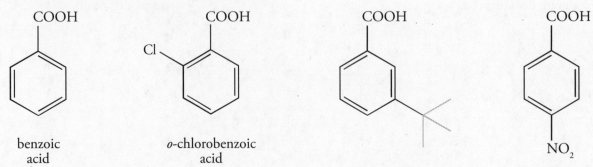

benzoic
acid

o-chlorobenzoic
acid

m-tert-butylbenzoic
acid

p-nitrobenzoic
acid

Electrophilic Aromatic Substitution: Reactivity of Aromatic Compounds

Even though aromatic compounds like benzene have π bonds, they are unusually stable and unreactive. For example, benzene does not react as alkenes do under ordinary electrophilic addition reaction conditions. Aromatic compounds will react, however, with *very* electrophilic reagents to undergo an overall substitution reaction for a hydrogen atom on the ring. These reactions are called **electrophilic aromatic substitution** reactions. Some examples are given below.

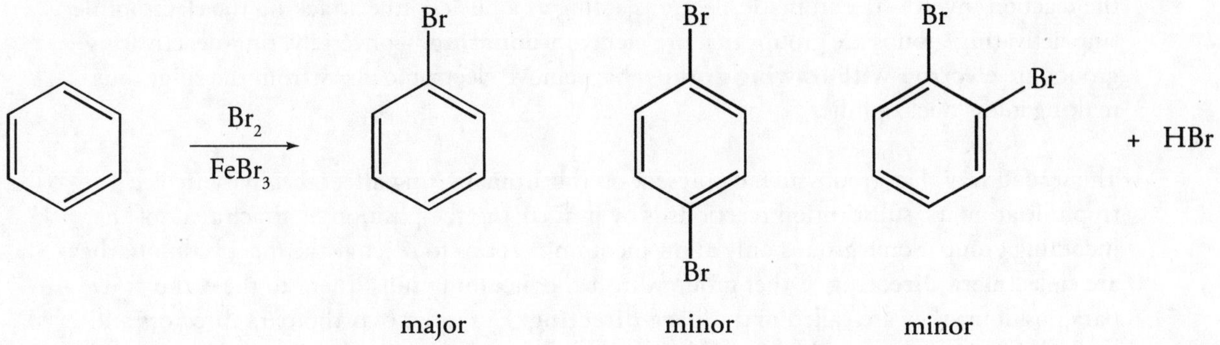

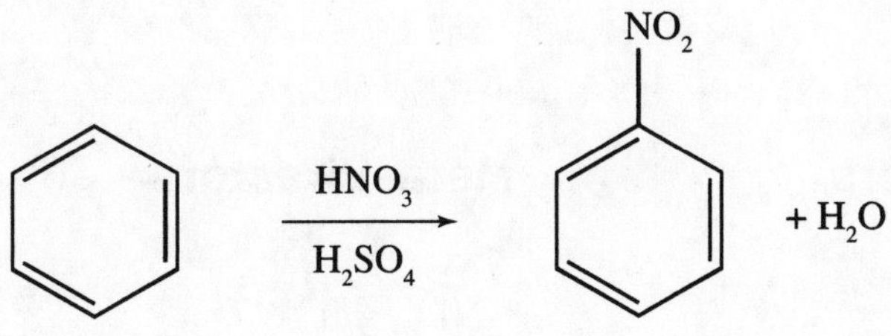

major   minor   minor

Let's now examine the mechanism of the electrophilic aromatic substitution reaction between benzene and bromine (Br_2) in the presence of catalytic $FeBr_3$ (see next page). In the first step of the reaction, a very reactive adduct between bromine and the catalyst forms. As is common in all types of electrophilic aromatic substitution reactions, this initial step provides the source of the electrophile (Br^+ in this example). In the second step, benzene acts as the nucleophile and attacks the electrophile in a substitution reaction. The resulting species is a cation and is no longer aromatic since it has an sp^3 hybridized carbon in the ring. Aromaticity can be restored to the intermediate by a simple deprotonation. Either bromide ion (Br^-) or $FeBr_4^-$ is a strong enough base to accomplish this last step in the reaction.

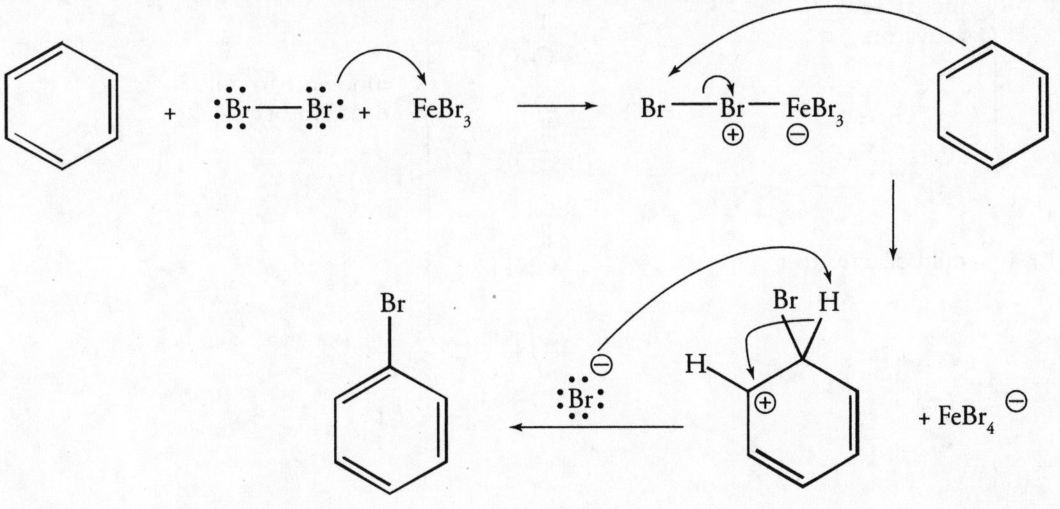

When a group is already present on the aromatic ring, it can affect the electrophilic aromatic substitution reaction in two important ways:

- First, the group already on the ring will affect the ease with which the reaction will take place (relative to the same reaction with an aromatic substrate that does not already have another group present). Groups that make it easier to introduce a new group to the aromatic compound are termed **ring-activating**. Groups that make it more difficult to introduce a new group to the aromatic compound are called **ring-deactivating**. Since the important step of the reaction involves the aromatic electrons acting as a nucleophile attacking the electrophile, ring-activating groups are groups that are **electron-donating**. Conversely, ring-deactivating groups are **electron-withdrawing groups** that remove electron density from the ring, thus making it less nucleophilic.

- The second way that groups already present on the aromatic ring affect reactivity in electrophilic aromatic substitution reactions is by influencing the position of attachment of the incoming group. Some groups only allow incoming groups to react at the meta position; they are called **meta-directing**. Other groups direct the incoming substituent to the ortho and para positions; they are called **ortho/para-directing**. Examples of ortho/para-directors and meta-directors are arranged in the table below, and their activating/deactivating natures are also indicated.

Ortho/para-Directors

$-NR_2$ ⎫
$-OH$ ⎬ very strong activators

$-OR$ ⎫
$$-NHCR \quad (O \parallel)$$ ⎬ moderate activators
$$-OCR \quad (O \parallel)$$
$-R$ ⎭

$-Cl, Br, I$ mild deactivators

Meta-Directors

$-NR_3^{\oplus}$
$-NO_2$ ⎬ very strong deactivators
$-C\equiv N$

$-SO_3H$
$$-CR \quad (O \parallel)$$
$$-C-OH \quad (O \parallel)$$ ⎬ moderate to mild deactivators
$$-COR \quad (O \parallel)$$
$$-CNH_2 \quad (O \parallel)$$
$-NH_3^{\oplus}$

Note that all of the substituents that have lone pairs of electrons on the atom of attachment to the aromatic ring are ortho/para-directing groups, and the substituents that do not have lone pairs of electrons on the atom of attachment to the aromatic ring are meta-directing groups, with a single exception; alkyl groups do not have a lone pair of electrons on the atom of attachment, but are ortho/para-directors. This should make sense, however, since alkyl groups are known to be electron-donating groups (this is why 3° carbocations are more stable than 1° carbocations).

Example 27-4: Predict the major product of each of the following reactions:

A.

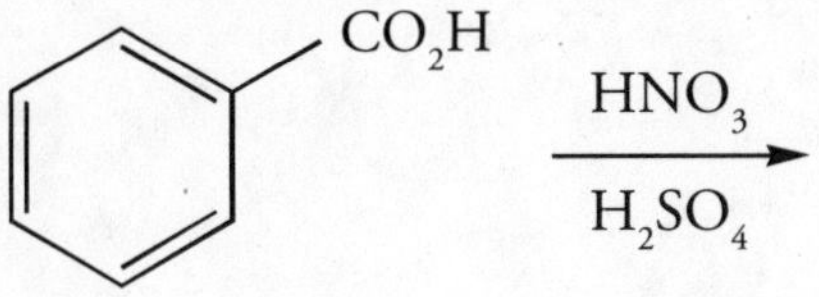

$$\xrightarrow[\text{H}_2\text{SO}_4]{\text{HNO}_3}$$

B.

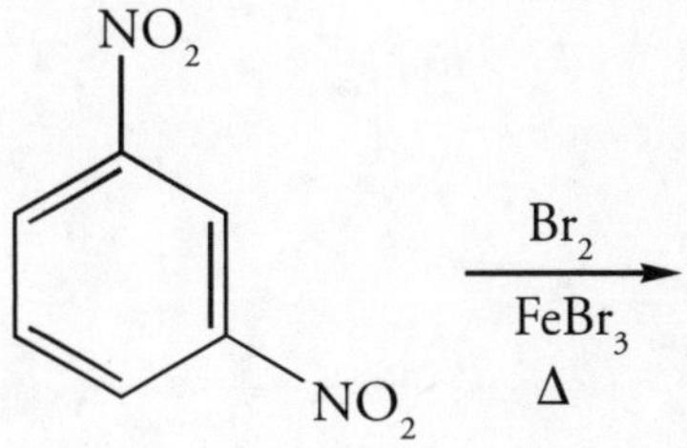

$$\xrightarrow[\substack{\text{FeBr}_3 \\ \Delta}]{\text{Br}_2}$$

C.

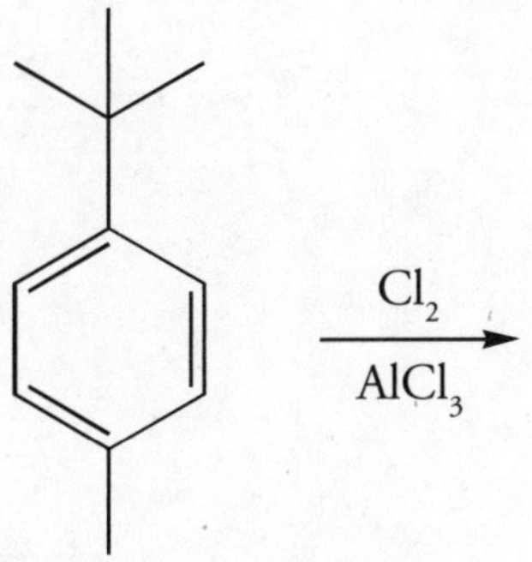

$$\xrightarrow[\text{AlCl}_3]{\text{Cl}_2}$$

D.

$$\xrightarrow[\text{FeBr}_3]{\text{Br}_2}$$

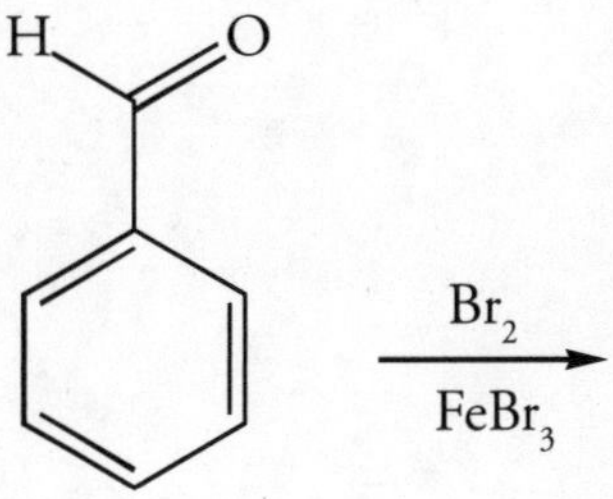

Solution:

A.

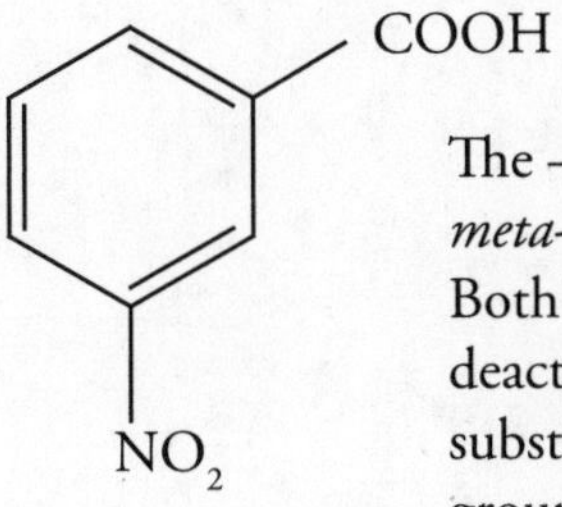

The –COOH group is a *meta*-director.
Both –COOH and –NO$_2$ are deactivating, so further substitution of an –NO$_2$ group does not occur.

B.

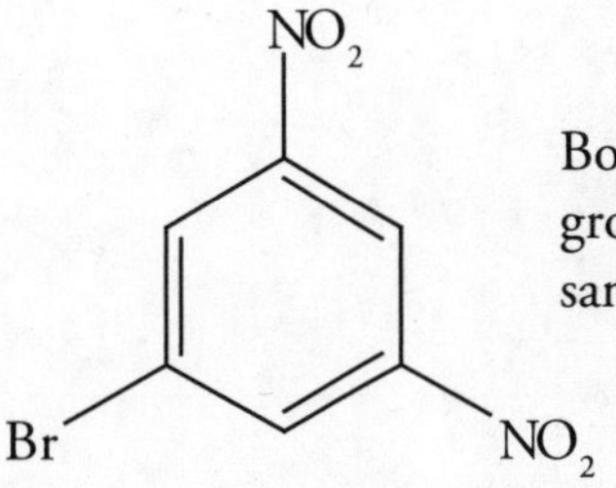

Both –NO$_2$ groups direct to the same position.

C.

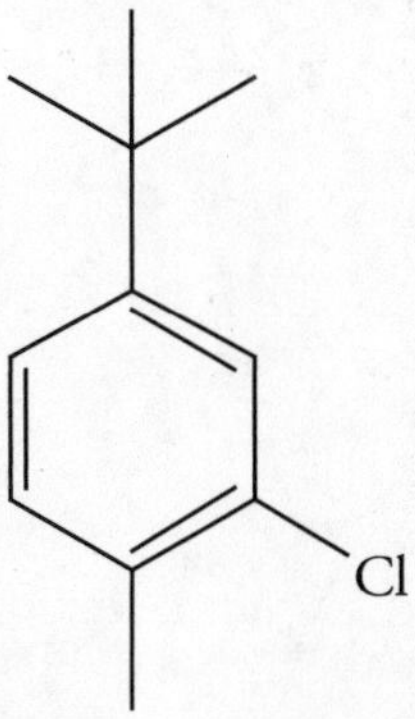

Both groups (–CH$_3$ and *tert*-butyl) are *ortho/para*-directors, but the –Cl ends up *ortho* to the methyl for steric reasons.

D.

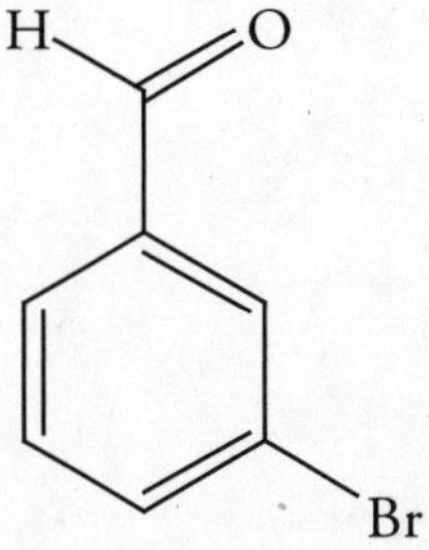

The –CHO group is a *meta*-director and is ring-deactivating.

Chapter 28
Nucleophilic Addition and Cycloaddition Reactions

We'll next examine two broad classes of reactions: first, reactions of carbonyl containing compounds and second, cycloaddition reactions. Simple carbonyl-containing organic compounds display two types of reactivity. The first is deprotonation of the α-carbon atom. The second is nucleophilic addition to the C=O double bond. We will see in this chapter how these two reactivity modes interrelate. We'll then look at the reactivity of α,β-unsaturated carbonyl containing compounds and carboxylic acids and their derivatives. Lastly, we will discuss the Diels–Alder reaction as a typical cycloaddition reaction.

28.1   ALDEHYDES AND KETONES

Two very important classes of oxygen-containing organic compounds are aldehydes and ketones. Here are three common examples you should recognize for the DAT:

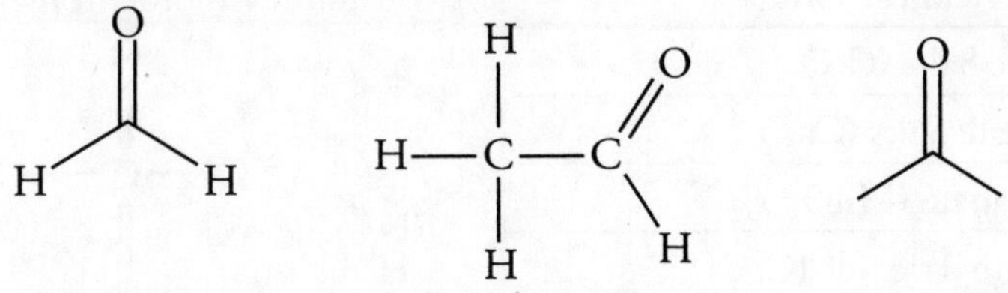

Formaldehyde   Acetaldehyde   Acetone

We begin the discussion of these functional groups by looking at a common way carbonyls are formed—oxidation of an alcohol:

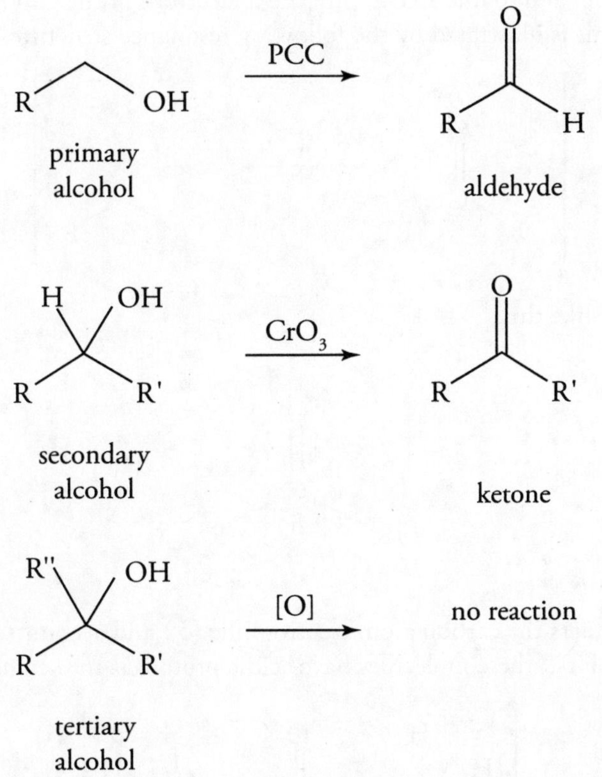

Note: Since the oxidizing agent removes a hydrogen from the carbon, tertiary alcohols are not able to react to form carbonyls since they have no hydrogen at the reactive site.

Oxidizing agents are able to absorb electrons (and be reduced). Below are some common oxidizing agents that appear on the DAT.

Aqueous Oxidants	Anhydrous Oxidant
Chromic Acid (H_2CrO_4)	Pyridinium Chlorochromate (PCC) 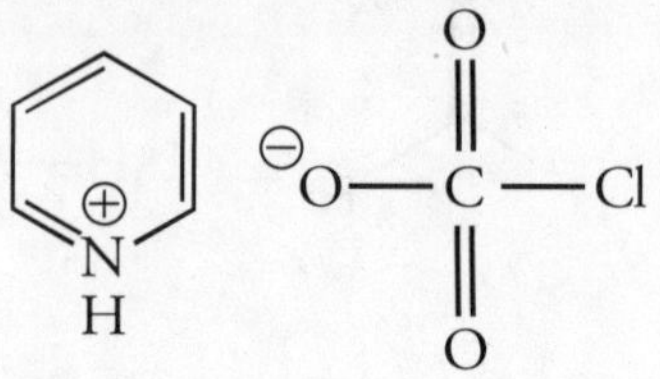
Chromate Salts (CrO_4^{2-})	
Dichromate Salts ($Cr_2O_7^{2-}$)	
Permanganate (MnO_4^-)	
Chromium Trioxide (CrO_3)	

Now that we understand how aldehydes and ketones are formed, let's look at their reactivities. The key to understanding the chemistry of aldehydes and ketones is to understand the electronic structure and properties of the carbonyl group. The C=O double bond is very polarized because oxygen is much more electronegative than carbon, and so it is able to pull the π electrons of the C=O double bond toward itself and away from carbon. This is illustrated by the following resonance structures:

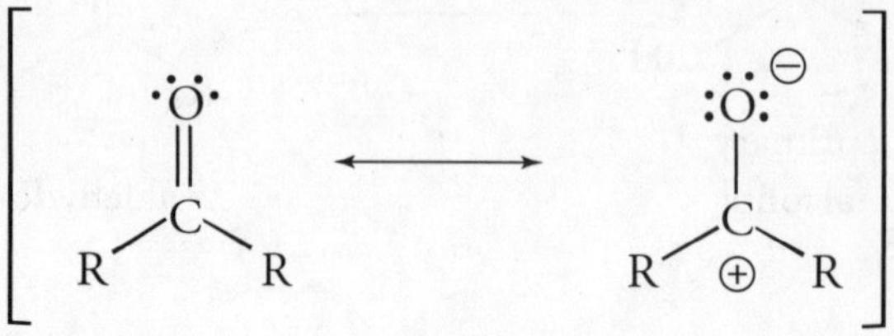

So overall, carbonyls react like this:

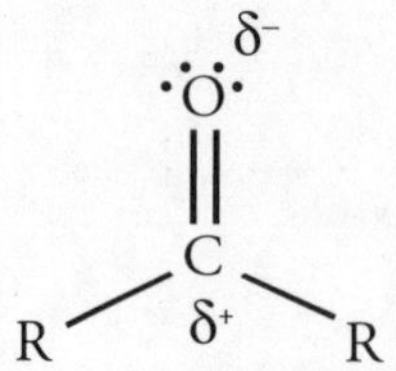

This bond polarization renders the carbon atom electrophilic (δ^+) and accounts for two kinds of reactions of aldehydes and ketones. First, these molecules have acidic protons α to (i.e., next to) the carbonyl group.

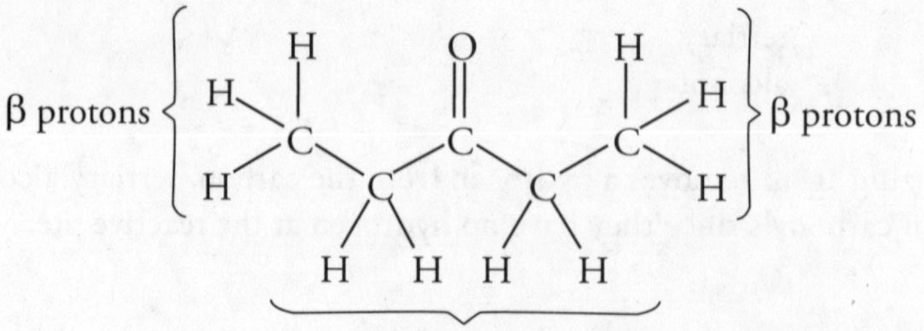

An α-proton is acidic because the electrons left behind upon deprotonation can delocalize into the π system of the carbonyl. Second, the electrophilic carbon of the carbonyl group makes aldehydes and ketones susceptible to nucleophilic attack. In the aldol condensation, which we will study in some detail, both of these types of reactivity are involved in a single reaction.

Acidity and Enolization

The first type of reaction that is commonly observed with aldehydes and ketones is the result of the relative acidity of protons that are α to the carbonyl group. These α-protons are sufficiently acidic that they can be removed by a strong base [such as hydroxide ion (OH⁻) or an alkoxide ion (OR⁻)] to yield a resonance stabilized carbanion. This carbanion can be easily formed because the electrons that are left behind on the carbon can be delocalized into the carbonyl π system. In this way, the negative charge can be delocalized onto the electronegative oxygen atom. A resonance-stabilized carbanion of this type is referred to as an **enolate ion**. An enolate ion is negatively charged and nucleophilic. The nucleophilic character of an enolate ion lies predominately at the carbon at which the proton was abstracted, not the oxygen atom of the carbonyl. This is why the α-carbon atom of enolates is the nucleophile in most common enolate reactions.

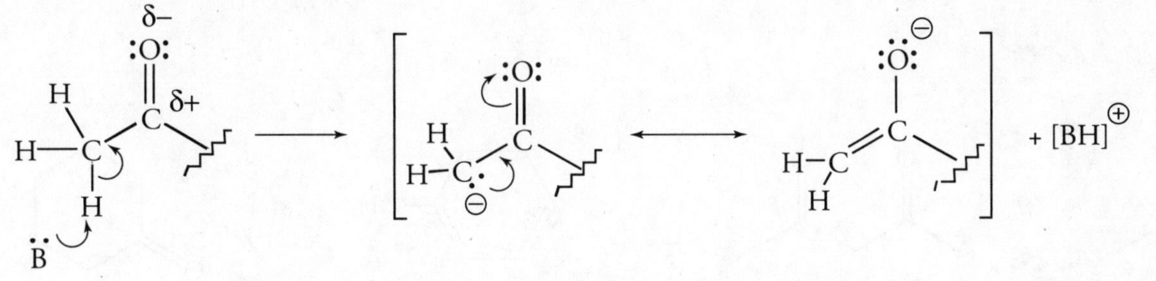

resonance forms of enolate anion

An example that demonstrates the acidity of α-protons is the exchange reaction that occurs between the α-proton of Compound I (below) and deuterium from D_2O. Compound I has a single α-proton that is α to *two* carbonyl groups in comparison to the six other α-protons in the molecule that are α to only *one* carbonyl group. It is this lone α-proton that exchanges with a deuterium of D_2O over the course of a couple of days, even in the absence of a base. Being next to two carbonyl groups greatly enhances the acidity of this α-proton and allows it to exchange (although slowly) with a deuterium from D_2O. The mechanism of this exchange, which essentially consists of protonation of the intermediate enolate ion, is shown in the following figure:

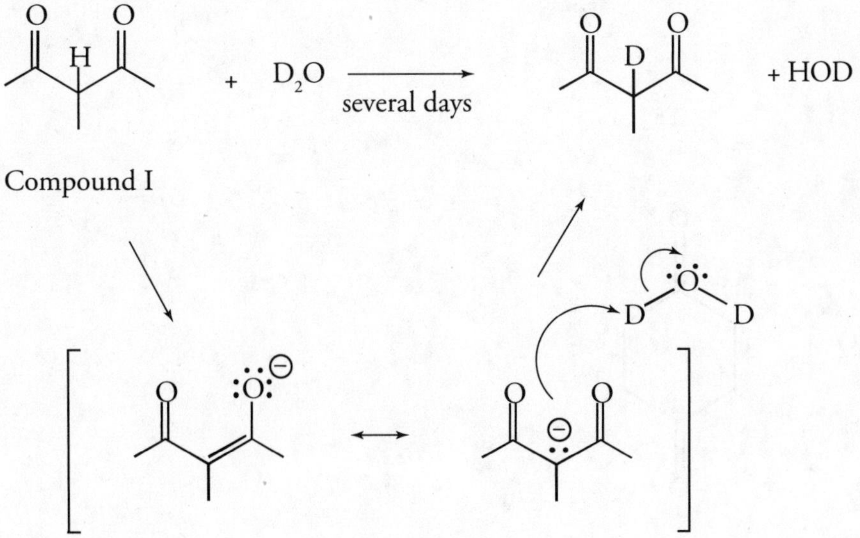

Compound I

Example 28-1: For each of the following pairs of compounds, identify the one with the more acidic proton. Review Sections 25.6 and 26.5 if you need a refresher on Ochem acidity.

A.

vs.

B.

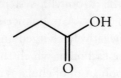

vs.

C.

vs.

D.

vs.

E.

vs.

F.

vs.

G.

vs.

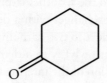

Solution:

A.

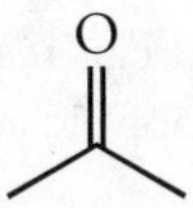

B.

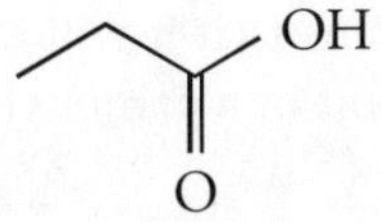

C.

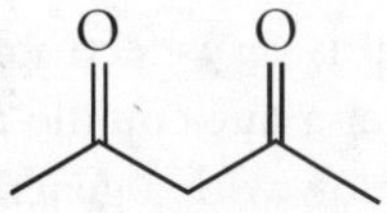

D.

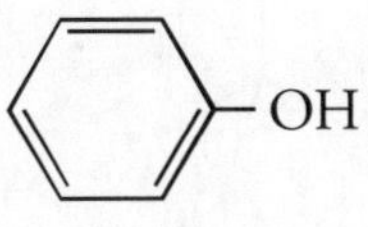

E.

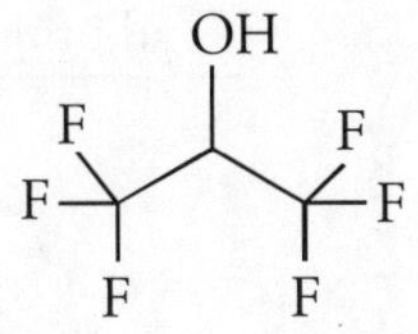

F.

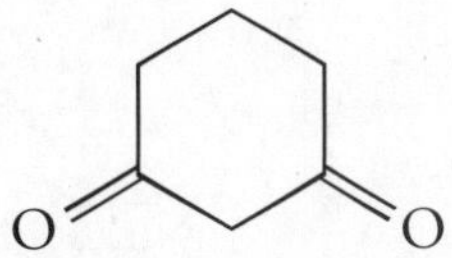

G.

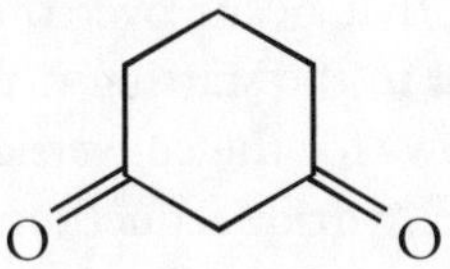

Since fluorine is the most electronegative atom, it will have a very strong inductive effect.

Keto-Enol Tautomerism

A ketone is converted into an enol by deprotonation of an α-carbon atom and subsequent protonation of the carbonyl oxygen. These two forms are very similar to one another and differ only by the position of a proton and a double bond. This is referred to as **keto-enol tautomerism**. Two molecules are **tautomers** if they are readily interconvertible constitutional isomers in equilibrium with one another.

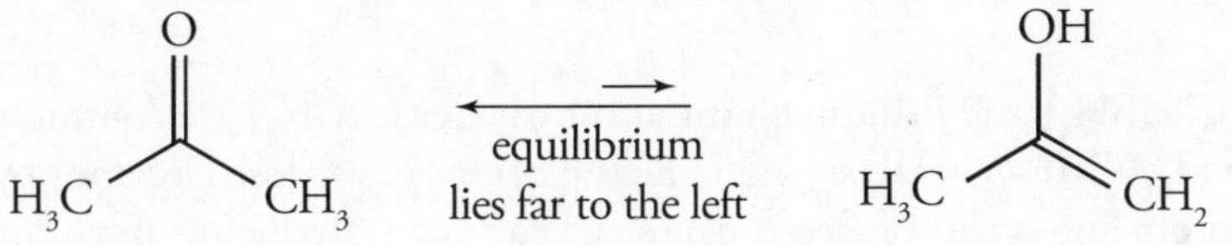

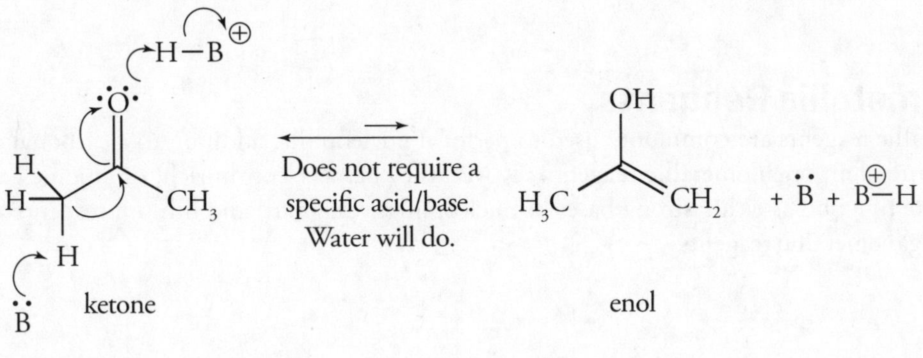

Nucleophilic Addition Reactions to Aldehydes and Ketones

Because of the polarized nature of the C=O double bond in aldehydes and ketones, the carbon of the carbonyl group is very electrophilic. This means that it will attract nucleophiles and can readily be reduced. The attack of a nucleophile upon the carbon of a carbonyl group, called a nucleophilic addition reaction, is shown below with a generic nucleophile (Nu:).

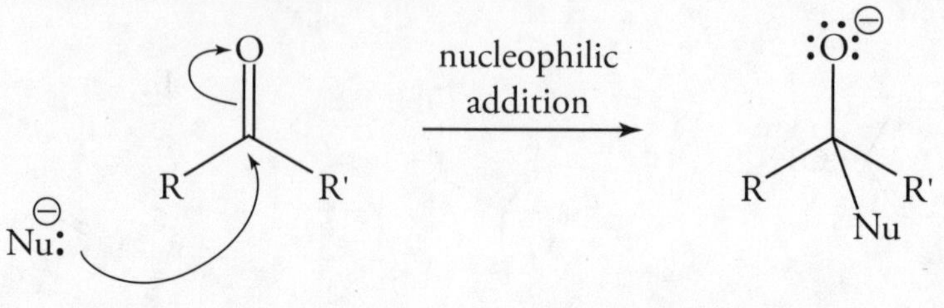

Nucleophilic addition reactions are defined by the bonding changes that occur over the course of the reaction, just as in electrophilic additions. In these reactions, a π bond in the starting material is broken, and two σ bonds in the product result. This very general reaction allows for the conversion of aldehydes or ketones into a variety of other functional groups such as alcohols via hydride reduction:

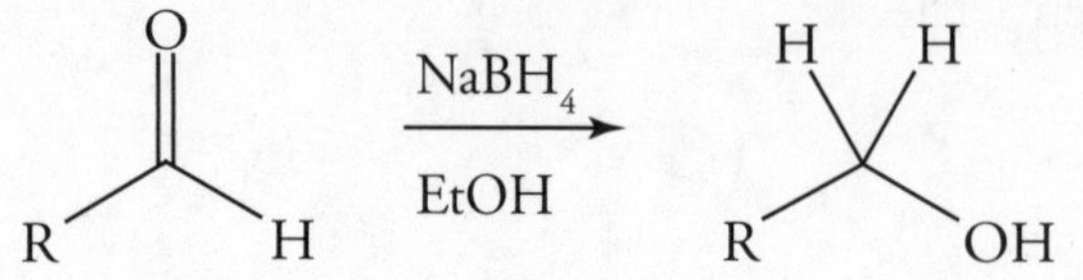

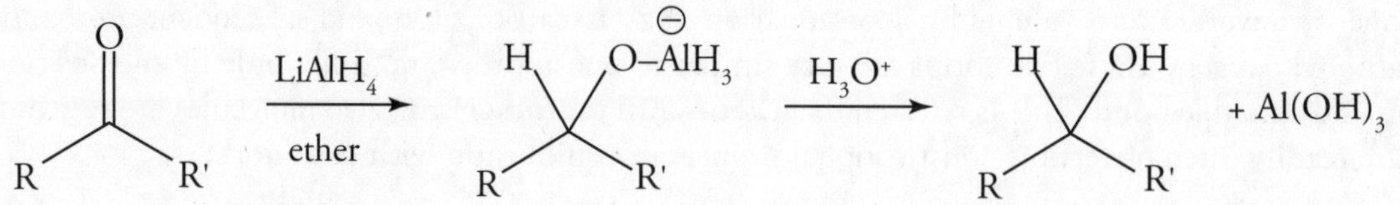

Note: Sodium borohydride ($NaBH_4$) and lithium aluminum hydride ($LiAlH_4$) are common reducing agents seen on the DAT. In general, strong reducing agents easily lose electrons by adding hydride (a hydrogen atom and a pair of electrons) to the carbonyl. Reducing agents often have many hydrogens attached to other elements with low electronegativity.

Organometallic Reagents

Organometallic reagents are commonly used to perform nucleophilic addition to a carbonyl carbon. The basic structure of an organometallic reagent is R^-M^+. They act as electron rich, or anionic carbon atoms and therefore function as either strong bases or nucleophiles. Grignard and lithium reagents are the most common organometallic reagents.

Grignard reagents are generally made via the action of an alkyl or acyl halide on magnesium metal, as depicted below. To avoid unwanted protonation of the very basic Grignard reagent, the reaction is carried out in an aprotic solvent such as diethyl ether.

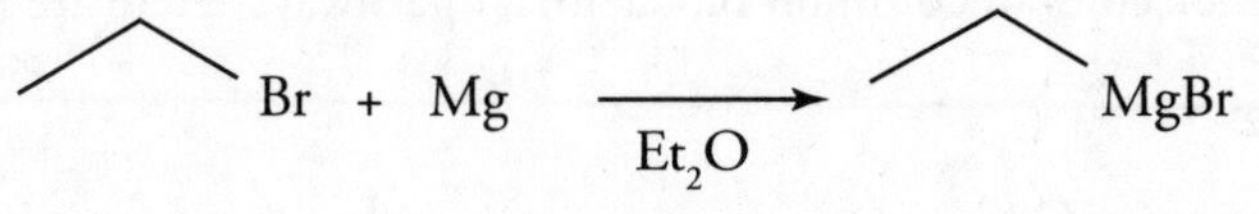

$$\text{Br} + \text{Mg} \xrightarrow{\text{Et}_2\text{O}} \text{MgBr}$$

The carbonyl containing compounds are then added to the Grignard reagents in order to yield alcohol products. In the reaction below, the methyl magnesium bromide acts as a nucleophile and adds to the electrophilic carbonyl carbon. An intermediate alkoxide ion is formed that is rapidly protonated to produce the alcohol during an aqueous acidic workup step.

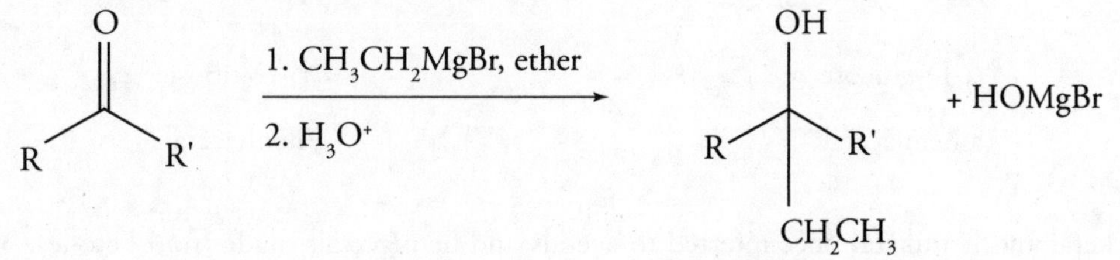

$$\underset{R \quad\quad R'}{\overset{O}{\|}} \xrightarrow[\text{2. H}_3\text{O}^+]{\text{1. CH}_3\text{CH}_2\text{MgBr, ether}} \underset{R \quad\quad R' \\ \quad\quad \text{CH}_2\text{CH}_3}{\overset{OH}{|}} + \text{HOMgBr}$$

Organolithium reagents are generally made by the reduction of alkyl halides with Li metal as depicted below. The reagents are prepared by reacting alkyl halide and lithium in a 1:2 molar ratio. Organolithium reagents react as bases or nucleophiles in the same manner as Grignard reagents.

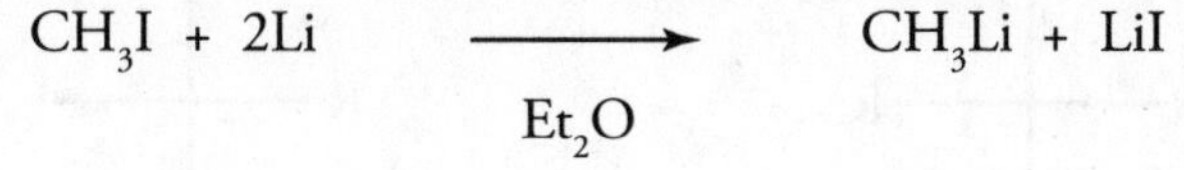

$$\text{CH}_3\text{I} + 2\text{Li} \xrightarrow{\text{Et}_2\text{O}} \text{CH}_3\text{Li} + \text{LiI}$$

Wittig Reaction

While the mechanism of the Wittig reaction is not important for the DAT and is fairly different from the standard nucleophilic addition reaction mentioned above, it is important to be able to recognize this reaction. **Wittig reagents** are also known as **phosphonium ylides** (pronounced "ill'-ids"), and react with aldehydes and ketones to form alkenes, as seen in the reaction below. Since the reaction involves both an addition and an elimination step in its mechanism, there is still a π bond in the product.

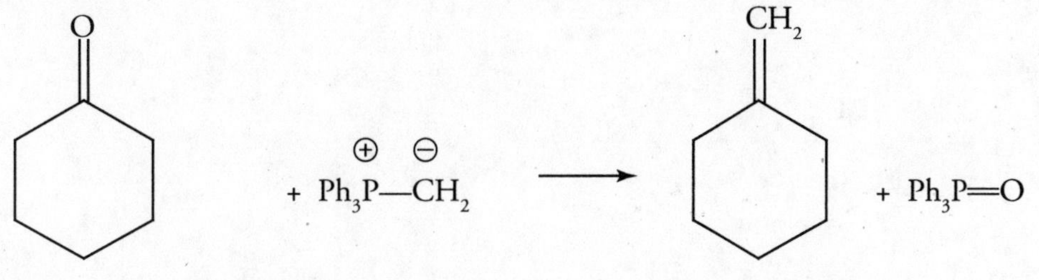

$$\underset{}{\overset{O}{\|}} + \text{Ph}_3\overset{\oplus}{\text{P}}-\overset{\ominus}{\text{CH}}_2 \longrightarrow \underset{}{\overset{CH_2}{\|}} + \text{Ph}_3\text{P}{=}\text{O}$$

Because the hydrocarbon is losing bonds to oxygen, this is a reduction reaction.

Acetals and Hemiacetals

Acetals and hemiacetals, which are of fundamental importance in biochemical reactions that occur in living organisms, can be synthesized from nucleophilic addition reactions to aldehydes or ketones. There are many examples of these molecules in common biochemical pathways. Here are two:

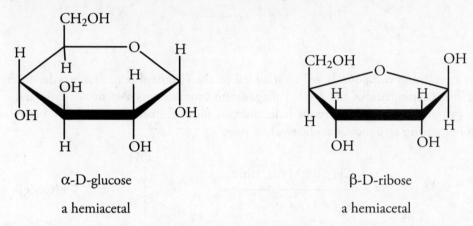

α-D-glucose

a hemiacetal

β-D-ribose

a hemiacetal

The terms ketal and hemiketal once referred to acetals and hemiacetals made from ketones, but this nomenclature has been abandoned by IUPAC. Before we learn the chemistry of acetals and hemiacetals, we must be able to identify them. Here are their general structures:

acetals

hemiacetals

Here are some specific examples:

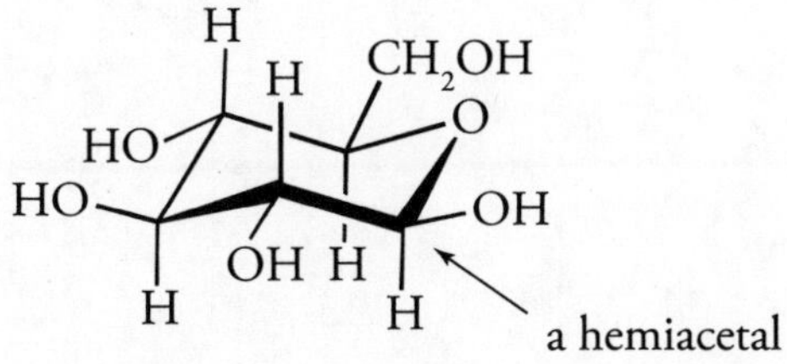

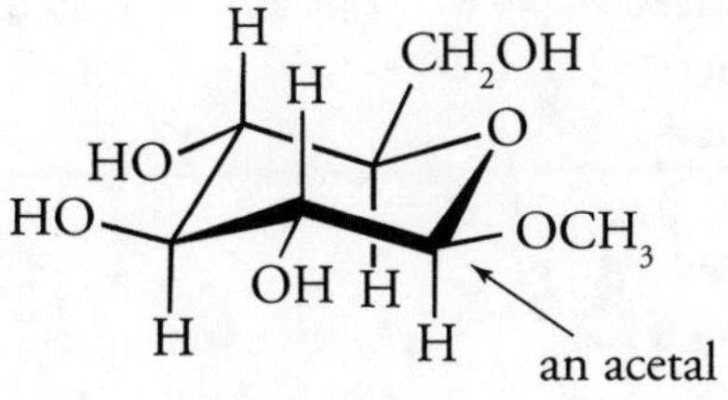

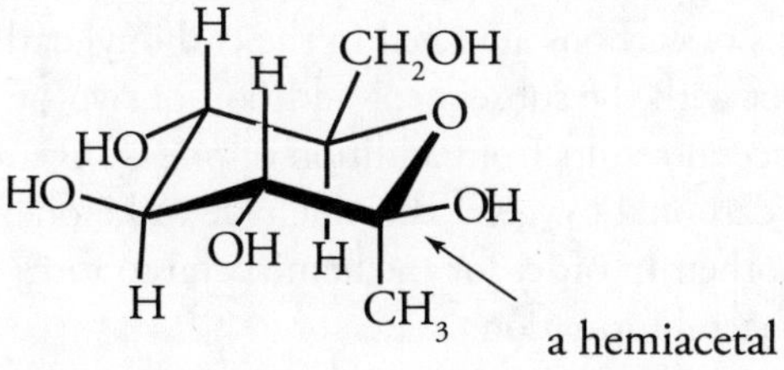

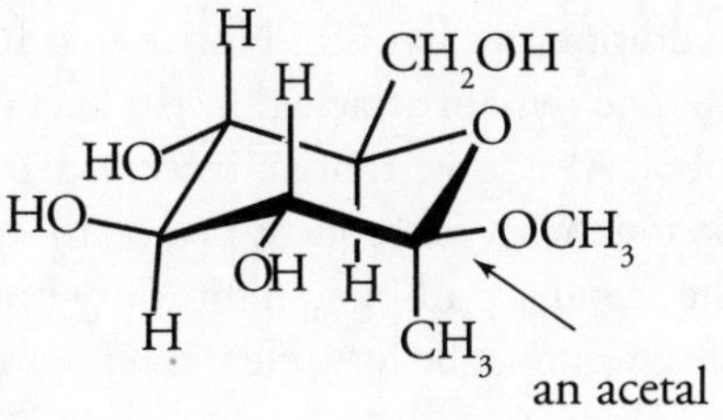

a hemiacetal

an acetal

a hemiacetal

an acetal

Example 28-2: For each of the following compounds, identify whether it's an acetal, hemiacetal, or neither:

A.

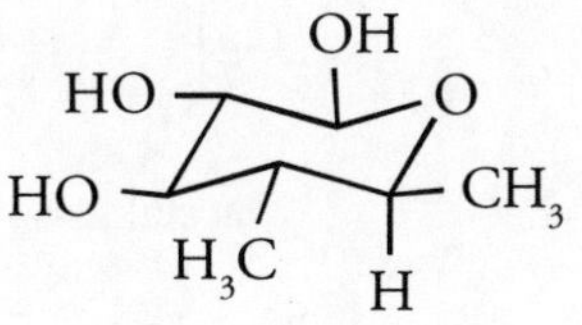

B.

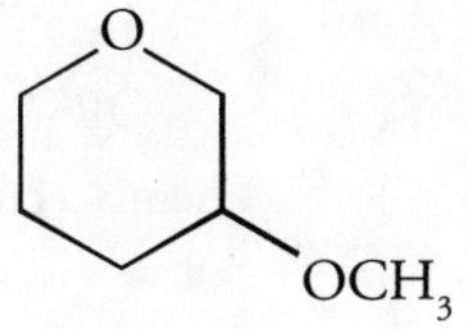

C.

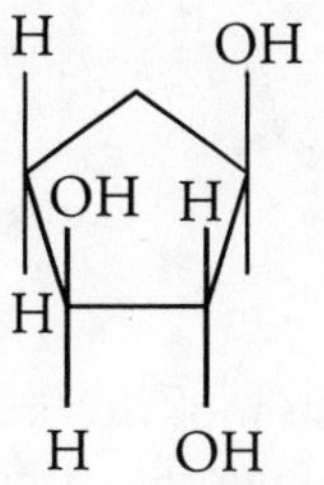

D.

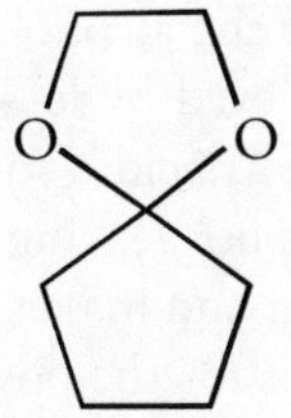

E.

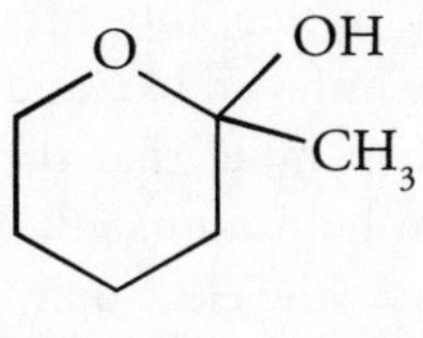

F.

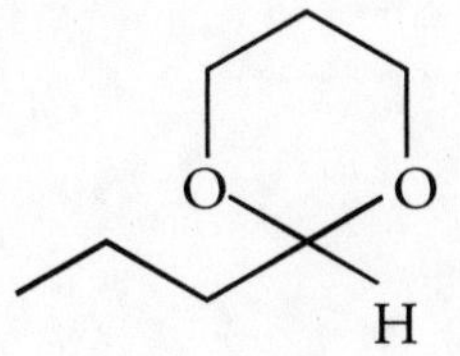

G.

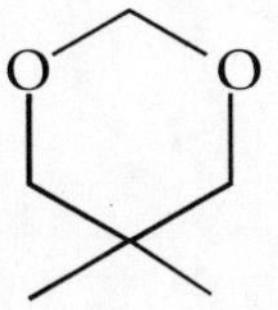

Solution:

A. hemiacetal
B. neither
C. neither
D. acetal
E. hemiacetal
F. acetal
G. acetal

Acetals are formed when aldehydes or ketones react with alcohols in the presence of acid. This occurs by a nucleophilic addition mechanism. Notice that hydrogens or carbons attached to the carbonyl carbon of the aldehyde or ketone remain attached in the acetal product with the subsequent addition of two –OR groups from the alcohol. Also, note that an intermediate hemiacetal results from addition of one –OR group to an aldehyde or ketone with subsequent protonation of the carbonyl oxygen. The aldehyde or ketone, the hemiacetal, and the acetal are all in equilibrium with one another. In order for the hemiacetal to form the acetal, a molecule of water must be lost. Here is a summary of acetal formation:

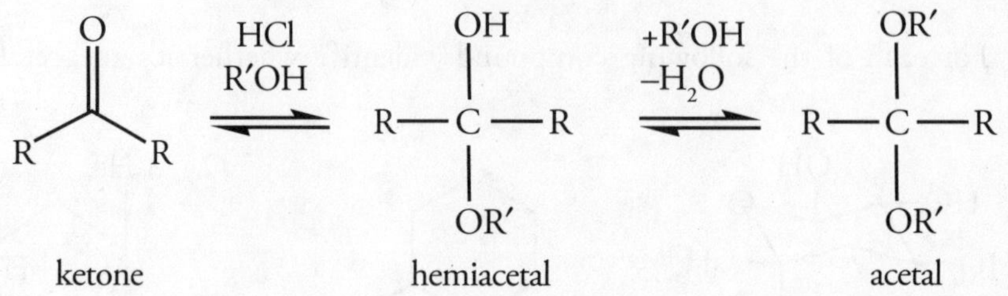

The mechanism of this important reaction is shown below. In the first step, the carbonyl oxygen is protonated, making the carbonyl carbon even more susceptible to nucleophilic attack by the oxygen of the attacking alcohol molecule. Following nucleophilic attack, the oxygen of the alcohol nucleophile is positively charged. This positive charge is unfavorable, and neutrality is achieved by loss of a proton which yields the intermediate hemiacetal. Remember that the reaction mixture is acidic so that a lone pair of electrons on the hemiacetal –OH can be protonated, which converts a poor leaving group into a good leaving group. Once again, this increases the electrophilicity of the carbon and makes it more susceptible to a second nucleophilic attack by an alcohol molecule. All that remains is for the positively charged oxygen from the attacking alcohol to lose a proton which yields the acetal product.

Overall Reaction

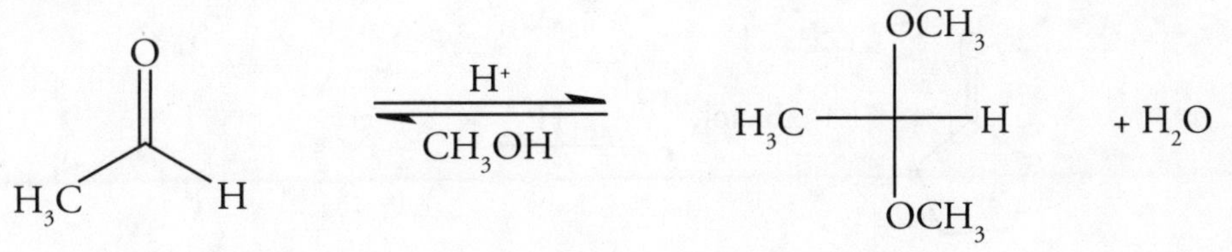
O
H+
CH3OH
H3C
H
OCH3
H3C
H
+ H2O
OCH3

Acetal Formation Mechanism

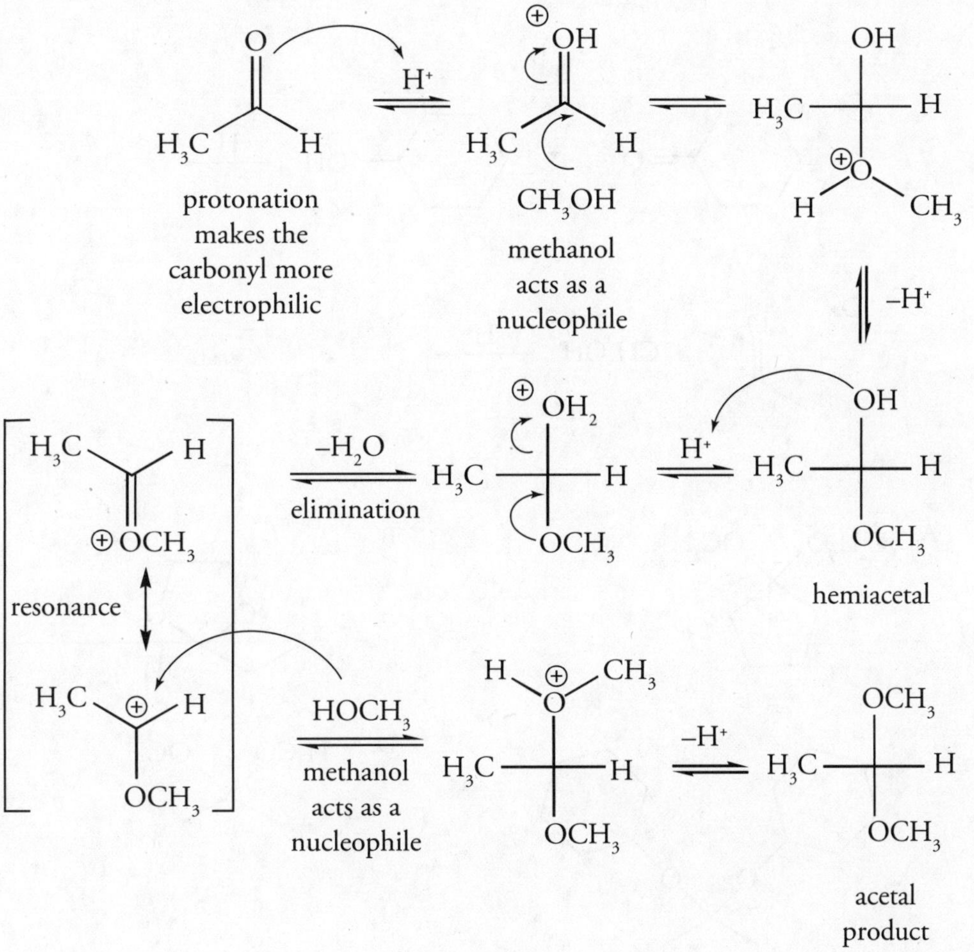
protonation
makes the
carbonyl more
electrophilic
methanol
acts as a
nucleophile
–H+
hemiacetal
–H2O
elimination
H+
resonance
HOCH3
methanol
acts as a
nucleophile
–H+
acetal
product

Example 28-3: Predict the acetal product from the following reactions:

A.

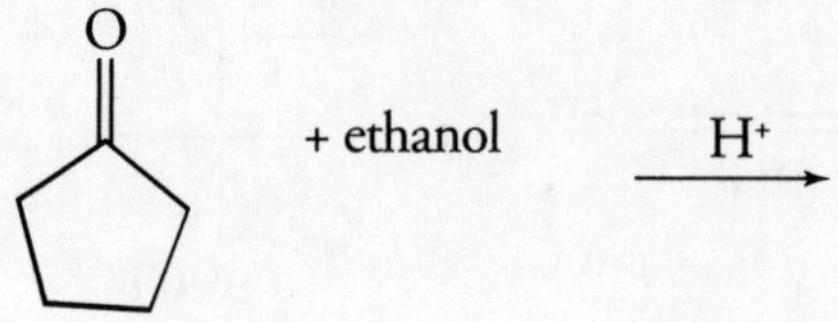
O
+ ethanol
H+

B.

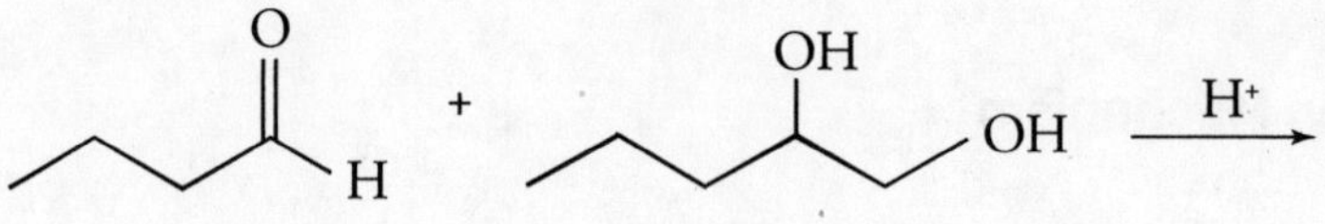
O
H
+
OH
OH
H+

C.

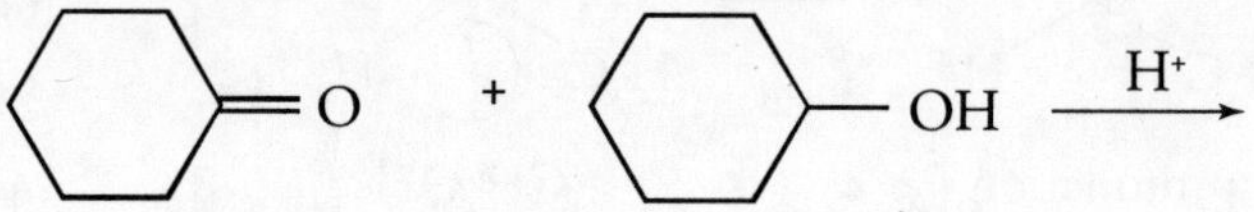
O
+
OH
H+

D.

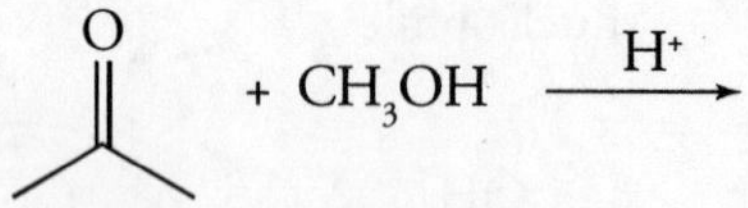
O
+ CH3OH
H+

Solution:

A.

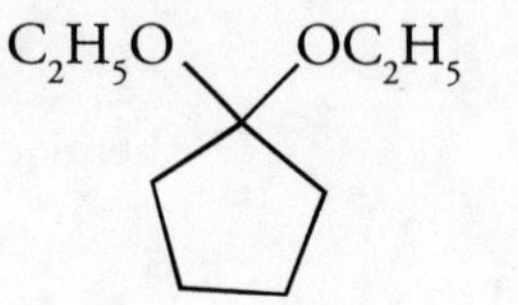
C2H5O
OC2H5

B.

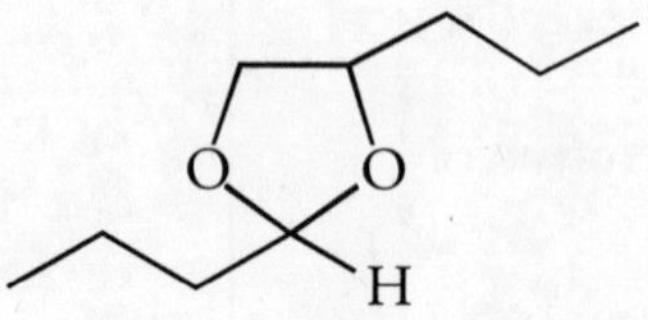
O
O
H

C.

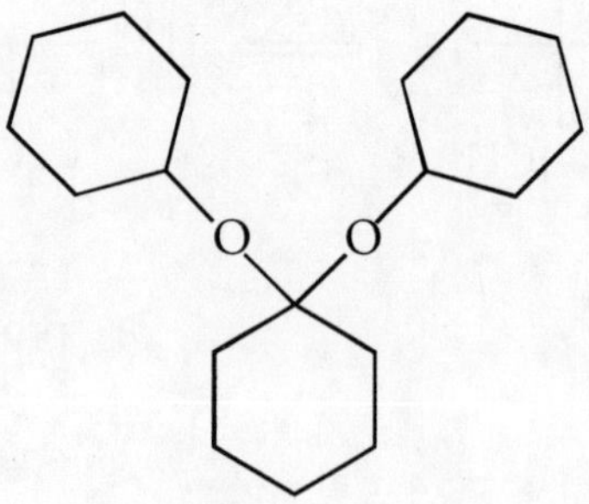
O
O

D.

H3CO
OCH3

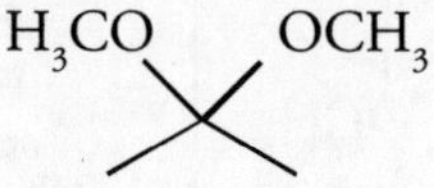

Imine Formation

A reaction that closely resembles acetal formation is the reaction of aldehydes or ketones with primary amines (R–NH_2). In this reaction, which is catalyzed by a weakly acidic buffer system (like an acetic acid/acetate buffer, pH about 4–5), an aldehyde or ketone reacts with a primary amine (R–NH_2) to form an imine. As in the acetal formation reaction, whatever is originally attached to the carbonyl carbon (other than the oxygen) stays attached in the product (an alkyl group or a hydrogen) and a molecule of water is produced. A brief examination of the reaction mechanism will help illustrate these common features.

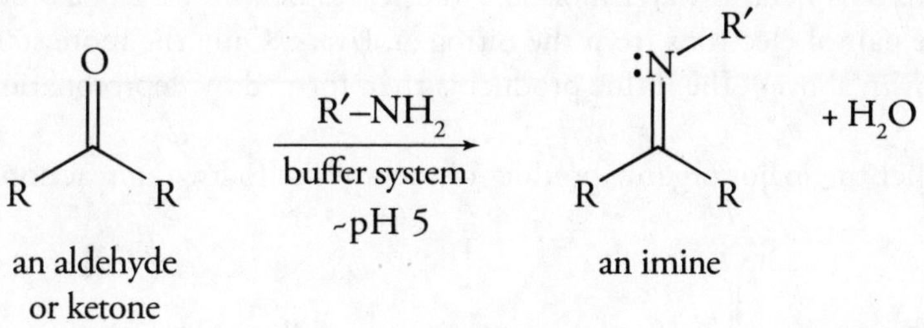

an aldehyde
or ketone

an imine

Imine Formation Mechanism

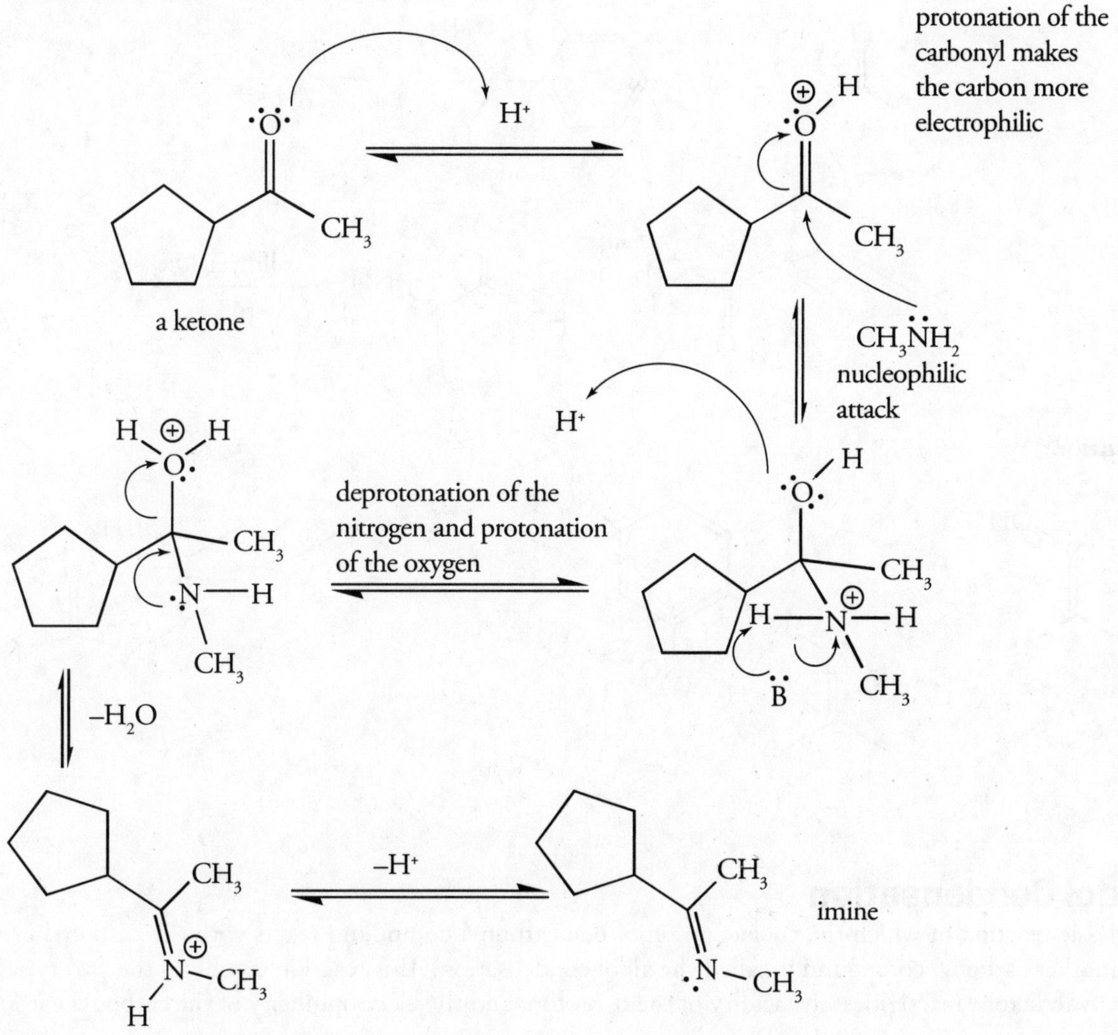

a ketone

protonation of the carbonyl makes the carbon more electrophilic

CH_3NH_2
nucleophilic attack

deprotonation of the nitrogen and protonation of the oxygen

$-H_2O$

imine

$-H^+$

In the first step of this reaction, a lone pair of electrons on the carbonyl oxygen is protonated by the acidic medium. As in acetal formation, protonation of the carbonyl oxygen makes the carbonyl carbon more electrophilic and therefore more susceptible to nucleophilic attack. This time, the nucleophile is an amine

(R–NH$_2$), so the nucleophilic nitrogen attacks the electrophilic carbon, resulting in a tetrahedral intermediate. The tetrahedral intermediate is then deprotonated at the nitrogen and protonated at the oxygen, thus converting a poor leaving group (–OH) into a good leaving group (–OH$_2^+$). Next, the oxygen departs with its electrons as a neutral water molecule and leaves behind a carbocation that is stabilized by resonance by the lone pair of electrons from the nitrogen. (*Note*: Only the more stable resonance form is shown in the mechanism above.) The imine product is then formed by deprotonation.

Example 28-4: Predict the major organic product of each of the following reactions:

A.

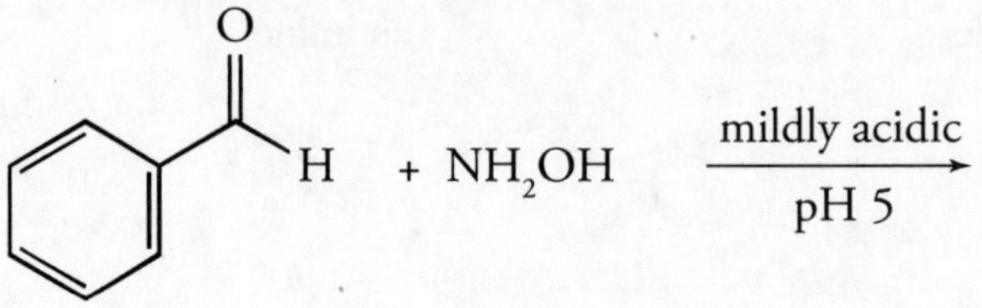

B.

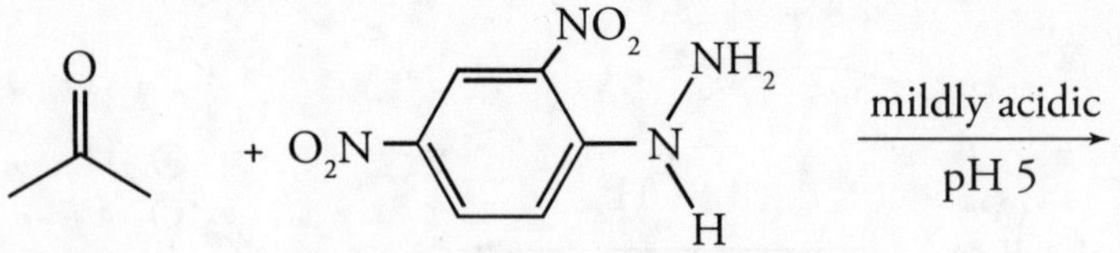

C.

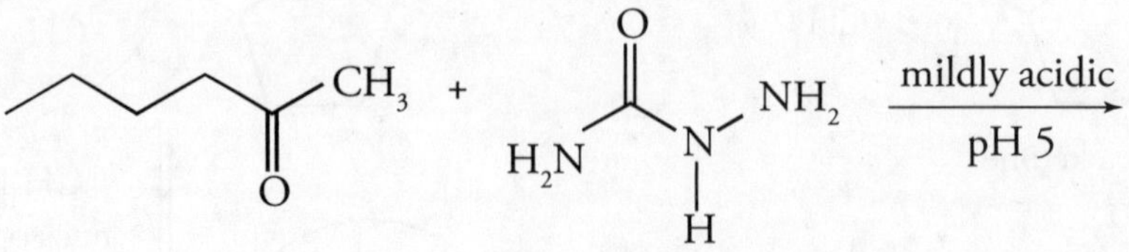

Solution:

A.

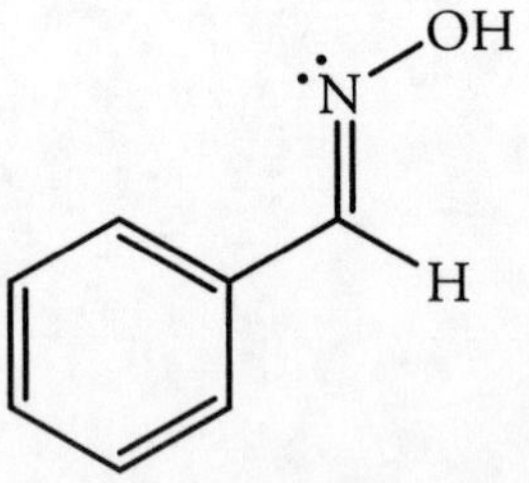

B.

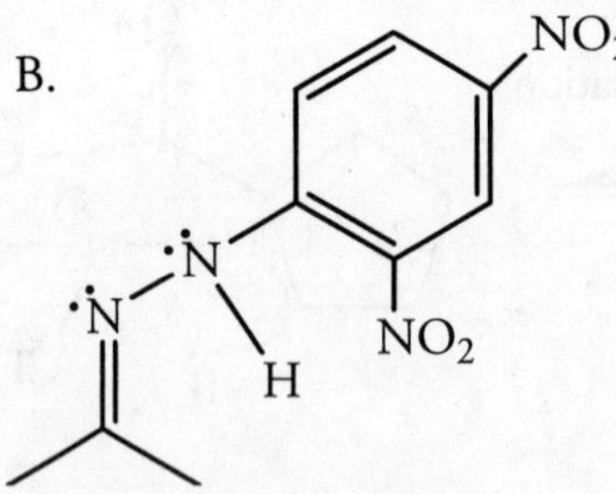

C.

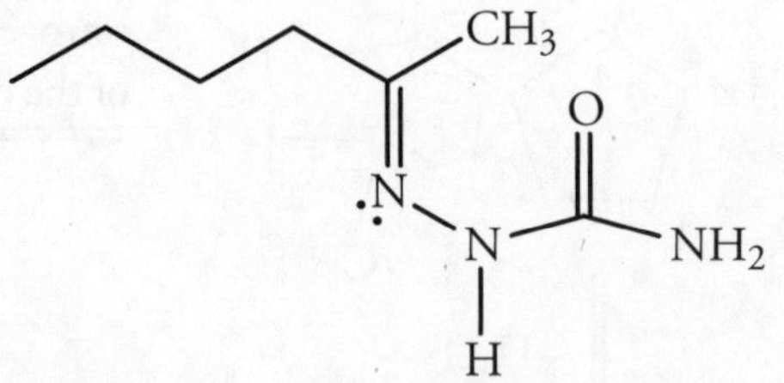

Aldol Condensation

A classic reaction in which the enolate anion of one carbonyl compound reacts with the carbonyl group of another carbonyl compound is called the aldol condensation. This reaction combines the two types of aldehyde/ketone reactivities: the acidity of the α-proton, and the electrophilicity of the carbonyl carbon.

In the first step of this reaction, a strong base removes an α-proton from the aldehyde, resulting in the formation of a resonance-stabilized enolate anion. This corresponds to the first type of reactivity of aldehydes and ketones, deprotonation of the α-carbon atom. Remember, the enolate anion is nucleophilic and usually reacts at the carbon atom which was deprotonated. Next, the α-carbon of the enolate anion attacks the carbonyl carbon of another aldehyde molecule, thereby generating an alkoxide ion that is subsequently protonated by a molecule of water. This results in the formation of a general class of molecules referred to as β-hydroxy carbonyl compounds. There are three important points to note about this reaction. First, it requires a strong base (typically hydroxide, OH⁻ or an alkoxide ion RO⁻) to remove an α-proton adjacent to the carbonyl group. Second, one of the aldehydes or ketones must act as a source for the enolate ions while the other aldehyde or ketone will come under nucleophilic attack by the enolate carbanion. Third, the aldol condensation does not require the two carbonyl groups that participate in the reaction to be the same. When they are different, it is called a **crossed aldol condensation** reaction. In order to avoid obtaining a complex mixture of products in a crossed aldol condensation, it is often the case that one of the carbonyl compounds is chosen such that it does not have any acidic α-protons, and therefore cannot act as the nucleophile (enolate ion), it must be the electrophile.

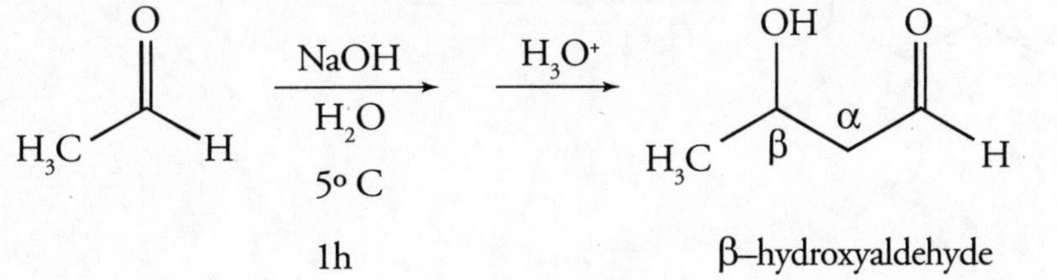

Aldol Mechanism

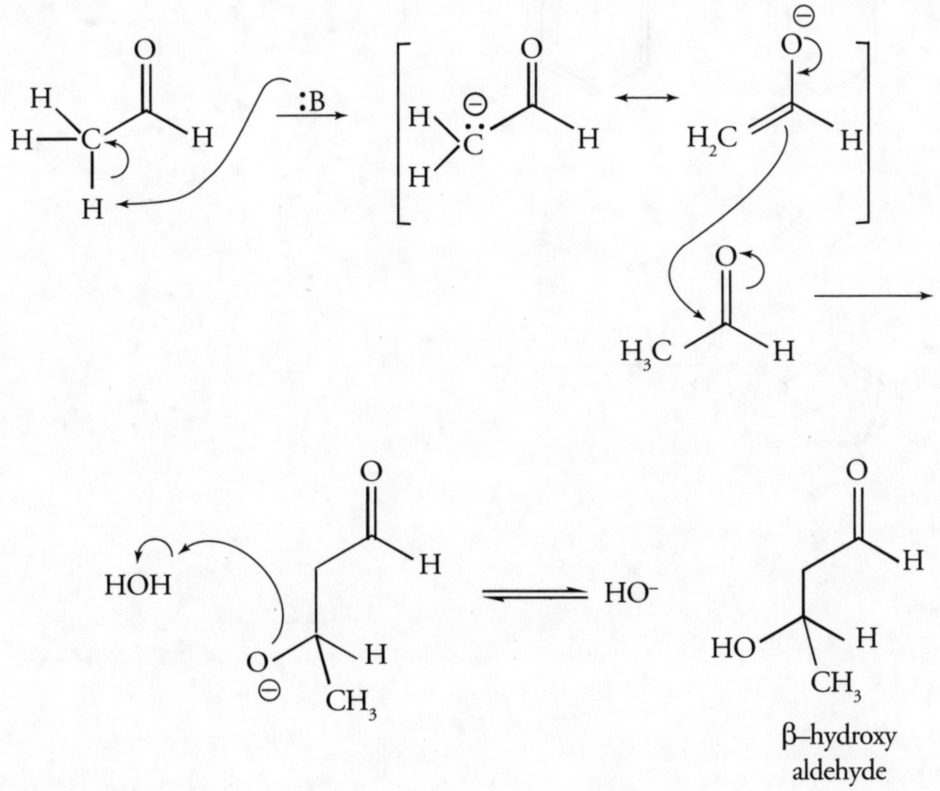

If the β-hydroxyaldehyde or ketone products are heated, they will undergo an elimination reaction (dehydration) to form an α,β-**unsaturated carbonyl compound**. Notice that the newly formed carbon-carbon π bond is in conjugation with the carbonyl group; this stabilizes the molecule.

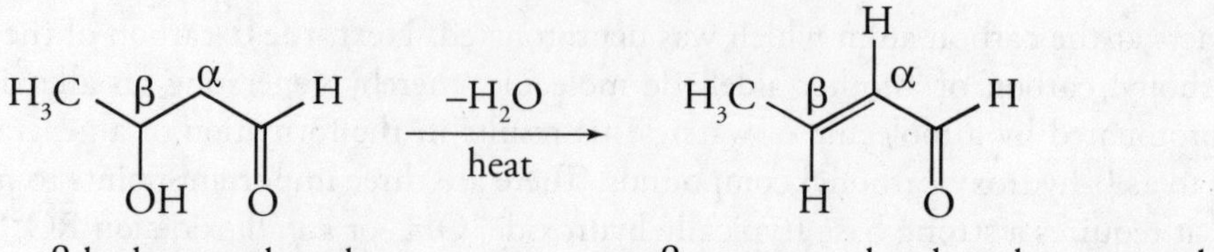

β-hydroxy carbonyl   α,β-unsaturated carbonyl compound

Example 28-5: Predict the condensation products of each of the following reactions. Show both the β-hydroxy carbonyl product and the elimination product.

A.

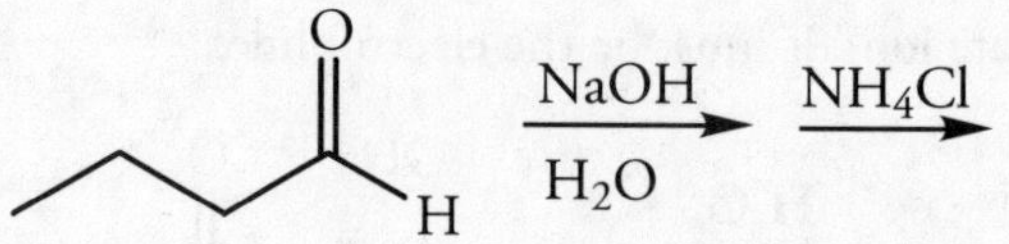

B.

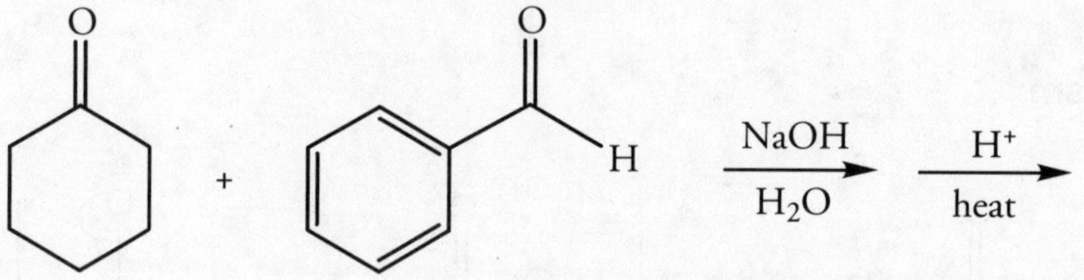

C.

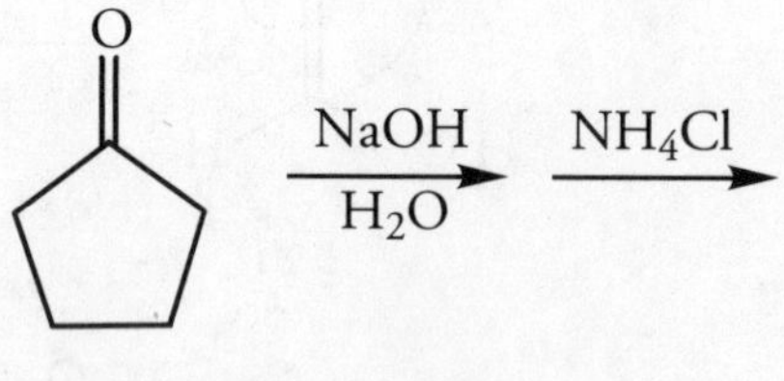

D.

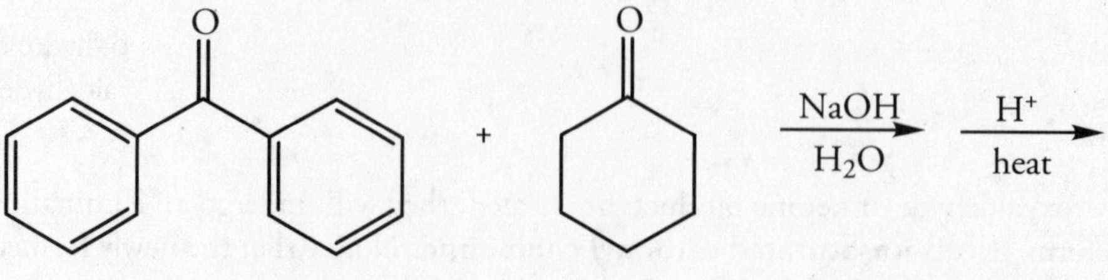

Solution:

A.

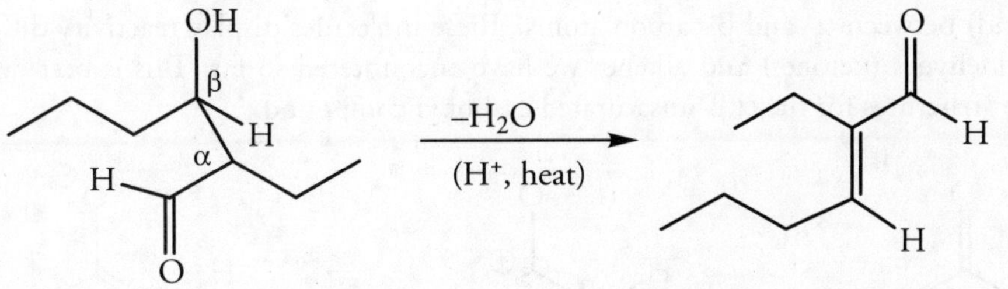

B.

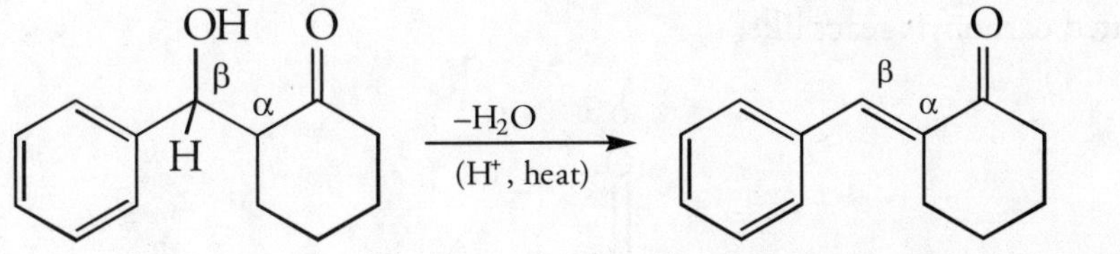

α,β-unsaturated carbonyl compound

C.

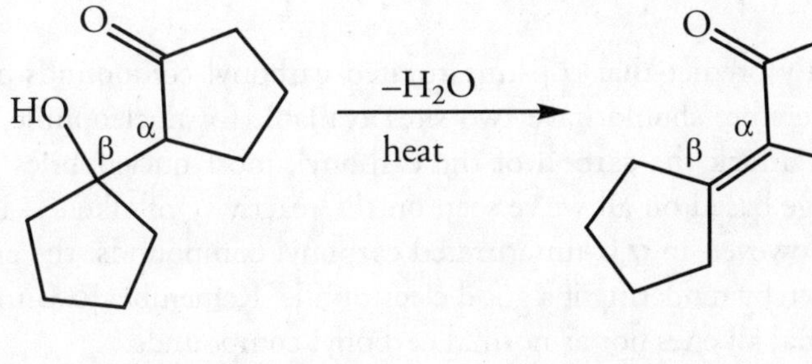

D.

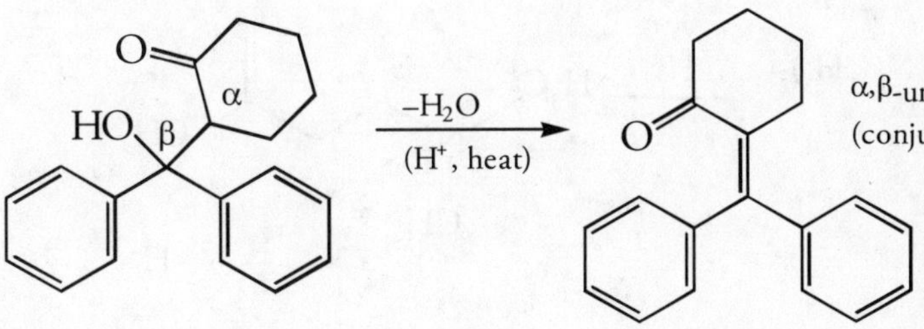

α,β-unsaturated resonance-stabilized
(conjugated) carbonyl compound

Conjugate Addition to α,β-Unsaturated Carbonyl Compounds

Products of aldol condensations are not ordinary aldehydes (or ketones); they have a unit of unsaturation (a C=C double bond) between α- and β-carbon atoms. These molecules display reactivity different from that of both the aldehydes (ketones) and alkenes we have encountered so far. This is best described by drawing resonance structures for the α,β-unsaturated carbonyl compound.

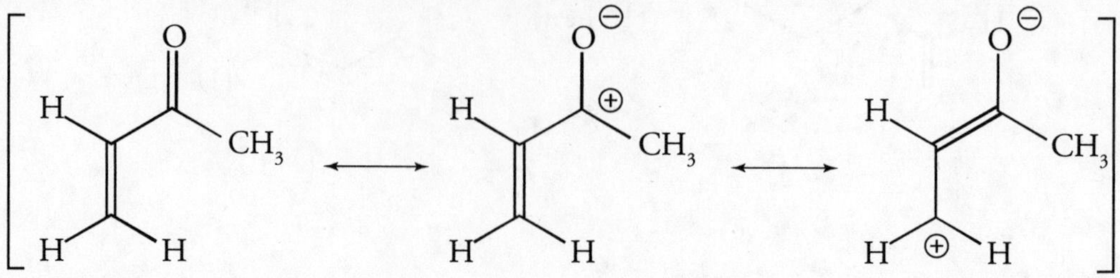

So, overall, α,β-unsaturated carbonyls react like:

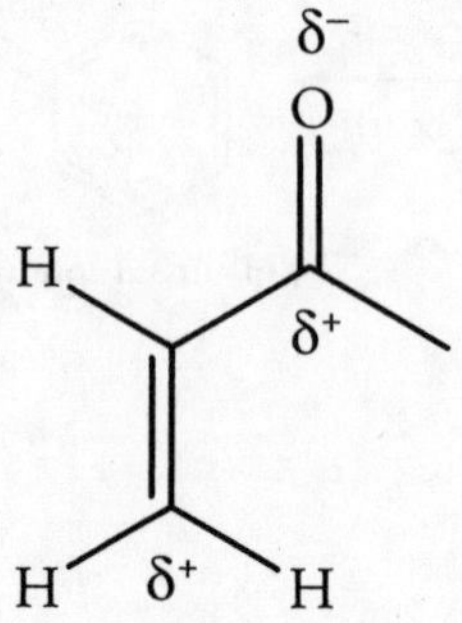

The resonance forms shown above clearly predict that α,β-unsaturated carbonyl compounds could have two sites of electrophilicity (δ⁺), and therefore should have two sites available for nucleophilic attack. Although some nucleophilic reagents will attack the carbon of the carbonyl, most nucleophiles attack the β-carbon atom. This should seem strange based on all we've seen on the reactivity of alkenes. Recall that alkenes usually react as nucleophiles. However, in α,β-unsaturated carbonyl compounds, the alkene is in conjugation with the carbonyl group, thereby rendering it a good electrophile. Remember, α,β-unsaturated carbonyl compounds act neither as normal alkenes nor as normal carbonyl compounds.

As an example of the reactivity of α,β-unsaturated carbonyl compounds, we'll look at the acid catalyzed addition of dimethylamine to methyl vinyl ketone.

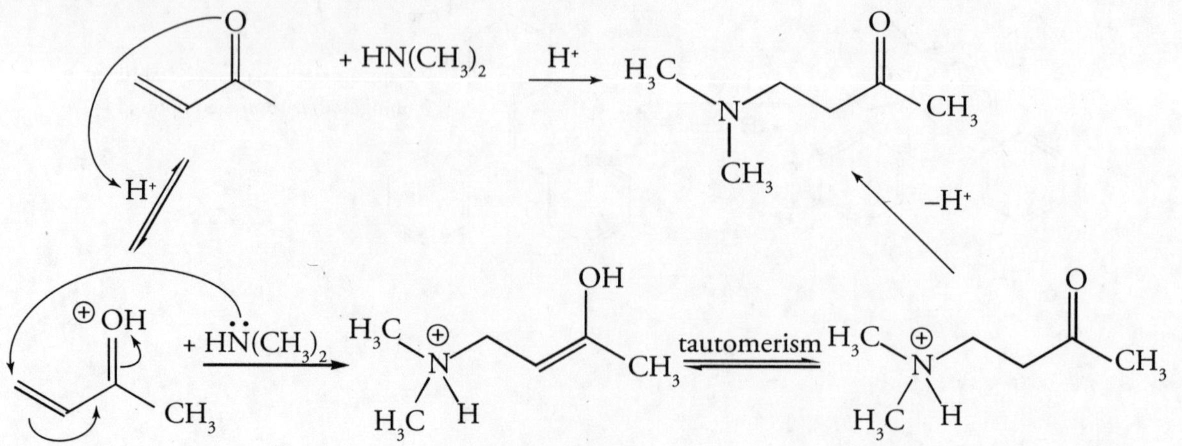

In the first step of the reaction, the carbonyl oxygen atom is protonated, thus making the β-carbon more electrophilic. In the second step, the nitrogen atom of dimethylamine attacks the β-carbon atom of the protonated methyl vinyl ketone, generating an enol intermediate. Since enols are not stable, the enol intermediate tautomerizes to the ketone. The ammonium ion is then deprotonated to form the product of the reaction. The overall reaction involves the addition of $-N(CH_3)_2$ and $-H$ from $HN(CH_3)_2$ across the C=C double bond of the α,β-unsaturated unit of methyl vinyl ketone. Reactions where the nucleophile becomes attached to the β-carbon atom of an α,β-unsaturated carbonyl compound are termed **1,4-addition** (or **conjugate addition**) reactions.

Example 28-6: Predict the product of each of the following conjugate addition reactions:

A.

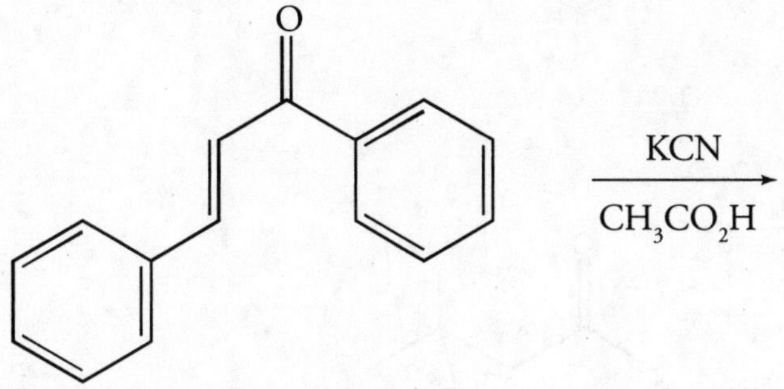

$$\xrightarrow[CH_3CO_2H]{KCN}$$

B.

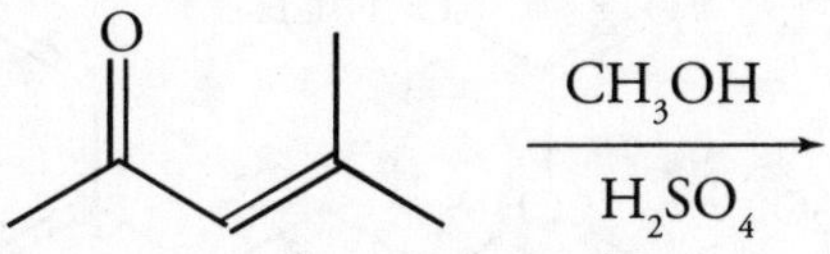

$$\xrightarrow[H_2SO_4]{CH_3OH}$$

C.

$$\xrightarrow[\text{base}]{CH_2(CO_2CH_2CH_3)_2}$$

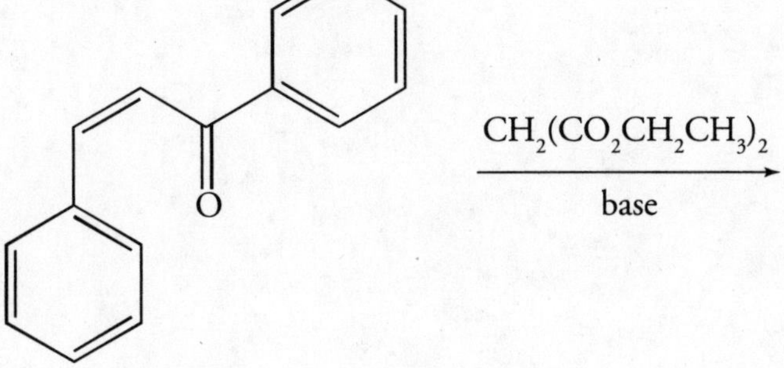

Solution:

A.

B.

C.

28.2   CARBOXYLIC ACIDS

Carboxylic acids are of fundamental importance in many biological systems. Fatty acids, for example, are long chain carboxylic acids that play important roles in both cellular structure and metabolism. In the following sections, we'll explore the basic physical properties and common chemical reactions of carboxylic acids and their derivatives.

Acidity of Carboxylic Acids

This is our last section on Ochem acidity; we've talked about this concept in Sections 25.6, 26.5, and 18.1. Here we will add the last layer and summarize what you need to know for the DAT. As we've already learned, the acidity of carboxylic acids results from the resonance stability of the carboxylate anion. When the carboxylic acid donates its acidic proton, the oxygen becomes negatively charged and this resulting negative charge can be delocalized into the adjacent π system. Two resonance structures of equivalent energy can be drawn. Remember that resonance structures of equivalent energy result in stability.

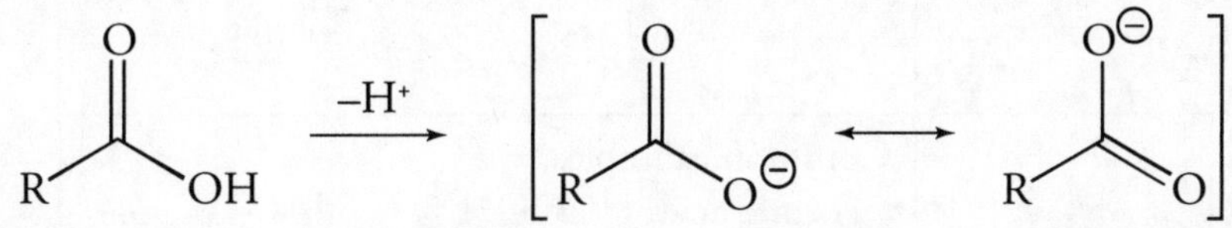

Electron-withdrawing groups increase acidity of carboxylic acids by increasing stability of the negative charge of the carboxylate anion. This is known as an **inductive effect** (as opposed to a resonance effect) and it exerts its effect by withdrawing electrons through σ bonds (single bonds). Inductive effects decrease with increasing distance; the closer the electron withdrawing group is to the acid, the greater the effect. The following order of acidity for the isomers of fluorobutanoic acid should help clarify this point.

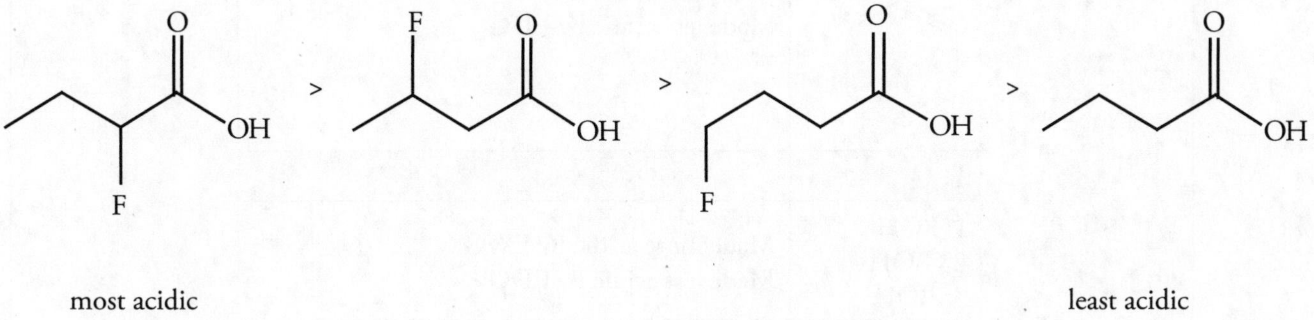

most acidic   least acidic

28.2

Now that you've seen all the Ochem acidity content you need to know for the DAT, let's summarize everything together. This table is a summary of Sections 25.6, 26.5, 28.1, and 28.2:

Acid Strength	Compound	Additional Details/Examples	Conjugate Base Strength
Strongest Acid (Good Proton Donor)	Strong acids	• Hydroiodic acid, HI • Hydrobromic acid, HBr • Hydrochloric acid, HCl • Perchloric acid, $HClO_4$ • Sulfuric acid, H_2SO_4 • Nitric acid, HNO_3	**Weakest Conjugate Base (Most Stable, Least Reactive)**
	Sulfonic Acids 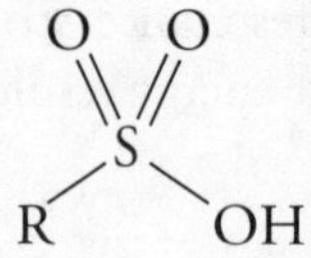		
	Carboxylic acids	Common examples: • Formic acid, HCOOH • Acetic acid, CH_3COOH Made more acidic by EWG (inductive effects)	
	Phenols 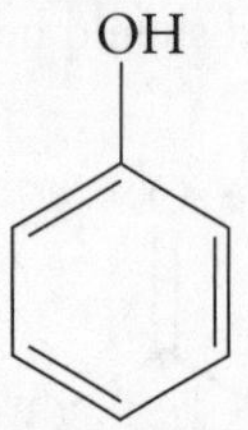	Made more acidic by EWG Made less acidic by EDG	
	H_2O		
	1° ROH 2° ROH 3° ROH	Made more acidic by EWG Made less acidic by EDG	
	Carbonyl αH	e.g., CH_3COCH_3	
	Alkyne	e.g., HC≡CH	
	H_2		
	NH_3		
Weakest Acid (Poor Proton Donor)	Alkene	e.g., $H_2C{=}CH_2$	**Strongest Conjugate Base (Least Stable, Most Reactive)**
	Alkane	e.g., $H_3C{-}CH_3$	

Example 28-7: Rank the following nine compounds in order of decreasing acidity.

A.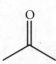

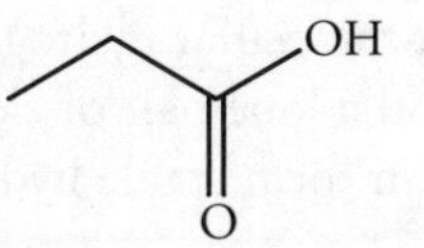

B. H—Cl

C. (phenol structure with OH)

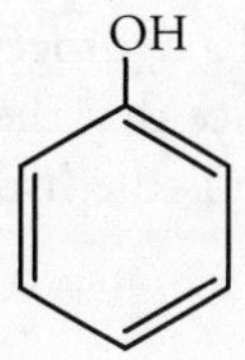

D. (monofluorinated carboxylic acid, F in β position)

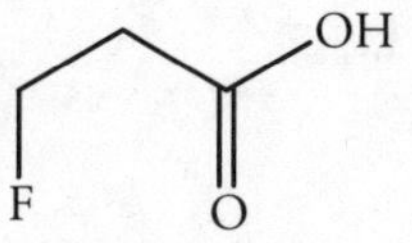

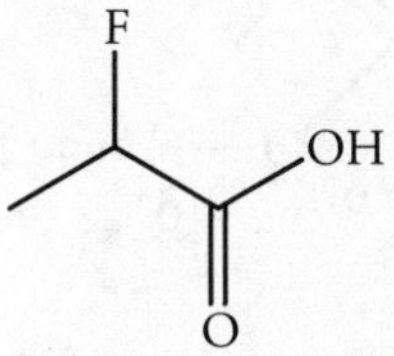

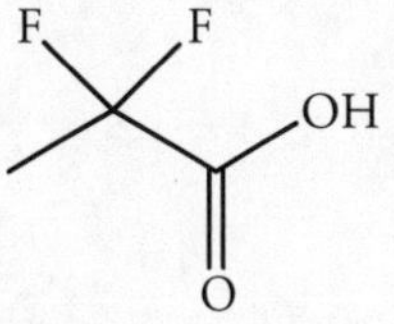

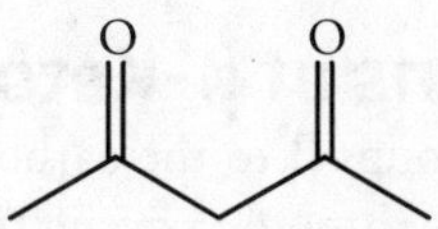

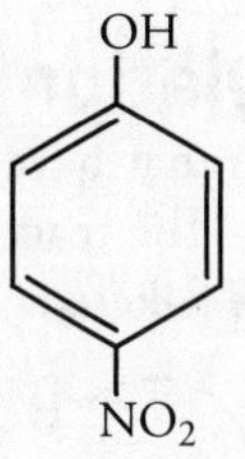

E. (monofluorinated carboxylic acid, F in α position)

F. (difluorinated carboxylic acid)

G. (acetone structure)

H. (diketone structure)

I. (phenol with NO₂ group)

Solution:

B.	>	F.	>	E.	>	D.	>	A.
strong acid		difluorinated carboxylic acid		monofluorinated carboxylic acid in α position		monofluorinated carboxylic acid in β position		carboxylic acid

>	I.	>	C.	~	H.	>	G.
	phenol with electron withdrawing nitro group		phenol		diketone with 2 α protons adjacent to 2 carbonyls		ketone

Hydrogen Bonding

Carboxylic acids form strong hydrogen bonds because the carboxylate group contains both a hydrogen bond donor and a hydrogen bond acceptor. This can be seen in the inter-molecular hydrogen bonding of acetic acid. Notice that the acidic proton is the hydrogen bond donor and a lone pair of electrons on the carbonyl oxygen is the hydrogen bond acceptor. For this reason, they can form stable hydrogen bonded dimers.

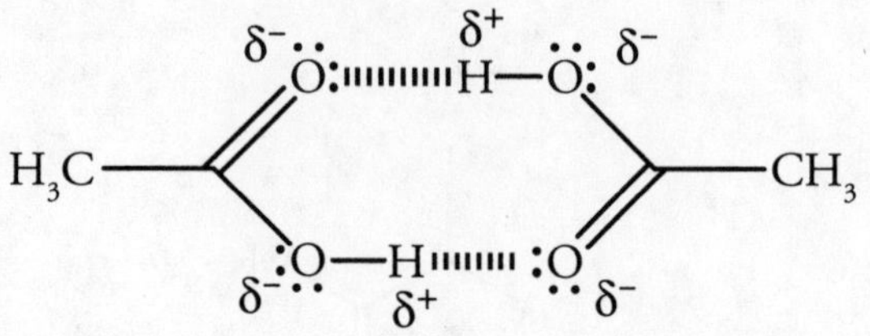

Decarboxylation Reactions of β-Keto Acids

Carboxylic acids that have carbonyl groups β to the carboxylate are unstable because they are subject to decarboxylation. The reaction proceeds through a cyclic transition state and results in the loss of carbon dioxide from the β-keto acid.

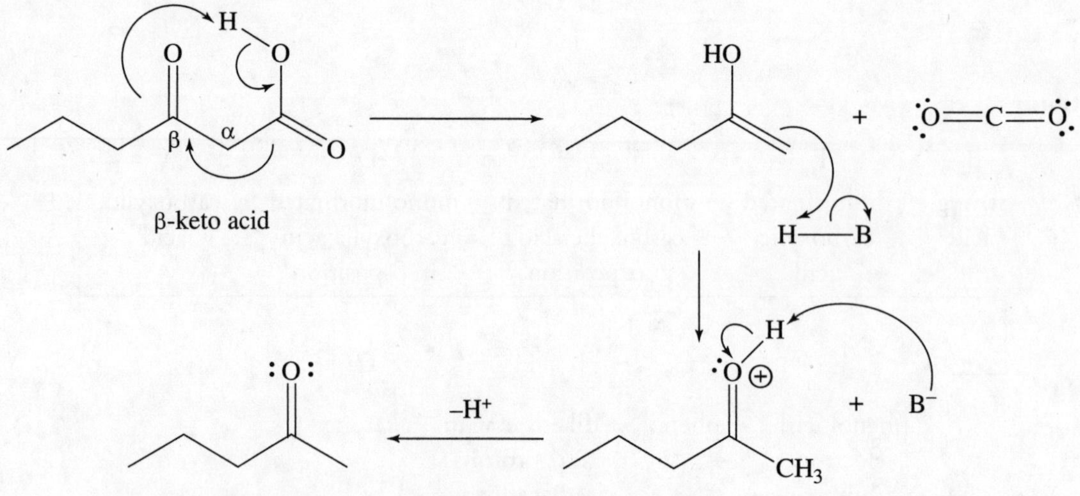

β-keto acid

28.3   CARBOXYLIC ACID DERIVATIVES

Carboxylic acid derivatives (CADs) include acid chlorides, acid anhydrides, esters, and amides. The general chemical structures for these acid derivatives are:

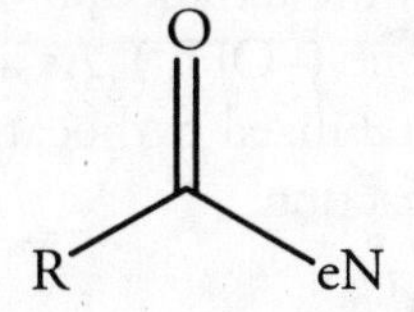

(eN = electronegative group)

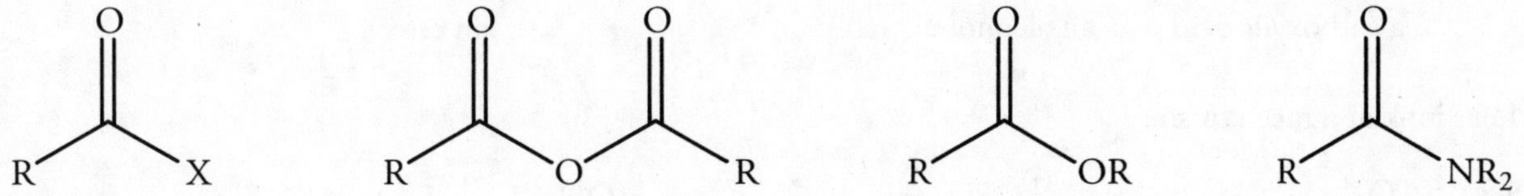

| X = halogen | acid | ester | amide |
| acid halide | anhydride | | |

Like aldehydes and ketones, acid derivatives often undergo nucleophilic addition reactions (see below). This is because they are very electrophilic at the carbonyl carbon atom. However, unlike reactions with aldehydes and ketones, nucleophilic addition reactions to carboxylic acid derivatives are usually followed by elimination. This is because the tetrahedral intermediate formed upon attack of the nucleophile on the carbonyl carbon has both a negatively charged oxygen atom (the former carbonyl oxygen), and a good leaving group (the eN-group of the carboxylic acid derivative). This elimination by the electrons on the oxygen atom regenerates the carbonyl, thereby displacing the leaving group (eN⁻). This is called a **nucleophilic addition-elimination reaction**.

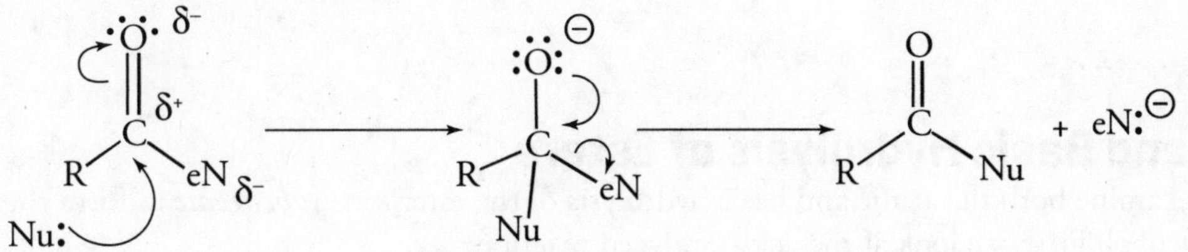

| Acid derivative | Tetrahedral intermediate | New acid derivative |

Esterification Reactions

An **esterification reaction** occurs when a carboxylic acid reacts with an alcohol in the presence of a catalytic amount of acid. The protonation of the carbonyl oxygen makes the carbonyl carbon more electrophilic, and nucleophilic attack by the oxygen of the alcohol results in a tetrahedral intermediate that is neutralized by deprotonation. An oxygen of the tetrahedral intermediate is then protonated and converts a poor leaving group ($-OH$) into a good one ($-OH_2^+$). As a result, the water molecule departs with its electrons, and leaves behind a resonance-stabilized carbocation. Deprotonation of the carbonyl oxygen yields the ester product. Here is a general reaction:

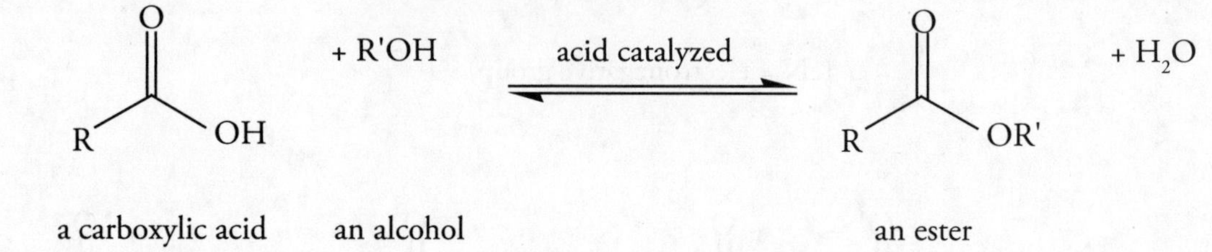

a carboxylic acid   an alcohol   an ester

Let's look at a mechanism:

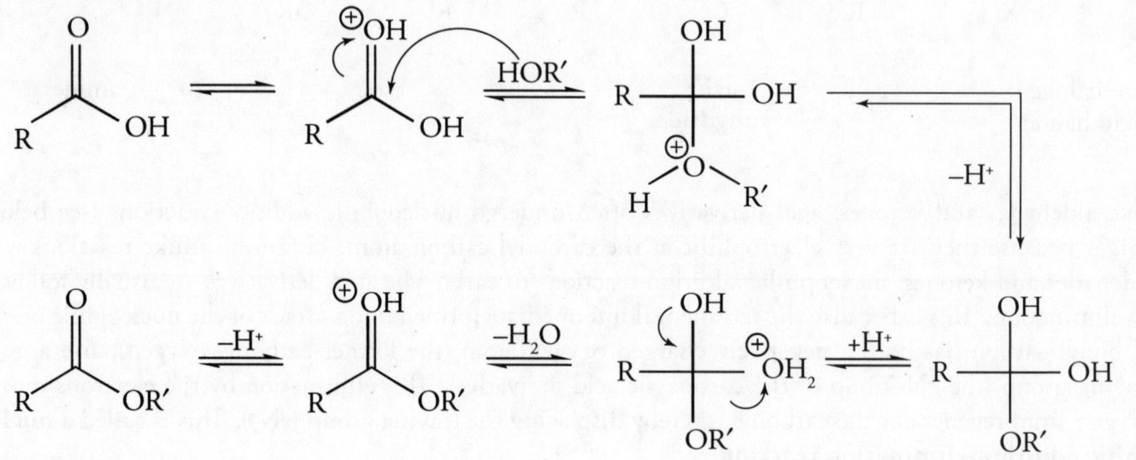

Acidic and Basic Hydrolysis of Esters

Let's now examine both the acidic and basic hydrolysis of the ester *methyl benzoate* to form the carboxylic acid and alcohol. First, we look at the acid-catalyzed reaction:

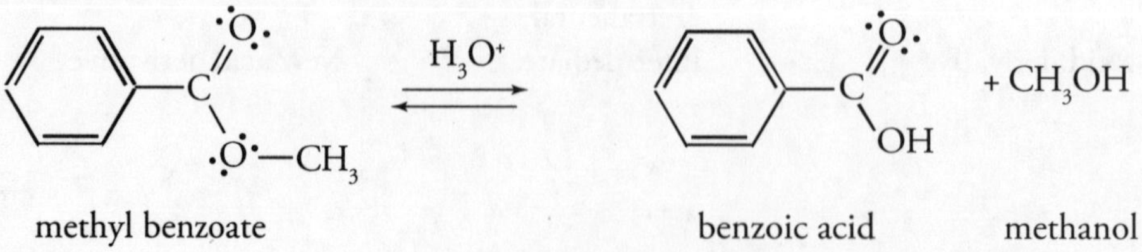

methyl benzoate   benzoic acid   methanol

In the first step of this reaction, the carbonyl oxygen is protonated. As before, the protonation of the carbonyl oxygen makes the carbon even more electrophilic and therefore susceptible to nucleophilic attack by a water molecule. Nucleophilic attack by a water molecule, followed by deprotonation, leads to the formation of a tetrahedral intermediate. In any nucleophilic addition-elimination reaction of an acid derivative, there will always be a tetrahedral intermediate. Here is the first part of the acid-catalyzed ester hydrolysis mechanism: Here is the first part of the acid-catalyzed ester hydrolysis mechanism:

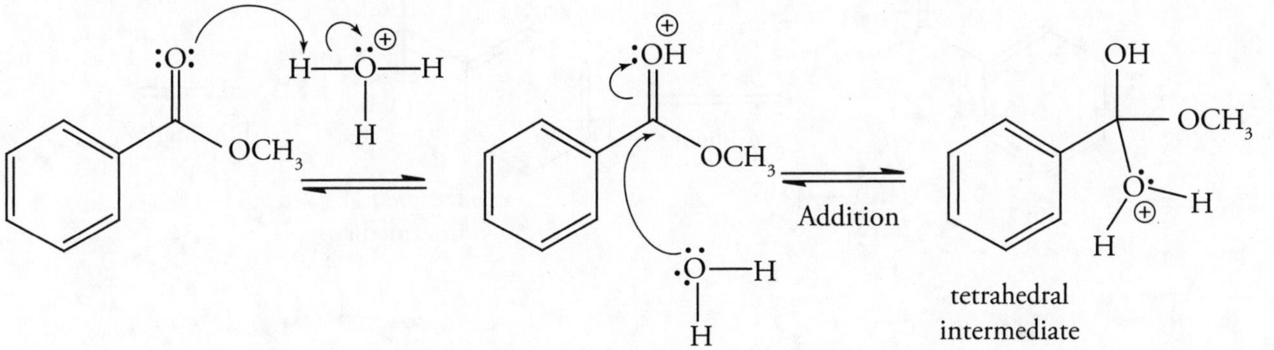

Next, the leaving group of the tetrahedral intermediate is protonated under the acidic reaction conditions. Notice that protonation of the hydroxyl oxygens can also occur. This leads to the reverse reaction. Protonation of the leaving group converts a poor leaving group (RO^-, an alkoxide ion) into a good one (ROH, a neutral alcohol molecule). The alcohol leaves and yields a protonated acid that only has to undergo a deprotonation to give the carboxylic acid product. Here is the rest of the mechanism for acid-catalyzed ester hydrolysis:

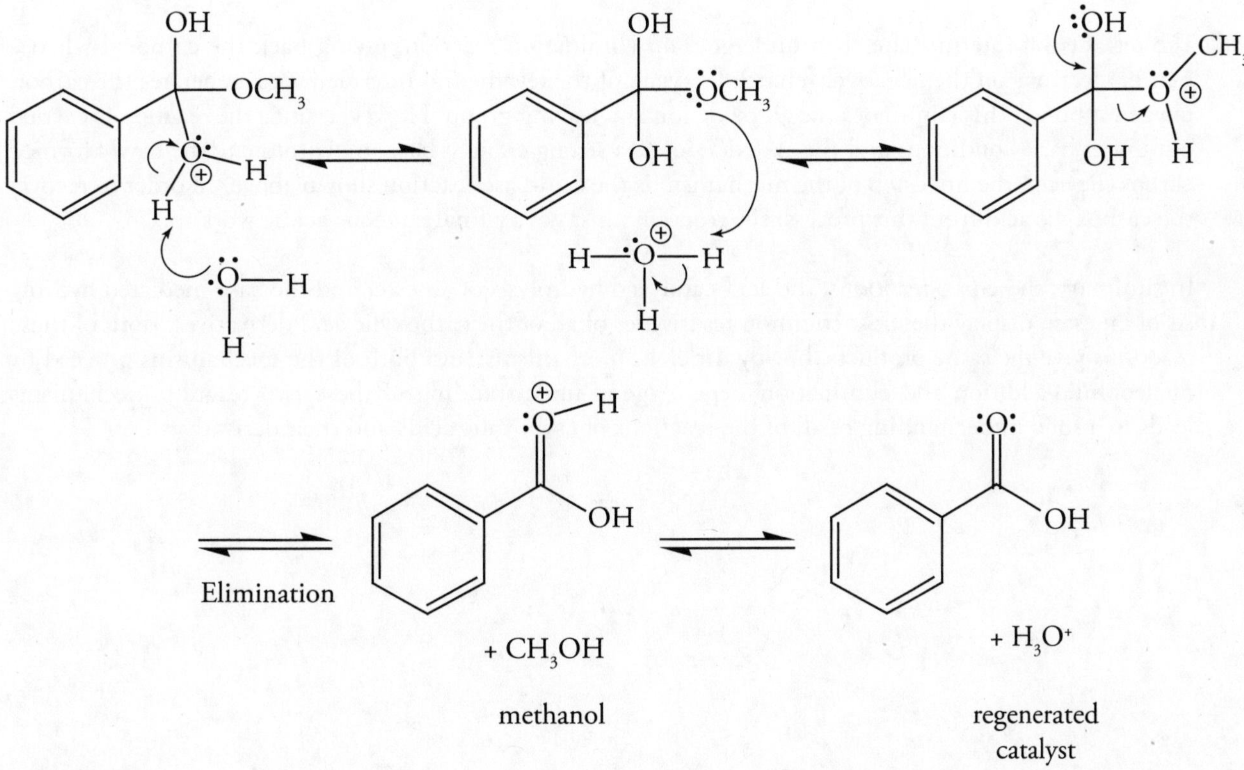

We now consider the corresponding *base*-mediated hydrolysis of methyl benzoate. In the first step of the reaction, the strongly nucleophilic hydroxide ion directly attacks the electrophilic carbonyl carbon. The nucleophilic attack results in the formation of a tetrahedral intermediate. Let's look at the mechanism for base-mediated ester hydrolysis:

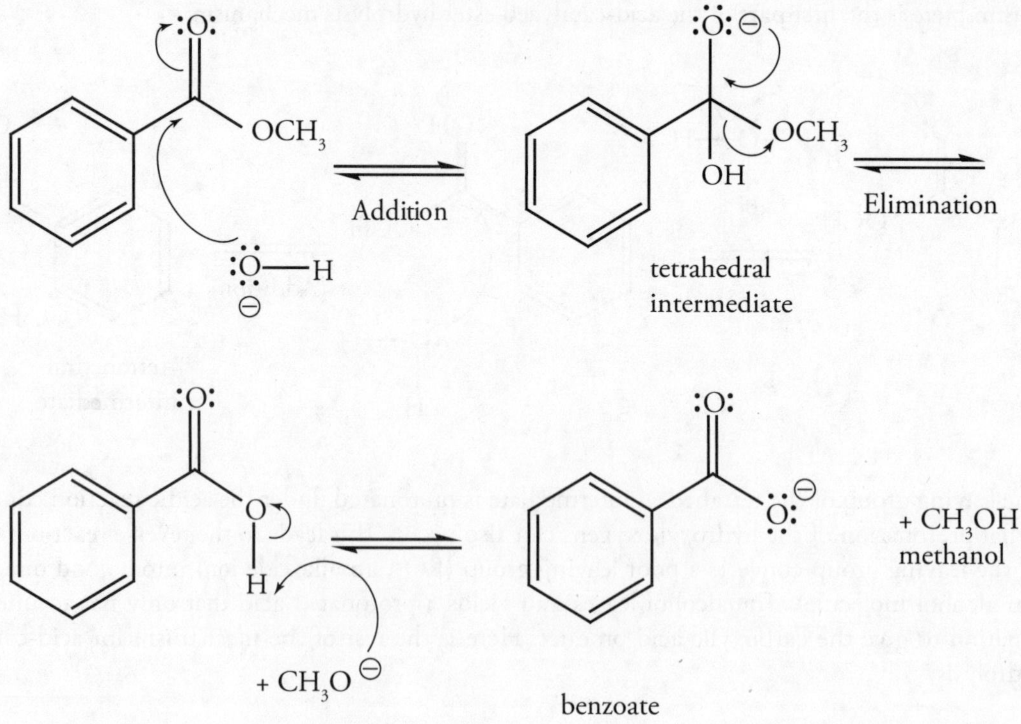

tetrahedral
intermediate

Addition

Elimination

+ CH$_3$OH
methanol

+ CH$_3$O$^{\ominus}$

benzoate

The tetrahedral intermediate then undergoes an elimination reaction, giving back the carbonyl when a pair of electrons on the negatively charged oxygen of the tetrahedral intermediate regenerates the carbon-oxygen π bond. This eliminates the alkoxide ion as a leaving group. However, since the reaction is carried out under basic conditions and the alkoxide ion is a strong enough base to deprotonate the newly formed carboxylic acid, the final step of the mechanism is the acid-base reaction shown above. In order to recover the carboxylic acid from this process, the reaction must have a final aqueous acidic workup.

In summary, these two reactions, the acid-catalyzed hydrolysis of an ester and the base-mediated hydrolysis of an ester, display the most common reactivities of all of the carboxylic acid derivatives. Both of these reactions give the same products, but by different mechanisms; and both of the mechanisms proceed by nucleophilic addition and elimination steps. A good understanding of these two reaction mechanisms leads to a solid understanding of all of the reactions of carboxylic acids and their derivatives.

Synthesis of the Carboxylic Acid Derivatives

Now that we understand the how the electronic structure of the carboxylic acid derivatives relates to their reactivity, the synthesis of carboxylic acid derivatives should be straightforward. For the most part, we shall only be concerned with the interconversion of one derivative to another. By the end of this section, you should be able to convert any carboxylic acid derivative into any other!

Acid Halides

Carboxylic acid halides are made from the corresponding carboxylic acid and either $SOCl_2$ or PX_3 (X = Cl, Br). This is very similar to the way alkyl halides are prepared from alcohols (Section 26.5).

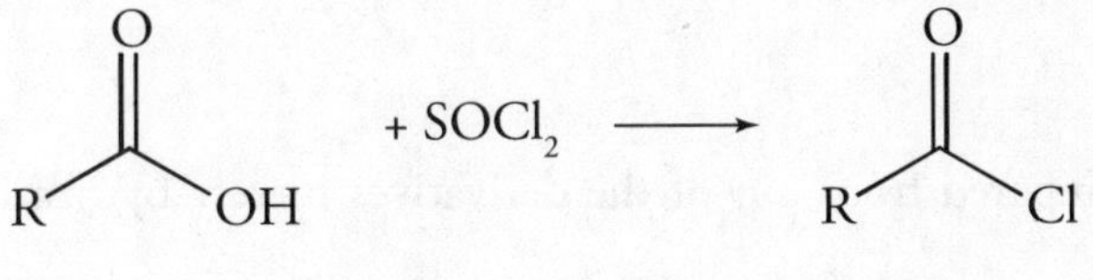

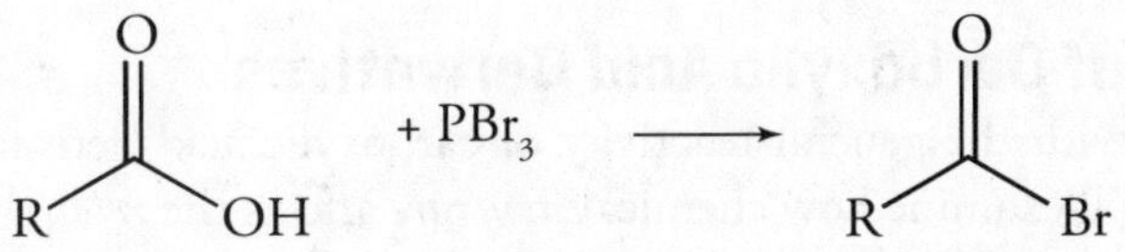

Acid Anhydrides

As their name implies, anhydrides (meaning "without water") can be prepared by the condensation of two carboxylic acids with the loss of water.

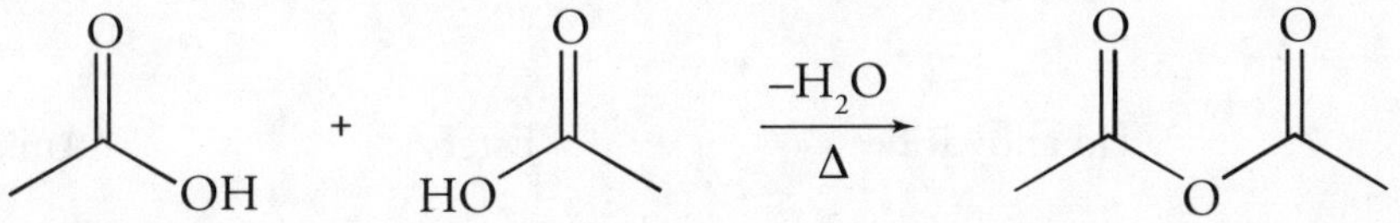

Acid anhydrides are also prepared from addition of the corresponding carboxylic acid (or carboxylate ion) to the corresponding acid halide.

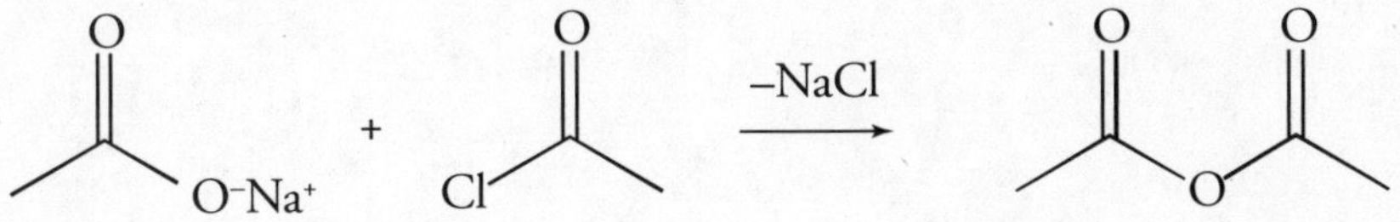

Esters

Esters are most easily synthesized from the corresponding carboxylic acid and an alcohol, as we saw earlier. This reaction is referred to as **esterification**. Esters can also be prepared from an acid halide or an anhydride and a corresponding alcohol.

Amides

Amides can be prepared from the corresponding acid halide, anhydride, or ester with the desired amine. They *cannot* be prepared from the carboxylic acid directly. This is because amines are very basic, and carboxylic acids are very acidic; an acid-base reaction occurs much faster than the desired addition-elimination reaction.

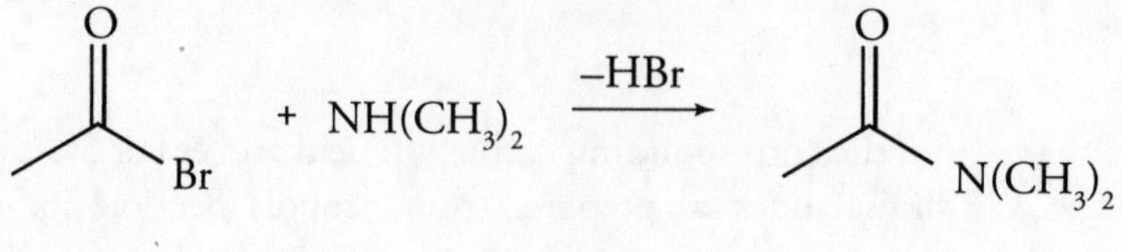

Carboxylic Acids

Carboxylic acids can be prepared from *any* of the derivatives merely by heating the derivative in acidic aqueous solutions.

Relative Reactivity of Carboxylic Acid Derivatives

Now that we are familiar with the general reactivity of carboxylic acid derivatives, nucleophilic addition-elimination reactions, we will examine how chemical *structure* affects the *relative* chemical reactivity of common acid derivatives. The order of reactivity in nucleophilic substitution reactions for acid derivatives is:

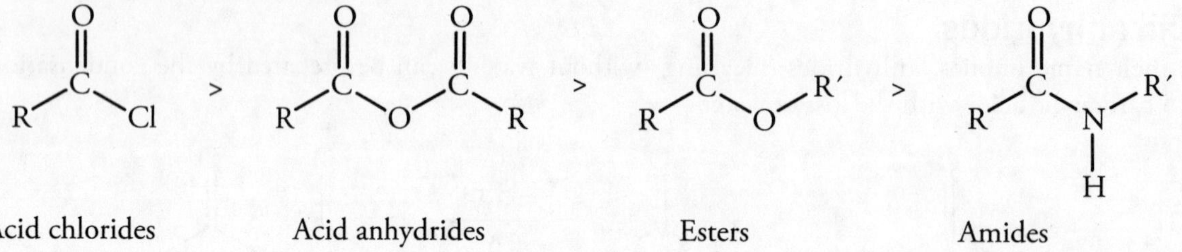

| Acid chlorides | Acid anhydrides | Esters | Amides |

If we examine the leaving groups of these acid derivatives, it is clear that the reactivity of acid derivatives in nucleophilic substitution reactions decreases with increasing basicity of the leaving group.

Acid Derivative   Leaving Group

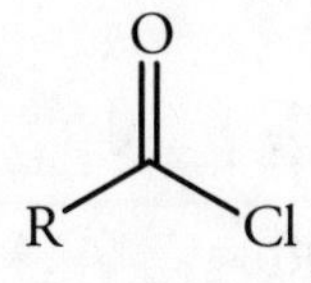

acid chloride

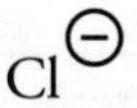

Chloride anion is a very good leaving group. It is a very weak base since it is the conjugate base of the strong acid HCl ($pK_a = -7$).

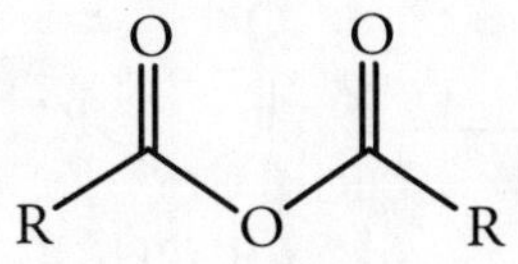

acid anhydride

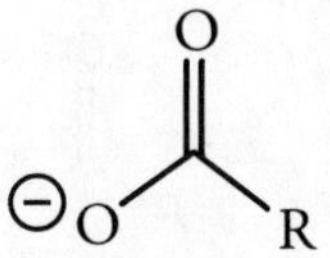

This is a fairly good leaving group. It is the conjugate base of the weakly acidic carboxylic acid ($pK_a = 4-5$).

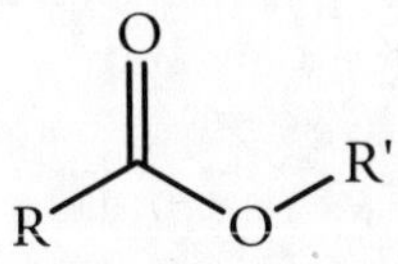

ester

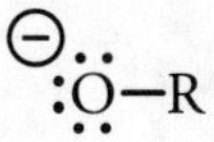

An alkoxide ion is a rather poor leaving group. It is moderately basic since it is the conjugate base of alcohol, which is a fairly weak acid ($pK_a = 15-19$).

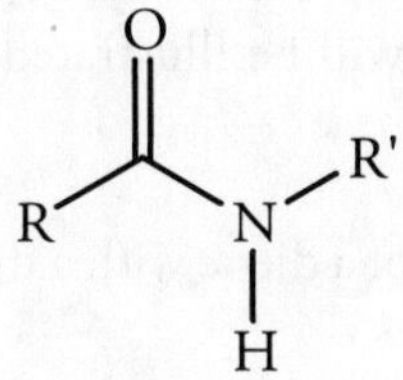

amide

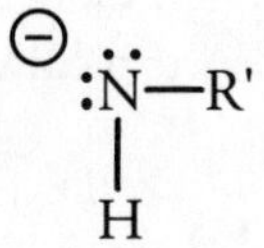

This is a horrible leaving group. It is strongly basic since it is the conjugate base of an amine, which is a terrible acid ($pK_a = 35-40$).

Acid chlorides are so reactive in nucleophilic addition-elimination reactions that they are readily hydrolyzed in cold water.

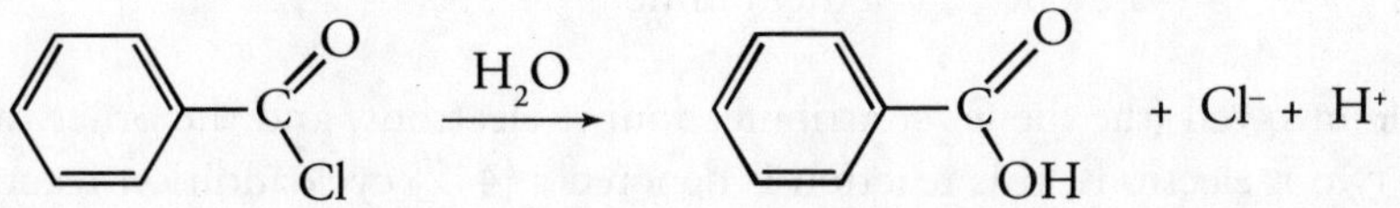

However, in order to hydrolyze amides and esters, heating with aqueous acid or base is required.

Here is a summary of the important CAD reactions you should recognize for the DAT:

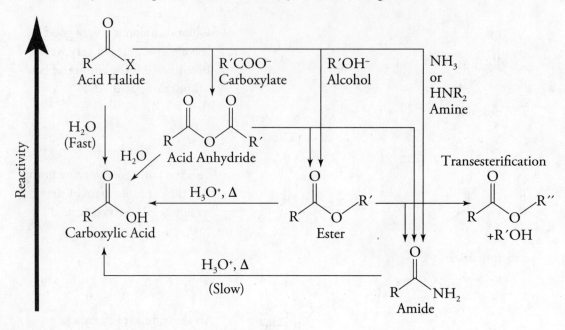

28.4   CYCLOADDITION REACTIONS

Concerted reactions are reactions that occur in one step without the formation of any intermediates. They usually occur with a high degree of stereoselectivity. Concerted reactions often occur via cyclic transition states by the reorganization of σ and π bonds. A typical concerted reaction will be illustrated with the **Diels-Alder reaction**.

In a Diels–Alder reaction, a cyclohexene ring is formed from the cycloaddition of a diene with a dienophile:

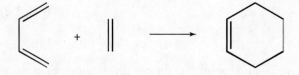

a diene   a dienophile

Since one molecule involved (the diene) contributes four π electrons, and the other molecule (the dieno-phile) contributes two π electrons, this reaction is denoted a [4+2] cycloaddition reaction. Although this reaction occurs both stereoselectively and regioselectively, these finer points are beyond the scope of the DAT, so we will not discuss them further in this text.

Example 28-8: Predict the product of the following Diels-Alder cycloaddition reactions:

A.

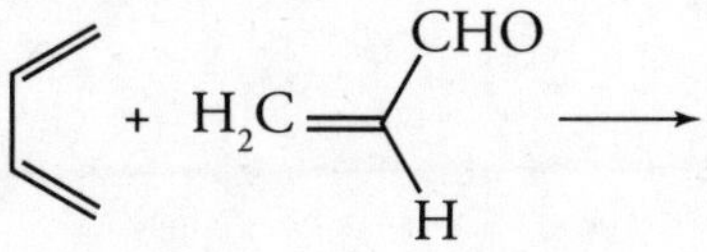

$$\text{diene} + H_2C = \overset{CHO}{\underset{H}{C}} \longrightarrow$$

B.

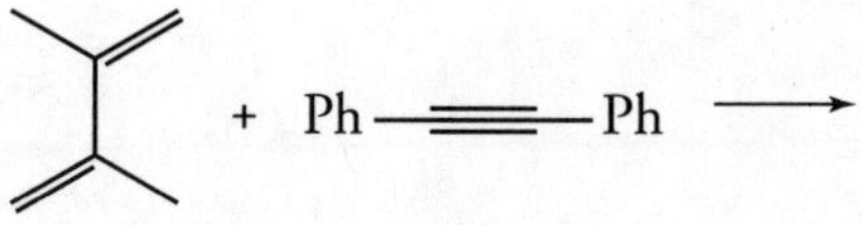

$$\text{diene} + Ph-\!\!\!\equiv\!\!\!-Ph \longrightarrow$$

C.

$$\text{diene} + \text{maleic anhydride} \longrightarrow$$

28.4

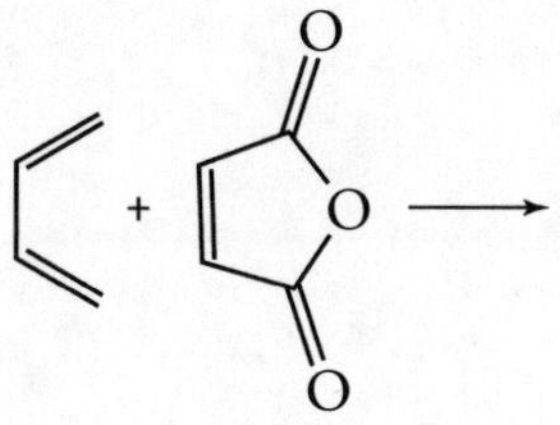

Solution:

A.

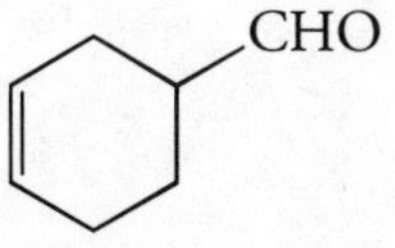

cyclohexene–CHO

B.

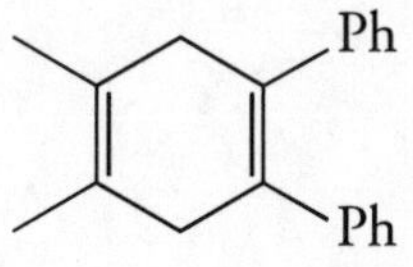

dimethyl diphenyl cyclohexadiene

C.

fused bicyclic anhydride

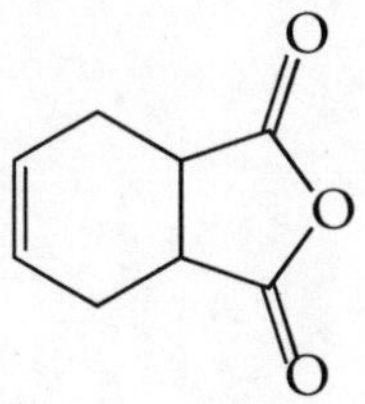

Want More Practice?
Scan the QR code below to
register your book for online
chapter summaries, drills,
practice tests, and more!

Chapter 29
Ochem Lab Techniques

29.1 SEPARATIONS

Extractions

One of the more useful techniques in experimental organic chemistry is solvent extraction. Isolation of natural products from marine organisms, plants, and other natural sources is facilitated by exploiting the particular solubilities of organic compounds in various solvents. Complex mixtures of organic compounds can be separated using careful choice of solvents based on the differential solubilities of the various components of the mixture. We'll see that the acid/base properties of organic molecules play an important role in the extraction process.

Extraction allows the chemist to separate one substance from a mixture of substances by adding a solvent in which the compound of interest is highly soluble. If the solution containing the compound of interest is shaken with a second solvent (completely immiscible with the first) and allowed to separate into two distinct phases, the compound of interest will distribute itself between the two phases based upon its solubility in each of the individual solvents. This is called a **liquid-liquid extraction**. The ratio of the substance's solubilities in the two solvents is called the **distribution** (or **partition**) **coefficient**.

The simplest liquid-liquid extraction is accomplished when an organic compound is extracted with water. A simple water extraction can remove substances that are highly polar or charged, including inorganic salts, strong acids and bases, and polar, low molecular weight compounds (less than five carbons) such as alcohols, amines, and carboxylic acids.

A second class of organic extraction involves the use of acidic or basic water solutions. Organic compounds that are basic (e.g., amines) can be extracted from mixtures of organic compounds upon treatment with dilute acid (usually 5–10% HCl). This treatment will protonate the basic functional group, forming a positively charged ion. The resulting cationic salts of these basic compounds are usually freely soluble in aqueous solution and can be removed from the organic compounds that remain dissolved in the organic phase.

Extraction of Organic Amines

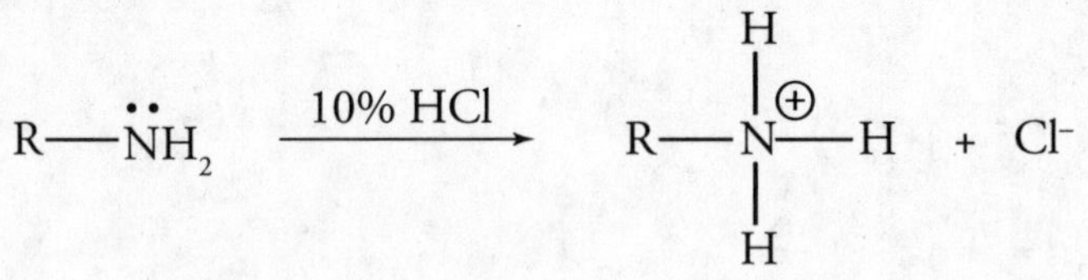

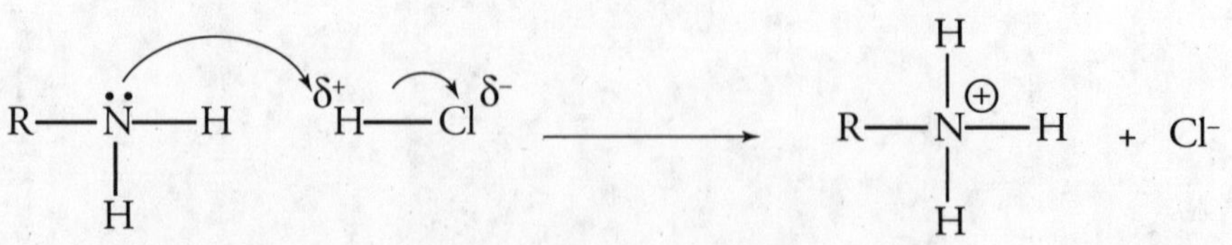

On the other hand, extraction with a dilute weak base—typically 5 percent sodium bicarbonate ($NaHCO_3$) —results in converting organic acids into their corresponding anionic salts.

Extraction of Carboxylic Acids

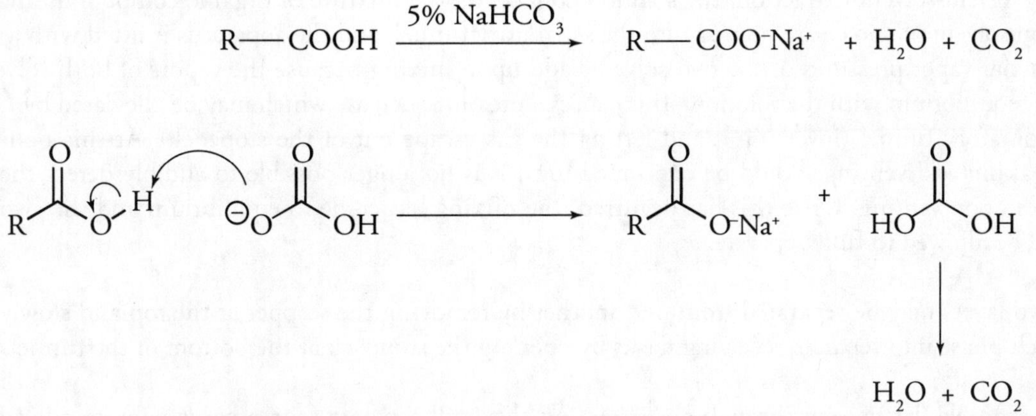

$$R-COOH \xrightarrow{5\% \ NaHCO_3} R-COO^- Na^+ \ + \ H_2O \ + \ CO_2$$

These anionic salts are generally soluble in aqueous solution and can be removed from the organic compounds that remain dissolved in the organic phase. Dilute sodium hydroxide could also be used for this kind of extraction, but it is basic enough to also convert phenols into their corresponding anionic salts. When phenols are present in a mixture of organic compounds and need to be removed, a dilute sodium hydroxide solution (usually about 10%) will succeed in converting phenols into their corresponding anionic salts. The anionic salts of the phenols are generally soluble in the aqueous phase and can therefore be removed from the organic phase.

Extraction of Phenols

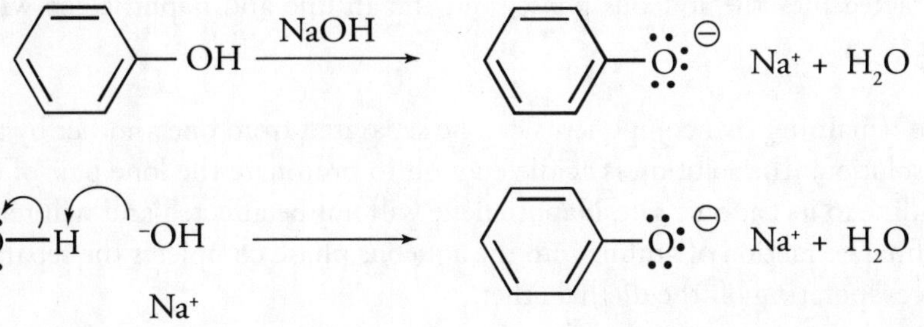

(*Note:* NaOH will also extract carboxylic acids.)

The apparatus in which these extractions are typically carried out is called a **separatory funnel**. To perform a solvent-solvent extraction, the solution containing the mixture of organic compounds and the extraction solvent of choice are poured into the separatory funnel, and the apparatus is fitted with a stopper. The partial vapor pressures of the two solvents add upon mixing because the vapors of both solvents are now in equilibrium with the solution. This causes a pressure increase which may be alleviated by "venting" the separatory funnel (inverting it and letting the gas escape out of the stopcock). At this point, vigorous shaking and venting should be continued until it is no longer possible to audibly detect the escape of gases upon venting. Once this has occurred, the mixing has come to equilibrium and the two phases should be allowed to fully separate.

The two layers may be separated from one another by removing the stopper at the top and slowly collecting each phase into separate receiving flasks by opening the stopcock at the bottom of the funnel.

As an example, let us step through an extraction that will separate four organic compounds from one another. The original mixture consists of *para*-cresol, benzoic acid, aniline, and naphthalene, all of which are dissolved in diethyl ether. This mixture is first extracted with an equal volume of aqueous sodium bicarbonate. The weakly basic bicarbonate is sufficiently basic to deprotonate benzoic acid and convert it to an anionic salt, but not strong enough to deprotonate *para*-cresol (a phenol). Likewise, a bicarbonate extraction will not affect aniline (a base itself) or naphthalene (a hydrocarbon). Thus, *para*-cresol, aniline, and naphthalene will remain dissolved in the ether phase, while the benzoic acid, now in its anionic salt form, will be extracted into the aqueous layer.

The ether layer, which now contains three components, is extracted with a sodium hydroxide solution. The strongly basic hydroxide ion is strong enough to deprotonate *para*-cresol and convert it to its anionic salt form. The basic conditions will not affect aniline or naphthalene so *para*-cresol is the only compound that is extracted into the aqueous phase, and the aniline and naphthalene will remain dissolved in the ether layer.

Finally, the remaining two components can be separated from one another by an acidic extraction with a 10% HCl solution. The solution is acidic enough to protonate the lone pair of electrons of aniline and to convert aniline to its cationic salt. Naphthalene will not be affected and will remain dissolved in the ether layer. The final extraction of aniline into the aqueous phase completes the separation. Naphthalene can be isolated by evaporating off the diethyl ether.

These steps are summarized on the following page.

All four components dissolved in diethyl ether

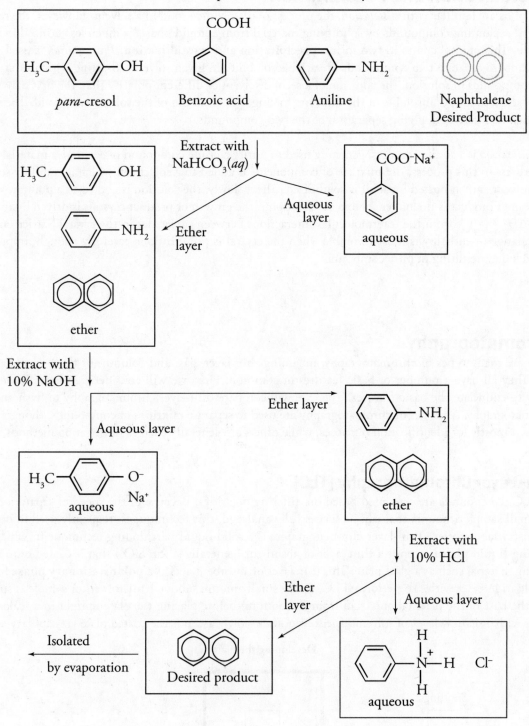

Crystallization and Precipitation

Most of us are familiar with *dissolution*, the process of dissolving a solid in a solvent. However, the reverse process, separating compounds by solidifying material from a liquid phase, is much less utilized in everyday life. This process comes in two forms, **precipitation** and **crystallization**. *Precipitation* is used when one wants to separate two compounds of variable solubility in given solvents. Starting with a mixture of two compounds in solution, the addition of a second solvent of different polarity than the first may make one of the two solutes insoluble in the mixture, forcing it to crash out of the solution as a solid. The solids can then be filtered off, giving separation of the two compounds.

Crystallization is a similar process, generally used to purify a crude compound or separate a material from impurities. In this process, the mixture of components is added to a solvent in which it is mildly soluble. This solvent is then heated until all is solubilized. Then, slowly, the solution is cooled to a point at which the desired product is no longer soluble. At this point, the growth of product crystals is driven by the negative $\Delta H_{\text{crystallization}}$, from the intermolecular interactions between molecules in the crystal (lattice energy). This change in enthalpy is most favorable when the crystal is pure. If done carefully enough, impurities are excluded, resulting in pure compound.

Chromatography

There are many types of chromatography, including thin layer, gas, and column (or flash) chromatography. They all have a number of basic features in common. First, we will consider thin-layer chromatography to enunciate the basic features. Then we will compare thin-layer chromatography to flash and gas chromatography. All types of chromatography are used to separate mixtures of compounds, though some are used mostly for identification purposes, while others are generally used as purification methods.

Thin-Layer Chromatography (TLC)

In TLC, compounds are separated based on differing polarities. Because of the speed of separation and the small sample amounts that can be successfully analyzed, this technique is frequently used in organic chemistry laboratories. Thin-layer chromatography is a solid-liquid partitioning technique in which the **moving liquid phase** ascends a thin layer of absorbent (generally silica, SiO_2) that is coated onto a supporting material such as a glass plate. This thin layer of absorbent acts as a **polar stationary phase** for the sample to interact with. To perform TLC, a very small amount (about 1 microliter) of sample is spotted near the base of the plate (about 1 cm from the bottom) before placing the plate upright in a sealed container with a shallow layer of solvent. The solvent then slowly ascends the coated plate via capillary action.

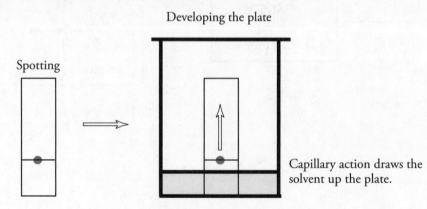

Developing the plate

Spotting

Capillary action draws the solvent up the plate.

As the solvent slowly ascends the plate via capillary action, the components of the spotted sample are partitioned between the moving liquid phase and the stationary solid phase. This process is referred to as **developing**, or **running**, a thin layer plate. Each component of the sample experiences many equilibrations between the moving and the stationary phases as the development proceeds.

Separation of the compounds occurs because different components travel along the plate at different rates. The more polar components of the mixture interact more with the polar stationary phase and travel at a slower rate. The less polar components have a greater affinity for the solvent than the stationary phase and travel with the mobile solvent at a faster rate than the more polar components. The thin layer plate is then removed and allowed to dry when the solvent front approaches a few centimeters from the top of the plate. If the compounds in the mixture that was spotted are colored, we would see a vertical series of spots on the plate; however, it is more likely that the components are not colored and need to be detected by some other means. Visualization methods include shining ultraviolet light on the plate, placing the thin layer plate in the presence of iodine vapor, and a host of other chemical staining techniques.

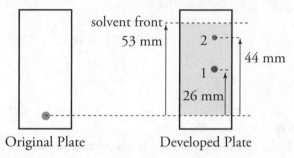

Once the separated components have been visualized, R_f values can be computed. This "ratio to front" value (R_f) is simply the distance traveled by an individual component divided by the distance traveled by the solvent front. For example, from the illustration above, we would find

$$R_f(\text{Compound 1}) = \frac{26 \text{ mm}}{53 \text{ mm}} = 0.49 \qquad R_f(\text{Compound 2}) = \frac{44 \text{ mm}}{53 \text{ mm}} = 0.83$$

(Note that R_f is always positive and never greater than 1.)

Column (Flash) Chromatography

While TLC is a good technique for separating very small amounts of material in order to assess how many compounds make up a mixture, it's not a good technique for isolating bulk compounds. A common technique known as column or flash chromatography employs the idea behind TLC toward just such a goal. Shown below is a chromatography column. This column is filled with silica gel (predominantly SiO_2, as in the TLC plate). The silica gel is saturated with a chosen organic solvent, and the mixture of compounds is then added to the top and allowed to travel down through the silica-packed column. Excess solvent is periodically added to the top of the column, and the flow of solvent (along with the separated compounds) is collected from the bottom. Just as is the case in TLC, polar compounds will spend more time adsorbed on the polar solid phase, and as such travel more slowly down the column than nonpolar compounds. Therefore, compounds can be expected to leave the column, and be collected in order of polarity (least polar to most polar).

Column Chromatography

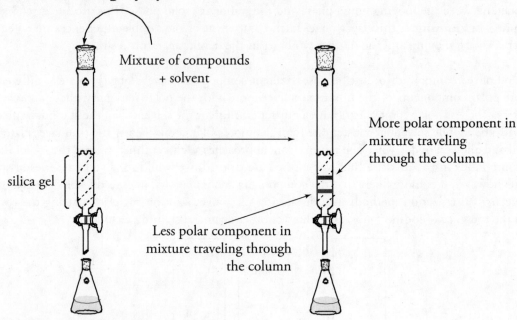

Mixture of compounds + solvent

silica gel

More polar component in mixture traveling through the column

Less polar component in mixture traveling through the column

Gas Chromatography

Gas chromatography (GC) is a form of column chromatography in which the partitioning of the components to be separated takes place between a **moving gas phase** and a **stationary liquid phase**. This partitioning, or separation, between mixtures of compounds occurs based on their *different volatilities*. In a typical gas chromatograph, a sample is loaded into a syringe and injected into the device through a rubber septum. The sample is then vaporized by a heater in the injection port and carried along by a stream of inert gas (typically helium). The vaporized sample is quickly moved by the inert gas stream into a column composed of particles that are coated with a liquid absorbent. As the components of the sample pass through the column, they interact differently with the absorbent based on their relative volatilities. Each component of the sample is subjected to many gas-liquid partitioning processes which separates the individual components.

As each component exits the column, it is burned, and the resulting ions are detected by an electrical detector that generates a signal that is recorded by a chart recorder. The chart recorder printout enables us to determine the number of components and their relative amounts.

Let's now take a closer look at the separation process by examining a typical GC column. In order to examine the separation process we will consider a mixture of two individual components. As the mixture enters the column, it begins to interact with the stationary phase, which is composed of support material coated with a liquid absorbent. The liquid absorbents can range from hydrocarbon mixtures that are very nonpolar to polyesters that are polar. As the mixture passes through the column, the components equilibrate between the carrier gas and the liquid phase. The less volatile components will spend more time dissolved in the liquid stationary phase than the more volatile components that will be carried along by the carrier gas at a faster rate. It is this equilibrium between the components (the absorbed liquid phase and the carrier gas mobile phase) that results in the separation of the mixture. If the interactions of the substrates with the column are similar (this is usually the case with most GC columns), the more volatile components emerge from the column first, while the less volatile components emerge from the column later.

Distillations

Distillation is the process of raising the temperature of a liquid until it can overcome the intermolecular forces that hold it together in the liquid phase. The vapor is then condensed back to the liquid phase and subsequently collected in another container.

Simple Distillation

A simple distillation is performed when trace impurities need to be removed from a relatively pure compound, or when a mixture of compounds with significantly different boiling points needs to be separated.

Fractional Distillation

Fractional distillation is a different type of distillation process that is used when the difference in boiling points of the components in the liquid mixture is not large. A fractional distillation column is packed with an appropriate material, such as glass beads or a stainless-steel sponge. The packing of the column results in the liquid mixture being subjected to many vaporization-condensation cycles as it moves up the column toward the condenser. As the cycles progress, the composition of the vapor gradually becomes enriched in the lower boiling component. Near the top of the column, nearly pure vapor reaches the condenser and condenses back to the liquid phase where it is subsequently collected in a receiving flask.

Example 29-1: A chemist wishes to separate a mixture of Compounds A and B. He decides to distill the mixture; however, he is unsure of their respective boiling points. After several minutes of heating, he collects the distillate, takes a small sample, and injects it into a gas chromatograph. The output is:

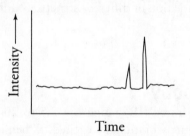

What can this chemist conclude about the separation, and how could it be improved?

Solution: Based on the data from the GC, his separation was only partial (because two different peaks are recorded). Because the second peak is larger than the first, the distillate consists primarily of one of the two compounds, but their boiling points may have been similar enough that a complete separation was not possible. Perhaps the chemist should try fractional distillation.

29.2 SPECTROSCOPY

A basic understanding of the general principles of spectroscopy will enable you to answer important questions regarding the structure of organic molecules. In this chapter, we'll examine the general principles of both infrared (IR) spectroscopy and nuclear magnetic resonance (NMR) spectroscopy with the goal of interpreting the spectra of simple organic molecules.

Most types of spectroscopy that we will discuss are examples of absorption spectroscopy. A short explanation of the molecular events involved in absorption spectroscopy will help you remember the details of IR and NMR spectroscopy. Molecules normally exist in their lowest energy form, called their **ground state**. When a molecule is exposed to light it *may* absorb a photon, provided that the energy of this photon matches the energy between two of the fixed electronic energy levels of the molecule. When this happens, the molecule is said to be in an **excited state**. Molecules tend to prefer their ground state to an excited state, but in order for them to return to their ground state, they must lose the energy they have gained. This loss of energy can occur by the emission of heat, or less commonly, light. In absorption spectroscopy, scientists induce the absorption of energy by a sample of molecules by exposing the sample to various forms of light, thereby exciting molecules to a higher energy state. They then measure the energy released as the molecules relax back to their ground state. This measured energy can reveal structural features of the molecules in the sample.

There are many different forms of light, as displayed in the electromagnetic spectrum. In principle, any of these forms of light could be used to do absorption spectroscopy on molecules, and, in fact, many are! The different forms of light induce different transitions in ground state molecules to different excited states of the molecules and allow for the acquisition of different structural information about the molecules.

Infrared (IR) Spectroscopy

Electromagnetic radiation in the infrared (IR) range λ = 2.5 to 20 µm has the proper energy to cause bonds in organic molecules to become vibrationally excited. When a sample of an organic compound is irradiated with infrared radiation in the region between 2.5 and 20 µm, its covalent bonds will begin to *vibrate at distinct energy levels* (wavelengths, frequencies) within this region. These wavelengths correspond to frequencies in the range of 1.5×10^{13} Hz to 1.2×10^{14} Hz. In IR spectroscopy, vibrational frequencies are more commonly given in terms of the **wavenumber**. Wavenumber ($\bar{v}$) is simply the reciprocal of wavelength:

$$\bar{v} = \frac{1}{\lambda} = \frac{1}{c}v$$

and is therefore directly proportional to both the frequency (since $\lambda v = c = 3 \times 10^{10}$ cm/sec) and the energy of the radiation (since $E = hv$). That is, the higher the wavenumber, the higher the frequency and the greater the energy. Wavenumbers are usually expressed in *reciprocal centimeters*, cm^{-1}, and DAT IR spectra will typically cover the range from 4000 to 1000 cm^{-1}.

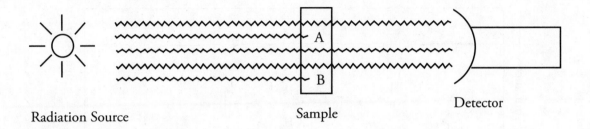

Radiation Source | Sample | Detector

When a bond absorbs IR radiation of a specific frequency, that frequency is not recorded by the detector and is thus seen as a peak in the IR spectrum (since low transmittance corresponds, naturally, to absorbance):

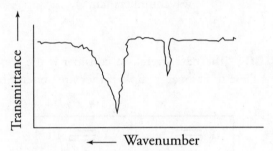

Important Stretching Frequencies

In order to do well on the DAT, it is important that you know the stretching frequencies of the common functional groups. The most important ones are listed below.

The Double Bond Stretch

VERY STRONG AND SHARP

Carbonyls
Centered around
1700 cm^{-1}

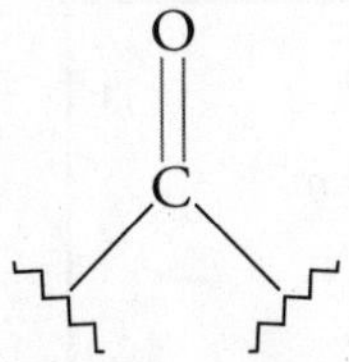

Centered around
1650 cm^{-1}

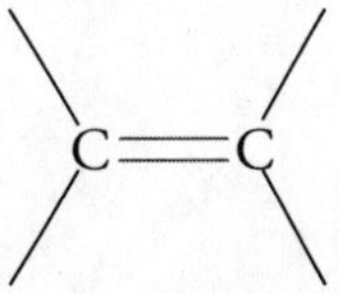

We'll begin by examining the carbonyl, or C=O, stretch. The carbonyl stretch is centered around 1700 cm^{-1} and is very **strong** and very **intense**. *Strength* is reflected in the percent absorbance (or transmittance). *Intensity* is reflected in the sharpness or distinctiveness ("V" shape) of the spike appearing on the spectrum. The carbonyl stretch is one of the most important absorptions, and you should commit its location to memory. In any spectrum, always look for this stretch first. If it is *not* present, you can eliminate a wide range of compounds that contain a carbonyl group, including aldehydes, ketones, carboxylic acids, acid chlorides, esters, amides, and anhydrides. On the other hand, if the carbonyl stretch *is* present, you know that one of the carbonyl-containing functional groups is indeed present.

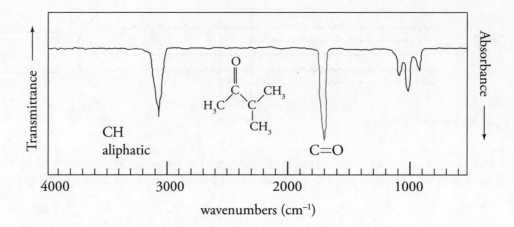

The Triple Bond Stretch

The next stretch to consider is the triple bond. This is an easy one because few molecules possess these functional groups. If they are present, however, the following characteristic stretches will be seen:

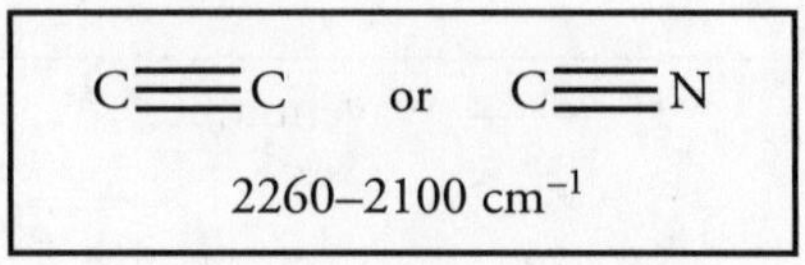

$$C \equiv C \quad \text{or} \quad C \equiv N$$

2260–2100 cm^{-1}

The O—H Stretch

Next we come to the hydroxyl stretch. *The O–H stretch is strong and very broad.* **Strength** is reflected as the degree of absorption a peak displays in the spectrum. **Broadness** is reflected as a wide "U"-shaped appearance on the absorption spectrum, as opposed to a "V," or spiked shape. The broadness is due to hydrogen bonding. Like the carbonyl stretch that occurs at 1700 cm^{-1}, one should always look for the O–H stretch at 3600–3200 cm^{-1}. Amines also have stretches in this region although they vary in intensity. The C–O stretch of the alcohol appears in the 1260–1000 cm^{-1} range of the spectrum, but is a much less important stretch for the DAT.

$$O—H$$

3600–3200 cm^{-1}

Alcohols

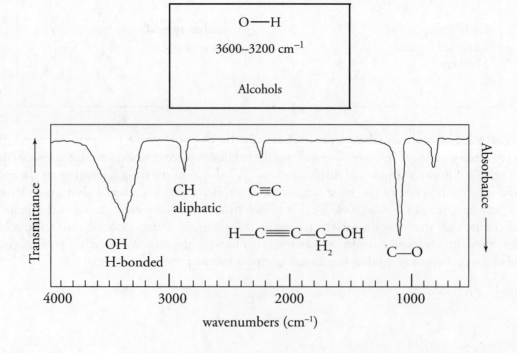

The C—H Stretches   Finally we come to the C–H stretching region (3300–2850 cm^{-1}). Since the vast majority of organic compounds contain C–H bonds, you will almost always see absorbances in this region. Even with the great number of these stretches, there are a few helpful characteristic absorptions in this region. Note that aliphatic C–H bonds stretch at wavenumbers a little less than 3000 cm^{-1}, and aromatic C–H bonds stretch at wavenumbers slightly greater than 3000 cm^{-1}.

C———H   for sp^3 carbon: 3000–2850 cm^{-1}

C———H   for sp^2 carbon: 3150–3000 cm^{-1}

C———H   for sp carbon: 3300 cm^{-1}

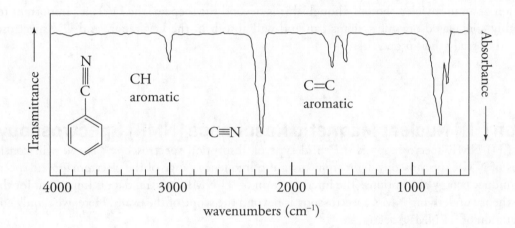

Summary of Relevant Infrared (IR) Stretching Frequencies

Bond	Frequency (Wavenumber) Range (cm^{-1})	Intensity
C=O	1735–1680	strong
C=C	1680–1620	variable
C≡C	2260–2100	variable
C≡N	2260–2220	variable
C—H	3300–2700	variable
N—H	3150–2500	moderate
O—H	3650–3200	broad

Ultraviolet/Visible (UV/Vis) Spectroscopy

UV/Vis spectroscopy is another type of absorption spectroscopy used in organic chemistry. It is very similar to IR, but instead focuses on the slightly shorter, more energetic wavelengths of radiation in the ultraviolet and visible area of the spectrum. Whereas infrared wavelengths are strong enough to induce bending and stretching of covalent bonds, the wavelengths in the UV and visible ranges are strong enough to induce electronic excitation, promoting ground state valence electrons into excited states.

In general, UV/Vis spectroscopy is used with two kinds of molecules. It is very useful in monitoring complexes of transition metals. The easy promotion of electrons from ground to excited states in the closely spaced *d*-orbitals of many transition metals gives them their bright color (by absorbing wavelengths in the visible region), and since many of these promotions involve energies in the UV range, these promotions allow study of these species.

More importantly in organic chemistry, UV/Vis spectroscopy is used to study highly conjugated organic systems. Molecular orbital theory tells us that when molecules have conjugated π-systems, orbitals form many bonding, non-bonding, and anti-bonding orbitals. These orbitals can be reasonably close together in energy, and in fact, close enough to allow promotion of electrons between electronic states through absorption of an ultraviolet photon. Though this is beyond the scope of the DAT, it's important to know that highly conjugated organic systems can and will absorb in the UV range, and UV spectroscopy is often used to study their properties.

Proton (¹H) Nuclear Magnetic Resonance (NMR) Spectroscopy

Proton (¹H) NMR spectroscopy is the third type of absorption spectroscopy that we will consider. In all types of NMR spectroscopy, light from the radio frequency range of the electromagnetic spectrum is used to induce energy absorptions. The interpretation of ¹H NMR spectral data is important for the DAT, but the theory underlying NMR spectroscopy is beyond the scope of the exam. Here, we'll only cover the interpretation of ¹H NMR spectra.

Four essential features of a molecule can be deduced from its ¹H NMR spectrum. First, the number of sets of peaks in the spectrum tells one the number of chemically nonequivalent sets of protons in the molecule. Second, the chemical shift values of those sets of peaks give information about the environment of the protons in that set. Third, the mathematical integration of the sets of peaks indicates the relative numbers of protons in each set. Fourth, the splitting pattern of each set of peaks tells how many protons are interacting with the protons in that set. These four key features of ¹H NMR spectroscopy are explained in the next four sections.

Chemically Equivalent Protons

Determining which protons are **equivalent** in an organic molecule is the first important skill to master with respect to NMR spectroscopy. Equivalent protons in a molecule are those that have *identical electronic environments*. Such protons have identical locations in the ¹H NMR spectrum. Nonequivalent protons will have different locations in the ¹H NMR spectrum. One must be able to determine which protons (or, usually, groups of protons) are equivalent to which other groups, so that you can predict how many distinct NMR signals there will be in a molecule's ¹H NMR spectrum. Protons are considered equivalent if they can be interchanged by a free rotation or a symmetry operation (mirror plane or rotational axis). Check yourself on the following examples:

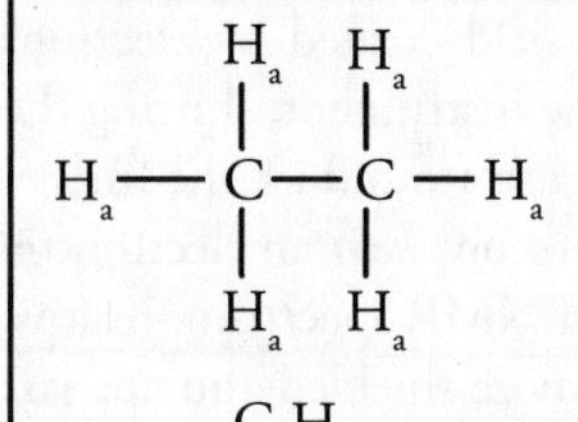

C_2H_6	6 protons	1 NMR signal

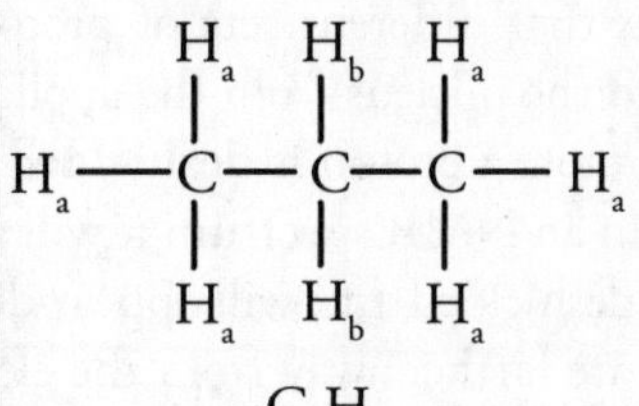

C_3H_8 — 6 H_a protons, 2 H_b protons, 2 NMR signals

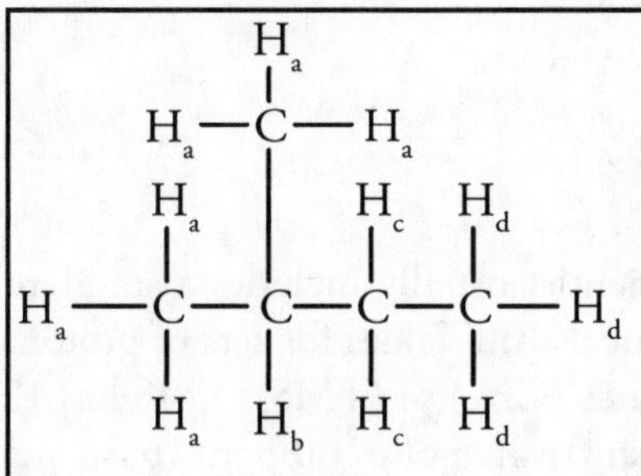

C_5H_{12} — 6 H_a protons, 1 H_b proton, 2 H_c protons, 3 H_d protons, 4 NMR signals

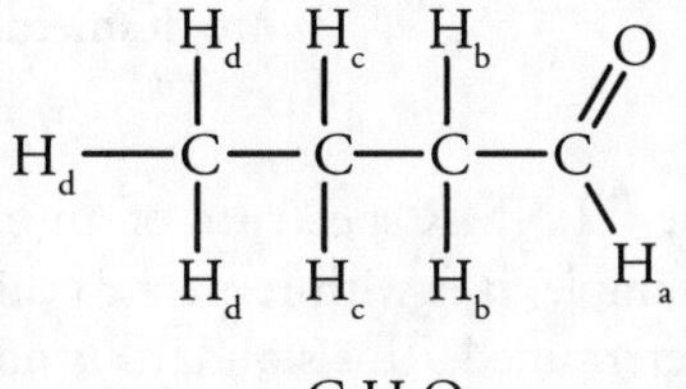

C_4H_8O — 1 H_a proton, 2 H_b protons, 2 H_c protons, 3 H_d protons, 4 NMR signals

Example 29-2: A hydrocarbon C_5H_{12} shows only one peak on its NMR spectrum. Identify its structure.

Solution: Compute the degrees of unsaturation: $n = [2(\#C) + 2 - (\#H)]/2$. In this case, $n = 0$, so there are no double bonds or rings. Because there is only one peak in the NMR, all protons are equivalent, and thus our molecule must be:

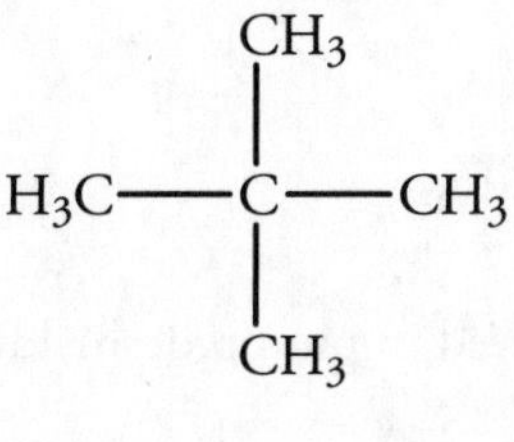

$$H_3C - \underset{\underset{CH_3}{|}}{\overset{\overset{CH_3}{|}}{C}} - CH_3$$

Example 29-3: C_5H_{10} also has an NMR spectrum showing only one peak. Identify.

Solution: Here, $n = [2(\#C) + 2 - (\#H)]/2 = 1$, so the molecule has a double bond or ring. All C_5H_{10} variations with a double bond have more than one type of proton. But in cyclopentane, all hydrogens are equivalent due to the presence of a five-fold axis of symmetry:

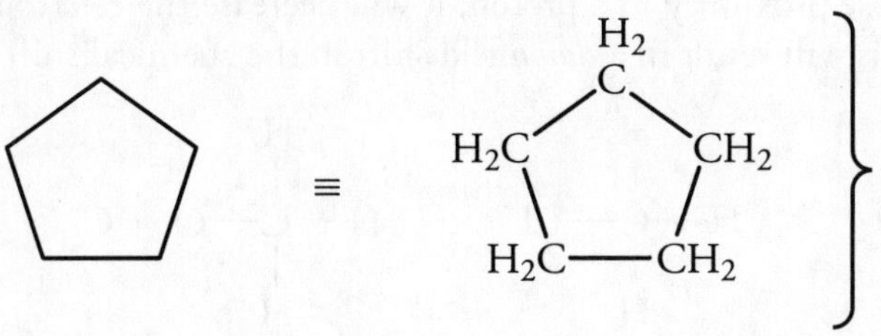

All protons are equivalent.

The Chemical Shift

The location of the resonance (set of peaks) in the ^1H NMR spectrum is referred to as its **chemical shift value**. Differences in the chemical shift values for different sets of protons in a molecule are the result of the differing electronic environments that different sets of protons experience. The magnetic field created by electrons near a proton will **shield** the nucleus from the applied magnetic field created by the instrument, shifting the resonance **upfield**. The more a proton is **deshielded** (i.e., the fewer electrons there are around it), the further **downfield** (to the left) in an NMR spectrum it will appear. For example, a set of protons *near* an electronegative group is said to be deshielded and will appear downfield (to the left) in the ^{1}H NMR spectrum, relative to a set of protons that are farther away from the electronegative group, which is more shielded and appears more upfield (to the right) in the ^{1}H NMR spectrum.

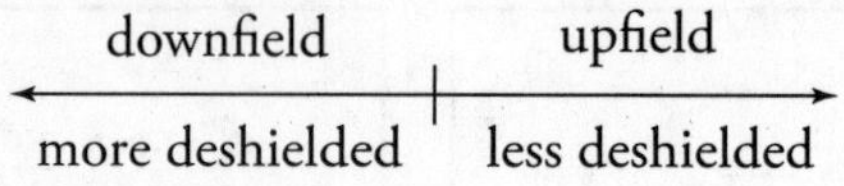

When obtaining the ^{1}H NMR spectrum of an organic molecule, a scientist usually includes a standard reference with the sample. It is with respect to this standard that chemical shift values for sets of protons in a molecule are determined. This standard is normally *tetramethylsilane,* $(CH_3)_4Si$ (TMS). TMS has 12 chemically equivalent protons that are arbitrarily assigned a chemical shift value of $\delta = 0$ ppm (**p**arts **p**er **m**illion). It turns out that the protons of TMS are very shielded compared to most other protons in common organic molecules, so the resonances of almost all protons will appear to the left (downfield, or more deshielded) of the TMS peak. The inclusion of TMS as a standard allows chemists to reliably compare their results with one another.

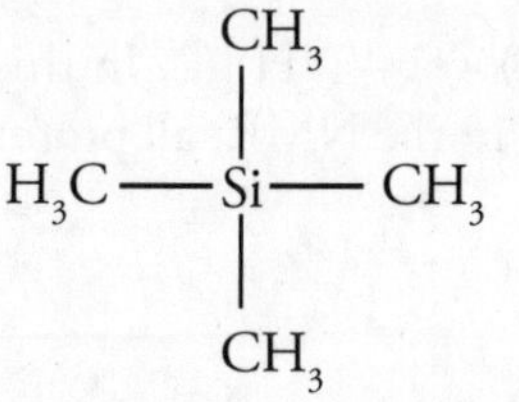

12 equivalent protons are assigned a chemical shift of $\delta = 0$ ppm.

Tetramethylsilane (TMS)

We now briefly examine the factors involved in proton deshielding. These include:

1. the electronegativity of the neighboring atoms,
2. hybridization, and
3. acidity and hydrogen bonding.

Electronegativity Effects on Chemical Shift Values

If an electronegative atom is in close proximity to a proton, it will decrease the electron density near the proton and thereby deshield it. This will result in a *down*field shift in the chemical shift value. Examples:

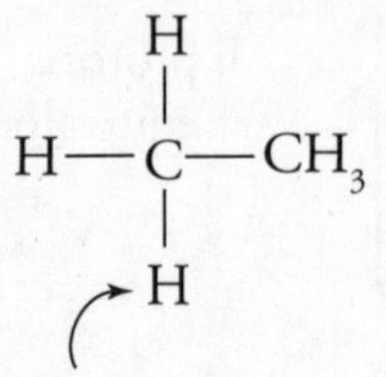

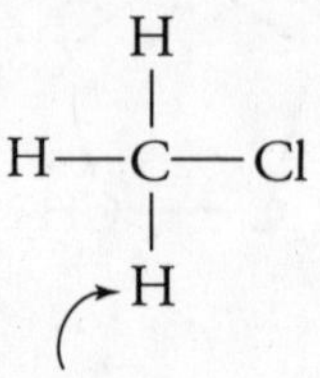

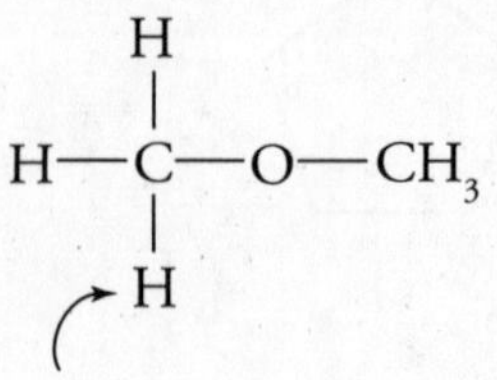

The spectrum of methyl acetate below shows how the two electronegative groups in the molecule (the O of the ester and the carbonyl) contribute to shifting both methyl signals downfield.

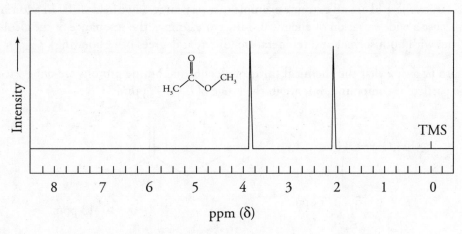

Hybridization Effects on Chemical Shift Values

The **hybridization effect** occurs as a result of the varying bond characteristics of carbon atoms *connected* to the hydrogens. The greater the *s* orbital character of a C–H bond, the less electron density on the hydrogen. Thus, when considering the hybridization effect alone, the greater the *s* orbital character, the more deshielded the set of protons is, which will result in a downfield shift for the peak corresponding to that set of protons. Here are two examples:

$$H_3C—C≡C—H$$

$$δ = 2 \text{ ppm}$$

$$δ = 6 \text{ ppm}$$

Hybridization effects alone would indicate the alkyne proton to be more deshielded than the alkene proton. However, due to a more complicated physical phenomenon (anisotropy), this turns out not to be the case. Another very characteristic chemical shift you should remember is that of the aromatic protons ($δ = 6–8$ ppm). A peak in an NMR spectrum in this region is highly indicative of an aromatic compound (usually a substituted benzene).

$$δ = 6–8 \text{ ppm}$$

Acidity and Hydrogen Bonding Effects on Chemical Shift Values

Protons that are attached to **heteroatoms** (oxygen and nitrogen, for example) are quite deshielded. Acidic protons on a carboxylic acid are an extreme example of a very large downfield shift. In addition, hydrogen bonding can cause a wide variation of chemical shift. For example, the resonance of the alcohol proton in methanol varies with both solvent and temperature (different degrees of H bonding).

You should also be aware that the chemical shifts of alcohol and amine protons are quite variable depending upon the particular compound, but are in the range of δ = 1–5 ppm.

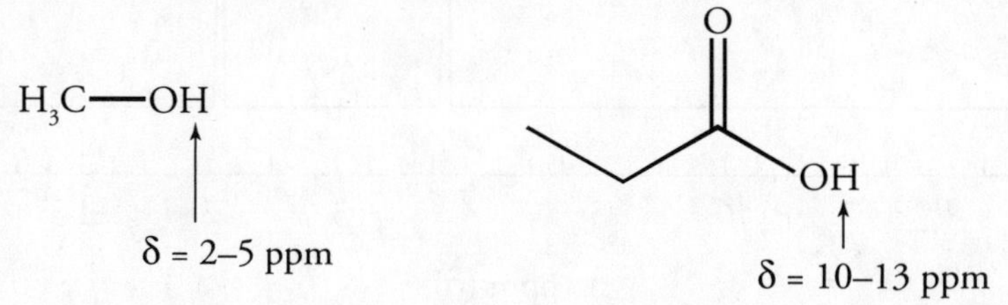

$$H_3C\text{—}OH$$

δ = 2–5 ppm

δ = 10–13 ppm

As with IR stretching frequencies, memorizing some commonly encountered ^{1}H NMR chemical shift values will be helpful. Below is a correlation chart for some common chemical shifts:

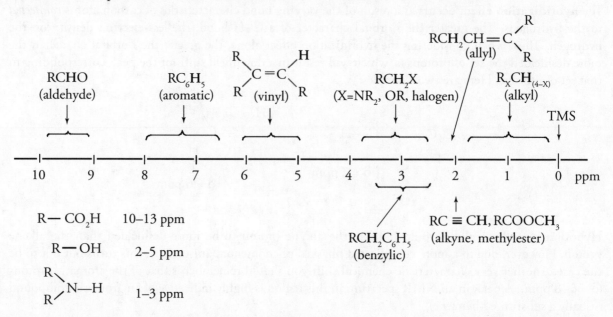

Integration

The third important piece of information obtained from the ^{1}H NMR spectrum of a molecule is the mathematical integration. As the NMR instrument obtains a spectrum of the sample, it performs a mathematical calculation, called an **integration**, thereby measuring the area under each absorption peak (resonance). The calculated area under each peak is proportional to the relative number of protons giving rise to each peak. Thus, the integration indicates the relative number of protons in each set in the molecule.

Splitting

The fourth and final aspect of NMR spectroscopy that you should be familiar with is the **spin-spin splitting phenomenon**. This occurs when protons interact with other protons that are not equivalent to it. Protons that are not equivalent can interact because the magnetic field felt by a proton is influenced by surrounding protons. This effect tends to fall off with distance, but it can often extend over two adjacent carbons. Nearby protons that are nonequivalent to the proton in question will cause a splitting in the observed ^1H NMR signal. The degree of splitting depends on the number of adjacent hydrogens, and a signal will be split $n + 1$ times, where n is the number of neighboring (interacting) protons. The important information one must determine is how a proton or a group of chemically equivalent protons will be split by their hydrogen neighbors.

This is best demonstrated by an example:

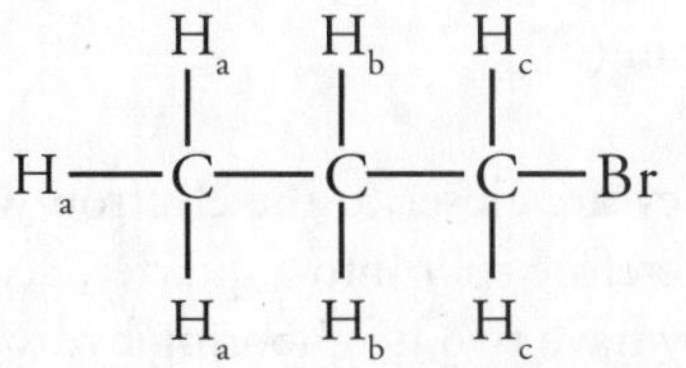

Three distinct types of hydrogens:
3 H_a hydrogens
2 H_b hydrogens
2 H_c hydrogens

H_a protons split into three peaks due to the two neighboring, but different, H_b protons.

H_b protons split into six peaks due to the five neighboring, but different, H_a and H_c protons.

H_c protons split into three peaks due to the two neighboring, but different, H_b protons.

Note that, for DAT purposes, the H_a and H_c protons neighboring H_b do not have to be equivalent in order to add them together to get $n = 5$.

$n + 1$ RULE

n = Number of neighboring nonequivalent hydrogens	Splitting ($n + 1$)
0	1—Singlet
1	2—Doublet
2	3—Triplet
3	4—Quartet
4	5—Quintet (or multiplet)
5	6—Sextet (or multiplet)

Consider the NMR spectrum of CH_3CH_2I:

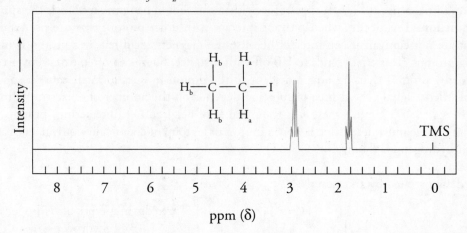

The α-hydrogens are farther downfield because they are closer to the electron-withdrawing iodine atom. They have three neighboring hydrogens and are therefore split into a quartet, according to the $n + 1$ rule. The β-hydrogens are split into a triplet because they have two neighboring hydrogens.

Example 29-4: How many ^1H NMR signals would you expect to find for the following molecules? What is the splitting pattern of each signal? Also indicate which protons would be shifted the farthest downfield.

A.

B.

C.

D.

Solution:

A. Three signals. C1's equivalent protons (which will be the farthest downfield) are split by two Hs on C2 to make a triplet. C2's protons (which are a bit more shielded than C1's) are split by a total of five Hs on C1 and C3 to make a sextet, or multiplet. C3's protons are split by two Hs on C2 to make a triplet.

B. One signal; all are equivalent, therefore no splitting.

C. Four signals. C1's equivalent protons are split by two Hs on C2 to make a triplet and appear the farthest downfield. C2's protons are split by a total of three Hs on C1 and C3 to make a quartet, which is more shielded. C3's proton is split by eight neighboring protons to make a multiplet. C4 and C5 have equivalent protons, split by C3's proton and forming the most shielded signal, a doublet.

D. Three signals. The most downfield proton signal is from the one on C3 (the one bearing the Br). It is split by three Hs on C4 to make a quartet. Slightly more shielded are the Hs on C4, split by the one H on C3 to yield a doublet. The remaining Hs on the *tert*-butyl group are equivalent (nine total), are the most shielded, and have no neighbors, making them appear as a singlet.

Carbon (^{13}C) Nuclear Magnetic Resonance (NMR) Spectroscopy

Carbon (^{13}C) spectroscopy is the third type of absorption spectroscopy that is important for the DAT. Many of the same principles discussed for ^{1}H NMR also apply to ^{13}C NMR; there are, however, a few important differences.

Carbon (^{13}C) Chemical Shifts

The range of chemical shifts for ^{13}C nuclei is much larger than the range for ^{1}H nuclei. Typically, the ^{13}C can span a range of about 200 ppm. The same effects that shield and deshield ^{1}H nuclei affect ^{13}C nuclei as well. The following chart should give you a general idea of ^{13}C shifts:

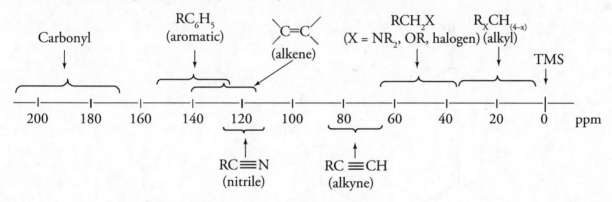

For example, the ^{13}C NMR spectrum of an ester is shown below.

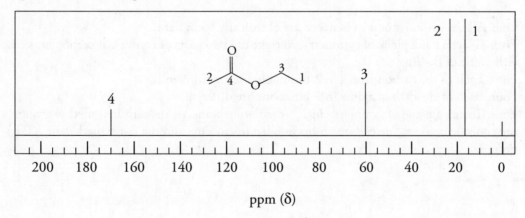

ppm (δ)

Integration

Unlike ^{1}H NMR, ^{13}C NMR spectra cannot be integrated meaningfully. The area under each peak is *not* exactly proportional to the number of carbons giving rise to that peak; however, the height of each peak does roughly correspond to the number of hydrogens that are attached to a particular carbon. The more hydrogens attached to a particular carbon, the taller the peak. So, a CH_3 peak would be taller than a CH_2 peak, which would be taller than a CH peak, and so on.

Splitting

Carbon NMR data are usually collected such that no splitting of the peaks occurs. Therefore, each ^{13}C peak will appear as a singlet.

Example 29-5: How many ^{13}C signals would you expect to find for each of the following molecules?

A.

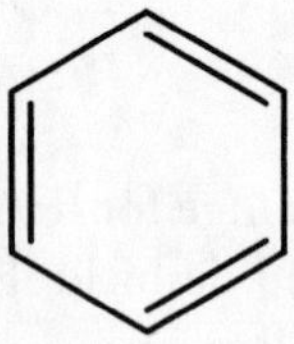

B.

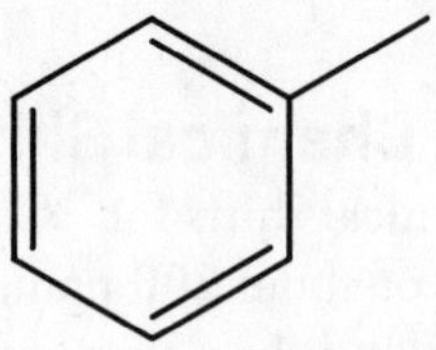

C.

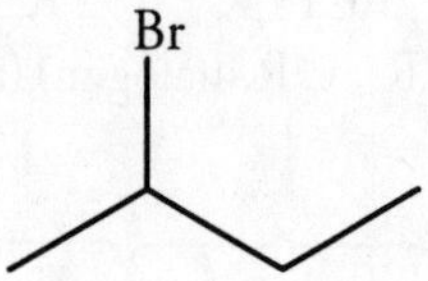

D.

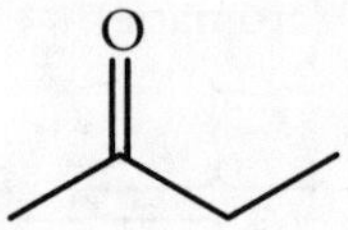

E.

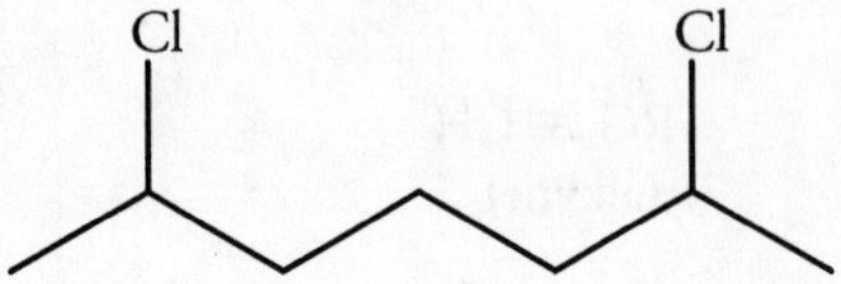

Solution:

A. One. All the carbon atoms in benzene are chemically equivalent.
B. Five. Toluene has a plane of symmetry, so there are two pairs of equivalent carbon atoms on either side of the ring.
C. Four. Each of the carbon atoms in 2-bromobutane are different.
D. Four. Each of the carbon atoms in 2-butanone are different.
E. Four. There's a plane of symmetry in 2,6-dichloroheptane, so the terminal methyl groups are equivalent, as are the carbon atoms bonded to chlorine and the outer methylene (CH_2) groups.

Perceptual Ability Test (PAT)

Chapter 30
Introduction to the PAT

30.1 INTRODUCTION TO THE PAT

The Perceptual Ability Test (or the PAT) is the second section of the DAT. It requires you to answer a total of 90 questions—broken down into six sections of 15 questions each—in 60 minutes! Since that is an average of just 40 seconds per question, you will not have the chance to look carefully at many of the questions, nor will you have the chance to ponder the answer choices.

Furthermore, the PAT is probably unlike anything you have done before, so gaining familiarity with it is an important first step toward doing well. Although the PAT is the only section of the DAT that is not included in the Academic Average, it is an important individual score for many dental schools. You can usually score a respectable 20 in this section by only getting 70–75 questions right. Therefore, you should not worry if you cannot answer every question. Instead, you should concentrate on four big things to maximize your performance on the PAT:

1. Practice as much as you can.
2. Through this practice, discover which sections you are good at, and which are more challenging for you.
3. On the exam, spend less time on the questions that are more challenging for you.
4. Do not leave any blanks.

There are six sections of the PAT, each containing 15 questions:

Part	Section	Questions	Answer Choices	Summary
1	Apertures	1–15	A–E	Passing a three-dimensional figure through an aperture (or opening)
2	Orthographic Projections	16–30	A–D	Identifying front, top, or side views of solid three-dimensional objects
3	Angle Ranking	31–45	A–D	Ranking four angles in order from smallest to largest measure
4	Hole Punching	46–60	A–E	Punching and counting holes in a folded square sheet of paper
5	Cube Counting	61–75	A–E	Painting the outside of a stack of cubes and counting the painted faces
6	Form Development	76–90	A–D	Folding a flat pattern into a three-dimensional figure

Notice that half of the PAT sections (Parts 2, 3, and 6) have 4 answer choices per question, while the other half (Parts 1, 4, and 5) have 5 answer choices per question.

Each of these sections has its own challenges, and different people will have different preferences. For example, many people find Hole Punching easier and Form Development very hard. Others may actually enjoy Cube Counting but struggle with Apertures. Through practice, you will learn what your preferences are. Many people rank the relative difficulty of the sections as follows:

Easy:	Cube Counting
Medium:	Angle Ranking and Hole Punching
Difficult:	Apertures, Orthographic Projections, and Form Development

This ranking is by no means universal. It is up to you to make your own ranking. This is important, because it will affect the order in which you approach questions on the PAT. You should always do the sections that you find easier—and get the most correct answers on—first. Then tackle questions that you find harder and answer correctly less frequently. For example, a lot of people do the PAT sections in this order: Cube Counting, Angle Ranking, Hole Punching, Apertures, Form Development, Orthographic Projections. You may even decide to completely skip an entire section of 15 questions, and devote all the time you save to improving your performance on the other sections. This is not a bad idea, particularly if there's a section in which you consistently struggle and have low accuracy. Alternatively, you can aim to complete each of the six sections, but skip a few very challenging questions in each.

30.2   PAT STRATEGIES

Skipping Questions and Guessing Answers

As discussed in Chapter 1, the DAT is not created to be completed. Very few successful DAT-takers complete every question or even spend time on every question. One of the easiest ways to see score improvements in the PAT is to skip a small number of questions and spend time on others you are more likely to get right. Remember, accuracy over speed! That said, you should never leave blanks on the DAT, and the best option for guessing is to use your Letter of the Day (which we also discussed in Chapter 1; go back there now if you need a refresher on these core DAT strategies!). However, there is another option for the PAT. You may find it more beneficial to pick your first impression. Some people find they have relatively high accuracy doing this; others do not and should stick with the Letter of the Day. You should sit down with a PAT section and try out each strategy, so you can pick the one that works best for you.

Two-Pass Technique

Each PAT question will fall into one of three categories:

Category 1	"Now" Questions	You can answer the question accurately within 10–30 seconds.
Category 2	"Later" Questions	You can answer the question accurately, but it takes a little longer, say 40–60 seconds.
Category 3	"Never" Questions	You could spend 2 painful minutes or more on the question and still not feel like you've answered it correctly.

Your approach to the PAT section should involve two passes through the section. On the first pass, do something to every question: answer your Now questions, mark your Later questions for a revisit on your second pass, and fill in an answer on the Never questions. Do not spend time reading or trying to work through these never questions. Use one of the two guessing strategies described above.

With study and practice, you will feel confident about your answers to approximately 50–60 questions on your first pass, and then have 15–20 minutes left. On the second pass, you should take as much time as you need to be accurate, but if a question begins to frustrate you, you should guess and move on. Think of the points on your second pass as a bonus. Time will probably run out before you finish, so you should not be surprised or disappointed when it does; make sure you have an answer selected for every question before time runs out. When you take practice exams, make sure you follow and practice this Two-Pass Technique strictly. Learning which questions to work on the first pass and which to mark for the second pass will pay off on the real DAT.

Pacing

We've already talked about how you should work the sections you feel more confident on before you do the sections you are not as comfortable with. In addition, your pace through the questions and sections will change. Some sections you will be able to move quickly through and others will take more time. Although you have 40 seconds per question (on average), some you will answer in 10 seconds and others will take up to 60–90 seconds. Generally, you shouldn't spend more than two minutes on any given question.

Finally, many people find they slow down as they progress through a 15-question section of the PAT. This is because the sections usually go from easy to hard. If there is a section you find difficult, it can be a good idea to aim to answer the first few questions in this section and then guess using your Letter of the Day on all the rest (rather that writing off the entire section). This is a great way to use the easy-to-hard setup for your benefit.

Improving Your Score

The following chapters break down each section of the PAT and give you strategies for working the questions. The first step is to know and understand the rules for each section. After the rules, there are section-specific strategies and techniques to master through practice. You must be aware of the typical trap answers that question writers will use to trick you into choosing a wrong answer, as well as how to use the noteboards and POE on each question type.

Chapter 31
Apertures

Chapter 31
Apertures

743

Apertures questions are also known as keyhole questions. These will always be the first 15 questions of the PAT, and every question will have five answer choices for you to pick from.

The goal of the Apertures section is to place a three-dimensional object through an opening (the word "aperture" means "opening"). This is similar to a common child's toy called a "shape sorter." You are given one three-dimensional drawing per question and five possible openings in the answer choices. For example:

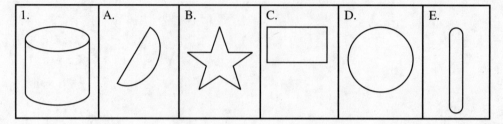

In this question, D is the correct answer. The cylinder is turned so that the base is passed through the aperture.

31.1 THE RULES

Here are the rules you should follow in Apertures questions:

1. A three-dimensional object will be shown on the left and will be followed by outlines of five apertures.
2. Consider how the object looks from all directions (rather than from a single direction as shown); select the opening the object could pass through if the proper side were inserted first.
3. Prior to passing through the aperture, the irregular solid object may be turned in any direction. It may be started through the aperture on a side not shown.
4. Once the object is started through the aperture, it may not be twisted or turned. It must pass completely through the opening.
5. The opening is always the exact shape of the appropriate external outline of the object.
6. Both objects and apertures are drawn to the same scale. Thus it is possible for an opening to be the correct shape but too small or too large for the object. In all cases, however, differences are large enough to judge by eye.
7. There are no irregularities in any hidden portion of the object. However, if the figure has symmetric indentations, the hidden portion is symmetric with the part shown.
8   For each object there is only one correct aperture.

Take note of the third rule. The object may be turned, rotated, flipped (or all of the above) before attempting to pass it through the opening. However, according to rule four, once the object begins its trip through the opening it cannot be turned, rotated, or flipped any more.

Example 31-1:

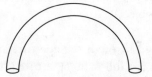

This object could be inserted end-first into a circular aperture, but as you approach the bend it would get stuck unless you were to turn it again as you were passing in through the aperture. This cannot be done on the PAT:

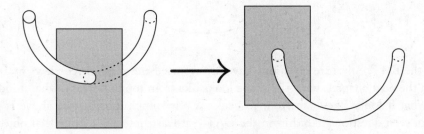

However, an object can be turned in any direction before passing through the aperture. For example, this object can be rotated sideways to fit through a small, circular aperture such as:

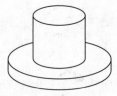

Example 31-2:

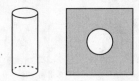

This object (we will call it the disc with cylinder on top) can be turned and slotted through any of these apertures:

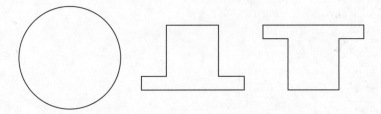

If you pass the base disc through first or the cylinder side first, the aperture on the left would be correct. If you were to pass the object through sideways, then the middle figure would be correct. Also, if you flip the disc with cylinder on top over first and then pass it through sideways, it would be as seen in the third figure. Note whether it is bottom first or top first, the same aperture would be correct (remember, we are only concerned with the outline of the object).

Technically, the object can also be passed through the aperture at any angle. For example, the disc with cylinder on top could also pass through the following aperture if it is not turned at all:

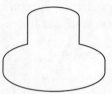

However, on the DAT, Aperture questions have always used the same three views of an object you will learn about in the next chapter: what the shape looks like from top to bottom, what it looks like from side to side, and what it looks like from front to back. While something like the above is theoretically possible, we've not seen questions like this on the DAT—at least not so far. Note that objects and apertures are drawn to the same scale (and without perspective). If an opening is narrower on the top than at the bottom, then the original object must really be narrower at the top than at the bottom. Below is a sample of a highway. The drawing on the left is with perspective; the drawing on the right is without perspective.

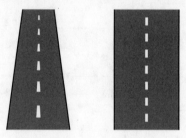

Perspective   No perspective

On the Apertures section of the PAT, the writers never use perspective. If an object appears smaller in the background than in the foreground, it is truly smaller on one side than the other. However, objects are usually drawn rotated a little to one side, so you can see two views of the object (the front and one side) at the same time; this is called an isometric projection.

31.2 STRATEGIES

Three Views

Because of the way the DAT presents the answer choices in Apertures questions, you can do some process of elimination by thinking about what the shape would look like from its three views (top to bottom, side to side, front to back). Compare this to the answer choices you're given, and you can usually eliminate at least a few bad options. If you can't do this right now, don't worry too much about it. We're going to revisit the concept of top/front/end in the next chapter!

The Dark Side of the Object

It often turns out that the answer to an Aperture question looks like one face of the object. Often this will be a side that is facing away from you (or the "dark side" of the object). There are some examples below. These examples show a 3-dimensional object, its 2-dimensional view from the indicated side (middle image), and an aperture the object could fit through from this vantage point (right image with gray perimeter). In each of these, the left image could be the question stem of an Apertures question, and the right image would be the correct answer.

Example 31-3:

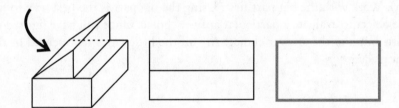

Example 31-4:

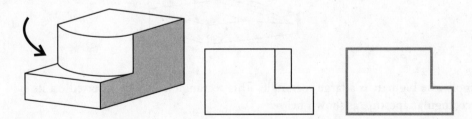

Example 31-5:

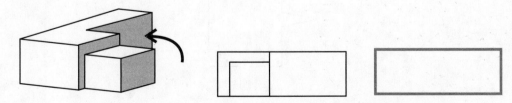

Example 31-6:

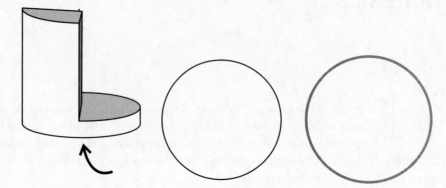

Example 31-7:

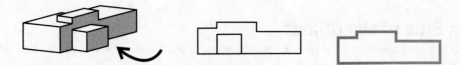

Big Part, Little Parts

Often the object will be made up of one big part with a few smaller features (for example, ridges added or trenches cut out). Work with the big part first. Using the big part is the best way to figure out how to begin orienting the object to evaluate a particular answer choice. Once you have figured this out, you can focus on specific attributes of the answer choice: Are all the little parts represented in the aperture? Are they all in the right places?

Example 31-8:

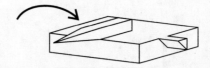

In this example, the big part is a large rectangle. This rectangle could be inserted on its side (as shown) through a rectangular aperture as shown below:

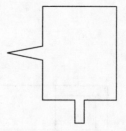

After taking into account the big part (the rectangle), then decide what shapes the little parts (or details) will require; here we have the pointed wedge on top and the triangular wedge on the side. Be aware of the orientation of these shapes once the big part is inserted through the aperture. For example, the little part on the right side of the 3D shape above will require a rectangular aperture, not a triangular aperture. The pointed part of this little arm (pointing down in the shape above) will not matter when passed through the opening as we've drawn it. Beware that mixing up parts of shapes like this is a very common trap in Apertures questions. You must keep track of the relative orientation of big and little parts of shapes.

By way of summary:

Work with the big part of a shape first and do POE. Then figure out how to orient the object for the answer choices and ask yourself:

- Do the answer choices have all the little parts they should?
- Are they in the right places?
- Do they have the right dimensions?

The same object can also be passed through the following aperture:

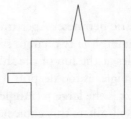

Here, again, the large rectangle is the primary concern. However, the little parts will be in a different orientation because the shape was rotated before being passed through the opening.

The Outline of the Object

Remember, we are only concerned with the outline of the object as it passes through the aperture. A cylinder sticking straight out from a block won't affect the outline of the object if the cylinder is passed through first or if the face opposite the cylinder is passed through first.

Example 31-9:

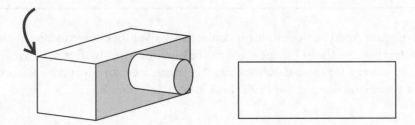

The cylinder protruding from the right side of the rectangular solid (above) will not affect the aperture if the cylinder side or the side opposite the cylinder is introduced through the aperture first.

When questions focus on the perimeter of a shape, you'll need a systematic plan of attack. Find a good starting place, like a distinctive region you'll be able to quickly find in each answer choice. Then walk around the outline of the object and do process of elimination (POE) as you go around each answer choice. These perimeter questions are common on the DAT and could test you on features such as curves, indents or protruding pieces. The answer choices usually all look really similar except for subtle differences in the presence, placement, or dimensions of these features.

You'll likely see at least a few perimeter Apertures questions on test day. Many versions of the test have four to six questions like this. Let's work through an example:

Example 31-10:

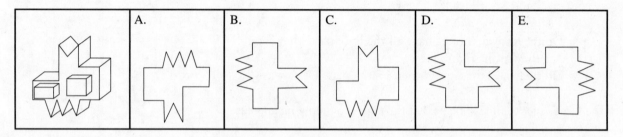

Based on the answer choices, this is a classic perimeter Apertures question. This means you should focus on the perimeter of the rear shape and ignore the two cubes stuck to the front of the 3D shape. Find a noticeable start spot (e.g., the two triangles at the top of the shape) and walk around the answer choices doing POE. The dip between the two triangles is too deep in A (eliminate this choice); this feature looks OK in the rest of the answer choices. Next is the large rectangle at the right side of the shape in the question stem; this rectangle is too thin in B (eliminate this choice) but looks good in C, D, and E. Next are the triangles at the bottom of the shape; these are shifted over in choice E (eliminate this choice) but look good in C and D. The last part of the 3D shape is the smaller rectangle at the left side. This is too short in C (eliminate this choice) and by POE, the correct answer is D. Notice that the small rectangle on the left side is also too large in B (another reason to eliminate this choice). Here is a summary of your POE reasons:

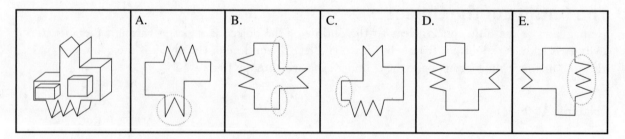

One version of perimeter Apertures questions is commonly called rock or gemstone questions. These are challenging questions because the 3D shape given in the question stem is often very irregular and hard to imagine in 3D. The strategy for these questions stays the same: look for distinctive features, work around the perimeter in a systematic way, rely on POE. Let's look at an example.

Example 31-11:

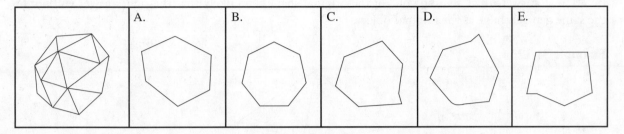

This question will require some careful comparisons between the 3D rock in the question stem and the answer choices. On your first pass, eliminate B and D. The shape is too irregular to match choice B and doesn't have any curved edges (as in D). Next, let's focus on the perimeter; the rock has a six-sided pyramid at the top of the shape. This is present at the top of choice A, the right side of choice C, and the bottom of choice E. However, the bottom of choice A is too wide, and this aperture doesn't have enough edges (eliminate A). The top of choice E is too wide and too flat to match the rock (eliminate E). By POE, the correct answer must be choice C. The rock is going through the aperture in this direction, with the aperture in gray dotted lines:

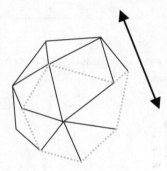

These questions can be a large waste of time, so if you're doing these questions on test day (vs. answering using your Letter of the Day), keep your eye on the clock!

Trap Answers

Be wary of answers that "remind you" of the original shape. It is likely that the right answer will not be the same general shape as the original object.

Example 31-12:

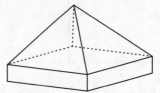

Many people focus on the triangle part of this shape right away. There might be trap answers that are basic triangles without the rectangular solid on the bottom:

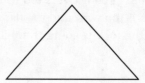

This is not correct. The correct right answer may be either of the two following apertures. The dark side of the object is the bottom, which is a square:

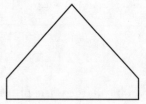

Another trap pattern here is that the DAT will present apertures that combine aspects of the top/front/end views of a 3D shape. If you can spot this pattern, it can be an easy strike-out and time-saver.

Best Fit

You want the answer choice that is the "best fit." That is, the edges of the object should be sliding perfectly through the aperture. For example, this object:

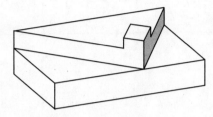

could pass through all apertures below, as demonstrated with a dotted line:

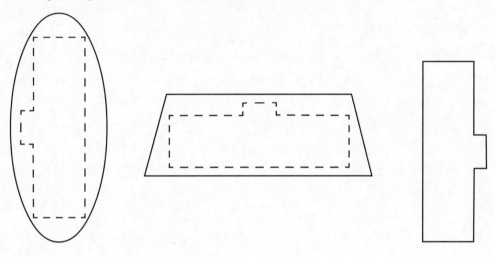

However, only the final aperture is the "best fit."

Pacing

Generally, you will come to a decision on these questions rapidly or, just as rapidly, find that you have very little idea what the answer is. If you're struggling, compare the answer choices to the shape in the question stem and see if this helps you eliminate any choices. If you still can't find the best answer, pick the Letter of the Day and move on.

Want More Practice?
Scan the QR code below to register your book for online chapter summaries, drills, practice tests, and more!

Chapter 32
Orthographic
Projections

Orthographic Projections questions are also known as view recognition, top/front/end, or T/F/E questions. These are always the second set of 15 questions on the PAT (questions 16–30) and will have four answer choices per question. In Orthographic Projections, you are again given a three-dimensional shape. However, you are only presented with two two-dimensional "views" of the shape, and you must determine what the third "view" of the shape should be. A lot of people think this means you must figure out what a three-dimensional object looks like based on only two two-dimensional views of the object, but if you have some solid strategies to use, this is not necessarily the case and can in fact be a giant waste of precious time. Many people find Orthographic Projections to be a difficult section of the PAT. If you find this to be the case, you could come back to this section after you have finished the others.

The following is a basic example of an orthographic projections question. In this example, you are given the Top View and Front View and are asked to find the correct End View:

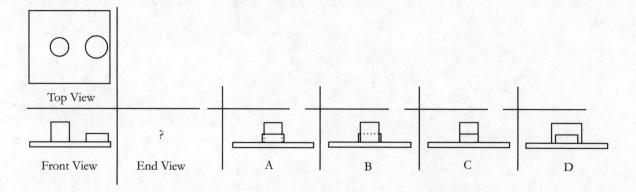

A is the correct answer, and once we review some strategies and techniques, you'll see why.

32.1   THE RULES

Here are the rules you should keep in mind for Orthographic Projections questions:

1.   There will always be three views of a 3D object: top, front, and end.
2.   All views are drawn without perspective.
3.   The Top View looks down on the shape (like a bird's-eye view) and is drawn in the upper left-hand corner. The projection looking at the object from the front (Front View) is shown in the lower left-hand corner. The projection looking at the object from the right side (called the End View) is shown in the lower right-hand corner. These views are always in the same positions and are labeled accordingly.
4.   Lines that cannot be seen on the surface in a particular view are dotted or dashed in that view.
5.   In each question, two views will be shown with four alternatives to complete the set.
6.   For each question, there is only one correct projection or view.

It is important to keep in mind the three-dimensional orientation of the three views:

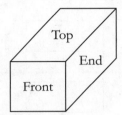

Most importantly, the End View is always from the right side of the figure.

Another important rule to keep in mind is the significance of dotted and solid lines. Solid lines are edges (or "features") that can be seen from the view shown (Top, Front, or End). Dotted or dashed lines are features that cannot be seen but are within or on the other side of the object. For example, let's work with a paper towel roll:

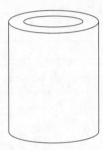

The views for this shape would be:

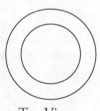   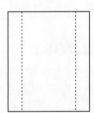   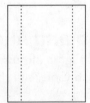

Top View   Front View   End View

The dotted lines in the Front and End Views are the hole down the center of the tube. Let's do another example:

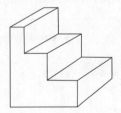

If you look at this object from the right (or the End View), the stairs would face you and the object would look like this:

However, if the stairs were turned away from you the two-dimensional representation would have dotted lines as seen here:

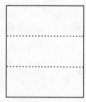

Note on both two-dimensional representations that the front edge of each step and the rear edge of each step line up and so only a single line (solid or dotted) is used.

32.2   STRATEGIES

Counting and Aligning Features

Counting and aligning features is the most important strategy for Orthographic Projections. A **feature** is a corner, edge, or hole, and the number and placement of features must line up between the three views, using these rules:

- Horizontal features in the Front View must match horizontal features in the End View
- Vertical features in the Top View must match vertical features in the Front View
- Horizontal features in the Top View must match vertical features in the End View

To demonstrate this strategy, let's use the paper towel roll again. Here are how the features line up:

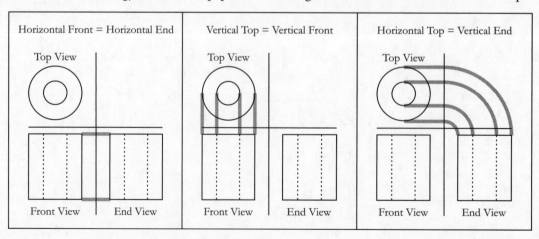

When you are taking the DAT, you can run your fingertip across the screen or hold the noteboard up to the screen to line up features. In either case, be sure not to touch the actual computer screen. If the number or placement of features doesn't match using these rules, the answer choice is wrong and can be eliminated. Also note that you don't have to count the very edge or external boundaries of the views; every shape has a perimeter. Focusing on internal features can save time.

Example 32-1:

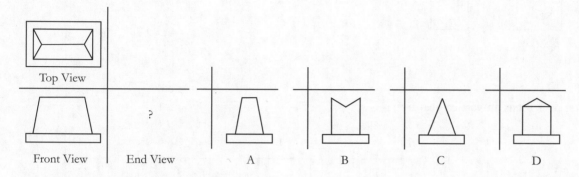

First let's deal with the horizontal features:

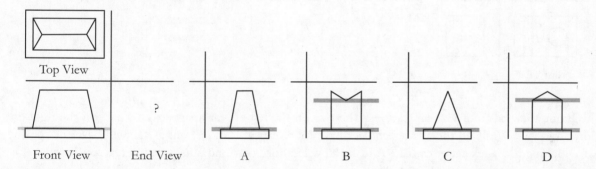

The Front View has one horizontal feature and B and D have two, so they cannot be the answer. Next, let's look at horizontal Top View features, as they become vertical End View features:

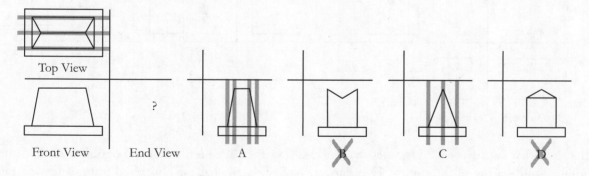

The Top View has three evenly spaced horizontal features, so the correct answer must have three evenly spaced vertical features. The correct answer must be C.

Example 32-2:

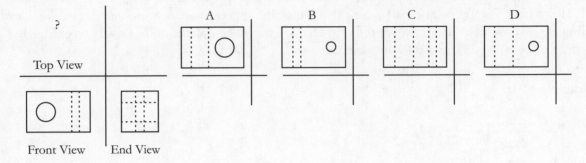

First, let's focus on vertical features:

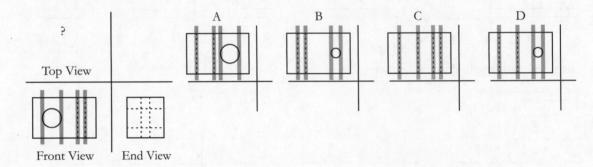

The Front View has four vertical features. The two on the left are far apart and the two on the right are closer together. While all the answer choices have four vertical features, only C and D have the spacing we're looking for. The answer can't be A or B. Now let's focus on End View vertical features because they turn into horizontal Top View features:

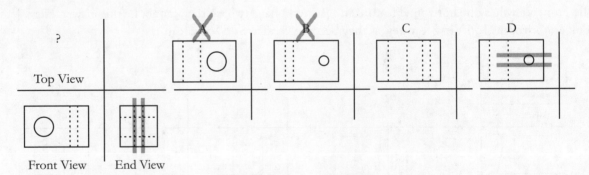

The End View has two vertical features that are close together. We need an answer option with the same number and spacing of features, so D is correct. Notice that C has no horizontal features (except the outside boundaries, which we are not counting to save time).

While counting and aligning features won't always lead you directly to the correct answer, it is a great strategy to help with POE and pacing. You may still need to do some visualizing of the figure, so let's review some other useful techniques.

Common Patterns

To master Orthographic Projections, it is also important to understand the views of some common shapes.

Example 32-3: End View

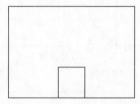

This could be one of several three-dimensional shapes (a few possibilities are shown):

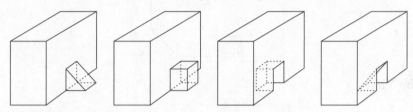

Example 32-4: Top View

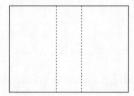

This could be the top view of any of the following three-dimensional shapes:

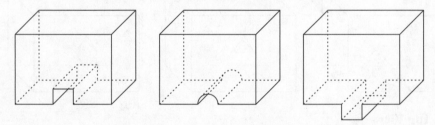

Also note that with any of these objects, the "tunnels" running through them (or the projections on the bottom of them) could be at an angle and the top two-dimensional representations would remain the same. For example:

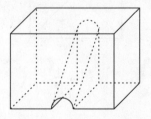

Additionally, the dotted lines could represent a "tunnel" running through the middle of the object. Here are some examples:

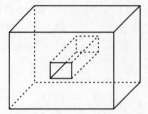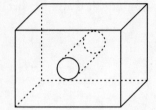

As mentioned earlier, these could also be at an angle:

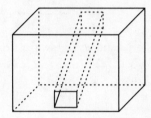

Example 32-5: Top View

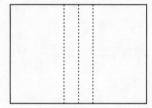

This two dimensional representation could be either a triangular cutout/tunnel or a diamond-shaped cutout as shown below:

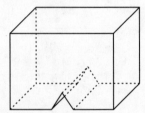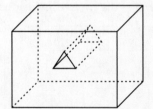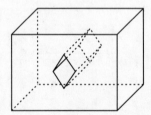

Example 32-6: Top View

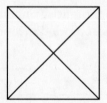

This could be either of the shapes below (pyramid or inverted pyramid):

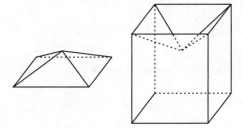

Section Strategies

For most students, Orthographic Projections are one of the most time-consuming and difficult of the PAT sections. It would be reasonable to just mark these questions on your first pass, then come back and try them out after all the other sections have been completed. However, if this is one of your better sections of the PAT, then you should spend time on these in your first pass. POE can be particularly useful on this section, because there will be some answers that are missing solid lines/dotted lines where they need to be and thus can be eliminated.

If counting aligning features isn't enough to answer a question, you have a few additional options:

- Try to figure out the shape or perimeter of the missing view, based on the views you are given, and how they fold together to form a 3D shape. Compare the answer choices to the perimeter you need and do POE.
- Determine which features you should be able to see (i.e., solid lines) and which you cannot (i.e., dotted lines). How many of each should there be? Count and then compare this to each answer choice you have left as a possibility; do POE. Where should they be located or placed? Again, compare the answer choices you have left to the question stem and do POE.
- Watch for symmetry. If one of the views has some lines of symmetry, it is common for the two other views to be the same as each other. This isn't true 100% of the time, but is a common pattern and something worth spotting on test day. Recognizing patterns of symmetry can help you zero in on good answer choices right away. Go back to the paper towel roll example we used at the start of this chapter. The top view has two lines of symmetry, a vertical line and a horizontal line; also notice that the Front and End Views of this shape are identical to each other. You will see more examples of symmetry in the practice problems at the end of this chapter.
- Fold the 2D views you're given together in your head and slot in each answer choice for the third view. Ask whether it matches what you know about the shape and what it looks like. This can be tricky and time-consuming, so only do this if you absolutely must to answer the question.

If none of these additional strategies help you, pick your Letter of the Day (or make your best guess) and move on.

Want More Practice?
Scan the QR code below to register your book for online chapter summaries, drills, practice tests, and more!

Chapter 33
Angle Ranking

33.1   THE RULES

Angle Ranking questions are also known as angle discrimination. Over the last few years, these questions have gotten much more difficult on the DAT. These are always the third set of 15 questions in the PAT (questions 31–45) and will have four answer choices per question.

Here are the rules you should follow in Angle Ranking questions:

1. You will be given four numbered angles, each formed by two lines.
2. Examine the interior angles; every angle is between 1° and 180°
3. You must rank the angles from smallest to largest.
4. In all cases, required comparisons will be different enough to be judged by eye.
5. For each question, there is only one correct ranking.

Rule number 2 means that every angle will be acute, right, obtuse, or a straight line. There are no reflex angles on the DAT.

While these instructions seem straightforward, the questions are not always the easiest. In some questions, the angles being compared have only a few degrees size difference! For each question, there are four angles given and there are four answer choices. As a result, not every possible ranking of the angles is an answer choice. You can use this to your advantage with aggressive POE.

33.2   STRATEGIES

Comparisons

There is no need to check every one of the four given angles against the other three. Do not stare at the screen for 40 seconds and try to compare all possible pairs of angles. Instead, use the answer choices to narrow down the number of comparisons to make and move quickly through this section. You can pick a pair of angles that are easy to compare, and eliminate any choice that has them listed backwards. Alternatively, you can start by identifying the smallest angle or the largest angle, and use that information to eliminate wrong choices. Next, use the remaining answer choices to help narrow down the number of additional comparisons you actually need to make. Typically, you will only need to make two comparisons: the first comparison (comparing two easy angles or selecting the smallest or largest angle) often eliminates two answer choices, and a second comparison will eliminate the final wrong choice. Only a few questions will require you to do three comparisons.

Big Angles vs. Small Angles

If the angles are large (obtuse), decide which one is closest to a straight line. That angle is the largest. The angle that is the farthest from being a straight line is the smallest.

Example 33-1: Big Angles

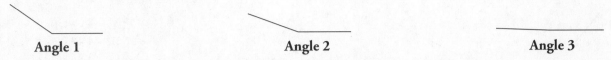

All three angles are obtuse. Angle 1 is the furthest from a straight line and closest to a right angle, so is the smallest. Angle 3 is the largest angle; it is almost a straight line. Angle 2 is a little less like a straight line, so is the second largest angle.

If angles are medium-sized, figure out which is closest to a right angle and compare to right angles to find which angles are largest/smallest.

Example 33-2: Medium-Sized Angles

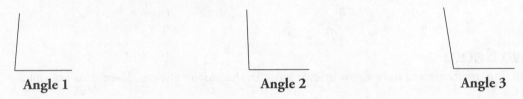

Notice that Angle 1, above, is not quite a right angle; therefore, it is the smallest angle. Angle 2 is almost a right angle (just slightly larger), so it is the second smallest angle. Angle 3 is definitely larger than a 90° angle, therefore, it is the largest angle.

To draw a small (acute) angle, the two arms must be close to each other and overlap at the vertex (where the two lines meet). This can make small angles look dark at the vertex. In fact, the smaller the angle, the more overlap, and the darker an angle looks. Not everyone can see this trend, so if this strategy doesn't work for you, don't stress about it. There are lots of other techniques in this chapter!

Example 33-3: Small Angles

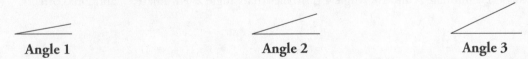

The smallest angle above (Angle 1) has the most overlap of lines near its vertex; it is darkest and smallest. Angle 2 has less overlap (so it is the second smallest angle) and Angle 3 has almost no overlap (it is the largest angle).

Angle Ranking questions often contain a mix of angles, such as an acute or two, one angle close to a right angle, then an obtuse or two. When different types of angles are used in one question, it is often sufficient to identify types of angles, pick the answer choice that matches that, and move on. Here is an example:

Example 33-4: Classifying Angles

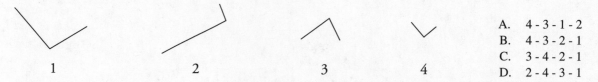

A. 4 - 3 - 1 - 2
B. 4 - 3 - 2 - 1
C. 3 - 4 - 2 - 1
D. 2 - 4 - 3 - 1

Angles 1 and 2 are obtuse (larger than 90°), angle 3 is acute (smaller than 90°), and angle 4 is a right angle (90°). This means the ranking from smallest to largest must be 3 – 4 – 1/2. Based on this, the correct answer must be C. Notice that to answer this question, you don't need to compare angles 1 and 2 to each other; in fact, these angles are only a few degrees different, which can be difficult to see by eye. Luckily, you don't need this comparison to succeed on this question; more on this shortly!

Two-by-Two Setup

Some Angle Ranking questions will have a two-by-two setup in the answer choices. Here is an example:

Example 33-5: Two-by-Two Answer Choices

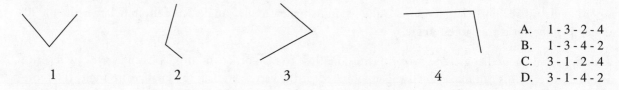

A. 1 - 3 - 2 - 4
B. 1 - 3 - 4 - 2
C. 3 - 1 - 2 - 4
D. 3 - 1 - 4 - 2

Look at the answer choices: the two smallest angles are 1 and 3. The larger angles are 2 and 4. This is a classic two-by-two setup. Focus on comparing 1 vs. 3 and 2 vs. 4 to answer this question quickly. Angle 3 is smaller than angle 1 (eliminate A and B). Angle 4 is smaller than angle 2 (eliminate C, and D is correct).

Different Lengths and Same Angles

Questions sometimes have portions of lines missing. You can hold your noteboard or hand up to the computer (without touching the computer) to "cut off" the longer line to make it easier to compare.

It is also possible that you could see two angles that are so similar in size that for all intents and purposes, they are the same as each other. Don't panic; you won't need to compare these two in order to get the question right. Similar angles have been cropping up on the DAT lately, and if you don't know to ignore them, they can be a giant waste of time. Here is an example:

Example 33-6: Challenging Comparisons

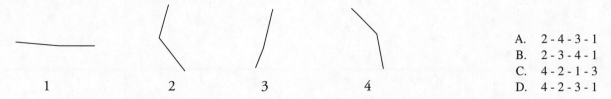

A. 2 - 4 - 3 - 1
B. 2 - 3 - 4 - 1
C. 4 - 2 - 1 - 3
D. 4 - 2 - 3 - 1

Angles 1 and 3 are very, very close in size. Don't focus on these two! Keep moving and work the answer choices instead. Angle 2 is smallest and closest to a right angle (eliminate C and D). Choices A and B both list angle 1 as the largest; you must compare angles 3 and 4 to answer this question. Angle 3 is larger than angle 4 (eliminate B, and A is correct). Notice that to answer this question, you don't need to compare angles 1 and 3 to each other; in fact, these angles are 2° different from each other, something very few people can see by eye.

Pacing and POE

Angle Ranking questions can be tricky but can also turn into a large waste of time if you're not careful. Work through this section efficiently using aggressive POE. Find the smallest and largest angles and eliminate answer choices that don't match what you've found. This alone might get you to the right answer. If not, use the answer choices that are left to drive your strategy and only do the work you need to in order to answer the question correctly.

Do not spend a long time staring at the computer screen when you're comparing angles. Look quickly, make a decision, and keep moving through the answer choices and question. Angles tend to start looking similar if you stare at them for a long time. If you're losing focus, look away from the computer for a second or two to reset your vision, then glance back down at the angles you're working. Most importantly, you must know when to move on.

Want More Practice?
Scan the QR code below to register your book for online chapter summaries, drills, practice tests, and more!

Chapter 34
Hole Punching

Part 4 of the PAT (questions 46 through 60) is Hole Punching. Hole Punching questions are also known as paper folding questions. These questions have five answer choices (A–E). Most people find these questions relatively doable once they find a strategy that works. If you are one of these people, you should count on answering most of the 15 questions in this section. In the worst-case scenario, you could mark the question and review it later in the section. Like the other subsections of the PAT, Hole Punching questions generally progress from easy to hard.

The questions in this section involve folding a piece of paper between one and four times, and then punching a hole in the folded paper; all this is given in the question stem. Your job is to mentally unfold the paper and determine where the holes are located in the unfolded sheet.

34.1   THE RULES

Here are the rules you should follow in Hole Punching questions:

1. A flat square of paper is folded from one to four times.
2. The paper is always folded toward you; it will never be folded away from you, or behind itself.
3. Broken (dashed or dotted) lines indicate the original position of the paper.
4. Solid lines indicate the position of the folded paper.
5. The paper is never turned, twisted, rotated, or flipped.
6. The folded paper always remains within the edges of the original square.
7. After the last fold a hole is punched in the paper.
8. There is always one fold per drawing except the last drawing, which contains the hole punch.
9. Your task is to unfold the paper mentally and determine the position of the holes on the original square and choose the corresponding answer choice.
10. There is only one correct pattern for each item.

34.2   STRATEGIES

Unfold the Paper

The most important strategy for this section involves working backward from the final picture, one fold at a time. You can use your noteboard for this, especially when you are new to these questions. By test day, you will be able to do most of this work mentally.

You should work backward from the final picture, one fold at a time. Unfold the last fold, and then ask where the hole(s) would be in the final picture. Unfold the next fold and ask where the hole(s) would be. In most questions, you will only have to undo two folds to find the correct answer. It can also be useful to do POE as you are unfolding the paper and working backward. To demonstrate this technique, we will use an example:

Example 34-1:

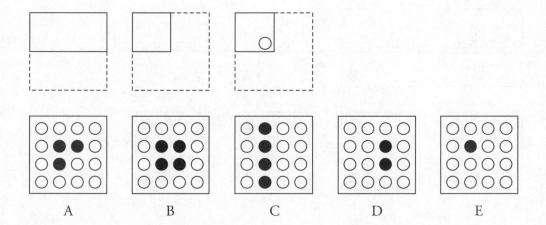

A B C D E

The unfolded solution looks like this:

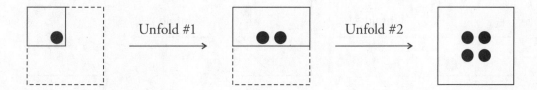

First, unfold the top half of the paper to the right. This duplicates the hole (eliminate C, D, and E). Next, unfold the paper from top to bottom. This duplicates both holes (eliminate A, and B is correct).

To use this strategy on the noteboard provided, you can do a quick sketch of the square, then mark each hole with a simple X:

Remember the noteboards are usually graph paper, so setting up 4×4 grids is quite doable. There is one additional trick to keep in mind. Sometimes the paper is folded internally to decrease the number of holes in the final picture. When you are unfolding:

- Keep and duplicate the hole if the paper is solid on the previous picture.
- Move the hole (do not duplicate) if the paper is dotted (hypothetical) in the previous picture.

Let's look at what this means. In Example 1 above, the first hole was kept and duplicated when the top half of the paper was unfolded from left to right. Both of these two holes were also kept and duplicated when the paper was unfolded from top to bottom.

Let's do another example to demonstrate the second bullet point of moving holes instead of duplicating them:

Example 34-2:

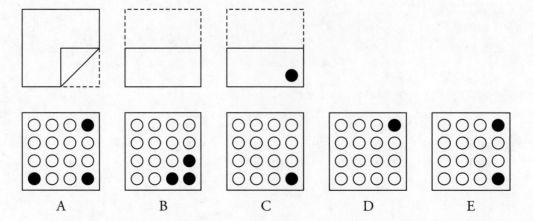

For the first unfold, the bottom half of the paper is unfolded to the top. Since the bottom right corner is a dotted (hypothetical) area, the hole is moved, not duplicated:

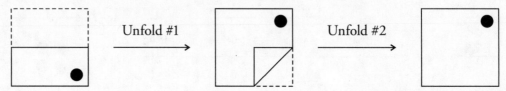

After the first unfold, eliminate B and C because they do not have a hole in the top right corner. After the final unfold, the answer must be D. There is no reason for a hole to be in the bottom left corner (eliminate choice A). If you accidentally kept and duplicated the hole during the first unfold, you would erroneously think E was correct.

How Many Holes?

Often the answer options have different numbers of holes punched. A second strategy involves determining how many holes would be in unfolded paper. Eliminate options with too many or too few holes. Another way to think about this is to ask how many thicknesses the paper is when the hole is punched. If the paper is three thicknesses when you punch, there must be three holes in the correct answer.

In Example 1 above, the paper was four thicknesses when it was hole punched, so there are four holes in the correct answer. In Example 2 above, the paper was only one thickness when it was punched (the bottom right corner was folded in at the beginning), so the correct answer has only one hole.

Strategies for Advanced Hole Punching

Over the last few years, Hole Punching questions have gotten harder. You may be wondering how this is possible, when you're stuck working in a 4 × 4 grid you can't leave, can only fold the paper up to four times, and have only 16 holes maximum to work with! Well, the DAT has started introducing some advanced folding patterns, including diagonal folds, folding off the 4 × 4 grid, and unfolds. They've also started creating examples where partial holes unfold to become full holes. Finally, some examples have lots of hole punches per question (not just one), which means you have more holes to keep track of. Let's look at a few advanced Hole Punching examples, so you can see how these patterns could show up on test day.

Example 34-3:

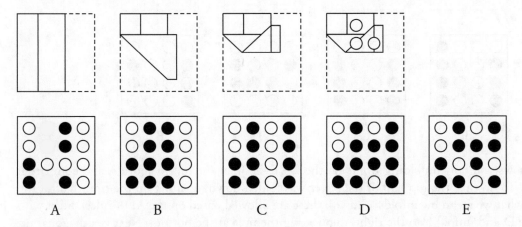

Before we solve this question, let's break down a few of the advanced patterns here. First, look at the image above choice A. The left side of the diagram is one column of the 4 × 4 grid. The section beside that and the section on the right are both one and a half columns. In other words, this is showing how the paper can be folded off the grid. Next, look how the paper rotates between the image above A and that above B; this is a classic diagonal fold. Finally, look at how many punches were added to this paper at the end; this is going to be a lot of holes to keep track of!

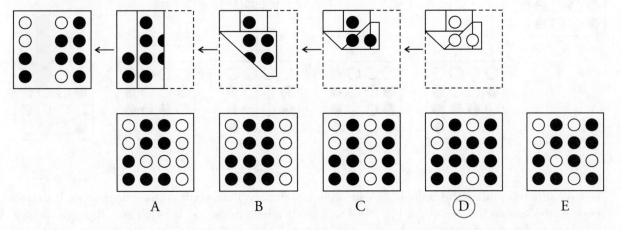

Now let's break this question down and figure out how to crack it. Working backward, the first unfold will take you from the image above choice C to the image above B. Unfold the paper down and add more holes to your diagram. In the image above C, you'll notice there is a half hole; watch how it becomes a full hole in the next step. To go from the image above B to that above A, diagonally unfold the paper down and to the left. This introduces two more half holes that will be filled out in the next step. As soon as you see the full column of punches in the second column, eliminate A and E. Finally, unfold to the right to form a full piece of paper (choice D is correct). Because the first fold was off the grid, B is not possible. Choice E is a common distractor if you do the diagonal unfold incorrectly or not at all.

Example 34-4:

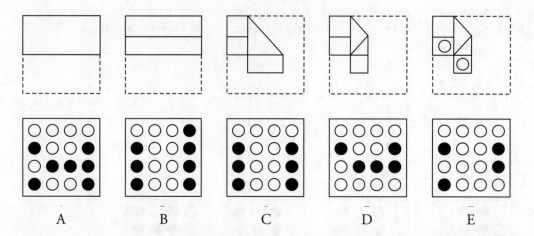

A   B   C   D   E

This question shows you how unfolding works on the DAT. Look at the image above A and compare it to that above B. To do this, the top half of the paper was folded down, opening up the front half of the paper; this was what we mean by unfolds (and yes, these are allowed based on the ADA rules). Start with the image above D and unfold it to the right, duplicating the hole at the bottom. Next is a diagonal un-fold, flipping the paper up and to the right. Notice you don't gain any holes when you do this; instead, you move around the holes you already have. Now is a good time for some POE; based on where you are right now, eliminate A, C, D, and E; choice B must be correct.

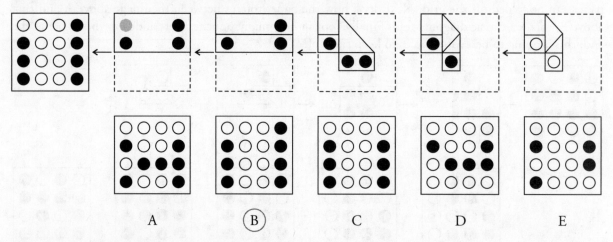

A   ⓑ   C   D   E

To make sure you understand unfolds, let's finish this example off. To get from the image above B to that above A, the bottom flap is unfolded up. This will create a hole in the top left that goes through the top layer of paper but not the whole stack; we've made this hole gray in the solution above. Finally, unfold the top half of the paper to form a full grid.

Example 34-5:

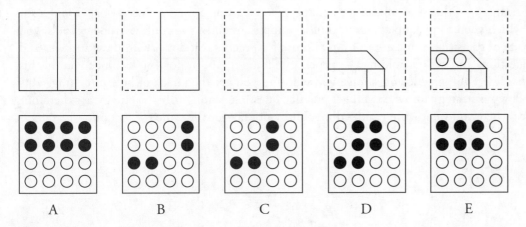

This is another example of unfolding and diagonal folds.

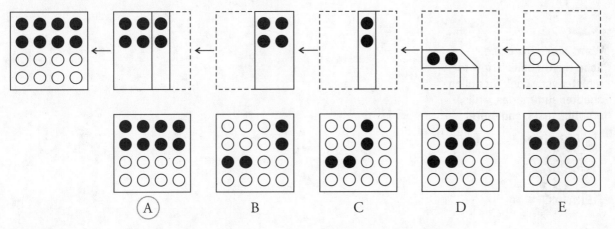

First, flip the paper up and to the right; the two holes move up (eliminate B). Next, unfold the paper to the right to get the image above B. Unfold to the left to get the image above A (eliminate C and D), and unfold the flap at the right to get a full grid (eliminate E, and A is correct).

What to Do If You Get Stuck

Sometimes you will be doing a Hole Punching problem and you will reach a point where you're not sure what to do next. If this happens, you have a few options:

- POE from where you are. Given what you have so far, where would the holes be in the final figure?
- Compare the remaining answer options. Many times, they only differ in one hole. When this is the case, focus on that hole and ask if it would be in the final picture.

Actually Do It!

One of the great things about the Hole Punching section is that you can actually do it on your own, quite easily. The final strategy for this section is exactly that—practice using a square piece of paper and a single hole punch (which you can pick up at a typical office supply store). In your online Student Tools, you will find a template of grids that you can print out and use for practice. Sit down with these supplies and a few practice questions and act out folding the paper, punching it, and unfolding it. Once you do this a few times with a few DAT practice questions, you will find you get the knack of hole punching. This is also a great follow-up strategy for when you get practice questions wrong. If you actually act them out, you will likely see where you went wrong and will hopefully not fall for the same trick again.

Want More Practice?
Scan the QR code below to register your book for online chapter summaries, drills, practice tests, and more!

Chapter 35
Cube Counting

Part 5 of the PAT (questions 61 through 75) is Cube Counting. These questions have five answer choices (A–E). You will find that these questions take time at first, but once you get the hang of it, most people find these questions are the easiest of the PAT section. Cube Counting is different from the other PAT question types in that you are given one figure and must answer one to four questions based on this figure.

35.1   THE RULES

Here are the rules you should keep in mind for Cube Counting questions:

1.   Each figure has been made by cementing together cubes of the same size.
2.   All cubes are connected to the rest of the stack in some way. Stacks and floating cubes are cemented together via faces. Cubes sitting on the ground can be connected by an edge.
3.   After being cemented each group is painted on all exposed sides.
4.   Assume every exposed face of every cube has been painted.
5.   The bottoms of cubes resting on the ground are not painted; the bottoms of floating cubes are painted.
6.   The only hidden cubes are those required to support other cubes or connect floating cubes to the stack via a face.
7.   The series of questions beside the figure will ask you how many cubes have no faces painted, one face painted, two faces painted, etc.

35.2   STRATEGIES

Counting Chart

The best way to answer Cube Counting questions is to figure out the entire stack of cubes and then answer all the questions. To do this, you should generate a counting chart on your noteboard:

0	1	2	3	4	5

As you count how many faces of each cube is painted, add a tick under the appropriate column. It is very important that you don't forget to count hidden cubes and the faces of visible cubes that are turned away. Hidden cubes are those required to support other cubes. Also note that there will never be a hidden cube with nothing on top of it.

To practice this strategy, let's use an example:

Example 35-1:

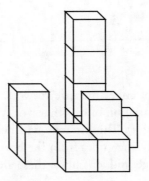

The counting chart for this stack of cubes looks like this:

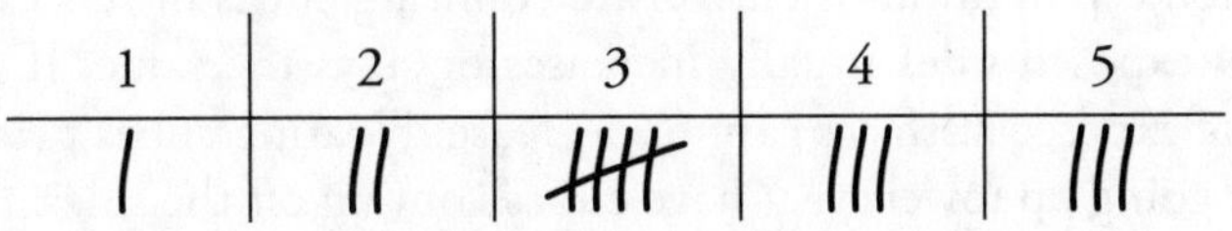

1	2	3	4	5
I	II	IIII	III	III

This is because the stack of cubes is counted like this:

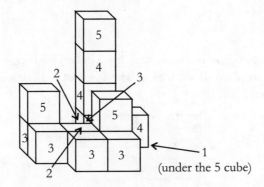

(under the 5 cube)

If you tend to forget hidden cubes, you should answer the questions from least faces to most faces. Questions about "no exposed surfaces," "one face," or "two faces" tend to ask about hidden cubes. Also keep in mind that the only way to have one face painted is to be at the base of a tower. The only way to have no exposed surfaces is to be sitting on the ground and surrounded by other cubes on all sides.

A version of this strategy involves writing first the numbers of exposed surfaces for each cube down on your Noteboard and then tallying them up. For the image above, this might look like this:

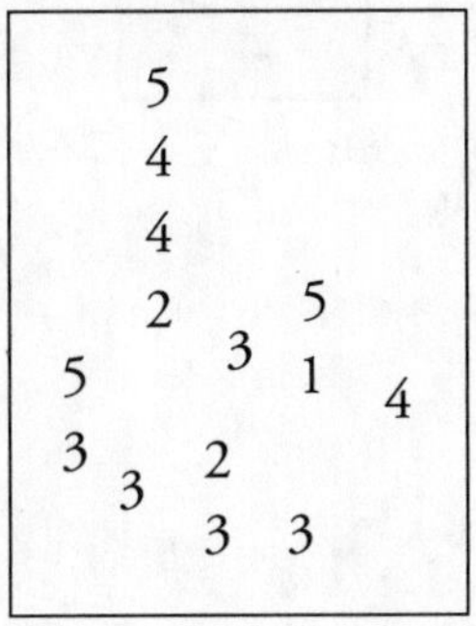

```
        5
        4
        4
        2      5
    5      3     1   4
    3   3   2
        3     3   3
```

In addition, if you find you sometimes skip cubes when you're analyzing the figure, consider taking a few seconds to total up the cubes. Count how many cubes there are in the image, total up your tally chart, and make sure the numbers match. Most cube stacks contain 15–22 cubes.

Work Systematically

When you are figuring out the stacks of cubes, be sure to work systematically. Work from left to right, back to front, and bottom to top (or a variation of this that works for you; the key is to find a pattern that works for you and to always be consistent). This strategy will help you work cubes more efficiently and will help you avoid missing cubes. Analyzing cubes from the bottom of the figure and working your way up is a great way to ensure you don't forget hidden cubes; these are often resting on the ground and under other cubes.

Another important trick to keep in mind when you are counting cubes in vertical stacks: as you move up a column, the number of exposed sides usually increases or stays the same. If the stack is a straightforward tower, the number of exposed surfaces cannot decrease. Floating cubes provide an exception to this, so be careful when you're going up towers that have cubes coming off the sides.

Parallel Lines

Sometimes you might struggle to figure out where exactly a cube is sitting. In Example 1 above, the cube on the farthest right is tricky to place. If we look at the stack of cubes from the top, some people can't figure out if the "floor plan" looks like this:

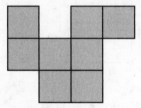

Or like this:

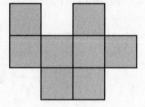

Different placements can affect how many sides are painted on several surrounding cubes, so it is important you have a strategy to correctly place cubes you can't see very well.

If you struggle to figure out where cubes are actually placed, you can use parallel lines and aligned lines to figure it out. In Example 1, the top of the tricky cube is aligned with top of the cube at the bottom of the stack:

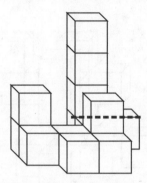

Therefore, the first floor plan was the correct one; the tricky cube on the right must be beside the tower at the back of the stack.

Patterns

The more you work with cubes, the more patterns you will see. Cubes that function as **tower caps** always have five faces painted. These are the cubes that are sitting on top of a tower of cubes, with no other cubes around them. Cubes that are **tower extenders** always have four faces painted. These are cubes that function to make a tower of cubes taller, and have no other cubes around them. Cubes that are **side sitters** always have four faces painted. These are cubes that look like they were added as an afterthought and are just plopped down at the edge of the stacks. They are joined to the stack by only one side. **Daring diagonals** are only connected to the rest of the stack via one edge. They always have 5 faces painted.

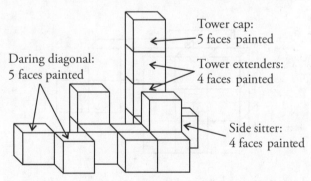

Floating Cubes

Over the last few years, the ADA has added floating cubes to their repertoire. Floating cubes are connected to the rest of the stack by cementing a side or top face to another cube. Because of this, they have an exposed bottom that must be counted because it can be painted. Here are some floating cube patterns you could see on test day:

Example 35-2:

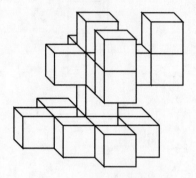

Example 35-3:

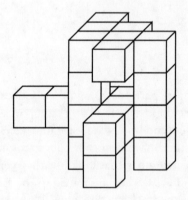

Example 35-4:

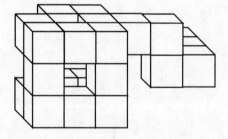

For each of these cube stacks, determine how many surfaces are exposed for each cube and generate a tally chart. Check your work at the end of this chapter.

You could see floating cubes connected by only a side face, at the front, rear, or side of the stack. You could also see more elaborate floating projections where several floating cubes are connected to come off into an arm-like section. Basically, if you could make the stack using actual cubes and strong cement, the pattern is possible. Stay flexible on test day and work with what you've got.

While these patterns seem weird and unusual, they don't break the Cube Counting rules set out by the ADA. In fact, all the strategies we've already discussed still apply to these cubes. Look for exposed surfaces and remember to check the bottoms of the floaters.

Unanswerable

If you get to a question and can't answer it, you made an error when you were generating your counting chart. You must go back and redo the stacks, and then redo all your questions. While this seems like a waste of time, it is very important. If you change one cube, it could change nearby cubes and your answer to other questions. If this happens to you, the best strategy is to go back to the beginning and regenerate your counting chart.

Answers and Explanations

EXAMPLE 35–2

This cube stack contains 18 cubes:

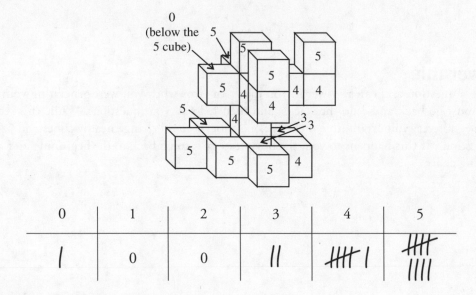

0	1	2	3	4	5
I	0	0	II	ⅢⅠ	ⅢⅢ

EXAMPLE 35–3

This cube stack contains 21 cubes:

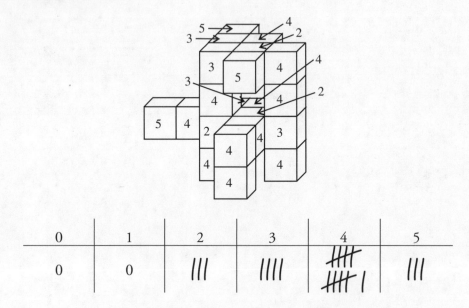

0	1	2	3	4	5
0	0	III	IIII	ⅢⅢⅠ	III

EXAMPLE 35–4

This cube stack contains 21 cubes:

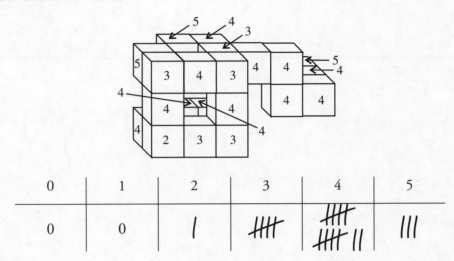

0	1	2	3	4	5
0	0	I	⊬⊬⊬	⊬⊬⊬ ⊬⊬⊬ II	III

Want More Practice?

Scan the QR code below to register your book for online chapter summaries, drills, practice tests, and more!

Chapter 36
3D Form Development

The sixth and final part of the PAT is called 3D Form Development; these questions are also known as pattern folding. Form Development questions (questions 76 through 90) are four-option multiple choice (A–D) and involve folding a flat pattern (the question stem) into a 3D shape (answer options). Most people consider this section a difficult one.

36.1 THE RULES

Here are the rules you should follow in Form Development questions:

1. A flat 2D pattern will be presented. This pattern is to be folded into a three-dimensional figure.
2. The outside of the figure must be the pattern visible in the question stem.
3. After being folded together, the figure can be rotated.
4. The correct figure is one of the four given at the right of the pattern.
5. There is only one correct figure in each set.

36.2 STRATEGIES

Find the Base

A good first step is to find the base of the 3D folded shape. Many times (but not always) the base is larger than the other faces. If the figure is symmetrical, the base may be near the center of the flat pattern. For example:

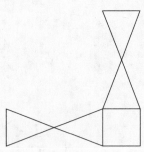

The base of this figure is the square and this pattern corresponds to a square-based pyramid:

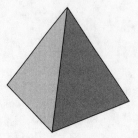

Dominant Faces

Many of these 3D shapes have dominant faces. Look for two faces the same size or shape in the 2D pattern. You can use these dominant faces to orient yourself when looking at shapes in the answer choices. You can also use them for counting and matching, which we'll discuss next. Dominant faces will be parallel if all the connecting faces have the same width; they will not be parallel if the connecting faces have varying widths. Finally, sometimes the dominant faces are split in two, if there are two different sizes of connectors. Let's look at an example:

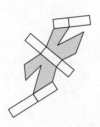
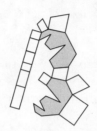
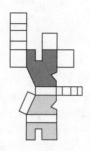

Dominant faces (in gray) will be parallel because all the connecting faces are the same width.

Dominant faces (in gray) will not be parallel because connecting faces have varying widths.

One dominant face (light gray) is split in two; the other (dark gray) is not. Connecting faces are a mix of narrow and wide.

Counting and Matching

A quick trick to Form Development questions involves taking inventory. For example, you could count the number of edges around the perimeter of a dominant face; then compare this to the figures in the answer choices. Eliminate any shape that doesn't have the same perimeter as the question stem. You could also look at the proportions and features in a dominant face. Again, compare to the figures in the answer choices and eliminate anything that doesn't match.

Finally, you can take inventory of faces. For example, if there are three small triangles in the 2D pattern, there must be three small triangular faces in the 3D shape, and they must have the same proportions as in the 2D pattern. If an answer choice contains four small square faces and these aren't in the question stem, eliminate that answer choice. If the 3D shape has a side of a certain size or shape, this must also be in the 2D pattern. Taking inventory and comparing the question stem and answer choices can be a fast way to use POE in Form Development. Like in all the other sections, if you eliminate three options, the remaining shape must be correct.

Let's look at an example. If you were working with this shape in an answer choice:

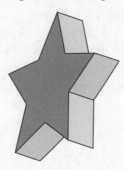

The 2D pattern would have to contain two stars that were the same shape (these are the dominant faces) and ten rectangles that are the same size; these would have to be the same size to ensure the dominant faces are parallel. The 2D pattern wouldn't contain any triangles or trapezoids.

Shading

Many Form Development problems include some shading or pattern. Sometimes this is a distractor, and other times it is the focus of the question. Questions that focus on shading require that the shaded sides are oriented correctly with respect to each other. Let's return to the square-based pyramid we used earlier.

Example 36-1:

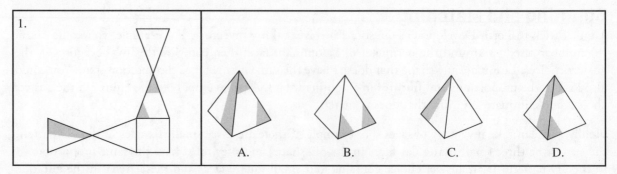

The base of this figure is the square, which is why all the answers are square-based pyramids. Since the only difference between the answer options is the shading pattern, this must be the focus of the question. The 2D pattern has one triangular face with a bottom corner and a top corner shaded. This pattern is not in answer choice B, which can be eliminated. When the pyramid is folded together, the long shaded edge of the triangle on the left will end up beside the face with two shaded corners; the long shaded face will be opposite the small shaded corner, not beside it (eliminate D). Overall C is best; the triangle with the two shaded triangles is at the back of this 3D shape. Remember the pattern at the left is the *outside* of the 3D shape. If you accidentally fold it so the pattern at the left is the inside of the pattern, you will be tempted to pick the distractor, option A (which is backward and incorrect). If you do not see this, make the 2D pattern out of a piece of paper and fold it up!

Focus on Small Features

Sometimes a small feature is the focus of Form Development questions. Watch out for angles of different sizes, tunnels, or holes in the 3D figure, small shading details (as we saw in Example 1 above), or small appendage or auxiliary parts. The placement and orientation of these small features can help you eliminate impossible answer choices and narrow down your options via POE.

Example 36-2:

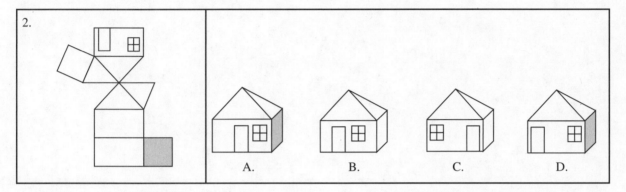

There are three small features in this question: the shaded wall, the window, and the door. The correct answer must have all three oriented correctly with respect to each other. In the 2D pattern, the window and the door are at opposite sides of the wall, therefore eliminate A (where they are together on one side) and B (where they are together in the middle). When the shape is folded together, the window will be beside the shaded side, at the back of the figure. When it is rotated so the window and door are at the front, the shaded side will be on the left (C is correct). The window and door are on the wrong side of D. Similar to the first example, if you accidentally fold the shape so the 2D pattern on the left is the *inside* of the shape (instead of the *outside*), you will mistakenly pick the distractor, option D (which is incorrect).

Practice with Common Shapes

Form Development questions often use common geometric shapes, such as cubes, triangular prisms, square-based pyramids, rectangle-based pyramids, triangular-based pyramids, or houses. Some examples are below. The roof of a house can be made of four triangles (which can or cannot all be the same dimensions) or two triangles and two rectangles. Before test day, spend some time thinking about what the patterns for each of these geometric shapes can look like. For example, to build a cube, you need six squares. In your online Student Tools, you will find some templates for these common shapes, so you can practice with them.

Want More Practice?
Scan the QR code below to register your book for online chapter summaries, drills, practice tests, and more!

Reading Comprehension Test (RCT)

Chapter 37
RCT

37.1 INTRODUCTION

The Reading Comprehension Test (RCT) on the DAT contains 50 questions that you must answer in 60 minutes. There are 3 passages, each of which has an average of 16–17 questions associated with it.[1] Each passage has about 1500 words, and between 7 and 20 paragraphs. The questions are not in any particular order with respect to the passage or difficulty; the first question could ask you about paragraph 15, and you could need the first few paragraphs to answer question 13. The first question could be very challenging, and the last question could be quite straightforward and quick. The passages are extremely dense with information and are usually (but not always!) about a science or health-related topic. The reading level of the passages is similar to what you'll be expected to read in first-year dental school. Additionally, most students find they do not have time to complete the section comfortably and must rush, at least to some extent, to complete the section in the allotted time.

No Outside Knowledge

One peculiar aspect of the RCT is that it does not test your knowledge of any particular subject area. While the Survey of Natural Sciences, for example, is supposed to test your knowledge of biology, general chemistry, and organic chemistry, the RCT is supposed to test your ability to "read, comprehend, and analyze…basic scientific information," according to ADA. What this means, in practical terms, is that everything you need to know is in the passage. If the passage says it, it's true. If the passage doesn't say it, you can't use it as the basis for an answer. Don't bring in specialized knowledge from outside the passage when answering questions. The ADA, in their characteristic manner, puts this in the following fashion: "Prior understanding of the science topics is not a prerequisite to answering the test items."

It is particularly important to keep this in mind because some RCT passage topics may be familiar to you. There have been passages on neurotransmitters, protein synthesis, oncology, sensory biology, and the microbiology of food poisoning. If you have prior knowledge of a topic, it can be tempting to answer questions based on that knowledge. This is risky because you don't know when the passage was written, and often the passages contain obscure facts and exceptions to broadly accepted truths. If you answer based on what you know, without referring to the passage, you may fall for distractor answer choices and end up getting some questions wrong.

Also, while most passages are about topics that are at least somewhat related to the typical pre-dental curriculum, don't worry if a passage is about a topic you're unfamiliar with. Even if the passage is about pianos, environmental science, or quantum physics, all the information you need is in the passage. You don't have to be a consummate musician or professional piano tuner in order to answer RCT questions about a piano.

---

[1] Theoretically, you could see 10-20 questions per passage, but most sections of RCT have 16-17 questions per passage.

Self-Evaluation

So how do you study for a test that doesn't test your knowledge of something? Obviously, you can't approach studying for RCT the way you approach studying for SNS or QRT. You have to become familiar with the basic structure of the test, common question types, and the essentials of eliminating answers. Then you have to practice. And practice. And practice. But simply doing lots of passages will not, in itself, help you, at least not much. You also have to review your work carefully. If you miss a question (or spend too long on a question), you have to figure out why, and how you can avoid doing so in the future when you see a similar question. You must train yourself to answer questions effectively and efficiently.

Often, when students are studying for the RCT, if they miss a question, they will say to themselves (once they've checked the answer and seen where it comes from in the passage), ""Oh well, all I have to do next time is just read a little more carefully." And then, the next time, when they continue to miss questions, they will make the same comment to themselves: "I'll just read more carefully next time." This continues, over and over.

This is not a specific enough plan for improvement. Formulating a better plan depends on figuring out where in the process things went wrong. Perhaps the comment should go something like this: "I only read the first few words of this answer before making up my mind that it was right, choosing it, and moving on, but the entire second half of the answer was wrong. What I will do in the future is read answer choices all the way to the end before making up my mind, and I will focus more closely on the way answer choices end, and not just how they begin, in order not to make the same sort of mistake."

Notice this is still, in essence, "reading more carefully." However, it is specific enough that the student can probably do this, whereas "reading more carefully" is so vague that it is hard to accomplish. Be specific with your self-evaluation!

37.2   CORE STRATEGIES

For clarity, we will split the strategies for RCT into several parts. First, we'll break down your section strategy, then we'll talk about the passage, the questions, the answer choices, and finally, pacing.

Section Strategy

Let's start by reviewing your basic approach to RCT:

Step 1:   Choose an order for the passages.
The passages are not of uniform difficulty, and, as discussed earlier, most students do not find that they can finish the entire test comfortably (and lose points by rushing too much). Thus, it is recommended that you review the passages in an order that you choose, rather than the order that is presented in the test. You can usually tell how hard a passage is going to be by reading the title and first sentence or two and glancing at the questions.

Thus, take about a minute at the beginning of the section to read the titles and first few sentences of each passage. To get from one passage to the next, you must press "Next" through all of the questions; as you are doing this, take a quick glance at each question, just to note whether it looks like a common question or a rare question type (discussed later). Based on this, quickly determine an order in which to work the passages.

Step 2:   Work the passages in that order.
Begin with the first passage that you have chosen to do, and work it according to the Basic Approach for Passages given below. Then move to the second passage. If you have time, continue to the third passage.

Step 3:   Inspect the section.
When the 5-minute warning pops up, consider where you are in the section. Unless you are completely certain that you will finish all questions in the time allotted, now is a good time to use the Review screen to check what remains unanswered and enter your Letter of the Day for those questions. Then return to where you were in the section and continue to work.

Basic Approach for Passages

Becoming more specific in scope, here is the basic approach to analyzing passages:

Step 1:   Skim read and map the passage
On the RCT, the passages are extremely long, and there are a great many questions about each one, with a fairly restrictive time limit. Thus, if you spent a great deal of time reading each passage before you got to the questions, you would not have anywhere near enough time to work the questions. However, the passages are also extremely thick with information, and it's certainly not possible to remember all the details from a quick read. Thus, you must read the passage relatively quickly and focus on main points and locating information, not on the mess of details. Ideally, this step takes 2–4 minutes (closer to 2 minutes if you intend to finish 2.5–3 passages, close to 4 minutes if you intend to finish 2–2.5 passages).

As you are doing this, use your noteboard. For each paragraph, write the number of the paragraph and a few words on the topic of the paragraph. Your goal is to summarize what the paragraph is about. Generating this **passage map** will tell you quickly what information is where. There is a good reason for doing this: The answer is usually straightforward if you are looking at the relevant portion of the passage. However, none of the questions contain line or paragraph references, and they are not in any useful order. Thus, the primary goal of an initial reading of the passage is to read quickly and create a map that can guide you through the questions. Think of your passage map as a table of contents for the passage. It should tell you where to go when you're answering questions.

You will also have the option of highlighting the passage (anything from a single word to a full paragraph) and these yellow highlights will be retained as you navigate around the RCT section. You can use highlighted words or phrases to generate a passage map, but be critical in what you highlight. Again, your goal is to generate a table of contents for each paragraph, or a map of what is where.

Be aware that the primary skill the RCT is testing is **scanning**. Scanning is a particular type of reading that involves searching for a key word or phrase. For example, if a question asks about John Hunter, and John Hunter appeared only in one part of the passage, then the most reliable way to answer that question is to find "John Hunter" in the passage. If you have no idea where to look, you have to scan across the entire passage until you find the name. In this case, "John Hunter" is a **lead word**, a word or phrase that leads you to the appropriate part of the passage. In general, your passage map should allow you to confine your scanning to a small portion of the passage, which will help you save time.

Step 2:   Work the questions
Proceed through the questions more or less in order, marking questions if they look confusing or time-consuming or if you have no idea where in the passage to look for the answer. (Come back to these questions before you move on to the next passage.) For each question, read it carefully to make sure that you understand what it's asking. Remember that you can highlight key words in the question stem if this will help you keep track of what the question is asking. Next, refer back to the relevant part of the passage and figure out what the answer will need to say, and come back to the answer choices. RCT question types and strategies will be reviewed more later in this chapter.

Step 3:   Answer the question
Go through the five answer choices in two passes. On your first pass, work efficiently and eliminate the worst answer choices using the strike-out feature. Slow down on your second pass; review what the question is asking, what the passage says, and how the remaining answer choices are different from each other. Rely heavily on POE. This will be reviewed more in section 37.6.

37.3   WORKING THE QUESTIONS

Two Passes

RCT questions come in a range of difficulty. You'll be able to answer some questions quite quickly. These questions usually have short question stems and short answer choices; less text means less time reading! Knowing exactly where to go to find the answer to a question is another characteristic of a quick and doable question. In contrast, challenging RCT questions will take you more time and are usually longer. It may not be clear which part of the passage you need to use, or you may need to use five different paragraphs to find the information you need. These questions are the worst-case scenarios on test day. You should mark these questions and save them for your second pass through the questions or skip them completely and answer using your Letter of the Day. There will also be a whole bunch of questions somewhere in the middle. Some of these questions may be a little long but you know exactly where to go to answer them. Some questions may be short and sweet, but you don't know where to go to find the information you need. Answer some of these questions on your first pass and save the trickiest questions for your second pass.

In conclusion, you should do two passes through the questions associated with a passage. On your first pass, answer the most doable questions, mark trickier questions, click your Letter of the Day on the most challenging and longest questions. On your second pass, slow down and go back to target the questions you skipped on your first pass.

Question Strategy

Next, let's review fundamental question strategy and discuss some of the crucial aspects.

In working each question, you should:

1. Read the question carefully and make sure that you understand what it's asking.
2. Refer back to the relevant part of the passage and figure out what the answer will need to say/do.
3. Eliminate answers until only one remains.

Sometimes students struggle with reading the question carefully after having just read the passage so quickly. However, while you do not need to retain every last detail of the passage on an initial reading, you do need to notice every word of a question, because there's probably a reason why it is phrased in a peculiar way. Thus, you must change gears when you reach the questions.

The second step—finding the relevant part of the passage—is vital to a degree that is hard to overstate. The person who wrote the questions for the passage that you're reading was looking right at a particular part of the passage when they wrote the question and the right and wrong answers. At the time, it was clear to them what the answer was based on this part of the passage. In order for it to be clear to you which answers are right and which are wrong, you should be looking at the same part of the passage. Thus, *find it!* Determine lead words in the question stem, try to locate the relevant area of the passage from your notes, and then scan for those lead words in the passage. If the question stem doesn't tell you where to go in the passage, look through the answer choices. They may help you figure out where to go.

Once you've found the relevant portion of the passage, back up a few lines. You should not start reading at the lead word or key phrase you found. For a lot of questions, you'll need some context to understand how to answer them. Start reading carefully a sentence or two before and continue a sentence or two after the bit that was referenced. Sometimes, you'll end up reading most of a paragraph, and that is okay.[2] You're doing the work required to get the questions right. Keep in mind how much you read will also depend on the style of question. If the answer choices are one word, find the word you need in the passage, pick the right answer, and move on. If the answer choices are long sentences, you'll likely need to read more of the passage to find what you need. At first, you should practice answering questions in your own words (or in the passage's own words when the answer should be exactly what the passage says). Over time, it will become so automatic that you do not need to work on it consciously anymore.

Finally, even if one answer looks superficially tempting, you must not simply choose that answer and move on without at least glancing at the rest of the answers. Likewise, if two answers look tempting, don't just guess between them without forming a solid reason to eliminate one and choose the other. Distractor answer choices on the RCT often contain common words from the passage. This test is constructed such that many of the answers look vaguely similar to a right answer, but only one will have no flaws that make it right. POE is fundamental, perhaps more fundamental than any other single strategy on the RCT.

---

[2] A good general rule is to actively and carefully read up to 10 lines of the passage to answer a question. If you're reading more than that, you probably haven't zeroed in specifically enough.

37.4 CORE QUESTION TYPES

Most questions on the RCT will be retrieval, inference, or open-ended, so we'll talk about these question types first. We'll review additional question types in the next section.

By far, the most common type of question on the RCT is the **Retrieval** question, which asks something to the effect of, "What did the passage say about [x]?" The next most common are **Inference** questions, which ask, "What did the passage suggest about [x]?" With either type of question, the right answer can consist of the **exact words** of the passage about that subject or a **close paraphrase** of the passage, although the former is more common on Retrieval questions and the latter more common on Inference questions.

Retrieval

Let's look at an example of a Retrieval question. Consider the following excerpt (from a much longer passage) and example question about this portion:

The platypus was first reported to Europeans in 1798 by Vice-Admiral John Hunter, a British naval officer and second governor of New South Wales, Australia. In 1797, he watched a local Australian observe a platypus for over an hour and then kill it with a spear. After this, he sent a remarkably accurate description back to Britain. In 1799, George Shaw gave the platypus its scientific name, *Platypus anatinus* (which was changed later to *Ornithorhynchus anatinus*), and in 1800, Thomas Bewick, a British wood engraver, circulated an image of the strange creature.

At first, many thought it was an elaborate hoax...

1. Who gave the platypus the name *Platypus anatinus*?

   A. John Hunter
   B. Thomas Bewick
   C. George Shaw
   D. A local Australian
   E. Carl Linnaeus

Notice this question asks for something that the passage outright says, so we expect the exact words of the passage to be the right answer. According to the middle of the excerpt, "George Shaw gave the platypus its scientific name, *Platypus anatinus*," so the answer must be George Shaw (C is correct). Many of the questions on the RCT will be this straightforward.

Inference

As just mentioned, **Inference** questions are the second most common question type on the RCT. These question stems often use words like "imply," "infer," or "suggest." Inference questions require you to match meaning rather than match words. Consider the following example:

Among venomous mammals, most bite in order to deliver their venom into victims. This is the method employed by venomous shrews, solenodons, and moles. The slow loris can also deliver a toxin via a bite, although its status as "venomous" is not without controversy. The platypus, however, attacks with spurs on its legs to deliver its cocktail of poisons. The venom can kill smaller animals, and while it is not strong enough to be deadly to humans, it can cause extreme pain. In contrast to the bites of certain snakes and spiders, platypus stings do not cause necrosis...

2. Which of the following does the passage suggest about venomous mammals?

A. The bite of a venomous shrew causes extreme pain.
B. Some people dispute that the slow loris is venomous.
C. The platypus is more poisonous than other mammals.
D. The platypus uses its poison to kill prey during hunting.
E. A single poison is responsible for the effects of the platypus's sting.

In this case, because the question is more vague, it is hard to predict what the answer will be. The passage indicates many things about venomous mammals. Use POE. Eliminate A, because it garbles two parts of the passage: According to the second-to-last sentence, the bite of a platypus causes extreme pain, but no explicit connections are made between that effect and the effect of the bite of a venomous shrew (in the second sentence). Choice B matches the third sentence adequately, so leave it alone for the moment. Eliminate C, because no comparison of degree of poison was made in the passage, so to say that the platypus is "more poisonous" is not justified. Eliminate D, because no reference was made to hunting or any related behavior, so no such conclusion can be drawn (in fact, the platypus actually uses the spurs for self-defense). Eliminate E, because the passage describes the venom as a "cocktail" of poisons in the fourth sentence, which means that there is more than one. Thus, the answer must be B.

Notice that B is not particularly a logical leap away from the passage. The passage says about the slow loris that "its status as 'venomous' is not without controversy," and this answer says that some people dispute this. These are close paraphrases, even if they are not the same exact words. Bear in mind that the *meaning* is the most important thing, not the words. Many of the wrong answers repeat some of the words of the passage, but only one will mean the same thing as what the passage said.

It is particularly important to note that the right answer to this question is not much of a leap from the passage since the word "suggest" might make you think that you have license to make stuff up. Maybe the passage doesn't *say* that the platypus is more poisonous than other mammals, but doesn't it *suggest* it? Or maybe the passage doesn't say the bite of a venomous shrew causes extreme pain, but doesn't it *suggest* it? The answer is no. If the passage doesn't say it, it doesn't say it. The same is true of words such as "imply" and "infer," as well.

Think of it this way: This is a standardized test. They can't make things up. If you decided that their question was fraudulent and unfair and sued them, they would have to be able to stand in court before a judge and defend their question, and they know it. They don't write questions for which their only defense would be, "But Your Honor, doesn't B just *feel* cosmically right?" They write questions for which their defense would be, "Your Honor, if you read the third sentence of the paragraph, you will clearly see that answer choice B is supported more than any of the others." They would be able to rattle off specific reasons that the rest of the answers are wrong (such as "more poisonous" in C). You should hold yourself to the same standard: You must be able to point to the part of the passage that supports the answer you are about to choose, and, equally, find the wrong parts of the answers that you are eliminating.

Because you need to find something directly stated in the passage, answering retrieval questions will be doable once you've found your strategy and have had lots of practice. Inference questions are usually more challenging and take a bit more time.

Open-Ended Questions

You will also see **Open-Ended** questions on the DAT. These questions ask things like "Which of the following is true based on information in the passage?" Other common question stems are "Based on the passage, which of the following is FALSE?" or "Each of the following is supported by the passage EXCEPT:" These question stems give you no information on where to go in the passage, and often the answer choices are from different parts of the passage. Because of this, these questions require POE and take time. You may want to mark these questions and come back to them later, once you've worked with the passage a little more.

37.5 ADDITIONAL QUESTION TYPES

While the overwhelming majority (generally more than 80%) of questions on the RCT will be Retrieval, Inference, or Open-Ended, there are other questions that are asked with some frequency, and these deserve a close look here. The most common of these are New Information and Two Parts questions, of which you are likely to see a few on any given RCT (usually 1-3 per section). Most versions of the DAT have 1-2 Tone/Attitude and Meaning in Context questions per section. The others may or may not show up at all, but they are here for completeness.

New Information

Sometimes a question will provide new information in the question stem and ask you a question about the new information, in the context of what is already in the passage. This is a **New Information** question. In general, you must first determine how the information relates to the passage, and then you can use POE aggressively. Consider the following example:

Among venomous mammals, most bite in order to deliver their venom into victims. This is the method employed by venomous shrews, solenodons, and moles. The slow loris can also deliver a toxin via a bite, although its status as "venomous" is not without controversy. The platypus, however, attacks with spurs on its legs to deliver its cocktail of poisons. The venom can kill smaller animals, and while it is not strong enough to be deadly to humans, it can cause extreme pain. In contrast to the bites of certain snakes and spiders, platypus stings do not cause necrosis…

3. The New Guinean quoll is a very small mammal. Which of the following can be concluded about it on the basis of the information in the passage?

    A. It is not venomous.
    B. It sometimes bites humans.
    C. Its habitat overlaps with that of the platypus.
    D. It is closely related to the platypus.
    E. It could be killed by a platypus sting.

Notice the first sentence of the question stem provides the new information: The New Guinean quoll is a very small mammal. Now, find anything relevant in the passage. It is tempting just to latch onto the word "mammal" and read the first few sentences of the passage. However, this might be misleading. The word "small" may also be important, which relates to the portion, "The venom can kill smaller animals." Bear this in mind as you eliminate answers.

While A may be tempting (and true by outside knowledge), it goes beyond what the passage says. The passage lists certain poisonous mammals but never says that these are the only ones. Thus, based on the information given, the quoll could be poisonous (eliminate A). Also, eliminate B, because this is never mentioned anywhere; even the biting animals in the passage are not described as biting humans in particular. Eliminate C, because this part of the passage does not give enough information to determine the habitat of the platypus. (Strictly speaking, if the earlier excerpt were from the same part of the passage, we could determine that the habitat of the platypus includes Australia, and the name "New Guinean" implies that the habitat of this type of quoll includes New Guinea. These are near each other but not necessarily overlapping, so the answer is still wrong.) Eliminate D, because no biological or evolutionary relationship was described in the passage or question. At this point, hopefully it's E, because everything else is gone, and indeed it is: The passage indicated that the platypus's venom could kill small animals, and the question stem indicates that the New Guinean quoll is a small mammal. Thus, the quoll could be killed by a platypus sting. Read choice E quickly to make sure it is the best answer, then select it, and move on.

In general, the right answer will do what this answer does, namely, relate the passage and the new information in the question stem accurately. If the answer does not come from the passage or is not relevant to the new information in the question stem, it is likely wrong.

Two Parts

A **Two Parts** question usually provides a statement and a reason (though it can occasionally provide two separate statements) and asks both whether they are true and whether they are related. Begin with the first consideration: Is the first statement true or not? Once you've decided, do POE. Next, is the second statement true or not? Do POE again. Finally, determine whether the two statements are related. Let's look at a typical example:

At first, many thought it was an elaborate hoax, because of its exotic appearance and characteristics. Like a duck, the platypus has a long, flat, broad bill. Also like a duck, it has webbed feet, and when on land, it must walk on its knuckles to avoid damaging the webbing. Onlookers observe that when it walks, it looks more like a reptile, since its feet are lateral to its body instead of underneath. Like a beaver, it has a paddle-shaped tail. Its body, however, is shaped like an otter's body. As a result, when a skin of a dead platypus was shipped back to Britain as one of the first pieces of evidence that such animals existed, the first to see it speculated that it had been sewn together by a taxidermist. However, they soon found out that this animal was genuine, and its other odd abilities included laying eggs and manufacturing poison.

Among venomous mammals...

4. British experts still living in Europe were skeptical that early specimens of the platypus were genuine because it walks like a reptile, not like most mammals.

A. Both the statement and the reason are true, and they are related.

B. Both the statement and the reason are true, but they are unrelated.

C. The statement is true, but the reason is not true.

D. The statement is not true, but the reason is true.

E. Neither the statement nor the reason is true.

First, determine whether the first part (the statement) is true. It definitely is because the first sentence of the excerpt says so, and the last two sentences of the paragraph confirm it. Thus, you can eliminate D and E, since these say that the statement is not true. Next, check whether the second part (the reason) is true. It is true, too, since the fourth sentence of the excerpt indicates this. Thus, eliminate C, because it says that the reason is not true. Now, you must decide whether the two statements are related. The passage indicates that the British in Europe were inspecting the "skin of a dead platypus" and suspected that it had been "sewn together by a taxidermist." Thus, they had to have been looking at the bizarre features of the body, such as the duck bill and feet, the beaver tail, and the otter body. More specifically, it was a skin, not a live animal, so they could not see it walk. (The passage specifically notes that "[o]nlookers" are the ones who observe its strange gait, which does not include experts speculatively reconstructing the appearance of the body in motion from a skin. Granted, some scientists have tried to infer how animals walked from their dead remains, such as fossils, but we have no evidence that happened here.) Thus, its method of walking could not have been fuel for their skepticism. Eliminate A, and the answer must be B.

Notice, by the way, that if either of the statements had been false, you could have eliminated both A and B and would not have had to determine whether the statements were related. This is the reason to determine the statements' truth first and their relationship later. Indeed, some Two Parts questions do not even ask whether the statements are related.

Tone/Attitude

Occasionally, a **Tone/Attitude** question will ask about the author's tone or attitude toward something; this could be the topic of the passage, a paragraph, an example, or a piece of the passage. These question stems can be broad and test the big picture of the passage (as the example below) or can be more narrow and specific. It depends on what the question is asking about. The author's tone or attitude will be revealed in the author's word choice. Words that indicate positive or negative value judgments or indicate agreement or disagreement are tone words, and such words will help you answer these questions. Consider the following example:

Recent research has located these peculiar features within the genome of the platypus. Because the evolution of monotremes, including the platypus and the echidna, split from that of all other mammals before the development of many non-reptilian features, such as viviparity, many unusual characteristics of the platypus come from genetic similarities to reptiles. This promising research has opened up the possibility of deeper understanding both of the platypus itself, which has always been difficult to study due to the animal's shy and reclusive nature, and of its relation to other animals…

5. The author's attitude toward recent research on the platypus can best be described as:

   A. cynical.
   B. shy.
   C. confused.
   D. optimistic.
   E. apathetic.

The question asks for the author's attitude toward recent research, so search the passage for tone words. Until the last sentence of the excerpt, not much tone is indicated, but the final sentence describes the research as "promising" and points out that it "has opened up the possibility of deeper understanding" that "has always been difficult" to achieve. These are all good things, so the passage is generally positive towards the research and believes that it can do good things in the future. Next, evaluate the answer choices.

Eliminate A, which means skeptical of others' motives or the value of something, so it is completely off the mark. While B is a word that is used in the passage, it is used about the platypus, not about the author's attitude, so it is also wrong. Choice C may represent how you feel after reading a particularly dense RCT passage, but an author would almost never feel "confused" about their subjects (if they were confused, they would figure out what they're talking about before writing about it), so not only is it wrong here, but also it is probably never going to be the right answer on any question. Choice D is fine, so keep it on your first pass. Choice E means not caring or lacking interest, so it, too, is almost certainly never going to be the right answer to any question about the attitude of the author (authors care about their subjects, even if no one else does). Thus, D is the best answer.

Notice that this question asks about something that might not seem very concrete ("attitude"), but the answer must still be based on the words in the passage. Even a question about tone or attitude is not an excuse to make stuff up. The answer is in the passage, no matter how buried it is in a mass of details. It has to be there, somewhere, and your task is to find it.

Meaning in Context

These questions ask about the meaning of a word or phrase in the context of the passage. There are a few tricks to these questions. First, they're not asking you for a general definition; they're asking you how the author uses the word or phrase in the passage. Go back to the passage, find the term, then read a few lines above and a few lines below the term you're being asked about. Predict what it means or why it is there and focus on its use in the passage.

Second, it is possible you won't know exactly where the term is in the passage. With a 1500-word passage, of course this is going to happen. In an ideal world, you'll either remember where the term is, approximately where it is, or even better, you have the term highlighted. If you know where to go in the passage, Meaning in Context will be first-pass questions. If you have no idea where the term is, don't worry about it too much. Mark the question, highlight the term or write it down on your noteboard, and watch for the phrase as you answer the other questions. If you find it, go back to the Meaning in Context question and answer it. If you never find the term, don't worry about it. Answer the Meaning in Context question using your Letter of the Day and move on. It is not worth your time rereading 1500 words of text to get one question right. You are better off to skip one question and spend your time on other questions you can answer more quickly.

Rare Question Types

It is possible you will see an Insertion, Purpose, or Main Point question on test day. These rare question types tend to test higher-level comprehension than straight Retrieval and Inference questions. Where a Retrieval question typically asks you to fetch the exact wording of the passage and an Inference question typically asks you to fetch the meaning of a particular sentence, these more advanced questions often depend on understanding the author's point. This is still not a huge leap from the passage. Always bear in mind that the right answer must be based on the text of the passage, and it will generally agree in tone, scope, topic, and main point with what the author has already said. Focus on synthesizing or summarizing what you've read and what you know about the passage. Answering these questions on your second pass and near the end of the questions for this passage can be helpful. Finally, don't panic: These questions are rare, and you may not see even one on the test you take.

Insertion

Very rarely, you may be asked to insert something into some portion of the passage, usually a final sentence. This is an **Insertion** question, and your goal is to be as close to what the passage has already said as possible. The right answer will match with the rest of the passage as it can be; it will not take the passage in a crazy, new direction or contradict information already presented in the passage. You are trying to summarize and support what has already been said. Consider the following example:

...This promising research has opened up the possibility of deeper understanding both of the platypus itself, which has always been difficult to study due to the animal's shy and reclusive nature, and of its relation to other animals.

One result that has arisen in the past few years from such research is the discovery that platypus sex determination in some way resembles the system in birds. In any mammal, including the platypus, the homogametic sex is female, with two X chromosomes, and the heterogametic sex is male, with an X and a Y. In birds, the homogametic sex is male, with two Z chromosomes, and the heterogametic sex is female, with a Z and a W. However, the platypus's X chromosome shows remarkable homology with a bird's Z chromosome, suggesting that the differences between the sex chromosomes in other mammals, such as humans, and those in birds evolved later than was previously thought, after the split between monotremes and other mammals.

Other genetic studies have yielded similarly remarkable results, and experiments continue with remarkable speed.

6. Which of the following sentences would be best to insert at the end of the passage?

A. The confusion that early biologists had regarding the platypus also inspired the title of *Kant and the Platypus*, a book regarding how humans perceive the things around us.

B. It is also remarkable that when threatened, the platypus can also emit low growls as well as use its leg stinger.

C. However, such experiments should be considered with skepticism, given the ongoing uncertainty whether the platypus is in fact a hoax.

D. Although we have come a long way from the early British explorers who doubted the platypus's authenticity, research continues into this odd but fascinating creature.

The passage concludes with paragraphs regarding research into the platypus's genes, so the correct answer will likely relate to platypus gene research. The rest of the passage, as we've seen up to this point, had to do with how strange and exotic the platypus is and how this utterly flummoxed the first Europeans to encounter it, so there is a pretty good chance that this, too, will show up in the right answer. Given this, evaluate the answers.

Eliminate A, because while this relates somewhat to the beginning of the passage about the early biologists, this is a complete non sequitur from the end of the passage. It has nothing to do with the genetic research and instead brings up problems of perception. Eliminate B, even though it is probably not wise to argue with a growling platypus, because this sentence's only connection with the end of the passage is the fact that this is "remarkable" (which is a tenuous connection at best). Eliminate C, because it contradicts much of the rest of the passage. There is no "ongoing uncertainty whether the platypus is in fact a hoax" anymore; this was a problem in the early history of the study of the platypus, not now. The answer is D, because this relates both to the beginning of the passage about the confusion of the British explorers and to the end of the passage about the genetic research.

In general, on Insertion questions, relevance is the most crucial issue. Is the sentence still on topic, or does it veer off in a strange new direction? Does it match the sorts of things that were said before, or does it seem to contradict them? Keep to the central points of the passage and the point of view that the author has already expressed. In this way, even if the right answer says something that is not exactly what the passage has already said, your answer will still be based on the text of the passage, which it must be in order to be right. This is not an exercise in creative writing; it's a Reading Comprehension Test.

Purpose

Not surprisingly, Purpose questions ask about the purpose of something, such as the passage as a whole, a paragraph, an example, a phrase, a fact, or a word. To answer these questions, find it in the passage, predict the answer (in general terms), and do POE with the answer choices. Ask yourself "why is that there?" or "why did the author include that?" Consider the following example:

Few animals have caused the sheer amount of confusion and consternation that the platypus has. Even the name itself is strange. Although the casual layperson might expect the plural of "platypus" to be "platypi," in the same way that the plural of "cactus" is "cacti," this turns out to be incorrect. The word "cactus" is derived from the Greek cactos, which in Greek has a plural of cactoi that in Latin becomes cacti and is retained in English. The word "platypus," on the other hand, is derived from a Greek compound platypos that in Greek has a plural of platypodes. Thus, in English, we might count "one platypus," "two platypodes." However, this is so strange that English speakers sometimes discard this notion and use the English plural "platypuses" rather than the Greek. The fact that we can hardly even speak about the platypus without confusion is no surprise when one considers the unique history and biology of the animal, which is equally baffling.

The platypus was first reported to Europeans in 1798…

7. The author mentions the plural of the word "platypus" most likely in order to

A. lament the inconsistencies of the English language.
B. correct a common misunderstanding.
C. present himself as a linguistic expert.
D. argue in favor of the English plural "platypuses."
E. illustrate a confounding subject of study.

This question asks about the author's purpose in mentioning the plural of the word "platypus." The passage introduces the topic by mentioning how much "confusion and consternation" there has been around the platypus, and it concludes by mentioning, "the unique history and biology of the animal…is equally baffling." Thus, the point the passage makes about the plural is that it is confusing and strange in exactly the same way as the animal is. Now let's do some POE.

Eliminate A, because it misses the essential point of this example. The point the author makes is not about language, but about biology. The platypus's name is just one example of how strange it is. Eliminate B, because it also is about language, not biology. The author's point is not just that the plural of "platypus" is not "platypi"; their point is that the confusion surrounding this is much like the confusion about the nature of the animal itself. Eliminate C, because this, too, focuses excessively on linguistics, and besides, one does not have to be a linguistics expert to know one's etymology. Eliminate D, because the author never does this anywhere. By POE, the answer is E. This option is good because discussion of the plural shows one example of how strange the platypus is, which is what E brings up.

If the question is asking about the overall purpose of the passage, there are a couple of common patterns you could watch for:

- Educate: the writing style of these passages is usually similar to a textbook or academic article. They are often neutral in tone and aim to give an educational overview of a specific topic.
- Tell a story: these passages are narrative; think "once upon a time… and then… and then… and they lived happily ever after… the end." These passages usually have a neutral tone or author attitude.
- Compare/contrast: these passages focus on similarities and differences between two things. They point out things in common and differences. Compare/contrast passages can have any tone/attitude but are often neutral.
- Advocate/defend: in these passages, a viewpoint, theory, or concept is presented that the author agrees with. The focus is the author explaining why they're right. These passages are usually positive or supportive in tone.
- Criticize: in these passages, a viewpoint, theory, or concept is presented that the author disagrees with. The focus of a criticize passage is often the author explaining why someone or something is or may be wrong. These passages usually have a negative or critical tone.
- Correct the record: these passages are a mix of advocate/defend, compare/contrast or criticize. The author is essentially saying someone is wrong or might not be correct and what the author thinks is correct instead. These passages have a mix of tone/attitude, from negative/critical (of the other person/thing) to positive/supportive (what the author thinks instead).

Main Point

Main Point questions ask for the author's thesis, conclusion, or main point. Focus on the big picture of the passage and POE. The best answer will address the whole passage, however, focusing on the first and last paragraph may help identify it. Ask yourself why the author wrote the passage. What are they trying to convince you of?

Miscellaneous Question Types

From time to time, the RCT will ask questions that are not easy to categorize. If you see something unexpected in an RCT question stem, don't panic. Read the question stem carefully and highlight key words to keep track of what you must do. Use the passage as your source of truth and rely on POE.

37.6 PROCESS OF ELIMINATION

In the RCT, if there are five answer choices, knowing that four are wrong is a good way to find the correct answer, especially on harder questions.[3] Furthermore, while several of the answer choices may superficially look tempting, all but one will be flawed, so looking for the right answer is less reliable than finding four wrong answers. Like the other sections of the DAT, process of elimination (POE) is a crucial element of your strategy. Doing POE in your head is slow and likely to cause problems, so be sure to use the strike out function available on the computer (right click). Eliminate answers until only one remains, and choose the last answer standing (after reading it to make sure it makes sense).

When you are doing POE on challenging questions, use the **Two Pass Technique:** The first time you are going through the answer choices, eliminate the worst options. Keep anything you're not sure about, tempting answer choices, options that look good, and keep anything you don't understand. You can probably work relatively quickly on your first pass. When you're down to two or three tempting answer choices, go back and do a second pass: slow down, pay attention, and read carefully. You can use a **comparison strategy** to find the best answer. Compare the remaining choices to the passage, the question stem, and each other. One of these comparisons will help you see that one answer choice is the best one there and the others have something wrong with them.

There are several common patterns for wrong answer choices. Watch for these as you're doing POE on your practice passages. Spend some time thinking about which ones from the list below you find particularly tempting:

- Not supported: when an answer choice contains information that was not in the passage, goes beyond the passage, or requires background information.
- Not relevant: when an answer choice contains irrelevant information from the passage. These answer choices sometimes contain statements from the wrong part of the passage, or common words from the passage. Remember, just because a statement is true and from the passage, doesn't mean it actually answers the question.
- Wrong scope or tone: when an answer choice is too specific or too general to answer the question, or is too extreme. Look out for words like only, solely, no, none, all, always, never, every, must, etc.
- Partially correct: when an answer is partially correct, it can be really tempting. However, be sure you read answer choices through to the end. If they're partially wrong, they're all wrong and you should strike that option out.
- Contradicts the passage: sometimes an answer choice will contradict something in the passage, meaning it is not the correct answer. Read answer choices carefully: adding one small word (such as "no" or "not") or slightly modifying a word (such as changing "typical" to "atypical") can mean a statement says the exact opposite of what it did before.
- Wrong direction or opposite: be careful not to pick a true statement on a false question, or vice versa. Also be careful when you're doing POE on least, most, not, and except question stems. Highlighting these key words in the question stem may help you keep track of what the question is asking.

---

[3] Most RCT questions will have five answer choices to pick from, but some questions may have only three or four options. This is true in all sections of the DAT except PAT, which has a predictable number of answer choices in each of the sub-sections.

37.7 PACE IN RCT

Difficulty Level of Questions

Let's review how to rank RCT questions. You must remember that all questions are worth 1 point, no matter how long you spend working on them! Many questions in the RCT will be doable: You will be able to work quickly and confidently. You will use your passage map to find the content you need in the passage, and you will be able to find the right answer and move on. These questions are good to do right away (these are your "now" questions), because they boost your confidence and allow you to gain familiarity with the passage. They often have clear question stems and short answer choices.

Some retrieval questions will take more time: Sometimes the question stems give you clear information on where to go, but the answer choices are longer, and you need to carefully read each one and do POE. In other questions, the question stem gives you no information on where to go, so the answer is hard to find. Once you find it in the passage, however, you can answer the question really quickly. You should also slow down when working on inference questions, and remember to stay within the scope of the passage. The questions we're talking about here are your "later" questions. Mark them on your first pass through the passage and come back to them when you're done with the "now" questions.

Finally, some questions on the RCT are going to be just plain hard. They will take you a long time to answer or maybe you never feel completely confident about the answer you end up picking. These questions are often open-ended or application questions, include content from all over the passage, and require effective POE skills. These time-wasting questions are good candidates for "never" questions. Get used to recognizing these so you save them for last, or skip them completely.

No matter what, make sure you've answered all the questions for a given passage before you move on to another passage.

Skipping Questions in RCT

Some test-takers don't have time to answer every RCT question, and that is okay. Many students aim to complete 2 and a half passages with high accuracy, instead of rushing through all three passages and making silly mistakes. Another option is aiming to get through all three passages but skipping a couple (the hardest) questions on each. Either way, make sure you're working at a pace on test day that ensures you're getting questions you're working on correct. To do this, find and do the "now" questions on your first pass, and "later" questions on your second pass. Identify and skip the "never" questions and answer them using your Letter of the Day. Note, that you must skip the hardest questions; don't spend any time on these questions, just select your Letter of the Day and move on.

Want More Practice?
Scan the QR code below to register your book for online chapter summaries, drills, practice tests, and more!

Quantitative Reasoning Test (QRT)

Chapter 38
Math Introduction

38.1 SECTION FORMAT AND GENERAL STRATEGIES

The Quantitative Reasoning Test (QRT) on the DAT contains 40 questions that you must complete in 45 minutes. The questions are not arranged in any useful order (for example, they are not in order of difficulty). Additionally, most students find that they do not have time to complete the section comfortably and must either rush to complete all the questions in the allotted time or make strategic decisions about which questions to spend time on.

Two-Pass System

The above facts (time pressure and no order of difficulty) give rise to the first basic section strategy, the **Two-Pass System**. The Two-Pass System means to take two passes through a section. On the first pass, complete questions that you can answer quickly and easily; mark questions that are more challenging so you can come back to them later. If a question is painfully long, complicated, or confusing, answer it using your Letter of the Day and move on. On the second pass, come back for the marked questions that you know you can answer but are likely to take more time. By doing this, you will make sure that you get to all the questions that you definitely can answer; if you simply do the questions in the order that they are presented, you run the risk of putting too much time into an earlier but harder question (which you might get wrong anyway) and not getting to a question that you could have answered correctly if only you'd known it was there. In fact, this strategy should be used across all sections of the DAT, not just in QRT.

Determining whether you know how to do a question quickly generally takes no more than a few seconds of reading, so skipping questions will not waste time; in fact, it will save you time. If you take the section in two passes, you'll get the easy questions right first, and then you'll have a very good idea how much time you have left for the harder questions. Thus, you will be able to allot your time more effectively.

The Two-Pass System takes some practice, so don't worry if it seems awkward at first. It will improve your score if you use it a few times.

Calculator

An on-screen calculator can be called up in the same way that you call up the periodic table in the Survey of the Natural Sciences. The calculator looks like this:

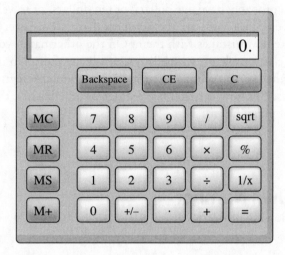

This is a basic four-function (not scientific or graphing) calculator. It can add, subtract, multiply, divide, take a square root, and take a reciprocal. However, it cannot do exponents, roots other than square roots, logs, or trig, and it does not know Order of Operations (it calculates as soon as you press buttons, rather than waiting for you to hit an "Enter" key). QRT is the only section of the DAT where a calculator will be available. In the SNS, you'll have to do all math mentally or using the Noteboard.

38.2 TEST CONTENT

QRT questions cover arithmetic, conversions, algebra, probability and statistics, word problems, geometry, and trigonometry. You will also see quantitative comparison and data sufficiency question formats on test day.

Note that some of this is not particularly specific. For example, "trigonometry" is tested, but what exactly that means is not specified. Does this just refer to the definitions of sine, cosine, and tangent? Does this also refer to more complex identities and laws? ADA is deliberately vague about this, which has provoked confusion and rumors among test takers. We have carefully studied the test and determined what it tests regularly. Those topics are covered in the later chapters that cover the content of the test.

It is certainly true, as you might expect from the discussion above, that knowing the content of the test is extremely important in order to do well. Much of the rest of our discussion of the math on the test will focus on content. However, content is not the only aspect of the test that you should be familiar with. While it is impossible to do well on the QRT without knowing certain mathematical facts and formulas, it is also important to make effective use of the knowledge that you already possess. We will discuss some of the most crucial techniques for doing this now. (The rest will be covered in later chapters.) The first is plugging in.

38.3 PLUGGING IN

Many questions on the test ask you to work with variables for everyday quantities. This is highly artificial and potentially confusing. In daily life, you probably don't walk around with *d* dollars in your pocket or travel *f* feet in *t* seconds. You probably have five dollars, or ten dollars, or travel ten feet in two seconds, or some actual, constant number. Since these are the numbers that you use every day, you're probably quite familiar with them and make few mistakes with them. On the other hand, you probably do algebra only when you're asked to do algebra problems, which is not nearly as often. No matter how good you are at algebra, it's easier to know whether you've made a mistake when you use regular old numbers than when you use algebraic expressions. But how can you use regular numbers when the test gives you an algebra problem? That's the magic of plugging in.

Plugging In Your Own Number

Let's say you're given the following problem.

1. If a, b, c, d, and e are nonzero numbers such that a is b percent of c and c percent of the square of d is e, then what percent of e is a, in terms of b and d ?

   A. $\dfrac{100d^2}{b}$

   B. $100b$

   C. $\dfrac{d^2}{b}$

   D. $\dfrac{d^2}{100b}$

   E. $\dfrac{100b}{d^2}$

You might (if you weren't a savvy test-taker) panic and guess on this question. It looks pretty horrible, after all. You could set up a whole bunch of equations with a whole bunch of variables, and if you make one little mistake anywhere, the whole problem is shot. However, take heart: you don't need to do any of that to solve this.

The whole point of algebraic formulas is that they relate variables that can have whatever value you could dream up. If the right answer is really right, it should work for *any* values of a, b, c, d, and e that fit the requirements they mention. Thus, you can just make up some values and run through the problem with those. If the answer doesn't work with the values that you chose, eliminate it.

Let's do that here. Since we're taking b percent of c to find a, let's make $b = 10$ and $c = 50$. This is doable enough: 10% of 50 is one-tenth of 50, which just removes the zero from the 50, so it's 5. With these numbers, then, $a = 5$.

The next portion of the problem says that c percent of the square of d is e. Now, c is already 50. Next, let's choose an easy square near these numbers, such as $d = 4$, so the square of d is 16. Thus, the question says that 50 percent of 16 is e. That means $e = 8$.

Now, the question is asking what percent of e is a, which might as well be saying what percent of 8 is 5. This is $\frac{5}{8}$, which you plug into the on-screen calculator to find that it is 62.5%. Thus, the answer to the question should be 62.5, if $a = 5$, $b = 10$, $c = 50$, $d = 4$, and $e = 8$.

At this point, the problem becomes pure calculation: plug these numbers into choice A and see if you get 62.5. You don't: choice A gives $\frac{100 \times 4^2}{10} = 160$. Likewise, B gives 1000, C gives 1.6, D gives 0.016, and E gives 62.5, so E is the right answer.

Okay, now for the bottom line. The point of this is that for just about any question that presents an algebraic expression, uses variables or unknown quantities, or uses the phrase "in terms of" (which, frankly, is meaningless here anyway—all of the answers are in terms of the right variables, so feel free to ignore that phrase entirely), you can make up your own numbers instead of working with their variables. The right answer will be right no matter what numbers you're using, so feel free to use the simplest, easiest numbers you can. Using regular numbers (constants) instead of variables is called **Plugging In**, and in this case, you're plugging in your own number (a number that you made up).

Notice, by the way, that this question is pretty darn hard unless you plug in. If you were to try to solve this with algebra, your first step would be to write down three equations: $a = \frac{b}{100}c$, $\frac{c}{100}d^2 = e$, and $\frac{x}{100}e = a$ (where x is the value you're actually solving for). From there, you would have to solve for x in terms of b and d by eliminating the other variables. This is challenging algebra and is going to take time to do correctly. The only thing challenging when Plugging In is making sure you use numbers that are easy enough to manipulate that you keep the problem from becoming even more unwieldy than it has to be.

On some other questions, it's not necessarily *hard* (in the sense of being complicated) to get the right answer, even if you don't plug in. However, such questions can be extremely *tricky*, since it's difficult to tell whether $\dfrac{x^2}{y}$ is okay or wildly wrong, whereas if you know that the answer should be about 20 and you get that the answer is 0.2, you know you've forgotten to multiply by 100 somewhere. The second crucial point is this: plugging in will make some questions easier to *work*, but its true significance is that it makes most questions easier to *check*. You're less likely to get wrong answers—or more likely to catch wrong answers if you get them—if you plug in.

Plugging In More Than Once

In general, when you make up numbers, it's possible to choose numbers where more than one answer works. You must check all five answer choices when Plugging In because you have to make sure that the answer that works is the *only* answer that works. If more than one answer works, try another number. A few tips to avoid having more than one answer work:

- Do plug in numbers that fit the constraints in the question (if it says "even" numbers, use an even number).
- Do plug in numbers that make the math easy. On most problems, this means 2, 3, 5, 10, or 100.
- Don't plug in 0 or 1. These numbers often lead to multiple answer choices working.
- Don't plug in numbers that appear in the question.
- Don't plug in the same number for more than one variable.

Bear in mind that these only apply to the first number you plug in. You may need to break several of these rules if you have to plug in again (discussed below).

Let's consider another example.

2. If x is an integer, which of the following must be an odd integer?

    A. $x + 2$
    B. $x - 3$
    C. $2x$
    D. $3x$
    E. $2x - 3$

To solve this, you might plug in. The only constraint on x is that it be an integer (not a fraction or a decimal), so let's try $x = 2$. In that case, A would be 4, which is not odd, so eliminate it. Choice B would be −1, which is odd, so keep it. Choice C would be 4, which is not odd, so eliminate it. Choice D would be 6, which is also not odd, so eliminate it. Choice E would be 1, which is odd, so keep that as well. With $x = 2$, both B and E work. They're not both correct; it's just that while both of them *could* be an odd integer, only one of them *must* be an odd integer, as the question stem says.

So try a different number, and since we're talking about odd and even and tried an even number before, try an odd number. Let's say $x = 3$. In that case, we don't have to check choices A, C, or D again; we already eliminated these options, and we know they don't *have* to be odd. You are down to choices B and E. Choice B is 0, which is not odd (it's even), so eliminate it. Choice E is 3, which is still odd, so it must be the right answer.

There are two points to this question. First, check all five answers when you're Plugging In! If you had just gone with the first answer that worked, you would've chosen B and gotten the question wrong.

Second, notice (and take seriously) words like "must" or "could." If a question asks what "must" be the case, then it's likely that many of the answers *could* work, given the right values of x, but only one of them *must* work with all values of x. On the other hand, if a question asks what "could" be the case, then it's likely that you need very particular values of x to make anything work at all, and with most values of x that you could choose, none of the answers will be right. You're just looking for an answer that *could ever* be right, which means that there might only be one value of x that ever makes it right, and your job is to find it. There's a pretty good chance you'll have to plug in more than once on questions that ask what *must* or *could* be true, and there's nothing worse than plugging in repeatedly but getting that B and E always work. You need to try different, weird numbers in order to differentiate between answers.

What are different, weird numbers? Well, for your second try at Plugging In on the same question, everything that we just said about not choosing numbers that break the question goes completely out the window. In fact, 0, 1, numbers in the question, and the same number for more than one variable are among the first things that you should try if you're working a question on which you have to plug in a second time. The acronym **ZONE-F** may be useful: try zero, one, negatives, extremes (very large and very small), and fractions, if you're trying to find different numbers to plug in that don't just give the same results as what you've already done.

Remember, this only applies when you're plugging in a second time on the same question, which you should only do if more than one answer worked on your first try.

Plugging In a Given Value

Sometimes questions will ask what the value of an expression is if a variable equals something (also known as **substitution**). For example, "What is the value of $x + 4$ when $x = 6$?" We substitute 6 for the x in the expression $x + 4$ and get $6 + 4$, which equals 10. This is plugging in, but the test has already given you the value to use. Consider the following examples.

3. Evaluate $2x + 7$ when $x = -3$.

    A.   −13
    B.   −1
    C.   1
    D.   8
    E.   13

Once we substitute −3 for x, we get $2(-3) + 7 = -6 + 7 = 1$. Thus, the answer is C.

4. If $f(x) = 3x^2 - x - 1$, what is $f(2)$?

    A.   9
    B.   11
    C.   13
    D.   15
    E.   33

Once we substitute 2 for x, we get $f(2) = 3(2^2) - 2 - 1 = 12 - 2 - 1 = 9$ (A is correct).

5. What is the value of $(3x)^2 - x - 1$ when $x = 2$?

    A.   9
    B.   11
    C.   13
    D.   15
    E.   33

Be sure to notice the difference between this expression and the one in the previous example. Substitute 2 for x and evaluate: $(3 \cdot 2)^2 - 2 - 1 = 6^2 - 2 - 1 = 33$ (E is correct).

6. Evaluate $2x + 3y$ when $x = 1$ and $y = -4$.

    A.   −14
    B.   −10
    C.   −5
    D.   6
    E.   14

We substitute 1 for x and −4 for y, then simplify: $2(1) + 3(-4) = 2 + (-12) = -10$. Thus, the answer is B.

Plugging In Points

On a graphical question, sometimes you can choose points from the graph to plug into an equation, and this will help you eliminate answers. Consider the following example.

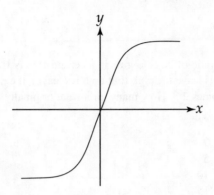

7. Which of the following equations represents the graph above?

A. $y = \dfrac{10x - 1}{\sqrt{x^2 + 1}}$

B. $y = \dfrac{10x^2 + 2}{\sqrt{x^4 + 1}}$

C. $y = \dfrac{x^2 + 1}{\sqrt{x^2 + 2}}$

D. $y = \dfrac{10x + 1}{\sqrt{x^2 + 1}}$

E. $y = \dfrac{10x}{\sqrt{x^2 + 1}}$

Okay, these are not normal equations. There is no way you're supposed to know, off the top of your head, the shapes of graphs of these equations. However, there is one point on the graph that you know: the origin. When $x = 0$ on this graph, $y = 0$. Thus, plug in this point! In A, when $x = 0$, $y = \dfrac{-1}{1}$, which is definitely not 0 (eliminate A). In B, when $x = 0$, $y = \dfrac{2}{1}$, which is also not 0 (eliminate B). In C, when $x = 0$, $y = \dfrac{1}{\sqrt{2}}$, which is still not 0 (eliminate C). In D, when $x = 0$, $y = \dfrac{1}{1}$, which continues to not be 0 (eliminate D). Presumably choice E is correct, but let's make sure. When you plug in $x = 0$, you get $y = \dfrac{0}{1}$, which is indeed equal to 0, so E must be the answer. It's the only option that contains the one identifiable point on the graph.

Whenever you have any question that involves a graph, remember you can plug in points.

38.3

Plugging In The Answers

For much the same reasons as making up a number can be useful, sometimes it can be useful to test answers to see if they are correct. This is called **Plugging In The Answers** (or PITA). For example, consider the following problem.

> 8. The ratio of boys to girls in a certain club is 1:2. When 5 girls leave the club (but no boys leave), the ratio becomes 2:3. How many girls were originally in the club?
>
> A. 2
> B. 5
> C. 10
> D. 15
> E. 20

Notice the answer choices are arranged in order. This is typically the case. Thus, start in the middle (for reasons that will become apparent in a moment if they are not already). The question is how many girls were originally in the club, and if there were 10 originally in the club (as C indicates), then the 1:2 ratio says that there would have been 5 boys in the club. So there were 5 boys and 10 girls, and then 5 girls left. That means that there are now 5 boys and 5 girls. That's a 1:1 ratio, not a 2:3 ratio, so C is not the right answer.

Next, we can tell that C is too small. A 2:3 ratio means that there are more girls than boys, so because 10 girls gave a 1:1 ratio, there are not enough girls (eliminate A, B, and C). Go for a larger number like 15 in answer choice D. If there were 15 girls originally, then the 1:2 ratio says that there would have been 7.5 boys. This seems pretty unlikely, but if you want to follow it all the way through, then after 5 girls left, there would have been 7.5 boys and 10 girls; this is 3:4 ratio, which is still not right (but is closer than 1:1 was).

It is likely at this point that choice E is the answer if C is too small and D is unlikely. If you want to be sure, you can run this one through as well: 20 girls would mean 10 boys originally, and then after the 5 girls leave, there would be 10 boys and 15 girls, which is a 2:3 ratio. Thus, choice E is in fact the right answer.

In general, regular numbers (not variables) in the answer choices are an indication that you can likely PITA. That is, when you see variables in the answer, you can probably try Plugging In, and when you don't, you can probably try PITA.

38.4   ESTIMATION

Answer choices on the DAT are often substantially different from each other, so even if you don't know exactly what the answer is, you can eliminate several options that are not even close. A reasonable estimate is sometimes as good as an exact answer, so **estimation** is another major technique. Some questions explicitly ask for an estimate, as in the following:

9. Which of the following is the best approximation of the

value of $\left(\sqrt{80} + \dfrac{11}{9}\right)^{3.01}$?

A. 1
B. 11
C. 108
D. 1075

To solve this, note first that the square root of 81 should be pretty close to the square root of 80, and the square root of 81 is not only an integer but also a number you either know or can calculate quickly. In other words, simplify $\sqrt{80} \approx \sqrt{81} = 9$. Also, 11 divided by 9 is going to be only slightly more than 9 divided by 9, and 9 divided by 9 is an integer and a quick calculation, so use that instead. In other words, $\dfrac{11}{9} \approx \dfrac{9}{9} = 1$. Thus, $\sqrt{80} + \dfrac{11}{9} \approx 9 + 1 = 10$, so the expression inside the parentheses should be pretty close to 10. (Since the square root of 80 is only *barely* less than the square root of 81, whereas 11 divided by 9 is somewhat more than 9 divided by 9, we can even say that it should be a little more than 10, although it makes no difference in this particular problem.) Now, that exponent is not a friendly one, but it is quite close to an integer, so just say that $3.01 \approx 3$, and you're left with $10^3 = 1000$. The only answer choice even close is D.

In general, when approximating, try to make expressions into integers by changing as little as possible. The square root of 80 is almost exactly equal to the square root of 81 (it differs by less than 1%), but it's not nearly as close to the square roots of 64 or 100, so using those to approximate would be substantially less accurate. Estimating will be a time-saving technique in QRT but will also help you answer questions faster in Gchem. Practicing this technique until you can do it well is worth your time.

In addition to questions that specifically ask for an estimate, some questions that don't mention approximating in any way can still be solved by this method. Consider the following example.

10. If log 2 = 0.301, log 3 = 0.477, and log 5 = 0.699, then what is the value of log 900?

A. 0.010
B. 0.100
C. 1.477
D. 2.186
E. 2.954

Okay, this looks like a monster. This is some sort of "rules of logarithms" question. Set that aside for a second, and focus on the end of the question, where it actually asks the important part. What is the value of log 900? That's the bit you have to answer.

Now, remember that a log is asking, "What power do I need to raise 10 to in order to get this number?" In other words, log 900 will be whatever the exponent has to be on a 10 to get 900. That is, if log 900 = x, then $10^x = 900$. So what do you have to raise 10 to in order to get 900? Well, to get 1000, you need to raise 10 to the 3. To get 900, you should raise 10 to somewhat less than 3 (not much less, since $10^2 = 100$, which is nowhere near 900). There's only one answer that's even close anyway: option E. All the other answers are far, far too small.

If you're curious how to get an exact answer (why is it 2.954, not 2.955 or some other number that is somewhat less than 3?), we'll cover that in the section on logs. The point for right now is that an estimate can get you the answer just as well as anything else, and this will frequently be true on the test.

Want More Practice?
Scan the QR code below to register your book for online chapter summaries, drills, practice tests, and more!

Chapter 39
Arithmetic

This chapter will overview arithmetic content you need to know for the QRT. However, the skills here will also help you save time in Gchem. Any time we talk about using the calculator, we're focusing on the QRT. Remember, you won't have access to a calculator for Gchem. For that reason, the skills in this chapter are crucial for not one, but two sections of the DAT. Make sure you're comfortable and confident with this content as soon as possible.

39.1 BASIC OPERATIONS

Integers are the counting numbers (1, 2, 3, …) along with their negatives (–1, –2, –3,…) and zero (0). Since any number greater than 0 is **positive**, counting numbers are positive integers. Since any number less than 0 is **negative**, negatives of the counting numbers are negative integers. Zero is neither positive nor negative. The nonnegative integers are, naturally, those integers that are not negative: 0, 1, 2, … Similarly, the nonpositive integers are 0, –1, –2,…

Note we say that 2 is greater than 1, but –2 is less than –1. The logic behind this is that "greater" means "farther to the right on a number line" (see below) and "less" means "farther to the left on a number line." On a number line, –2 would be on the left, then –1, then 1, then 2. So we can say that $-2 < -1 < 1 < 2$. It may be somewhat counterintuitive to describe –9999999 as "less" than –1; if so, you're thinking of the number's **magnitude** (its absolute value; more on that shortly), rather than its **value**.

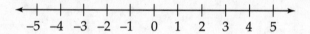

Addition

When two or more numbers are added, the result is called their **sum**. For example, the sum of 2, 3, and 4 is 9, since $2 + 3 + 4 = 9$. Addition is a **commutative operation**; this means that the order in which numbers are added makes no difference: $2 + 3 + 4$ is the same as $3 + 2 + 4$, or $2 + 4 + 3$, or $4 + 2 + 3$, or any other ordering.

Subtraction

When one number is subtracted from another, the result is called their **difference.** For example, the difference between 8 and 5 is 3, since $8 - 5 = 3$. Subtraction is *not* a commutative operation: the order in which the numbers are written does make a difference: $8 - 5$ is not the same as $5 - 8$. Further, notice that $8 - 5 = 3$, and $5 - 8 = -3$, which means that changing the order is the same as multiplying by –1. That is, $8 - 5 = 3$, and $5 - 8 = (-1)(3) = -3$. To distinguish between the two orders, sometimes the first is called the **positive difference** (because $8 - 5$ is positive) and the second is called the **negative difference** (because $5 - 8$ is negative).

Multiplication

When two or more numbers are multiplied, the result is called their **product.** For example, the product of 2, 3, and 4 is 24, since 2 × 3 × 4 = 24. Multiplication can be indicated in two other ways: 2 · 3 · 4 or (2)(3)(4). Multiplication is a commutative operation: the order in which the factors are written makes no difference: 2 × 3 × 4 is the same as 3 × 2 × 4, or 2 × 4 × 3, or any other ordering.

Division and Remainder

When one number is divided by another, the result is called their **quotient**. For example, the quotient of 14 and 7 is 2 since 14 ÷ 7 = 2. Division can be indicated by ÷ or by a slash, /, or by a horizontal bar. Therefore, all of the following are equivalent: $14 ÷ 7 = 14/7 = \dfrac{14}{7}$.

If an integer is divided by another integer, it is possible that the division doesn't yield an integer as the quotient. For example, when 14 is divided by 5, we get 2 with 4 "left over." In such a case, we usually say "the quotient is 2, with **remainder** 4." Division is *not* a commutative operation: the order in which the numbers are written *does* make a difference: 14 ÷ 7 is not the same as 7 ÷ 14.

It is also possible that one integer cannot be divided by another in one specific case: you cannot divide by zero. The value of $\dfrac{1}{0}$ (or anything else over 0) is undefined. For any other number in the denominator, the value will be defined (though it may yield a remainder or not).

Factors and Multiples

If the remainder is 0 when one integer is divided by another, we say that the first integer is **divisible by** (or a **multiple of**) the other integer. Here are some examples:

- 14 is divisible by 7 but not by 5. Another way of saying this is 14 is a multiple of 7 but not of 5.
- 32 is divisible by 8 but not by 9.
- Every integer is divisible by 1 and itself.
- The integer 12 is divisible by 1, 2, 3, 4, 6, and 12 but by no other positive integer.

The above list of integers that divide into 12 and yield no remainder are called the (positive) **factors** of 12. The factors of 7 are just 1 and 7. If an integer has exactly two **distinct** (different) positive factors (1 and itself), the integer is called a **prime.** Here are some examples:

- The numbers 7 and 37 are prime, but 9 and 39 are not (since 3 is a factor of both).
- The number 31 is prime, but 51 is not.
- The only even prime number is 2.

[Note: since the only positive factor of 1 is 1, we might say this fits the common, casual definition of a prime: "the only positive factors are 1 and itself." Nevertheless, we do not consider 1 prime, since it has only one *distinct* factor; 1 and 1 are not distinct from each other.] An integer with more than two distinct factors (any integer greater than 1 that is not a prime) is called a **composite.** For example: 5, 11, and 23 are primes, but 4, 15, and 21 are composites.

Factors and multiples are often confused for each other, though they are opposites. Since 7 goes into 14, 7 is a factor of 14, and 14 is a multiple of 7. *Multiples* of a number come from *multiplying* that number by an integer (hence the name), so the positive multiples of 7 are the results of multiplying 7 by 1, 7 by 2, and so on: 7, 14, 21, 28, 35, etc. *Factors* are the numbers that *divide* evenly into the number.

Is there any number that is both a factor of 10 and a multiple of 10? Well, the first multiple of any number is itself, and any number is a factor of itself. So 10 is both a factor of 10 (because it goes in evenly) and a multiple of 10 (because you can multiply 10 by 1 and get 10). The same would be true of any number: it is both a factor and a multiple of itself.

Knowing how larger numbers break down into their factors is something that can be exploited to facilitate quick multiplication and division. For instance, multiplying by 10 shifts the decimal place once to the right, ultimately tacking on a zero to the end of the number. Therefore, multiplying by 100, which breaks down into 10 times 10, amounts to making this rightward decimal shift twice, ultimately tacking on two zeroes to the end of the number. Therefore, when multiplying by a number that breaks down into factors of 10, we simply tack on to our number as many zeroes as are found in the number we are multiplying by. Similarly, dividing by a number that breaks down into factors of 10 shifts the decimal place to the left as many times as there are zeroes in the number we are dividing by. For example, $841 \times 100 = 84100$ and $\frac{841}{1,000} = 0.841$.

If we have to multiply or divide by other multiples of 10, like 20 or 30, we can break down those numbers into factors, like (2)(10) or (3)(10), respectively, and proceed to shift the decimal in the manner the factor(s) of 10 dictate and then divide or multiply by the remaining factor(s). For example, $33 \times 20 = 33 \times (2)(10) = 330 \times 2 = 660$ and $\frac{33}{30} = \frac{33}{(3)(10)} = \frac{3.3}{3} = 1.1$.

It's also worth noting that numbers like 0.1 or 0.01 can be thought of like the number 1 divided by an appropriate amount of 10s to shift the decimal. In other words, $0.1 = \frac{1}{10}$ and $0.01 = \frac{1}{100}$. Therefore, when multiplying by decimals like 0.1 or 0.01, you can instead divide by 10 or 100, respectively.

Lastly, when multiplying by a number greater than 1, we get back something larger than what we started with. Conversely, when multiplying by a number less than 1 (but greater than 0), we get back something smaller than what we started with. For example, $4 \times 10 = 40$ and $4 \times 0.1 = 0.4$. When dividing by a number greater than 1, we get back something smaller than what we started with. Conversely, when dividing by a number less than 1 (but greater than 0), we get back something larger than what we started with. For example, $\frac{4}{10} = 0.4$ and $\frac{4}{0.1} = \frac{4}{\frac{1}{10}} = 4 \times 10 = 40$.

Many of the patterns we've discussed here will help you do efficient math and quick POE on the test in both QRT and Gchem.

Sum and Product Properties

When you perform arithmetic operations on certain types of numbers, you predictably get certain types of numbers as a result. Product properties for positive and negative numbers should be memorized and are:

- positive $\times$ positive = positive
- negative $\times$ negative = positive
- negative $\times$ positive = positive $\times$ negative = negative
- anything $\times$ 0 = 0

The fourth rule is necessary because zero is neither positive nor negative, so it doesn't fit any of the other situations.

Exactly the same rules regarding positive and negative numbers hold for division as for multiplication (e.g. $\frac{negative}{negative}$ = positive). However, the rules for addition and subtraction are not always definite. It is always true that positive + positive = positive, and negative + negative = negative, but a positive plus a negative could be positive or negative. For example, $3 + (-2) = 1$, which is positive, but $3 + (-4) = -1$, which is negative. Subtraction works similarly, if you take subtraction to be the same as addition by a negative number. That is, $-3 - 2 = -3 + (-2)$, and a negative plus a negative is another negative.

In addition to the positive and negative rules, there are even and odd rules. These do not need to be memorized, as long as you remember that they exist. These are the rules:

- even + even = even
- odd + odd = even
- even + odd = odd + even = odd
- even × even = even
- odd × odd = odd
- even × odd = odd × even = even

The rules for subtraction are, of course, the same as the rules for addition. If you forget these rules at any point, you can derive them from the numbers 1 and 2. Since 1 + 2 = 3, an odd plus an even must be an odd. The crucial thing to realize is that this is *always* true: *any* odd plus *any* even is equal to another odd, whether it's 1 + 2 = 3, 3 + 4 = 7, or 33 + 56 = 89. Similarly, since (1)(2) = 2, an odd times an even is an even. Thus, don't bother remembering the even and odd rules; just remember that there *are* rules for addition, subtraction, and multiplication, and test examples as needed.

However, there are no even/odd rules for division. For example, $\frac{4}{2} = 2$, so an even divided by an even could be even, but $\frac{4}{4} = 1$, so an even divided by an even could be odd, or for that matter, $\frac{4}{8} = 0.5$, so an even divided by an even may not be an integer in the first place.

39.2   FRACTIONS, DECIMALS, AND PERCENTS

Fractions

Fractions are one way of expressing numbers between the integers, as well as expressing parts of a whole. For example, the number $\frac{2}{3}$ is between 0 and 1, and two-thirds of a pizza is part of a whole pizza. Also, remember that a fraction is simply a way of denoting a division. For example, $\frac{5}{4}$ means "5 divided by 4" and could equally be written 5 ÷ 4. The simplest arithmetic operation to perform with fractions is multiplication, since to multiply fractions, you multiply the numerators and multiply the denominators separately. For example, $\frac{2}{3} \times \frac{4}{7} = \frac{2 \times 4}{3 \times 7} = \frac{8}{21}$. Sometimes the result can be reduced. Reduce fractions if factors in the numerator and denominator are equal. For example, $\frac{2}{3} \times \frac{9}{4} = \frac{18}{12}$, but this can be reduced, because the numerator

and denominator are both divisible by 6. Thus, $\frac{18}{12} = \frac{3}{2} \times \frac{6}{6} = \frac{3}{2} \times 1$, since anything divided by itself is 1.

Since anything times 1 is itself, $\frac{18}{12}$ reduces to $\frac{3}{2}$. In fact, this whole process could have been shortened

by noticing that $\frac{2}{3} \times \frac{9}{4} = \frac{2}{4} \times \frac{9}{3} = \frac{1}{2} \times \frac{3}{1}$. When multiplying fractions, numerators and denominators can

be interchanged however you like (since multiplication is commutative) to cancel anything possible. This

makes numbers smaller, and smaller numbers are easier to handle (especially under time and test pressure)

than larger ones.

Dividing fractions works similarly. To divide fractions, multiply by the reciprocal. That is, $\frac{1}{3} \div \frac{1}{2}$, or,

equivalently, $\dfrac{\frac{1}{3}}{\frac{1}{2}}$, is equal to $\frac{1}{3} \times \frac{2}{1}$, which in turn equals $\frac{2}{3}$.

Just as fractions can be reduced by factoring out a form of 1 ($\frac{6}{6}$ when reducing $\frac{18}{12}$ above), so too fractions

can be changed in other ways by multiplying by a form of 1. For example, $\frac{4}{2} \times \frac{2}{2} = \frac{8}{4}$, since $\frac{2}{2} = 1$. This

is most frequently employed when adding or subtracting fractions, in which you must find a common

denominator and then add or subtract the numerators. For example, $\frac{1}{3} + \frac{1}{4}$ is an addition problem with

different denominators, so the first step is to change the denominators to the same numbers. The easiest

way to do this is just to use the other denominator as your guide: $\left(\frac{1}{3} \times \frac{4}{4}\right) + \left(\frac{1}{4} \times \frac{3}{3}\right) = \frac{4}{12} + \frac{3}{12}$. Now

they have the same denominator, so just add the numerators, and the result is $\frac{7}{12}$.

Any fraction can be added in this fashion, though some will need to be reduced afterwards. For example,

solving $\frac{1}{6} + \frac{1}{9}$ in the same fashion looks like this: $\frac{1}{6} + \frac{1}{9} = \left(\frac{1}{6} \times \frac{9}{9}\right) + \left(\frac{1}{9} \times \frac{6}{6}\right) = \frac{9}{54} + \frac{6}{54}$, and now that

they have a common denominator, you can just add 9 and 6, so the result is $\frac{15}{54}$. However, this can be

reduced. Factoring out a 3 yields $\frac{5 \times 3}{18 \times 3} = \frac{5}{18}$.

In summary, to do arithmetic with fractions, you must follow these rules:

- To add or subtract fractions, find a common denominator and then add or subtract the numerators.
- To multiply fractions, multiply the numerators and multiply the denominators.
- To divide fractions, multiply by the reciprocal.

Decimals

Like fractions, decimals are ways of expressing numbers between the integers, as well as expressing parts of a whole. For example, 2.5 is a number between 2 and 3, and half of a pizza could also be described as 0.5 of a pizza.

To add or subtract decimals, line up the decimal points. For example, $0.45 + 0.1$ can be added as follows:

$$\begin{array}{r} 0.45 \\ + \ 0.1 \\ \hline \end{array}$$

Then add digits just as you would add any other number. If a digit is not written in, assume that it is zero.

$$\begin{array}{r} 0.45 \\ + \ 0.1 \\ \hline 0.55 \end{array}$$

To multiply decimals, simply multiply as usual, then count the number of digits after the decimal point in the two numbers being multiplied and place the decimal point so that there are as many digits after the decimal point in the result. For example, 0.4×0.5 is just like 4×5, except that after you get 20, find that there is one digit after the decimal point in 0.4 and one in 0.5, so there should be two digits after the decimal point in the result, so the answer is 0.20, or 0.2. As another example, 0.3×0.12 is much like $3 \times 12 = 36$, except that you must have three digits after a decimal point, so $0.3 \times 0.12 = 0.036$. If you find yourself getting lost counting digits, approximate! You know that $0.3 \times 0.12 \approx 0.3 \times 0.1$, and $0.3 \times 0.1 = 0.03$, so the result should be slightly greater than 0.03, which is true of 0.036.

To divide by a decimal, multiply by 10 until you don't have a decimal anymore. For example, if you must divide $\dfrac{0.2}{0.05}$, multiply by 10 twice. Then you'll have $\dfrac{0.2 \times 10 \times 10}{0.05 \times 10 \times 10} = \dfrac{20}{5}$, and you can divide normally.

Of course, you can use the on-screen calculator on the QRT to do arithmetic with decimals. On the QRT, it is unlikely that a question will be phrased such that you must do arithmetic by hand with the decimals; this is not true of Gchem questions, which will require you to do mental or manual math calculations.

Indeed, you can use the on-screen calculator on the QRT to do arithmetic with fractions if you convert them to decimals by dividing. (That is, to convert $\dfrac{5}{4}$ to a decimal, use the calculator to divide 5 by 4.)

However, answer choices may be phrased in terms of fractions, so you may spend a great deal of time if you convert your fractions to decimals and then must also divide each of the answer choices to convert them to decimals as well. Also, be sure to have some idea what the answer is supposed to be before you start punching buttons. At least know whether you're supposed to get a number between 0 and 1, a number greater than 1 (and if so, nearest which integer), or a negative number (and again, if so, nearest which integer). If you do not, you run the risk of getting an answer that is wildly wrong because you simply clicked incorrectly. This is the main reason that it is worth having a general sense of how fractions and decimals work even if you do not have to do a lot of this by hand on test day.

Also, it is likely to be useful to be able to recognize decimal equivalents of the fractions from one-half to one-tenth (e.g. $\frac{1}{2} = 0.5$, $\frac{1}{3} = 0.\overline{3}$, and $\frac{1}{4} = 0.25$). While you can just use the calculator to divide 1 by 4 to determine that one-fourth is equal to 0.25, you may be able to take a shortcut if you see 0.25 and recognize it as a basic fraction.

Percents

A percentage is nothing more than an operation that says, "divide by 100." It is denoted by %. For example, the symbol 50% literally means $\frac{50}{100}$, which equals $\frac{1}{2}$. The symbol 125% means $\frac{125}{100}$, which equals 1.25 (or $\frac{5}{4}$). Many percent problems can be solved using the following equivalents between English and math:

Verbal statement	Equivalent algebraic expression/symbol
two-thirds of a number	$\frac{2}{3}x$ ("of" means multiply)
two out of three	$\frac{2}{3}$ ("out of" means divide)
five percent	$\frac{5}{100}$ or 0.05
is	=
what	x, y, or any other variable

Many percent problems can be solved using the English/math equivalents listed above. For example, what is 20 percent of 50? Translate this into math: $x = \dfrac{20}{100} \times 50$. Next, calculate, and the answer is 10.

A trickier example using the same principles might be: If x is two-fifths of y, what percent of x is y? Translate the first equation as $x = \dfrac{2}{5} \times y$, and the second as $\dfrac{z}{100} \times x = y$, where z is the answer that we're looking for. In this case, plug the first equation into the second, which yields $\dfrac{z}{100}\left(\dfrac{2}{5}y\right) = y$. Divide both sides by y, and you're left with $\dfrac{z}{100}\left(\dfrac{2}{5}\right) = 1$. Now, isolate the z, and $z = 250$.

Consider the following even trickier example.

11. If y is x percent of z, what percent of x is y ?

    A. z

    B. $\dfrac{xz}{100}$

    C. $\dfrac{100z}{x}$

    D. $10\sqrt{z}$

Now, before you go crazy writing down a whole bunch of algebraic equations, remember that there are techniques you can use to deal with excessive variables. In this case, let's plug in! The variable we're taking percents of is z, so let's say that $z = 200$. Then we should make x something easy, so let's say that $x = 50$, since 50 percent is an easy percent. In that case, $y = 100$. Now, the second part of the question is asking what percent of 50 is 100. Well, 100 is 200% of 50 (since it's twice as big). So the answer to the question is 200. Choice A works, so leave it. Choice B gives 100, not 200 (eliminate B). Choice C is no good either, since it comes out to 400 (eliminate C). Choice D comes out to an awful decimal that is somewhat more than 140, which isn't right either (eliminate D; A is correct).

Here are a few more examples.

12. What is 40% of 60?

    A.   12
    B.   24
    C.   30
    D.   40
    E.   90

40% of 60 is equivalent to $\dfrac{40}{100} \times 60$, which is 24 (B is correct).

13. 30 is what percent of 90?

    A. 10

    B. 30

    C. $33\frac{1}{3}$

    D. 40

    E. $66\frac{2}{3}$

Translate this sentence into a mathematical equation: $30 = \dfrac{x}{100} \times 90$. Dividing both sides by 90, we get $\dfrac{30}{90} = \dfrac{x}{100}$, so $x = 33\frac{1}{3}$ (C is correct).

Another topic within percents is **percent change.** The formula for percent change is that percent change $= \dfrac{\text{difference}}{\text{original}} \times 100$. The difference is the result of subtracting one value from the other, and the original is the smaller value for percent increase and the larger value for percent decrease. Consider the following example.

14. If the price of an item is originally $120 and this is reduced by $24, by what percent has it decreased?

    A. 20
    B. 24
    C. 30
    D. 50
    E. 96

The percent change will be given by $\dfrac{24}{120} \times 100$. This equals 20, so the percent decrease was 20% (A is correct).

39.3   EXPONENTS AND ROOTS

Exponent and Root Basics

Exponents provide a shorthand notation for a repeated multiplication. For example, if we wish to multiply the number 2 by itself six times, we could write $2 \times 2 \times 2 \times 2 \times 2 \times 2$, but it is much easier to write this expression using exponent notation: 2^6. This is read "2 to the sixth power," or "2 raised to the sixth," or most briefly, "2 to the 6." The 6 is the **exponent** and specifies how many times the **base** (2 in this case) is to be multiplied by itself. Here's another example: $5^4 = 5 \times 5 \times 5 \times 5$; the base is 5, and the exponent is 4.

Raising a base to a power 2 is referred to as "squaring" and to 3 is "cubing" (e.g. 3^2 is the square of 3 and 2^3 is the cube of 2). It would be helpful for the DAT (both Gchem and QRT sections) to recognize the squares of the integers up to 12 (that is, 1, 4, 9, 16, 25, 36, 49, 64, 81, 100, 121, and 144) and the cubes up to 5 (that is, 1, 8, 27, 64, 125). Even though you can use the on-screen calculator to determine what the square of 7 is, for example, recognizing 49 as a perfect square may save you time. The fact that the calculator can tell you that 49 is a square if you ask doesn't necessarily mean that you'll think to ask, unless you recognize the squares and cubes already.

A **root** is the opposite (technically, the inverse function) of an exponent. That is, since $2^2 = 4$, it is also true that $\sqrt{4} = 2$. A square root asks, "What do you have to square to get this number?" Since you square 2 to get 4, 2 is the square root of 4. Notice that this means the square root of a number bigger than 1 gets you something smaller than what you started with (like what we just saw with $\sqrt{4}$) and the square root of something smaller than 1 gets you something bigger than what you started with. For example, $\sqrt{0.81} = 0.9$. Other roots work similarly. For example, because $2^3 = 8$, it is also true that $\sqrt[3]{8} = 2$ (that is, the cube root of 8 equals 2).

Any even exponent will result in a nonnegative number, regardless of the base. For example, $(-2)^2 = 4$, because a negative times a negative is a positive. However, this is *not* true of odd exponents. For example, $(-2)^3 = -8$. Also, all roots (including even roots) refer to the positive root. That is, $\sqrt{4} = 2$, even though both -2 and 2 result in 4 when squared. This means that there is a difference between writing $x^2 = 4$ and $x = \sqrt{4}$. If $x^2 = 4$, then x could equal -2 or 2 (since both of them, when squared, give 4). However, if $x = \sqrt{4}$, then $x = 2$, since the square root refers only to the positive root. (This paragraph might be worth re-reading. This is our favorite example of absurdly finicky distinctions in math.)

Exponent and Root Rules

If you need to do arithmetic with numbers raised to some power, use the following rules:

- To multiply with the same base, add the exponents.
- To divide with the same base, subtract the exponents.
- To raise to another power, multiply the exponents.

One mnemonic for the rules above is MADSPM (Multiply → Add, Divide → Subtract, Power → Multiply).

For example, consider 2^3 and 2^4. Both expressions use exponents and have the same base (2, in this case). To compute $2^3 \times 2^4$, we could expand these numbers out: $(2 \times 2 \times 2) \times (2 \times 2 \times 2 \times 2)$. There are seven 2's multiplied, so this is the same as 2^7. However, a shorter way to do this would be to add the exponents: $2^3 \times 2^4 = 2^{3+4} = 2^7$.

Next, consider evaluating $\dfrac{2^4}{2^3}$. Expanded out, this would read $\dfrac{2 \times 2 \times 2 \times 2}{2 \times 2 \times 2}$, and since three 2s cancel in the numerator and denominator, this is equal to 2. The shorter way, using the second rule above, is to subtract the exponents: $\dfrac{2^4}{2^3} = 2^{4-3} = 2^1$, and 2^1 is just 2.

Finally, consider evaluating $(2^3)^4$. Expanded out, this would be $2^3 \times 2^3 \times 2^3 \times 2^3$, and according to the first rule, we can just add the exponents at this point, so the result is 2^{12}. The third rule states that we could've sidestepped writing all this out by just saying that $(2^3)^4 = 2^{3 \times 4} = 2^{12}$. Bear in mind, too, that exponents distribute to multiplied or divided terms. For example, $(2^3 \times 3^4)^5 = 2^{3 \times 5} \times 3^{4 \times 5} = 2^{15} \times 3^{20}$. This does *not* apply to added terms, however, since, for example, $(3 + 4)^2 \neq (3^2 + 4^2)$, which you can check by computing each of them; the left side is 49, but the right side is 25.

These rules also work for exponents that are not positive integers. For example, consider 2^0. We know that, for example, $\dfrac{2^3}{2^3} = 2^{3-3} = 2^0$, and we also know that anything divided by itself equals 1. Thus, 2^0 must equal 1. The same reasoning would apply for almost any base, so anything raised to the power zero must equal 1. (The one exception is zero, since division by zero is not defined, so $\dfrac{0^3}{0^3}$, which equals 0^0 for the same reasons as above, is undefined. Thus, 0^0 is undefined.)

Similarly, negative exponents follow these rules. If we had $\dfrac{2^3}{2^4}$ (instead of the reciprocal, which was discussed above), then by the rules above, this should equal 2^{-1}, but expanding this out would yield $\dfrac{2 \times 2 \times 2}{2 \times 2 \times 2 \times 2}$, and canceling three 2s in the numerator and denominator would leave just $\dfrac{1}{2}$. Thus, $2^{-1} = \dfrac{1}{2}$. By similar reasoning, any negative exponent just signifies a reciprocal, so, for example, $3^{-4} = \dfrac{1}{3^4}$.

Fractional exponents, likewise, follow these rules. From the rules above, $\left(2^{\frac{1}{2}}\right)^2 = 2^{\frac{1}{2} \times 2} = 2^1$. That is, if you square $2^{\frac{1}{2}}$, you get 2. Thus, $2^{\frac{1}{2}} = \sqrt{2}$ (since, by definition, if you square $\sqrt{2}$ you get 2). For the same reasons, any fractional exponent is a root. For example, $2^{\frac{1}{3}} = \sqrt[3]{2}$. For another example, $2^{\frac{2}{3}} = \sqrt[3]{2^2}$ (the denominator becomes the root, and the numerator stays an exponent). This means that, just as exponents distribute to multiplied or divided terms, so too do roots. For example, $\sqrt{\frac{4}{9}} = \frac{\sqrt{4}}{\sqrt{9}} = \frac{2}{3}$.

To summarize, four more exponent rules are:

- Exponents distribute to multiplied or divided terms (e.g. $(4 \times 5)^2 = 4^2 \times 5^2$).

- Anything to the zero is 1 (except 0^0, which is undefined).

- Negative exponents are reciprocals (e.g. $2^{-3} = \frac{1}{2^3}$).

- Fractional exponents are roots (e.g. $2^{\frac{1}{3}} = \sqrt[3]{2}$).

39.4 SCIENTIFIC NOTATION

In order to simplify writing very large or very small numbers, we use exponential (or scientific) notation. A number is said to be expressed in scientific notation when it appears in the following form: $y \times 10^n$, where y is between 1 and 10 ($1 \leq y < 10$) and n is a nonzero integer. For example, the number 5,600,000 would be written in scientific notation as: 5.6×10^6.

The exponent n indicates how the decimal point in y should be moved to obtain the given number. In this example, the fact that the exponent is +6 means that the decimal point in "5.6" should be moved 6 places to the *right* to obtain the given number: 5,600,000. A negative value of the exponent n indicates movement of the decimal point in y to the *left*; for example, the number 0.0000234 would be written in scientific notation as follows: 2.34×10^{-5}. Similarly, if we have a number that was expressed with a power of 10, say 84.1×10^{-3}, we can put that number into scientific notation by adjusting the location of the decimal while accounting for the effect that has on the power of 10. To put 84.1×10^{-3} into scientific notation, we need to have a lead value of 8.41, which means we need to move the decimal to the left once. Recall this is the same thing as dividing by 10; therefore, we must also multiply by 10 to preserve the magnitude of our number. We can do this without moving the decimal by multiplying our power of 10 by that factor of 10: here, this means 10^{-3} will become 10^{-2}. Finally, we can write our number in scientific notation as 8.41×10^{-2}.

As another example, let's express the product $350{,}000 \times 40{,}000{,}000$ in scientific notation. Since $350{,}000 = 3.5 \times 10^5$ and $40{,}000{,}000 = 4 \times 10^7$, the product is equal to $(3.5 \times 10^5)(4 \times 10^7) = (3.5)(4)10^{5+7} = 14 \times 10^{12} = 1.4 \times 10^{13}$.

Exponents are an implicit part of our usual system for writing numbers. The position of a digit in an integer indicates its value. Since we use a base–ten (decimal) number system, positions denote powers of ten as follows:

$$\cdots \quad \overline{10^3} \quad \overline{10^2} \quad \overline{10^1} \quad \overline{10^0}$$

The rightmost position is the units' (or ones') position; next to this is the tens' position, then the hundreds', then the thousands', and so on. Consider the number 543. The 5 in the hundreds' position means there are five 100's, the 4 in the tens' position means there are four 10's, and the 3 in the ones' position means there are 3 ones'. Therefore, 543 means $(5 \times 100) + (4 \times 10) + (3 \times 1)$.

$$\cdots \quad \overline{\frac{}{10^3}} \quad \overline{\frac{5}{10^2}} \quad \overline{\frac{4}{10^1}} \quad \overline{\frac{3}{10^0}} = (5 \times 10^2) + (4 \times 10^1) + (3 \times 10^0)$$

Note: Positions after the decimal point have values 10^{-1} (the tenths' digit), 10^{-2} (the hundredths), and so forth.

39.5   LOGARITHMS

Logarithms are another way to express exponents. If you know that $a^b = c$, you can also write this as $\log_a c = b$. (You can imagine, in converting the latter log into the former exponent, that the a moves over to the other side of the equation and pushes up the b, thus giving a^b.) The a is called the "base" either way, and if a log is written without a base expressed, the base is assumed to be 10. That is, $\log 5$ is exactly the same thing as $\log_{10} 5$. Converting between logs and exponents should allow you to calculate most normal log questions. Consider the following example.

15.   What is the value of $\log_5 125$?

    A.   1
    B.   2
    C.   3
    D.   5
    E.   125

If x is the answer, then $x = \log_5 125$. Convert this to an exponent, and you get $5^x = 125$. Now, what do you raise 5 to in order to get 125? Well, $5^3 = 125$, so C is the answer.

You should also be aware of the following properties of logs, which are equivalent to the MADSPM exponent rules that were just discussed.

- $\log(a) + \log(b) = \log(ab)$

- $\log(a) - \log(b) = \log\left(\dfrac{a}{b}\right)$

- $\log(a)^b = b\log(a)$

Consider the following example.

16. Given that log 2 = 0.301 and log 7 = 0.845, which of the following is log 56?

    A.   1.447
    B.   1.690
    C.   1.748
    D.   1.991
    E.   2.049

You can estimate that the answer to this question should be more than 1 but less than 2, since log 10 = 1 and log 100 = 2, and 56 is between 10 and 100, but that only eliminates E. Choice D looks awfully high, but what about A, B, and C? It may be a little hard to tell, especially given how close B and C are to each other. In that case, try to use a log rule. Prime factorizing 56 yields that $56 = 2^3 \times 7$. Thus, $\log 56 = \log(2^3 \times 7)$, and according to the multiplication rule, that can be changed to $\log(2^3) + \log(7)$. According to the power log rule, that can be turned into $3\log(2) + \log(7)$, and the question stem gives the values of these logs, so this becomes $3(0.301) + 0.845$. Use the on-screen calculator at this point, and the answer is C.

39.6   PROPORTIONS

Proportions are a common way to relate two quantities. They tell us how one quantity will change for a given change in another quantity. The two most common proportions you're likely to run into are "directly proportional" and "inversely proportional."

If two quantities are directly proportional to one another then, as one of the quantities changes by a certain factor, the other quantity must also change by that same factor. For example, if we're told that y varies directly with x, then if x is doubled, y will double. Similarly, if x is halved, y will also be halved. This can be interpreted as an equation: $y = kx$, where k is called "the constant of proportionality." We don't need to know the value of k to see that y and x are directly proportional because k is a constant. For example, whether $y = 2x$ or $y = 4x$, doubling x will still double y, and increasing x by a factor of 3 will still increase y by a factor of 3. Note that "increased by a factor of" means our quantity was multiplied by a given factor, and "decreased by a factor of" means our quantity was divided by a given factor. For example, if x is increased by a factor of 3, it means whatever the value of x was, it tripled; if x is decreased by a factor of 3, it means whatever the value of x was, it was divided by 3.

If two quantities are inversely proportional to one another, then as one of the quantities changes by a certain factor, the other quantity will change by the same factor, but in the opposite sense. For example, if we're told that y varies inversely with x, then if x is doubled, y will be halved. Similarly, if x is halved, y will be doubled. This can be interpreted as an equation: $y = \dfrac{k}{x}$.

We can also exploit proportions to help us interpret known equations. Let's look at a common Gchem example; the Ideal Gas Law tells us $PV = nRT$. Under isothermal (constant temperature) conditions, the right-hand side of this equation is a constant. Therefore, we can now write the equation like $PV = k$. If the volume changes by a certain factor, the pressure will have to change by the same factor in the opposite sense to compensate. For example, if we triple or increase the volume of our gas by a factor of 3, the pressure must decrease by a factor of 3. Therefore, being on the same side of the equation means P and V are inversely proportional to one another. After all, we can rewrite this equation as $P = \dfrac{k}{V}$, which is analogous to $y = \dfrac{k}{x}$. Similarly, if we instead had our gas under isobaric (constant pressure) conditions, we can write the Ideal Gas Law as $V = \dfrac{nR}{P}T$ or $V = kT$. Now, if the temperature changes by a certain factor, the volume will change by the same factor. For example, if the temperature is decreased by a factor of 10, the volume will also decrease by a factor of 10. Therefore, being on opposite sides of the equation means V and T are directly proportional to one another. After all, $V = kT$ is analogous to $y = kx$.

39.7 ORDER OF OPERATIONS

By convention, the order in which mathematical operations should be performed is anything in parentheses, then exponents, then multiplication and division, and then addition and subtraction. (Mnemonics for this include "Please Excuse My Dear Aunt Sally" and PEMDAS, which stand for Parentheses Exponents Multiplication Division Addition Subtraction.)

For example, consider $4 + 3 \times 2$. By the order of operations, multiplication should be performed first, so the next step is $4 + 6$, which equals 10. As another example, consider $(4 + 3)^2 - 3^3 \times 2$. First, do what's in parentheses, which yields $(7)^2 - 3^3 \times 2$. Next, do the exponents, which yields $49 - 27 \times 2$. Next, multiply, which yields $49 - 54$. Finally, subtract, which yields -5.

If you are doing operations within a step (such as several additions and subtractions), read left to right. For example, $5 - 4 + 2$ becomes $1 + 2 = 3$. If you do this right to left instead, you might be tempted to think you should do $4 + 2$, which would yield $5 - 6 = -1$; this is wrong. You would have to analyze this as $5 + (-4) + 2$ to do the operation on the right first, so it would become $5 - 2 = 3$, which still gives the right answer. If you don't want to have to worry about this sort of thing, just read left to right.

Want More Practice?
Scan the QR code below to register your book for online chapter summaries, drills, practice tests, and more!

Chapter 40
Algebra

Algebra is characterized by the application of laws of arithmetic to **variables**. Variables are letters that can stand for different (varying) values. (This is to be distinguished from **constants**, which are either regular numbers or letters that stand for set values that you don't know or aren't told.) Typical variables are x and y, and algebra is devoted to manipulating expressions containing these variables.

40.1   SOLVING EQUATIONS

The most important rule of algebra is: *whatever you do to one side of an equation, you must do to the other*. Think of an equation as a scale on which two things are balanced. To not destroy this balance, whatever we do to one side of the scale (take things away, add things, etc.), we must do to the other side.

For example, to solve $4x = 12$, divide both sides by 4, and you get that $x = 3$. To solve $x - 3 = 5$, add 3 to both sides, and you get that $x = 8$.

You may have to bring variables to one side of the equation and constants (regular numbers) to the other side. For example, to solve $2x - 14 = x - 6$, subtract x from both sides, and you get that $x - 14 = -6$. Then add 14 to both sides, and $x = 8$.

Here are a few more examples.

17. Solve: $3x + 2 = 7x - 6$.

     A. -1

     B. $-\dfrac{10}{8}$

     C. $\dfrac{10}{8}$

     D. 1
     E. 2

Subtract 2 from both sides to get $3x = 7x - 8$, then subtract $7x$ from both sides to arrive at $-4x = -8$. Finally, dividing both sides by -4 yields our result, $x = 2$ (E is correct).

18. Solve: $9 - 5x = 6 + 3(1 - x)$.

     A. -3
     B. 0

     C. $\dfrac{9}{8}$

     D. $\dfrac{9}{4}$

     E. 3

The right–hand side simplifies to $9 - 3x$, so the equation reads $9 - 5x = 9 - 3x$. We subtract 9 from both sides and get $-5x = -3x$. Adding $3x$ to both sides gives $-2x = 0$, and then dividing both sides by -2 yields our answer, $x = 0$. Thus, the answer is B.

19. If $3x + 2y = 6$, what is the value of $12x + 8y$?

    A. 6
    B. 12
    C. 24
    D. There is not enough information to tell.

If we are presented with one equation containing more than one variable, there is usually no way to find a unique answer. The equation $3x + 2y = 6$ presents precisely this problem; there are infinitely many possibilities for x and for y. But the question is specially constructed to allow us to answer it uniquely; it's really a substitution problem: $12x + 8y$ factors into $4(3x + 2y)$, which is equal to $4(6)$. Thus, the answer is C.

Important note: when solving equations, there are some things you simply cannot do, even if you respect the golden rule of doing the same thing to both sides: never multiply or divide both sides of an equation by zero, and never divide by a variable (or an expression containing a variable) that could equal zero. Both of these could lead to the omission of valid solutions or to the complete destruction of the equation. To see the damage violating this rule can cause, look back at the example above where we arrived at the equation $-5x = -3x$. If we had divided both sides by x, we would have gotten $-5 = -3$. Since this is a blatantly false statement, we would conclude that the equation had no solution. But clearly it does: $x = 0$.

40.2 ARITHMETIC WITH ALGEBRAIC EXPRESSIONS

The **distributive law** tells us $a(b+c) = ab+ac$. For example, the usual way of computing $2(3+5)$ would be to add 3 and 5 first, so you get $2(8) = 16$. However, this is the same as $2 \times 3 + 2 \times 5$, which becomes $6 + 10 = 16$. With pure arithmetic, there is little reason to distribute instead of adding what's in parentheses, but in algebra, there might be reason to do so.

For example, $2x + 3x = (2 + 3)x = 5x$. This is such a simple use of the distributive law that you may not have thought of it in this way before, but it is a use. There are many others. To add the like terms $2x$ and $3x$, we simply add the **coefficients** (2 and 3), and the same process can be used to combine any like terms. Two expressions, like $2x$ and $3x$, or $2x^2$ and $3x^2$, are called "like" terms if they contain the same variable(s) raised to the same power(s); that is, two terms are like terms if they differ only in their numerical coefficients. For example, $2x$ and $3x^2$ are *not* like terms because the first one contains the variable x to the first power (x by itself means x^1), but the second term contains x to the second power.

As another example, simplify the expression $4x + 7x - (-5x)$. These are like terms, so we combine the coefficients; the result is $(4 + 7 + 5)\, x = 16x$.

Let's look at another example. Similarly, simplify the expression $4x^2 + 7x - (-5x)$. Here, only $7x$ and $(-5x)$ are like terms. Combining them, we get $7x - (-5x) = 7x + 5x = 12x$. Since no further simplification is possible with the unlike term $4x^2$, the result is $4x^2 + 12x$.

20. Simplify: $(4a^2)(2a)(5a^3) - (6a^3)^2$.

    A. $4a^6$
    B. $36a^6$
    C. $40a^6$
    D. $40a^7 - 6a^6$
    E. $40a^7 - 36a^6$

The product $(4a^2)(2a)(5a^3)$ equals $(4)(2)(5)a^{2+1+3} = 40a^6$, and the other term is $(6a^3)(6a^3) = (6)(6)a^{3+3} = 36a^6$. Therefore, the difference of these like terms is $40a^6 - 36a^6 = 4a^6$ (A is correct). Note the exponent rules discussed earlier are used here.

Complicated distribution problems can be solved in the same way: multiply each term by each other term. For example, $(5 + x)(2 + y) = (5 \times 2) + (5 \times y) + (x \times 2) + (x \times y)$. This very long expression simplifies to $10 + 5y + 2x + xy$. One acronym for the various terms is FOIL: multiply the firsts, outsides, insides, and lasts. In this case, 5 and 2 were the first terms in each expression, 5 and y were the outside terms in the expressions, x and 2 were the inside terms in the expressions, and x and y were the last terms in each expression.

As you might imagine, for anything with more than two terms, distribution can get extremely complicated very quickly, but multiply each term by each other term, and you will get the answer (eventually).

40.3 FACTORING

To **factor** is to undo distribution. For example, if you see $3x(5 + y)$, distributing would mean expressing this as $15x + 3xy$. If you see $15x + 3xy$, factoring would mean noticing that $3x$ is a factor of both $15x$ and $3xy$, and pulling this out to yield $3x(5 + y)$. Distributing goes one direction; factoring goes the other.

For another example, consider the expression $2a + 4ab$. We notice that both terms have a factor of 2, so we can write $2a + 4ab = 2(a + 2ab)$, and we have successfully written the sum as a product. However, one of these factors, $a + 2ab$, could be factored further since it is a sum and both terms contain a factor of a. Performing this additional factoring step, $a + 2ab = a(1 + 2b)$, we have $2a + 4ab = 2(a + 2ab) = 2a(1 + 2b)$.

If we wish to factor an expression *completely,* we can do it step by step as we did here, or we could do it in one step by finding the **greatest common factor** (the **gcf**) right from the start. Consider the original expression $2a + 4ab$ again. Since 2 divides 4, and both terms have a factor of a, the gcf of $2a$ and $4ab$ is $2a$. We therefore factor this out and write $2a + 4ab = 2a(1 + 2b)$.

Notice that we have written a sum, $2a + 4ab$, as a product (of $2a$ and $1 + 2b$). This is the essence of factoring.

As another example, factor $9ab + 12ab^2 - 6a^3b$. The gcf of the terms is $3ab$. Therefore, $9ab + 12ab^2 - 6a^3b$ $= 3ab(3 + 4b - 2a^2)$. Since we have factored out the gcf, the expression has been factored completely.

21. Complete: The expression $8x^2 + 12x^3$ is the product of $2x$ and _____.

    A. $4x$
    B. $6x$
    C. $4x + 6x$
    D. x^2
    E. $4x + 6x^2$

Since the question is asking us to express a sum as a product, we know this is a factoring problem. Although the gcf of the two terms in this expression is $4x^2$, the question tells us to only factor out a $2x$. Doing so, we have $8x^2 + 12x^3 = 2x(4x + 6x^2)$. Therefore, the expression $8x^2 + 12x^3$ is the product of $2x$ and $4x + 6x^2$. The answer to the question is $4x + 6x^2$ (E is correct).

Common Quadratics

Distributing two expressions with two terms each can take a variety of forms, but the simplest (and therefore most common) ways this can play out are the products of $(x + y)$ and $(x - y)$ with each other. Let's look at an example:

- $(x + y)(x + y) = x^2 + 2xy + y^2$
- $(x - y)(x - y) = x^2 - 2xy + y^2$
- $(x + y)(x - y) = (x - y)(x + y) = x^2 - y^2$

Familiarity with the above is useful, even if they can be derived by distributing (specifically, FOILing) the expressions on the left. Any time you see x^2 and y^2 in the same problem, or the product xy, the first thing that should come to mind is that one of the above equations is probably being tested. Let's look at an example:

22. If $x + y = 4$ and $x^2 + y^2 = 10$, then what is the value of xy ?

    A. 0
    B. 1
    C. 3
    D. 4
    E. 6

To solve this, square the first equation. Thus, $(x + y)^2 = 16$. FOIL out the left side of this equation, and $x^2 + 2xy + y^2 = 16$. Now, the question also says that $x^2 + y^2 = 10$, so regroup the left side of the first equation and substitute, so $x^2 + y^2 + 2xy = 16$ becomes $10 + 2xy = 16$. Then subtract 10 from both sides, and $2xy = 6$, so $xy = 3$ (C is correct).

It might be worth noting as well that choice E is a trap for two reasons, both that $10 - 4 = 6$ (subtract the two numbers given in the problem) and that it is the value of $2xy$, so it is a partial answer. For that matter, the values of x and y are not hard to guess in this question. One of the variables is 1, and the other is 3, since these add to 4 and their squares add to 10. In some questions of this nature, guess and check is a possible strategy if all else fails.

Note also that $x^2 - y^2$ is the difference (result of subtraction) of two squares, so any time you see squares in a question, factoring of this nature may be necessary.

As another example, factor $4m^2 - n^2$. The first term is the square of $2m$, and the second term is the square of n. Therefore, we are given a difference of two squares, which is factored as follows: $4m^2 - n^2 = (2m)^2 - n^2 = (2m + n)(2m - n)$.

Let's try another problem: factor $8x^5 - 18xy^2$. First, let's factor out the gcf of $2x$: $8x^5 - 18xy^2 = 2x(4x^4 - 9y^2)$. Now notice we can factor further, because we have a difference of two squares: $4x^4 - 9y^2 = (2x^2)^2 - (3y)^2 = (2x^2 + 3y)(2x^2 - 3y)$. Therefore, $8x^5 - 18xy^2 = 2x(2x^2 + 3y)(2x^2 - 3y)$.

23. If $x > y > 0$, simplify $\sqrt{(x - y)^2 + 4xy}$.

    A. $x + y$

    B. $(x - y) + 2xy$

    C. $xy\sqrt{6}$

    D. $x^2 + 2xy + y^2$

First, expand $(x - y)^2$, so you get $\sqrt{x^2 - 2xy + y^2 + 4xy}$. Now, combine the xy terms, which results in $\sqrt{x^2 + 2xy + y^2}$. This factors into $\sqrt{(x + y)^2}$, which is $x + y$ (A is correct).

Simplifying Algebraic Fractions

To simplify algebraic fractions, pull out any common factors of the numerator and denominator and cancel. Let's simplify the following algebraic fraction (assuming that x doesn't equal 0 or 2): $\dfrac{x^2 - 4}{x^2 - 2x}$.

It may seem tempting to cross out the x^2 in the numerator and the x^2 in the denominator, but this would be incorrect here. Think of an example with regular numbers: $\dfrac{1 + 4}{1 + 2} = \dfrac{5}{3}$, but if you tried to cancel the 1s, you'd get $\dfrac{4}{2} = 2$, which is definitely not the same. Thus, only common factors (things multiplied, not things added) can be canceled. The problem is that neither the numerator nor the denominator of the fraction above is expressed as a product; therefore, factor: $\dfrac{x^2 - 4}{x^2 - 2x} = \dfrac{(x + 2)(x - 2)}{x(x - 2)}$. Now, since $(x - 2)$ is multiplied in the numerator and denominator, this part can be canceled, which leaves $\dfrac{x+2}{x}$, and this is as simple as the fraction can be made.

For another example, simplify: $\dfrac{6a+4b}{12a+8b}$. We cannot cancel anything in a fraction until we have factored both the numerator and the denominator. Doing so, we find $\dfrac{6a+4b}{12a+8b} = \dfrac{2(3a+2b)}{4(3a+2b)}$, and now we can cancel to get $\dfrac{2}{4} = \dfrac{1}{2}$.

Let's look at one more example of this: if $x \neq -3$, simplify: $\dfrac{2x^3 - 18x}{6x+18}$. We factor: $\dfrac{2x^3-18x}{6x+18} = \dfrac{2x(x^2-9)}{6(x+3)}$. However, the numerator can be factored further, and then terms cancel: $\dfrac{2x(x^2-9)}{6(x+3)} = \dfrac{2x(x+3)(x-3)}{(2)(3)(x+3)} = \dfrac{x(x-3)}{3}$. Notice, by the way, that both a 2 and an $x+3$ cancel in this step. At this point, the fraction is as simplified as it can be.

24. Simplify (assuming $x > 0$): $\dfrac{\sqrt{80x^7}}{\sqrt{5x^3}}$.

    A. $2x$
    B. $4x^2$
    C. $8x^3$
    D. $16x^4$
    E. $32x^5$

Combine the square roots, so that $\dfrac{\sqrt{80x^7}}{\sqrt{5x^3}} = \sqrt{\dfrac{80x^7}{5x^3}}$. Next, reduce: $\sqrt{\dfrac{80x^7}{5x^3}} = \sqrt{16x^4}$. Split the square root back apart, and $\sqrt{16x^4} = \sqrt{16}\sqrt{x^4} = 4x^2$. Thus, the answer is $4x^2$ (B is correct).

Solving Quadratics by Factoring

The basic principle we will be using in this section is the property of real numbers: If a product of real numbers is equal to zero, then at least one of the factors must be zero.

Let's solve the equation $x^2 - x = 2$. We can factor the left–hand side as $x(x-1)$, but there's nothing to be gained by this because there is no procedure (besides blind trial and error) to solve $x(x-1) = 2$. This equation says a certain product equals 2, but there's nothing special about the number 2 that's helpful in this context.

Instead, we take our original equation and move the 2 to the left–hand side to get $x^2 - x - 2 = 0$. The left–hand side is factorable, giving $(x - 2)(x + 1) = 0$. Now we have a product equaling zero, which means that one (or both) of the factors must be zero. That is, either $x - 2 = 0$ or $x + 1 = 0$ (or both), which means $x = 2$ or -1.

For another example, solve $x^3 = 9x$. Rewrite the equation as $x^3 - 9x = 0$ (remember, the key is to have a factored expression set equal to 0, so we always want to get 0 by itself on the right–hand side) and factor: $x(x^2 - 9) = 0$. Continue factoring: $x(x + 3)(x - 3) = 0$. Therefore, $x = 0, -3,$ or 3.

Let's keep practicing. If $y \neq 0$, find x if $xy = 2y^2$. Rewrite the equation as $xy - 2y^2 = 0$ and factor: $y(x - 2y) = 0$. This equation says $y = 0$ or $x - 2y = 0$. But since we were told that $y \neq 0$, it must be the case that $x - 2y = 0$; that is, x must equal $2y$.

Here are a couple more examples.

25. For what values of y does $2y^2 = 5y - 2$?

    A. 0 only

    B. 0 and 2 only

    C. $\frac{1}{2}$ only

    D. 2 only

    E. $\frac{1}{2}$ and 2 only

As usual, we rewrite the equation to leave 0 on the right–hand side: $2y^2 - 5y + 2 = 0$. Next, factor: $(2y - 1)(y - 2) = 0$. Finally, this means that $2y - 1 = 0$ or $y - 2 = 0$, so $y = \frac{1}{2}$ or 2 (E is correct). Note you could also PITA to answer this question.

26. For what positive value of x does $(x + 2)(x - 2) = 60$?

    A. $\sqrt{56}$

    B. $\sqrt{60}$

    C. 8

    D. $\sqrt{68}$

    E. 9

We expand the left–hand side: $x^2 - 4 = 60$. Next, move the 60 over and simplify: $x^2 - 64 = 0$. Finally, factor: $(x + 8)(x - 8) = 0$. This last equation says $x = -8$ or 8, so the positive solution is $x = 8$ (C is correct).

40.4   SIMULTANEOUS EQUATIONS

Simultaneous equations are two equations, each containing two unknowns (for example, x and y), for which we seek a solution that makes both equations true *simultaneously*. For example, consider the equations $2x + y = 8$ and $x - y = 1$. There are many values of x and y that make the first equation true, and many values of x and y that make the second equation true; but there is *only one* choice of x and y that makes both equations true at the same time. This is the solution we're looking for. For these two equations, we could add them, thereby eliminating y: the result is $3x = 9$, which immediately gives $x = 3$. Now, substitute $x = 3$ into either of the original equations and find the corresponding value of y. We get $y = 2$. Therefore, the solution which makes both equations true simultaneously is $x = 3$ and, $y = 2$.

Adding or subtracting equations is by far the most common way to solve simultaneous equations on the DAT. It is possible that you will have to multiply or divide by a number before or after you add or subtract the equations.

For example, if $3x + 2y = 13$ and $x + y = 6$, what is the value of y? In this case, multiply the second equation by 3 to get $3x + 3y = 18$. Now, subtract this equation from the first equation given: $(3x + 2y) - (3x + 3y) = 13 - 18$ gives $-y = -5$, so $y = 5$.

Let's try another example. If $7x + 13y = 2$ and $3x + 17y = 8$, what is the value of $x + 3y$? In this case, if you add the two equations, you get $10x + 30y = 10$. Then divide by 10, and you get that $x + 3y = 1$, which is the answer to the question.

Let's try one more problem. If $2x - 5y = 2$ and $-2x + 7y = 2$, what is the value of x? Adding the two equations gives $2y = 4$, so $y = 2$. Substituting this into either one of the original equations gives $x = 6$.

40.5   ABSOLUTE VALUE AND INEQUALITIES

Absolute Value

The **absolute value** of a number is its magnitude. Formally, if $x \geq 0$, then the absolute value of x, denoted $|x|$, is equal to x. If $x < 0$, then $|x| = -x$. In other words, if a number has a negative sign, the absolute value takes away the negative sign, and if not, it does nothing. Thus, $|2| = 2$, and $|-2| = 2$.

The above implies that there are two possible solutions to $|x| = 2$. Both $x = 2$ and $x = -2$ would solve the given equation. However, don't confuse this with $x = |2|$, which means that $x = 2$. Also, distinguish these two from $|x| = -2$, which has no solutions; it is impossible to take an absolute value of a real number and get a negative number.

Solving Inequalities

Examples of inequalities include 5 > 3, 2 < 9, 6 ≤ 6, –3 ≥ –4, and 8 ≠ 10. To solve an algebraic inequality, we observe the same rules as for solving equations: whatever we do to one side, we must do to the other, we never multiply or divide by zero, and we never divide by a variable. There is just one additional rule: *if we multiply or divide an equality by a negative number, we must switch the direction of the inequality.* That is, < would become > (and vice versa), and ≤ would become ≥ (and vice versa).

Let's look at a few examples. First, solve $3x + 2 < 7x - 6$. Subtract 2 from both sides to get $3x < 7x - 8$, then subtract 7x from both sides to arrive at $-4x < -8$. Finally, dividing both sides by –4 and reversing the inequality, we get $x > 2$. Thus, only numbers greater than 2 will satisfy the given inequality.

Next, solve $|2x + 1| > 11$. This says the absolute value of a quantity is greater than 11. Therefore, the quantity is either greater than 11 or less than –11; that is, $2x + 1 > 11$ *or* $2x + 1 < -11$. Solving the first inequality gives $2x > 10$, so $x > 5$. Solving the second inequality gives $2x < -12$ so $x < -6$. Therefore, the given inequality is satisfied by all values of x such that $x > 5$ or $x < -6$.

Finally, solve $|3x - 2| < 7$. This says the absolute value of a quantity is less than 7. Therefore, the quantity is greater than –7, but also less than 7; that is, $3x - 2 > -7$ and $3x - 2 < 7$. Solving the first inequality gives $x > -\frac{5}{3}$. Solving the second inequality gives $x < 3$. Therefore, the given inequality is satisfied by all values of x such that $-\frac{5}{3} < x < 3$.

40.6   FUNCTIONS

A function is just an instruction to do something to a number. Functions can be expressed in two major ways.

Function Notation

The usual way to express a function in math is with function notation. For example, a function f might be defined such that $f(x) = x + 3$. This function says to add 3 to whatever number is put into it. Thus, $f(2)$ means "take this 2 and add 3 to it." In symbols, we write that as $f(2) = 2 + 3 = 5$. This is a fairly simple function, but functions can be much more complicated. For example, if f is defined by $f(x) = \dfrac{\sqrt{x + 4}}{x^2 - 3x - 5}$, then the operations to do are much more involved, but they work exactly the same way. If you need to evaluate $f(2)$ for this function, then since the 2 is in the place of the x inside the parentheses, put the 2 in the place of x on the right side: $f(2) = \dfrac{\sqrt{2 + 4}}{2^2 - 3(2) - 5}$. At this point, it's a matter of arithmetic to reduce to $-\dfrac{\sqrt{6}}{7}$, which is what $f(2)$ equals in this case.

Of course, functions can be named with any letter, not just f, so you may see $g(x)$ or $h(x)$ or any other letter. These mean the same thing as $f(x)$, but it can be convenient to use different letters in certain circumstances, particularly if two functions are being defined. For example, consider the following problem:

27. If $f(x) = x + 7$ and $g(x) = 2x - 5$, for which of the following values of x will $f(x) = g(x)$?

    A.   1
    B.   2
    C.   5
    D.   7
    E.   12

40.6

There are two functions here, $f(x)$ and $g(x)$. The question wants values for which the functions are equal, so set them equal, and you get $x + 7 = 2x - 5$. Now solve for x by subtracting x from both sides (yielding $7 = x - 5$) and adding 5 to both sides, so that $x = 12$ (E is correct).

However, setting two functions equal to each other is not the only way to solve a problem of this nature. Consider the following:

28. If $f(x) = \dfrac{\sqrt{x+4}}{x^2 - 3x - 5}$ and $g(x) = \dfrac{3}{3x - 10}$, for which of the following values of x will $f(x) = g(x)$?

    A.   0
    B.   5
    C.   10
    D.   15
    E.   20

These functions are extremely complicated, and it's probably a bad idea to set them equal and try to solve $\dfrac{\sqrt{x+4}}{x^2 - 3x - 5} = \dfrac{3}{3x - 10}$ under the pressure of test day. Instead, PITA. Start as usual in the middle, with 10. Put 10 into f, and $f(10) = \dfrac{\sqrt{10 + 4}}{10^2 - 3(10) - 5} = \dfrac{\sqrt{14}}{65}$. However, $g(10) = \dfrac{3}{3(10) - 10} = \dfrac{3}{20}$, so for this value of x, the two functions are not equal. It may not be entirely clear whether this value of x is too big or too small, so just choose a direction and go with it. In this case, since 5 is a smaller and easier number to work with than 15 is, let's try B. Thus, $f(5) = \dfrac{\sqrt{5 + 4}}{5^2 - 3(5) - 5} = \dfrac{\sqrt{9}}{5}$. This can be reduced further, so $f(5) = \dfrac{3}{5}$. And trying the same number in g, we find that $g(5) = \dfrac{3}{3(5) - 10} = \dfrac{3}{5}$. Thus, $f(5) = g(5)$, so the answer is choice B.

Funny Symbols

Instead of using regular function notation, a question may invent some weird symbol to define a particular operation. For example, let's say they want to make up a symbol for doubling a number and then subtracting 3. They might write, "Let $x^* = 2x - 3$." Then the question could ask for the value of, say, 6^*. Well, 6^* is $2(6) - 3$, which equals 9. Just follow the rule they make up for the symbol they invent.

As another example, if $\langle n \rangle = n^2 + n - 1$, what is the value of $\langle -3 \rangle$? We simply plug in the given value:

$\langle 3 \rangle = (-3)^2 + (-3) - 1$. Next, evaluate, and this comes out to 5.

Let's look at a few more typical DAT questions like this.

29. Let $\lozenge x = 2x + 7$. For what value of x does
$\lozenge x = \lozenge(2x + 7)$?

   A. -7
   B. -3.5
   C. 0
   D. 1
   E. 3.5

First, evaluate the right side according to the given rule: $\lozenge(2x + 7) = 2(2x + 7) + 7$. (Note we put $2x + 7$ in for x in the original rule.) Now, simplify this to get $4x + 21$. Thus, the question is really asking, "For what value of x does $2x + 7 = 4x + 21$?" In that case, subtract $2x$ from both sides, which gives that $7 = 2x + 21$, and then subtract 21 from both sides, so that $-14 = 2x$. Divide by 2, and $x = -7$ (A is correct).

30. If $x \; \heartsuit \; y$ is defined as $2x + 5y$, then is it true that $x \; \heartsuit \; y = y \; \heartsuit \; x$?

   A. No, it is not ever true.
   B. No, unless $y = x$.
   C. Yes, unless $x = 0$.
   D. Yes, it is always true.

Want More Practice?
Scan the QR code below to register your book for online chapter summaries, drills, practice tests, and more!

Apply the rule to the left side and to the right side of the equation. This equation now says $2x + 5y = 2y + 5x$. Is that true? Presumably not, if x and y are different. To determine when it *would* be true, subtract $2x$ and $2y$ from both sides, and you get that $3y = 3x$, which, when divided by 3, shows that it is only true when $x = y$ (B is correct).

Chapter 41
Word Problems

41.1 TRANSLATING A VERBAL STATEMENT INTO AN ALGEBRAIC EXPRESSION

In order to apply the techniques of algebra to "real–life" problems, it is important to be able to translate verbal statements into algebraic expressions. For example, we might rewrite the statement "a number added to 4 yields 10" as $x + 4 = 10$. Study these examples, which build on the ones in the percent section earlier:

Verbal statement	Equivalent algebraic expression
a number increased by 2	$x + 2$
a number decreased by 5	$x - 5$
5 less than a number	$x - 5$
5 decreased by a number	$5 - x$ [*not* $x - 5$]
3 more than twice a number	$2x + 3$ [*not* $2(x + 3)$, which is "twice the sum of a number and 3"]
7 less than three times a number	$3x - 7$ [*not* $7 - 3x$, which is "7 decreased by three times a number"]
the square of 1 more than a number	$(x + 1)^2$ [*not* $x^2 + 1$, which is "1 more than the square of a number"]
two consecutive integers	n and $n + 1$
two consecutive even integers	n and $n + 2$ (where n is an even integer)
two consecutive odd integers	n and $n + 2$ (where n is an odd integer)
the sum of three consecutive integers	$n + (n + 1) + (n + 2)$
8 more than four times the cube of a number	$4x^3 + 8$

Note: the choice of letter really doesn't matter. Traditionally, the letter x is the most popular choice. The letter n is often used to denote a number that is known to be an integer, but this is certainly not a law. The expression $x + 2$ is equivalent to $y + 2$ or $z + 2$ or $n + 2$, or for that matter, $\square + 2$ or $\theta + 2$ (θ is the Greek letter theta).

To solve a word problem, we often need to translate the given question into a mathematical sentence (an equation or an inequality), solve the equation or inequality, then translate back.

For example, consider the following. A jar contains three types of jelly beans: red, blue, and yellow. The number of red jelly beans is 3 more than the number of blue, and the number of blue jelly beans is twice the number of yellow. If the jar contains 88 jelly beans, how many are yellow?

To solve this, let y denote the number of yellow jelly beans. Then the number of blue jelly beans is $2y$, and the number of red jelly beans is $2y + 3$. Then, since $y + 2y + (2y + 3) = 88$, we find that $5y = 85$, so $y = 17$.

Many word problems on the DAT fit into standard categories, and each of the major categories is discussed below.

41.2 COUNTING AND RATIOS

Most ratio problems depend heavily on determining how many members there are in each group represented in the ratio, and how many such groups there are in the total. Here is an example:

32. A university science class consists of juniors and seniors, with no other students. If the ratio of juniors to seniors is 3 to 5, and the total number of students in the class is 96, how many are seniors?

   A. 32
   B. 51
   C. 54
   D. 57
   E. 60

The problem gives a ratio of 3 to 5, which adds up to 8. This means that for every group of 3 juniors and 5 seniors, there are 8 students. Now, how many such groups of 8 are there in 96 total students? Well, 8 goes into 96 exactly 12 times. Thus, in our 96 students, there are 12 groups of 3 juniors and 5 seniors. That makes a total of 36 juniors and 60 seniors (E is correct).

If you would like a visual strategy to work through the steps above, allow us to introduce the Ratio Box.

Juniors	Seniors	Total

← Ratio
← Multiply by
← Actual number

Fill in the details from the problem. The ratio was 3 to 5, and the total number of actual students was 96.

Juniors	Seniors	Total
3 +	5 =	
		96

← Ratio
← Multiply by
← Actual number

Next, add up the ratio to get the total in the ratio line.

Juniors	Seniors	Total
3 +	5 =	8	← Ratio
×	×	×	← Multiply by
=	=	=
=	+	= 96	← Actual number

Now, determine how many times that total goes into the actual number. Eight goes into 96 12 times, so that's the "multiply by" number, all the way across:

Juniors	Seniors	Total
3 +	5 =	8	← Ratio
× 12 =	× 12 =	× 12	← Multiply by
=	=	=
+	= 96		← Actual number

Finally, multiply the numbers in the Ratio (top) line by the numbers in the middle line to get the Actual number line at the bottom:

Juniors	Seniors	Total
3 +	5 =	8	← Ratio
× 12 =	× 12 =	× 12	← Multiply by
= 36 +	= 60 =	= 96	← Actual number

Thus, the actual number of seniors is 60, as shown above.

The Ratio Box will solve most ratio problems on the DAT. Let's look at another example.

33. There are 35 children in a room, some of whom are boys
and the rest of whom are girls. Which of the following is
a possible ratio of boys to girls?

    A.   1:2
    B.   2:3
    C.   3:7
    D.   4:5
    E.   9:2

Sometimes PITA can be used for ratio problems. If the ratio of boys to girls were 1:2, as A suggests, then

there would be 3 children total in each group. However, 35 is not divisible by 3, so there would have to

be fractional children to make this ratio work; that is, there would have to be $11\frac{2}{3}$ boys and $23\frac{1}{3}$ girls

to have a 1:2 ratio with 35 children. This does not seem possible (eliminate A). However, in B, the ratio is

2:3, and this creates groups of 5. There would be 7 such groups in 35 children, which would yield 14 boys

and 21 girls. This would be fine, so B is the answer. (The rest of the ratios total to numbers that do not go

into 35, specifically 10, 9, and 11, so none of them are possible either.)

Occasionally, word problems involving differences and ratios together do not lend themselves to the Ratio
Box. For these, translate into algebra and solve, or PITA, if possible. Consider the following example:

34. On a certain day, a movie theater sold regular price
tickets, student discount tickets, and senior discount
tickets. It sold five more student discount tickets than
senior discount tickets, and twice as many regular price
tickets as senior discount tickets. If it sold 89 total
tickets of the three types, how many senior discount
tickets did it sell?

    A.   21
    B.   23
    C.   26
    D.   30
    E.   42

The fastest thing to do in this case is to PITA. The question asks how many senior discount tickets it sold,
so let's start in the middle as usual. If the theater sold 26 senior discount tickets, then it must have sold 31
student discount tickets, since there were 5 more of that type, and 52 regular price tickets, since there were
twice as many of that type. However, 26 + 31 + 52 = 109, which is too large, so C is not the answer, and
neither is D nor E, which are larger (eliminate C, D, and E). Try B next: 23 senior discount tickets means
28 student discount tickets and 46 regular price tickets, which adds up to 97 tickets, which is still too large
(eliminate B). Presumably the answer is A. If you have copious amounts of extra time on the QRT, you
could verify by adding 21 + 26 + 42, which is in fact 89. However, there is no need to do this. If four answers are incorrect, the remaining choice should be your answer. Select it and move on!

There is another way to answer this question. You could translate the statements into algebra. If the number of senior discount tickets is x, the number of student discount tickets is y, and the number of regular price is tickets is z, then the equations given in the question come down to $y = x + 5$, $z = 2x$, and $x + y + z = 89$. Plugging the first two equations into the third yields $x + (x + 5) + 2x = 89$. Collect like terms to get $4x + 5 = 89$. Subtract 5 from both sides, and $4x = 84$. Divide both sides by 4, and $x = 21$. If you do solve the problem algebraically, it would not be a bad idea to check by determining what the other numbers of tickets would be (26 and 42), and making sure that they fit the requirements in the problem and add up to the right number, just to make sure that you have not made an algebraic mistake.

41.3 AGE

Age problems lend themselves to translating into equations or PITA, depending on what exactly the question is asking.

35. Nicholas is 8 years older than Cindy. In four years, he
will be twice as old as Cindy will be then. How old is
Nicholas now?

    A. 4
    B. 8
    C. 12
    D. 16
    E. 20

PITA works well here. This question asks for Nicholas' age, so start in the middle as usual. If Nicholas were 12, then Cindy would be (8 years younger) 4 right now. In four years, they would be 16 and 8, respectively. Since the question says that Nicholas would be twice as old as Cindy this works (16 years old is twice as old as 8 years old), so C is the answer.

Algebraically, the solution would look something like this. Let c denote Cindy's age (in years) now; then Nicholas's age now is $c + 8$. In four years, Nicholas will be $c + 12$, and Cindy will be $c + 4$, and we are told that $c + 12 = 2(c + 4)$. Therefore, $c + 12 = 2c + 8$, which implies that $c = 4$. Thus, Nicholas is now $c + 8 = 4 + 8 = 12$ years old.

As you can see, this question can be solved either by PITA or via algebra. Some questions can only be solved by algebra, however. Let's look at an example:

36. Fifteen years ago, Tom was three times as old as Steven.
Today, he is only 6 years older than Steven. What was
the sum of their ages fifteen years ago?

    A. 3
    B. 12
    C. 18
    D. 24
    E. 42

Since this question asks for the *sum* of their ages, it would be hard to plug in the answers. If the sum of their ages is 18, as in choice C, then… um… we still don't know either of their ages individually, so this is useless. (In truth, you could use the Ratio Box to find that Tom would have been 13.5 and Steven would have been 4.5 and then check if these numbers work in the rest of the problem, but this is doing far more work than the question requires.)

Thus, write down two algebraic equations. Let Tom's age 15 years ago be t and Steven's age then be s. In that case, the first sentence boils down to $t = 3s$, and the second can be represented as $t + 15 = (s + 15) + 6$, since their ages now are $t + 15$ and $s + 15$. Plug the first equation into the second and simplify, so that $3s + 15 = s + 21$. Then subtract s and 15 from both sides, so that $2s = 6$. Divide both sides by 2, and $s = 3$. Plug this back into the first equation, and $t = 9$. The sum of their ages was $3 + 9 = 12$ (B is correct).

41.4 MONEY

Money problems, when not caused by a lack of it, can also be solved by PITA or translating into algebra. Consider the following example:

37. Laura has a pocketful of change consisting of nickels, dimes, and quarters. The number of dimes is 1 more than the number of nickels, and the number of quarters is 2 fewer than the number of dimes. If the total value of all the change is $1.85, how many coins does she have?

A. 5
B. 6
C. 15
D. 18
E. 20

Since it asks for the total number of coins, PITA would be hard, so let's solve algebraically. Let n denote the number of nickels. Then the number of dimes is $n + 1$, and the number of quarters is $(n + 1) - 2 = n - 1$. The value of the nickels is $5n$ cents, the value of the dimes is $10(n + 1)$ cents, and the value of the quarters is $25(n - 1)$ cents. Since $5n + 10(n + 1) + 25(n - 1) = 185$, we find that $40n - 15 = 185$, so $40n = 200$, which gives $n = 5$. Therefore, Laura has 5 nickels, 6 dimes, and 4 quarters, for a total of 15 coins (C is correct).

41.5   AVERAGES, RATES, AND MIXTURES

Averages and Rates

Given a list of values, their arithmetic **mean** is equal to their sum divided by how many values are in the list. Let's compute the arithmetic mean of 7, 8, 11, 14, and 20. First, we find the sum of the numbers of $7 + 8 + 11 + 14 + 20 = 60$. Next, we count: there are 5 numbers in the list. Finally, we divide: since $60 \div 5 = 12$, the arithmetic mean of the numbers in the list is 12.

The DAT QRT likes to ask this question with strange pieces of the puzzle, however. It is unlikely that you will be given a list of numbers and asked to average them. However, you might be given a number of numbers and their average, and one step in the problem might involve determining their total. In the discussion above, there were 5 numbers, and their average was 12. The product of 5 and 12 is 60, and this was the total. In general, the total of the numbers will always be the product of the number of numbers and their average. Similarly, the numbers added up to 60 and their average was 12, so, since 60 divided by 12 is 5, there had to have been 5 numbers. The rule implicit here is that the total divided by the average gives the number of numbers.

A visual summary of these three rules is the average pie:

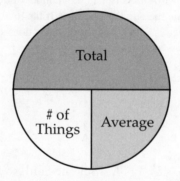

The average pie has three parts:

1.   The total goes in the top.
2.   The number of numbers (or number of things, more generally) goes in the lower left.
3.   The average goes in the lower right.

Any time you know any two of these numbers, you can find the third. To find the top, you multiply the two things on the bottom. To find either of the things in the bottom, divide the top by whatever you have in the bottom, and the result will be the other thing in the bottom.

For example, if you have 4 numbers, and their average is 12, what is their total?

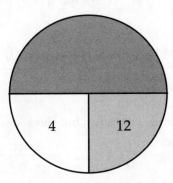

To find the total from these numbers, you must multiply them, and their product is 48, so the total of the 4 numbers must be 48.

Let's look at a second example. If you have some numbers that add up to 90, and their average is 3, how many numbers do you have?

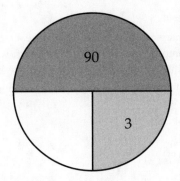

To find the number of things, you must divide 90 by 3, which results in 30. Thus, the number of things must be 30. Here is another problem:

38. Evan's golf scores for his last four rounds are 78, 82, 83, and 76. What must be his golf score in the fifth round to have an average of 80?

   A. 80
   B. 81
   C. 82
   D. 83
   E. 84

To have an average of 80, he must have a total score of 400 across 5 rounds, since 80 times 5 is 400 (draw an average pie to see this clearly). So far, he has a total of 319. Thus, he needs 81 more to get to 400. His final score must be 81 (B is correct).

For rate problems, bear in mind that distance = speed × time, and work = rate × time. Since rates are calculated in a similar way as averages, rate problems can be solved using a rate pie. Put the total on top (distance or work), the time required on the bottom left, and the rate on the bottom right of the rate pie. Also bear in mind that Plugging In can be useful for rate problems.

For example, consider the following. A runner completes the first lap of a 2–lap race at an average speed of 12 miles per hour and the second lap at an average speed of 15 miles per hour. What was the runner's average speed for the race?

The answer is not the average of 12 and 15. By definition, average speed is equal to total distance traveled divided by total time. The simplest thing to do here is to plug in for the unknown distance of the laps.

Let's say the laps were 60 miles each (long laps to run but short laps to calculate). This runner completed the first lap at a speed of 12 miles per hour. Since time = $\dfrac{\text{distance}}{\text{speed}}$, 60 miles at 12 miles per hour means divide 60 by 12, so the first lap takes 5 hours (draw the rate pie to see this clearly). For the second lap, divide 60 by 15, and it takes 4 hours. Thus, both laps together are 120 miles in 9 hours, which is a speed of $\dfrac{120}{9} = \dfrac{40}{3} = 13\dfrac{1}{3}$ miles per hour.

39. Two painters work together on a house. One painter could complete the job alone in 20 hours, while the other painter could complete the job alone in 15 hours. How many hours will it take them to complete the job working together?

A. 5

B. $6\dfrac{2}{3}$

C. $7\dfrac{5}{6}$

D. $8\dfrac{4}{7}$

E. 9

Plug in an amount for the unknown total work. Let's say painting the house requires painting 60 square feet (or square meters). Draw the rate pie to see this means that the first painter paints at a rate of 3 square feet per hour (which is pretty slow). The second painter paints at a rate of 4 square feet per hour (which is only marginally faster). Together, they would paint at a rate of 7 square feet per hour (just add the rates together to find the combined rate). Thus, since the whole thing is 60 square feet, it would take $\dfrac{60}{7} = 8\dfrac{4}{7}$ hours to finish together (D is correct).

Mixtures and Weighted Averages

Mixtures are one example of weighted averages, which appear in a few different forms on the DAT. In general, the formula for a weighted average is (fractional weight$_1$)(number$_1$) + (fractional weight$_2$)(number$_2$) + ... + (fractional weight$_n$)(number$_n$). This is the most generic, abstract, and probably incomprehensible way of phrasing the formula. One possible way that this formula might come up is in a mixture of liquids. Let's look at an example:

40. Katherine decided to take two solutions of salt water, one that is 12 parts per thousand salt and another that is 30 parts per thousand salt, and pour them together. However, she had twice as much of the less salty water than she had of the more salty water. How many parts per thousand of the result will be salt?

    A. 14
    B. 18
    C. 21
    D. 24
    E. 28

In this case, the numbers that we are averaging are 12 and 30. However, there is more of the less salty water, which means that the 12 should count for somewhat more than the 30 does. To account for this, note that two-thirds of the resulting mixture will come from the less salty water, while only one-third will come from the more salty water. These are the fractional weights. Thus, the weighted average is $\left(\frac{2}{3}\right)(12) + \left(\frac{1}{3}\right)(30)$, which simplifies to 8 + 10 = 18. Thus, the result will be 18 parts per thousand salt, (B is correct).

Mixtures and weighted averages can also be tested using temperature. Let's look at an example:

41. Two glasses of water are mixed together. Before mixing, the water in one of the glasses has a mass of 4 kilograms and a temperature of 10°C, and the water in the other of the glasses has a mass of 1 kilogram and a temperature of 90°C. After the water is thoroughly mixed, what will the resulting temperature of the mixture be?

    A. 19°C
    B. 26°C
    C. 30°C
    D. 50°C
    E. 100°C

In this case, temperatures are being averaged, and weighting has to do with the masses. There is some Gchem behind this question, such as the equation $q = mc\Delta T$. Whatever heat (q) is transferred from one sample will go to the other, so q lost from one equals the q gained in the other. Both samples are water, so c is equal for both. Thus, we know that $m\Delta T$ is the relevant product to consider here. One sample has a mass of 4 kilograms and is, therefore, four-fifths of the resulting mixture; the other has a mass of 1 kilogram and is, therefore, one-fifth of the resulting mixture. Therefore, the weighted average is $\left(\frac{4}{5}\right)(10) + \left(\frac{1}{5}\right)(90)$, which reduces to 26 (B is correct).

Mixtures and weighted averages can also be tested using interest. Let's look at an example:

42. Alison has $1000 invested in two different accounts, one of which pays 20% annual interest and the other of which pays 7% annual interest. One year, the annual interest she receives is $167.5. How much money does she have invested in the 7% interest account?

   A. $250
   B. $350
   C. $450
   D. $650
   E. $750

In this case, since we're looking for the fractions involved, it would probably be simplest to PITA, starting with the middle value as usual. If she has $450 invested in the 7% account, she gets 7% of $450 each year from that account, which is $31.5, and she has $550 left to invest in the 20% account, which would yield $110. The total of these two amounts is $141.5, which is not enough, so she needs less money in the 7% account and more money in the 20% account to get more interest (eliminate C, D, and E). Plugging-in choice B results in $24.5 from the 7% account and $130 from the 20% account. This totals $154.5, which is getting closer but is still not high enough (eliminate B, and by POE, the correct answer is A). On test day, you should pick option A and move on. For the sake of reviewing here, let's confirm A is correct. 7% of $250 is $17.5, while 20% of the remaining $750 is $150, which totals $167.5.

By the way, if you really felt like solving this with the weighted average equation, you could. The numbers that we're averaging are 7% (that is, 0.07) and 20% (that is, 0.2). Their weights are the amounts invested in the accounts. Call the amount in the 7% account x, so the amount in the 20% account is $(1000 - x)$. In that case, the equation comes out to $(0.07)(x) + (0.2)(1000 - x) = 167.5$. To solve, it's probably simplest to multiply everything by 100 to get rid of the decimals, which yields $7x + 20(1000 - x) = 16750$. Distribute, and $7x + 20,000 - 20x = 16750$. Collect like terms and bring the xs to the right and constants to the left, and you're left with $3250 = 13x$. Divide both sides by 13, and $x = 250$, which means that she invests $250 in the 7% account, as found above. This solution will take more time than PITA.

Weighted averages can show up in slightly different ways, too. Let's look at another problem:

43. A fruit drink is made by combining grape juice that costs
$1.80 per quart with apple juice at $1.20 per quart. If a
gallon (4 quarts) of a mixture of grape juice and apple
juice costs $5.70, how many quarts of grape juice are in
the mixture?

A. 0.5
B. 1
C. 1.5
D. 2
E. 2.5

First of all, since the grape juice costs $\dfrac{\$5.70}{4} = \$1.425$ per quart, which is closer to $1.20 than to $1.80,

eliminate D and E. This mixture is more apple juice than grape juice. Of the three answers remain-

ing, plug in the middle, or choice B. If the mixture was 1 part grape juice and 3 parts apple juice, the

weighted average equation would be $\left(\dfrac{1}{4}\right)(\$1.80) + \left(\dfrac{3}{4}\right)(\$1.20)$, which reduces to $1.35 per quart. This

is not expensive enough, so it's too much apple juice and not enough grape juice. The answer must be the

only one left with more grape juice than B, which is answer C. This is the more technique-based, POE

and PITA solution.

The algebraic solution would look like this: let g denote the number of quarts of grape juice in the
mixture and $4 - g$ denote the number of quarts of apple juice. The cost of the grape juice is $(1.8)g$, the cost
of the apple juice is $(1.2) \times (4 - g)$ and we're told that the total cost is 5.7 (all in dollars). Thus, $(1.8)g +
(1.2)(4 - g) = 5.7$. Simplifying, we get $(0.6)g + 4.8 = 5.7$, so $(0.6)g = 0.9$. This gives 1.5 quarts (C is correct).

41.6 GROUPS

There are essentially two kinds of group problems: some call for the group formula, and others call for the group grid. The group formula says that for two groups that share members, total = group 1 + group 2 – both + neither.

For example, consider the following:

44. If a room contains 50 college students, 30 of whom are majoring in chemistry, 30 of whom are majoring in biology, and 10 of whom are majoring in something else, how many double-majors in chemistry and biology must there be?

    A. 10
    B. 20
    C. 30
    D. 40

According to the group formula, given that group 1 is the chemistry majors, group 2 is the biology majors, and "both" refers to the double-majors, 50 = 30 + 30 – both + 10 in this case. That means that 50 = 70 – both, so there must be 20 double-majors. Put another way, if there are some double-majors, we're counting them twice when we count 30 chem majors and 30 bio majors. If 10 people aren't majoring in either, that leaves 40 people left who are majoring in chem, bio, or both. If there are 30 and 30 but that only comes to 40 people, we must be counting 20 of them twice, so there must 10 chem-only, 10 bio-only, and 20 double-majors.

The group grid comes into play when groups cut across each other repeatedly. For example, consider the following:

45. A room contains 50 college chemistry and biology majors, with no double-majors, 30 of whom are majoring in chemistry. Half of the students are 22 years old, and half of the chemistry majors are not 22 years old. How many 22-year-old biology majors are in the room?

    A. 10
    B. 15
    C. 25
    D. 30
    E. 45

This calls for a grid. We need to keep track of chemistry, biology, 22 years old, and not 22 years old, and these groups cut across each other. Thus, draw the following:

	22 Years Old	Not 22 Years Old	Total
Chem			30
Bio			
Total	25		50

There are 50 total students and 30 total chemistry majors. Since half the students are 22 years old, that means that 25 students are 22 years old. Now, 30 chemistry majors means 20 biology majors, and 25 students who are 22 years old means 25 students who are not 22 years old, so fill those in as well. The question also says that half of the chemistry majors are not 22 years old, too, which is 15.

	22 Years Old	Not 22 Years Old	Total
Chem		15	30
Bio			20
Total	25	25	50

If there are 15 chemistry majors who are not 22 years old and 25 students altogether who are not 22 years old, then there must be 10 biology majors who are not 22 years old. If there are 20 biology majors altogether and 10 of them are not 22 years old, then 10 of them must be 22 years old.

	22 Years Old	Not 22 Years Old	Total
Chem	15	15	30
Bio	10	10	20
Total	25	25	50

Thus, the answer to the question is A.

Want More Practice?
Scan the QR code below to register your book for online chapter summaries, drills, practice tests, and more!

Chapter 42
Advanced Arithmetic

42.1 CONVERSIONS

Converting Time, Length, and Weight

A **conversion** is a rewriting of a measurement in one set of units in terms of a different set of units. For example, "1 foot = 12 inches" is a conversion, since it takes a measurement in feet and converts it to inches. For the DAT QRT, you must know how to convert American units of length (inches, feet, yards, and miles), time (seconds, minutes, hours, days), and weight (ounces, pounds, tons). Here are the conversions:

- 1 foot = 12 inches
- 1 yard = 3 feet
- 1 mile = 5280 feet
- 1 minute = 60 seconds
- 1 hour = 60 minutes
- 1 day = 24 hours
- 1 pound (lb.) = 16 ounces (oz.)
- 1 ton = 2000 pounds

You may be asked to convert a number of inches to yards, or days to seconds, or any of the like. For example, how many yards are in 2.5 miles? To solve this, begin with the 2.5 miles and convert to feet as follows: $2.5 \text{ miles} \times \dfrac{5280 \text{ feet}}{1 \text{ mile}}$. Notice that the miles in the denominator cancel the miles in the original quantity, and the units come out in feet (13200 feet, specifically). Next, multiply by another conversion factor to get to yards: $13200 \text{ feet} \times \dfrac{1 \text{ yard}}{3 \text{ feet}} = 4400 \text{ yards}$. Again, feet cancel, and the units come out in yards. Thus, there are 4400 yards in 2.5 miles.

Notice this works because 5280 feet = 1 mile, so multiplying by $\dfrac{5280 \text{ feet}}{1 \text{ mile}}$ is multiplying by something over itself, and anything over itself is equal to 1. Multiplying by 1 doesn't change the value of the number, though, just as with changing the denominator of a fraction, it can change the way that the number is expressed. That is, 2.5 miles and 4400 yards are different ways of expressing the same quantity, and multiplying by a form of 1 converts from one to the other.

Prefixes

You will also need to memorize the following metric prefixes:

Prefix	Letter	Magnitude
micro	μ	10^{-6}
milli	m	10^{-3}
centi	c	10^{-2}
kilo	k	10^{3}
mega	M	10^{6}

Thus, just as one meter can be written as 1 m, one millimeter can be written as 1 mm and is equal to 10^{-3} meters. The same goes for microseconds (1 μs = 10^{-6} s), kilometers (1 km = 10^{3} m), or any other measurement with these prefixes.

For example, let's convert a speed of 60 miles per hour into meters per minute, given that 1 mile = 1.6 km.

To do this, note that the abbreviation "k" stands for "kilo-," a prefix which means "one thousand." Thus, a kilometer is to 1000 meters. Therefore, $\dfrac{60 \text{ mile}}{1 \text{ hour}} \times \dfrac{1.6 \text{ km}}{1 \text{ mile}} = \dfrac{96 \text{ km}}{1 \text{ hour}}$. This means 60 miles per hour is the same as 96 kilometers per hour. Next, in the same fashion, convert kilometers to meters and hours to minutes: $\dfrac{96 \text{ km}}{1 \text{ hour}} \times \dfrac{1000 \text{ m}}{1 \text{ km}} \times \dfrac{1 \text{ hour}}{60 \text{ min}} = \dfrac{1600 \text{ m}}{1 \text{ min}}$. (Notice that hours must be in the numerator in the conversion factor to cancel the hours in the denominator in the original quantity.) Thus, 60 miles per hour is equivalent to 1600 meters per minute.

Using a Given Formula

You may also be asked to convert units with a formula provided. For example, consider the following:

47. What is the temperature in Celsius if it is 77°F? Note: if C is temperature in Celsius and F is temperature in Fahrenheit, then $C = \dfrac{5}{9}(F - 32)$.

   A. 20°
   B. 25°
   C. 45°
   D. 109°
   E. 196°

Plug the provided value into the given equation. This gives $C = \dfrac{5}{9}(77 - 32)$, which simplifies to 25° (B is correct). You do not have to be familiar with such a formula to use it, so if you see something new or unexpected on test day, don't worry. Plug in values and keep moving.

42.2   STATISTICS, PROBABILITY, AND ARRANGEMENTS

Mean, Median, Mode

There are three statistical words that begin with M that you'll have to know about for the DAT test. The first (and most common) is mean, also called **arithmetic mean** or **average**, which has been discussed already; go back to section 41.5 if you need a review. The two others are called the median and the mode.

The **median** of a list of numbers is the number in the middle of the list when the numbers are arranged in order. For example, the median of the collection of numbers 7, 8, 11, 14, and 20 is 11 because that's the one that's in the middle when they're written in ascending order. You may need to properly arrange the values yourself. For example, "What is the median of the values 63, 35, 76, 21, 54, 21, and 5?" First, we must arrange the numbers in order (increasing or decreasing); for example: 5, 21, 21, 35, 54, 63, 76. Now we see that 35 is the middle value, so it's the median. (Median = middle.)

If the collection contains an even number of values, then there is no middle value. In this case, take the average (arithmetic mean) of the two middle values. For example, the median of the values 3, 16, 23, 37, 44, 45 is the average (arithmetic mean) of 23 and 37, which is (23 + 37) ÷ 2 = 30.

The **mode** of a list of values is the value that appears the most times. For example, the mode of the values 1, 4, 1, 4, 2, 1, 3, 5, 6, 2 is 1 because it appears three times, which is more times than any other value in the list. In other words, the mode is the most common value in the collection. (Mode = most.)

Variance, Standard Deviation

Given a set of numerical data, **variance** is one way of measuring the dispersion of values from the central value. The central value used to determine variance is the arithmetic mean. Consider the following list of data values; they represent outcomes of throwing a fair die eight times: 2, 4, 5, 1, 2, 6, 1, 3 The arithmetic mean of the values is (2 + 4 + 5 + 1 + 2 + 6 + 1 + 3)/8 = 24/8 = 3. To compute the variance of this set of data, determine the square of the difference between each value in the given data set and the mean, and compute the sum of these squares. Next, divide the sum above by the number of values in the data set, and the result is the variance. In this case, the sum of squares of differences between each value in the data set and the mean is $(2 - 3)^2 + (4 - 3)^2 + (5 - 3)^2 + (1 - 3)^2 + (2 - 3)^2 + (6 - 3)^2 + (1 - 3)^2 + (3 - 3)^2 =$ 24. Now, dividing this by 8, we find the variance 24/8 = 3. Note the usual definition of *variance* calls for dividing the sum of the squares of the difference between each value in the data set and the mean by $n - 1$, where n is the number of values in the data set. Dividing by n, as we've done, gives what is properly called the **population variance**. The DAT seems to use this latter definition. In any case, whether we divide by n or by $n - 1$, the results are typically quite close, allowing you to select the correct answer on a multiple-choice question, regardless of the definition used.

Standard deviation is the square root of variance. Thus, for the data set given above (eight throws of the die), we calculated that the variance is 3. Therefore, the standard deviation is $\sqrt{3}$, which is approximately 1.7.

However, while the above is given for completeness, it is extraordinarily unlikely that you will have to *compute* the variance or standard deviation of given data on test day. It is more likely that you will have to work with the *concepts* of variance and standard deviation. Standard deviation is often used to describe a **normal distribution** of data, which looks like the following:

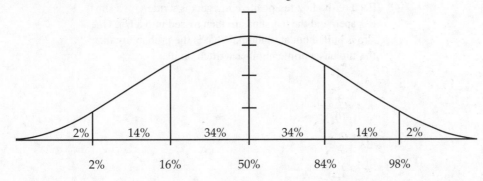

A normal distribution is a bell curve as drawn above. The mean value is in the middle, and the most common values are near the middle; extreme values are far less common. Standard deviation is a measuring stick for this: we can say any particular value is one standard deviation away from the mean, two standard deviations away from the mean, etc. For example, if the mean of some particular set of values is 5 and the standard deviation is 2, then the value 3 would be one standard deviation below the mean (because 5 − 2 = 3) and the value 9 would be two standard deviations above the mean (because 5 + 2 + 2 = 9).

As the diagram above indicates, for data that fits a normal distribution, only about 2% of values are more than two standard deviations below the mean, about 14% of values are between one and two standard deviations below the mean, and about 34% of values are between zero and one standard deviation below the mean. The curve is symmetric about the mean, so exactly the same percentages hold for the other side.

Standard deviation is thus a measure of the width of the bell curve. If one curve has a mean of 5 and a standard deviation of 2, then 68% of values are between 3 and 7. (That's 34% between 3 and 5 and 34% between 5 and 7.) However, if another curve has a mean of 5 and a standard deviation of 5, then 68% of values are between 0 and 10; that is, the second curve would be much wider than the first.

Basic Probability

The probability of an event occurring is the number of ways that event could occur divided by the total number of outcomes possible. In other words, Probability $= \dfrac{\text{Number of outcomes you want}}{\text{Number of outcomes possible}}$.

Consider rolling a standard, fair die. It has six sides, all of which are equally likely to turn up. Since there are six possible outcomes, all equally likely, the probability of any one of them happening is $\dfrac{1}{6}$. What is the probability of rolling an even number? In this case, there are three desired outcomes: rolling 2, 4, or 6.

Again, there are six possible outcomes, so the probability of rolling an even number is $\frac{3}{6}$, which is equal

to $\frac{1}{2}$. Let's look at another example:

48. Each of the first ten positive integers is written on a slip of paper, and the ten slips are then tossed into a hat. One slip is pulled out at random. What is the probability that the slip has a prime number written on it?

A. $\frac{3}{10}$

B. $\frac{2}{5}$

C. $\frac{1}{2}$

D. $\frac{2}{3}$

E. 1

Assuming all ten numbers are equally likely to be selected, we divide the number of desired outcomes by

the total number of possible outcomes. Among the first ten positive integers, the only primes are 2, 3, 5,

and 7 (four desired outcomes). Thus, the probability of pulling out a prime number is $\frac{4}{10} = \frac{2}{5}$ (B is cor-

rect).

Decks of cards also represent a convenient way of asking probability questions. If a question begins, "An ordinary deck of playing cards is shuffled, and a card is randomly chosen," a variety of questions could follow. Consider each of the following: What is the probability the card selected is a heart? What is the probability it is red? What is the probability the card drawn is the jack of hearts? What is the probability of not selecting a face card?

First, an ordinary deck contains 52 cards. Since there are 13 hearts, the probability the card selected is a

heart is $\frac{13}{52} = \frac{1}{4}$. Since two suits are red (hearts and diamonds), there are 13 + 13 = 26 red cards, so the

probability a red card is selected is $\frac{26}{52} = \frac{1}{2}$. Since there is only one jack of hearts, the probability this

particular card is chosen is $\frac{1}{52}$. There are three face cards per suit: jack, queen, and king. Since there are

four suits (hearts, diamonds, spades, and clubs), there are (3)(4) = 12 face cards. Therefore, 52 − 12 = 40

of the cards are not face cards: the probability of not selecting a face card is $\frac{40}{52} = \frac{10}{13}$.

Finally, coins are also a common source of probability questions. For example, a fair coin is tossed twice. What is the probability of getting tails on both tosses? To solve this, first note that the probability of getting tails on each toss is one half. This means the probability of getting a tail on two tosses is $\frac{1}{2} \times \frac{1}{2} = \frac{1}{4}$.

Factorials

If you see 2! written in an arithmetic expression, this is not a really surprising or emphatic 2; this is a **factorial**. In particular, $2! = 2 \times 1$, and $3! = 3 \times 2 \times 1$, and so on. In other words, to compute a factorial, multiply by all of the integers starting from the number and counting down to 1. The one exception to this is 0!, which is defined as 1.

Since $3! = 3 \times 2 \times 1$ and $2! = 2 \times 1$, we can also say that $3! = 3 \times 2!$. In general, $x! = (x - 1)!$. This can be useful to remember because computing factorials of even relatively small numbers, such as 6 or 7, can be very clunky with the DAT on-screen calculator, and factorials much larger than that will overflow the calculator. Thus, if you are asked to calculate the value of, for example, $\frac{100!}{98!}$, there is no way that you can calculate 100!, then calculate 98!, and then divide. Instead, notice that $\frac{100 \times 99 \times 98!}{98!}$, and then cancel the 98! in the numerator with the 98! in the denominator. Thus, the value is $100 \times 99 = 9900$.

Permutations, Combinations, and Other Arrangements

Some questions may ask how many ways something can be done. Sometimes you can simply list out all of the possibilities. For example, how many ways are there to arrange the letters A, B, and C? Organize the list by first letter, so that there are ABC, ACB, BAC, BCA, CAB, and CBA. There are 6 ways to do this.

However, sometimes there are far too many different possibilities to list out the different arrangements. In this case, you will need a method for calculating them. For most of these problems, you can write out blanks for each of the things that are actually being done (for example, decisions or choices made) and fill each blank with the number of ways of doing that thing. Finally, multiply the numbers.

Let's look at an example. If you must choose a shirt, pants, and shoes, and if there are 7 shirts, 3 pairs of pants, and 4 pairs of shoes to choose from, how many outfits can you choose? Draw out three slots (one for the shirt, one for the pants, and one for the shoes):

_____   _____   _____

Shirt   Pants   Shoes

Then put 7 in the shirts slot, 3 in the pants slot, and 4 in the shoes slot, because these are the number of options in each case.

$$\underline{\quad 7 \quad} \qquad \underline{\quad 3 \quad} \qquad \underline{\quad 4 \quad}$$

Shirt   Pants   Shoes

Now multiply, and you'll get the answer.

$$\underline{\quad 7 \quad} \quad \times \quad \underline{\quad 3 \quad} \quad \times \quad \underline{\quad 4 \quad}$$

Shirt   Pants   Shoes

Thus, the number of different outfits is $7 \times 3 \times 4 = 84$. Sometimes this kind of problem is called "choosing one thing from multiple sources," since you can imagine having a pile of shirts (one source), a pile of pants (another source), and a pile of shoes (another sources), and choosing one thing from each of these piles.

What if we were choosing multiple things from the same source? Consider the following example. If you must choose which shirts to wear for next Monday, Tuesday, and Wednesday, and you will wear a different shirt each day, then how many different sequences of shirts could you choose from the 7 shirts that you own? In this case, there are three decisions being made (one for Monday, one for Tuesday, and one for Wednesday), so draw out three slots; the answer will be the product of three numbers.

Next, you have 7 options for the first day, since there are 7 shirts to choose from and you could wear any of them. For the second day, though, you've already worn one shirt, so it's no longer available and you only have 6 options left. For the third day, you've already worn two shirts, so you only have 5 options left. This means that the number of possibilities is $7 \times 6 \times 5 = 210$. This is sometimes called "choosing multiple things in order from the same source without replacement." The "without replacement" part just means that once you've taken a shirt out of the pile, you don't put it back; you can't wear the same shirt several days in a row. If you could, the answer would just be $7 \times 7 \times 7 = 343$. This is also called a **permutation**.

However, if order didn't matter, things would be slightly different. For example, if you accidentally spilled coffee on three different shirts out of your 7 shirts, how many different groups of shirts could have been spilled on? In this case, we start in the same way, with three slots that are filled as $7 \times 6 \times 5$, but this does not quite give the final answer yet. In this case, there's no first shirt or second shirt or third shirt. If you spill coffee on your red shirt and your blue shirt and your green shirt, that's the same as spilling on blue and red and green, or green and blue and red, or any other rearrangement of these same shirts. Thus, these different groups aren't really different, and we're overcounting if we just multiply $7 \times 6 \times 5$.

To solve this problem, divide by the number of ways of rearranging three items in different orders, which, according to the discussion above, must be $3 \times 2 \times 1$ (you have three options for which shirt will go first, two for which will go second, and only one left to go last). In other words, the number of ways of spilling coffee on three shirts out of seven is $\dfrac{7 \times 6 \times 5}{3 \times 2 \times 1}$. Before you start pressing a bunch of calculator buttons, notice that the denominator is 6, which cancels the 6 in the numerator, and you get $7 \times 5 = 35$.

If the items you're choosing don't go in any particular order but are just a group of things, then you multiply as described above, but then divide by the factorial of the number of slots you had. That is, if there were three things actually being chosen, you'd divide by 3!. If there were 4 things actually being chosen, you'd divide by 4!. This is called "choosing multiple things from the same source without replacement, when order doesn't matter." This is also called a **combination**.

There's one final case to consider. We've looked at choosing multiple things from the same source and choosing one thing from multiple sources. Choosing one thing from one source is pretty self-explanatory. If you have 7 shirts, and you have to choose one, you have 7 options. But what if you're choosing multiple things from multiple sources?

For example, let's say you were donating some of your clothes to charity. You have to choose four shirts, one pair of pants, and two pairs of shoes to donate, and you have 7 shirts, 3 pairs of pants, and 4 pairs of shoes to choose from. How many different groups of clothing could you donate?

In this case, take each source separately. For the shirts, you're donating four, and there's no particular order (if it's donated, it's donated, whether it's donated first or second or whatever), so the number of options is $\dfrac{7 \times 6 \times 5 \times 4}{4 \times 3 \times 2 \times 1}$, which, if you cancel the 4 in the denominator with the 4 in the numerator and the rest of the denominator with the 6 in the numerator, comes out to 7×5. Thus, there are 35 options for shirts.

For pants, you're only donating one, so there are 3 options (you could call this $\dfrac{3}{1}$, since there's no order here, either, but that's the same thing). For shoes, you're donating two, and there's no particular order, so the number of options is $\dfrac{4 \times 3}{2 \times 1}$, which reduces to 2×3, so there are 6 options for shoes. Finally, multiply all of the options for all of the types of clothing, so the number of different groups of clothing you could donate is $35 \times 3 \times 6 = 630$. Let's look at another example:

49. A personal code for your ATM card consists of six characters: any letter or any numerical digit. How many possible personal codes are there?

   A. 216
   B. 60,466,176
   C. 1,402,410,240
   D. 1,838,265,625
   E. 2,176,782,336

Since there are twenty-six letters (A through Z) and ten digits (0 through 9), there are 26 + 10 = 36 possible characters; the total number of ways the six decisions can be made is $36 \times 36 \times 36 \times 36 \times 36 \times 36 = 2,176,782,336$ (E is correct). Fortunately, the on-screen calculator makes this less labor-intensive than it would have been when everything had to be done by hand.

42.2

Let's work through a final example. What if you want your personal ATM code to have no repeated characters? Now how many possible codes are there? In this case, there are 36 ways to make the first decision, but only 35 for the second because, to avoid a repeat, we can't use the same choice we made for the first character. Then there are only 34 possible choices for the third character, 33 for the fourth, 32 for the fifth, and 31 for the sixth. Thus, the total number of codes that don't have any repeated characters is 36 × 35 × 34 × 33 × 32 × 31 = 1,402,410,240. The answer would have been C in that case.

Want More Practice?
Scan the QR code below to register your book for online chapter summaries, drills, practice tests, and more!

Chapter 43
Plane Geometry

43.1 ANGLES

Terms

When two line segments (or rays, which are half lines) meet at a point (called the **vertex**), they form an **angle**. The symbol for an angle is $\angle$.

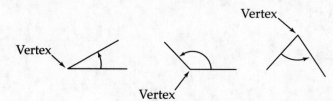

We can refer to an angle by the letter we assign to its vertex, or, if this would be ambiguous, by three letters, where the middle one is the vertex, and the other two are on the sides of the angle. For example, we have $\angle A$:

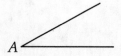

However, which of the angles in the following diagram would be $\angle A$?

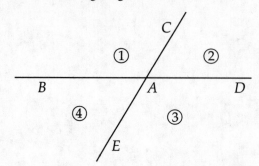

There is an ambiguity here because there are many angles with vertex A, so if we didn't refer to the angles by number, we'd have to use a three-letter notation. Angle 1 is *BAC* or *CAB*, 2 is *CAD* or *DAC*, and so on.

The size (i.e., measure) of an angle can be expressed in degrees (denoted °). One **degree** is equal to $\frac{1}{360}$ of a complete revolution. If two angles have the same measure, we say that they are **congruent**; the word "congruent" is a generic term used in geometry to describe figures that have the same shape and size. In the figure below, we can estimate the measure of each angle: x is about 30°, y is about 135°, and z is about 75°.

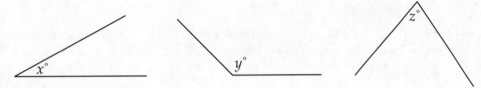

An angle of 90° is, by definition of a degree, $\frac{1}{4}$ of a complete revolution; such an angle is called a **right angle**. Two lines that meet in a right angle are said to be **perpendicular** to one another. If angles A and B are perpendicular, we can express this as $A \perp B$.

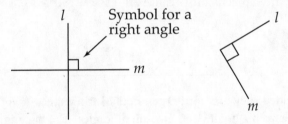

An angle less than 90° is called an **acute** angle:

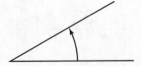

An angle greater than 90° but less than 180° is called an **obtuse** angle:

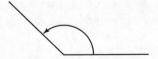

A 180° is called a **straight** angle:

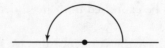

An angle greater than 180° but less than 360° is called a **reflex** angle:

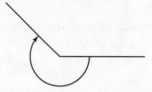

Two angles whose sum is 90° are said to be **complementary** (or to be complements of one another). In the figure below, angles 1 and 2 are complements because $\angle 1 + \angle 2 = 90°$.

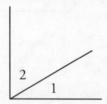

Two angles whose sum is 180° are said to be **supplementary** (or to be supplements of one another). In the figure below, angles 1 and 2 are supplements because $\angle 1 + \angle 2 = 180°$.

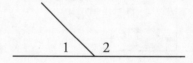

When two lines cross (provided they are not perpendicular), they create two kinds of angles: big angles and small angles. There are two big angles and two small angles. The big angles are equal, and the small angles are equal. Any big angle plus any small angle equals 180°. In other words:

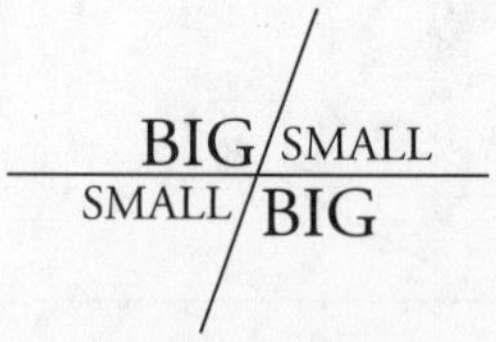

If two lines lie in the same plane and never intersect, the lines are said to be **parallel**. If angles A and B are parallel, we can express this as $A \| B$. If two lines are parallel and are intersected by a third line (provided it's not perpendicular), they again create big angles and small angles, and the same rules apply as above: All the big angles are equal, all the small angles are equal, and any big angle plus any small angle equals 180°:

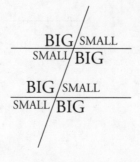

43.2 TRIANGLES

A **polygon** is a closed figure one can draw with straight lines. The simplest polygon is a **triangle**, a three-sided polygon.

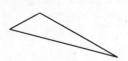 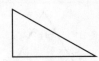 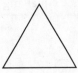

The corners of a triangle (or of any polygon) are known as the **vertices**; each one is called a **vertex**. Given a triangle, the sum of the lengths of any two sides must be greater than the length of the third side, and the difference must be less than the length of the third side. This fact is known as the **triangle inequality** (or the Third Side Rule). For example, for the triangle below, the lengths of whose sides are labeled a, b, and c, it must be true that $a + b > c$, that $b + c > a$, and that $a + c > b$. Equally, it must be true that $a - b < c$, that $b - c < a$, and that $a - c < b$.

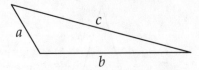

The sum of measures of the three interior angles of any triangle is 180°. Therefore, in the figure below, $x + y + z = 180$:

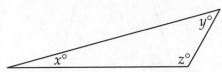

Perimeter and Area

The **perimeter** of a polygon is the sum of the lengths of its sides. Thus, for a triangle with sides of lengths a, b, and c, the perimeter is $a + b + c$. The **area** of a polygon is a measure of the region the shape encloses.

For a triangle, the area can be found from the formula $A = \dfrac{1}{2}bh$, where b is the base of the triangle (any of its sides) and h is the height of the triangle (the perpendicular distance from the base to one of the vertices).

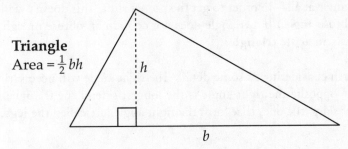

Triangle
Area $= \frac{1}{2}bh$

Scalene, Isosceles, and Equilateral

A triangle in which all the sides are equal is called **equilateral**. In any polygon, the length of a side corresponds to the size of the opposite angle (big sides are opposite big angles, small sides are opposite small angles, and equal sides are opposite equal angles), so a triangle with three equal sides must also have three equal angles. Three equal angles that add up to 180° must each equal 60°.

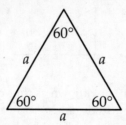

A triangle in which two sides are equal is called **isosceles**. The angles opposite the equal sides are also equal.

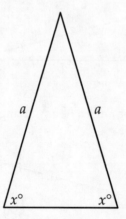

If none of the sides or angles are equal, then the triangle is called **scalene**.

Acute, Obtuse, and Right Triangles

We reviewed the important types of angles (acute, right, obtuse, and reflex) in Chapter 33; go back there now if you need a review. Let's look at how these angles show up in triangles on the DAT. A triangle that contains an obtuse angle is called an **obtuse triangle**, and a triangle that contains a right angle is called a **right triangle**. (No triangle can contain more than one obtuse or right angle, since the interior angles must add up to 180°. Two right angles would already add up to 180°, so the third angle would have to be 0°—that is, not be an angle at all—in order to get the proper sum. This doesn't work, so triangles contain at most one right or obtuse angle.) If a triangle does not contain an obtuse or right angle, then all of its angles are acute, and it is an **acute triangle**.

Right triangles are worth considering in some detail. The right angle will necessarily be the largest angle, and, therefore, the side opposite the right angle is the longest side of the triangle; it is called the **hypotenuse**. The two smaller sides (the ones that form the right angle) are called the **legs**.

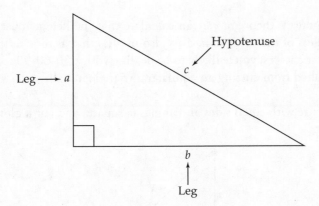

In any right triangle, the sum of the squares of the legs is equal to the square of the hypotenuse. Thus, in the figure above, $a^2 + b^2 = c^2$. This is known as the **Pythagorean Theorem**. Any three positive integers a, b, and c that satisfy this equation can be the lengths of the sides of a right triangle (with c, the largest number, being the hypotenuse); such sets of three numbers are called **Pythagorean triples**.

The smallest Pythagorean triple is 3, 4, 5, since $3^2 + 4^2 = 5^2$; this forms the **3-4-5 right triangle**. Furthermore, any multiple of a 3-4-5 right triangle (or of any right triangle) will be another right triangle. For example, if we double a 3-4-5 right triangle, we get a 6-8-10 right triangle (which is a right triangle because $6^2 + 8^2 = 10^2$). Other than multiples of the 3-4-5 triple, the next smallest Pythagorean triple is 5-12-13, which is found in the **5-12-13 right triangle**.

It is certainly true that you can square numbers using the DAT on-screen calculator to determine the third side of a right triangle. However, it is worth remembering these two triples, partly because it is faster to recall these ratios than to have to re-derive them on test day but also as a technique in itself. If you see a length of 5 in a geometry figure, it's likely you're going to have to make a 3-4-5 or a 5-12-13 right triangle out of it. Similarly, as soon as you see a 3 or 4 in a geometry figure, start trying to draw a 3-4-5 right triangle, and likewise with a 12 or a 13 and a 5-12-13 right triangle.

In addition to the 3-4-5 and 5-12-13 right triangles, are two additional special triangles that you should be familiar with. Take an equilateral triangle and cut it in half, as you see below:

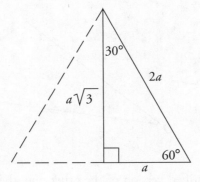

Since one 60° angle has been cut in half, it becomes a 30° angle. One angle is unchanged, so it remains 60°. The final angle is perpendicular to the base, so it is 90°. This triangle is called a **30-60-90 right triangle**, after the angles. Since it is an equilateral triangle cut in half, if the base is a, the hypotenuse must be $2a$ (since the base is half a side of the original triangle, and the hypotenuse is a full side of the original triangle). From the Pythagorean Theorem, we can calculate that the height must be $a\sqrt{3}$. This ratio is always maintained, regardless of the value of a. This also implies that as soon as you see a $\sqrt{3}$ in a problem, especially in the answer choices, you're likely to be dealing with a 30-60-90 right triangle somewhere. The 30-60-90 triangle resulted from cutting an equilateral triangle in half.

If you have a four-sided figure with equal sides and angles (a square) and cut it along its diagonal, you get a **45-45-90 right triangle**.

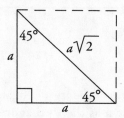

The angles were all 90° angles, and one remains, but two have been sliced in half, so those two are 45° each. The base and height are both a, if a was the side length of the original square, and from the Pythagorean Theorem, we can calculate the hypotenuse is $a\sqrt{2}$. This ratio of sides is also always maintained in 45-45-90 right triangles. This suggests that whenever you see a $\sqrt{2}$ in a problem, especially in the answer choices, you should start looking for a 45-45-90 right triangle.

Similarity

Consider two triangles, $\triangle ABC$ and $\triangle DEF$, with $\angle A = \angle D$, $\angle B = \angle E$, and $\angle C = \angle F$. These triangles have the same shape but not necessarily the same size; one is simply a magnified version of the other. We say the triangles are **similar** and express this fact as follows: $\triangle ABC \sim \triangle DEF$ (the $\sim$ means "is similar to"). The order in which the vertices of the triangles are written in the similarity expression is important. A corresponds to D, B corresponds to E, and C corresponds to F; therefore, once we write, say, the first triangle as $\triangle ABC$ (the vertex A followed by B followed by C), we *must* write the second one in the corresponding order: $\triangle DEF$.

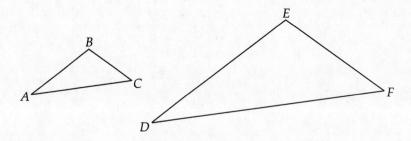

Since one triangle is simply a magnified version of the other one, the ratio of lengths of corresponding sides is a constant. This means, for example, if side DF is twice the length of side AC, then side EF is twice the length of side BC, and side DE is twice the length of side AB. In general, if $\triangle ABC \sim \triangle DEF$, then

$\dfrac{DE}{AB} = \dfrac{EF}{BC} = \dfrac{DF}{AC}$. That is, the ratio of sides is a constant. If this constant is C, then the perimeter of the

larger triangle is C times greater than the perimeter of the smaller triangle and the area is C^2 times greater.

This same idea can be applied to any pair of polygons, not just to triangles. For example, the following two pentagons are similar: $ABCDE \sim PQRST$.

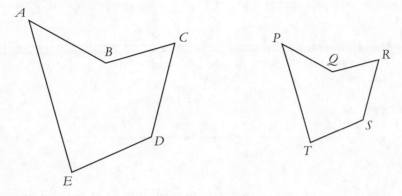

43.3   QUADRILATERALS

A **quadrilateral** is a polygon with four sides. The sum of the interior angles in a quadrilateral is 360°. Thus, in the figure below, $w + x + y + z = 360°$.

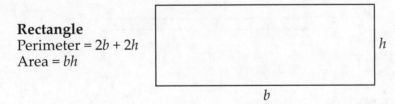

$$w + x + y + z = 360°$$

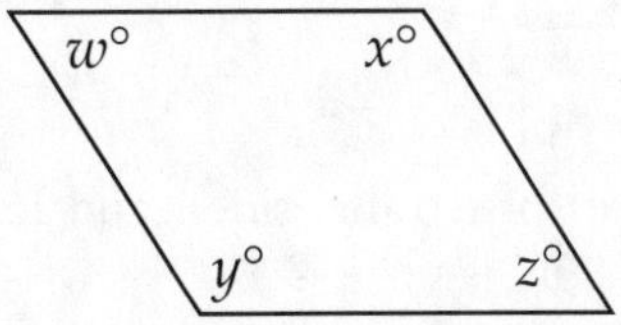

Two common special quadrilaterals (4-sided polygons) are the rectangle and the square. A **rectangle** is a 4-sided polygon, all of whose angles are right angles. It follows from this that opposite sides are equal. Thus, if two of sides have length b, and the other two sides have length h, then the perimeter is $2b + 2h$, or equivalently, $2(b + h)$. The area of a rectangle is given by the formula $A = bh$, where b is the base of the rectangle (any of its sides) and h is its height (a side perpendicular to the base).

Rectangle
Perimeter = $2b + 2h$
Area = bh

A **square** is a rectangle, all of whose sides are equal. The perimeter of a square of side length b is $4b$, and the area is b^2.

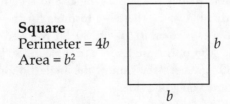

Square
Perimeter = $4b$
Area = b^2

Rectangles and squares are special cases of a more general quadrilateral: the **parallelogram**. The figure gets its name from the fact that opposite sides are parallel, from which it follows that opposite sides are equal as well. The area of a parallelogram is found by dropping a perpendicular line to the base and multiplying base times height.

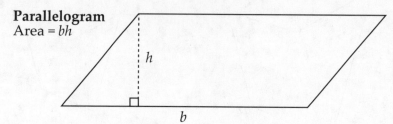

Parallelogram
Area = bh

The formula is the same as for a rectangle, and you can see this must be true because the triangle at the left could be transferred to the right side, giving a rectangle of base b and height h:

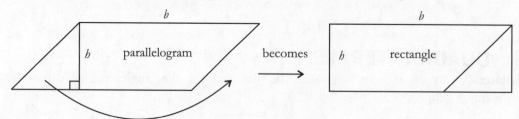

A **trapezoid** has only one pair of parallel sides, and its area can be found from the following formula: $A = \dfrac{b_1 + b_2}{2} h$. That is, since it has effectively two bases, average the two bases and multiply by the height.

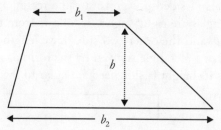

Other Polygons

Polygons that have more sides than quadrilaterals have include **pentagons** (5 sides), **hexagons** (6 sides), **heptagons** (7 sides), **octagons** (8 sides), **nonagons** (9 sides), and **decagons** (10 sides). There are no good general formulas for their areas or perimeters. To find the area of a many-sides polygon, you must divide it up into smaller, more recognizable shapes (such as triangles and rectangles), and to find the perimeter, you must add up all the side lengths. However, there is a formula for the sum of the interior angles of an n-sided polygon. The sum of the angles is equal to $(n - 2)180°$. If you find yourself forgetting this formula, remember the following. Since the sum of the angles in a triangle is 180°, and the sum of the angles in a quadrilateral is 360° (which is 180° greater), the sum of the angles in a pentagon is 540° (which is 180° greater). Keep adding 180° each time you add a side.

43.4   CIRCLES

A **circle** is the set of all points in a plane that are at a fixed distance from some given point. This given point is called the center of the circle, and the fixed distance is called the **radius** (denoted *r*).

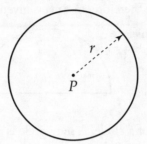

A line that just touches a circle at exactly one point is called a **tangent** to the circle. If the radius is drawn to the point of tangency, it will always be perpendicular to the tangent line.

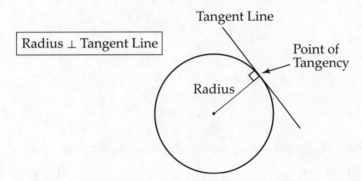

Any line segment with endpoints on the circle and which passes through the center is called a **diameter**. Note that the diameter is twice the radius: *d* = 2*r*.

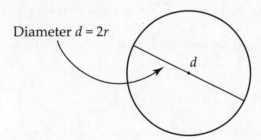

The distance around a circle—its perimeter—is called its circumference, and is given by the equation $C = 2\pi r$. Because $2r = d$, the circumference is equivalently given by $C = \pi d$. The number π is called *pi* and is approximately equal to 3.14. The formula for the area of a circle is $A = \pi r^2$.

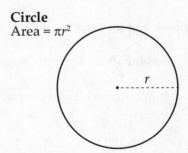

A **semicircle** is half a circle. Its length, naturally, is half the circumference of the full circle. If we form a closed figure by drawing in the diameter connecting the endpoints of a semicircle, the figure encloses an area equal to half that of the full circle. Therefore, its area is given by $A = \frac{1}{2}\pi r^2$.

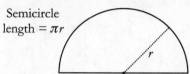

Semicircle
length $= \pi r$

An **arc** is any single connected portion of a circle. A semicircle is a special case of an arc. If the endpoints of an arc are labeled A and B, and if we let P denote the center of the circle, then the measure of the arc AB is the same as the measure of $\angle APB$.

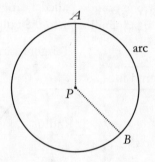

The length of an arc is proportional to its degree measure. In general, that means that $\dfrac{\text{arc length}}{\text{circumference}} = \dfrac{\text{central angle}}{\text{angle of a full circle}}$. In degrees, that becomes $\dfrac{\text{arc length}}{2\pi r} = \dfrac{\text{central angle}}{360°}$. For example, if the degree measure of an arc is 120°, then, since $\dfrac{120°}{360°} = \dfrac{1}{3}$, the arc length is one-third the circumference of the circle. That is, if the circumference is 3, then we get that $\dfrac{\text{arc length}}{3} = \dfrac{120°}{360°}$, so the arc length = 1. Another example: if the degree measure of an arc is 90°, then the arc length is one-fourth the circumference of the circle.

The same idea applies to finding the area of a sector of a circle. If you think of a circular region as a pizza, then a **sector** is a slice. The boundaries of a sector are two radii and an arc. The area is given by the formula $\dfrac{\text{sector area}}{\pi r^2} = \dfrac{\text{central angle}}{360°}$, where πr^2 is the total area of the circle. For example, if the area of the circle were 8 and the degree measure of the arc were 90°, then the sector area would be given by $\dfrac{\text{sector area}}{8} = \dfrac{90°}{360°}$, which comes out to sector area = 2. By the way, the area of a circle does not have to have π in it, provided that the radius does. A circle with area 8 would, from $A = \pi r^2$, have a radius equal to $\sqrt{\dfrac{8}{\pi}}$.

Consider the following example:

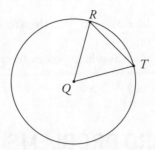

50. In the circle above, Q is the center. If the length of the minor arc connecting R and T is 2π and the measure of $\angle RQT$ is 90°, then which of the following is the length of line segment QT? Note: the figure above is not necessarily drawn to scale.

A. 2
B. $\sqrt{8}$
C. $\sqrt{12}$
D. 4
E. $\sqrt{18}$

There are two things to notice before we begin solving anything. The phrase **minor arc** just means the most direct connection along the circumference (in this case, going clockwise). This is to be contrasted with **major arc**, which would mean the arc going the other way.

More importantly, the note that indicates the figure is "not necessarily" **drawn to scale** tells us the figure is drawn wrong! Unless the DAT specifically says otherwise, the figures it supplies are accurate, so you could use them to estimate and eliminate answers. However, if this note is present (and yes, they do put them in questions and phrase it like this), the figure is *deliberately misleading*. It's not just that it's as close as they could get it, but they're just letting you know that it's a little off; the figure is deliberately drawn to entice you into a wrong answer. Believe what you read, not what you see, if you're told that the figure is not to scale.

Now, let's apply the formula. We know the central angle is 90°, and we know that the arc length is 2π. Substitute these values in the arc length formula as follows:

$$\frac{\text{arc length}}{\text{circumference}} = \frac{\text{central angle}}{\text{angle of full circle}}$$

$$\frac{2\pi}{2\pi r} = \frac{90}{360}$$

$$\frac{1}{r} = \frac{90}{360}$$

$$90r = 360$$

$$r = 4$$

It also happens that the segment QT is a radius, so this is what we're solving for (D is correct).

Notice that QT looks like it's only slightly smaller than the arc in the provided figure; however, if you draw the figure correctly, QT will look like it's $\frac{1}{2}$ to $\frac{2}{3}$ of the arc. Drawing the figure can help you spot that the provided figure is not drawn to scale and help you POE via ballparking.

43.5 GEOMETRIC WORD PROBLEMS

You may also have to solve a word problem involving geometry on the QRT. Generally, draw whatever visual situation is presented in the text, and the question will turn into a question like what has been discussed above. Consider the following question:

51. A rectangular painting has dimensions 15 inches by 12 inches. It is surrounded by a rectangular frame of constant width. If the outer perimeter of the frame is 70 inches, how wide is the frame, in inches?

    A. 1
    B. 1.5
    C. 2
    D. 2.5
    E. 3

First, draw a picture:

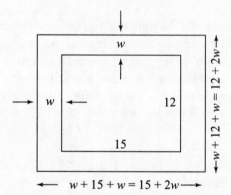

Want More Practice?
Scan the QR code below to register your book for online chapter summaries, drills, practice tests, and more!

Let w denote the width (in inches) of the frame. The length of the painting plus frame is thus $15 + 2w$ inches, and the width is $12 + 2w$ inches. The perimeter is therefore $2(15 + 2w) + 2(12 + 2w)$. Set this equal to 70 and solve for w: $(30 + 4w) + (24 + 4w) = 70$. Then, $54 + 8w = 70$, so $8w = 16$, which gives $w = 2$ inches (C is correct).

Chapter 44
Solid and Coordinate Geometry

44.1   SOLID GEOMETRY

Volume

So far we have been dealing with figures that lie flat in a plane: they are either 1-dimensional (that is, have only length, like lines) or 2-dimensional (have length and width, like rectangles). We now move to 3-dimensional **solids,** figures that have length, width, and height. The most fundamental solid is a **box.** (Its official name is the *rectangular parallelepiped,* which is reason enough to just call it a box.)

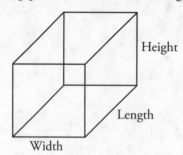

The measure of the size of the 3-dimensional region enclosed by a solid is called its **volume** (denoted V). For a box, the volume is the length times the width times the height, or $V = l \times w \times h$. If the length, width, and height are all equal, then the box is called a **cube.** If each edge of a cube has length l, then its volume is given by $V = l^3$.

Note that the volume of the box is equal to the area of its base ($l \times w$) times the height. This same general principle applies to any **prism** (a solid with two parallel bases and straight faces connecting them; basically, a 2D shape stretched into 3D by straight lines). For example, a **cylinder** is a solid whose base is a circle. If it has radius r, then the area of its base is πr^2 so its volume is given by $V = \pi r^2 h$.

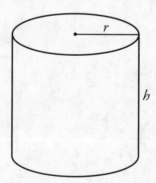

If the solid has a 2D shape for its base and with smooth, straight lines coming to a point at the top, then the volume is the area of the base multiplied by the height and divided by 3. For example, a **cone** with a circular base has a volume given by $V = \frac{1}{3}\pi r^2 h$. This is exactly the same as the formula for the volume of a cylinder, except for the $\frac{1}{3}$, which divides the volume by 3.

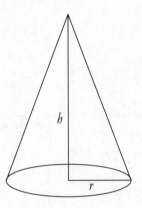

Surface Area

Let's say we were to paint the outside of the box, how much surface area would we cover? (Do you feel like you're back in PAT cube counting?) A closed box has 6 faces, each of which is a rectangle. Therefore, its total surface area is equal to the sum of the area of the six faces. One pair of opposite faces each has area lw, another pair of opposite faces each has area lh, and the third pair of opposite faces each has area wh. Therefore, the total surface area of a box is given by $SA = 2lw + 2lh + 2wh$.

In the case of a cube, all six faces are equal squares. If each edge has length l, then the formula above simplifies to the following: $SA = 6l^2$.

For any general solid, the surface area is found by adding up the areas of each of the faces. For example, a cylinder has a circle for the top and bottom bases, and it has a round part for the height, so the total surface area will be the sum of the areas of the circles on the top and bottom and the round part. Each of the circles has an area of πr^2. Since the round part is the circumference of the circles stretched out by the height of the cylinder—if this were a can and had a label around the round part, and if that label were torn off and flattened, the base of the label would be the circumference of the circle and the height of the label would be the height of the cylinder—the round part has an area of Ch, where C is the circumference of the circle, which in turn is equal to $2\pi r$. Thus, the total surface area of the cylinder is given by $SA = 2\pi r^2 + 2\pi rh$.

44.2   COORDINATE GEOMETRY

Coordinates

Take two number lines and cross them perpendicularly at their zero marks:

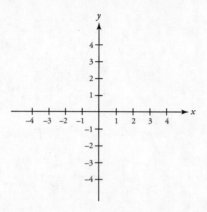

This is the **coordinate plane,** and the two lines are called the **coordinate axes.** The horizontal axis is called the **x-axis,** and the vertical one is called the **y-axis**, and they divide the plane into four **quadrants.** All the analysis done in the coordinate plane rests on the following observation: every point in the plane can be located by means of two numbers, called its **coordinates.** The first number tells us where to go along the horizontal x-axis, and the second number then tells us where to go vertically (that is, parallel to the y-axis). Verify the coordinates of each of the points shown below:

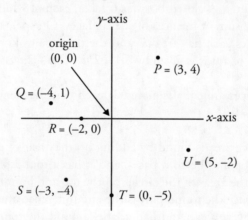

Distance Between Two Points

After plotting points in the plane, the next simplest operation involves computing the distance between two given points. If the points lie on the same horizontal or vertical line, count along the line joining them, which amounts to finding the difference between the x-coordinates (in the case of a horizontal line) or the difference between the y-coordinates (in the case of a vertical line).

Let's find the distance between points A and P and the distance between points B and P in the figure below. Since A and P lie on the same horizontal line (because their y-coordinates are the same), the distance between them is found simply by calculating the difference between their x-coordinates: $3 - (-5) = 8$. Thus, the distance between A and P is 8. Similarly, since points B and P lie on the same vertical line (because their x-coordinates are the same), the distance between them is found simply by calculating the difference between their y-coordinates: $4 - (-2) = 6$. Thus, the distance between B and P is 6.

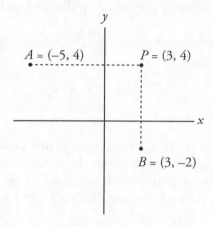

The question now is: What if the two given points are not on the same horizontal or vertical line? For example, what is the distance between the points A and B in the figure above? To solve this, note that we can form a right triangle with the two points A and B as the endpoints of the hypotenuse.

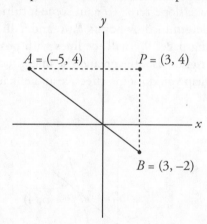

The lengths of the legs of the right triangle have already been found (they are the distances between A and P and between B and P), namely 6 and 8. Thus, the Pythagorean Theorem will give the length of the hypotenuse. Since $6^2 + 8^2 = 100$, the hypotenuse must equal the square root of 100, which is 10. That is, the distance between A and B is 10. (Note also that you could avoid calculating anything if you notice this is a 6-8-10 right triangle, which is a 3-4-5 right triangle doubled.)

This same procedure can be used every time we need the distance between two points that do not lie on a horizontal line or on a vertical line: sketch the right triangle, find the lengths of the legs, then use the Pythagorean Theorem. In general, the distance formula is $d = \sqrt{(x_2 - x_1)^2 + (y_2 - y_1)^2}$, which comes from doing this calculation on the generic points (x_1, y_1) and (x_2, y_2) and finding the distance d, but this is rather complicated and drawing a right triangle on your Noteboard is probably easier.

Slope

The coordinate plane can be used to graph equations, such as that of a straight line. In order to specify a line, we need to know two things: a point that it passes through and its steepness. The steepness is called the **slope** and it is defined as follows. Given any two points on a line, label one of them (x_1, y_1) and the other (x_2, y_2). The slope of the line, denoted traditionally by the letter m, is given by this ratio:

$$m = \frac{y_2 - y_1}{x_2 - x_1}$$

If the line is vertical, then x_1 will equal x_2, and this fraction would have a zero denominator. Therefore, vertical lines have undefined slope. If the line is horizontal, then y_1 will equal y_2, and this fraction would equal zero; thus, horizontal lines have slope zero. To gain some intuition with the concept of slope, let's find the slope of some of the lines determined by points P, R, and T in the figure below, and points Q, S, and U in the figure on the following page. We will see lines with positive slope rise to the right, while lines with negative slope fall to the right. Also, the greater the magnitude of the slope, the steeper the line. Knowing these general trends can help you do some effective and efficient POE on test day!

Consider lines RP and TP:

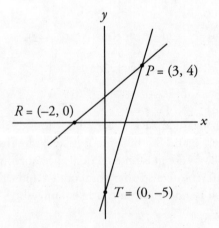

Since both lines rise to the right, we expect both to have positive slopes. Furthermore, since line TP is steeper than line RP, we expect the slope of TP to be greater than the slope of RP. Since $m_{TP} = \frac{4 - (-5)}{3 - 0} = 3$

and $m_{RP} = \frac{4 - 0}{3 - (-2)} = \frac{4}{5}$, both of our predictions are indeed true.

Now consider lines QS and QU:

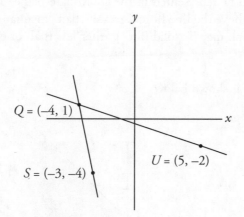

Since both lines fall to the right, we expect both to have negative slopes. Furthermore, since line QS is steeper than line QU, we expect the slope of QS to be more negative than the slope of QU. Since

$$m_{QS} = \frac{-4-1}{-3-(-4)} = -5 \text{ and } m_{QU} = \frac{-2-1}{5-(-4)} = -\frac{1}{3}, \text{ both of these predictions are true.}$$

Lines in the Coordinate Plane

The equation of a non-vertical line in the coordinate plane can be written in the form $y = mx + b$. Here, m is the slope of the line and b is the value of the y-coordinate at the point where the line crosses the y-axis (b is called the **y-intercept**). Two lines with equal slopes are parallel, and two lines whose slopes are negative reciprocals of each other are perpendicular. For example, consider the line L whose equation is $y = 3x + 4$. Its slope is 3. So every line parallel to this line must also have slope 3 and have the form $y = 3x + b$ for some value of b. If one knows a point—any point—on this line then the value of b can be determined. Every line perpendicular to L has slope $-\frac{1}{3}$, so every line perpendicular to L has an equation of the form $y = -\frac{1}{3}x + b$, and if a particular point on the line is known, then the value of b can be determined.

Inequalities in the Coordinate Plane

Like equations, inequalities can be represented in the coordinate plane. These look much like equations, but they will contain shading above the line (for a "greater than" inequality) or below the line (for a "less than" inequality). Also, the graph may be solid (for "greater/less than or equal to") or dashed (for strictly "greater/less than").

For example, the graph of $y \leq x$ is shown below.

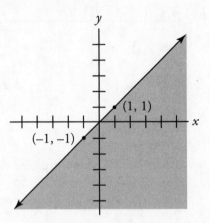

In contrast, the graph of $y > x$ is shown below.

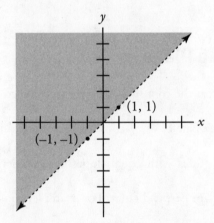

Other than shading and sometimes dashed lines, graphing inequalities is exactly like graphing equations. Remember that you can always plug in points if you are confused. For example, in the above inequality, the point (2,3) should be on the graph, since $y = 3$ and $x = 2$ obeys the inequality $y > x$. Find this point, and it appears in the shading, so this point is in fact included. However, the point (3,2) should not be included. Find this point, and it is in the white space; it is not included. Plugging in points like these can help to distinguish whether the graph you are looking at fits the equation you think it does. This is another good example of how Plugging In can help you save time and effort on the DAT!

Other Graphs in the Coordinate Plane

While there are infinitely many other possible graphs that could be drawn in the coordinate plane, there is one other specific example you should know for the QRT: the graph of a **quadratic**. The graph of $y = x^2$ looks like this:

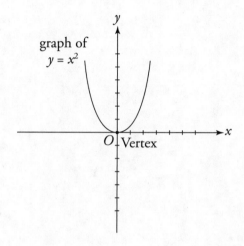

graph of
$y = x^2$

A graph of any equation of the form $y = ax^2 + bx + c$ will have the same shape as the above, although it may either open up (as this one does) or open down (like a frownie face); it may be wider, narrower, shifted up or down, or shifted left or right. The lowest point (or highest, if the graph opens down) is called the **vertex**, and the graph is symmetric about the vertex. That is, it looks exactly the same to the left of the vertex as it does to the right of the vertex.

For any other graph in the coordinate plane, you should plug in points to solve whatever problem you're asked. You are not expected to be intimately familiar with intricacies of cubics and the infinite other possible graphs.

Want More Practice?
Scan the QR code below to
register your book for online
chapter summaries, drills,
practice tests, and more!

Chapter 45
Trigonometry

45.1   DEFINITIONS OF TRIGONOMETRIC FUNCTIONS

Trigonometry is the study of various aspects of triangles. While we've already discussed the Pythagorean Theorem and how to find the area and perimeter of triangles, there are certain functions that apply to triangles that still need to be explained.

The three basic trigonometric functions are sine (sin), cosine (cos), and tangent (tan), and they describe the ratio of sides of a right triangle given a certain angle. Specifically, let *ABC* be a right triangle and the measure of $\angle A$ be θ, as shown below.

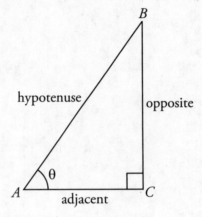

For the above triangle, the basic trig functions are defined as followed:

SOHCAHTOA

$$\sin\theta = \frac{\text{opposite}}{\text{hypotenuse}} \qquad \cos\theta = \frac{\text{adjacent}}{\text{hypotenuse}} \qquad \tan\theta = \frac{\text{opposite}}{\text{adjacent}}$$

From these definitions, it must also be true that $\tan\theta = \dfrac{\sin\theta}{\cos\theta}$, since $\dfrac{\sin\theta}{\cos\theta} = \dfrac{\frac{\text{opposite}}{\text{hypotenuse}}}{\frac{\text{adjacent}}{\text{hypotenuse}}}$. The hypotenuse in the numerator and the denominator cancel, leaving $\dfrac{\text{opposite}}{\text{adjacent}}$, which is the definition of tangent.

Functions have also been defined that are reciprocals of the three basic trig functions. These are cosecant (csc), secant (sec), and cotangent (cot):.

Reciprocal Trigonometry Functions

$$\csc\theta = \frac{1}{\sin\theta} = \frac{\text{hypotenuse}}{\text{opposite}} \qquad \sec\theta = \frac{1}{\cos\theta} = \frac{\text{hypotenuse}}{\text{adjacent}} \qquad \cot\theta = \frac{1}{\tan\theta} = \frac{\text{adjacent}}{\text{opposite}}$$

These functions apply to any right triangle, following the same definitions. Of course, if we were considering the angle at B instead of A, opposite and adjacent sides would be reversed: the base would be the opposite side and the height would be the adjacent side.

Consider the following examples:

52. What is the sine of the smallest angle in a 3-4-5 right triangle?

   A. $\dfrac{2}{3}$

   B. $\dfrac{3}{5}$

   C. $\dfrac{3}{4}$

   D. $\dfrac{3}{5}$

   E. 1

The smallest angle in this triangle is the angle that is opposite the leg of length 3. The sine of this angle is "opposite over hypotenuse," which equals $\dfrac{3}{5}$ (B is correct).

53. If $\cos 35° = c$, what is the value of $\csc 55°$?

   A. c

   B. c^2

   C. $\sqrt{1 - c^2}$

   D. $\dfrac{1}{c}$

   E. $\dfrac{1}{\sqrt{1 - c^2}}$

Cosine of 35° is equal to sine of 55°, because the angles 35° and 55° are complements. That is, the "adjacent" angle for the 35° angle will be the "opposite" angle for the 55° angle, so $\dfrac{\text{adjacent}}{\text{hypotenuse}}$ for the 35° angle will be the same as $\dfrac{\text{opposite}}{\text{hypotenuse}}$ for the 55° angle. Therefore, sin 55° = c also. Since cosecant is the reciprocal of the sine, we have $\csc 55° = \dfrac{1}{c}$ (D is correct).

54. In triangle *ABC*, angle *C* is a right angle. If *BC* = 6 and *A* = 40°, what is the hypotenuse?

    A.   6 sin 40°
    B.   6 cos 40°
    C.   6 tan 40°
    D.   6 sec 40°
    E.   6 csc 40°

First, draw the triangle on your Noteboard:

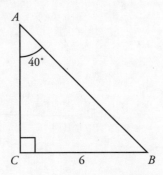

Since we're trying to relate an angle, its opposite side (*BC*), and the hypotenuse, we know we want sine. In particular, $\sin(40°) = \dfrac{6}{\text{hypotenuse}}$. Solve for the hypotenuse, and you get hypotenuse $= \dfrac{6}{\sin(40°)}$. This is equivalent to saying that the hypotenuse equals 6 csc 40° (E is correct).

45.2   EXACT VALUES

Trig Values from Special Triangles

Values of trig functions of certain angles can be calculated from the 45-45-90 and 30-60-90 right triangles mentioned earlier. Let's start with the 30-60-90 right triangle:

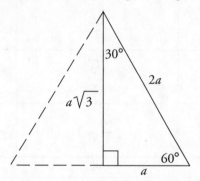

In this triangle, $\sin 30° = \dfrac{a}{2a}$, since the side opposite to the 30° angle is a and the hypotenuse is $2a$. This fraction reduces to $\dfrac{1}{2}$. Now, here's the point: sine should have the same value for any triangle, so if $\sin 30° = \dfrac{1}{2}$ for this triangle, then $\sin 30°$ *always* equals one-half. Likewise, since $\sin 60° = \dfrac{a\sqrt{3}}{2a}$ in this triangle, which reduces to $\dfrac{\sqrt{3}}{2}$, we can conclude that, in general, $\sin 60° = \dfrac{\sqrt{3}}{2}$. Next, let's look at the 45-45-90 right triangle:

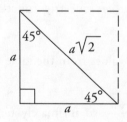

In this triangle, there are two 45° angles, and for either one, $\sin 45° = \dfrac{a}{a\sqrt{2}}$. This reduces to $\dfrac{1}{\sqrt{2}}$, which is usually multiplied by $\dfrac{\sqrt{2}}{\sqrt{2}}$ to get $\dfrac{\sqrt{2}}{2}$. Thus, $\sin 45° = \dfrac{\sqrt{2}}{2}$.

Values of cosine can be found from the same triangles. Values of sine and cosine of 0° and 90° will be derived in the section on the unit circle (coming up shortly), but the following table includes them to complete the pattern of exact values.

Values of sine and cosine

θ	$\sin \theta$	$\cos \theta$
0°	$\dfrac{\sqrt{0}}{2} = 0$	$\dfrac{\sqrt{4}}{2} = 1$
30°	$\dfrac{\sqrt{1}}{2} = \dfrac{1}{2}$	$\dfrac{\sqrt{3}}{2}$
45°	$\dfrac{\sqrt{2}}{2}$	$\dfrac{\sqrt{2}}{2}$
60°	$\dfrac{\sqrt{3}}{2}$	$\dfrac{\sqrt{1}}{2} = \dfrac{1}{2}$
90°	$\dfrac{\sqrt{4}}{2} = 1$	$\dfrac{\sqrt{0}}{2} = 0$

The pattern you should notice is that sine and cosine of these values is the square root of an integer over 2, in which that integer starts at 0 and counts up to 4 for sine and goes the other way for cosine. Make sure you see this pattern in the table above. Some of the values can be simplified, and some cannot. For example, the square root of 0 is 0, so sin 0° = 0, but the square root of 2 is not an integer, so sin 45° cannot be simplified; its value is approximately 0.7, but that is just an approximation. Likewise, the value of sin 60° is approximately 0.87, but again, this is just an approximation.

Values of Other Trig Functions

You can compute exact values of the other four trig functions from the table above. For example, $\tan 30° = \dfrac{\sin 30°}{\cos 30°}$, so plug in the exact values from the table above, and $\tan 30° = \dfrac{\frac{1}{2}}{\frac{\sqrt{3}}{2}}$, which simplifies to $\dfrac{1}{\sqrt{3}}$. This is often rationalized to $\dfrac{\sqrt{3}}{3}$, so, ultimately, $\tan 30° = \dfrac{\sqrt{3}}{3}$. It is better to remember the pattern of values for sine and cosine in the table above and derive values of other trig functions (if you ever need them) from sine and cosine. However, if you'd rather memorize a big table (and have the extra mental space to do this), here are the rest of the values:

θ	$\tan \theta$	$\csc \theta$	$\sec \theta$	$\cot \theta$
0°	0	undefined	1	undefined
30°	$\dfrac{\sqrt{3}}{3}$	2	$\dfrac{2\sqrt{3}}{3}$	$\sqrt{3}$
45°	1	$\sqrt{2}$	$\sqrt{2}$	1
60°	$\sqrt{3}$	$\dfrac{2\sqrt{3}}{3}$	2	$\dfrac{\sqrt{3}}{3}$
90°	undefined	1	undefined	0

If you are ever asked to work with a trig function of an angle that is not listed above (such as 40°), it may be possible to derive it from definitions. If not, the function should not actually be computed (that is, the answer choices will literally say 5 cos 40° and the like), unless a special identity is given to compute it (which will be discussed later).

Consider the following example:

55. What is the measure of the acute angle whose sine equals its cosine?

    A. 0°
    B. 30°
    C. 45°
    D. 60°
    E. 90°

Since sin θ = opp/hyp and cos θ = adj/hyp, the value of sin θ can equal the value of cos θ only when opp = adj. If two legs of a right triangle are equal, then the triangle is an isosceles right triangle; that is, a 45-45-90 triangle. Therefore, θ = 45°. Alternatively, recall that sin(45°) = $\dfrac{\sqrt{2}}{2}$ and cos(45°) = $\dfrac{\sqrt{2}}{2}$. Either way, the answer is C.

45.3 FINDING TRIANGLE AREA USING TRIG

We already know that the area of a triangle is given by $A = \dfrac{1}{2}bh$. However, while the base of a triangle is one of its sides, the height does not have to be (and for a non-right triangle, the height is *not* one of the sides). With trig, though, we can find the area of a triangle from two sides and the angle between them.

Consider this figure:

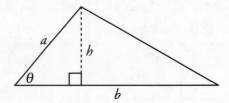

If you were given a, b, and θ in this triangle and need to find the area, you could use sine to relate the opposite side (the height) to the hypotenuse (a) in the small right triangle on the left. That is, $\sin\theta = \dfrac{h}{a}$, so the height must be given by $h = a\sin\theta$. This means the usual formula, $A = \dfrac{1}{2}bh$, could be rewritten as $A = \dfrac{1}{2}b\big(a\sin\theta\big)$, or, rearranging for aesthetic reasons, $A = \dfrac{1}{2}ab\sin\theta$. Note the base can be *any* of the sides, and a can be any of the other sides, so the formula for the area of a triangle is always this for any two sides and the angle between them.

45.4   INVERSE TRIGONOMETRIC FUNCTIONS

Just like any other function, a trig function can be undone by an inverse function. As usual for inverse functions, these functions are represented by a $^{-1}$ on the function. For example, if $\sin 30° = \dfrac{1}{2}$, then taking the inverse sine of both sides should yield $30° = \sin^{-1}\left(\dfrac{1}{2}\right)$. These inverse trig functions are sometimes indicated with the prefix "arc," so equivalently, $30° = \arcsin\left(\dfrac{1}{2}\right)$. As far as geometric meaning, you can think of an inverse sine as saying, "the angle whose sine is," as in, $\sin^{-1}\left(\dfrac{1}{2}\right)$ is referring to the angle whose sine is $\dfrac{1}{2}$, which we know from the table above is the angle $30°$.

Bear in mind this $^{-1}$ represents doing an inverse function; although the notation may look like an exponent, this is a completely different operation. For example, as just mentioned, $\sin^{-1}(0.5) = 30°$, which involves an inverse function, but $(\sin(0.5°))^{-1}$, which involves an exponent, is equal to $\dfrac{1}{\sin(0.5°)}$, which is approximately 0.0087. You will get a very, very wrong answer if you mix up an inverse function, in which the $^{-1}$ is right on the sin, cos, or other trig function, with an exponent, in which the $^{-1}$ is elsewhere in the expression.

45.5   RADIAN MEASURE

Just as angles can be measured in degrees, so too can they be measured in **radians**. Radians and degrees are two different units of angle measurement, just as feet and meters are two different units of length measurement. To convert between radians and degrees, use the following equation: π radians = 180°. Thus, if you have an angle that has a measure of $\frac{\pi}{3}$ radians (which is often just written as $\frac{\pi}{3}$, since any angle without a degree symbol on it is assumed to be measured in radians), you can determine how many degrees it is by multiplying $\frac{\pi}{3}$ radians $\times \frac{180°}{\pi\,\text{radians}}$. Radians cancel, and the fraction reduces to 60°.

Everything about trigonometry that was discussed above is exactly the same in radians or in degrees. For example, $\sin\left(\frac{\pi}{3}\right) = \sin 60°$, as you might expect. In this case, you might wonder why anyone would go to the trouble of defining radians in the first place. The entire reason for the existence of radians is that they make finding arc length easier. Remember that arc length is proportional to central angle size, according to an equation that was discussed earlier. In degrees, this was a somewhat complicated calculation. In radians, it is more straightforward.

For example, if a circle has a radius of 3 and a central angle of $\frac{\pi}{4}$, find the arc length. According to the equation given previously, $\dfrac{\text{arc length}}{\text{circumference}} = \dfrac{\text{central angle}}{\text{angle of a full circle}}$. In radians, if the central angle is θ, this comes out to $\dfrac{\text{arc length}}{2\pi r} = \dfrac{\theta}{2\pi}$. (Recall that a full circle is 360°, which is 2π radians.) Thus, solving for the arc length, it turns out that arc length = $\theta \times r$. In other words, if the radius is 3 and the central angle is $\frac{\pi}{4}$, then the arc length is $\frac{3\pi}{4}$. If the central angle had been 2 (which would be a strange but possible angle in radians), then the arc length would be 6. Multiply the central angle by the radius to get the arc length, if your central angle is in radians.

For additional practice, let's write the measures of the angles 90°, 120°, 135°, and 150° in radians. An angle of 90° is half of 180°, so in radians, 90° = $\frac{\pi}{2}$. Now, since 30 = 180/6, we have 30° = $\frac{\pi}{6}$ radians; also, the fact that 45 = $\frac{180}{4}$ implies that 45° = $\frac{\pi}{4}$ radians; and since 60 = $\frac{180}{3}$, we have 60° = $\frac{\pi}{3}$ radians.

These four conversions are worth memorizing because then multiples of 30°, 45°, 60°, and 90° can be converted quickly to radians, as follows: $120° = 2 \times 60° = \dfrac{2\pi}{3}$ in radians; likewise, $135° = 3 \times 45° = \dfrac{3\pi}{4}$ and $150° = 5 \times 30° = \dfrac{5\pi}{6}$.

Consider the following example, which implicitly uses radians:

56. What are the maximum and minimum values of the function $f(x) = 3 \cos (x + \pi)$?

A. −1 and 1
B. −2 and 2
C. −3 and 3
D. −π and π

According to the values given for $\cos \theta$, $\cos \theta$ is never less than −1 nor greater than 1. In this case, we are multiplying $\cos \theta$ (where $\theta = x + \pi$), by 3. Therefore, the maximum value of $f(x)$ is +3, and the minimum value is −3 (C is correct).

Note: when the graph of $f(x)$ is sketched, it will oscillate between 3 and −3. Half the difference between its greatest and smallest values is called the **amplitude** of the function, which in this case is 3. Here, it is the numerical coefficient before the $\cos \theta$ term in $f(x)$. Amplitude of sine works the same way.

45.6 UNIT CIRCLE

Trig Functions of Large Angles

The definitions of trig functions can be extended to an angle of any size. Consider a triangle drawn inside a unit circle (a circle with radius 1):

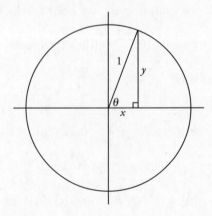

The top vertex is at a point (x, y), where x is the length of the base of the triangle and y is the length of the height of the triangle. From our basic definitions, $\sin \theta = \dfrac{y}{1}$, since y is the opposite side and the hypotenuse is 1. Thus, the y-coordinate of the point is the same as the value of $\sin \theta$. By similar reasoning, the x-coordinate of the point is the same as the value of $\cos \theta$. This is true no matter the value of θ, even if it goes beyond 90°.

Consider the following example:

45.6

57. What is the value of $\sin 210°$?

    A. $-\dfrac{\sqrt{2}}{2}$

    B. $-\dfrac{1}{2}$

    C. $\dfrac{1}{2}$

    D. $\dfrac{\sqrt{2}}{2}$

    E. $\dfrac{\sqrt{3}}{2}$

Since the angle is not between 0° and 90°, draw it on your Noteboard in standard position in the x-y plane:

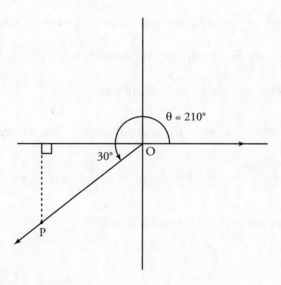

Notice that 210° is 30° past 180°. First of all, this means it must be negative, since the y-value is negative, (eliminate C, D, and E). This also means the y-value will be just as far below 0 as the y-value of 30° is above 0. That is, $\sin 210° = -\sin 30°$. Since $\sin 30° = \dfrac{1}{2}$, it must also be true that $\sin 210° = -\dfrac{1}{2}$ (eliminate B, and A is correct).

Pythagorean Identities

The unit circle also gives grounds for one more identity. Consider the Pythagorean Theorem as it applies to a triangle in the unit circle.

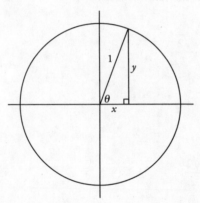

In this picture, we know that $x = \cos \theta$ and $y = \sin \theta$. From the Pythagorean Theorem, we also know that $x^2 + y^2 = 1$. Putting these together we get that $\sin^2 \theta + \cos^2 \theta = 1$. Note that math convention dictates $(\sin \theta)^2$ be written as $\sin^2 \theta$, probably to avoid ambiguity if parentheses were not written, since $\sin \theta^2$ could mean $(\sin \theta)^2$ or $\sin(\theta^2)$. This is the first **Pythagorean Identity**, and it's the only one that must be memorized for the DAT, since the other two can be derived from it.

The other two Pythagorean Identities come from dividing each side by either $\sin^2 \theta$ or $\cos^2 \theta$. The latter gives $\dfrac{\sin^2 \theta}{\cos^2 \theta} + \dfrac{\cos^2 \theta}{\cos^2 \theta} = \dfrac{1}{\cos^2 \theta}$, which reduces to $\tan^2 \theta + 1 = \sec^2 \theta$, while the former gives $\dfrac{\sin^2 \theta}{\sin^2 \theta} + \dfrac{\cos^2 \theta}{\sin^2 \theta} = \dfrac{1}{\sin^2 \theta}$, which reduces to $1 + \cot^2 \theta = \csc^2 \theta$.

Consider the following pair of examples:

58. What is the value of $\sin^2 26° + \cos^2 26°$?

   A. 0

   B. $2 \sin^2 26°$

   C. $\sin^4 26°$

   D. $\dfrac{1}{2}$

   E. 1

For *any* value of θ, $(\sin \theta)^2 + (\cos \theta)^2$ is equal to 1. This is the fundamental Pythagorean Identity. Thus, the answer is E.

59. If $\sin \theta = s$ and $90° < \theta < 180°$, what is the value of $\cot \theta$?

   A. $-\sqrt{\dfrac{1}{s^2} - 1}$

   B. $-\sqrt{\dfrac{1}{1 - s^2}}$

   C. $-\sqrt{\dfrac{1}{s^2 - 1}}$

   D. $\sqrt{\dfrac{1}{1 - s^2}}$

   E. $\sqrt{\dfrac{1}{s^2} - 1}$

If $\sin \theta = s$, then by the first Pythagorean Identity, $s^2 + \cos^2 \theta = 1$, so, in the process of solving for $\cos \theta$, we get that $\cos^2 \theta = 1 - s^2$ and since θ is between 90° and 180°, the value of cosine must be negative (this quadrant is left of the *x*-axis, so the *x*-value is negative, so $\cos \theta$ is negative). This means that $\cos \theta = -\sqrt{1 - s^2}$.

Next, since $\cot \theta = \dfrac{1}{\tan \theta}$ and since $\tan \theta = \dfrac{\sin \theta}{\cos \theta}$, it must also be true that $\cot \theta = \dfrac{\cos \theta}{\sin \theta}$. Plugging in

the values that we know, $\cot \theta = \dfrac{-\sqrt{1 - s^2}}{s}$. This can be reduced by bringing the denominator under the

square root, so $\cot \theta = -\sqrt{\dfrac{1 - s^2}{s^2}}$. Continue simplifying, which yields $-\sqrt{\dfrac{1}{s^2} - \dfrac{s^2}{s^2}} = -\sqrt{\dfrac{1}{s^2} - 1}$. Thus,

the answer is that $\cot \theta = -\sqrt{\dfrac{1}{s^2} - 1}$ (A is correct).

45.6

45.7   OTHER IDENTITIES

You may be given an identity in a problem and asked to use it to compute something. If this happens, don't worry if the identity is unfamiliar. That's why it is being given to you. If it were an identity that you were supposed to know already, you would not be supplied the equation in the problem.

Consider the following example:

60. What is the value of sin 75° ?
    Note: the addition formula for sine says, $\sin(\alpha + \beta) = \sin \alpha \cos \beta + \sin \beta \cos \alpha$.

   A. $\dfrac{\sqrt{2}}{2}$

   B. $\dfrac{\sqrt{6}}{2}$

   C. $\dfrac{1 + \sqrt{2}}{4}$

   D. $\dfrac{\sqrt{6} + 1}{2}$

   E. $\dfrac{\sqrt{6} + \sqrt{2}}{4}$

Don't worry if you've never seen the addition formula for sine before. The only question is, how does it apply here? Presumably you are supposed to rephrase sin 75° as $\sin(\alpha + \beta)$, since that is what the formula expresses. (Don't worry about the Greek letters, either; think of them as x and y, if you prefer.) Now, what plus what equals 75°? Many values would not be very useful, such as 50° + 25°, since sin 50° is not a value that you are supposed to know any more than sin 75° is. However, 45° + 30° is useful, since these are both angles for which you know the sine and cosine.

Next, apply the formula. Since sin 75° = sin(45° + 30°), you can also write sin 75° = sin 45° cos 30° + sin 30° cos 45°. Now, plug in the exact values you know, so $\sin 75° = \left(\dfrac{\sqrt{2}}{2} \right)\left(\dfrac{\sqrt{3}}{2} \right) + \left(\dfrac{1}{2} \right)\left(\dfrac{\sqrt{2}}{2} \right)$.Multiply the fractions, and the next step reads $\sin 75° = \dfrac{\sqrt{6}}{4} + \dfrac{\sqrt{2}}{4}$. Since this already has a common denominator, you can add the numerators directly (E is correct).

Want More Practice?
Remember to register your book online for chapter summaries, drills, practice tests, and more!

There are dozens of identities in trigonometry, and you cannot possibly memorize all of them. (To give some idea how many there are, there are addition and subtraction identities for each of the three basic trig functions, as well as double, triple, and half-angle identities, power reduction identities, and product identities, among other things. That's nearly two dozen right there!) Thus, if you are asked a trigonometry question and given a bizarre identity, use the given identity and don't worry about it too much. This is another good example of the DAT requiring you to be flexible.

Chapter 46
Quantitative
Comparison and
Data Sufficiency

In 2018, the ADA introduced two new types of math questions, called Quantitative Comparison (QC or quant comp) and Data Sufficiency (DS). These question types will only make up a handful of the questions on the QRT; however, knowing the format of these questions and how to approach them can help save time and improve accuracy when tackling them. These questions don't test new content areas; there is no new content in this chapter! Instead, quantitative comparison and data sufficiency questions use a unique format to test content we've already reviewed in previous chapters.

46.1   QUANTITATIVE COMPARISON

These questions ask you to compare two quantities and pick an answer choice that appropriately describes the relationship between the two quantities. These questions have four answer choices instead of five, and they'll consist of the following, potentially in varied order:

  A.   Quantity A is always greater than B.
  B.   Quantity B is always greater than A.
  C.   Quantities A and B are always equal.
  D.   The relationship cannot be determined from the information given.

Your job is to compare the two quantities and choose the single best answer. Because there are only four choices on QC questions, after you use POE to eliminate all the answer choices you can, your odds of guessing correctly are even better. Think about it this way: eliminating even one answer on a QC question will give you a one-in-three chance of guessing correctly.

QC Strategies

QC questions test the same arithmetic, statistics, algebra, and geometry content as do other QRT problems. To solve these problems, you can use the same techniques you use on other DAT questions. Plugging In and ballparking (estimation) can be valuable techniques for these question types. It is also worth noting you don't necessarily need to know the exact values of A and B; it's enough to know how the quantities compare to each other. For instance, if A is positive and B is negative, then A is always greater than B. In this case, you could confidently pick answer choice A, even though you don't have specific values for quantities A and B.

If a QC question contains only numbers, the answer can't be answer choice D. Any QC problem that contains only numbers and no variables must have a single solution. Therefore, on these problems, you can eliminate option D immediately because the larger quantity can be determined. For example, if you're asked to compare $\frac{3}{2}$ and $\frac{3}{4}$, you can determine which fraction is larger, so the answer cannot be choice D.

You don't always have to calculate the exact value of each quantity before you compare them. After all, your mission is to compare two quantities. It's often helpful to treat the two quantities as though they were two sides of an equation. Anything you can do to both sides of an equation, you can also do to both quantities. You can add the same number to both sides, you can multiply both sides by the same positive number, and you can simplify a single side by multiplying it by one. If you can simplify the terms of a QC question, you should always do so. In general, compare instead of doing calculations, and do only as much work as you need to.

QC Examples

Let's look at a few examples:

61.

A	B
$\dfrac{1}{16} + \dfrac{1}{7} + \dfrac{1}{4}$	$\dfrac{1}{4} + \dfrac{1}{16} + \dfrac{1}{6}$

A. Quantity A is greater.
B. Quantity B is greater.
C. The two quantities are equal.
D. The relationship cannot be determined from the information given.

Don't do any calculating! Remember: do the minimum work required to answer the question! The first thing you should do is eliminate D. After all, there are only numbers here. After that, get rid of numbers that are common to both columns (think of this as simplifying). Both columns contain a $\dfrac{1}{16}$ and a $\dfrac{1}{4}$, so because we're talking about addition, they can't make a difference to the outcome. With them gone, you're merely comparing a $\dfrac{1}{7}$ in column A to a $\dfrac{1}{6}$ in column B. Now we can eliminate C as well—after all, there is no way that $\dfrac{1}{7}$ is equal to $\dfrac{1}{6}$. Comparing the two fractions, we know B must be the answer.

62. If you have $x^2 - 4x + 4 = 0$, and:

A	B
x	+2

A. Quantity A is always greater than B.
B. Quantity B is always greater than A.
C. Quantities A and B are always equal.
D. The relationship cannot be determined from the information given.

Although quantity A is listed as a variable, x, it can be solved for based on the equation in the question stem. Factoring the quadratic in the question stem gives:

$$x^2 - 4x + 4 = 0$$
$$(x - 2)^2 = 0$$
$$x = 2$$

If $x = 2$, then so does quantity A. Therefore, quantities A and B are always equal (C is correct).

63. If you have $x^2 - 9 = 0$, and:

A	B
x	+2

    A.   Quantity A is always greater than B.
    B.   Quantity B is always greater than A.
    C.   Quantities A and B are always equal.
    D.   The relationship cannot be determined from the information given.

Again, quantity A is a variable. Factoring the quadratic gives:

$$x^2 - 9 = 0$$
$$(x + 3)(x - 3) = 0$$
$$x = 3 \text{ or } x = -3$$

If $x = 3$, then quantity A = 3 and A > B. But if $x = -3$, then A = -3 and A < B. Therefore, the relationship between quantities A and B cannot be determined from the information given (D is correct).

46.2 DATA SUFFICIENCY

Data Sufficiency (DS) questions present you with a question and two statements, then ask you to assess which statement or statements, if any, are sufficient to answer the question. Note that you're not asked to actually answer the math problem; you're asked if you *can* solve the math problem. So, you don't need to spend time fully answering the problem. Like QC problems, DS questions also test the same arithmetic, statistics, algebra, and geometry content as do other QRT problems.

The answer choices will likely consist of the following: read these carefully:

    A.   Statement (1) ALONE is enough to answer the question, but statement (2) ALONE is not sufficient to answer the question.
    B.   Statement (2) ALONE is enough to answer the question, but statement (1) ALONE is not sufficient to answer the question.
    C.   BOTH statements (1) and (2) TOGETHER are sufficient to answer the question, but NEITHER statement ALONE is sufficient.
    D.   EACH statement ALONE is sufficient to answer the question.
    E.   Statements (1) and (2) TOGETHER are not sufficient to answer the question, and additional data are needed.

It's worth noting that sometimes there are only four answer choices on the QRT. If that happens with a DS question, it's likely that either answer choice C or D, as listed above, would be removed. Regardless, you should still approach the question using the same steps and apply POE the same way.

Notice there are two words the answer choices keep repeating—alone and sufficient. This means you're supposed to evaluate the statements on their own, at least at first. Moreover, your task is to determine whether you have sufficient information to answer the question. This is how DS questions differ from problem-solving. In many QRT questions, you are asked to give a numerical answer to the question. In fact, if you see five numerical answer choices, you can assume the question can be solved. For DS questions, however, you're not being asked to solve the question but to decide *whether* the question can be solved. It may, in fact, turn out the statements do not provide sufficient information to answer the question.

Let's look at an example:

64. What is the value of y?

1. y is an even integer such that −1.5 < y < 1.5

2. Integer y is not prime

A. Statement (1) ALONE is sufficient, but statement (2) alone is not sufficient.
B. Statement (2) ALONE is sufficient, but statement (1) alone is not sufficient.
C. BOTH statements TOGETHER are sufficient, but NEITHER statement ALONE is sufficient.
D. EACH statement ALONE is sufficient.
E. Statements (1) and (2) TOGETHER are not sufficient.

Option A indicates that we should first look at Statement (1) by itself to see if it is sufficient to answer the question. In fact, the best way to work Data Sufficiency problems is to look at one statement at a time. So, ignore Statement (2) for now.

There are three integers between −1.5 and 1.5: −1, 0, and 1. Of those, only 0 is even. So, Statement (1) does provide sufficient information to answer the question. Next, assess Statement (2). The second statement tells us only that y is not prime. Possible values for y include 1, 4, 6, 8, and many more. Do we know the value of y? No way. So, Statement (2) is not sufficient. Because (1) is sufficient and (2) is not, the answer to this question is option A.

46.2

DS Answer Choices

Now that you've seen and worked a DS question, it's time to learn how to make this weird question type your own. The first step is to understand what each of the answer choices means.

By making small changes to the example you've just seen, we can provide examples of each of the answer choices. Next to each example, you'll find a graphic that provides a quick and dirty way to understand and remember each answer choice. Here's the example for choice A again:

A. Statement (1) ALONE is sufficient, but statement (2) ALONE is not sufficient.

What is the value of y ?

1.   y is an even integer such that −1.5 < y < 1.5.

2.   Integer y is not prime.

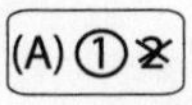

(A) ①✗

Now, let's make some changes to the statements, to get an example of choice B:

B. Statement (2) ALONE is sufficient, but statement (1) ALONE is not sufficient.

What is the value of y ?

1.   Integer y is not prime.

2.   y is an even integer such that −1.5 < y < 1.5.

(B) ✗②

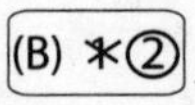

As you can see from this example, B is pretty much the flip side of A. In this case, the first statement provides no help in determining the value of y, but the second statement tells us that y = 0.

A few more changes produce an example of choice C:

C. BOTH statements TOGETHER are sufficient, but NEITHER statement ALONE is sufficient.

What is the value of y ?

1.   y is an even integer.

2.   −1.5 < y < 1.5

(C) ✗✗

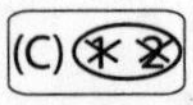

The first statement tells us y is even, but there are a lot of even integers. The second statement gives us a range of values for y, but, by itself, we don't even know that y is an integer from the second statement. So, neither statement is sufficient on its own. But, when we put them together, we know that $y = 0$.

Now, let's get an example of choice D:

> D. EACH statement ALONE is sufficient.
>
> What is the value of y ?
>
> 1. y is an even integer such that $-1.5 < y < 1.5$.
>
> 2. For any integer $a \neq 0$, $ay = 0$.

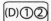

As pointed out in previous examples, the information in Statement (1) allows us to conclude that $y = 0$. The information in the second statement also tells us that y is 0 because the only way for the product of ay to equal 0 is if either a or y is 0. Since a can't be 0, y must be 0. Note how the statements independently allow us to arrive at the conclusion that $y = 0$ for D.

Finally, let's look at an example of choice E:

> E. Statements (1) and (2) TOGETHER are not sufficient.
>
> What is the value of y ?
>
> 1. y is an even integer.
>
> 2. Integer y is not prime.

For this example, there's no way to determine the value of y. The first statement doesn't work because y could be any even integer. The second statement also doesn't help because y can be any integer that isn't prime. Even when we combine the statements, we don't know the value of y because any even integer except 2 fits the conditions. So, E is the no-way, no-how answer.

Below, you'll find the full graphic for all the answers choices. You may find it helpful to keep this graphic handy until you are completely comfortable with what each answer choice means.

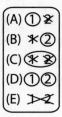

POE in DS

DS questions should be tackled in steps, using POE. Evaluate the statements one at a time before you think about combining them. Many people mistakenly pick choice C—you need both statements together—when it would have been possible to answer the question with only information in the first statement or the second statement. Generally, people make this mistake when they read both statements right after reading the question stem. In fact, this mistake is the most common mistake that test-takers make when working DS questions.

To avoid this common mistake, read the question stem and only the first statement; ignore the second statement. Once you have evaluated Statement (1), forget about it and move on to evaluating Statement (2).

What happens when you evaluate the statements one at a time? Something magical, that's what! POE comes roaring back. Consider the following partial example:

What is the value of x ?

1. $x + 7 = 12$

We don't even have Statement (2), but we can still do a lot with this partial question. (Don't worry. There won't be any partial questions on the real test!) First, you want to see if the statement is sufficient to answer the question. In this case, you could subtract 7 from both sides of the equation to discover that $x = 5$. We'll take this as an opportunity to remind you, however, that you don't really need to solve the equation—you just need to know that you *can* solve the equation. After all, to pick an answer to the problem, you just need to know if you have sufficient information.

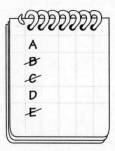

Since Statement (1) is sufficient in this case, which answer choices can be eliminated? From the chart on the previous page, you can see that there are only two answer choices—A and D—that have Statement (1) circled to indicate Statement (1) is sufficient. You don't need to worry about choices B, C, or E; eliminate these options! If the first statement is sufficient, the answer to the problem must be A or D. You're down to 50/50 just based on looking at the first statement!

Now, check out this example:

What is the value of x ?

1. x is an integer.

Now, what are the possible answers? If you said B, C, or E, you are well on your way to getting this Data Sufficiency stuff under control. If you said something else, take a look at the steps outlined previously. In this case, the first statement is insufficient to determine the value of x. So, you want the answer choices that have 1 crossed off, and that is B, C, or E.

Practice with AD/BCE

In the following activity, each question is followed by only one statement. Based on the first statement, decide if you are down to AD or BCE. See the solutions on the next page.

1. What is the value of x ?

    1. $y = 4$

    2. ????

2. Is y an integer?

    1. $2y$ is an integer.

    2. ????

3. A certain room contains 12 children. How many more boys than girls are there?

    1. There are three girls in the room.

    2. ????

4. What number is x percent of 20 ?

    1. 10 percent of x is 5.

    2. ????

AD/BCE Drill Solutions

1. **BCE** Statement (1) gives a value for y but no information on the value of x. Since the problem asks for a value of x, Statement (1) is insufficient.

2. **BCE** Statement (1) states that $2y$ is an integer. Consider what values of y are possible. The value of y could be an integer, such as 2, but it could also be a fraction, such as $\frac{1}{2}$. Statement (1) is insufficient.

3. **AD** The question states that there are 12 children in the room. Statement (1) provides the number of girls, so both the number of boys and the difference between the number of boys and the number of girls can be determined. Since the difference can be determined, Statement (1) is sufficient.

4. **AD** Statement (1) can be rewritten as the equation $\left(\frac{10}{100}\right) x = 5$, which can be used to solve for x.

   If the value of x is known, the question can be answered. Statement (1) is sufficient.

From AD or BCE to the Answer

Every time you start a Data Sufficiency question, you should read the question, read only the first statement, and review the answer choices. If the first statement is sufficient, your possible answers are A or D. If the first statement is insufficient, your possible answers are B, C, or E. You can always get rid of either two or three answer choices just by evaluating the first statement. The AD/BCE split is so important that you'll want to write down AD or BCE on your noteboard as you work DS questions.

But what happens next? How do you get to the answer? Let's take a look.

If $x + y = 3$, what is the value of xy ?

1. x and y are integers.

2. x and y are positive.

A.   Statement (1) ALONE is sufficient, but statement (2) ALONE is not sufficient.
B.   Statement (2) ALONE is sufficient, but statement (1) ALONE is not sufficient.
C.   BOTH statements TOGETHER are sufficient, but NEITHER statement ALONE is sufficient.
D.   EACH statement ALONE is sufficient.
E.   Statements (1) and (2) TOGETHER are not sufficient.

As always, ignore Statement (2) and look only at Statement (1). If x and y are integers and $x + y = 3$, do we know what they are? Not really—x could be 1 and y could be 2 (in which case, xy would be 2). But x could also be 0 (yes, 0 is an integer) and y could be 3 (in which case, xy would be 0). Because Statement (1) alone is not sufficient, we are down to BCE.

Now, ignore Statement (1) and look at Statement (2). By itself, this statement doesn't begin to give us values for x and y—x could be 1 and y could be 2, but x could just as easily be 1.4 and y could be 1.6. Because there is still more than one possible value for xy, eliminate choice B.

We're down to choice C or E. Now it's finally time to look at both statements at the same time. See how late in the process we combine the statements? Get into the habit of physically crossing off choice B before you think about combining the statements. That's how you can avoid making the most common DAT Data Sufficiency mistake of putting the statements together too early.

Because we know from the first statement that x and y are integers, and from the second statement that they must be positive, do we now know specific values for x and y?

Well, we do know that there are only two positive integers that add up to 3: 2 and 1. (Remember, zero is an integer but it is neither positive nor negative.)

Do we know if $x = 1$ and $y = 2$, or vice versa? Not really, but frankly, it doesn't matter in this case. The question is asking us the value of xy.

Because neither statement by itself is sufficient, but both statements together are sufficient, the correct answer is choice C.

Here's a handy flowchart that shows you what to do for any Data Sufficiency problem. You should keep the flowchart next to you and consult it as you first start practicing DS questions. After you have done 10 or 20 questions, you'll probably find that you have learned the basic POE process well enough that you don't need the chart anymore. However, if you ever find yourself having trouble with Data Sufficiency, pull out the chart again and do some more problems, using it as a guide.

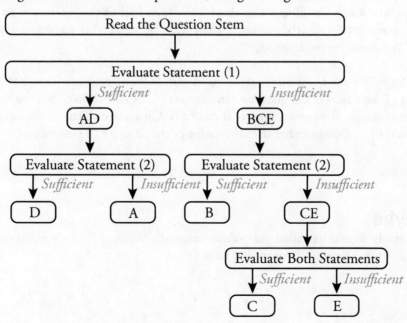

Yes/No Data Sufficiency

These DS questions are pretty unique. Let's look at an example:

> Did candidate x receive more than half of the 30,000
> votes cast in the general election?
>
> 1. Candidate y received 12,000 of the votes cast.
>
> 2. Candidate x received 18,000 of the votes cast.

When all is said and done, the answer to this question is either yes or no. Start by ignoring Statement (2) and evaluating Statement (1). Does Statement (1) alone answer the question? If you were in a hurry, you might think so. Many people assume that there are only two candidates in the election. They reason that if candidate y got 12,000 votes, then candidate x must have received 18,000 votes. However, there's no reason to assume that there are only two candidates. Statement (1) is insufficient. Write BCE down on your Noteboard. Does Statement (2) alone answer the question? Yes, it's pretty clear that candidate x received more than half of the votes. So, the correct answer is B.

Let's look at a more challenging example:

> Did candidate x receive more than half of the 30,000
> votes cast in the general election?
>
> 1. Candidate y received 12,000 of the votes cast.
>
> 2. Candidate x received 13,000 of the votes cast.

As always, start by ignoring Statement (2) so that you can properly evaluate Statement (1) alone. As in our previous example, Statement (1) is insufficient, so write down BCE on your Noteboard. Statement (2) seems pretty straightforward. Candidate x received fewer than half of the votes cast. At this point many people say, "Since candidate x clearly got fewer than half the votes, this statement doesn't answer the question, either." But those people are wrong!

Broken down to its basics, the question we were asked was, "Did he get more than half of the vote—yes or no?" Statement (2) *does* answer the question. The answer is, "No, he didn't." So, the answer is the same as that of the first example. The correct answer is choice B. On a yes/no Data Sufficiency problem, if the statement answers the question in either the affirmative or the negative, it is sufficient.

Yes/No/Maybe

Yes/no questions really should be called yes/no/maybe questions. Even if that's not their "official" name, it's still worthwhile to think about them in that fashion.

Let's look at one last example to see why:

> Did candidate x receive more than half of the 30,000
> votes cast in the general election?
>
> 1. Candidate *y* received 12,000 of the votes cast.
>
> 2. Candidate *x* received at least 13,000 of the votes cast.

Since the first statement of this question is the same as that of the previous two examples, we know that it is insufficient; write BCE down on your Noteboard. Now, let's tackle Statement (2). Based on Statement (2), candidate *x* could have received exactly 13,000 votes, which would make the answer to the question "No, he did not receive more than half the votes cast." However, he could have also received 16,000 votes, and that would make the answer to the question, "Yes, he did receive more than half the votes cast." So, based on Statement (2), the best we can really say is that candidate *x* may have received more than half the votes. "Maybe" isn't good enough—we need a definitive yes or no answer. This means Statement (2) is insufficient (eliminate B). What if we combine the statements? We still have the same problem. We've accounted for at least 25,000 of the votes between the two candidates, but we don't know about the other 5,000. All of those votes could have gone to candidate *x*, making the answer to the question "yes." However, there could have been a third candidate who received those 5,000 votes. In that case, *x* would have received only 13,000 votes and the answer to the question is "no." Combining the statements doesn't give us a definitive answer. If the answer is sometimes "yes" and sometimes "no," the statement is not sufficient (eliminate C, and E is correct).

DS Core Strategy

Let's review your core DS strategy. These questions should be tackled in steps, using POE. First, assess whether Statement (1) alone provides sufficient information to answer the question. According to answer choices B, C, and E, Statement (1) alone doesn't provide sufficient information to answer the question. Therefore, if Statement (1) does provide sufficient information to answer the question, then the correct answer must either be answer choice A or D. Next, assess Statement (2). If it is sufficient to answer the question on its own, the correct answer is D; otherwise, the correct answer is A.

If, instead, Statement (1) alone is insufficient to answer the question asked, you can eliminate choices A and D, leaving you with options B, C, and E. Again, assess whether Statement (2) alone provides sufficient information to answer the question asked. If it does, pick choice B. Otherwise, you can eliminate option B, leaving you with C and E. Finally, assess whether both Statements (1) and (2) together provide sufficient information to answer the question. If they do, pick choice C; otherwise, pick E. We call this the **AD/BCE approach** since the assessment of Statement (1) will leave you with either AD or BCE as remaining answer choices.

Let's look at one last example:

65. If x and y are positive integers and $\dfrac{x}{y} = 3$, what is the value of x?

1. $3 < y < 7$

2. y is odd

Simplifying any algebraic expressions in the question is often a good way to start. For instance, rearranging $\dfrac{x}{y} = 3$ to state $x = 3y$ gives a slightly more straightforward way to assess whether there is sufficient information to solve for x.

To find a unique, positive integer value for x, this expression requires a unique, positive integer value for y. Looking at Statement (1) alone first, y is limited to the positive integer values of 4, 5, or 6. Three possible values for y means there are three possible values for x: Statement (1) alone is insufficient to answer the question (eliminate A and D).

Next, looking at Statement (2) alone, y is restricted to odd, positive integers meaning there are an infinite number of possible values for y. Remember, you're assessing Statement (2) alone and ignoring Statement (1). Statement (2) alone is insufficient to answer the question (eliminate B).

Looking at both statements together, the only odd, positive integer value between 3 and 7 is 5. Therefore, there is only one possible value for y, which is what is required to solve for x (eliminate E, and C is correct). Again, you don't need to know that $x = 15$ to know that there will be a unique, positive integer value for x; it's enough to know that you can solve for that unique, positive integer value for x, and that allows you to confidently pick answer choice C.

DS Additional Strategies

In addition to working the AD/BCE approach, there are additional techniques you can use on test day for DS questions.

Pieces of the Puzzle

Your familiarity with math content can give you an advantage when working a DS question. Most people read the question and then immediately read the statements. But that's not how you would normally work a math problem. Normally, you would read the problem and then ask yourself, "What do I already know?" and "What do I need?"

You should always attempt to do the same thing when working a DS question. Before proceeding to the statements, take stock of the information you already know. Then, see if you can determine what sort of information the statements need to provide so that you could solve the problem. We call this approach **Pieces of the Puzzle**. In a sense, DS questions are just like jigsaw puzzles. When you work a jigsaw puzzle, you know what piece you are looking for based on the shapes of the pieces that fit around it. In DS questions, you'll often know what sort of information you need from the statements based on what you already know from the question stem.

DS and Geometry

For DS questions, be very careful when using figures in the question stem. The figures are drawn so they represent information in the question stem, but they need not accurately represent information in the statements. This means you should base your conclusions about whether you have sufficient information on the statements rather than any figures provided with a DS question.

When DS questions are about geometry, you can often make very effective use of the Pieces of the Puzzle approach; this approach works very well in situations in which you can use formulas and take stock of facts.

DS, Equations, and Variables

DS questions are particularly well suited to testing your knowledge of equation rules and variables. Let's review some important information:

1. When working with equations, you generally need as many equations as there are variables in those equations.
   - A single equation with two variables cannot be solved, but two distinct equations with the same two variables can be solved, using simultaneous equations.
   - For example, $x = y + 1$ cannot be solved, but $x = y + 1$ and $2x = -y - 6$ can be added together, eliminating one variable so the other may be solved.
2. Just because there is only one variable doesn't mean that an equation has just one solution.
   - Generally, equations have as many solutions as the greatest exponent in the equation. So, an equation with a squared term will typically have two solutions.
   - Simple equations with a variable raised to an odd power may have only one solution.
   - For example, if $x^2 = 4$, then x could equal either 2 or –2. If $x^3 = 8$, then x can only equal 2.
3. Sometimes, it's possible to get an answer even if there is only a single equation with two variables—*if* the problem asks for an expression that contains both variables.
4. Sometimes you can also get an answer if there is only a single equation with two variables if both of those variables can only take on integer values.

Plugging In on Yes/No Questions

It is a good idea to have a strategy for these questions and to do lots of practice. When Yes/No questions involve variables, you can plug into the statement and use those numbers to see if you always get the same answer to the question. Here is a checklist for using Plugging In with Yes/No DS questions:

- First, try plugging in a normal number for your variable. The number you pick must satisfy the statement itself. If it doesn't, plug in another number. The number will yield an answer to the question—either yes or no. But you're not done yet.
- Now try plugging in a different number for your variable. This time, you might try one of the "weird" numbers, such as 0, 1, a negative number, or a fraction. If the number still answers the question the same way, then you can begin to suspect that the statement yields a consistent answer and that you're down to AD.
- If you plug in a different number and get a different answer this time (a "yes" after getting a "no" or a "no" after getting a "yes"), then the statement does NOT definitively answer the question, and you're down to BCE.
- Repeat this checklist with Statement (2).

Want More Practice?
Scan the QR code below to register your book for online chapter summaries, drills, practice tests, and more!

NOTES

NOTES

NOTES

NOTES

NOTES

NOTES

NOTES

NOTES

NOTES

BIOLOGY

MACROMOLECULES

	Structure	Function
Proteins	Polymers of amino acids (20) 4 levels of structure	Enzymes, hormones, receptors, transporters, antibodies, etc.
Carbohydrates	Polymers of mono-saccharides such as glucose, fructose, galactose	Energy Oxidized in cell respiration Stored in glycogen or starch
Lipids	Hydrophobic Glycerol + fatty acids Steroid/cholesterol derivatives	Phospholipids in membranes Triglycerides store energy Steroid hormones
Nucleic Acids (DNA and RNA)	Polymers of nucleotides A = T and C ≡ G	Hereditary/genetic material

THE CELL

The plasma membrane: selective permeability barrier consisting of phospholipid bilayer, proteins, and cholesterol.

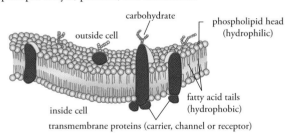

ORGANELLES

- **Ribosome:** protein synthesis via translation
- **Nucleus:** houses the genome
- **Mitochondria:** cell respiration and energy production
- **Rough ER and Golgi:** protein trafficking and modification
- **Lysosome:** autophagy and degradation
- **Peroxisome:** degradation and detoxification
- **Smooth ER:** lipid synthesis
- **Chloroplast:** photosynthesis
- **Vacuole:** water storage
- **Cytoskeleton:** structural support

TRANSMEMBRANE TRANSPORT

- **Simple diffusion:** hydrophobic molecules diffuse across the membrane, down their gradient
- **Facilitated diffusion:** hydrophilic molecules through a channel across the membrane, down their gradient
- **Active transport:** energy is used to move molecules across the membrane, against their gradient

CELL RESPIRATION

GLUCOSE CATABOLISM

Cellular Process	Location	O₂ condition	Major substrates	Net products
Glycolysis	Cytosol	Both	Glucose	2 Pyruvate, 2 ATP, 2 NADH
Fermentation	Cytosol	Anaerobic	Pyruvate, NADH	Lactic acid or Ethanol, NAD⁺
Pyruvate decarboxylation	Mitochon-drial matrix	Aerobic	Pyruvate	2 Acetyl-CoA, 2 NADH
Citric acid (Krebs) cycle	Mitochon-drial matrix	Aerobic	Acetyl-CoA	6 NADH, 2 FADH₂, 2 GTP
Electron transport chain	Inner mitochondrial membrane	Aerobic	NADH, FADH₂, O₂	NAD⁺, FAD, H₂O
Oxidative phosphorylation	Inner mitochondrial membrane	Aerobic	ADP, Pᵢ (H⁺ gradient)	Euk: 30 ATP Prok: 32 ATP

PHOTOSYNTHESIS

- Light energy is converted into chemical energy (ATP/NADPH), which is then used to produce sugars.
- Occurs in chloroplasts.

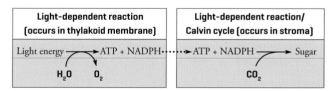

MOLECULAR GENETICS

NUCLEIC ACID

- **Basic unit:** nucleotide (five-carbon sugar, nitrogenous base, phosphate group(s)).
- Sugar in DNA is deoxyribose; sugar in RNA is ribose.
- 2 types of bases: double-ringed purines (adenine, guanine) and single-ringed pyrimidines (cytosine, thymine, uracil).
- DNA double helix; antiparallel strands joined by hydrogen bonding between base pairs (A = T, G ≡ C).
- RNA is usually single-stranded: A pairs with U, not T.

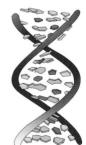

MUTATIONS

Point: one nucleotide is substituted for another. Includes missense, non-sense, and silent mutations.

Missense: one amino acid substituted for another.

Nonsense: introduces a premature stop codon in the sequence (truncated protein).

Silent: no change in amino acid sequence.

Frameshift: insertions or deletions of nucleotides not in multiples of three shift the reading frame; the protein can be nonfunctional, of a different length, or not produced.

DNA Replication

- **Semiconservative replication:** parent strand + newly synthesized strand.

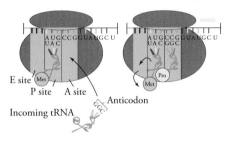

- Key enzymes are helicase (unwinds the DNA), primase (lays down RNA primer), and DNA polymerases (synthesize DNA).

EUKARYOTIC PROTEIN SYNTHESIS

- **Transcription:** RNA polymerase synthesizes hnRNA using DNA, "antisense strand" as a template.
- **Post-transcriptional processing:** splicing of introns and addition of 5' cap and 3' polyA tail (hnRNA → mRNA); mRNA is then exported out of the nucleus.
- **Translation** occurs on ribosomes in the cytoplasm.

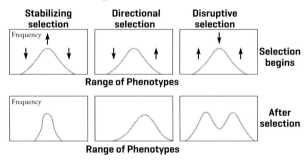

Post-translational modifications: (i.e., disulfide bonds) made before the polypeptide becomes a functional protein.

PROKARYOTIC PROTEIN SYNTHESIS

- Occurs simultaneously with transcription because no mRNA processing is required.
- Ribosome is slightly smaller than eukaryotic ribosome.
- mRNA can be polycistronic (code for several different proteins).

GENE EXPRESSION CONTROL

- Epigenetics: DNA methylation, histone modification, RNA interference
- Control of: transcription, RNA processing, RNA transport and localization, mRNA degradation, translation, protein activity

CLASSICAL GENETICS

- **Genotype:** the combination of alleles an individual possesses
- **Phenotype:** physical characteristics of an individual, resulting from their genotype

Law of independent assortment: alleles of unlinked genes assort independently during meiosis.
- For $Rr \times Rr$: genotypic ratio is 1:2:1, phenotypic ratio is 3:1.
- For $AaBb \times AaBb$: gametes produced are *AB, Ab, aB,* and *ab,* and phenotypic ratio is 9:3:3:1

Statistical calculations
- probability of A **and** B = prob (A) × prob (B)
- probability of A **or** B = prob (A) + prob (B) − prob (A and B)

INHERITED DISORDERS IN PEDIGREES
- **Autosomal recessive:** skips generations
- **Autosomal dominant:** appears every generation
- **X-linked (sex-linked):** no male-to-male transmission, and more males affected; can be recessive (red/green colorblindness or hemophilia) or dominant.

POPULATION GENETICS
- **Equation for allele frequency:** $p + q = 1$
- **Equation for genotype frequency:** $p^2 + 2pq + q^2 = 1$

For a population to be in Hardy-Weinberg equilibrium it must be large, be randomly mating, and have no mutation, no natural selection, and no migration.

EVOLUTION

- **Evolution** is driven by natural selection: organisms with advantageous traits survive and reproduce while organisms with disadvantageous traits die out.
- **Fitness** refers to the ability of an organism to successfully pass on its alleles to future generations.

Stabilizing selection	Directional selection	Disruptive selection	
			Selection begins
			After selection

↑ = Phenotypes being selected FOR
↓ = Phenotypes being selected AGAINST

- **Speciation:** creation of new species.
- **Reproductive isolation** is caused by prezygotic barriers that prevent formation of a viable zygote or postzygotic barriers that prevent development, survival, or fertility of the hybrid organism.
- **Homologous structures** in two different organisms have similar functions as a result of common ancestry.
- **Analogous structures** in two different organisms have similar functions but do not share a common ancestry.

DIVERSITY OF LIFE
- **Domain Bacteria:** "true," mostly mesophilic bacteria
- **Domain Archaea:** extremophilic bacteria
- **Domain Eukarya:**
  - **Kingdom Protista:** includes organisms that are plant-like (algae), animal-like (protozoa), and fungus-like (absorptive protists)
  - **Kingdom Fungi:** saprophytes made of hyphae; e.g. yeast, truffles, and mushrooms
  - **Kingdom Plantae:** most have roots, stems, and leaves; perform alternation of generations

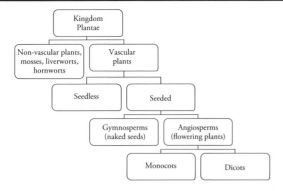

Kingdom Animalia: most diverse kingdom, includes many phyla such as poriferans, cnidarians, worms, mollusks, arthropods, echinoderms and chordates

Vertebrates include fish, amphibians, reptiles, birds, and mammals.

Animal Behavior and Interaction:

- **Commensalism:** one organism benefits, the other is unaffected
- **Mutualism:** both organisms benefit
- **Parasitism:** one organism benefits, the other is harmed
- **Innate behavior:** preprogrammed, known from birth
- **Learned behavior:** acquired through interaction with the environment

Viruses
- Acellular structures of double or single-stranded DNA or RNA in a protein coat
- Lytic cycle: virus kills the host
- Lysogenic cycle: virus enters host genome

BODY CONTROL AND COMMUNICATION

NERVOUS SYSTEM
- **Neutrons** are the basic cellular unit; they relay signals via an action potential.
- Synapse: junction between a neuron and another neuron/effector organ. Two types: electrical (uses gap junction) and chemical (uses neurotransmitters).
- **Central nervous system:** brain and spinal cord.
- **Peripheral nervous system:** somatic nervous system (voluntary, controls skeletal muscle) and autonomic nervous system (involuntary, controls cardiac and smooth muscle).
- **Two branches of autonomic system:** sympathetic (fight or flight) and parasympathetic (rest and digest).

ENDOCRINE SYSTEM
- **Direct hormones** directly stimulate their effector organs.
- **Tropic hormones** stimulate release of hormones from other endocrine glands.
- Hormones released from the adrenal cortex and the gonads are steroid hormones. All other hormones are peptide hormones.
- Mechanisms of hormone action:
  - **Peptide hormones** bind to their receptor on the PM and activate second messengers like cAMP.
  - **Steroid hormones** diffuse across the PM and bind to their receptor in the cytoplasm; the hormone/receptor complex then translocates to the nucleus and regulates transcription of genes.

CIRCULATORY SYSTEM

- Includes the heart (a muscular pump) and blood vessels
- **Heart:**
  - Made of cardiac muscle fibers
  - Has 2 atria (top) and 2 ventricles (bottom)
  - Has its own pacemaker cells (SA node), which spontaneously depolarize and trigger contraction of the heart.
- **Blood vessels:**
  - Arteries: carry blood away from the heart; have thick smooth muscle wall; high pressure vessels
  - Veins: carry blood toward the heart; contain one-way valves; low pressure vessels
  - Capillaries: site of gas, nutrient, and waste exchange
- **Blood** is 55% plasma (water, ions, sugars, proteins), 45% red blood cells (carry oxygen), and ~1% white blood cells (immunity) and platelets (blood clotting).
- Oxygen is carried through the blood bound to hemoglobin in RBCs
- Carbon dioxide is converted into bicarbonate and dissolves in plasma

IMMUNE SYSTEM

Acquired	**B-cells [Humoral immunity]**	Plasma cells	Make and secrete antibodies (IgG, IgA, IgM, IgD, IgE), which induce antigen phagocytosis
		Memory cells	Remember antigens, speed up secondary response
	T-cells [Cell-mediated immunity]	Cytotoxic T-cells	Destroy cells directly
		Helper T-cells	Activate B- and T-cells, and macrophages
		Memory cells	Remember antigens, speed up secondary response
Innate			Includes skin, passages lined with cilia, macrophages, low pH in the stomach and vagina, inflammatory response, and interferons (proteins that help prevent the spread of a virus).

RESPIRATORY SYSTEM

- Two major functions: gas exchange and pH regulation.
- **Conduction zone:** site of air movement (ventilation) only; consists of the nose, pharynx, larynx, trachea, bronchi, and most bronchioles
- **Respiratory zone:** site of gas exchange (respiration); consists of respiratory bronchioles, alveolar ducts, and alveoli

DIGESTION

- **Mouth:** functions to grind food (mastication) and digest carbohydrates (via salivary amylase)
- **Esophagus:** moves food from mouth to stomach
- **Stomach:** stores food, breaks down proteins (via pepsin)
  - Gastrin stimulates secretion of acid in the stomach
- **Small intestine:** site where most digestion and absorption occurs
  - CCK stimulates bile release
  - Secretin stimulates: HCO_3^- release
  - Enterokinase activates trypsin from trypsinogen
- **Large intestine:** site of reabsorption of water and electrolytes, production of vitamin K by colonic bacteria, stores feces

Accessory digestive organs:

- **Liver:** synthesizes and secretes bile for fat emulsification
- **Gallbladder:** stores and concentrates bile
- **Pancreas:** produces digestive enzymes for breakdown of all macromolecules (amylase, trypsin and other proteases, lipase, nucleases) and secretes HCO_3^-

RENAL SYSTEM

- Functions of the kidneys include:
  - urine formation
  - BP and pH regulation
  - ion and water balance
- Basic functional unit: **nephron**
- Blood filtration occurs at **glomerulus**
- Modification of the filtrate (**reabsorption** and **secretion**) occurs along the PCT, loop of Henle, DCT, and collecting duct.
- Low BP → Posterior pituitary secretes ADH → more water reabsorption in DCT and collecting ducts
- Low BP → kidneys release renin → activates angiotensinogen → produces angiotensin II → vasoconstriction and release of aldosterone → increased BP

MUSCULOSKELETAL SYSTEM

SARCOMERE

- Contractile unit of the fibers in a skeletal muscle cell
- Contains thin actin and thick myosin filaments

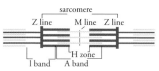

SKELETAL MUSCLE CONTRACTION

- ACh release from a neuron leads to action potential
- Ca^{2+} in the sarcoplasm increases
- Troponin/tropomyosin shift to expose myosin binding sites on actin
- Myosin and actin interact and cause muscle contraction
- Sarcomeres, H zone, and I band shorten

BONE FORMATION AND REMODELING

- Regulated by PTH and calcitonin
- Osteoblasts: builds bone
- Osteoclasts: break down bone
- Osteon is the unit of compact bone

REPRODUCTION

Cell division

- G_1: cell growth, organelle and protein synthesis, metabolism
- S: DNA replication
- G_2: similar to G_1
- M: mitosis via PMAT

SEXUAL REPRODUCTION

Meiosis I

- Replicated homologous chromosomes (each has two chromatids) pair up to form a tetrad in prophase I.
- Crossing over leads to genetic recombination in prophase I.
- Recombined homologous chromosomes are separated into haploid daughter cells.

Meiosis II

- Similar to mitosis.
- Recombined sister chromatids are separated into haploid daughter cells that have a single copy of one set of chromosomes, 23 in humans.

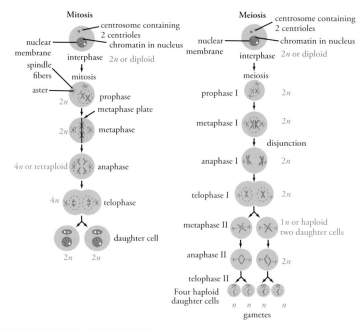

Examples of meiosis in humans:

- Spermatogenesis in males: making sperm in seminiferous tubules of testes
- Oogenesis in females: making ova in ovaries

FOUR STAGES OF EARLY DEVELOPMENT

Cleavage: mitotic divisions of the zygote to form a morula

Implantation: blastocyst (trophoblast and inner cell mass) implant into the endometrial layer of uterus

Gastrulation: formation of 2 or 3 primary germ layers

Neurulation: formation of the nervous system from germ cell layers

Organogenesis: formation of all other major organs

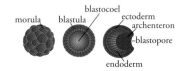

SKIN

Functions in thermoregulation by piloerection and vasoconstriction when cold, and sweating and vasodilation when warm.

GENERAL CHEMISTRY

ATOMIC STRUCTURE

Atomic weight: the weight in grams of one mole (mol) of a given element and is expressed in terms of g/mol.

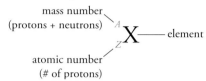

mass number
(protons + neutrons) — $^A_Z X$ — element
atomic number
(# of protons)

A **mole** is a unit used to count particles and is represented by **Avogadro's number:** 6.022×10^{23} particles

$$\text{Moles} = \frac{\text{grams}}{\text{atomic or molecular weight}} = \frac{n}{M}$$

Isotopes: for a given element, multiple species of atoms with the same number of protons (same atomic number) but different numbers of neutrons (different mass numbers).

Planck's quantum theory: energy emitted as electromagnetic radiation from matter exists in discrete bundles called quanta.

Bohr atom: electrons reside in discreet energy levels around a nucleus. Electrons can absorb energy and move to higher levels of energy or shed energy as photons and settle to lower energy states.

Quantum numbers:

#	Character	Symbol	Value
1st	Shell	n	n
2nd	Subshell	l	From zero to $n-1$
3rd	Orbital	m_l	Between l and $-l$
4th	Spin	m_s	$\frac{1}{2}$ or $-\frac{1}{2}$

The four subshells corresponding to $l = 0, 1, 2,$ and 3 are known as $s, p, d,$ and f, respectively.

ELECTRONIC CONFIGURATION

Electrons are filled in order, from left to right, along the periodic table. The shell in which electrons fall is dictated by their block, and their row. For s and p electrons, $n =$ # of row, for d electrons, $n =$ row # $- 1$, and for f electrons $n =$ row # $- 2$.

Hund's rule: every orbital in a subshell gets one electron (with the same spin) before any orbital gets a second electron.

Valence electrons: electrons of an atom in its outer energy shell, available for bonding.

NUCLEAR CHEMISTRY

Unstable nuclei decay, becoming new stable nuclei through the emission of a number of different particles (α, β, γ, etc). In any nuclear chemistry reaction total mass and total atomic number in the reactants must equal the total mass and atomic number of the products.

Summary of Radioactive Decay		
$N\downarrow Z\downarrow$	Alpha Decay	$^A_Z X \xrightarrow{\alpha} {}^{A-4}_{Z-2}Y + {}^4_2\alpha$
$N\downarrow Z\uparrow$	Beta Minus Decay	$^A_Z X \xrightarrow{\beta^-} {}^{A}_{Z+1}Y + {}^0_{-1}e^-$
$N\uparrow Z\downarrow$	Beta Plus Decay	$^A_Z X \xrightarrow{\beta^+} {}^{A}_{Z-1}Y + {}^0_{+1}e^+$
$N\uparrow Z\downarrow$	Electron Capture	$^A_Z X + {}^0_{+1}e^- \xrightarrow{EC} {}^{A}_{Z-1}Y$
	Gamma Decay	$^A_Z X^* \xrightarrow{\gamma} {}^A_Z X + \gamma$

$N =$ # of neutrons; $Z =$ atomic number/# of protons; $A = N + Z$

Half life $t_{1/2}$: the amount of time it takes for a sample to decay to half its original mass.

MOLECULAR GEOMETRY AND SHAPE

Geometric Family	# Electron Pairs on Central Atom	Shape		Bond Angles
Linear	0	Linear		180°
Trigonal Planar	0	Trigonal Planar		120°
	1	Bent		116°
Tetrahedral	0	Tetrahedral		109.5°
	1	Trigonal Pyramidal		107°
	2	Bent		104.5°
Trigonal Bipyramidal	0	Trigonal Bipyramidal		90° 120° 180°
Octahedral	0	Octahedral		90° 180°

BONDING AND CHEMICAL INTERACTIONS

Formal charges

$$\text{Formal Charge} = \text{Valence electrons} - \frac{1}{2}N_{bonding} - N_{nonbonding}$$

INTERMOLECULAR FORCES

1. **Hydrogen bonding:** between H and lone pair of electrons in N, O, F
2. **Dipole-dipole interactions:** between δ^+ and δ^- in a polar molecule
3. **Dispersion forces:** present in all molecules; due to transient unequal sharing of electrons in a bond.

GASES

1 atm = 760 mm Hg = 760 torr
STP: 273K, 0°C, 1 atm, 1 mole of gas = 22.4 L, used for gases

Standard state: 298 K or 25°C, 1 atm, 1 M, used in thermodynamics, equilibrium, electrochemistry

Boyle's law

$$PV = k \text{ or } P_1V_1 = P_2V_2$$

Law of Charles and Gay-Lussac

$$\frac{V}{T} = k \text{ or } \frac{V_1}{T_1} = \frac{V_2}{T_2}$$

Avogadro's principle

$$\frac{n}{V} = k \text{ or } \frac{n_1}{V_1} = \frac{n_2}{V_2}$$

Ideal gas law

$$PV = nRT$$

GRAHAM'S LAW OF DIFFUSION AND EFFUSION

Diffusion occurs when gas molecules diffuse through a mixture.

Effusion is the flow of gas particles under pressure from one compartment to another through a small opening. Both diffusion and effusion have the same formula.

$$\frac{r_1}{r_2} = \left(\frac{M_2}{M_1}\right)^{\frac{1}{2}}$$

SOLUTIONS

UNITS OF CONCENTRATION

Percent composition by mass: $= \dfrac{\text{Mass of solute}}{\text{Mass of solution}} \times 100(\%)$

Mole fraction: $\dfrac{\text{\# of mol of compound}}{\text{total \# of mols in system}}$

Molarity: $\dfrac{\text{\# of mol of solute}}{\text{liter of solution}}$

Molality: $\dfrac{\text{\# of mol of solute}}{\text{kg of solvent}}$

PHASES AND PHASE CHANGES

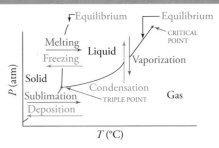

Colligative properties: physical properties derived solely from the number of particles present, not the nature of those particles. These properties are usually associated with dilute solutions.

Van't Hoff factor (i): the number of particles a given substance will form in solution. For binary salts (e.g., NaCl) $i = 2$.

Freezing point depression $\Delta T_f = k_f \, im$

Boiling point elevation $\Delta T_b = k_b \, im$

Osmotic pressure $\Pi = iMRT$

Vapor-pressure depression (Raoult's law) $P_A = X_A P°_A$; $P_B = X_B P°_B$

Solutions that obey Raoult's law are called ideal solutions.

KINETICS

For $xA + yB \rightarrow C$, Rate $= k\,[A]^x[B]^y$

- Rate = determined experimentally; units = M/sec
- k = rate constant; unit varies
- $x + y$ = reaction order

Factors that affect reaction rates: [R] in rate limiting step, T, catalysts

Catalysts: ↑ reaction rate, ↓ E_a, not consumed

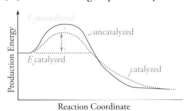

EQUILIBRIUM

Law of mass action $\qquad a\,A + b\,B \rightleftharpoons c\,C + d\,D$

$$K_c = \frac{[C]^c[D]^d}{[A]^a[B]^b}$$

K_c is the equilibrium constant. c stands for concentration.

Properties of the Equilibrium Constant

- K: don't include pure (s) and (l)
- K_{eq} for a specific system at a given T
- K_{eq} changes if temperature changes
- If $K_{eq} \gg 1$, then [P] $\gg$ [R]
- If $K_{eq} \ll 1$, then [P] $\ll$ [R]
- If $K_{eq} = 1$, then [P] = [R]

Reaction quotient (Q): once a reaction commences, standard state conditions no longer hold. For the reaction,

$$a\,A + b\,B \rightleftharpoons c\,C + d\,D \qquad Q = \frac{[C]^c[D]^d}{[A]^a[B]^b}$$

A(g) + B (g) ⟶ C (g) + heat	
Will Shift to the Right	**Will Shift to the Left**
1. if more A or B added	1. if more C added
2. if C taken away	2. if A or B taken away
3. if pressure applied or volume reduced	3. if pressure reduced or volume increased
4. if temperature reduced	4. if temperature increased

ACIDS AND BASES

	Acid	**Base**
Arrhenius	Produces H^+ in (aq) solution	Produces OH^- in (aq) solution
Bronsted-Lowry	Donates H^+	Accepts H^+
Lewis	Accepts e^-	Donates e^-

Properties of Acids and Bases

$$pH = -\log[H^+]$$
$$pOH = -\log[OH^-]$$
$$H_2O(l) \rightleftharpoons H^+(aq) + OH^-(aq)$$
$$Kw = [H^+][OH^-] = 10^{-14}$$
$$pH = pOH = 14$$

Weak Acids and Bases

$$HA(aq) + H_2O(l) \rightleftharpoons H_3O^+(aq) + A^-(aq)$$
$$K_a = \frac{[H_3O^+][A^-]}{[HA]}$$
$$K_b = \frac{[B^+][OH^-]}{[BOH]}$$
$$pH = pK_a + \log\frac{[\text{conjugate base}]}{[\text{weak base}]}$$
$$pOH = pK_b + \log\frac{[\text{conjugate base}]}{[\text{weak base}]}$$

Neutralization:

$$\underset{\text{(acid)}}{HA} + \underset{\text{(base)}}{BOH} \longrightarrow \underset{\text{(salt)}}{BA} + \underset{\text{(water)}}{H_2O}$$

Titration and Buffers

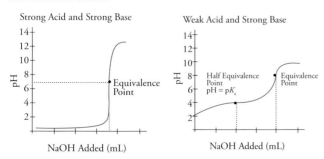

Titration is a technique used to determine concentration of an acid or a base using a solution of known concentration to neutralize it.

THERMOCHEMISTRY

Specific heat

$$Q = mc\Delta T$$

- Q is heat absorbed or released; units: joules or calories
- m = mass, c = specific heat, ΔT = change in temperature
- Can only be used when phase is not changing
- $Q > 0$ = heat is absorbed
- $Q < 0$ = heat is released

Heat of transformation: the quantity of heat required to change the phase of 1 kg of a substance.

$$q = n \times \Delta H_{\text{phase change}}$$
$$q = m \times \Delta H_{\text{phase change}}$$

Phase changes are isothermal processes

First law of thermodynamics: $\Delta E = q + w$

- **Enthalpy (H):** change in heat energy at constant pressure
- **Standard heat of formation (ΔH_f°):** change in enthalpy when one mole of a compound is formed from its elements in their standard states
- **Standard heat of reaction (ΔH_{rxn}°)** = (sum of ΔH_{rxn}° of products) – (sum of ΔH_{rxn}° of reactants)
- **Hess's law:** enthalpies of reactions are additive
- **Bond dissociation energy:** energy required to break a particular type of bond in one mole of gaseous molecules
- **Entropy (S):** measure of the disorder, or randomness, of a system. $\Delta S_{\text{universe}} = \Delta S_{\text{system}} + \Delta S_{\text{surroundings}}$
- **Gibbs free energy:** $\Delta G = \Delta H - T\Delta S$
- $\Delta G < 0$ = spontaneous reaction
- $\Delta G > 0$ = nonspontaneous reaction
- $\Delta G = 0$ = reaction is in equilibrium

REDOX REACTIONS AND ELECTROCHEMISTRY

Oxidation: loss of electrons, gain O, loss of H

Reduction: gain of electrons, loss of O, gain H

Redox tricks: LEO GER or OIL RIG

Oxidizing agent: causes another atom to undergo oxidation, and is itself reduced.

Reducing agent: causes another atom to be reduced, and is itself oxidized.

Galvanic cell: electrons flow **spontaneously** from anode (–) to cathode (+). E_{cell} = **positive**

Electrolytic cell: electrons are forced to flow from anode (+) to cathode (–) using external power source (**non-spontaneous**). E_{cell} = **negative**.

ORGANIC CHEMISTRY

NOMENCLATURE

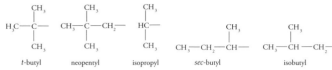

t-butyl   neopentyl   isopropyl   sec-butyl   isobutyl

Functional Group	Suffix	Functional Group	Suffix
Carboxylic Acid	-oic acid	Ketone	-one
Ester	-oate	Thiol	-thiol
Acyl halide	-oyl halide	Alcohol	-ol
Amide	-amide	Amine	-amine
Nitrile/ Cyanide	-nitrile	Imine	-imine
Aldehyde	-al	Ether	-ether
Alkene	-ene	Alkyne	-yne

ISOMERS

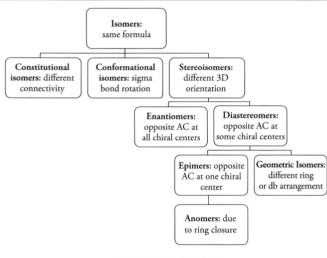

Newman Projections:

staggered and anti   gauche and staggered   eclipsed   totally eclipsed

Conformations of Cyclohexane:

chair   boat   twist boat

BONDING

Bond order	Single	Double	Triple
Bond type	Σ	Σ	Σ
		π	2π
Hybridization	sp^3	sp^2	sp
Angles	109.5°	120°	180°
Example	C–C	C=C	C≡C

STABILIZATION

Induction: electron deficient groups (radicals and C⁺) are more stable when substituted with EDG

Electron rich groups (C⁻) are more stable when less substituted, or by EWG.

Resonance: delocalization of π electrons and charge leads to stabilization.

Charge must be adjacent to π bond for resonance to occur.

ALKANES

REACTIONS

Free radical halogenation

- initiation (↑# radicals)
- propagation (no change # radicals)
- termination (↓# radicals)

Combustion

$$C_3H_8 + 5\,O_2 \rightarrow 3\,CO_2 + 4\,H_2O + heat$$

Types of Carbons: 1° → CH₃, 3°, 2°

ALKYL HALIDES SYNTHESIS

$$+OH + HBr \rightarrow +OH_2^+ + Br^-$$

$$Br^- + +OH_2^+ \rightarrow +Br + H_2O$$

OH + ClSO₂ (TsCl) → OTs — NaI → I + ⁻OTs

SUBSTITUTIONS REACTIONS

$$X + Nu^- \rightarrow Nu + X^-$$

S$_N$1	S$_N$2
2 steps, rearrangements possible	1 step, backside attack
3° > 2° >1° > methyl	Methyl > 1° > 2° > 3°
Racemic products	Optically active and inverted products
Rate = k[RX]	Rate = k[Nu⁻][RX]
Strong nucleophile not required	Favored with strong nucleophile
Favored in polar protic solvents	Favored in polar aprotic solvents

ELIMINATION REACTIONS

$$X + Base \xrightarrow{\Delta} + BH^+ + X^-$$

E1	E2
2 steps, rearrangements possible	1 step, antiperiplanar H and LG
3° > 2° > 1°	3° > 2° >1°
Zaitsev (most substituted) product forms; trans > cis	Stereochemistry of double bond determined by starting conformation
Rate = k [substrate]	Rate = k [substrate][base]
Favored with heat and weak base	Favored with heat and strong base; small base gives most substituted db; bulky base gives least substituted db

ALKENES

Electrophilic addition of HX (Markovnikov)

Free radical addition (anti-Markovnikov)

most stable radical

Electrophilic addition of X_2

Bromonium ion   *anti* addition

Electrophilic addition of H_2O (Markovnikov)

Hydroboration (anti-Markovnikov, *syn* orientation)

1. BH_3
2. H_2O_2, OH^-

Catalytic reduction

Oxidation with $KMnO_4$

cold dilute $KMnO_4$

Oxidation with O_3

1) O_3, CH_2Cl_2
2) Zn/H_2O

ALKYNES

Reduction with Lindlar's catalyst or Na in liquid ammonia

$CH_3C \equiv CCH_3$ 2-butyne $\xrightarrow[\text{Quinoline (Lindlar's Catalyst)}]{H_2, Pd/BaSO_4}$ *cis*-2-butene

$CH_3C \equiv CCH_3$ 2-butyne $\xrightarrow{Na, NH_3(l)}$ *trans*-2-butene

ALCOHOLS

- Higher boiling points than alkanes
- Weakly acidic hydroxyl hydrogen

Synthesis

- Addition of water to double bonds
- S_N1 and S_N2 reactions
- Reduction of carboxylic acids, aldehydes, ketones, and esters
  - Aldehydes and ketones with $NaBH_4$
  - Esters and carboxylic acids with $LiAlH_4$

REACTIONS

E1 dehydration reactions in strongly acidic solutions

$\xrightarrow[\Delta]{H_2SO_4}$

Hydride Shift

Minor, Hoffman

Major, Zaitsev   Minor, Hoffman

Oxidation

- PCC oxidizes a primary alcohol to an aldehyde.

$\xrightarrow{PCC}$

- CrO_3, $KMnO_4$, and dichromate salts oxidize secondary alcohols to ketones, and primary alcohols to carboxylic acids.

$\xrightarrow[H_2SO_4]{Na_2Cr_2O_7}$

- Tertiary alcohols cannot be oxidized without breaking a carbon to carbon bond.

ALDEHYDES AND KETONES

The dipole moment of carbonyl compounds causes an elevation of boiling point, but not as high as alcohols since there is no hydrogen bonding.

Synthesis

- Oxidation of primary or secondary alcohols
- Ozonolysis of alkenes

Nucleophilic addition

Commonly used $Nu^- = RMgBr$, ROH, RNH_2

When $Nu^- = H^-$, this reaction is a reduction.

Aldol condensation

An aldehyde acts both as nucleophile (enolate) and electrophile (keto form).

$\xrightarrow[H_2O]{NaOH}$ H_3O^+ $\xrightarrow[\text{heat}]{-H_2O}$

β-hydroxyaldehyde   α,β-unsaturated carbonyl compound

Oxidation and reduction

$\xrightarrow[NaBH_4]{LiAlH_4}$

$\xrightarrow{KMnO_4, CrO_3}$

CH_3CH CH_3COH

CARBOXYLIC ACIDS

Carboxylic acids have pK_a's of around 5 due to resonance stabilization of the conjugate base. Electronegative atoms increase acidity with inductive effects. Boiling point is higher than alcohols because of the ability to form two hydrogen bonds.

Synthesis

Oxidation of primary alcohols with $KMnO_4$

Organometallic reagents with CO_2 (Grignard)

Reactions

Formation of soap by reacting carboxylic acids with NaOH; arrange in micelles

nonpolar tail   polar head

Reduction to alcohols

R—C—OH   →   R—C—OH   →   aldehyde
carboxylic acid

→   R—C—H   →   R—C—H
alcohol

CARBOXYLIC ACID DERIVATIVES

All derivatives go through addition-elimination mechanisms when they are interconverted:

Addition   Elimination   Nu + LG

All derivatives can be synthesized from an appropriate nucleophile and a more reactive derivative.

Relative reactivity of derivatives

acid halide > acid anhydride > ester > amide

Amide Synthesis: Amine + acid chloride, anhydride, or ester

Ester Synthesis: Alcohol + acid chloride or anhydride

Acid Anhydride Synthesis: Carboxylate + acid halide

Acid Halide Synthesis: can only be synthesized from a carboxylic acid directly.

$$RCOOH + SOCl_2 \longrightarrow$$

Other reagents: PCl_3 or PBr_3

LAB TECHNIQUES

Extractions separate based on solubility.
- RNH_2 extracted with HCl
- RCOOH extracted with $NaHCO_3$
- PhOH extracted with NaOH

Chromatography separates based on polarity.
- High polarity = low R_f values
- Low polarity = high R_f values

Gas chromatography separates based on boiling point.
- High boiling point comes off column late
- Low boiling point comes off column early

Distillation separates based on boiling point.
- Simple distillation works when solvents have very different BPs
- Fractional distillation is used when solvents have similar BPs

Spectroscopy: IR

Functional group	Wave number
C=O	1720 cm^{-1}
C=C	1650 cm^{-1}
O–H	3200-3600 cm^{-1}
C≡C, C≡N	2100-2260 cm^{-1}

^{1}H NMR: spectrum tells four things about structure.

1. # of nonequivalent Hs = # signals
2. # of nonequivalent neighboring Hs = splitting pattern (follows $n + 1$ rule where n = # neighboring Hs)
3. chemical environment of Hs = chemical shift
4. # of Hs in each signal = integration

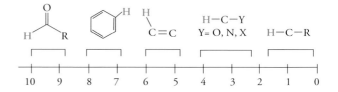

PERCEPTUAL ABILITY

APERTURES

Questions: 1 to 15
Answer choices: A–E
Rank: Medium

What You're Given

One three-dimensional shape.

What You Need To Do

Find an opening this shape can pass through.

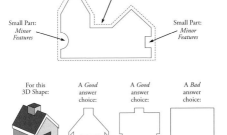

RULES

- You can rotate the object before passing it through the opening.
- Once you've started putting it through the opening, you can't turn or twist the shape any more.
- The shape in the question stem and the apertures in the answer choices are drawn to the same scale and without perspective.
- There are no hidden parts on the 3D shape.

STRATEGIES

- Focus on the dark side of the object: what do the sides that you can't see very well look like?
- Focus on big parts: what is the overall shape or perimeter of the object? Then focus on small parts: where would the smaller feature(s) need to be? Are they in the correct location? With the correct orientation and scale?
- Match the outline of the object perfectly. You're not looking for the biggest opening the shape can fit through. You're looking for the most accurate and specific, or the best fit.
- Focus on the perimeter of the shape, from the side, front and top

ORTHOGRAPHIC PROJECTIONS

Questions: 16 to 30
Answer choices: A–D
Rank: Difficult

What You're Given

Two two-dimensional views of a 3D object.

What You Need To Do

Figure out what the third view would look like.

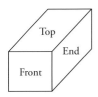

RULES

- The same three views are always used: **Top, Front, and End**
- End is always what the shape looks like from the right side
- Any two views will be given and you need to find the third
- **Solid lines** represent features (corner, edge, or hole) that you can see
- **Dotted lines** represent internal or rear features that you cannot see but know are there

The views for this shape:

Look like this:

Top View

Front View

End View

STRATEGIES

- Count and align internal features:
  - Horizontal features in the Front View must match horizontal features in the End View
  - Vertical features in the Top View must match vertical features in the Front View
  - Horizontal features in the Top View must match vertical features in the End View

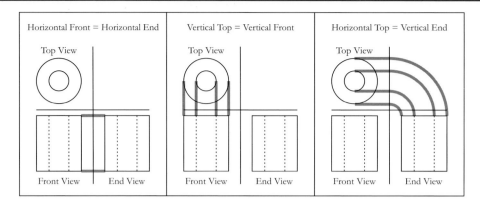

- Compare features, focusing on dotted and solid lines. Ask yourself if the feature would be visible or not.
- Fold the shape together by folding the Top View down on top of the Front View, and the End View over to the right. The correct answer will complete the 3D shape.

ANGLE RANKING

Questions: 31 to 45	**What You're Given**	**What You Need To Do**
Answer choices: A–D		
Rank: Medium	Four angles of varying degrees and arm lengths.	Rank them from smallest to largest.

STRATEGIES
- Find the biggest angle and POE
- Find the smallest angle and POE
- Compare two obviously different angles, rank them with respect to each other, then POE
- Classify angles as acute, right, or obtuse
- Have points of reference:
  - Compare large angles (obtuse) to a straight line:

    180°   <180°

  - Compare medium-sized angles to a right angle (90°):

    <90°   90°   >90°

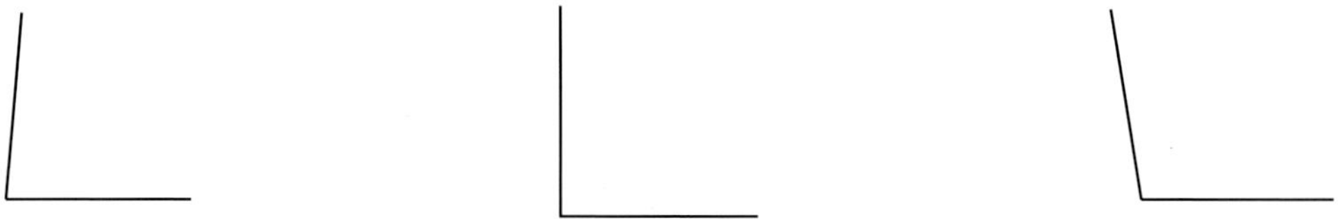

  - Use pixel overlap to compare small angles (acute):

    The most pixel overlap   **Some pixel overlap**   **The least pixel overlap**
    at vertex = Smallest angle   **at vertex = Middle-sized angle** **at vertex = Largest angle**

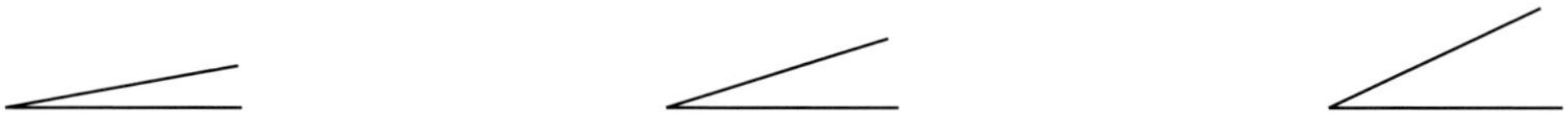

HOLE PUNCHING

Questions: 46 to 60
Answer choices: A–E
Rank: Medium

What You're Given
A pattern for folding a square piece of paper, which ends with a hold punch.

What You Need To Do
Mentally unfold the paper and determine the number and locations of the holes.

RULES

- The paper is never turned, twisted or flipped
- The paper will always be folded towards you (not behind itself)

STRATEGIES

- Unfold the Paper
  - Work backward from the final picture, one fold at a time, placing the hole(s) as you go; keep track of your work on your Noteboard
  - Eliminate answer choices as you work
  - Keep and duplicate the hole if the paper is solid on the previous picture
  - Move the hole (do not duplicate) if the paper is dotted (hypothetical) in the previous picture
  - For example, for this pattern:

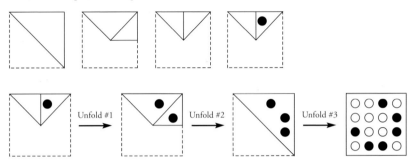

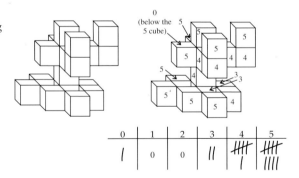

- Determine how many holes the correct answer must have: how thick was the paper when it was punched?
- Use the answer choices to focus on holes that are different between remaining answer choices.

CUBE COUNTING

Questions: 61 to 75
Answer choices: A–E
Rank: Easy

What You're Given
A stack of cubes that have been painted on the outside.

What You Need To Do
Figure out how many cubes have one face painted, two faces painted, etc.

RULES

- All cubes are connected to the rest of the stack in some way. Stacks and floating cubes are cemented together via faces. Cubes sitting on the ground can be connected by an edge.
- After being cemented each group is painted on all exposed sides.
- Assume every exposed face of every cube has been painted.
- The bottoms of cubes resting on the ground are not painted; the bottoms of floating cubes are painted.
- The only hidden cubes are those required to support other cubes or connect floating cubes to the stack via a face.

STRATEGIES

- Determine how many sides are painted for each cube in the stack; write numbers and/or create a tally chart on your Noteboard
- Work systematically (i.e. from left to right, back to front, bottom to top)
- Don't forget to count hidden cubes
- Use parallel lines to figure out exactly where hard-to-see cubes are sitting
- Watch for patterns:
  - As you move up a vertical stack, the number of painted faces usually increases or stays the same
  - Know some common cube types, such as tower cap, tower extender, side sitters, and daring diagonals
- If you have an unanswerable question, you have made an error in your counting chart. Erase and start again rather than trying to problem solve.

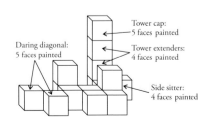

Questions: 76 to 90	**What You're Given**	**What You Need To Do**
Answer choices: A–D	A two-dimensional pattern.	Fold it into a three-dimensional shape.
Rank: Difficult		

RULES

- The outside of the shape is what you see in the 2D pattern
- The shape can be rotated after it is folded together

STRATEGIES

- Use the answer choices to guide you; compare them to the question stem
- Counting and matching: compare the 2D pattern with the answer options
  - If there is an odd-sized face in the 3D shape, this same shape must be somewhere in the 2D pattern
  - If the 2D pattern has three small triangles, the 3D shape must as well
- Find the base of the shape
- Find dominant faces to orient yourself
  - Are they parallel or not?
- If all the answer choices have the same overall shape, focus on shading or face patterns
  - How will faces align in the shape?
  - Which faces will be beside each other?
  - Which faces will be across from each other?

READING COMPREHENSION TEST (RCT)

- **Rank the passages:** look at topic and readability so you work on the easiest passage first and save the hardest one for last
- Skim read the passage in 2-4 minutes
- Generate a passage map by writing down the topic of each paragraph
- Annotate as you read: highlight key words in the passage
- Answer straight forward and short questions first
- Leave harder or open-ended questions for later
- Make sure you understand what the question is asking; read the question stem carefully
- Go back to the passage (using your annotations and passage map) and answer questions based on information in the passage
- Do **process of elimination (POE):** eliminate incorrect answer choices by striking them out
- **Retrieval questions:** the correct answer will be exact words from the passage or a close paraphrase
- **Inference questions:** the correct answer will be something implied by the passage (but maybe not directly stated)
- Stick to the content, tone, and scope of the passage when answering questions
- **Know when to move on:** if you're spinning your wheels, cut your losses, answer the question with your letter of the day, and move on
- Make sure you have an answer selected for all 50 questions before time is up!

QUANTITATIVE REASONING TEST (QRT)

GLOBAL TECHNIQUES

- Two-pass system
- P.I. or P.I.T.A.
- Rounding/Estimation
- AD/BCE for data sufficiency questions

ALGEBRA

- To solve simultaneous equations, usually you must add or subtract one equation from the other.
- **Common Quadratics**
  - $(x + y)(x + y) = x^2 + 2xy + y^2$
  - $(x - y)(x - y) = x^2 - 2xy + y^2$
  - $(x + y)(x - y) = x^2 - y^2$
- To solve inequalities, solve just like equations, except that if you multiply or divide by a negative number, you must reverse the direction of the inequality.
- **Exponent Rules**
  - MADSPM
  - $x^0 = 1, x \neq 0$
  - $x^{a/b} = \sqrt[b]{x^a}$
  - $x^{-a} = \dfrac{1}{x^a}$
- **Logarithm Rules**
  - $a^b = c \Leftrightarrow b = \log_a c$
  - $\log a + \log b = \log(ab)$
  - $\log a - \log b = \log(a/b)$
  - $\log a^b = b \log a$
- **Absolute Value:** the magnitude of a number (its value without a negative sign).
- To solve ratio problems, use the Ratio Box.
- To solve mixture and weight average problems, use the weighted average formula.
- **Direct variation:** $y = kx$, k is constant
- **Indirect variation:** $y = \dfrac{k}{x}$, k is constant

NUMERICAL CALCULATIONS

- To add or subtract fractions, find a common denominator and then add or subtract the numerators.
- To multiply fractions, multiply the numerators and multiply the denominators.
- To divide fractions, multiply by the reciprocal of the fraction that was in the denominator.
- To add or subtract decimals, line up the decimal points.
- To multiply decimals, simply multiply as usual. Then count the number of digits after the decimal point in the two numbers being multiplied, and place the decimal point so that there are as many digits after the decimal point in the result.
- percent change $= \dfrac{difference}{original} \times 100$
- When putting a number in scientific notation, each shifting of the decimal point once to the left (right) means increasing (decreasing) the exponent on the factor of 10 by 1.

CONVERSIONS

- T (in K) $= T$(in °C) + 273.15
- 1 minute = 60 seconds
- 1 hour = 60 minutes
- 1 day = 24 hours
- 1 pound (lb.) = 16 ounces (oz.)
- 1 ton = 2000 pounds
- 1 foot = 12 inches
- 1 yard = 3 feet
- 1 mile = 5,280 feet

PROBABILITY AND STATISTICS

- **Arithmetic mean:** the normal average. To solve average problems, use the Average Pie.
- **Median:** the middle number or the average of the two middle numbers (when numbers are arranged in order).
- **Mode:** the number that occurs most frequently.
- **Variance and standard deviation:** describe the spread of the

data. A larger variance or standard deviation means that the values are farther apart from each other than a smaller variance or standard deviation indicates.

- **Factorial:** written with a !, means multiply by the integers decreasing to 1.

- **Permutations, combinations, and other arrangements:** to determine how many ways something can be done, write out blanks for each thing to be done and the number of ways each can be done. (If the things are not in any particular order, divide by integers starting with the number of blanks and counting down.) Then multiply.

- Probability = $\dfrac{\text{\# of outcomes you want}}{\text{\# of outcomes possible}}$

GEOMETRY

- When two non-perpendicular lines cross, they form two types of angles: big angles and small angles. The big angles are equal, and the small angles are equal. Big + Small = 180°. Adding another line in parallel to the first two creates more equal angles.

- $m = \dfrac{y_2 - y_1}{x_2 - x_1}$

- $y = mx + b$, b is the y-intercept

- $d = \sqrt{\left(x_2 - x_1\right)^2 - \left(y_2 - y_1\right)^2}$

- Area of a triangle = $\dfrac{1}{2} bh$

- Area of a triangle = $\dfrac{1}{2} ab \sin \theta$

- Area of a rectangle = bh

- Area of a trapezoid = $\dfrac{1}{2} (b_1 + b_2)h$

- **Pythagorean Theorem:** $a^2 + b^2 = c^2$
    - $3^2 + 4^2 = 5^2$
    - $5^2 + 12^2 = 13^2$
    - $7^2 + 24^2 = 25^2$

- **Special Triangles** (angles and sides)
    - 30°:60°:90° and $1:\sqrt{3}:2$
    - 45°:45°:90° and $1:1:\sqrt{2}$

- $\dfrac{\text{central angle}}{360°} = \dfrac{\text{arc length}}{2\pi r} = \dfrac{\text{sector area}}{\pi r^2}$

- The sum of the angles inside a polygon with n sides is given by $(n - 2)180°$.

- S.A. of a box = $2lw + 2lh + 2wh$

- S.A. of a cylinder = $2\pi r^2 + 2\pi rh$

- Volume of a box = lwh

- Volume of a cylinder = $\pi r^2 h$

- Volume of a cone = $\dfrac{1}{3}\pi r^2 h$

TRIGONOMETRY

- SOHCAHTOA

- $\tan \theta = \dfrac{\sin \theta}{\cos \theta}$

θ	0°	30°	45°	60°	90°
$\sin \theta$	$\dfrac{\sqrt{0}}{2}$	$\dfrac{\sqrt{1}}{2}$	$\dfrac{\sqrt{2}}{2}$	$\dfrac{\sqrt{3}}{2}$	$\dfrac{\sqrt{4}}{2}$
$\cos \theta$	$\dfrac{\sqrt{4}}{2}$	$\dfrac{\sqrt{3}}{2}$	$\dfrac{\sqrt{2}}{2}$	$\dfrac{\sqrt{1}}{2}$	$\dfrac{\sqrt{0}}{2}$
$\tan \theta$	$\dfrac{\sqrt{0}}{\sqrt{4}}$	$\dfrac{\sqrt{1}}{\sqrt{3}}$	$\dfrac{\sqrt{2}}{\sqrt{2}}$	$\dfrac{\sqrt{3}}{\sqrt{1}}$	$\dfrac{\sqrt{4}}{\sqrt{0}}$

- $\csc \theta = \dfrac{1}{\sin \theta}$

- $\sec \theta = \dfrac{1}{\cos \theta}$

- $\cot \theta = \dfrac{1}{\tan \theta}$

- π radians = 180°

- $\sin^2 \theta + \cos^2 \theta = 1$